BREAST CANCER – CARCINOGENESIS, CELL GROWTH AND SIGNALING PATHWAYS

Edited by **Mehmet Gunduz** and **Esra Gunduz**

Breast Cancer – Carcinogenesis, Cell Growth and Signaling Pathways
Edited by Mehmet Gunduz and Esra Gunduz

Published by InTech
Janeza Trdine 9, 51000 Rijeka, Croatia

Technical Editor Sonja Mujacic

Cover Designer InTech Design Team

Additional hard copies can be obtained from orders@intechopen.com

Breast Cancer – Carcinogenesis, Cell Growth and Signaling Pathways,
Edited by Mehmet Gunduz and Esra Gunduz
p. cm.
ISBN 978-953-307-714-7

For EU product safety concerns:
IN TECH d.o.o., Prolaz Marije Krucifikse Kozulić 3, 51000 Rijeka, Croatia,
info@intechopen.com or visit our website at intechopen.com.

Meet the editors

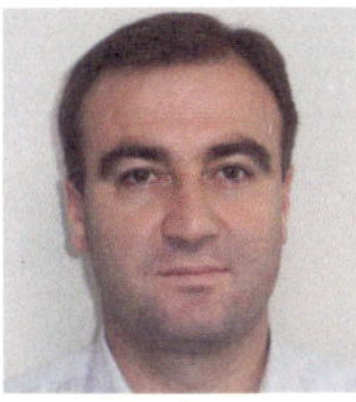

Dr. Mehmet Gunduz graduated from the Faculty of Medicine of Hacettepe University in Ankara, Turkey in 1990. From 1995 until 2009 he studied and worked in Japan, both at Wakayama Medical University and Okayama University Graduate School of Medicine, Dentistry and Pharmaceutical Sciences at various academic levels (from PhD candidate to Assistant Professor). During this period, he led a discovery and identification of roles of several cancer-related genes such as ING1 and 3. He has also been a visiting scientist in MD Anderson Cancer Center University of Texas, Houston, USA. Since March 2011, he is holding the position of a Professor at the Departments of Otolaryngology and Medical Genetics in School of Medicine Fatih University in Ankara. He has over 150 publications in internationally indexed journals, and over 160 presentations at various levels in national and international meetings. He also served as a reviewer for a number of journals.

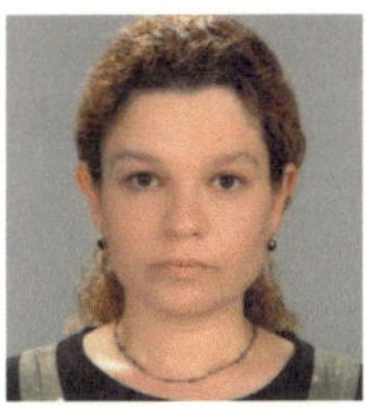

Dr. Esra Gunduz is Associate Professor of Medical Genetics at Fatih University Medical School, Ankara, Turkey. She completed her PhD program in 2005 at Okayama University Graduate School of Medicine, Dentistry and Pharmaceutical Sciences, Japan. She was awarded by the Japan Society for the Promotion of Science (JSPS) as a post-doctoral fellow in 2006. In 2009 she was appointed as Assistant Professor at Fatih University, and in 2010 she was promoted to Associate Professor at the same faculty. Her research focuses mainly on tumor suppressor genes. In her lab she leads various ongoing projects for her research teams. She contributed to the literature with forty articles in peer reviewed journals and over sixty presentations both in national and international meetings.

Contents

Preface

Cancer is the leading cause of death in most countries and continues to increase mainly because of the aging and growth of the world population as well as habitation of cancer-causing behaviors such as smoking and alcohol. Based on statistics of the GLOBOCAN 2008, about 12.7 million cancer cases and 7.6 million cancer deaths are estimated to have occurred in 2008 (Siegel et al. Ca Cancer J Clin 61:212-236, 2011). Breast cancer is the most frequently diagnosed cancer and the leading cause of cancer death among females, accounting for 23% of the total cancer cases and 14% of the cancer deaths. Thus cancer researches, especially breast cancer, are important to overcome both economical and physiological burden. The current book on breast cancer aims at providing information about recent clinical and basic researches in the field. The book includes chapters written by the well-known authors, who are worldwide experts in their research areas. The book basically covers topics related to carcinogenetic mechanisms, such as roles of estrogen receptors, tumor suppressors, signaling pathways including EGFR family and Wnt in breast cancer. We hope that the book will serve as a good guide for the scientists, researchers and educators in the field.

Prof. Dr. Mehmet Gunduz
Assoc. Prof. Dr. Esra Gunduz
Fatih University Medical School
Turkey

Part 1

Signaling Pathways (EGFR)

1

EGFR-Ligand Signaling in Breast Cancer Metastasis: Recurring Developmental Themes

Nicole K. Nickerson[1], Jennifer L. Gilmore[1], Kah Tan Allen[1], David J. Riese II[2], Kenneth P. Nephew[1,3] and John Foley[1,3,4]
[1]*Medical Sciences Program, Indiana University School of Medicine, Bloomington, IN*
[2]*Harrison School of Pharmacy, Auburn University, Auburn, AL*
[3]*Indiana University Cancer Center Indiana University School of Medicine, Indianapolis, IN*
[4]*Department of Dermatology, Indiana University School of Medicine, Indianapolis, IN*
United States of America

1. Introduction

1.1 ErbB receptors, ligands and signaling

Breast cancer affects nearly 1 out of 9 women worldwide. The quality of treatment for breast cancer has improved to the point that close to 80% of patients in countries with advanced healthcare delivery systems survive the disease (1). Yet over 20% of breast cancer patients succumb to the disease, and the majority of these have metastatic breast cancer cells that occupy and compromise the function of distal organs (1). There has been an intensive effort to improve treatments for metastatic breast cancer. Novel treatment strategies have arisen from the study of the molecular and cellular biology of breast cancer cell lines. These studies have produced a group of agents called targeted therapeutics because they are often directed at a single molecule rather than a general process such as DNA replication or cytoskeletal function. The ErbB family represents a target that is present in breast cancer. Therapeutics to ErbB2 have been used to treat aggressive breast cancer for over a decade with considerable success (2). However, therapeutics that primarily target the EGFR have not been used extensively in breast cancer, and there are some improved agents for the receptor that are just entering the clinic. Recent conclusions from studies of metastatic breast cancer suggest new possibilities for the use of EGFR therapeutics. This review will describe the members of the EGFR signaling family, discuss the cellular context in which they function in development, and correlate this with the biological role of these molecules in breast cancer metastasis.

1.2 ErbB family members

The ErbB family consists of 4 receptors: ErbB1 or more commonly called EGFR, ErbB2/Her2, ErbB3 and ErbB4 (3). Signaling is generated when EGFR and ErbB4 bind to their ligands. In contrast, the ErbB2 extracellular binding domain fails to bind any of the 15 agonists, and in ErbB3 the kinase domain is not functional. Upon ligand stimulation, EGFR and ErbB4 receptors can transduce their signals as homodimers or heterodimers; however,

the signal generation from ErbB2 or ErbB3 require heterodimerization with another ErbB family member (3).
The ErbB receptors are stimulated by 15 ligands but the situation is complicated because several of these agonists can bind more than one receptor. The EGFR exclusive agonists are epidermal growth factor (EGF), transforming growth factor alpha (TGF-α), amphiregulin (AREG) and Epigen (Epi) (3, 4). ErbB4 is specifically bound and activated by Neuregulins (NRG) 3, 4, 5 (3, 4). Heparin-binding EGF-like growth factor (HB-EGF), epiregulin (EREG), and β-cellulin (BTC) bind and activate both the EGFR and ErbB4 (3, 4). NRG 1 and 2 binds both ErbB3 and ErbB4 and NRG 1 can bind the EGFR with low affinity (3, 4).
All of the ErbB agonists are synthesized as plasma membrane bound integral membrane proteins (5). In some cases, the transmembrane ligands stimulate ErbB signaling on adjacent cells through a juxtracrine mechanism which may mediate the stromal-epithelial interactions (6) (7). Most ErbB signaling requires proteolytic cleavage termed ectodomain shedding for the ligand to be released and available to bind receptors that may be on the same cell (autocrine signaling), or on neighboring cells (paracrine signaling) (5). The proteases that mediate the process are from the "a disintegrin and metalloproteinase " or (ADAM) family (8, 9). There are 40 members of the ADAM protein family that function in cell adhesion and ectodomain shedding. These ADAMs are integral membrane proteins in which the extracellular region contains a protease as well as a disintegrin domain that modulates integrin binding (9). ADAMs can be activated by a wide range of stimuli that signal through G-protein-coupled receptors and these signals are often transduced by Src (10). The shedding of AREG, EREG, HB-EGF, Epigen, TGFα and NRG 1&2 is typically catalyzed by the single family member ADAM 17, whereas BTC and EGF are cleaved by ADAM 10 (8). In addition, ADAM 17 cleaves many other cytokines, growth factors, receptors, adhesion molecules and extracellular matrix proteins, suggesting its activity may be a key determinate of cellular behavior (9). Nevertheless, emerging data suggest that EGFR ligands can be shed by other proteases such as the ADAM thrombospondin (ADAMTS) family that is structurally related to the ADAM family, but is secreted and the disintgrin domain is replaced by a thrombospondin domain that binds to matrix (11, 12). Also, it is likely that other metalloproteinases secreted from cells in a paracrine relationship are capable of releasing ligands (13).
Over the past two decades the expression of ErbB receptors, ligands, and their activating proteases in normal breast and breast cancers have been intensively studied. Various mRNA detection methods and immunohistochemistry studies have concluded that the entire ErbB family is expressed in various breast cancers. In fact, it appears the vast majority of the family is expressed in the mammary epithelia (14-16). Since newer therapeutics that target the EGFR are being considered for use in cases of advanced breast cancer, in the rest of this review we will focus on how this receptor is activated and describe its role in development and cancer progression.

1.3 EGFR homodimer signaling

EGF was the first ligand identified and due its abundance in the mouse salivary gland and relative ease of purification from this source (17). EGF has historically been used for receptor binding, signaling, trafficking, and cell fate studies resulting in a model of receptor signaling that is in many ways considered to be the prototype for receptor tyrosine kinases (18-20). The binding of EGF to the EGFR exposes the dimerization arm in the extracellular domain that permits interaction with another EGFR receptor or hetrodimerization with other ErbBs. Ligand binding also induces a conformational change in the receptor that activates the intracellular kinase domain, which in turn can phosphorylate tyrosine residues on the adjacent C-terminal tail of the dimerized ErbB receptor. The 10 phosphorylated tyrosine residues serve as docking sites for adapter proteins or other signal transduction components, resulting in activation of Ras, MAPK, src, STAT 3/5 and PLCγ/PKC and the PI3 kinase-AKT-pro survival pathway. Activation of these signaling pathways by ErbB dimers has profound impact on proliferation, resistance to apoptosis, differentiation, as well as motility/migration associated behaviors. Not all tyrosine phosphorylation of EGFR C-terminal tail results in stimulation of downstream signaling pathways. For example, phosphorylation of the 974 residue triggers enodcytosis of the receptor, and phospho 1045 binds to Cbl, mediating ubquitination of the receptor and subsequent proteosomal degradation (4, 21). Trafficking studies suggest that ~50% of EGF stimulated EGFR is degraded, whereas the remainder is recycled back to the plasma membrane (22). Thus, activation of the EGFR by EGF directly stimulates a broad group of cellular signaling pathways, many of which converge on elements of the ERK/MAPK pathway (3), but this signaling is dampened by receptor turnover. The rapid turnover of the EGF stimulated EGFR is believed to limit stimulation of cellular proliferation, permitting a balance with various differentiation-inducing stimuli present in a normal tissue (3, 22, 23). In cancers, autocrine EGFR homodimer signaling is substantially attenuated, shifting the cell fate balance towards proliferation and survival rather than differentiation, apoptosis and senescence.

1.4 Attenuating EGFR signaling with heterodimerization

Probably the most well understood attenuation of EGFR signaling occurs when the receptor heterodimerizes with the ErbB 2 receptor (24, 25). It is believed that EGFR heterodimerization with ErbB2 frequently occurs in a number of breast cancers (26, 27). Despite being unable to bind ligand, the ErbB2 dimerization arm is constitutively exposed, which allows this receptor to more efficiently dimerize with other liganded ErbB family members (4). The resulting ErbB2 containing heterodimers attenuate EGFR signal transduction in several ways (28-32). First, the affinity of this ErbB2 complex for ligands is enhanced. Second, the ErbB2 phosphotyrosine domains bind most adapter proteins with higher affinity than those of the ErbB homodimers, resulting in more efficient signal transduction. Third, ErbB2/EGFR heterodimers are slowly endocytosed, and are more frequently recycled to the plasma membrane than the EGF stimulated homodimers. By virtue of its strong interactions with adapter proteins and altered trafficking downstream of endocytosis, an EGFR/ErbB2 heterodimer can amplify and extend the duration of EGFR ligand signaling, leading to proliferation and survival at the expense of other cell fates (28-31).

In contrast to the fairly well established understanding of ErbB2 containing heterodimers, there have been few studies on the EGFR heterodimerized with ErbB4 or ErbB3. Co-immuno precipitation experiments have confirmed the presence of the ErbB4/EGFR in a lung epithelial cells and type II pneumocytes; however, the specific function of this complex was not determined (33, 34). Co-expression of ErbB4 and EGFR plasmids in model NIH 3T3 fibroblasts or CHO lines, provided evidence of dimerization of these receptors, and suggested that this complex could induce cellular transformation in the presence of EGF or NRG1. Further analysis of the CHO system found that the ErbB4/EGFR heterodimer specifically induced B-Raf kinase activity, which was speculated to induce transformation by increasing the activity of the ERK/MAPK pathway (35). Recently, ErbB3/EGFR heterodimers have been identified in pancreatic cancer cell lines (36, 37). It appeared that the ErbB3/EGFR complex may be a more effective stimulus of proliferation in pancreatic cancer cell lines than EGFR homodimers (36). Additionally, these studies suggest the ligand AREG is able to stimulate activity of the ErbB3/EGFR heterodimer (36, 37). Unfortunately, the comprehensive binding, signal transduction and trafficking studies completed for ErbB2 containing receptor complexes have not been completed for EGFR/ErbB4 or ErbB3 heterodimers. This information, coupled with the identification of the specific cell types and tumors that express heterodimers and the function of these complexes will be important considerations for expanded use of ErbB targeted therapeutics.

1.5 Other EGFR ligands

As studies of receptor binding, conformation, phosphorylation, and trafficking are completed for each ligand, it is becoming clear that each agonist induces signaling that can be viewed as a variation of the basic EGF-EGFR homodimer scenario. This attenuated signaling produced by each ligand has the potential to induce subtle differences in downstream signaling, which would be expected to result in altered gene expression and cellular behavior. In the preceding section, the emerging differences in signaling are detailed for each of the ligands that bind the EGFR.

1.5.1 TGFα

Next to EGF, the most intensively studied ligand has been TGFα. Similar to EGF, TGFα exclusively binds to and activates the EGFR. Binding studies suggest that TGFα binds to the receptor with similar affinity as EGF (32). However, conclusions from structural studies involving ligand-receptor complex data indicates there are subtle differences in the conformation of the extracellular ligand-binding domain (sub domain II) induced by TGFα as compared to EGF (4). It is unclear whether this conformational change induced by TGFα could generate alterations in EGFR kinase activity or accessibility of C-terminal tyrosines. Although not comprehensively studied at this point, some of our early studies with breast cancer cell lines suggest that TGFα does not induce the extensive receptor phosphorylation observed with mouse salivary gland derived EGF (Fig 1). Additionally, it has been long recognized that TGFα induces different trafficking of the receptor than EGF (38). Close to 100% of receptors internalized after TGFα treatment are recycled to the plasma membrane (22). At physiological pH of 7.4 in the extracellular environment, TGFα and EGF have similar binding affinities for the EGFR (22, 38). However, at pH close to 5 such as in the endosome, TGFα has decreased affinity for the EGFR (22, 38). It appears that dissociation of the ligand from the EGFR in the endosome permits the receptor to be recycled back to the plasma membrane where it can be reengaged by ligand. It is thought that the three additional histidines found in the receptor binding domain of TGFα provide a greater sensitivity to pH for agonist-receptor interactions (38). In fact, mutations that add histidines to this region of EGF decreased ligand-receptor binding at low pH (39, 40). Together, the altered ligand induced receptor conformation, phosphorylation and trafficking appear to result in TGFα being a more potent stimulator of proliferation of EGFR expressing cell lines than EGF.

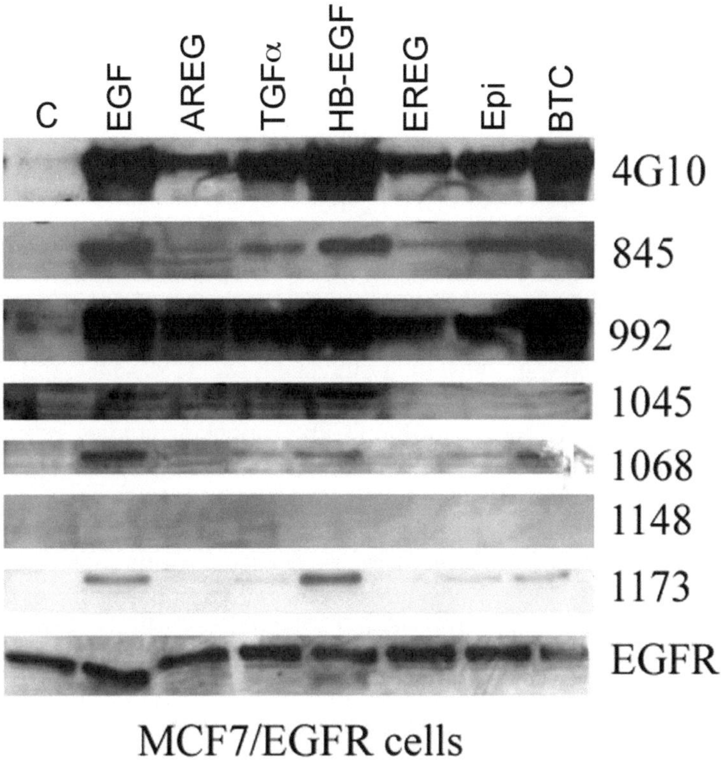

Fig. 1. EGFR phosphorylation after ligand stimulation.
The human breast cancer cell line MCF7 was engineered to overexpress high levels of the EGFR after retroviral transduction. Cells were grown to 80% confluence and placed on ice for 30 minutes. Ligands (R&D, Minneapolis) were applied for 10 minutes to the media and then the media was removed, cells washed and proteins extracted. The EGFR was concentrated with Concanavalin A beads and extracted with Laemmli sample and applied to gels and western blotted with specific antibodies to phosphorylated tyrosines listed on the left. The various ligands used are listed on the top of the figure (C) represents vehicle treated cells.

1.5.2 AREG

The differential impact on breast cancer cell behavior that AREG exhibits compared to EGF has drawn considerable attention to the concept that various EGFR ligands have discrete functions (41-43). Among the ErbB receptors, AREG appears to exclusively bind and activate the EGFR. In addition, the ligand contains a heparin-binding domain N-terminal to the receptor binding region (44, 45). It appears that interaction with heparin-sulfated proteoglycans on the plasma membrane enhances the ability of exogenous AREG to activate the EGFR (46). What has been a matter of controversy has been the relative strength of AREG binding to the EGFR as compared to other ligands. The initial identification of human AREG by Shoyab and colleagues, reported the fully processed ligand isolated from breast cancer cells had reduced affinity for the human EGFR, as compared to salivary gland derived mouse EGF (44). In contrast, subsequent studies with human recombinant ligands

found that AREG has similar affinity for the EGFR as EGF and TGFα (47, 48). Inducing further complexity, additional analyses of ligand receptor interactions have suggested that recombinant AREG does not induce efficient dimerization of the EGFR, as compared to recombinant EGF and TGFα (49). Interestingly, proteolytic processing of AREG in mammalian cells may eliminate the C-terminal portion of the ligand binding domain that is required for high affinity for the receptor (50). In addition, the terminal portion of the receptor binding domain in all other EGFR ligands contains a leucine, whereas a methionine is found in AREG, and this is speculated to reduce affinity for the receptor (50).
More recent studies have focused on the distinct downstream signaling and cellular behavior induced by AREG. Unlike exogenous EGF treatment, AREG stimulation of model cell lines and breast cancer cell lines is unable to induce efficient phosphorylation of many of the tyrosine residues in the C-terminal tail of the EGFR (22, 43, 51, 52) and (Fig. 1). Notably, the Cbl binding 1045 tyrosine residue is not efficiently phosphorylated by AREG and this ligand fails to induce rapid turnover of the EGFR. Trafficking studies indicate that AREG liganded EGFR is rapidly internalized, but then is recycled back to the plasma membrane. In addition, AREG binding to the EGFR is very resistant to acidic pH suggesting that the ligand does not disengage in the endosome as does TGFα (22). It appears that AREG may be unique among the ligands in that it induces EGFR trafficking through Rab 4 and Rab 11 containing endosomes (22, 43). AREG induces prolonged phosphorylation of ERK relative to EGF (41, 52). This altered signaling appears to be the basis of AREG stimulating the loss of cell-cell adhesion and increase motility/migration associated behaviors in breast and other epithelial cells (41, 53). AREG overexpression has also been found to selectively activate interleuken-1 induced NFκβ signaling in breast epithelial cells (41-43).

1.5.3 Epigen

This was the last ErbB family member identified in 2000, and it has not been as intensively studied as other ligands. The ligand activates the EGFR and does not activate ErbB3 or ErbB4 when these receptors are expressed in isolation (54, 55). However, epigen can activate ErbB4 and ErbB3 when these receptors are co-expressed with ErbB2 (54, 55). Epigen appears to have ~100 fold less affinity for the EGFR relative to recombinant human EGF. Not surprisingly, we found that epigen induced modest phosphorylation of breast cancer cells (Fig. 1). The binding of epigen to the EGFR appears to be sensitive to pH similar to TGFα. Modeling suggests that additional histidines in the receptor binding domain are responsible for the dissociation of the ligand from the EGFR at low pH (54, 55). In comparison with EGF, epigen induced significantly weaker ubiquitylation and degradation of EGFR, and once internalized, it appears that the receptor is efficiently recycled to the plasma membrane. As expected for lower affinity ligands, epigen is a more potent mitogen than EGF and displays prolonged MAPK signaling (54, 55).

1.5.4 HB-EGF

Exogenous HB-EGF is a high affinity ligand for the EGFR but it also binds and activates ErbB4 (32). Exogenous HB-EGF does not as robustly stimulate phosphorylation of ErbB4 as it does the EGFR (56). In addition, pro-HB-EGF serves as the diptheria toxin receptor in human cells (6). Similar to EGF, exogenous HB-EGF induces extensive EGFR tyrosine phosphorylation in most cell types studied (22, 56), and we found this to be the case for breast cancer cells (Fig. 1). Upon binding to and activation by HB-EGF, the EGFR is rapidly endocytosed and the majority of ligand engaged receptors are trafficked to lysosomes and degraded (22). The binding of HB-EGF to the EGFR was resistant to low pH. HB-EGF shows similar effects on cell proliferation and migration to those exhibited by EGF (57).

As its name implies, HB-EGF has a heparin-binding region N-terminal to the EGF domain. This domain has been shown to interact with heparin sulfated plasma membrane proteins such as the tetraspanin, CD9 and the extracellular matrix binding/cell differentiation marker protein CD44 (6, 57). In particular the heparin-mediated interaction between HB-EGF and CD9 appear to be crucial to juxtacrine signaling by the proligand (58). Finally, the associations between the heparin binding domain and cell membrane associated heparin sulfated proteoglycans appear to be crucial to localizing HB-EGF to regions of cell-cell contact. Furthermore, the interaction with these heparin-sulfated proteoglycans prevented proteolytic cleavage of the pro-ligand, whereas exogenous heparin increased shedding of HB-EGF (7, 58). In contrast to the impact of shed ligand, juxtacrine signaling by the pro HB-EGF appears to be antiproliferative (58).

1.5.5 β-cellulin

Exogenous β-cellulin is a high affinity ligand for the EGFR and ErbB4 (32). In general, exogenous β-cellulin phosphorylates the EGFR to a similar extent as EGF in model cell types, and this is what we observed with breast cancer cells (Fig. 1) (22, 59). This exogenous ligand also stimulates total ErbB4 phosphorylation to an extent similar to NRG1, but there may be differences in phosphorylation of specific tyrosine residues (60). Upon binding to and activation by β-cellulin, the EGFR is rapidly endocytosed and trafficked to lysosomes where the majority of it is degraded (22). The binding of β-cellulin to the EGFR was resistant to low pH. Exogenous β-cellulin was slightly less efficient than EGF at inducing proliferation in some specific cell types (60). There have been some reports that β-cellulin binds to heparin and may participate in juxtacrine signaling (61).

1.5.6 EREG

Unlike the other dual receptor ligands HB-EGF and BTC, EREG is a low affinity ligand for the EGFR (32). EREG typically induces much less phosphorylation of the EGFR than EGF in model cell lines (62-65). In breast cancer cells, we found that the epiregulin induced phosphorylation of the various tyrosines on the EGFR to an extent similar to AREG and the low affinity ligand epigen (Fig. 1). EREG is not as effective as NRG or BTC in stimulating ErbB4 phosphorylation (62-65). The ligand appears to preferentially activate heterodimers and efficiently induces EGFR heterodimers with all three other receptors (65). Upon binding to and activation by EREG, the EGFR is rapidly endocytosed, but then is recycled back to the plasma membrane, and its binding to the receptor was resistant to low pH (22). Exogenous EREG was more efficient than EGF at inducing proliferation in some cell types (63, 65). Also EREG does not induce as great of activation of the MAPK pathway as EGF, but the duration of MAPK phosphorylation was increased relative to the prototype ligand (63, 65).

Thus, the expression of specific EGFR ligands could influence the progression of breast cancer in several ways. First, three of the ligands (HB-EGF, BTC and EREG) could induce ErbB4 signaling on breast cancer cells themselves or their microenvironment, whereas the other 4 ligands EGF, TGFα, AREG and epigen would only induce EGFR signaling. Second, if juxtacrine EGFR signaling between breast cancer cells may require interaction with heparin sulfate proteoglycans, only HB-EGF and AREG would be likely mediators of this signaling.

Juxacrine EGFR signaling might be antiproliferative and also only occur in breast cancer that lacked active sheddases that released HB-EGF and AREG. Third, EGFR signaling induced by soluble ligands appears to be dependent on the relative ratio of receptor degradation versus recycling to the plasma membrane. For example, those ligands whose binding leads to rapid receptor degradation (EGF, HB-EGF and BTC) would activate high levels of downstream signal transduction, but this would likely be of short duration. In contrast, the ligands that induce recycling of the internalized receptor to the plasma membrane would produce longer duration EGFR signaling. In the context of autocrine signaling in breast cancer cells, the longer duration EGFR signaling is likely to more efficiently induce mitogenesis. What remains to be determined is whether the duration of EGFR signaling differentially impacts other cellular behaviors relevant to breast cancer progression such as resistance to apoptosis, and the stimulation of invasive/motile behaviors. Finally, in the context of paracrine signaling it is not clear how EGFR turnover influences the supportive functions of stromal and immune cells of the tumor microenvironment.

2. EGFR/ErbB signaling in development

2.1 ErbB signaling and mammary gland development

The majority of research on mammary gland development is performed in the mouse model due to its biologically and histologically similarity with humans, and the power of transgenic knockout murine models (66). Embryonic mammary gland development in the mouse begins around embryonic day 10.5 (E 10.5), where bilateral milk lines are formed from front to hind paws. Between E11.5 and E12.5, five placodes on each milk line develop with eventual epithelial bud formation at each placode. These epithelial buds remain quiescent until E15.5, where minor branching permits the migration of mammary epithelia into the fat pad, and mesenchymal differentiation forms the overlying nipple epidermis. This rudimentary mammary gland will remain quiescent until after birth (67). The majority of mammary gland growth and development occurs in postnatal life during puberty and pregnancy, and ErbB signaling impacts this phase.

The primary hormone that drives post-natal mammary gland development is the nuclear steroid hormone, estrogen. Estrogen stimulates proliferation of luminal cells within the mammary ducts, causing ductal elongation and branching (68). Progesterone also increases cellular proliferation of the mammary ducts, and acts synergistically with estrogen during periods of high hormone levels such as pregnancy (68). Prolactin, a non-steroid hormone released from the pituitary gland, is active in mammary gland development, late in pregnancy, stimulating alveolar development and triggering milk production during lactation (69).

The mouse mammary gland begins pubertal outgrowth between 3-4 weeks of age, and is complete at 8-12 weeks of age. The gland requires both longitudinal ductal growth, as well as ductal branching to fully infiltrate the mammary fat pad. Pubertal growth is directed by the cells within structures called terminal end buds (TEBs), which are a bulbous expansion of the epithelia. The TEBS are found at the distal end of each growing duct, and consist of 3 to 4 cell layers, including cap cells that make up the 'basal' layer and multiple layers of interior luminal-like body cells that line the duct. Signaling within the cells of the TEBs and the surrounding stroma will determine the extent of continued ductal branching (70) (71). From this point, the mammary gland will show minimal growth with each estrous cycle. Upon pregnancy, estrogen and progesterone drive another large spurt of growth resulting in extensive ductal branching. Progesterone also works with prolactin to signal differentiation of the secretory or alveolar cells throughout the duct system, which produces the large volumes of milk post parturition (72, 73). Termination of lactation will eventually lead to involution, where large-scale apoptosis will eliminate the secretory alveoli and remodel the remaining ducts of the mammary gland, returning the structure to a state similar to that of the virgin gland.

2.1.1 Role of EGFR in mammary gland growth

In virgin mice, EGFR, ErbB2, and ErbB3 are present in the developing ductal structure while there is minimal ErbB4. During pregnancy, this pattern changes to greatly increase expression of ErbB4 in the mammary epithelium, while ErbB4 levels will again regress during lactation and involution (74). Even though three of the receptors are present during growth, there is minimal ErbB phosphorylation observed until ductal morphogenesis begins. During pubertal growth, phosphorylated EGFR and ErbB2 are detected, which suggested that these receptors may mediate the impact of estradiol (E2) on the gland (75).

The EGFR$^{-/-}$ mice die within 8-days after birth and show a wide range of dysfunctional epithelia, but their mammary glands were similar to their wild-type littermates. Transplantation of pre-pubertal glands from EGFR$^{-/-}$ mice into cleared fat pads of wild-type littermates failed to infiltrate the structure, but glands from wild-type mice produced normal ductal systems (76). In contrast, when a purified mammary epithelium from the EGFR$^{-/-}$ mouse was implanted into cleared fat pads with mammary stroma from wild-type mice it produced a normal ductal tree, whereas the opposite combination of wild-type epithelium and EGFR$^{-/-}$ stroma failed to penetrate the fat pad. Thus, postnatal mammary ductal growth is dependent on the presence of the EGFR in mammary stromal fibroblasts. It appears that signaling by the receptor triggers the production of stromal growth factors important to TEBs in ductal elongation (76).

The EGFR ligands EGF, TGFα, and AREG, are found in different locations within the TEB during ductal growth. Using immunohistochemical techniques, TGFα is found exclusively in the basal cap cell layer while the luminal cells express only EGF (70). AREG has been found in both the basal cap cells and the luminal cell layers of TEBs (77). Luekette and colleagues produced knockout mice for each of these ligands separately or as double and triple knockouts. While all three mice null for the individual ligands and their various crosses were fertile, not all had distinct mammary phenotypes. Double-knockout mice for EGF and TGFα, but which contained AREG, displayed normal ductal growth and TEB formation. Mice that were single-knockout for AREG or a triple-knockout for all ligands displayed almost a complete lack of ductal growth into the fat pad at 8-12 weeks (78). In the AREG$^{-/-}$ mice, mammary epithelial failed to fill the fat pad even after multiple pregnancies, strongly suggesting that AREG-EGFR signaling mediated the impact of estrogen on mammary ductal growth. This suggests that EGF and TGFα are dispensable for mammary gland growth, while AREG plays a vital role in glandular development. Recombination grafts indicated that estrogen stimulated pubertal mammary gland growth will not occur without AREG signaling to the stroma (79). The AREG gene is regulated by estrogen receptor alpha (ERα), which apparently accounts for its requirement in postnatal mammary gland development (80, 81). Whether there are any ligand specific effects of the AREG ligand in mammary development have not been explored.

Studies performed with mice deficient for ADAM-17 have shown cardiac insufficiencies, a constellation of epithelial defects and die soon after birth similar to the phenotype of EGFR -/- mice. The ADAM17$^{-/-}$ mice have small, immature mammary glands with minimal branching or ductal growth (82). To verify the requirement of ADAM-17, the defective growth of ADAM-17-null mammary epithelia can be rescued in the presence of exogenous AREG, EGF, or TGFα (82). In conclusion, estrogen induced growth of the mammary pad requires mammary epithelial cell ADAM-17 to shed AREG which then, is necessary to stimulate EGFR signaling in the stromal fibroblasts.

2.1.2 Breast epithelial stem cell and ErbB signaling

Potential mammary gland stem and progenitor cells have been identified using a series of methodologies used to identify the hierarchy of cells that produces that mature hematopoetic system. A single human mammary gland stem cell has been shown to regenerate all the cellular components of the human mammary gland, as well as produce milk proteins in immunocompromised mice (83-86). This work, coupled with mouse work has given rise to an epithelial hierarchy illustrated in figure 2. In this hierarchy, the mammary stem cells give rise to " the common or bipotent" progenitor; the bipotent progenitor gives rise to a luminal progenitor, as well as a cell type that gives rise to mature myoepthelial cells; and the luminal progenitor produces derivatives that ultimately differentiate into mature duct and alveolar cells (83-86).

The reproducible isolation of stem and progenitor cells from mammary epithelia has permitted profiling the various cell types for the expression of the receptors involved in post-natal mammary gland growth and breast cancer progression (85). The subpopulation containing putative mammary multipotent stem cells appear to lack expression of estrogen and progesterone receptors, whereas the EGFR is expressed in ~12% of this fraction. Nearly 50% of the luminal progenitor inclusive population expressed high levels of EGFR. The relatively small subset of the differentiated luminal cell segment (ductal and alveolar cells) express the EGFR (83-86). Of possible significance is that both the mammary stem cell and luminal progenitor population are routinely propagated in a media supplement containing EGF. Whether this implies that propagation of these stem and progenitor cells are dependent on EGFR signaling or simply that there is a requirement for generalized receptor tyrosine kinase activity remains to be determined.

Taken together, the post-natal development of the mammary gland is regulated in large part by the EGFR. EGFR signaling in stromal fibroblasts is required for the estrogen-stimulated invasion mammary epithelium into the stromal fat pad that establishes the adult virgin mammary gland. It appears that the stromal EGFR signaling is mediated primarily by the estrogen-controlled ligand, AREG. Interestingly, the EGFR and its ligands are expressed in the mammary epithelia, but the recombination experiments suggest that autocrine receptor activity in this compartment is dispensable for the establishment of the adult mammary gland. At this time, it is not clear if autocrine EGFR signaling in a mammary epithelial stem or progenitor cells might be required for maintenance of the organ throughout adult life.

2.2 EGFR signaling and cardiac development

Careful reexamination of the EGFR-/- mice along with observations from the Waved-2 mice (these express a mutant form of the receptor with only 10% kinase activity) found defective

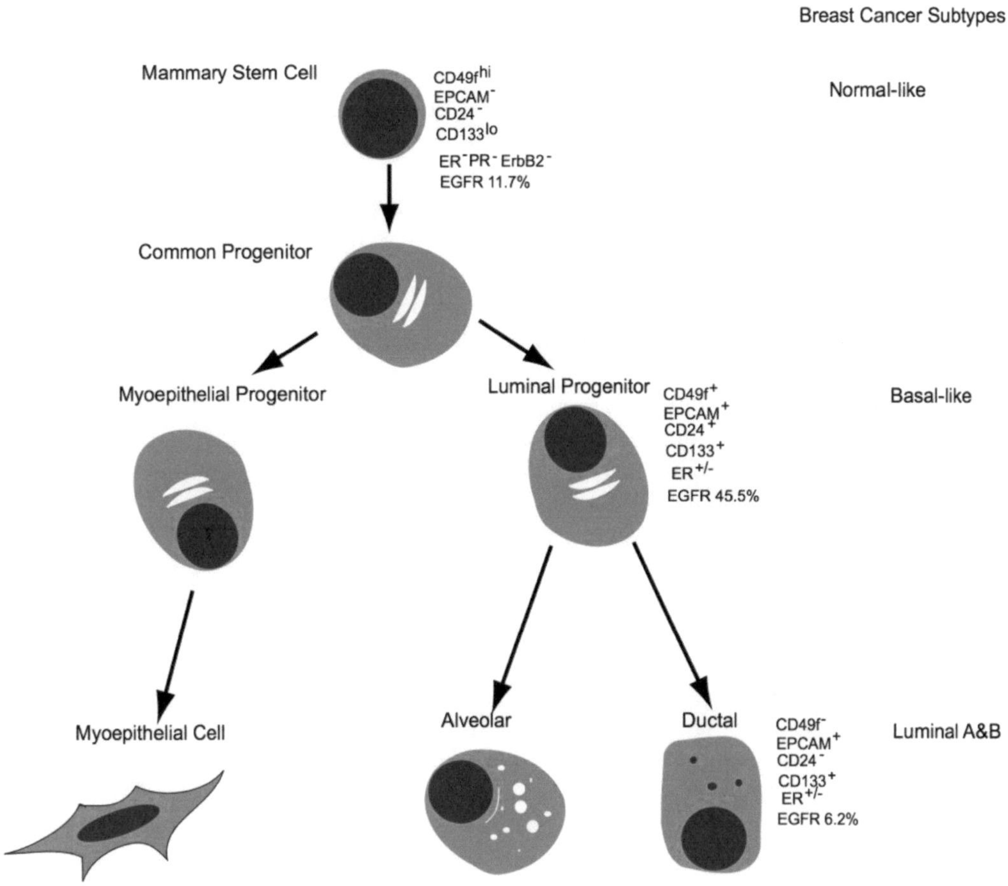

Fig. 2. Hierarchy of mammary epithelial cells.
The various cells of the mammary epithelium and their relationships are represented. To the right, is the expression pattern of the various cell surface markers. Below this is the ErbB and ERα expression along with breast cancer cell types the various cells are related to.

cardiac valve morphogenesis and maturation (94, 96). HB-EGF KO mice also exhibit defective maturation of cardiac valves, suggesting that this may be the relevant ligand that induces EGFR signaling in this process. Also, the HB-EGF-/- cardiac defect was phenocopied in the ADAM-17, suggesting that this protease released the ligand during cardiac development (97).

In the context of cellular behaviors, it appears that the EGFR signaling system plays a role in differentiation. In the EGFR, HB-EGF and ADAM-17 KO mice which have hyperplastic valves it appears that the impact of this signaling is distinct from a proliferation and migration defect observed with the other ErbB knockouts. It is thought that HB-EGF-EGFR signaling decreases BMP expression, the factor which drives cardiac valve maturation, and hence is a differentiation factor (97).

2.3 EGFR signaling and nervous system

In the mouse, EGFR is highly expressed during brain development (E-7 to E-17) and is present on multipotent precursors of both neurons and glia, as well as developing astrocytes and some neurons (98, 99). The initial reports of the EGFR knockout did not identify a nervous system defect. However, reexamination of the KOs with extended post natal survival due to breeding of the knockout allele onto other mouse strains was able to identify brain defects (98). Among the defects identified were smaller or thinner forebrain regions, including the cerebral cortex, olfactory bulb and neocortex (98). Both HB-EGF and TGFα are expressed in portion of the fore brain during late embryonic and early postnatal life (98, 100). Modest histological defects were observed in the prefrontal cortex of mice with a conditional KO of HB-EGF in the forebrain, and these mice displayed behavior and defects in dopamine metabolism that have been observed in schizophrenia (98).

The defects observed in the forebrain of the EGFR-KO mice appear to result from disruption of the cellular interactions required to support neurons. There was substantial neuronal apoptosis in the early postnatal forebrain regions affected (98). However, this occurred in EGFR-expressing and non-receptor bearing neurons. In addition, there was a delay in the appearance of glial fibrulary acidic protein (GFAP) positive astrocytes in the glial limitans and white matter tracks of the fore brain. Although EGFR ligands can stimulate both the proliferation of astrocytes and recruitment of these cells from multipotent precursor cells, the major defect of the knockout mice appears to have a defect in the migration these glial cells from germinal centers. It is speculated that the delay in formation of contacts between neurons and astrocytes results in a deficiency of trophic support, resulting in neuronal cell death in the forebrain (98, 99).

EGFR expression is high in developing astrocytes, but the receptor is not present in mature astrocytes of the healthy adult brain. Upon injury or disease, EGFR expression is up regulated in reactive astrocytes (101). Reactive astrocytes lengthen processes produce plasma membrane pseudopodia and increase expression GFAP in response to all forms of CNS injury or disease (102). Stimulation of the EGFR on reactive astrocytes results in the upregulation of motility chemokines and extracellular matrix remodeling genes that are likely to contribute to glial scarring (101). Intriguingly, the use of EGFR tyrosine kinase inhibitors reduced nerve loss and lead to greater nerve fiber regeneration in optic nerve crush a model of a glial scarring (101). Thus, EGFR signaling in astrocytes facilitates neuronal survival during development, but receptor activity in reactive astrocytes actually contributes to neuron loss in pathologies.

2.4 EGFR signaling and bone

Bone phenotypes had not been reported in the original characterization ErbB receptor KO mice. However, work on the problem of malignancy-associated hypercalcemia had long established that TGFα increased the formation of bone resorbing osteoclasts in bone marrow cultures and whole animals (103, 104). The EGFR is expressed on both chondrocytes and cells of the osteoblast lineage in animals and humans (105). However, the function of the receptor was not established until a human EGFR gene-knockin mouse was created (106). This human EGFR transgene had a limited expression in mouse tissues that normally express the receptor, probably due to the presence of the Neo gene in the first intron of the construct. The human EGFR was expressed in the heart and nervous system and provided a rescue of the murine EGFR KO, but the receptor was not expressed in epithelia and bone. The human EGFR knockin mice were growth retarded and the skeletal phenotype appeared to be largely due to premature hypertrophy of the growth plate cartilages. Although routine histology did not reveal defects in the bones, growth of the knockin osteoblasts *in vitro* resulted in the increased formation of calcified nodules, which represent the end point of differentiation for these cells. Thus, in both cartilage and bone, EGFR signaling inhibits differentiation and helps maintain chondrocytes and osteoblasts in a proliferative state. At this point, it is unknown if any other ErbB receptors play a functional role in bone development or physiology.

Further insight into the role of EGFR in bone resulted from a study of global changes in osteoblast gene expression induced by the main serum calcium regulator, PTH. Activation of the PTH receptor on osteoblasts rapidly upregulates AREG mRNA expression 10 to 20-fold, as well as increasing the TGFα and HB-EGF ligands (107, 108). In addition, PTH signaling induces shedding of ADAM-17 controlled ligands in the kidney (109). Further experiments indicated that addition of exogenous AREG to osteoblasts stimulated their proliferation. However ligand-EGFR signaling also inhibited osteoblast differentiation and dramatically decreased mineralization of osteoblast cell lines. Consistent with the role for AREG in stimulating the proliferation of osteoblasts, 4-week-old AREG-knockout mice exhibited less trabecular bone in the tibia than wild type littermates (107). These experiments suggested that EGFR signaling may mediate the impact of PTH on the recruitment and expansion of cells committed to the osteoblast lineage, but excessive signaling by this system could prevent these cells from undergoing terminal differentiation and forming mineralized bone. The inhibition of osteoblast differentiation and subsequent mineralized bone matrix deposition by-EGFR signaling may contribute to the uncoupling of bone formation from the accelerated bone resorbtion

3. EGFR and breast cancer

3.1 ErbB and EGFR expression in primary tumors

The development of platforms capable of simultaneously evaluating gene expression from a large portion of the genome have lead to identification of gene expression profiles that correlate with various established and some novel classes of breast cancer. These profiles have produced further insights into the impact of ErbB family members in breast cancer progression. Based on these studies, breast cancers are now divided into the following subclasses: ErbB2 amplified, luminal A, luminal B, normal breast-like, and basal (110-112). The ErbB2 amplified, basal and luminal B subtypes had substantially worse prognosis than the normal breast-like and luminal A.

3.1.1 ErbB2 amplified tumors

Among the molecular subclasses of breast cancer, the ErbB2 amplified, has the most well established functional role for an ErbB member in disease development and progression. The ErbB2 amplified tumors typically express ErbB3 and cell line experiments suggest the

ErbB2/ErbB3 heterodimers stimulate proliferation of these cells through the PI3 kinase-AKT pathway (113). Despite the identification of the ErbB2 co-receptor, the precise ligand activating the ErbB3 has not been established. In addition, the correlation between high ErbB2 expression and poor prognosis suggests that ErbB2 contributes to metastasis and how the receptor contributes to these processes, is still under investigation (110-112).

3.1.2 ER+ tumors: luminal A&B

Luminal A tumors express ERα along with GATA binding protein 3, X-box binding protein 1, trefoil factor 3, and other estrogen-regulated genes and high levels of the luminal keratins K8 and 18 (110-112). Luminal B tumors tend to express the above markers at slightly reduced levels, but have an upregulated cassette of genes, including proliferation related genes such as Myb and components involved in DNA replication. There is no specific ErbB family member included in luminal A or B signature. Further evaluations of ERα+ tumors have indicated that the majority of these tumors lack ErbB2 and EGFR expression, but close examination of data from microarray and PCR studies suggest there are occasional luminal type tumors that express these receptors (16, 110-112). A large fraction of ERα+ tumors also contain ErbB4 (110-112), and there is some indication this receptor may be involved in a reciprocal regulatory loop with ERα signaling (114). Surprisingly, AREG was not in the original gene set that defined ERα+ luminal tumors. A follow up interrogation of data that was used to relate disease outcome to cancer subclasses identified a correlation between higher levels of AREG expression, ERα, and the luminal A subclass (115). Also, this analysis indicated that ADAM-17 levels were low in the luminal A class relative to other tumor subtypes. These observations suggest that although most ERα+ luminal A breast cancers express AREG, they lack the EGFR; therefore, autocrine signaling by this ligand receptor system should not be present in most of these tumors. Because the tumor cells express low levels of ADAM-17 it is unclear whether AREG could even participate in paracrine signaling between luminal A breast cancer cells and the tumor stroma. There is a possibility that other proteases produced by the tumor cell or microenvironment lead to shedding of AREG by luminal A breast cancers but whether this signaling impacts progression is unclear.

3.1.3 Normal-like breast cancers

The gene expression signature of these tumors clustered with the normal breast samples. These tumors had a signature that was not associated with epithelial cell types. They instead express high levels of collagen receptors, lipoprotein lipase and glycerol-3-phosphate dehydrogenase normally found in stromal cells or adipocytes. High levels of AREG and moderate levels of ADAM-17 were observed in occasional samples from this group of tumors, but the EGFR was absent. At this time there is no evidence that ErbB signaling plays any role in the biology of these tumors (110-112).

3.1.4 Basal tumors

These tumors lack the expression of the estrogen, progesterone and ErbB2 receptor-for this reason they are often called triple receptor negative tumors-and these cancers express some markers consistent with the myoepithelial cells that are in contact with the basement membrane. These tumors express high levels of the epithelial markers kertatin 5 and 14 (basal keratins), P cadherin as well as troponin (110-112). Basal breast cancers are correlated with poor survival, high rates of distant metastasis and are generally high grade, large tumors. Once the category became established, antibody labeling studies indicated that 50 to 70% of the basal cancers expressed high levels of EGFR immunoreactivity (116). Low levels of EGFR expression is correlated with reduced numbers of distant metastasis (117). These tumors also frequently express elevated levels of TGFα and ADAM-17 (115).

Within basal breast cancers there could be a fraction that exhibits autocrine TGFα-EGFR signaling. The correlation of ADAM-17, TGFα and EGFR with poor prognosis implicates some role for this signaling system in metastasis. At this time, functional testing of TGFα in basal breast cancer models has not been completed. One major question that remains is: does TGFα participate in autocrine tumor cell signaling or paracrine tumor-stroma interactions. Future studies will identify which prometastatic cellular behaviors are activated by TGFα-EGFR signaling, providing insight into whether receptor-targeted therapeutics might provide benefit in a metastasis prevention paradigm.

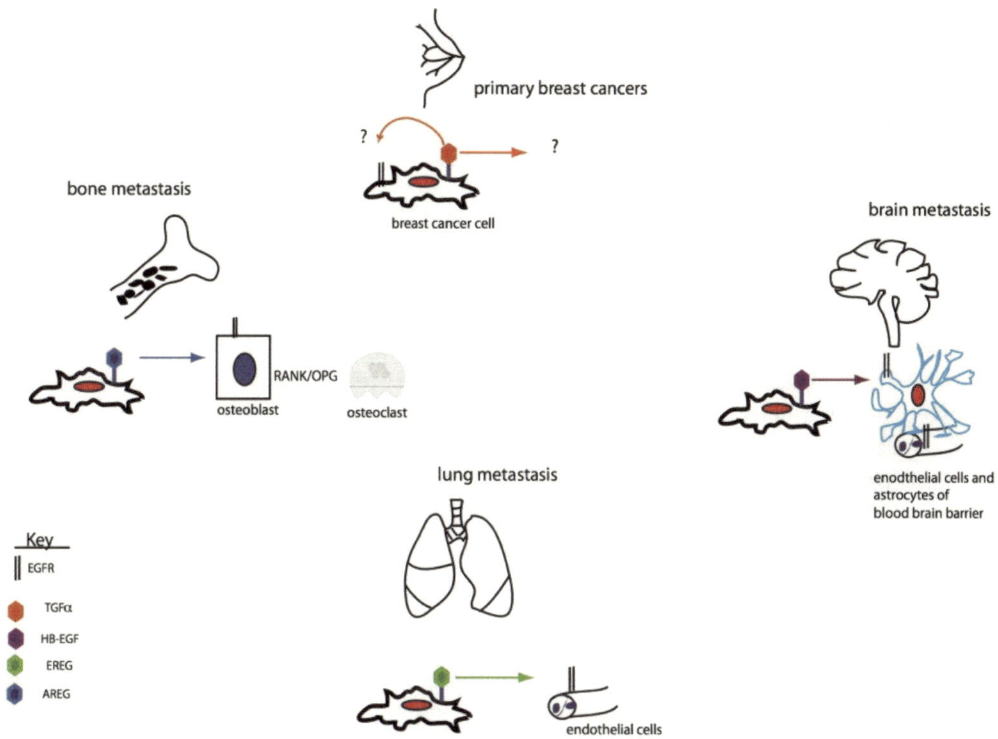

Fig. 3. Summary of EGFR-ligand signaling in models of basal breast cancer metastases. The specific ligand involved in primary tumors and metastatic site are indicated by the colored hexagons. The cell type that responds to the signal is also indicated. Paracrine signaling interactions appear to be important to metastases, whereas the relative role of autocrine versus paracrine signaling has not been explored in primary basal breast cancer.

3.2 ErbB signaling in breast cancer metastasis

Metastasis requires a set of cellular behaviors that are distinct from primary tumor formation. To spread from the site of the primary tumor to distant organs cancer cells must:

1) move out of the primary tumor and invade through local connective tissue; 2) enter capillaries (intravasation); 3) survive in the blood stream; 4) exit the blood stream (extravasation) and invade into a new organ; 5) survive in the new organ possibly as a micro metastasis; 6) adapt to the new organ and grow as a macrometastasis (virulence) (118, 119). These steps can be viewed as two generalized processes: 1) invasion, which is movement of cancer cells through normal tissue and entry into the blood stream, and 2) colonization, which is escape from the blood stream and growth in a distant organ. Substantial progress is being made in identifying metastasis genes that mediate these generalized steps of the process. Metastasis genes are thought dispensable for primary tumor initiation and growth, but are crucial to the novel processes involved in the spread of cancer (119). In general, genes that facilitate invasion for carcinomas such as breast cancer are associated with EMT. Some of the genes involved in invasion are expressed in primary tumors. Colonization is considered to be the most inefficient part of the metastatic process and the growth of a cancer cells in a novel organ is likely to require novel changes in gene expression. Thus, the expression of colonization/virulence-associated metastasis genes are thought to be limited tumors within the specific target organ, rather than being present in most primary tumors (118, 119). Due to less availability, comprehensive gene expression studies of metastases have lagged behind the studies of primary tumors. As a result, alternative strategies for identifying gene signatures that are functionally involved with metastasis have been developed. For breast cancer metastases, Massague and colleagues selected *in vitro* various subclones of the aggressive breast cancer cell line MDA-MB-231. They found that many of the subclones had differing capacities to colonize various organs after intracardiac injection into mice (12, 119-123). Gene expression profiles were generated from the subclones that colonized specific organs, and these were compared to signatures from subclones that colonized the other organs. These signatures were then compared to larger data bases generated from human primary tumors that had ultimately metastasized to the organ of interest producing a refined signature. Subsequent functional analysis of these gene signatures has resulted in the identification of specific EGFR ligands as breast cancer metastasis genes.

3.2.1 EREG and lung metastases

The identification of a lung metastatic signature was derived from subclones of the MDA-MB-231 (LM) breast cancer cells that produced lesions in the lung after intracardiac injection. Among the genes that emerged from this analysis was the ErbB ligand, EREG (121, 123). Knockdown of EREG alone failed to slow the growth of LM as primary tumors in the mammary fat pad or in lung. However, knockdown of EREG in conjunction with cyclooxigenase 2 (COX2), MMP1 and MMP2 (these genes had also been identified as upregulated in the LM signature) had a dramatic impact on both primary tumor growth and subsequent metastasis to lungs. The decreased primary tumor growth in the cells with reduced levels of EREG, COX2, MMP1 and MMP2 appeared to result from reduced angiogenesis. The LM cells recruited abundant dilated tortuous and leaky blood vessels, and the repression of these 4-genes resulted in reduced capillary branching, length and dye effusion. However, VEGF levels were not reduced in the quadruple knockdown tumors relative to controls. Also, no differences were observed in pericyte recruitment to the capillaries between the LM cells and the quadruple knockdowns, suggesting that capillary defects were the result of altered endothelial cell behavior. Also, these multiple knockdowns exhibited reduced ability to colonize lungs after intravenous injection as compared to the parental LM cells. Close evaluation of the lungs of animals injected with the quadruple knockdown cells found abundant cells trapped in the vasculature, suggesting a failure in extravasation. The deficiencies in quadruple knockdown extravasation were also observed with an *in vitro* assay. Consistent with the knockdown studies, single therapeutic agents that targeted EGFR (such as cetuximab, an EGFR blocking antibody), COX2 (celecoxib) or MMPs (GM6001) also had modest impact on behavior of the LM cells grown as primary tumor and their spontaneous metastases to the lung. However, combinations of two agents slowed the growth of primary tumors and reduced subsequent lung colonization. The efficacy of cetuximab suggests that EREG is stimulating this the EGFR and not ErbB4. The fact that LM cells lacked upregulation of VEGF production, (an EGFR regulatory target in most cancer cells) was interpreted as evidence that EREG functioned in paracrine signaling with endothelial cells rather than being engaged in autocrine signaling.

Although microvasculature defects do not appear to be a major component of the various EGFR-/- or other ErbB-knockout mice, studies of normal and tumor capillaries *in vitro* suggest signaling by family members has an influence on angiogenesis. Intriguingly, ErbB receptor expression is altered in tumor capillary endothelial cells as compared to those in normal vessels. ErbB 2, 3, 4 but minimal EGFR is found in most normal endothelial cells in culture (124). In contrast, tumor endothelial cells acquire the EGFR and down regulate ErbB3 expression both *in vitro* and *in vivo*. Endothelial cells in culture also express EGFR and ErbB4 ligands HB-EGF and NRG-1 (124-126). It is thought that HB-EGF signaling through both the EGFR and Erbb4 helps recruit pericytes to capillaries to stabilize the structures (125). The addition of exogenous EGF to tumor endothelial cells *in vitro* increases their proliferation (124). Shedding of HB-EGF and activation of the EGFR leads to down regulation of tight junction proteins and migration of normal endothelial cells (127). Also, NRG-1-ErbB4 signaling stimulates endothelial cell proliferation, migration and angiogenesis in animals; however, NRG-1 inhibits proliferation of tumor derived endothelial cells (124, 126). In light of the impact of EGFR signaling on tumor endothelial cells, breast cancer cell upregulation of EREG would contribute to the recruitment of a leaky vasculature that is common to aggressive tumors. In addition, EREG-EGFR/ErbB4 signaling might contribute to intrasavation and extrasavation by down regulation adhesion molecules between endothelial cells within capillaries. The question that remains is whether the low affinity ligand EREG might be more efficient at stimulating proliferation, migration and downregulation of junctional complexes than the high affinity ligand, HB-EGF normally present in endothelial cells.

3.2.2 HB-EGF and brain metastasis

A brain metastasis signature was derived using methods similar to those described for lung metastasis (120, 128). Among the genes that emerged as upregulated in brain metastatic cells was the ErbB ligand, HB-EGF (120). Treating mice cardiac-injected with brain seeking sublines MDA-MB-231 and CN34-BrM2C with cetuximab resulted in reduced numbers of brain metastases. Knockdown of both EREG and HB-EGF, or cetuximab treatment, reduced migration of MDA-MB-231 and CN34-BrM2C through consecutive monolayers of endothelial cells and astrocytes in a model of blood brain barrier extravasation. Brain endothelial cells and astrocytes both express the EGFR (100, 127). Activation of the EGFR has been shown to down regulate components of tight junctions in brain endothelial cells (127). This coupled with EGFR signaling induced upregulation of motility, chemokines and extracellular matrix remodeling genes in astrocytes would likely aid in extrasavation of breast cancer cells through the blood brain barrier into the parenchyma. Beyond this EGFR signaling produces reactive astrocytes that are components of the microenvironment of brain metastases. This raises the question of whether breast cancer generated EGFR ligands could play a role in breast cancer cell virulence in the brain by generating increased numbers of reactive astrocytes (129). HB-EGF is the EGFR ligand most abundantly expressed in the brain and endothelial cells, suggesting it may be the most well suited agonist to mediate in paracrine interactions among cancer cells, capillaries and the brain parenchyma.

3.2.3 AREG and bone metastasis

Tumor cell colonization of bone may be a less complex process than that of lung and brain because the capillaries in bone called sinusoids, have large openings in them to facilitate entrance of bone marrow derivatives into the circulation (119). It is thought that cancer cells may be able to exit through these openings dispensing with the intricacies of extravasation from continuous capillaries.

The growth of breast cancer macrometastases is described as a vicious cycle (130, 131). In this cycle, breast cancer cells exploit the natural renewal process based on the paracrine interactions between the bone forming osteoblast and the bone resorbing osteoclast. In normal bone, osteoblasts regulate osteoclast numbers and activity by releasing chemokines that recruit osteoclast precursors and then differentiate and activate them with a cell surface ligand for the receptor for activation of NFκβ (RANKL). Osteoblasts also produce a soluble decoy receptor osteoprotegrin (OPG) that prevents RANKL from engaging its receptor; therefore, the level of the ratio of OPG to RANKL controls osteoclastogenesis. Once activated, osteoclasts adhere to the bone surface and secrete proteases and acid that degrades mineralized matrix. Growth factors including TGFβ and IGF-1 are released from the bone matrix, and this in turn stimulates new bone matrix formation by osteoblasts. This is a regenerating system that is in balance within the local environment; however, the rate of turnover and formation can be modulated by a series of endocrine hormones including PTH and calcitonin. Within the bone marrow, breast cancer cells produce a series of cytokines and growth factors including IL-11 and PTH-related protein (PTHrP) that increase the levels of RANKL relative to OPG leading to increased osteoclastogenesis. The increased bone resorption and resulting high level of growth factors enhance the survival of breast cancer cells, and also TGFβ increases gene expression of IL-11 and PTHrP, which begets more osteoclasts.

Profiling bone metastasis subclones of MDA-MB-231 cells resulted in an 11-gene signature (122). Several of the genes identified were factors like IL-11 that directly altered the RANKL/OPG ratio or connective tissue factor that enhanced osteoblast proliferation. Ectopic expression of a single gene from the profile had very little impact on the ability of modestly osteolytic 231 subclones to grow within in the bone of immunocompromised mice. However, the combination of 3 of the genes from the signature induced destructive growth in bone after intracardiac injection. Among the genes identified in the signature that produced increased osteolysis when overexpressed as part of a 3 gene cassette were the proteases, MMP1 and ADAMTS-1 (12). It was unclear what the role of these molecules would play in bone metastasis. Eventually, a careful evaluation of aggressively osteolytic MDA-MB-231 lines that were engineered to overexpress ADAMTS-1 and MMP1 were found to shed dramatically increased levels of AREG. Conditioned media from the ADAMTS-1 and MMP1 engineered MDA-MB-231 lines caused an increased RANKL/OPG ratio in primary murine bone cell cultures (12, 132). The conditioned media from the MDA-MB-231-ADAMTS-1 and MMP1 cells activated osteoclastogenesis in the primary bone cell cultures, and this could be inhibited by the EGFR inhibitors gefitinib or cetuximab. Remarkably, these agents (Gefitinib 100mg/kg daily or Cetuximab 100 mg/kg weekly) completely prevented the formation of osteolytic lesions by the MDA-MB-231 ADAMTS-1+MMP1 line delivered by either the intracardiac or intratibial injection method (12). These findings clearly support the notion that EGFR signaling on cells of the osteoblast is a major regulator of the RANKL/OPG ratio, but point out the requirement for appropriate protease expression to make EGFR ligands accessible to the bone microenvironment. These experiments provide an explanation of how bone resorbtion could be uncoupled from bone formation by breast cancer cells because stimulation of the EGFR should block osteoblast differentiation and matrix production.

To some extent, the identification of a role for AREG in bone metastasis is confounding given that its expression is associated with ERα+ breast cancers that generally have good prognosis (115). The MDA-MB-231 cells are ERα- and have a phenotype that is similar to basal cancers. So we interrogated the breast cancer transcriptome datasets GSE2034(133), GSE2603 (123), and GSE12276 (120) from the NCBI Gene Expression Omnibus to evaluate AREG expression in ERα- tumors. We found that AREG expression was lower in the ERα-negative tumors that ultimately metastasized to bone as compared to those that did not (134). A similar pattern of expression has been reported for the classical bone metastasis virulence factor PTHrP. Low expression of the peptide is observed in the primary tumors that ultimately metastasize to bone (135-137). PTHrP gene expression is thought to be activated by TGFβ when breast cancer cells enter the bone microenvironment (138). In contrast to PTHrP, the enhanced activity or expression of the proteases that cleave AREG would be sufficient to increase its expression in the bone microenvironment without activating gene expression. Consistent with this concept, high expression ADAMTS-1 and MMP1 protein have been observed in primary breast cancer tumors that ultimately metastasized to bone (12). Thus, the complex post-genomic regulation of EGFR ligand processing and receptor interactions provides mechanism beyond transcription where the amplitude of signaling of this system can be increased to contribute to colonization. Given that AREG appears to be the physiological mediator of EGFR signaling in the bone, it may be ideally suited to uncouple bone formation from bone resorbtion, which is a component of osteolytic predominant bone metastases that arise from breast cancers.

3.3 Conclusions: EGFR ligand function in breast cancer

EGFR ligands and receptors are frequently expressed together on epithelial cells and the cancers that are derived from these tissues, including the breast. Addition of exogenous EGFR ligands to breast epithelial or cancer cells typically has a profound impact on proliferation or migratory behavior, leading to the concept that autocrine receptor signaling would contribute to tumor progression. Despite this perspective, the unraveling of the developmental breast, heart and brain phenotypes of the various family member KOs suggest that EGFR, ligand and ADAM-17 function as part of a complex paracrine-signaling network. In addition, *in vitro and in vivo* models based on MDA-MB-231 cells where EGFR ligands have been found to function as metastasis genes, suggest they signal in a paracrine fashion to key elements of the microenvironment. On the basis of these conclusions, we speculate that TGFα expression in primary basal breast cancers may also be engaged in paracrine signaling with cells in the microenvironment. This conclusion suggests that the efficacy of EGFR targeted therapeutics will depend upon their uses in combination with other compounds that target the tumor microenvironment in primary basal tumors, as well as those that have metastasized to the lung, brain and bone.

4. References

[1] Llombart-Cussac A. Improving decision-making in early breast cancer: who to treat and how? Breast Cancer Res Treat2008 Dec;112 Suppl 1:15-24.

[2] Brufsky A. Trastuzumab-based therapy for patients with HER2-positive breast cancer: from early scientific development to foundation of care. Am J Clin Oncol2010 Apr;33(2):186-95.

[3] Yarden Y, Sliwkowski MX. Untangling the ErbB signalling network. Nat Rev Mol Cell Biol2001 Feb;2(2):127-37.

[4] Wilson KJ, Gilmore JL, Foley J, Lemmon MA, Riese DJ, 2nd. Functional selectivity of EGF family peptide growth factors: implications for cancer. Pharmacol Ther2009 Apr;122(1):1-8.

[5] Daub H, Weiss FU, Wallasch C, Ullrich A. Role of transactivation of the EGF receptor in signalling by G-protein-coupled receptors. Nature1996 Feb 8;379(6565):557-60.

[6] Iwamoto R, Mekada E. Heparin-binding EGF-like growth factor: a juxtacrine growth factor. Cytokine Growth Factor Rev2000 Dec;11(4):335-44.

[7] Prince RN, Schreiter ER, Zou P, Wiley HS, Ting AY, Lee RT, Lauffenburger DA. The heparin-binding domain of HB-EGF mediates localization to sites of cell-cell contact and prevents HB-EGF proteolytic release. J Cell Sci2010 Jul 1;123(Pt 13):2308-18.

[8] Sahin U, Weskamp G, Kelly K, Zhou HM, Higashiyama S, Peschon J, Hartmann D, Saftig P, Blobel CP. Distinct roles for ADAM10 and ADAM17 in ectodomain shedding of six EGFR ligands. J Cell Biol2004 Mar 1;164(5):769-79.

[9] Tousseyn T, Jorissen E, Reiss K, Hartmann D. (Make) stick and cut loose--disintegrin metalloproteases in development and disease. Birth Defects Res C Embryo Today2006 Mar;78(1):24-46.

[10] Zhang Q, Thomas SM, Lui VW, Xi S, Siegfried JM, Fan H, Smithgall TE, Mills GB, Grandis JR. Phosphorylation of TNF-alpha converting enzyme by gastrin-releasing peptide induces amphiregulin release and EGF receptor activation. Proc Natl Acad Sci U S A2006 May 2;103(18):6901-6.

[11] Wagstaff L, Kelwick R, Decock J, Edwards DR. The roles of ADAMTS metalloproteinases in tumorigenesis and metastasis. Front Biosci2011;16:1861-72.

[12] Lu X, Wang Q, Hu G, Van Poznak C, Fleisher M, Reiss M, Massague J, Kang Y. ADAMTS1 and MMP1 proteolytically engage EGF-like ligands in an osteolytic signaling cascade for bone metastasis. Genes Dev2009 Aug 15;23(16):1882-94.

[13] Chokki M, Eguchi H, Hamamura I, Mitsuhashi H, Kamimura T. Human airway trypsin-like protease induces amphiregulin release through a mechanism involving protease-activated receptor-2-mediated ERK activation and TNF alpha-converting enzyme activity in airway epithelial cells. Febs J2005 Dec;272(24):6387-99.

[14] Pawlowski V, Revillion F, Hebbar M, Hornez L, Peyrat JP. Prognostic value of the type I growth factor receptors in a large series of human primary breast cancers quantified with a real-time reverse transcription-polymerase chain reaction assay. Clin Cancer Res2000 Nov;6(11):4217-25.

[15] McIntyre E, Blackburn E, Brown PJ, Johnson CG, Gullick WJ. The complete family of epidermal growth factor receptors and their ligands are co-ordinately expressed in breast cancer. Breast Cancer Res Treat2010 Jul;122(1):105-10.

[16] Revillion F, Lhotellier V, Hornez L, Bonneterre J, Peyrat JP. ErbB/HER ligands in human breast cancer, and relationships with their receptors, the bio-pathological features and prognosis. Ann Oncol2008 Jan;19(1):73-80.

[17] Edwin F, Wiepz GJ, Singh R, Peet CR, Chaturvedi D, Bertics PJ, Patel TB. A historical perspective of the EGF receptor and related systems. Methods Mol Biol2006;327:1-24.

[18] Riese DJ, 2nd, Stern DF. Specificity within the EGF family/ErbB receptor family signaling network. Bioessays1998 Jan;20(1):41-8.

[19] Lemmon MA. Ligand-induced ErbB receptor dimerization. Exp Cell Res2009 Feb 15;315(4):638-48.

[20] Riese DJ, 2nd, Gallo RM, Settleman J. Mutational activation of ErbB family receptor tyrosine kinases: insights into mechanisms of signal transduction and tumorigenesis. Bioessays2007 Jun;29(6):558-65.

[21] Schulze WX, Deng L, Mann M. Phosphotyrosine interactome of the ErbB-receptor kinase family. Mol Syst Biol2005;1:2005 0008.

[22] Roepstorff K, Grandal MV, Henriksen L, Knudsen SL, Lerdrup M, Grovdal L, Willumsen BM, van Deurs B. Differential effects of EGFR ligands on endocytic sorting of the receptor. Traffic2009 Aug;10(8):1115-27.

[23] Avraham R, Yarden Y. Feedback regulation of EGFR signalling: decision making by early and delayed loops. Nat Rev Mol Cell Biol2011 Feb;12(2):104-17.

[24] Bublil EM, Yarden Y. The EGF receptor family: spearheading a merger of signaling and therapeutics. Curr Opin Cell Biol2007 Apr;19(2):124-34.

[25] Citri A, Yarden Y. EGF-ERBB signalling: towards the systems level. Nat Rev Mol Cell Biol2006 Jul;7(7):505-16.

[26] Slamon DJ, Clark GM, Wong SG, Levin WJ, Ullrich A, McGuire WL. Human breast cancer: correlation of relapse and survival with amplification of the HER-2/neu oncogene. Science1987 Jan 9;235(4785):177-82.

[27] Salomon DS, Brandt R, Ciardiello F, Normanno N. Epidermal growth factor-related peptides and their receptors in human malignancies. Crit Rev Oncol Hematol1995 Jul;19(3):183-232.

[28] Earp HS, Dawson TL, Li X, Yu H. Heterodimerization and functional interaction between EGF receptor family members: a new signaling paradigm with implications for breast cancer research. Breast Cancer Res Treat1995 Jul;35(1):115-32.

[29] Wada T, Qian XL, Greene MI. Intermolecular association of the p185neu protein and EGF receptor modulates EGF receptor function. Cell1990 Jun 29;61(7):1339-47.

[30] Wang Z, Zhang L, Yeung TK, Chen X. Endocytosis deficiency of epidermal growth factor (EGF) receptor-ErbB2 heterodimers in response to EGF stimulation. Mol Biol Cell1999 May;10(5):1621-36.

[31] Hendriks BS, Wiley HS, Lauffenburger D. HER2-mediated effects on EGFR endosomal sorting: analysis of biophysical mechanisms. Biophys J2003 Oct;85(4):2732-45.

[32] Jones JT, Akita RW, Sliwkowski MX. Binding specificities and affinities of egf domains for ErbB receptors. FEBS Lett1999 Mar 26;447(2-3):227-31.

[33] Liu W, Volpe MA, Zscheppang K, Nielsen HC, Dammann CE. ErbB4 regulates surfactant synthesis and proliferation in adult rat pulmonary epithelial cells. Exp Lung Res2009 Feb;35(1):29-47.

[34] Zscheppang K, Korenbaum E, Bueter W, Ramadurai SM, Nielsen HC, Dammann CE. ErbB receptor dimerization, localization, and co-localization in mouse lung type II epithelial cells. Pediatr Pulmonol2006 Dec;41(12):1205-12.

[35] Hatakeyama M, Yumoto N, Yu X, Shirouzu M, Yokoyama S, Konagaya A. Transformation potency of ErbB heterodimer signaling is determined by B-Raf kinase. Oncogene2004 Jun 24;23(29):5023-31.

[36] Frolov A, Schuller K, Tzeng CW, Cannon EE, Ku BC, Howard JH, Vickers SM, Heslin MJ, Buchsbaum DJ, Arnoletti JP. ErbB3 expression and dimerization with EGFR influence pancreatic cancer cell sensitivity to erlotinib. Cancer Biol Ther2007 Apr;6(4):548-54.

[37] Liles JS, Arnoletti JP, Tzeng CW, Howard JH, Kossenkov AV, Kulesza P, Heslin MJ, Frolov A. ErbB3 expression promotes tumorigenesis in pancreatic adenocarcinoma. Cancer Biol Ther2010 Sep;10(6):555-63.

[38] Waterman H, Sabanai I, Geiger B, Yarden Y. Alternative intracellular routing of ErbB receptors may determine signaling potency. J Biol Chem1998 May 29;273(22):13819-27.

[39] French AR, Sudlow GP, Wiley HS, Lauffenburger DA. Postendocytic trafficking of epidermal growth factor-receptor complexes is mediated through saturable and specific endosomal interactions. J Biol Chem1994 Jun 3;269(22):15749-55.

[40] Reddy CC, Niyogi SK, Wells A, Wiley HS, Lauffenburger DA. Engineering epidermal growth factor for enhanced mitogenic potency. Nat Biotechnol1996 Dec;14(13):1696-9.

[41] Willmarth NE, Ethier SP. Autocrine and juxtacrine effects of amphiregulin on the proliferative, invasive, and migratory properties of normal and neoplastic human mammary epithelial cells. J Biol Chem2006 Dec 8;281(49):37728-37.

[42] Streicher KL, Willmarth NE, Garcia J, Boerner JL, Dewey TG, Ethier SP. Activation of a nuclear factor kappaB/interleukin-1 positive feedback loop by amphiregulin in human breast cancer cells. Mol Cancer Res2007 Aug;5(8):847-61.

[43] Willmarth NE, Baillo A, Dziubinski ML, Wilson K, Riese DJ, 2nd, Ethier SP. Altered EGFR localization and degradation in human breast cancer cells with an amphiregulin/EGFR autocrine loop. Cell Signal2009 Feb;21(2):212-9.

[44] Shoyab M, McDonald VL, Bradley JG, Todaro GJ. Amphiregulin: a bifunctional growth-modulating glycoprotein produced by the phorbol 12-myristate 13-acetate-

treated human breast adenocarcinoma cell line MCF-7. Proc Natl Acad Sci U S A1988 Sep;85(17):6528-32.
[45] Shoyab M, Plowman GD, McDonald VL, Bradley JG, Todaro GJ. Structure and function of human amphiregulin: a member of the epidermal growth factor family. Science1989 Feb 24;243(4894 Pt 1):1074-6.
[46] Stoll SW, Johnson JL, Bhasin A, Johnston A, Gudjonsson JE, Rittie L, Elder JT. Metalloproteinase-mediated, context-dependent function of amphiregulin and HB-EGF in human keratinocytes and skin. J Invest Dermatol2010 Jan;130(1):295-304.
[47] Barnard JA, Graves-Deal R, Pittelkow MR, DuBois R, Cook P, Ramsey GW, Bishop PR, Damstrup L, Coffey RJ. Auto- and cross-induction within the mammalian epidermal growth factor-related peptide family. J Biol Chem1994 Sep 9;269(36):22817-22.
[48] Cook PW, Mattox PA, Keeble WW, Pittelkow MR, Plowman GD, Shoyab M, Adelman JP, Shipley GD. A heparin sulfate-regulated human keratinocyte autocrine factor is similar or identical to amphiregulin. Mol Cell Biol1991 May;11(5):2547-57.
[49] Neelam B, Richter A, Chamberlin SG, Puddicombe SM, Wood L, Murray MB, Nandagopal K, Niyogi SK, Davies DE. Structure-function studies of ligand-induced epidermal growth factor receptor dimerization. Biochemistry1998 Apr 7;37(14):4884-91.
[50] Adam R, Drummond DR, Solic N, Holt SJ, Sharma RP, Chamberlin SG, Davies DE. Modulation of the receptor binding affinity of amphiregulin by modification of its carboxyl terminal tail. Biochim Biophys Acta1995 Apr 6;1266(1):83-90.
[51] Gilmore JL, Scott JA, Bouizar Z, Robling A, Pitfield SE, Riese DJ, 2nd, Foley J. Amphiregulin-EGFR signaling regulates PTHrP gene expression in breast cancer cells. Breast Cancer Res Treat2007 Sep 20.
[52] Stern KA, Place TL, Lill NL. EGF and amphiregulin differentially regulate Cbl recruitment to endosomes and EGF receptor fate. Biochem J2008 Mar 15;410(3):585-94.
[53] Chung E, Graves-Deal R, Franklin JL, Coffey RJ. Differential effects of amphiregulin and TGF-alpha on the morphology of MDCK cells. Exp Cell Res2005 Sep 10;309(1):149-60.
[54] Kochupurakkal BS, Harari D, Di-Segni A, Maik-Rachline G, Lyass L, Gur G, Kerber G, Citri A, Lavi S, Eilam R, Chalifa-Caspi V, Eshhar Z, Pikarsky E, Pinkas-Kramarski R, Bacus SS, Yarden Y. Epigen, the last ligand of ErbB receptors, reveals intricate relationships between affinity and mitogenicity. J Biol Chem2005 Mar 4;280(9):8503-12.
[55] Strachan L, Murison JG, Prestidge RL, Sleeman MA, Watson JD, Kumble KD. Cloning and biological activity of epigen, a novel member of the epidermal growth factor superfamily. J Biol Chem2001 May 25;276(21):18265-71.
[56] Elenius K, Paul S, Allison G, Sun J, Klagsbrun M. Activation of HER4 by heparin-binding EGF-like growth factor stimulates chemotaxis but not proliferation. Embo J1997 Mar 17;16(6):1268-78.

[57] Higashiyama S, Abraham JA, Miller J, Fiddes JC, Klagsbrun M. A heparin-binding growth factor secreted by macrophage-like cells that is related to EGF. Science1991 Feb 22;251(4996):936-9.

[58] Nishi E, Klagsbrun M. Heparin-binding epidermal growth factor-like growth factor (HB-EGF) is a mediator of multiple physiological and pathological pathways. Growth Factors2004 Dec;22(4):253-60.

[59] Shing Y, Christofori G, Hanahan D, Ono Y, Sasada R, Igarashi K, Folkman J. Betacellulin: a mitogen from pancreatic beta cell tumors. Science1993 Mar 12;259(5101):1604-7.

[60] Sweeney C, Lai C, Riese DJ, 2nd, Diamonti AJ, Cantley LC, Carraway KL, 3rd. Ligand discrimination in signaling through an ErbB4 receptor homodimer. J Biol Chem2000 Jun 30;275(26):19803-7.

[61] Tada H, Sasada R, Kawaguchi Y, Kojima I, Gullick WJ, Salomon DS, Igarashi K, Seno M, Yamada H. Processing and juxtacrine activity of membrane-anchored betacellulin. J Cell Biochem1999 Mar 1;72(3):423-34.

[62] Komurasaki T, Toyoda H, Uchida D, Morimoto S. Epiregulin binds to epidermal growth factor receptor and ErbB-4 and induces tyrosine phosphorylation of epidermal growth factor receptor, ErbB-2, ErbB-3 and ErbB-4. Oncogene1997 Dec 4;15(23):2841-8.

[63] Sasaki E, Arakawa T, Fujiwara Y, Kawada N, Fukuda T, Higuchi K, Komurasaki T, Kobayashi K. Epiregulin stimulates proliferation of rabbit gastric cells in primary culture through autophosphorylation of the epidermal growth factor receptor. Eur J Pharmacol1997 Nov 12;338(3):253-8.

[64] Riese DJ, 2nd, Komurasaki T, Plowman GD, Stern DF. Activation of ErbB4 by the bifunctional epidermal growth factor family hormone epiregulin is regulated by ErbB2. J Biol Chem1998 May 1;273(18):11288-94.

[65] Shelly M, Pinkas-Kramarski R, Guarino BC, Waterman H, Wang LM, Lyass L, Alimandi M, Kuo A, Bacus SS, Pierce JH, Andrews GC, Yarden Y. Epiregulin is a potent pan-ErbB ligand that preferentially activates heterodimeric receptor complexes. J Biol Chem1998 Apr 24;273(17):10496-505.

[66] Cardiff RD, Wellings SR. The comparative pathology of human and mouse mammary glands. J Mammary Gland Biol Neoplasia1999 Jan;4(1):105-22.

[67] Hens JR, Wysolmerski JJ. Key stages of mammary gland development: molecular mechanisms involved in the formation of the embryonic mammary gland. Breast Cancer Res2005;7(5):220-4.

[68] Fendrick JL, Raafat AM, Haslam SZ. Mammary gland growth and development from the postnatal period to postmenopause: ovarian steroid receptor ontogeny and regulation in the mouse. J Mammary Gland Biol Neoplasia1998 Jan;3(1):7-22.

[69] Nandi S. Endocrine control of mammarygland development and function in the C3H/ He Crgl mouse. J Natl Cancer Inst1958 Dec;21(6):1039-63.

[70] Snedeker SM, Brown CF, DiAugustine RP. Expression and functional properties of transforming growth factor alpha and epidermal growth factor during mouse mammary gland ductal morphogenesis. Proc Natl Acad Sci U S A1991 Jan 1;88(1):276-80.

[71] Watson CJ, Khaled WT. Mammary development in the embryo and adult: a journey of morphogenesis and commitment. Development2008 Mar;135(6):995-1003.
[72] Brisken C, Kaur S, Chavarria TE, Binart N, Sutherland RL, Weinberg RA, Kelly PA, Ormandy CJ. Prolactin controls mammary gland development via direct and indirect mechanisms. Dev Biol1999 Jun 1;210(1):96-106.
[73] Brisken C, Park S, Vass T, Lydon JP, O'Malley BW, Weinberg RA. A paracrine role for the epithelial progesterone receptor in mammary gland development. Proc Natl Acad Sci U S A1998 Apr 28;95(9):5076-81.
[74] Schroeder JA, Lee DC. Dynamic expression and activation of ERBB receptors in the developing mouse mammary gland. Cell Growth Differ1998 Jun;9(6):451-64.
[75] Sebastian J, Richards RG, Walker MP, Wiesen JF, Werb Z, Derynck R, Hom YK, Cunha GR, DiAugustine RP. Activation and function of the epidermal growth factor receptor and erbB-2 during mammary gland morphogenesis. Cell Growth Differ1998 Sep;9(9):777-85.
[76] Wiesen JF, Young P, Werb Z, Cunha GR. Signaling through the stromal epidermal growth factor receptor is necessary for mammary ductal development. Development1999 Jan;126(2):335-44.
[77] Kenney NJ, Huang RP, Johnson GR, Wu JX, Okamura D, Matheny W, Kordon E, Gullick WJ, Plowman G, Smith GH, et al. Detection and location of amphiregulin and Cripto-1 expression in the developing postnatal mouse mammary gland. Mol Reprod Dev1995 Jul;41(3):277-86.
[78] Luetteke NC, Qiu TH, Fenton SE, Troyer KL, Riedel RF, Chang A, Lee DC. Targeted inactivation of the EGF and amphiregulin genes reveals distinct roles for EGF receptor ligands in mouse mammary gland development. Development1999 Jun;126(12):2739-50.
[79] Ciarloni L, Mallepell S, Brisken C. Amphiregulin is an essential mediator of estrogen receptor alpha function in mammary gland development. Proc Natl Acad Sci U S A2007 Mar 27;104(13):5455-60.
[80] Rho JY, Wada-Kiyama Y, Onishi Y, Kiyama R, Sakuma Y. Expressional regulation of neuronal and cancer-related genes by estrogen in adult female rats. Endocr Res2004 May;30(2):257-67.
[81] Britton DJ, Hutcheson IR, Knowlden JM, Barrow D, Giles M, McClelland RA, Gee JM, Nicholson RI. Bidirectional cross talk between ERalpha and EGFR signalling pathways regulates tamoxifen-resistant growth. Breast Cancer Res Treat2006 Mar;96(2):131-46.
[82] Sternlicht MD, Sunnarborg SW, Kouros-Mehr H, Yu Y, Lee DC, Werb Z. Mammary ductal morphogenesis requires paracrine activation of stromal EGFR via ADAM17-dependent shedding of epithelial amphiregulin. Development2005 Sep;132(17):3923-33.
[83] Asselin-Labat ML, Vaillant F, Shackleton M, Bouras T, Lindeman GJ, Visvader JE. Delineating the epithelial hierarchy in the mouse mammary gland. Cold Spring Harb Symp Quant Biol2008;73:469-78.

[84] Eirew P, Stingl J, Raouf A, Turashvili G, Aparicio S, Emerman JT, Eaves CJ. A method for quantifying normal human mammary epithelial stem cells with in vivo regenerative ability. Nat Med2008 Dec;14(12):1384-9.

[85] Lim E, Vaillant F, Wu D, Forrest NC, Pal B, Hart AH, Asselin-Labat ML, Gyorki DE, Ward T, Partanen A, Feleppa F, Huschtscha LI, Thorne HJ, Fox SB, Yan M, French JD, Brown MA, Smyth GK, Visvader JE, Lindeman GJ. Aberrant luminal progenitors as the candidate target population for basal tumor development in BRCA1 mutation carriers. Nat Med2009 Aug;15(8):907-13.

[86] Asselin-Labat ML, Sutherland KD, Barker H, Thomas R, Shackleton M, Forrest NC, Hartley L, Robb L, Grosveld FG, van der Wees J, Lindeman GJ, Visvader JE. Gata-3 is an essential regulator of mammary-gland morphogenesis and luminal-cell differentiation. Nat Cell Biol2007 Feb;9(2):201-9.

[87] Jackson-Fisher AJ, Bellinger G, Breindel JL, Tavassoli FA, Booth CJ, Duong JK, Stern DF. ErbB3 is required for ductal morphogenesis in the mouse mammary gland. Breast Cancer Res2008;10(6):R96.

[88] Jackson-Fisher AJ, Bellinger G, Ramabhadran R, Morris JK, Lee KF, Stern DF. ErbB2 is required for ductal morphogenesis of the mammary gland. Proc Natl Acad Sci U S A2004 Dec 7;101(49):17138-43.

[89] Tidcombe H, Jackson-Fisher A, Mathers K, Stern DF, Gassmann M, Golding JP. Neural and mammary gland defects in ErbB4 knockout mice genetically rescued from embryonic lethality. Proc Natl Acad Sci U S A2003 Jul 8;100(14):8281-6.

[90] Lee KF, Simon H, Chen H, Bates B, Hung MC, Hauser C. Requirement for neuregulin receptor erbB2 in neural and cardiac development. Nature1995 Nov 23;378(6555):394-8.

[91] Erickson SL, O'Shea KS, Ghaboosi N, Loverro L, Frantz G, Bauer M, Lu LH, Moore MW. ErbB3 is required for normal cerebellar and cardiac development: a comparison with ErbB2-and heregulin-deficient mice. Development1997 Dec;124(24):4999-5011.

[92] Kramer R, Bucay N, Kane DJ, Martin LE, Tarpley JE, Theill LE. Neuregulins with an Ig-like domain are essential for mouse myocardial and neuronal development. Proc Natl Acad Sci U S A1996 May 14;93(10):4833-8.

[93] Gassmann M, Casagranda F, Orioli D, Simon H, Lai C, Klein R, Lemke G. Aberrant neural and cardiac development in mice lacking the ErbB4 neuregulin receptor. Nature1995 Nov 23;378(6555):390-4.

[94] Sanchez-Soria P, Camenisch TD. ErbB signaling in cardiac development and disease. Semin Cell Dev Biol2010 Dec;21(9):929-35.

[95] Schroeder JA, Jackson LF, Lee DC, Camenisch TD. Form and function of developing heart valves: coordination by extracellular matrix and growth factor signaling. J Mol Med2003 Jul;81(7):392-403.

[96] Sibilia M, Wagner EF. Strain-dependent epithelial defects in mice lacking the EGF receptor. Science1995 Jul 14;269(5221):234-8.

[97] Jackson LF, Qiu TH, Sunnarborg SW, Chang A, Zhang C, Patterson C, Lee DC. Defective valvulogenesis in HB-EGF and TACE-null mice is associated with aberrant BMP signaling. Embo J2003 Jun 2;22(11):2704-16.

[98] Kornblum HI, Hussain R, Wiesen J, Miettinen P, Zurcher SD, Chow K, Derynck R, Werb Z. Abnormal astrocyte development and neuronal death in mice lacking the epidermal growth factor receptor. J Neurosci Res1998 Sep 15;53(6):697-717.

[99] Kornblum HI, Zurcher SD, Werb Z, Derynck R, Seroogy KB. Multiple trophic actions of heparin-binding epidermal growth factor (HB-EGF) in the central nervous system. Eur J Neurosci1999 Sep;11(9):3236-46.

[100] Kornblum HI, Hussain RJ, Bronstein JM, Gall CM, Lee DC, Seroogy KB. Prenatal ontogeny of the epidermal growth factor receptor and its ligand, transforming growth factor alpha, in the rat brain. J Comp Neurol1997 Apr 7;380(2):243-61.

[101] Liu B, Neufeld AH. Activation of epidermal growth factor receptors in astrocytes: from development to neural injury. J Neurosci Res2007 Dec;85(16):3523-9.

[102] Kang W, Hebert JM. Signaling pathways in reactive astrocytes, a genetic perspective. Mol Neurobiol2011 Jun;43(3):147-54.

[103] Ibbotson KJ, D'Souza SM, Ng KW, Osborne CK, Niall M, Martin TJ, Mundy GR. Tumor-derived growth factor increases bone resorption in a tumor associated with humoral hypercalcemia of malignancy. Science1983 Sep 23;221(4617):1292-4.

[104] Ibbotson KJ, D'Souza SM, Smith DD, Carpenter G, Mundy GR. EGF receptor antiserum inhibits bone resorbing activity produced by a rat Leydig cell tumor associated with the humoral hypercalcemia of malignancy. Endocrinology1985 Jan;116(1):469-71.

[105] Shupnik MA, Ip NY, Tashjian AH, Jr. Characterization and regulation of receptors for epidermal growth factor in mouse calvaria. Endocrinology1980 Dec;107(6):1738-46.

[106] Sibilia M, Wagner B, Hoebertz A, Elliott C, Marino S, Jochum W, Wagner EF. Mice humanised for the EGF receptor display hypomorphic phenotypes in skin, bone and heart. Development2003 Oct;130(19):4515-25.

[107] Qin L, Partridge NC. Stimulation of amphiregulin expression in osteoblastic cells by parathyroid hormone requires the protein kinase A and cAMP response element-binding protein signaling pathway. J Cell Biochem2005 Oct 15;96(3):632-40.

[108] Qin L, Qiu P, Wang L, Li X, Swarthout JT, Soteropoulos P, Tolias P, Partridge NC. Gene expression profiles and transcription factors involved in parathyroid hormone signaling in osteoblasts revealed by microarray and bioinformatics. J Biol Chem2003 May 30;278(22):19723-31.

[109] Cole JA. Parathyroid hormone activates mitogen-activated protein kinase in opossum kidney cells. Endocrinology1999 Dec;140(12):5771-9.

[110] van 't Veer LJ, Dai H, van de Vijver MJ, He YD, Hart AA, Mao M, Peterse HL, van der Kooy K, Marton MJ, Witteveen AT, Schreiber GJ, Kerkhoven RM, Roberts C, Linsley PS, Bernards R, Friend SH. Gene expression profiling predicts clinical outcome of breast cancer. Nature2002 Jan 31;415(6871):530-6.

[111] van de Vijver MJ, He YD, van't Veer LJ, Dai H, Hart AA, Voskuil DW, Schreiber GJ, Peterse JL, Roberts C, Marton MJ, Parrish M, Atsma D, Witteveen A, Glas A, Delahaye L, van der Velde T, Bartelink H, Rodenhuis S, Rutgers ET, Friend SH, Bernards R. A gene-expression signature as a predictor of survival in breast cancer. N Engl J Med2002 Dec 19;347(25):1999-2009.

[112] Sorlie T, Perou CM, Tibshirani R, Aas T, Geisler S, Johnsen H, Hastie T, Eisen MB, van de Rijn M, Jeffrey SS, Thorsen T, Quist H, Matese JC, Brown PO, Botstein D, Eystein Lonning P, Borresen-Dale AL. Gene expression patterns of breast carcinomas distinguish tumor subclasses with clinical implications. Proc Natl Acad Sci U S A2001 Sep 11;98(19):10869-74.

[113] Wiseman SM, Makretsov N, Nielsen TO, Gilks B, Yorida E, Cheang M, Turbin D, Gelmon K, Huntsman DG. Coexpression of the type 1 growth factor receptor family members HER-1, HER-2, and HER-3 has a synergistic negative prognostic effect on breast carcinoma survival. Cancer2005 May 1;103(9):1770-7.

[114] Zhu Y, Sullivan LL, Nair SS, Williams CC, Pandey AK, Marrero L, Vadlamudi RK, Jones FE. Coregulation of estrogen receptor by ERBB4/HER4 establishes a growth-promoting autocrine signal in breast tumor cells. Cancer Res2006 Aug 15;66(16):7991-8.

[115] McGowan PM, McKiernan E, Bolster F, Ryan BM, Hill AD, McDermott EW, Evoy D, O'Higgins N, Crown J, Duffy MJ. ADAM-17 predicts adverse outcome in patients with breast cancer. Ann Oncol2008 Jun;19(6):1075-81.

[116] Burness ML, Grushko TA, Olopade OI. Epidermal growth factor receptor in triple-negative and basal-like breast cancer: promising clinical target or only a marker? Cancer J2010 Jan-Feb;16(1):23-32.

[117] Viale G, Rotmensz N, Maisonneuve P, Bottiglieri L, Montagna E, Luini A, Veronesi P, Intra M, Torrisi R, Cardillo A, Campagnoli E, Goldhirsch A, Colleoni M. Invasive ductal carcinoma of the breast with the "triple-negative" phenotype: prognostic implications of EGFR immunoreactivity. Breast Cancer Res Treat2009 Jul;116(2):317-28.

[118] Chaffer CL, Weinberg RA. A perspective on cancer cell metastasis. Science2011 Mar 25;331(6024):1559-64.

[119] Nguyen DX, Bos PD, Massague J. Metastasis: from dissemination to organ-specific colonization. Nat Rev Cancer2009 Apr;9(4):274-84.

[120] Bos PD, Zhang XH, Nadal C, Shu W, Gomis RR, Nguyen DX, Minn AJ, van de Vijver MJ, Gerald WL, Foekens JA, Massague J. Genes that mediate breast cancer metastasis to the brain. Nature2009 Jun 18;459(7249):1005-9.

[121] Gupta GP, Nguyen DX, Chiang AC, Bos PD, Kim JY, Nadal C, Gomis RR, Manova-Todorova K, Massague J. Mediators of vascular remodelling co-opted for sequential steps in lung metastasis. Nature2007 Apr 12;446(7137):765-70.

[122] Kang Y, Siegel PM, Shu W, Drobnjak M, Kakonen SM, Cordon-Cardo C, Guise TA, Massague J. A multigenic program mediating breast cancer metastasis to bone. Cancer Cell2003 Jun;3(6):537-49.

[123] Minn AJ, Gupta GP, Siegel PM, Bos PD, Shu W, Giri DD, Viale A, Olshen AB, Gerald WL, Massague J. Genes that mediate breast cancer metastasis to lung. Nature2005 Jul 28;436(7050):518-24.

[124] Amin DN, Hida K, Bielenberg DR, Klagsbrun M. Tumor endothelial cells express epidermal growth factor receptor (EGFR) but not ErbB3 and are responsive to EGF and to EGFR kinase inhibitors. Cancer Res2006 Feb 15;66(4):2173-80.

[125] Iivanainen E, Nelimarkka L, Elenius V, Heikkinen SM, Junttila TT, Sihombing L, Sundvall M, Maatta JA, Laine VJ, Yla-Herttuala S, Higashiyama S, Alitalo K, Elenius K. Angiopoietin-regulated recruitment of vascular smooth muscle cells by endothelial-derived heparin binding EGF-like growth factor. FASEB J2003 Sep;17(12):1609-21.

[126] Russell KS, Stern DF, Polverini PJ, Bender JR. Neuregulin activation of ErbB receptors in vascular endothelium leads to angiogenesis. Am J Physiol1999 Dec;277(6 Pt 2):H2205-11.

[127] Chen F, Hori T, Ohashi N, Baine AM, Eckman CB, Nguyen JH. Occludin is regulated by epidermal growth factor receptor activation in brain endothelial cells and brains of mice with acute liver failure. Hepatology2011 Apr;53(4):1294-305.

[128] Yoneda T, Williams PJ, Hiraga T, Niewolna M, Nishimura R. A bone-seeking clone exhibits different biological properties from the MDA-MB-231 parental human breast cancer cells and a brain-seeking clone in vivo and in vitro. J Bone Miner Res2001 Aug;16(8):1486-95.

[129] Fitzgerald DP, Palmieri D, Hua E, Hargrave E, Herring JM, Qian Y, Vega-Valle E, Weil RJ, Stark AM, Vortmeyer AO, Steeg PS. Reactive glia are recruited by highly proliferative brain metastases of breast cancer and promote tumor cell colonization. Clin Exp Metastasis2008;25(7):799-810.

[130] Guise TA, Mohammad KS, Clines G, Stebbins EG, Wong DH, Higgins LS, Vessella R, Corey E, Padalecki S, Suva L, Chirgwin JM. Basic mechanisms responsible for osteolytic and osteoblastic bone metastases. Clin Cancer Res2006 Oct 15;12(20 Pt 2):6213s-6s.

[131] Guise TA, Mundy GR. Cancer and bone. Endocr Rev1998 Feb;19(1):18-54.

[132] Zhu J, Jia X, Xiao G, Kang Y, Partridge NC, Qin L. EGF-like ligands stimulate osteoclastogenesis by regulating expression of osteoclast regulatory factors by osteoblasts: implications for osteolytic bone metastases. J Biol Chem2007 Sep 14;282(37):26656-64.

[133] Wang Y, Klijn JG, Zhang Y, Sieuwerts AM, Look MP, Yang F, Talantov D, Timmermans M, Meijer-van Gelder ME, Yu J, Jatkoe T, Berns EM, Atkins D, Foekens JA. Gene-expression profiles to predict distant metastasis of lymph-node-negative primary breast cancer. Lancet2005 Feb 19-25;365(9460):671-9.

[134] Foley J, Nickerson NK, Nam S, Allen KT, Gilmore JL, Nephew KP, Riese DJ, 2nd. EGFR signaling in breast cancer: bad to the bone. Semin Cell Dev Biol2010 Dec;21(9):951-60.

[135] Henderson M, Danks J, Moseley J, Slavin J, Harris T, McKinlay M, Hopper J, Martin T. Parathyroid hormone-related protein production by breast cancers, improved survival, and reduced bone metastases. J Natl Cancer Inst2001 Feb 7;93(3):234-7.

[136] Powell GJ, Southby J, Danks JA, Stillwell RG, Hayman JA, Henderson MA, Bennett RC, Martin TJ. Localization of parathyroid hormone-related protein in breast cancer metastases: increased incidence in bone compared with other sites. Cancer Res1991 Jun 1;51(11):3059-61.

[137] Southby J, Kissin MW, Danks JA, Hayman JA, Moseley JM, Henderson MA, Bennett RC, Martin TJ. Immunohistochemical localization of parathyroid hormone-related protein in human breast cancer. Cancer Res1990 Dec 1;50(23):7710-6.
[138] Yin JJ, Selander K, Chirgwin JM, Dallas M, Grubbs BG, Wieser R, Massague J, Mundy GR, Guise TA. TGF-beta signaling blockade inhibits PTHrP secretion by breast cancer cells and bone metastases development. J Clin Invest1999 Jan;103(2):197-206.

2

EGF Regulation of HRPAP20: A Role for Calmodulin and Protein Kinase C in Breast Cancer Cells

Manasi N. Shukla, Donna J. Buckley and Arthur R. Buckley
Division of Pharmaceutical Sciences, James L. Winkle College of Pharmacy, University of Cincinnati, Cincinnati, OH, United States of America

1. Introduction

The breast cancer cell genome is remarkably unstable, most likely due to early dysfunction of DNA replication, repair or recombination (Roskelley and Bissel, 2002). Accumulation of genetic alterations in the cells and/or stroma lead to development of a genetically diverse cell population characterized by uncontrolled cell proliferation (Witz, 2002; Gupta et al., 2006). Therefore, identification of genes that may be responsible for pre-disposition or facilitate progression of the disease may contribute to improvement of currently available therapeutic approaches in treatment of breast cancer.

We previously reported the identification, cloning and functional characterization of HRPAP20, which encodes for protein designated Hormone Regulated Proliferation-Associated Protein 20 (accession number: NM_ 014165; Karp et al., 2004). Our observations indicated that HRPAP20 is a regulator of proliferation, survival, and invasion in hormone-responsive breast cancer cells. Moreover, highly invasive, hormone unresponsive breast cell lines, such as MDA-MB-231 and tumor specimens of invasive breast adenocarcinomas from patients exhibited constitutively elevated levels of HRPAP20 (Karp et al., 2007). Results from an independent study conducted by another group suggested that HRPAP20 is a promising marker of tamoxifen resistance in women with ER alpha-positive breast tumors (Tozlu-Kara et al., 2007). Together, these observations suggested that elevated HRPAP20 may facilitate breast cancer progression toward a more malignant phenotype.

Other studies from our group suggested that an interaction between HRPAP20 and calmodulin (CaM) may contribute to HRPAP20-mediated biological effects in tumor cells. Furthermore, a basic amino acid residue (K73) within the putative CaM-binding domain of HRPAP20 appeared to be important for CaM-binding to the protein. CaM has been shown to influence cell cycle control and proliferation in human breast cancer cells by activating CaM-kinase II (CaMK II) and MAPK-mediated signaling pathways (Cheung , 1980; Wang et al., 1983; Rodriguez-Mora et al., 2005). The recent identification of the ErbB2/HER2/Neu, ER-α, and androgen receptor (AR) as CaM-binding proteins, has opened new areas of investigation in the regulation of signaling by CaM, particularly in hormone-responsive cancer (Cifuentes et al., 2004; Li et al., 2006; Maximciuc et al., 2006).

Overexpression or constitutive activation of the epidermal growth factor receptor (EGFR) is frequently associated with the development and progression of a number of human cancers, including breast cancer (Garcia et al., 2006). HER-2, a member of this receptor tyrosine kinase family is overexpressed in 20% -30% of aggressive breast cancers, making it an appealing target for prognosis and therapy of the disease (Meric-Bernstam et al., 2006). These and other observations have shed light on the fact that the complex role of EGF signaling in development and progression of breast cancer is incompletely understood, and suggests that gaps exist in our knowledge of its signaling mechanisms. Therefore, experiments were conducted to evaluate a potential role of HRPAP20 in EGF-mediated signaling in hormone-dependent breast cancer cells.

Protein kinase C (PKC) is a signaling intermediate that has been linked to EGF stimulation in cancer cells. The PKC family of at least 12 serine/threonine protein kinase isoforms, has been extensively studied in the regulation of intracellular signaling in response to stimuli such as growth factors and hormones (Dekker et al., 1994; Nishizuka et al., 1995; Newton 1995, and 1997; Mellor et al., 1998). The classical and novel isoforms of PKC are targets for phorbol ester compounds, such as TPA, which are a widely studied tumor promoters that mimic the actions of diacylglycerol on PKC activation (Barry et al., 2001). Altered expression and activity of several PKC isoenzymes has been observed in numerous cancers including those affecting the lung, colon, and breast (Gordge et al., 1996; McCracken et al., 2003; Gokmen-Polar et al., 2001). It has been reported that PKC-α, -δ and -ε activate several substrates that promote breast tumor cell migration and invasion (Pan et al., 2005; Tan et al., 2006; Ways et al., 1995). Therefore, it appears that PKC isoforms have distinct roles, which relate to their unique localization and/or access to substrates upon activation (Nakagawa et al., 2005). Here we show results from experiments conducted to evaluate whether HRPAP20 is a substrate for PKC. We also demonstrate whether specific PKC isoforms activated by EGF stimulation are possibly involved in HRPAP20 phosphorylation and invasion. The observations presented in this chapter support the hypothesis that HRPAP20 is an important regulator of tumor cell signaling, which may direct malignant progression in breast cancer.

2. Experimental procedures

2.1 Cell culture and treatments

The human mammary adenocarcinoma cell line MCF-7 was maintained in DMEM supplemented with 10% FBS and penicillin/streptomycin. MCF-7 cells were serum starved for 24 hrs in DMEM supplemented with 1% ITS+ (BD Biosciences, Bedford, MA) or 0.1% BSA. Quiescent MCF-7 cells were treated with EGF (100 ng/ml) or TPA (20 nM). Treatment of MCF-7 cells with Gö6976 (1µM) or Rottlerin (10µM) was carried out 60 min prior to stimulation with EGF (100 ng/ml for 30 min). All cells were harvested by washing with ice-cold PBS and centrifugation.

2.2 HRPAP20 plasmid construction and site-directed mutagenesis

The full length HRPAP20 cDNA was ligated into the mammalian expression vector pcDNA3.1 using the restriction sites Hind III (5′ end) and Eco-RI (3′ end). The construct was sequenced and used for transfection of MCF-7 cells. For bacterial expression of recombinant HRPAP20-GST fusion protein, the restriction sites Bam-H1 and Eco-RI were engineered on the 5′ and 3′ terminals of the protein frame of HRPAP20 respectively. This oligonucleotide was generated by PCR and ligated into the bacterial expression vector PGEX-4T1 (Amersham Biosciences, Piscataway, NJ). The vectors pcDNA 3.1 and PGEX-4T1 encoding

HRPAP20 were used as templates for site-directed mutagenesis. Alanine substitutions were performed using the Quick-Change point-mutation kit (Stratagene, La Jolla, CA.). The following primers were synthesized to generate the variant HRPAP20 oligonucleotides. K73A: 5′-GAGATGTATATGTCAATTCCGCAGATCCGGTGCCTTCCT-3′. R66A: 5′-ACAAGCTGTTGTCCTTACTAGCAGATGTATATGTCAATTCC-3′. Reverse primers were synthesized complementary to the forward primers. The HRPAP20 sequence harboring both K73A and R66A site-mutations was generated by using HRPAP20/K73A as a template using primers encoding for the R66A mutation. A PCR reaction using cycling conditions recommended by the manufacturer was performed. Digestion of the parental plasmid template was accomplished using Dpn I. The site mutants were transformed into E-coli, and colonies selected on ampicillin-containing soft agar. The individual colonies were grown and the plasmid constructs isolated using Qiagen plasmid Mini-prep kit protocol. All constructs were sequenced at the University of Cincinnati DNA core facility to confirm the amino acid substitutions. The appropriate plasmids were then used for stable transfection of cells, or for bacterial expression of variant HRPAP20-GST fusion proteins.

2.3 Recombinant HRPAP20-GST protein expression and purification

Recombinant HRPAP20-GST fusion protein was produced by transformation of the Escherichia coli strain BL21-Star/p-RARE with the plasmid vector PGEX-4T1 encoding for wild-type or variant HRPAP20. The construct was sequenced at the University of Cincinnati's DNA Core Facility prior to transformation. Bacteria transformed with the empty vector alone were used to express recombinant GST alone, which was used as an assay control. The transformants were grown in complete LB broth, and IPTG (5mM) was used to induce protein expression at 27˚C. Following 4 hrs of induction, the cells were lyzed by freeze-thawing (3X) and sonication (60V, 5 cycles). Sonicates were centrifuged and GST or HRPAP20-GST fusion proteins in the supernatants were purified using glutathione-agarose (Amersham). Bound GST or HRPAP20-GST protein was eluted by reduced glutathione (20mM) and quantitated using Bradford reagent (Biorad, Hercules, CA). The purity and molecular weights of the proteins were confirmed by SDS-PAGE followed by Coomassie blue staining.

2.4 CaM-Sepharose binding analysis

The assay was performed as described previously (Boehning et. al, 2004; Karp et al., 2007). Briefly, 20 µl of CaM-Sepharose-4B beads (1.3 mg/ml, Amersham) were equilibriated with Buffer A. The equilibriated beads were then blocked for 1 h at room temperature with 1% BSA, followed by washing 1X with 500 µl of buffer A. Binding of HRPAP20-GST to CaM was evaluated by incubating 5 µg of HRPAP20-GST (wild-type or variant) or GST-only with CaM-Sepharose for 1 h at 4°C in buffer A ± $CaCl_2$ (5 mM). Bound protein was eluted using SDS sample buffer, followed by SDS-PAGE analysis. Immunoblotting with α-GST or α-HRPAP20 was used to identify HRPAP20 binding to CaM.

2.5 *In vitro* PKC kinase assay employing HRPAP20 as a substrate

The assay was performed as described in (Li and McNulty et al., 2005). Briefly, 5 µg of the fusion protein HRPAP20-GST or GST in 100 µl of PKC buffer containing 20 mM HEPES (pH: 7.4), 1.67 mM $CaCl_2$,10 mM $MgCl_2$, 1 mM DTT, 1mM ATP and 10 µCi of [γ-^{32}P] ATP was used for the kinase reaction. Myristoylated peptide PKC inhibitor (Promega, Madison, WI) was used at a concentration of 100 mM. The kinase reaction was initiated by adding 1 µl of PKC (Promega), followed by incubation at 30 °C for 30 min. A duplicate set of the above reactions with the substitution of [γ-^{32}P] ATP with non-radioactive ATP was performed in parallel for immunoblotting analysis. The reactions were stopped by placing on ice. The fusion proteins were isolated using glutathione agarose, followed by washing, elution and SDS-PAGE. The resolved proteins were transfered to PVDF membranes and subjected to autoradiography, or immunoblotting with α-GST. The immunoblotted membranes were subsequently stripped and reprobed with α-HRPAP20.

2.6 Immune-complex kinase assay

Cells were harvested and lyzed using phosphorylation lysis buffer containing 50 mM HEPES (pH: 7.5), 150 mM NaCl, 200 µM sodium orthovanadate, 10 mM sodium pyrophosphate, 100 mM sodium fluoride, 1 mM EDTA, 1.5 mM $MgCl_2$, 10% glycerol, 1% Triton X-100, and protease inhibitors (Rahman et al., 2001). Lysates were immunoprecipitated using α-PKC-A3 (Santa Cruz Biotechnology, Santa Cruz, CA) and protein-G agarose. Immune-complexes were washed with kinase wash buffer: Tris HCl (50 mM , pH 7.4), NaF (10 mM), sodium orthovanadate (1 mM), EDTA (0.5 mM), EGTA (0.5 mM), magnesium chloride (2 mM), leupeptin (10 µg/ml), PMSF (1mM) as previously described (Arya et al., 2004). 5 µg of recombinant HRPAP20-GST or GST protein, in a kinase reaction buffer containing 20 mM Tris-HCl (pH: 7.4), 10 mM $MgCl_2$ and 1 mM DTT was incubated with ATP (1 µM), γ-^{32}P-ATP (10 µCi) for 30 min at 30°C. The reactions were terminated by placing on ice, followed by SDS-PAGE and autoradiography as described in previous section.

2.7 Cell transfection

MCF-7 cells were transfected with wild-type HRPAP20, R66A, K73A+R66A, or empty vector (pcDNA 3.1) alone, according to manufacturer's protocol using Lipofectamine® (Invitrogen, Carlsbad, CA). Following transfection, all cells were subjected to G418 selection (250 µg/ml) to generate stably transfected cell lines. Cells were transiently transfected with wild-type and dominant-negative PKC-δ constructs or empty vector pcDNA3.1, and used in experiments 72 hrs after transfection (previously described in Kruger et al., 2003).

2.8 Co-immunoprecipitation/immunoblotting (co-IP/IB)

Following treatments, cells were harvested using ice-cold PBS and centrifugation; then lysed in a buffer containing 10 mM Tris (pH 7.4), 0.15 M NaCl, 5 mM EDTA and 1% Triton X-100. The lysates were pre-cleared with normal rabbit serum and protein G (Upstate, Lake Placid, NY), then immunoprecipitated using α-HRPAP20 antiserum (Karp et. al, 2004) and protein G. The immunoprecipitates, together with lysates, were resolved using 12% SDS-PAGE gels, then immunoblotted with α-CaM (Upstate, Charlottesville, VA.). The membranes were subsequently stripped using a buffer containing 62.5 mM Tris (pH 6.8) and 2% SDS, then reprobed with α-HRPAP20.

2.9 Cell invasion analysis

The invasive capacity of the breast tumor cell lines was measured utilizing an in vitro transwell assay (Repesh et al., 1989, Karp et al., 2007). Briefly, 2.5 x 10^5 cells, in DMEM containing 0.1% BSA, were added to the upper well of transwell chambers (Corning Inc.,

Corning, NY) containing an 8 μm porous membrane, previously coated with type I collagen, fibronectin, and Matrigel ® (Becton Dickinson Biosciences, San Diego, CA). Lower chambers contained DMEM containing 0.1% BSA and 10% FBS as a chemoattractant. Following 24 hrs, invading cells were fixed with 4% paraformaldehyde, stained with crystal violet, and counted microscopically (20X magnification) in five random fields/membrane.

3. Results

3.1 EGF regulates the interaction between HRPAP20 and CaM in MCF-7 cells

We previously showed that HRPAP20 interacts with Ca^{2+}/CaM in purified preparations and in MCF-7 cells (Karp et al., 2007). To determine whether this interaction was influenced by mitogenic stimulation such by EGF, co-immunoprecipitation/ immunoblotting (co-IP/IB) experiments were conducted using MCF-7 cells. As shown in Fig. 1, CaM co-immunoprecipitated with HRPAP20 in lysates from control cell suggesting that the two proteins existed as a complex in unstimulated cells (time 0) consistent with our previous observations. Stimulation with EGF (100 ng/ml) rapidly disrupted the HRPAP20:CaM ($p<0.05$). Thus, mitogenic stimulation appeared to cause dissociation of the protein complex that was observed in unstimulated cells. These observations suggest that HRPAP20 may function as a signaling intermediate coupled to activation of the EGFreceptor.

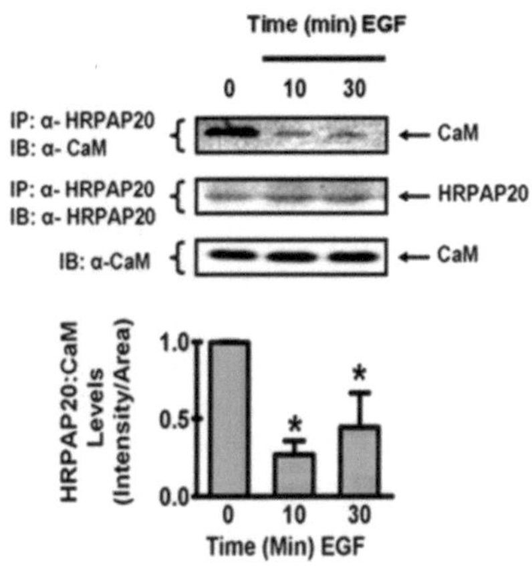

Fig. 1. EGF stimulation disrupts HRPAP20:CaM in MCF-7 cells. MCF-7 cells, previously cultured for 24 hr in serum-free medium, were treated with h-EGF (100 ng/ml). The cells were harvested at the indicated times following EGF stimulation. Cell lysates were immuno precipitated with α-CaM (upper panel). Membranes were stripped and reprobed with α-HRPAP20 (middle panel). 10% of total protein used for immunoprecipitation was resolved in parallel as an input control and Immunoblotted with α-CaM (lower panel). Densitometric analysis of three separate experiments is presented. *$p<0.05$ vs CTL.

HRPAP20:CaM interaction requires basic residues K73 and R66 in MCF-7 cells. Experiements were conducted to determine which amino acid residues within HRPAP20 were required for its interaction with CaM. Studies by others (Bagchi et al., 1992) showed that certain basic residues within the CaM-binding domains of several interacting proteins were required for their interaction. K73, R66, and V70 (hydrophobic) were identified as potential critical residues within HRPAP20 for its interaction with CaM based upon comparison with other binding proteins (Fig. 2).

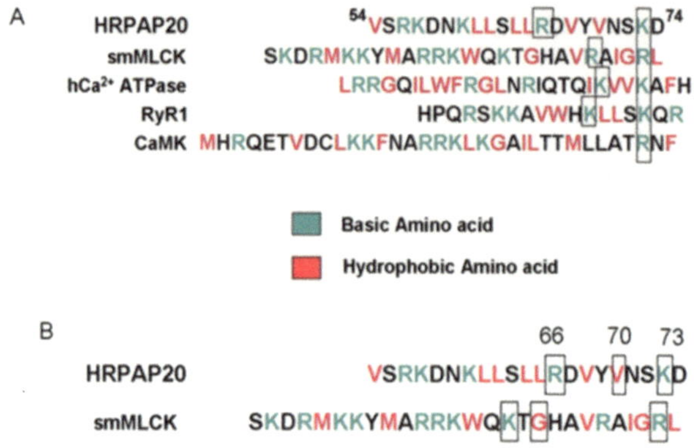

Fig. 2. Sequence of the HRPAP20 CaM-binding domain. (A) The amino acid sequence of HRPAP20 (residues 54-74) consisting of the predicted CaM-binding motif, was aligned with those of other well-characterized CaM-binding proteins. While there is no sequence conservation observed in most of the CaM-binding domain, they are characterized by a typical positioning of a C-terminal basic residue, preceded by 2-3 hydrophobic residues. (B) Sequence alignment of the CaM-binding motif of HRPAP20 with that present in smMLCK indicating positions of basic and hydrophobic residues on smMLCK that are critical for CaM-binding (Bagchi et al., 1992). Analogous residues within HRPAP20 are boxed and the positions numbered.

Previously, we showed that alanine (ala) substitution of K73 resulted in diminished CaM-binding of HRPAP20 in MCF-7 cells (Karp et al., 2007). Using site-directed mutagenesis, we generated a series of HRPAP20 variants harboring ala substitutions at these residues (HRPAP20-K73A, HRPAP20/R66A or HRPAP20/K73A+R66A, and HRPAP20/V70A). The proteins were expressed as GST-fusion proteins, then the purified recombinant proteins were evaluated by CaM-Sepharose pull-down analysis to assess their capacity to bind to CaM. The results indicated that HRPAP20-K73A exhibited ~50% reduction in CaM-binding compared to the wild-type protein (Fig. 3). Moreover, ala substitutions at K73 and R66 in combination inhibited the HRPAP20:CaM interaction to the same extent as R66A, indicating that each of these residues may contribute to CaM-binding (Fig. 3). Alanine substitution of the hydrophobic residue V70 did not significantly affect CaM-binding of HRPAP20, suggesting that this residue may not be required for in HRPAP20:CaM complex formation (results not shown).

To determine whether the HRPAP20/R66A or HRPAP20/K73A+R66A exhibited a diminished interaction with CaM in MCF-7 cells, we conducted co-IP/IB experiments using cells stably transfected with HRPAP20, R66A, K73A+R66A, or the empty vector as a control. The results demonstrated that CaM co-immunoprecipitated using α-HRPAP20, in MCF-7/HRPAP20 cells, consistent with our previous observations. In contrast, significantly reduced CaM binding was observed in cells transfected with HRPAP20/R66A or HRPAP20/K73A+R66A compared to the level observed in wildtype HRPAP20 (Fig. 4A and D). The membranes from Fig. 4A were subsequently stripped and reprobed with

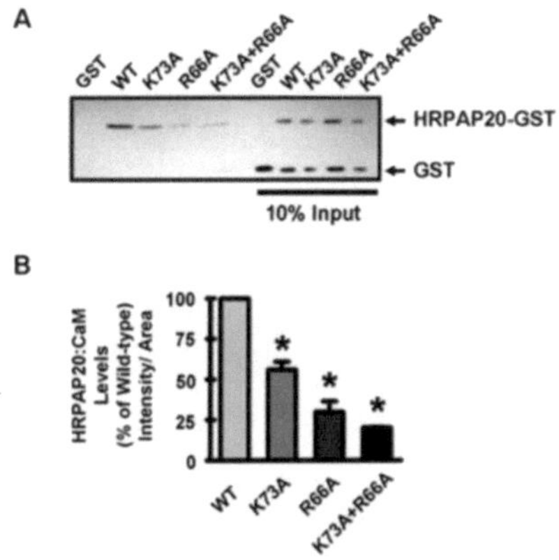

Fig. 3. K73 and R66 regulate HRPAP20:CaM interact1on in vitro. (A) 5 µg of recombinant HRPAP20-GST [wildtype-WT, or HRPAP20 harboring the substitutions K73A, R66A, or K73A+R66A] or GST alone were incubated with CaM-Sepharose in the presence of Ca^{2+} (5 mM). Eluted proteins were resolved bySDS-PAGE, then immunoblotted with α-GST. 10% of each protein used in pull-down assays was evaluated in parallel as an input control. (B) Cumulative results of densitometric analysis of three separate experiments is presented. *$p<0.05$ vs. WT.

α-HRPAP20 to confirm HRPAP20 immunoprecipitation in each of the samples (Fig. 4B). Equal concentrations of lysate protein from each of the transfectants were immunoblotted using α-CaM as an additional control (Fig. 4C). Together, these results suggested that the basic residues K73 and R66 in the CaM-binding motif of HRPAP20 may regulate its interaction with CaM in MCF-7 breast cancer cells.

Shown in Fig. 4E are results from in vitro invasion analysis of cells transfected with HRPAP20 and and its variants. Here wildtype HRPAP20 significantly ($p<0.01$) increased invasion through Matrigel® coated filters in transwell chambers. In contrast, invasion observed by the cells expressing the HRPAP20 variants R66A or K73A+R66A did not differ from empty vector-transfected controls. These observations indicated that even a partial disruption of the HRPAP20:CaM interaction by mutation of the basic residues K73 and R66 blocked HRPAP20-mediated increase in invasion. Therefore, it is suggested that K73 and R66 are likely required to maintain integrity of the HRPAP20:CaM complex, which appears to be a requisite for MCF-7 invasion.

3.2 HRPAP20 is a substrate for PKC

We previously showed that HRPAP20 is a phosphoprotein and that pharmacological inhibition of PKC reduced its phosphorylation in Nb2-11 cells (Karp et al., 2004). Experiments to evaluate whether HRPAP20 is phosphorylated by PKC were conducted utilizing recombinant HRPAP20-GST fusion protein and catalytically active rat brain PKC, in the presence of cofactors and ^{32}P-ATP. As shown in Fig. 5A, HRPAP20 was phosphorylated in the presence of PKC (lane 1), but not in its absence (lane 2). Addition of a myristoylated peptide substrate, serving as a competitive inhibitor of PKC, inhibited PKC-mediated phosphorylation of HRPAP20 (lane 3). An equal amount of recombinant GST

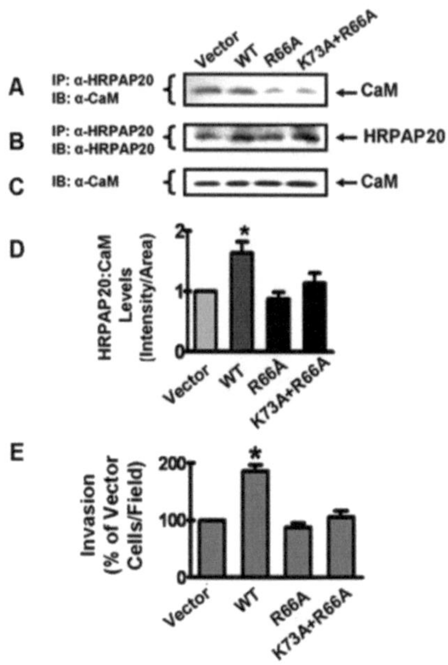

Fig. 4. Effect of HRPAP20 amino acid substitution (R66A, K73A+R66A) on HRPAP20:CaM association and invasion in MCF-7 cells. (A) MCF-7 cells, transfected with empty vector (Vector), wildtype HRPAP20 (WT), HRPAP20/R66A (R66A) or HRPAP20/K73A+R66A (K73A + R66A) were immunoprecipitated with α-HRPAP20 and immunoblotted with α-CaM. (B) Membranes were stripped and reprobed with α-HRPAP20. (C) 10% of total protein used for immunoprecipitation was resolved in parallel as an input control and immunoblotted with α-CaM. (D) Densitometric analysis of three separate experiments is presented. *$p<0.01$ WT vs Vector; $p<0.05$ WT vs K73A. (E) Cumulative results obtained from three separate in vitro invasion experiments. *$p<0.01$ WT vs Vector.

incubated with PKC represents a control reaction demonstrating the inability of PKC to phosphorylate GST (lane 4). To ensure equal loading of samples, duplicates of the above reactions with the substitution of ^{32}P-ATP with non radioactive ATP were resolved in parallel and subjected to immunoblotting with α-HRPAP20 (Fig. 5B) or α-GST (Fig. 5C). Together, these results suggest that HRPAP20 is a substrate for PKC in vitro.

3.3 HRPAP20 is phosphorylated by EGF-activated PKC

There is abundant evidence indicating an important role for EGFR and its ligands in the development and progression of human neoplasia (Johnston et al., 2006; Ji et al., 2006; Speake et al., 2005; D'Alessio et al., 2010). To evaluate whether PKC-mediated HRPAP20 phosphorylation is an event that occurrs downstream of EGF stimulation, immune-complex kinase assays were performed utilizing PKC immunoprecipitated from lysates of EGF-treated MCF-7 cells and HRPAP20-GSTas a substrate. The reactions were performed in the presence of ^{32}P-ATP, but in the absence of cofactors. As illustrated in Fig. 6A and B, HRPAP20 phosphorylation was significantly elevated upon its incubation with PKC immunoprecipitated from EGF-treated cells, compared to the level observed in control samples from untreated cells. These results suggest that PKC, activated by EGF stimulation catalyzed HRPAP20 phosphorylation.

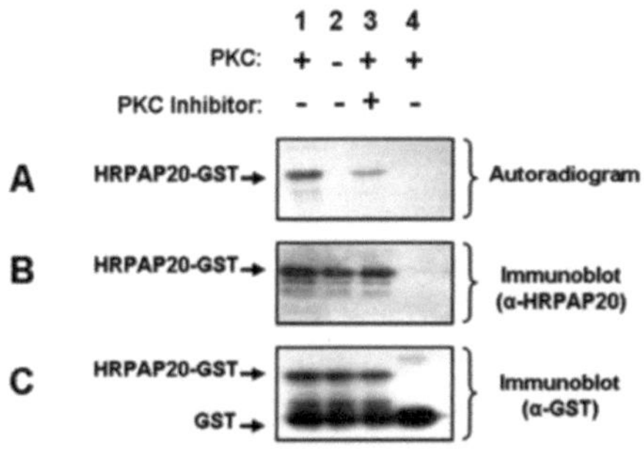

Fig. 5. Phosphorylation of HRPAP20 by PKC. (A) Recombinant HRPAP20-GST (lanes 1-3) or GST alone (lane 4) were incubated at 30°C in the presence (+) or absence (-) of purified rat brain PKC or a PKC inhibitor (myristoylated PKC peptide inhibitor, 100 μM) in the presence of [γ-^{32}P] ATP. Samples were resolved by SDS-Page followed by autoradiography. (B) Duplicates of reactions in (A), but without [γ-^{32}P] ATP, were immunoblotted with α-HRPAP20. (C) Membranes from (B) were stripped, then reprobed with α-GST.

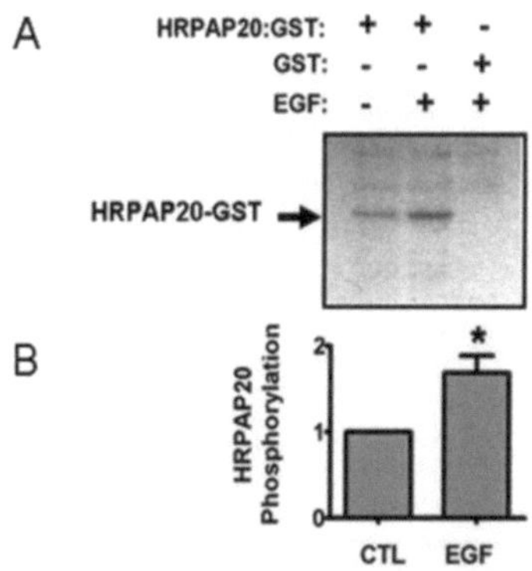

Fig. 6. HRPAP20 is phosphorylated by PKC activated subsequent to EGF stimulation in MCF-7 cells. (A) PKC from quiescent or EGF-treated MCF-7 cells was immunoprecipitated, then incubated with recombinant HRPAP20-GST or GST in the presence of γ-^{32}P-ATP, followed by SDS-PAGE and autoradiography. A representative autoradiograph indicating the level of HRPAP20 phosphorylation is shown. (B) Cumulative results from three independent experiments analyzed by densitometry are presented. *$p<0.01$ vs CTL.

3.4 PKC-δ phosphorylates HRPAP20 subsequent to EGF stimulation and is required for invasion in MCF-7 cells

The role of various PKC isoforms in the process of tumor progression in the mammary epithelium is only partially understood. However, several studies support a role for PKC-δ in breast tumor progression (McCracken et al., 2003; Nabha et al., 2005). Moreover, PKC-δ has been shown to regulate the activation of MMP-9 in breast tumor cells; an effect also observed in MCF-7 cells stably expressing elevated levels of HRPAP20 (Karp et al., 2007). Therefore, experiments were conducted to determine whether PKC-δ phosphorylated of HRPAP20 following EGF stimulation in this cell line. Quiescent MCF-7 cells were subjected to treatment with Gö6976, a pharmacological inhibitor of classic PKC isozymes, or Rottlerin, with specificity directed toward the PKC-δ isoform. The results from immunecomplex kinase analysis indicated that while Gö6976 did not affect EGF-stimulated HRPAP20 phosphorylation, Rottlerin nearly completely blocked this effect (Fig. 7A). These results suggested that PKC-δ, activated by EGF stimulation, may be responsible for the downstream phosphorylation of HRPAP20.

To further investigate whether PKC-δ catalyzed HRPAP20 phosphorylation, MCF-7 cells were transiently transfected with constructs encoding a constitutively active wild-type (WT) PKC-δ, a kinase inactive/dominant negative PKC-δ (DN), or with the empty vector. Transfectants were treated with EGF and evaluated using immune-complex kinase analysis. The results indicated that EGF stimulated substantial HRPAP20 phosphorylation in cells expressing WT-PKC-δ (Fig. 7B). However, expression of DN- PKC-δ almost completely abolished this effect. Together, these results support the hypothesis that PKC-δ mediates phosphorylation of HRPAP20 and that this effect may underlie EGF stimulated actions.

To determine whether HRPAP20 phosphorylation affected cell invasion in vitro, invasion analysis was conducted using MCF-7 cells co-transfected with HRPAP20 and dominant negative PKC-δ. As shownin Fig. 7C, co-expression of dominant negative PKC-δ with HRPAP20, caused a significant reduction of MCF-7 cell invasion, compared to the level observed in cells transfected with HRPAP20 alone. These results suggested that activated PKC-δ is required to regulate HRPAP20, ultimately resulting in stimulating increased invasiveness in breast cancer cells.

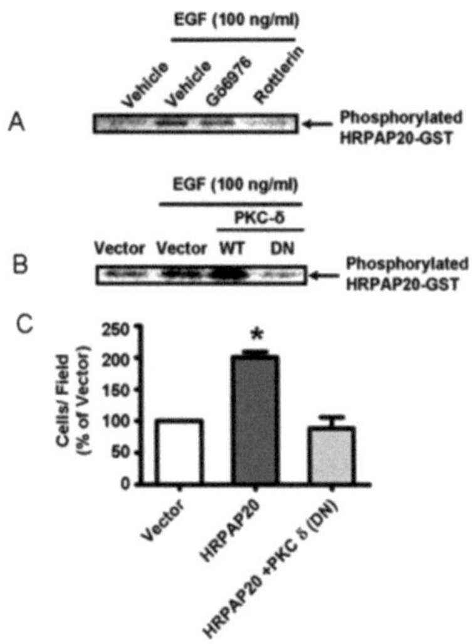

Fig. 7. PKC-δ catalyzes EGF-stimulated HRPAP20 phosphorylation and contributes to invasion. (A) Quiescent MCF-7 cells were pre-treated with PKC inhibitors Gö6976 (1 µM) or Rottlerin (10 µM), followed by the addition of EGF (100 ng/ml). PKC was immunoprecipitated and incubated with recombinant HRPAP20-GST in the presence of γ-^{32}P-ATP. A representative autoradiograph showing HRPAP20 phosphorylation is presented. (B) MCF-7 cells were transiently transfected with empty vector (Vector), wild-type (WT) or dominant negative PKC-δ (DN). Cells were then treated with EGF, followed by immunecomplex kinase analysis. (C) MCF-7 cells were transfected with empty vector (Vector), HRPAP20, or HRPAP20 and PKC-δ (DN), then evaluated by in vitro invasion assay. Cumulative results from three independently performed experiments are presented. *$p<0.01$ (HRPAP20 vs. Vector or HRPAP20 + DN-PKC-δ).

3.5 Effect of phosphorylation on HRPAP20: CaM interaction

Numerous previous studies have reported that post-translational modification may alter protein-protein interactions. Therefore, whether HRPAP20 phosphorylation affected its interaction with CaM was investigated. Experiments were conducted using MCF-7 cells treated with the phorbol ester, TPA, an activator of PKC. The HRPAP20:CaM interaction in these cells was evaluated by co-IP analysis. As demonstrated in Fig. 8A, TPA rapidly stimulated a significant ($p<0.01$) reduction in HRPAP20:CaM complex suggesting that PKC-catalyzed phosphorylation of HRPAP20 may reduce its binding capacity to CaM. Moreover, this observation correlated with the pattern of HRPAP20:CaM disruption observed upon EGF stimulation in these cells.

Furthermore, CaM Sepharose pull-down experiments were conducted to determine whether PKC-mediated phosphorylation of HRPAP20 affected its CaM-binding in vitro. The results obtained indicated that HRPAP20, phosphorylated by PKC prior to incubation with CaM, exhibited markedly reduced HRPAP20:CaM complex formation, in contrast to that observed with the native protein (Fig. 8B). This observation is consistent with our previous results suggesting that PKC likely regulates HRPAP20:CaM association. Taken together, the results suggest that HRPAP20 may modulate signaling involved in growth factor/hormone-responsive cancers by associating with PKC and CaM.

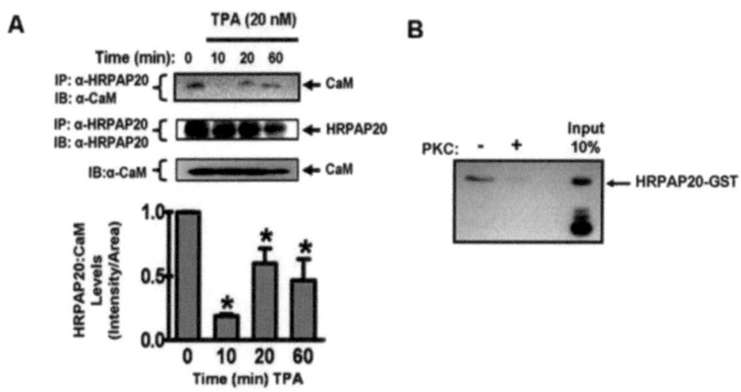

Fig. 8. HRPAP20:CaM is likely regulated by PKC-catalyzed phosphorylation. (A) Serum starved MCF-7 cells were treated with TPA (20 nM). Cells were harvested at the indicated time points, followed by immunoprecipitation of lysates using α-HRPAP20, then immunoblotted with α-CaM (upper panel). Membranes were stripped and reprobed with α-HRPAP20 (middle panel). 10% of total protein used for immunoprecipitation was resolved in parallel as an input control and immunoblotted with α-CaM (lower panel). Densitometric analysis of three separate experiments is presented. *$p<0.05$ vs. 0 min. (B) 5 µg of recombinant HRPAP20-GST was phosphorylated in vitro using rat brain PKC, then subjected to CaM- pulldown assay. A representative immunoblot using α- is shown.

4. Discussion

Tumor cell responses to extracellular stimuli includes activation of kinase pathways and alteration of protein-protein interactions, ultimately resulting in modulation of biological responses leading to progression of the disease. Since previous observations implicated a role for HRPAP20 in breast tumor proliferation and invasion, it was important to investigate the mechanisms by which this protein participated in tumor cell signaling.

Previously we showed that HRPAP20 and CaM interacted in vitro and in MCF-7 cells (Karp et al., 2007). We therefore sought to investigate whether this interaction contributed to tumor signaling and whether it was subject to regulation by growth factor stimulation.

Recent studies have broadened the view of signal transduction to encompass a complex networks, which allow interaction between discrete signaling pathways with EGFR as a key unit for integration of multiple stimuli (Prenzel et al., 2000). CaM has been shown to bind to the EGFR, as well as modulate EGF-stimulated signaling leading to tumor progression. It was therefore important to investigate whether HRPAP20 was subject to regulation downstream of EGFR activation in tumor cells. Using co-IP/IB, we showed that HRPAP20 resides within a complex with CaM in quiescent MCF-7 cells. Stimulation with EGF caused a significant reduction in HRPAP20:CaM association. These results suggest that the HRPAP20:CaM complex is likely regulated by EGF, and may serve as a potentially important step in growth factor-stimulated cell signaling.

To investigate which specific amino acid residues within HRPAP20 participate in its interaction with CaM, we compared the sequence of the CaM-binding domain of HRPAP20 to binding domains present in other CaM interacting proteins. This assessment revealed that several basic and hydrophobic amino acids were interspersed within the HRPAP20 CaM-binding motif at positions analogous to those found to be important for other CaM-binding proteins (Bagchi et al., 1992; Fitzsimons et al., 1992). Following generation of HRPAP20 variants harboring ala substitutions at suspected key locations, experiments were conducted to evaluate HRPAP20:CaM binding of the altered proteins. Results from these suggested that the basic residues, K73 and R66, located near the C-terminus of the CaM-binding domain of HRPAP20, may be critical for its interaction with CaM.

Bioinformatic analysis of the wildtype and variant HRPAP20 amino acid sequences indicated that both K73A and R66A substitutions most likely altered the length and stability of α-helices within the protein. Notably, K73 was predicted to be responsible for a bend in the strand following the α-helix that constituted the CaM-binding motif of HRPAP20 (www.igb.uci.edu/tools/scratch.html; http://npsa-pbil.ibcp.fr/cgi-bin/secpred_hnn.pl; NNPredict Query server; and http://distill.ucd.ie/porter/). Moreover, alanine substitution of R66 reduced the number of its residue contacts, hence potentially destabilizing the helix and potentially affecting its ability to bind CaM.

To investigate whether abrogation of HRPAP20:CaM interaction by R66A or K73A+R66A substitutions affected tumor cell invasion, we compared the invasive capacity of MCF-7 cells transfected with either wildtype HRPAP20 or its variants. In contrast to the wildtype protein, HRPAP20/R66A or HRPAP20/K73A+R66A failed to increase invasion. Therefore, consistent with our previous observations, the results suggest reports an upstream requirement for CaM-binding of HRPAP20 that is coupled to tumor invasiveness.

Protein phosphorylation has been known to play a significant role in the regulation of numerous aspects of cellular function such as growth, metabolism, motility, survival, and apoptosis. Moreover, numerous protein-protein interactions have been shown to be regulated by phosphorylation (Cho et al., 2004). Since HRPAP20 appears to complex with CaM and contains three consensus motifs for PKC catalyzed phosphorylation, it was hypothesized that HRPAP20 function may be regulated by CaM-binding and phosphorylation. EGF has been reported to activate PKC in MCF-7 cells (Mueller et al., 1997). Increased levels of PKC expression and activation have been associated with malignant transformation in a number of cell lines including breast, lung and gastric carcinomas (O'Brian et al., 1989; Takenaga et al., 1986; Schwartz et al., 1993). These observations suggest that PKC contributes to tumor progression and may serve as a therapeutic target for treatment of breast cancer.

We proposed that EGF stimulation in MCF-7 cells may subsequently induce HRPAP20 phosphorylation, following activation of PKC. To test this hypothesis, we conducted immune-complex kinase assays utilizing recombinant HRPAP20 and PKC immunoprecipitated from MCF-7 cells treated with/without EGF. Indeed, the results generated suggest that PKC immunoprecipitated from EGF-treated MCF-7 cells catalyzed HRPAP20 phosphorylation. Therefore, it appeared likely that EGF stimulation, which subsequently activates PKC, may lead to downstream phosphorylation of HRPAP20.

Results provided by others have suggested that the PKC-δ isoform is a positive regulator of metastatic progression and a survival factor in breast cancer (McCracken et al., 2003). Several reports now suggest that PKC-δ plays an important role in EGFR-mediated breast tumor progression as an important contributor to the later stages of cell migration (Kruger et al., 2003). Results presented here from immune-complex kinase assays suggested that while PKC-δ inhibition by rottlerin abrogated EGF-stimulated HRPAP20 phosphorylation, inhibition of conventional PKC isoforms with Gö6976 had no effect. This suggests that PKC-δ but not -α, -β, or -γ may mediate EGF-induced HRPAP20 phosphorylation. To further investigate HRPAP20 phosphorylation, immune-complex kinase assays were conducted using PKC immunoprecipitated from MCF-7 cells transiently transfected with wildtype or dominant negative PKC-δ. The results indicated that while expression of wildtype PKC-δ enhanced EGF-mediated HRPAP20 phosphorylation, the dominant negative PKC-δ variant failed to produce this effect. Together, the results strongly indicate that PKC-δ, activated upon EGF stimulation, may be responsible for HRPAP20 phosphorylation.

In breast cancer cell lines and fibroblasts, EGF stimulation has been shown to induce chemotactic migration with significant involvement of PKC α, ζ, δ and ε (Rabinovitz et al., 1999; Joberty et al., 2000; Iwabu et al., 2004). To determine whether PKC-δ is required for the observed HRPAP20-mediated increase in MCF-7 cell invasion, in vitro invasion experiments were conducted using cells co-expressing HRPAP20 and the dominant negative PKC-δ construct. It was observed that cells co-expressing DN PKC-δ with HRPAP20, failed to increase invasion above levels found in empty vector transfectants. These observations suggest that HRPAP20 phosphorylation by PKC-δ may be required for breast tumor cell invasion. Together, the results suggest that HRPAP20 may participate in EGF-stimulated signaling pathways in tumor cells, and that the effects of HRPAP20 may be regulated at least in part by CaM and PKC-catalyzed phosphorylation.

Phosphorylation has been shown to affect the CaM-binding affinity of several proteins. The myristoylated alanine rich C kinase substrate (MARCKS) protein and its homologue, MARCKS related protein (MRP), have been shown to bind CaM in a Ca^{2+}-dependent manner. Importantly, their interaction with CaM was diminished upon phosphorylation by PKC (Porumb et. al, 1997; Mc Ilroy et al., 1991). Several hormones produce an increase in intracellular Ca^{2+}, which facilitates CaM-binding to its target proteins and the consequent activation of PKC. These and the previous observations implicate that activation of PKC by various external stimuli may result in release of its substrates from CaM-bound pools by virtue of their phosphorylation. On the other hand, this may, in effect, result in the increase in intracellular levels of freely accessible CaM, leading to amplification of CaM-dependent processes.

Based on these observations and results indicating that HRPAP20 was a substrate for PKC downstream of EGF stimulation, we investigated whether phosphorylation affected CaM-binding of HRPAP20. Our results indicated that TPA caused a disruption of the HRPAP20:CaM complex in MCF-7 cells, in a manner similar to that observed upon EGF stimulation. In addition results from CaM-Sepharose pull-down assays illustrated that the phosphorylated form of HRPAP20 exhibited diminished CaM-binding in vitro, compared to the unphosphorylated protein.
We suggest that EGF stimulation, which activates PKC, may subsequently result in HRPAP20 phosphorylation. Furthermore, our observations clearly indicate that PKC-catalyzed phosphorylation of HRPAP20 regulates HRPAP20:CaM complex formation, and may potentially serve as an activation intermediate that leads to tumor invasion. Finally, our results suggest that a requirement of PKC-δ together with elevated HRPAP20 as factors that enhance breast cancer cell invasion. These observations provide additional clues with regard to the mechanism of regulation of HRPAP20 function and invasion in breast cancer. Thus, further studies on the role of HRPAP20 in tumor progression may reveal a hitherto unsuspected target for therapy of breast cancer.

5. Acknowledgements

We thank Dr. Jae-Won Soh at the Biomedical Research Center for Signal Transduction Networks, Inha University, Incheon, Korea, for generously providing constructs encoding wildtype and dominant negative PKC-δ.

6. References

Bagchi, I. C., Q. H. Huang, et al. (1992). "Identification of amino acids essential for calmodulin binding and activation of smooth muscle myosin light chain kinase." J Biol Chem 267(5): 3024-9.

Barry, O. P. and M. G. Kazanietz (2001). "Protein kinase C isozymes, novel phorbol ester receptors and cancer chemotherapy." Curr Pharm Des 7(17): 1725-44.

Cheung, W. Y. (1980). "Calmodulin plays a pivotal role in cellular regulation." Science 207(4426): 19-27.

Cho, S., S. G. Park, et al. (2004). "Protein-protein interaction networks: from interactions to networks." J Biochem Mol Biol 37(1): 45-52.

Cifuentes, E., J. M. Mataraza, et al. (2004). "Physical and functional interaction of androgen receptor with calmodulin in prostate cancer cells." Proc Natl Acad Sci U S A 101(2): 464-9.

D'Alessio, A., A. De Luca, et al. (2010). "Effects of the combined blockade of EGFR and ErbB-2 on signal transduction and regulation of cell cycle regulatory proteins in breast cancer cells." Breast Cancer Res Treat 123(2): 387-96.

Dekker, L. V. and P. J. Parker (1994). "Protein kinase C--a question of specificity." Trends Biochem Sci 19(2): 73-7.

Fitzsimons, D. P., B. P. Herring, et al. (1992). "Identification of basic residues involved in activation and calmodulin binding of rabbit smooth muscle myosin light chain kinase." J Biol Chem 267(33): 23903-9.

Garcia, R., R. A. Franklin, et al. (2006). "EGF induces cell motility and multi-drug resistance gene expression in breast cancer cells." Cell Cycle 5(23): 2820-6.

Gokmen-Polar, Y., N. R. Murray, et al. (2001). "Elevated protein kinase C betaII is an early promotive event in colon carcinogenesis." Cancer Res 61(4): 1375-81.

Gordge, P. C., M. J. Hulme, et al. (1996). "Elevation of protein kinase A and protein kinase C activities in malignant as compared with normal human breast tissue." Eur J Cancer 32A(12): 2120-6.

Gupta, G. P. and J. Massague (2006). "Cancer metastasis: building a framework." Cell 127(4): 679-95.

Iwabu, A., K. Smith, et al. (2004). "Epidermal growth factor induces fibroblast contractility and motility via a protein kinase C delta-dependent pathway." J Biol Chem 279(15): 14551-60.

Ji, H., D. Li, et al. (2006). "The impact of human EGFR kinase domain mutations on lung tumorigenesis and in vivo sensitivity to EGFR-targeted therapies." Cancer Cell 9(6): 485-95.

Joberty, G., C. Petersen, et al. (2000). "The cell-polarity protein Par6 links Par3 and atypical protein kinase C to Cdc42." Nat Cell Biol 2(8): 531-9.

Johnston, J. B., S. Navaratnam, et al. (2006). "Targeting the EGFR pathway for cancer therapy." Curr Med Chem 13(29): 3483-92.

Karp, C. M., H. Pan, et al. (2004). "Identification of HRPAP20: a novel phosphoprotein that enhances growth and survival in hormone-responsive tumor cells." Cancer Res 64(3): 1016-25.

Karp, C. M., M. N. Shukla, et al. (2007). "HRPAP20: a novel calmodulin-binding protein that increases breast cancer cell invasion." Oncogene 26(12): 1780-8.

Kruger, J. S. and K. B. Reddy (2003). "Distinct mechanisms mediate the initial and sustained phases of cell migration in epidermal growth factor receptor-overexpressing cells." Mol Cancer Res 1(11): 801-9.

Li, L. and D. B. Sacks (2007). "Functional interactions between calmodulin and estrogen receptor-alpha." Cell Signal 19(3): 439-43.

Maximciuc, A. A., J. A. Putkey, et al. (2006). "Complex of calmodulin with a ryanodine receptor target reveals a novel, flexible binding mode." Structure 14(10): 1547-56.

McCracken, M. A., L. J. Miraglia, et al. (2003). "Protein kinase C delta is a prosurvival factor in human breast tumor cell lines." Mol Cancer Ther 2(3): 273-81.

McIlroy, B. K., J. D. Walters, et al. (1991). "Phosphorylation-dependent binding of a synthetic MARCKS peptide to calmodulin." J Biol Chem 266(8): 4959-64.

Mellor, H. and P. J. Parker (1998). "The extended protein kinase C superfamily." Biochem J 332 (Pt 2): 281-92.

Meric-Bernstam, F. and M. C. Hung (2006). "Advances in targeting human epidermal growth factor receptor-2 signaling for cancer therapy." Clin Cancer Res 12(21): 6326-30.

Mueller, H., R. Liu, et al. (1997). "Selective modulation of protein kinase A and protein kinase C activities in epidermal growth factor (EGF)-stimulated MCF-7 breast cancer cells." Biol Chem 378(9): 1023-9.

Nabha, S. M., S. Glaros, et al. (2005). "Upregulation of PKC-delta contributes to antiestrogen resistance in mammary tumor cells." Oncogene 24(19): 3166-76.

Nakagawa, M., J. L. Oliva, et al. (2005). "Phorbol ester-induced G1 phase arrest selectively mediated by protein kinase Cdelta-dependent induction of p21." J Biol Chem 280(40): 33926-34.

Newton, A. C. (1995). "Protein kinase C: structure, function, and regulation." J Biol Chem 270(48): 28495-8.

Newton, A. C. (1997). "Regulation of protein kinase C." Curr Opin Cell Biol 9(2): 161-7.

Nishizuka, Y. (1995). "Protein kinase C and lipid signaling for sustained cellular responses." FASEB J 9(7): 484-96.

O'Brian C. (1989). "Elevated protein kinase C expression in human breast tumor biopsies relative to normal breast tissue." Cancer Res. 49(12):3215-7

Pan, Q., L. W. Bao, et al. (2005). "Protein kinase C epsilon is a predictive biomarker of aggressive breast cancer and a validated target for RNA interference anticancer therapy." Cancer Res 65(18): 8366-71.

Porumb, T., A. Crivici, et al. (1997). "Calcium binding and conformational properties of calmodulin complexed with peptides derived from myristoylated alanine-rich C kinase substrate (MARCKS) and MARCKS-related protein (MRP)." Eur Biophys J 25(4): 239-47.

Prenzel, N., E. Zwick, et al. (2000). "Tyrosine kinase signalling in breast cancer. Epidermal growth factor receptor: convergence point for signal integration and diversification." Breast Cancer Res 2(3): 184-90.

Rabinovitz, I., A. Toker, et al. (1999). "Protein kinase C-dependent mobilization of the alpha6beta4 integrin from hemidesmosomes and its association with actin-rich cell protrusions drive the chemotactic migration of carcinoma cells." J Cell Biol 146(5): 1147-60.

Rodriguez-Mora, O. G., M. M. LaHair, et al. (2005). "Calcium/calmodulin-dependent kinase I and calcium/calmodulin-dependent kinase kinase participate in the control of cell cycle progression in MCF-7 human breast cancer cells." Cancer Res 65(12): 5408-16.

Roskelley, C. D. and M. J. Bissell (2002). "The dominance of the microenvironment in breast and ovarian cancer." Semin Cancer Biol 12(2): 97-104.

Schwartz, G. K., J. Jiang, et al. (1993). "Protein kinase C: a novel target for inhibiting gastric cancer cell invasion." J Natl Cancer Inst 85(5): 402-7.

Speake, G., B. Holloway, et al. (2005). "Recent developments related to the EGFR as a target for cancer chemotherapy." Curr Opin Pharmacol 5(4): 343-9.

Takenaga, K. and K. Takahashi (1986). "Effects of 12-O-tetradecanoylphorbol-13-acetate on adhesiveness and lung-colonizing ability of Lewis lung carcinoma cells." Cancer Res 46(1): 375-80.

Tan, M., P. Li, et al. (2006). "Upregulation and activation of PKC alpha by ErbB2 through Src promotes breast cancer cell invasion that can be blocked by combined treatment with PKC alpha and Src inhibitors." Oncogene 25(23): 3286-95.

Tozlu-Kara S. et al. (2007). "Oligonucleotide microarray analysis of estrogen receptor alpha-positive postmenopausal breast carcinomas: identification of HRPAP20 and TIMELESS as outstanding candidate markers to predict the response to tamoxifen". J Mol Endocrinol. 2007 Oct;39(4):305-18.

Wang, K. C., B. Mutus, et al. (1983). "On the mechanism of interaction between calmodulin and calmodulin-dependent proteins." Can J Biochem Cell Biol 61(8): 911-20.

Ways, D. K., C. A. Kukoly, et al. (1995). "MCF-7 breast cancer cells transfected with protein kinase C-alpha exhibit altered expression of other protein kinase C isoforms and display a more aggressive neoplastic phenotype." J Clin Invest 95(4): 1906-15

Witz, I. P. (2002). "The tumour microenvironment--introduction." Semin Cancer Biol 12(2): 87-8.

3

Endocytic Trafficking of the Epidermal Growth Factor Receptor in Transformed Cells

Brian P. Ceresa
University of Oklahoma Health Sciences Center
United States of America

1. Introduction

The epidermal growth factor receptor (EGFR) is the prototypical receptor tyrosine kinase. It is localized to the plasma membranes of cells with an extracellular ligand binding domain and an intracellular kinase domain. Through the binding of extracellular ligands, the receptor undergoes a conformational change that alters the biochemical properties of proteins (effectors) within the cell. Ultimately, these changes result in modulation of the rate of cell growth, protein and DNA synthesis, cell motility, and cell proliferation. The EGFR is necessary for the proper development of organisms, as indicated by the fact that genetic knockout of the receptor results in animals that are embryonic lethal or die shortly after birth. This developmental role is also observed in adult animals, as pharmacological inhibition of the EGFR disrupts tissue homeostasis.

In addition to these developmental roles, there is a strong association between overexpression and/or hyperactivation of the EGFR and cancer. Currently, there are several small molecule inhibitors and neutralizing, humanized antibodies against the EGFR that successfully treat EGFR-positive cancers (*i.e.* non-small cell lung carcinomas, colon, and head and neck cancers). Breast cancer is among those cancers that are characterized by enhanced EGFR levels and activity. However, the aforementioned pharmacologic agents have been of little success in the treatment of breast cancers. Therefore, a more detailed understanding of the cellular and molecular biology of EGFR function is required in order to successfully attenuate the growth and metastasis of EGFR-positive cells.

Cells have numerous endogenous mechanisms to that regulate the specificity and duration of EGFR signaling. Endogenous regulatory mechanisms are logical pharmacological targets to inhibit EGFR activity because of their intrinsic ability to modulate signaling. One of the most important regulators of EGFR signaling is the endocytic pathway. The endocytic pathway can control both the duration of signaling and the spatial placement of the receptor. Historically, endocytosis has been considered a mechanism for the negative regulation of EGFR, as it decreases the number of cell surface receptors and inactivates the ligand:receptor complex by targeting it for lysosomal degradation. More recently, it has been appreciated that signaling of the EGFR varies based on the subcellular localization of the receptor. Specifically, in a given cell, the liganded EGFR can promote cell proliferation at some cellular locations (*i.e.* plasma membrane), whereas at others (*i.e.* the limiting membranes of endosomes) the receptor can induce apoptosis. Thus, a potential molecular etiology of EGFR overexpression in transformed cells is disrupted normal endocytic

trafficking of the EGFR. Slowed kinetics of receptor degradation will increase the steady-state levels of the EGFRs over time. If this hypothesis holds true, the endocytic pathway is a logical target for pharmacological manipulation to prevent the progression of such cells.
This chapter will explore the basic cell biology of the EGFR and the endocytic mechanisms that regulate its signaling. To be discussed are the workings of the endocytic pathway, strategies used to understand the relationship between endocytic trafficking and EGFR signaling, and data indicating how trafficking regulates signaling. These mechanisms will be dissected and potential points for attenuating the enhanced EGFR activity will be discussed.

2. The EGFR

The EGFR is an approximately 180 kDa transmembrane protein that is oriented on the plasma membrane such that the amino terminus half of the protein is extracellular and the carboxyl terminus portion is intracellular. Thus, by virtue of its orientation, the amino terminus of the EGFR detects and binds ligands; the carboxyl terminal kinase domain converts the conformational change induced through ligand binding into intracellular, biochemical signals. The EGFR is also known as ErbB1, and is part of the larger ErbB family of receptor tyrosine kinases that is comprised of ErbB1, ErbB2, ErbB3 and ErbB4. This family shares many features such as membrane topology, mechanism of activation and signaling, and downstream effectors. However, each member is unique in its tissue expression, its activating ligands, magnitude and duration of effector signaling, and membrane trafficking (Hynes and MacDonald, 2009).
There have been seven ligands that have been reported to be able to activate the EGFR – epidermal growth factor (EGF), heparin binding epidermal growth factor (HB-EGF), betacellulin (BTC), transforming growth factor-α (TGF-α), amphiregulin (AR), epiregulin, and epigen (Harris *et al.*, 2003). The regulated secretion of these ligands is an important determinant of when a receptor gets activated. Further, overexpression of certain ligands, namely TGF-α, has been associated with an increase in receptor activity and enhanced cell proliferation (Matsui et al., 1990; Sandgren et al., 1993).
Based on the available data, it is commonly held that all ligands initiate signaling in the same fundamental manner (Figure 1). Briefly, ligand binding to an EGFR monomer induces a conformation change in the receptor that exposes a dimerization motif (cysteine rich domain). Through association with another EGFR or related family member (ErbB2, ErbB3, or ErbB4), a dimeric receptor forms, and initiates activation of the intracellular kinase domain (Dawson et al., 2005). In turn, the kinase domain phosphorylates tyrosine residues on the very carboxyl terminus of the protein. These newly formed phosphotyrosines serve as docking site for downstream signaling molecules (effectors). The EGFR-stimulated effector activity alters the intracellular biochemistry and results in cellular changes, such as cell proliferation, differentiation, and migration.
There is a long list of effector molecules reported to be downstream of the activated EGFR. Two of the major questions for scientists that study EGFR biology and pathology are 1) to identify which receptor:effector interactions occur under physiological and pathological conditions and which ones are an artifact of cell culture models and 2) to determine which effectors are necessary and sufficient for a specific cell physiology/pathology. Asking these questions is confounded by the fact that receptor:effector interactions can arise as an unintended consequence of receptor overexpression. This is true in model systems that are generated by the scientist as well as naturally occurring cell transformation. As discussed

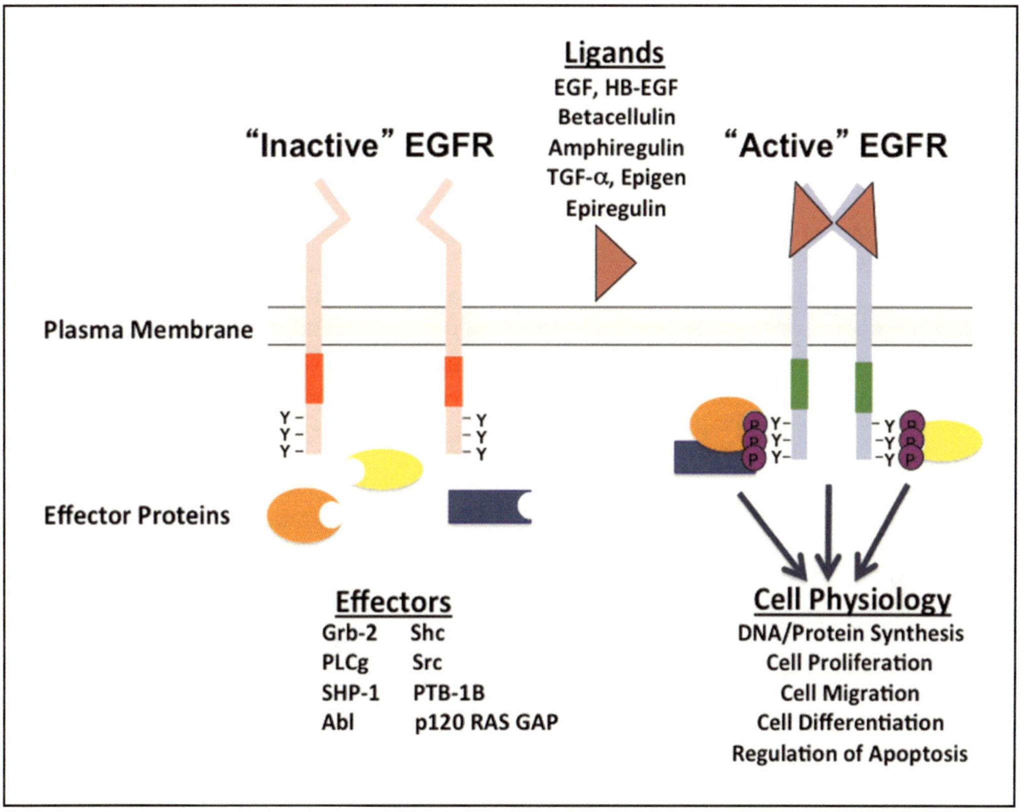

Fig. 1. Schematic of EGFR Activation. Binding of one of the EGFRs endogenous ligands induces a conformational change in the receptor that permits dimerization and kinase activity. Kinase active receptor than transphosphorylates the receptor with which it is associating. The resulting phosphotyrosines serve as docking sites for down stream signaling molecules.

below, many cancers are characterized by overexpression of the EGFR. Therefore, interactions that do not occur in a biological setting may be very relevant in a pathological condition.

There are numerous lines of evidence that indicate the EGFR plays important physiological roles in tissue development and homeostasis (Jorissen *et al.*, 2003). It is expressed on the surface of virtually every cell in the body. Mice that have been engineered to knock out the EGFR gene are either embryonic lethal or die shortly after birth, indicating its role in pre-natal development (Miettinen *et al.*, 1995; Sibilia and Wagner, 1995; Threadgill *et al.*, 1995). Patients taking EGFR inhibitors as part of an anti-cancer chemotherapeutic regimen, experience complications such as colitis, dermatitis, and corneal abrasions, indicating the receptor contributes to the homeostasis of those tissues (Tullo et al., 2005; Zhang et al., 2007). This is supported by the genetically engineered deletion of EGFR ligands (*i.e.* EGF, transforming growth factor-α (TGF-α), or amphiregulin) have revealed roles in maintaining development of tissue, such as mammary glands, eyes, hair, and epidermis (Luetteke *et al.*, 1999) and provide evidence of the receptors' role in tissue homeostasis.

3. EGFRs in cancer

In addition to roles in tissue development and homeostasis, the driving force behind the study of the EGFR has been its role in cancer. The EGFR is overexpressed and/or hyperactivated in many cancers including, but not limited to, cancers of the breast, ovary, colon, lung, head and neck, pancreas, and brain (Rowinsky, 2004). Further, overexpression of the EGFR in many cancers correlates with poor patient prognosis (Nicholson *et al.*, 2001). There are a number of events that can cause the increase in EGFR activity that is associated with cancer. These include gene amplification, activating mutations of the receptor's kinase domain, and deletions of the extracellular domain that regulate the receptor's ligand-binding dependent activity (Hynes and MacDonald, 2009; Uberall et al., 2008). Despite this strong association, it remains unclear whether overexpression/hyperactivation of the EGFR is the root cause of cell transformation or a cell becoming transformed is what leads to the overexpression/hyperactivation of the EGFR.

Regardless of the cause of increased EGFR activity, there are several anti-cancer therapies that specifically target the EGFR that have been approved by the United States Food and Drug Administration (FDA). These drugs fall in two classes. First, humanized monoclonal antibodies target the extracellular portion of the receptor and antagonize the binding of endogenous EGFR ligands. These antibodies are 528 mouse IgG_{2a}, the 225 mouse IgG_1, and the C225 humanized monoclonal antibody. The second class of drugs are small molecule inhibitors of the EGFR kinase domain [Iressa (gefitinib) and Tarceva (erlotinib)]. Both classes of drugs are able to prevent the progression of cancer by inducing apoptosis specifically in those cells with increased EGFR activity. Therapeutic use of these drugs has been approved for non-small-cell lung cancer, squamous cell carcinoma of the head and neck, and colorectal cancers (Baselga and Arteaga, 2005).

One issue that remains unresolved is the limited therapeutic efficacy of EGFR inhibitors in the treatment of breast cancers. This is true, despite the fact that EGFR overexpression is associated with some breast cancers. To date, only Tykerb (lapatinib) is approved for the treatment of breast cancer. However, it should be noted that Tykerb inhibits both the EGFR and its receptor tyrosine kinase family member, ErbB2, and is only approved for use in conjunction with the aromatase inhibitor Femara (letrozole) (Cameron et al., 2010). Despite the limited success of EGFR inhibitors in treating breast cancers, the evidence from other cancers indicates the receptor still has potential as a therapeutic target. In order to develop better anti-cancer chemotherapeutic agents that target the EGFR in breast cancer, a more detailed understanding of EGFR signaling is required.

4. EGFR endocytic pathway

Not only are the effectors with which the EGFR interacts important, but also the quality of interaction. Both the duration and magnitude of effector activity are what determine how cell physiology is modified. A tremendous body of literature supports the idea that the regulation of signaling is the critical determinant in how receptor specific signals are produced. This is the most logical explanation for how a number of different cell surface receptor (*i.e.* EGFR, insulin receptor, and platelet derived growth factor receptor) can share an overlapping set of effector molecules, yet each produces a receptor-specific change in cell physiology.

One of the principle mechanisms by which EGFR signaling is regulated is ligand-mediated endocytosis. Internalization of the EGF:EGFR complex can be either clathrin-dependent or clathrin-independent. Clathrin-dependent endocytosis is the most well studied as it is the predominant route of receptor internalization in response to physiological concentrations of ligand.

By all accounts, all of the endogenous EGFR ligands can promote internalization of the EGFR, through a series of well-defined steps (Figure 2). Following binding of ligand, the ligand:receptor complex translocates along the plasma membrane to a domain that is enriched on the intracellular face with clathrin. The clathrin lattice invaginates to form a clathrin-coated pit that pinches off generating an intracellular clathrin-coated vesicle. Once inside the cell, clathrin is shed from the vesicle, giving rise to an intermediate vesicle. The intermediate vesicle fuses with and delivers the ligand:receptor complex to the early endosome. This compartment is where sorting of the cargo occurs. The predominant route of trafficking of the EGF:EGFR complex is into a late endosome/multivesicular body, by way of vesicle maturation. Alternative routes include recycling to the plasma membrane, trafficking to the nucleus, and delivery to the endoplasmic reticulum (Liao and Carpenter, 2007; Masui et al., 1993; Wang et al., 2010). For those receptors that get delivered to the late endosome/multivesicular body, that compartment fuses with the lysosome that degrades the ligand and receptor in the protease rich environment.

Each endocytic compartment has a number of distinguishing features. First, as the compartments get further away from the plasma membrane, they become more acidic and increase in density. In addition, each endocytic location has a unique protein composition. These three features have proven to be important in understanding ligand:receptor interactions, receptor trafficking, and receptor signaling. Further, researchers continue to utilize these features to distinguish one compartment from another. For instance, the different densities of the endosomes can be use to separate compartments by sedimentation centrifugation (Vanlandingham and Ceresa, 2009). Endosome specific proteins can be used as markers to identify which intracellular compartment the receptor resides (Vanlandingham and Ceresa, 2009).

It is important to note that following endocytosis, not all ligands target the EGFR for lysosomal degradation. A recent, comprehensive study of the trafficking of EGFR ligands was performed using human laryngeal carcinoma (Hep2) cells as a model (Roepstorff et al., 2009). In this study, six of the endogenous EGFR ligands were analyzed for their ability to induce receptor internalization, lysosomal degradation, and recycling. Following ligand treatment, the authors used indirect immunofluorence to monitor receptor co-localization with early and late endosome markers [early endosome autoantigen 1 (EEA1) and Lysosome associated membrane protein 1 (Lamp1)]. In addition, biochemical assays were used to assess the kinetics of ligand stimulated EGFR degradation and recycling. The data from the manuscript indicate that two ligands TGF-α and epiregulin lead to receptor recycling. HB-EGF and betacellulin, like EGF, target the receptor for degradation. Interestingly, amphiregulin treatment yields a phenotype that is somewhere in between - recycling with slower kinetics.

While the molecular basis for these differences in receptor trafficking are not entirely clear for all ligands, one ligand has been particularly well studied, particularly in the context of cancer. As stated above, treatment with TGF-α induces EGFR internalization and recycling to the plasma membrane. Once back at the plasma membrane, the receptor can be re-stimulated with available ligand and another round or signaling can occur (McClintock and Ceresa, 2010). The question becomes: what are the properties of TGF-α that promote

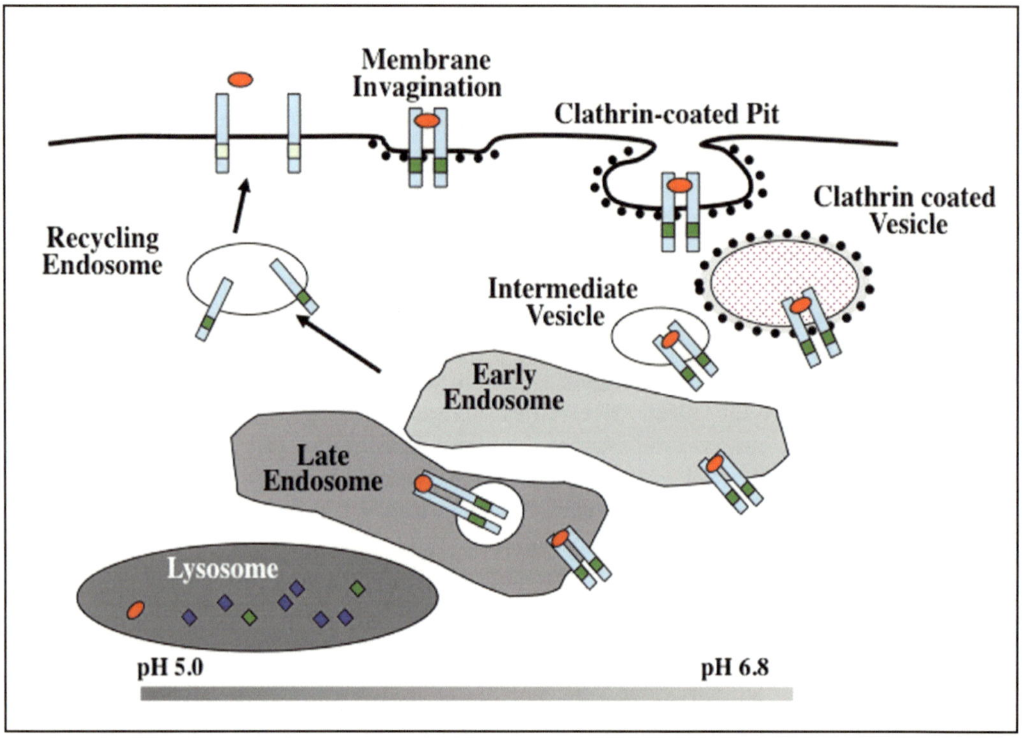

Fig. 2. Schematic of EGFR Endocytic Trafficking.

receptor recycling, whereas EGF (and others) does not? It is widely held that the difference lies in the pH sensitivity of ligand binding. Both EGF and TGF-α bind the EGFR with comparable affinity at neutral, physiological pH (pH 7.3-7.4). At pH 6.8, 50% of TGF-α will dissociate from the receptor. EGF requires a pH of 5.9 for 50% of ligand dissociation (Rutten et al., 1996). This is biologically important because the pH of the early endosome is ~6.8 (Gruenberg and Maxfield, 1995), therefore significant dissociation occurs. The loss of ligand likely converts the receptor back into a kinase-inactive conformation and is accompanied by dephosphorylation of the receptor. This would prevent association with the c-Cbl ubiquitin ligase that ubiquitylates the receptor, thereby targeting it to the lysosome for degradation.

Since EGFR endocytosis frequently culminates in the targeted destruction of the ligand:receptor complex in the lysosome, it is logical to assume this route of membrane trafficking would negatively regulate signaling. However, the role of endocytosis is more complex. Data exist that support the endocytic pathway positively regulating EGFR signaling, as well. It is clear that endocytic trafficking provides temporal regulation of receptor signaling.

4.1 Endocytosis as a negative regulator of EGFR signaling

Formal proof that endocytosis negatively regulates EGFR signaling came from the laboratory of Michael Rosenfeld (Wells *et al.*, 1990). In order to understand the role of endocytosis in signaling, Wells et al. generated mutant EGFRs that were deficient in the ability to internalize. They stably expressed these receptors in NR6 cells (derived from NIH3T3 cells) that are devoid of endogenous EGFRs. Once they established that ligand mediated endocytosis of these receptors was blocked, they examined EGF-mediated cell transformation using a colony formation assay. A dose response curve of EGF-mediated cell transformation revealed the EGFRs defective in the ability to internalize required lower doses of EGF to undergo transformation and produced more transformed cells. From these data, it was generally accepted that endocytosis is a negative regulator of EGFR signaling.

There have been numerous of additional lines of evidence to support this model, particular in cancer models. Importantly, several come from naturally occurring cancers. For instance, one common EGFR mutation, EGFRvIII, demonstrates the relationship between receptor internalization and signaling. EGFRvIII is associated with cancers of the brain, lung, prostate, and ovary. The receptor itself is a truncation mutant that is devoid of amino acids 6-273, which encompasses the ligand binding domain and dimerization arm (Wikstrand et al., 1995). Grandal et al. compared the levels of internalization and receptor phosphorylation in NR6 cells expressing either EGFRvIII or wild type EGFR (Grandal et al., 2007). While EGFRvIII can be internalized, its rate of degradation is much slower than the EGFR. These delayed kinetics correspond to prolonged signaling. While the authors do not perform a detailed analysis of signaling, there is clearly enhanced signaling based on their association with cancer.

A second example demonstrates how other ErbB family members can both delay EGFR degradation and enhance its signaling. Like the EGFR, ErbB2 is frequently overexpressed in cancers, notably breast cancers (Guerin et al., 1988). Several groups have examine how ErbB2 (and other ErbB family members) impinge on EGFR trafficking. Worthylake et al. performed a detailed biochemical characterization of EGFR ligand binding, cell surface expression, recycling and degradation with and without ErbB2 present (Worthylake et al., 1999). Using mammary epithelial cells (MTSV1 and derivative lines) as a model, they examined the EGFR and ErbB2 when the two receptors were expressed at a 9:1 and 1:1 ratio. One of their major findings was that ErbB2 inhibits the downregulation of the EGFR.

Similarly, Offterdinger and Bastiaens examined if expression of ErbB2 affected the signaling of the EGFR (Offterdinger and Bastiaens, 2008). Using Chinese Hamster Ovary (CHO) cells that express EGFRs, but low levels of ErbB2, the authors stably transfected the cells with ErbB2. Using single cell assays, the two cells line were transiently transfected with an EGFR that had been tagged with green fluorescent protein (GFP). With this model, they observed expression of ErbB2 attenuated the rate of EGFR-GFP internalization, it also prolonged the phosphorylation of the EGFR. Since kinase dead ErbB2 had similar affects on trafficking and signaling, the authors concluded that the increased phosphorylation was not due to ErbB2 kinase activity, but rather decreased EGFR degradation/phosphorylation in the presence of ErbB2.

Additionally, there are a number of cancers that have been associated with defects in the endocytic trafficking of the EGFR and other cell surface receptors. Mutations and deletions of proteins involved in trafficking have been reported to be associated with acute myeloid leukemia (AML), hepatocellular carcinomas (HCC), breast and prostate cancer (Mosesson et al., 2008). It general, these protein aberrations result in a delay in the kinetics of receptor degradation and yield a higher level of receptor signaling, consistent with endocytosis negatively regulating signaling.

4.2 Endocytosis as a positive regulator of EGFR signaling

In the last fifteen years, a second role for the endocytic pathway to regulate EGFR signaling has come to light. This secondary mechanism is the spatial regulation conferred by placing the active receptor in the same microenvironment as downstream signaling molecules (or effectors). The first evidence for this came from the laboratory of Sandra Schmid. Vieira et al, expressed a dominant negative mutant of the large guanine nucleotide-binding protein, dynamin, in HeLa cells, which prevents endocytosis of the EGFR via clathrin-coated pits. EGFR stimulation of cells expressing this dominant negative protein retains the liganded EGFRs at the plasma membrane (Vieira *et al.*, 1996). This approach removes the potential confounding effects of receptor mutagenesis or differences in expression levels in stable cell lines. The data from this study revealed that the activity from some effectors was enhanced when endocytosis blocked (EGFR phosphorylation, Shc, Grb2). Conversely, other effectors required endocytosis for maximal activity, namely, mitogen activating protein kinase (MAPK) and phosphatidyl inositol 3'-kinase (PI3K). This finding introduced the idea that endocytosis could be a positive regulator of signaling.

This finding was not without controversy. Subsequent groups reported that the expression of dominant negative dynamin inhibited MAPK activity. Thus, it was suggested that the attenuated MAPK activity was not due to a failure of the active EGFR to reach the endosome and stimulate MAPK, but rather a dynamin-dependent activation of MAPK (Johanessen et al., 2000). In addition, it has been suggested that blocking normal endocytic trafficking may affect the ligand binding properties to the EGFR (Ringerike et al., 1998).

However, since the initial report, there have been several additional lines of evidence that endocytosis provides spatial regulation to EGFR signaling. Two separate studies from the Lauffenburger's group provide compelling support. To examine the spatial regulation of EGFR:effector interactions, the authors exploited the different trafficking itineraries used by TGF-α as compared to EGF. By comparing the effects of the two ligands, they were able to alter the ratio of active EGFR at the plasma membrane and within the cell. They discovered that EGFRs at the plasma membrane preferentially activated phospholipase Cγ1 (Haugh et al., 1999b). Although these data indicate that endocytosis negatively regulates PLCγ1 activity, it also supports the idea that receptor:effector interactions are spatially regulated . Evidence that the spatial regulation of signaling is a positively regulator came from the follow-up publication. Using a similar approach, the authors were able to demonstrate that p21ras was actively activated from within the cell (Haugh et al., 1999a).

The detailed kinetic analysis performed in these studies is not trivial. One of the strengths of this work is that the signaling is studied in the context of wild type EGFRs that are expressed at the physiological concentrations receptors (Chen et al., 1996). Further, there was not perturbation of the endocytic pathway. Thus, these data likely provide the most accurate snapshot of what occurs physiologically.

Regardless of exactly how endocytic trafficking affects EGFR signaling, it is clearly an important mechanism. Understanding this process will undoubtedly generate important insights regarding the etiology of cancer and, potentially, the treatment of cancers.

4.3 Deciphering the role of endocytosis in EGFR signaling

There is plenty of direct and indirect evidence to indicate the endocytic trafficking regulates EGFR signaling, but a deeper understanding of the molecular mechanism is necessary. For instance, elucidating the molecular mechanism(s) will provide insight into how to specifically manipulate the pathway and modulate signaling as desired. There are a number of fundamental questions that need to be answered. Does endocytosis regulate EGFR signaling spatially, temporally, or both? Are the regulatory processes unique for individual cells and tissues? Do variations in receptor expression (as often occur in cancers) affect the regulation?

Temporal regulation of signaling refers to the duration of signaling, and would be consistent with endocytosis serving strictly as a negative regulator. How this might occur is not entirely clear. There has been much speculation in the literature whether this occurs by: 1) promoting receptor dephosphorylation, thereby eliminating its ability to interact with downstream effectors, 2) sequestration into the intraluminal vesicles of the late endosome/multivesicular body which prevents interactions with cytosolic effector proteins, or 3) degradation of the receptor. Alternatively, it may be that a combination of the three events (or possibly others) may contribute to signal attenuation.

In contrast, if endocytosis provides spatial regulation to signaling, it could either positively or negatively regulate signaling, depending of the effector protein and its subcellular location. Spatial regulation suggests the co-localization of the receptor and effector. Since this could occur at any point along the pathway (*i.e.* plasma membrane, early endosome, late endosome), its effect on signaling could be positive or negative. If receptor:effector communication is occurring at the plasma membrane, then endocytosis negatively regulate those interactions; conversely, receptor:effector interaction at intracellular locales, such as the early endosome, would be positively regulated by endocytosis.

It is important to note that the model of spatial regulation of EGFR signaling is predicated on the fact that there is compartmentalization of effector proteins. Only if an effector is concentrated at a given subcellular locale will endocytosis be able to confer specificity. If an effector is ubiquitously expressed throughout the cell, either in normal or pathological conditions, then spatial regulation cannot be achieved. This is an important consideration when examining cancer cells with aberrant protein expression. The unregulated signaling may be a consequence of lost spatial regulation of signaling.

As mentioned above, it cannot be ruled out that the endocytic pathway plays both positive and negative roles, depending on the effector. In fact, such a model may help explain the diversity in the cell biology that can be mediated by the receptor. For instance, signals that promote cell migration may be negatively regulated by endocytosis whereas those that control cell proliferation may require endocytosis.

Understanding the contribution of the endocytic pathway to EGFR signaling has important implications for a number of reasons. First, it will reveal the fundamental mechanisms of cell surface receptor signaling. It is likely this regulatory process is not unique to the EGFR or receptor tyrosine kinases. Thus, understanding this regulatory process has implications for other cell surface receptors and may guide the development of novel therapeutic agents for diseases other than cancer. Second, understanding the molecular mechanisms that regulate EGFR signaling will provide potentially useful clues to how the EGFR contributes to the pathology that underlies many cancers. These findings may provide new insights into the causes and potential prevention of cancer. Finally, the intricacies of signaling need to be appreciated in order to develop novel therapeutics that target the EGFR. Currently, the EGFR inhibitors (antibodies and tyrosine kinase inhibitors) are only effective against a subset of EGFR-positive cancers. A better of understanding of EGFR signaling will aid in the targeted design of therapeutics for a broader spectrum of cancers.

5. Strategies for deciphering the role of endocytic trafficking in EGFR signaling

Membrane trafficking and signal transduction are two very dynamic processes. Studying these events in real time has proven difficult. As a result, most investigators use a strategy of disrupting endocytic trafficking or at least dramatically slowing it, and determining how signaling is affected. To this end, investigators have relied heavily on two fundamentally different strategies: mutagenesis of the receptor itself or perturbation of the endocytic pathway. Here we discuss the basic components of these strategies and the strengths and weaknesses of each approach.

5.1 Receptor mutagenesis to inhibit EGFR endocytic trafficking

Endocytosis-deficient, mutant EGFRs allows one to examine the EGFR directly, without disrupting proteins that are also used by other receptors that share the endocytic pathway. Therefore, the effects seen in response to EGF treatment are truly from the EGFR and do not represent a change in the fundamental properties of the cell. One technical limitation to this approach is that in order to accurately study two different receptor populations (*i.e.* wild type and an endocytosis-deficient mutant), the two receptors need to be stably expressed in cells that are devoid of the EGFRs. First, all cell line are not amenable to stable transfection, therefore the repertoire of cell lines can be limited. Second, in making stable cell lines, it is difficult to control the level of protein expression. Differences in receptor expression will affect the total level of activated receptor in response to ligand as well as number of effectors that are activated downstream. Thus, it could be hard to determine if the difference in signaling reflect changes in endocytic trafficking or receptor expression. Finally, as with all mutagenesis strategies, there is the potential that mutation of the receptor inhibits one function (such as endocytosis), there will an unexpected change in another (for instance, signaling).

In addition to the technical limitations to using mutant EGFRs, there is an even greater biological limitation. The molecular mechanisms the regulate EGFR endocytic trafficking are complex and multi-faceted. Despite the EGFR being arguably the most studied receptor in the field of endocytic trafficking, there are constantly new mechanisms of internalization being identified. Often newly discovered mechanisms are redundant with a previously identified mechanisms. The multiple mechanisms for regulating internalization are consistent with the notion EGFR endocytosis is critical to the proper function of the cell.

The complexity of EGFR endocytosis is illustrated by a recent study by Goh et al. (Goh et al., 2010). In this study, the authors used a combination of receptor mutagenesis and RNA interference (RNAi) to completely block EGFR endocytosis in porcine aortic endothelial (PAE) cells. PAE cells were chosen because they do not express the EGFR or any of its ErbB family members. Ultimately, the authors demonstrate that there are at least four completely redundant or partially interrelated mechanisms for EGFR endocytosis. When all four processes were targeted, the result was a signaling-capable EGFR with normal kinetics of kinase activation and tyrosine phosphorylation.

5.2 Disruption of endocytic trafficking by inhibition of stage-specific regulatory proteins

An alternative approach for understanding how the endocytic pathway affects EGFR signaling is to disrupt the machinery that guides the ligand:receptor complex through the endocytic pathway. Entry and exit from each endocytic location is highly regulated by a set of proteins that are unique for that endocytic stage. Knock down or expression of dominant negative forms of those proteins can be used to alter EGFR trafficking. For instance, as described above, internalization of the receptor is regulated by the large GTPase dynamin. Expression of dominant negative dynamin (Damke et al., 1994) or knock down of dynamin expression by RNAi (Huang et al., 2004) prevents EGFR endocytosis.

It should be noted that there are several proteins that are required for the internalization of the EGFR. Expression of dominant negative mutants or knock down of many of these proteins of proteins will impair the kinetics of EGFR endocytosis. For instance, work by the Sorkin laboratory has shown that knock down of clathrin heavy chain, Grb2, and dynamin II will all cause a decrease in EGFR endocytosis to some extent (Huang *et al.*, 2004). Further, since each step along the endocytic pathway is regulated by a variety of small molecular weight G-proteins, endosomal sorting complex required for transport (ESCRT), and adaptor proteins, the activity and expression of these proteins can also be targeted to inhibit intracellular trafficking. Considerable work has been done analyzing how the RAB family of proteins contributes to EGFR trafficking; therefore modulation of RAB expression or activity can alter movement of the receptor into and out of various endocytic compartments (Ceresa, 2006).

While this approach eliminates the complications like variable levels of receptor expression and potential conformational changes in the receptor, there are other caveats. First, many of the proteins used to regulate EGFR endocytic trafficking are shared with other receptors. Therefore, knocking down at protein to prevent EGFR endocytosis, will likely affect the internalization of other receptors. This likely will not be a problem if the focus is on receptor:effector communication, because the basal activity can be established by examining cells in the absence of an EGFR ligand. However, the analysis of whole cell physiology may be more complex, depending on what receptors are present in the cell, their basal activity, and the cell physiology that is being examined. Second, one must keep in mind that disrupting endocytic trafficking, only inhibits the kinetics of the pathway. It is not an absolute block. Therefore, receptors may accumulate at one endocytic stage, but in all likelihood, still be able to proceed to the next compartment, albeit at a dramatically slowed rate.

The third issue is more likely to be a problem. Disrupting endocytic trafficking can alter the steady-state distribution of the receptor . It is often under appreciated that the EGFR internalizes in the absence of ligand, albeit at a much slower rate than in the presence of ligand. Approximately, 2-3% of the EGFR constitutively internalizes every minute. Following internalization, these unliganded receptors recycle back to the plasma membrane (Herbst *et al.*, 1994).

The cause of unliganded EGFR internalization has not been determined experimentally, but may reflect receptors that spontaneously form an "active" conformation in the absence of ligand or receptors that randomly localize to a clathrin enriched membrane domain as the clathrin-coated pit forms. While the molecular determinants guiding unliganded receptors to internalize is not fully understood, it is clear that unliganded and liganded EGFRs trafficking through the same endocytic machinery. Therefore, when the endocytic trafficking is disrupted, receptors that constitutively internalize will accumulate within the endocytic pathway where the block is in place. This may, or may not, affect the total number of EGFRs in the cell. However, it has been shown for mutants of RAB5 to change the amount of cell surface EGFR (Dinneen and Ceresa, 2004).

This caveat is particularly important when using strategies that block receptor internalization (*i.e.* knock down of dynamin, clathrin heavy chain, Grb2), as an increase in cell surface receptors may result. In this case, one would need to be cautious when enhanced signaling is observed to determine whether it is the result of the block in endocytosis or increased number of ligand:receptor complexes. Similarly, if reagents were used to block

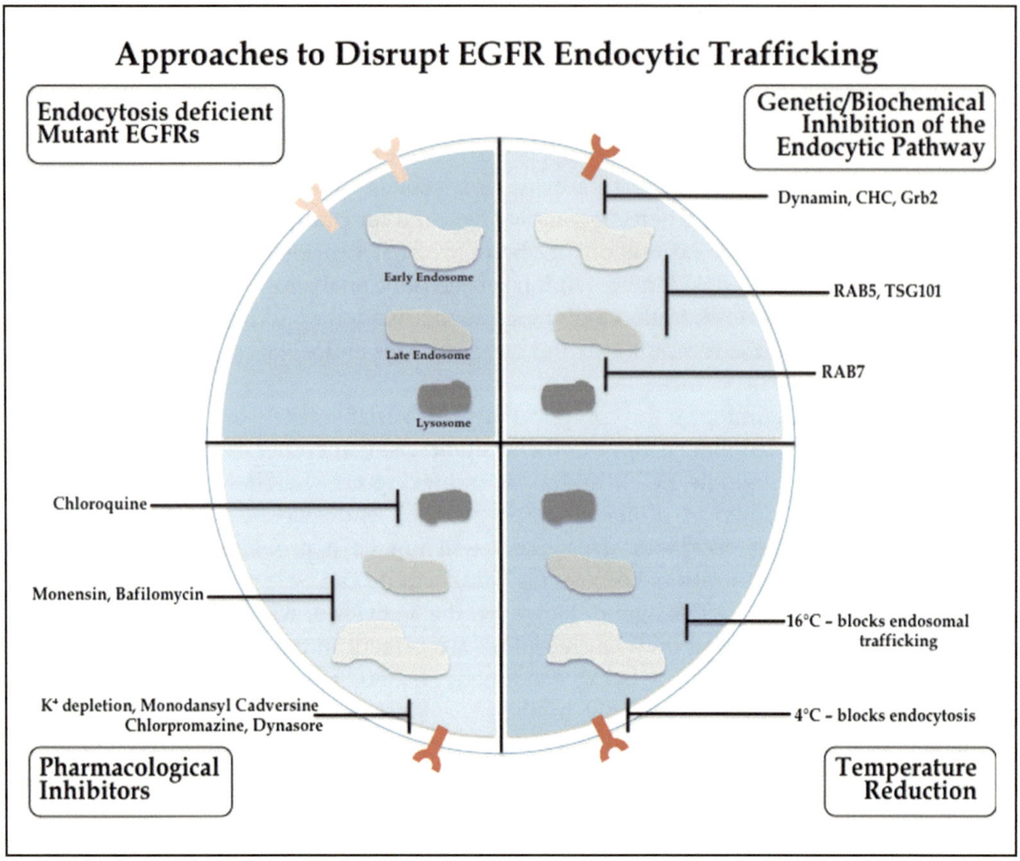

Fig. 3. Summary of Different Strategies Used to Study the Relationship between EGFR Endocytic Trafficking and Signaling.

endocytic trafficking within the cell (*i.e.* knock down of RAB5, RAB7, or TSG101), there may be an intracellular accumulation of receptors and a decrease in cell surface receptors. Under this scenario, the challenge is to understand whether decreases in signaling are due to the endocytic trafficking or decreased ligand:receptor complexes.

5.3 Pharmacological inhibitors of the endocytic machinery

Pharmacological inhibitors of the endocytic pathway offer an alternative strategy for studying EGFR endocytic trafficking. There are a limited number of such agents available. To date, these compounds have been primarily used for studying endocytic trafficking. Only recently have they been used to study how trafficking affects signal transduction.

As with most aspects of the endocytic pathway, the knowledge and reagents are greatest at the plasma membrane and decrease as one progresses to the lysosome. This is true for pharmacological inhibitors as well. At the plasma membrane, there are a number of pharmacological options available. One of the earliest strategies was intracellular potassium depletion. Work by Larkin et al. demonstrated that depletion of intracellular potassium reduced the formation of clathrin-coated pits and dramatically reduce low density lipoprotein internalization (Larkin et al., 1983). This strategy is particularly attractive because the technique is relatively easy to perform and the endocytic inhibition is readily reversible. Since that report, other agents have been used including, chlorpromazine (inhibitor of clathrin assembly/disassembly) (Feugaing et al., 2007), monodansyl cadversine (Ray and Samanta, 1996), and most recently the dynamin inhibitor, dynasore (Hill et al., 2009).

One of the most well described inhibitors of intracellular trafficking is the ionophore, monensin. Monensin functions by inhibiting early endosome acidification. When monensin-treated cells are incubated with EGF, the receptor accumulates in the early endosome, and rates of receptor degradation and recycling are dramatically reduced (King, 1984). A similar drug, bafilomycin, disrupts trafficking in a similar manner (Presly et al., 1997). Intracellular endocytic trafficking can also be inhibited by the anti-malarial drug, chloroquine. Due to its properties as a weak base, it accumulates in the lysosome and inhibits trafficking to that compartment (Anderson et al., 1984).

5.4 Temperature reduction to inhibit endocytic trafficking

Membrane trafficking is temperature dependent. Exploiting this property can be a useful, non-invasive strategy for disrupting endocytic trafficking. Carrying out experiments at 4°C will effectively reduce all endocytosis, whereas a 16°C incubation prevents movement out of the early endosome. Both inhibitions are reversible by restoring cells to physiological temperatures (37°C). Further, temperature reduction is readily applicable to all cells.

Many of the same advantages of pharmacological inhibitors are seen with temperature reduction. The effects on membrane trafficking are rapid and reversible, which minimizes the changes in the steady-state distribution of the receptor. The biggest disadvantage is in studying EGFR-signaling. Most receptor:effector communication is temperature dependent. While receptor:effector interactions would likely still occur at lower temperature (although it would take longer to reach steady-state), the kinetics of activation would be altered, thereby making the interpretation of signaling difficult.

As with most of cell biology, the best approach is multiple approaches. Complementing receptor mutagenesis and endocytic inhibitors will provide the strongest case that differences in signaling are due to changes in trafficking.

6. Ligand based strategies for studying EGFR endocytosis

Given the limitations of using a receptor based and a cell-based strategies, an alternative approach is to use a modified ligand to disrupt trafficking. An emerging strategy is to conjugate EGF (or another EGFR ligand) to an immobilized matrix. For instance, EGF can be covalently bound to polystyrene beads that are too large to internalize or a tissue culture dish. This strategy allows the ligand to bind and activate the receptor, but the conjugated matrix (polystyrene bead or tissue culture dish) physically impedes receptor internalization.

There are several advantages to this approach. First, there is no limitation to what EGFR-expressing cell type can be studied. This is particularly important since often times cell lines that are good models for studying EGFR endocytic trafficking are not good models for studying receptor signaling. In addition, previous methods favored the used of cell lines that are receptive to the introduction of cDNA, siRNA, and viral transduction. Second, since the endocytic inhibitor affects only liganded receptors, a homogenous population of

Approach	Advantages	Disadvantages
Endocytosis Deficient, Mutant EGFR	•Specific for the EGFR	•Requires stable cell line •Difficulty getting comparable receptor numbers •Numerous endocytic processes
Biochemical/Genetic Disruption of Endocytic Machinery	•Can examine endogenous receptors at physiological levels •Can examine an array of endocytic locations	•Other cell surface receptors are affected •Can change the steady-state distribution of EGFRs • Difficult to define endocytic compartments
Pharmacological Inhibitors	•Act Quickly •Can Use in a range of cell lines	•Questions of specificity on endocytic location •Disrupt trafficking of multiple receptors
Temperature Reduction	•Act Quickly •Can Use in a range of cell lines	•Disrupt trafficking of multiple receptors •Decreases Receptor and Effector enzyme activity
Tethered Ligands	•Can Use in a range of cell lines •Specific for activated EGFR	•May select for high affinity receptors

Table 1. Advantages and Disadvantages to Various Methods for Studying EGFR Endocytic Trafficking.

receptors is being examined, and there are no concerns that some receptors have escaped the endocytic inhibition. Finally, since the endocytic inhibitor is the ligand, there are no changes in the steady-state distribution of the receptor or compensatory mechanisms developed by the cell.

The use of EGF-beads has some limitations as well. First, by design, the EGF-beads have multiple molecules of EGF bound to them. Therefore, there could be multiple ligand:receptor interactions with one EGF-bead. While this will not likely affect the kinetics of ligand association, the increased stability may affect the kinetics of ligand dissociation. This may affect the duration of ligand binding. Second, it is unknown how the conjugation process affects ligand binding and subsequent biological activity. As illustrated in Figure 4, the EGF molecule is conjugated to a carboxylate modified polystyrene bead via zero length crosslinker. Depending on which amino group is the site of conjugation that may affect the ability of the ligand to bind to the receptor. Although all studies using modified EGF clearly demonstrate at least some of the immobilized ligand retains its biological activity, it is not always clear to what extent. Finally, the bead itself has unintended consequences. While the large physical size of the bead provides a means for blocking entry through clathrin-coated pits, it may also sterically hinder the formation of EGF:EGFR complexes within a subdomain of the cell.

At this point it is difficult to discern which issues are theoretical and which are practical. From a biochemical perspective, we attempted to circumvent these issues by comparing

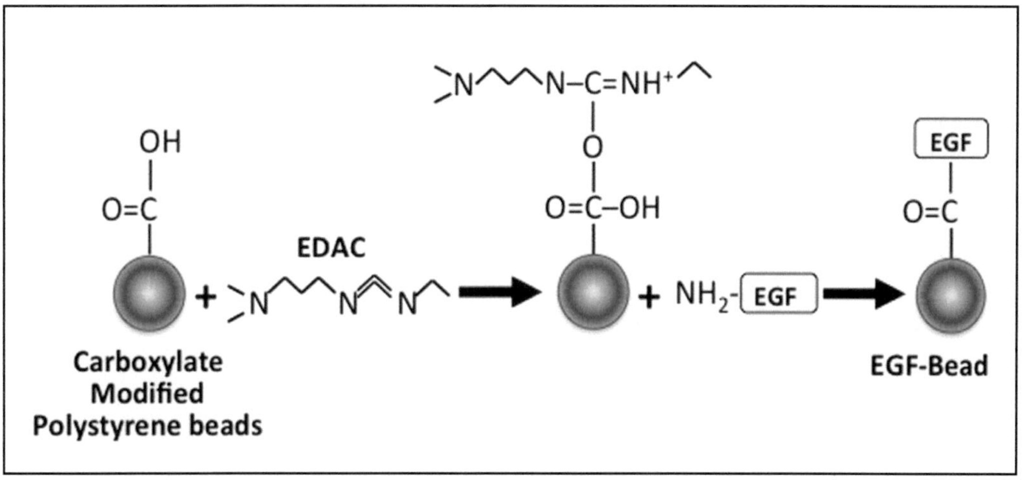

Fig. 4. Schematic of the Synthesis of EGF-beads. 900 nm polystyrene beads modified with carboxylate groups are reacted with 1-Ethyl-3-[3-dimethylaminopropyl]carbodiimide hydrochloride (EDAC) to form an active O-acylisourea intermediate that readily couples to the terminal amino group in EGF (Verveer *et al.*, 2000).

cells that had comparable levels of EGFR phosphorylation. Therefore, the basis for comparison was activated receptors at the cell surface (stimulated by EGF-beads) or within the cell (EGF stimulated).

6.1 Studying of EGFR-mediated cell signaling with immobilized EGF

The initial studies with immobilized EGF were not designed to study differences in EGFR signaling from the plasma membrane as compared to inside the cell. They were designed to understand how signaling was propagated at the plasma membrane. A study by Verveer et al. demonstrated that a liganded EGFR could propagate phosphorylation along the plasma membrane to other EGFRs that were not bound to a ligand (Verveer *et al.*, 2000).

The authors of this study used a microscopy-based assay that allowed the measure of receptor phosphorylation in real time. Briefly, cells expressing a green fluorescence protein (GFP)-tagged EGFR were microinjected with a Cyanine 3 (Cy3) labeled anti-phosphotyrosine antibody. When the receptor is phosphorylated, the anti-phosphotyrosine antibody binds and places the Cy3 in close enough proximity (nanometers) to the GFP conjugated to EGF for fluorescent energy transfer (FRET). From these studies, it was concluded that both soluble EGF and EGF-beads could propagate signaling along the plasma membrane of cells.

Secondary to the authors intent, this study demonstrated that EGF-beads could: 1) bind to the EGFR and 2) be retained at the plasma membrane. In addition to the insights about EGFR signal propagation provided by this study, it also provided an important foundation for future studies analyzing the temporal and spatial basis of EGFR signaling.

A second study using EGF-beads, also took a single cell approach (Kempiak *et al.*, 2003). The goal of this study was to assess the localized signaling of the EGFR using chemotaxis as the physiological readout. The authors demonstrate that EGF beads, like EGF, can induce a chemotactic response as visualized by video microscopy. Further, cell surface receptors could initiate the cell migration by triggering cytoskeletal reorganization as measured by staining with rhodamine phalloidin. The authors examined selected signaling pathways and found that phosphorylation of Akt was about three time greater following treatment with EGF-beads as compared to EGF.

It is worth re-stating that the goal of these two studies was not to distinguish cell surface versus intracellular EGFR signaling. Rather, both studies set up out to examine localized EGFR signals initiated from the plasma membrane. Therefore, they provide important information regarding cell surface receptor signaling, but are limited in what they reveal about what occurs within the cell.

6.2 Using EGF immobilized to a solid support to study EGFR-mediated cell migration

Although the EGF-beads are a useful way to study EGFR from the plasma membrane, variations on this theme have proven useful as well. Most notably, EGF that has been immobilized to the bottom of tissue culture dishes has proven to be an effective tool in studying cell migration. Bioengineering groups seeking to develop new methods for drug delivery performed these studies. Although EGFR is closely associated with the development of cancer, it has also been shown to be instrumental in wound healing and tissue homeostasis as well. Thus, cancer biologists should take notice of these engineering studies, as the tools developed for *in vitro* models of wound healing may provide important mechanistic insights into EGFR-mediated changes in cell biology and well as useful tools for studying the fundamental cell biology of the EGFR.

Early studies by Chen et al. used covalently linked EGF to a polystyrene dish using photo irradiation. Briefly, EGF was coupled with N-(4-azidobenzoyloxy)succinimide and the resulting solution was coated on a polystyrene dish, and the water was allowed to evaporate. Ultraviolet light was used to crosslink the modified EGF to the dish (Chen *et al.*, 1997).

To test the new ligand, Chinese Hamster Ovary (CHO) cells or mouse fibroblasts were plated on top of the immobilized EGF and monitored for cell growth by ^{3}H-thymidine incorporation. The rate of cell growth was approximately three fold higher with the immobilized EGF as compared to soluble EGF.

A modification of this approach was used by Stefonek and Masters (Stefonek and Masters, 2007). While these authors used the same basic model of immobilizing EGF to the bottom of a tissue culture dish, they did so with a concentration gradient. Using photo-patterning, precise control of the spatial localization of the EGF was achieved. Human keratinocytes (HaCaT cells) were plated on this EGF matrix and monitored for cell migration over the course of 16 days. These studies demonstrated that cells migrated toward the higher concentrations of immobilized EGF. Migration was approximately five fold greater than the control conditions. Both groups considered their findings to support the model that endocytosis negatively regulates EGFR signaling. Restricting endocytosis, prevents receptor degradation, and prolongs signaling, thereby enhancing cell migration.

Our understanding of EGFR signaling is enhanced by these studies for several reasons. First, in both studies with immobilized EGF are looking at EGFR-mediated responses in large populations of cells, rather than events in one cell. In doing so, these studies lay the groundwork for providing a biochemical analysis of changes in signaling. Second, they examine changes in cell biology that are of interest to a cancer biologist. Cell migration and proliferation are two key EGFR-mediated signaling events that need to be attenuated in the successful treatment of cancer. Finally, as bioengineering groups, the authors introduce the biologists to ways of modifying ligands in a manner that does not compromise their biologic activity.

However, in terms of understanding the spatial and temporal regulation of signaling, these studies are limited in their scope. These studies provide evidence, at least in these physiological assays that indicate endocytosis is a negative regulator of signaling. This finding supports the original report by Wells et al, in which mutant, endocytosis resistant EGF were more potent and efficacious activator of cell transformation (Wells *et al.*, 1990). However, it is not clear from these experiments whether all signaling pathways are enhanced or just a subset. Further, since all physiological responses being analyzed are enhanced, it is unclear whether some responses are positively regulated by endocytosis.

6.3 A biochemical analysis of EGFR signaling using EGF-beads

Work done by Hyatt and Ceresa combined the flexibility of EGF-beads with the biochemical analysis provided by immobilized EGF, to analyze EGFR signaling (Hyatt and Ceresa, 2008). This study, in contrast to the previous ones, specifically seeks to understand 1) whether EGFR signaling was spatially regulated, and 2) if so, how? Thus, in this work, the authors used EGF-beads to stimulate cells and examined cell physiology in response to activated EGFRs at the plasma membrane and within the cell.

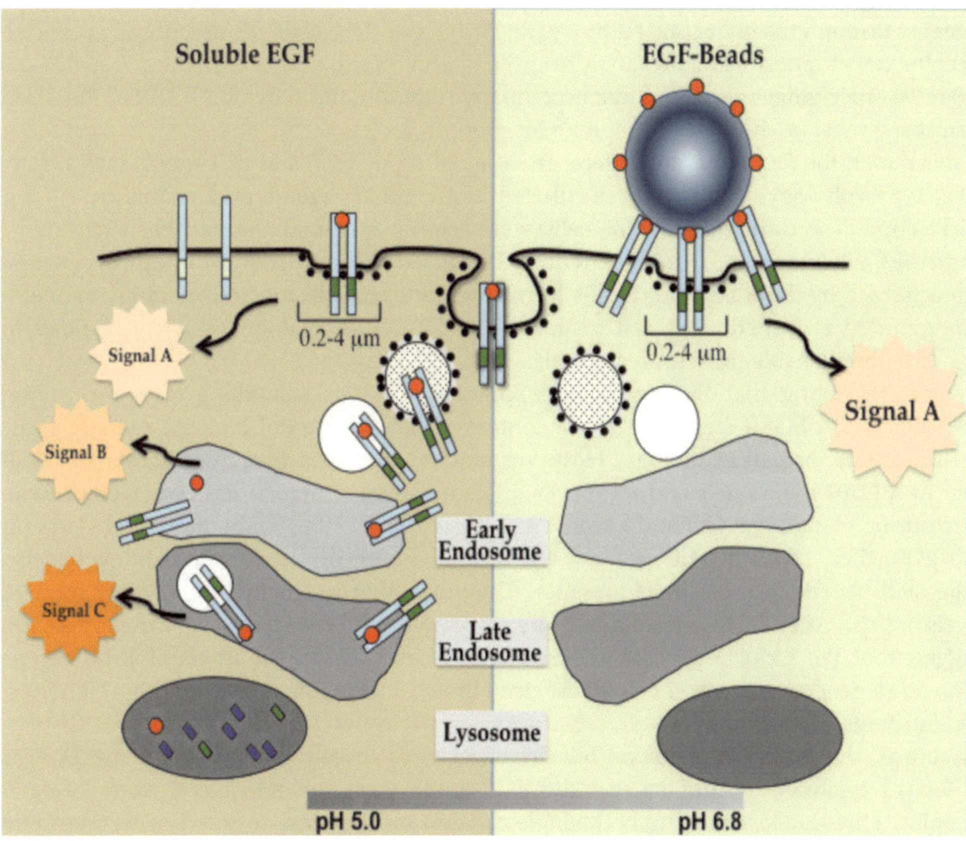

Fig. 5. Depiction of How Soluble EGF and EGF-beads elucidate Differences in EGFR Signaling.

MDA-MB-468 cells were used to study signaling by cell surface and intracellular receptors. MDA-MB-468 cells were first described by Cailleau et al, as part of a series of metastatic breast cancer cell lines derived at the MD Anderson Cancer Center in Houston, Texas (Cailleau *et al.*, 1978). Cell lines derived from metastatic breast cancer tumors were examined for common features as well as for developing model systems for studying the cell biology of transformed cells. Despite a number of similarities, each cell line has some unique features. In the case of the MDA-MB-468 cells, one of its distinguishing features is the overexpression of EGFR. It is reported that MDA-MB-468 cells express ~ 1.3×10^6 EGFRs/cell (Filmus *et al.*, 1985). This is about 15-25 times what is regarded as a physiological level of receptors (50-100,000 EGFRs/cell).

The high level of EGFRs makes it amenable for studying the spatial regulation of signaling for a number of reasons. First, the high levels of receptors provide a dynamic range of response following stimulation with ligand. This increases the signal-to-noise ratio. Second, cell lines with high levels of EGFR have slowed kinetics of endocytic trafficking. This has been demonstrated both in cell lines that naturally overexpress EGFR (*i.e.* cancer cell lines), as well as cells that have by stably transfected with receptors to increase their expression (French et al., 1994; Stoscheck and Carpenter, 1984). It is commonly held that the delay in trafficking is the result of saturation of the machinery that moves the ligand:receptor complex through the endocytic pathway. Regardless of the cause, the absence of appreciable receptor degradation facilitates analyzing the spatial regulation of signaling. In MDA-MB-468 cells, any changes signaling that accompany retaining the activated EGFR at the plasma membrane must be due to the receptor's location.

In this paper, the first apparent difference in signaling by EGF and EGF-beads was a change in cell morphology. Cells were incubated with either ligand and examined by light microscopy. The differences in the cells were readily apparent. As had been reported by numerous other groups, treatment with EGF caused the induction of apoptosis that was characterized by the transition of cells from spread-out cobblestone morphology to one that was rounded up. In contrast, cell treated with EGF-beads, maintained a morphology that was indistinguishable from untreated cells.

It is worth noting that EGF-mediated apoptosis is not is something that is commonly associated with EGFR signaling in the context of developmental biology, maintenance of healthy tissue, or cancer biology. However, among cell lines that overexpress the EGFR, such as MDA-MB-468 cells and A431 cells, EGF-mediated apoptosis has been well described (Armstrong et al., 1994; Gill and Lazar, 1981; Kottke et al., 1999; Tikhomirov and Carpenter, 2004). Further, indirect evidence for the role of apoptosis in cancer biology has been suggested by Tikhomirov and Carpenter. They note that in the literature, more moderate levels of ErbB receptor tyrosine kinases are associated with more invasive carcinomas. They suggest that the induction of apoptosis in cell lines with higher levels of ErbB receptor expression generates a cancer cell whose growth and metastasis is self limiting (Tikhomirov and Carpenter, 2004).

Of course, the easiest explanation for the differences in cell survival following EGF and EGF-bead treatment would be that the EGF-beads were not adequately stimulating the receptor. This was tested using both single cell and biochemical approaches. A time course of EGF-bead stimulation resulted in cells with anti-phosphoEGFR staining along the plasma membrane of the cell. This is evidence that 1) the EGFR was activated and 2) the EGFR was retained at the plasma membrane, two key features of the EGF-beads if a meaningful analysis of signaling is to be made. Further, when cell lysates were prepared from EGF-beads treated dishes of cells, a comparable level of EGFR phosphorylation was observed as seen with treatment with soluble EGF.

These data provide evidence that endocytosis is required for the induction of apoptosis, however, it does not determine whether distinct signals are occurring at the plasma membrane. To answer this question, the authors measured cell proliferation as a function of ^{3}H-thymidine incorporation. In cells treated with soluble EGF, there was a dose dependent decrease in ^{3}H-thymidine incorporation, which likely reflects the fact that the cells are undergoing apoptosis in response to EGF. Cells treated with EGF-beads had an approximately three-fold increase in ^{3}H-thymidine incorporation.

In addition, the authors demonstrate that intracellular, but not cell surface, EGFRs activate the caspase-3, an executioner caspase in the apoptotic pathway. Further, inhibition of caspase-3 prevents the induction of apoptosis, but does not enhance the proliferative effects of the cell surface EGFRs.

Together, these data provide evidence that cell surface and intracellular EGFRs, not only signal differently, but the induce reciprocal effects. Often such reciprocal effects indicate an important regulatory mechanism in biology. This work stimulates a number of important questions. Can the induction of the EGFR-mediated apoptosis be engineered into a therapeutic treatment for cancer? What are the effector proteins being activated at the cell surface versus inside the cell? How are these differences in signaling manifest in cell lines with physiological levels of receptors?

7. Future studies in the temporal and spatial regulation of EGFR signaling

Over the last approximately 25 year, the complex relationship between EGFR signaling and membrane trafficking has been increasingly exposed. While it is widely accepted that endocytic trafficking can both positively and negatively regulate EGFR signaling, it remains unclear exactly to what extent. The field has faced technical limitations that accompany studying two dynamic processes. Further, since both processes branch out into multiple directions, the complexity increases. Through normal, physiological membrane trafficking, the EGFR can be found on the plasma membrane, in endosomes, lysosomes, the nucleus, and endoplasmic reticulum. Similarly, the activated EGFR can signal to multiple downstream effectors. Therefore, identifying which signaling events occur at which subcellular locations is anything but a trivial undertaking.

Thus far, the most fruitful approaches have been ones that have attempted to disrupt or at least dramatically slow down endocytic trafficking. The myriad approaches have been discussed in this chapter. Essentially, these approaches allow the investigator to take a snapshot of signaling. Despite the caveats of such approaches, to date, it has proven to be the most effective strategy.

Although tremendous progress has been made, it appears that we have only begun to understand how these processes come together much more needs to be done. For example, a more comprehensive map of EGFR:effector communication at the cell surface and within the cell. Definitively proving that a receptor:effector interaction occurs is a major undertaking, and requires substantial experimentation to establish such a model. To date, there are only a limited number of effectors whose activity has been studied. Although many of these effectors have well-established roles in EGFR signaling, this does not preclude the need to study other effectors. Further, a systematic analysis of plasma membrane versus intracellular signaling for a large cohort of known EGFR effectors would be helpful for developing a model that predicts how receptor:effector communication occurs.

Once cell surface versus intracellular EGFR signaling is established, signaling from various locations within the cell needs to be understood. At this point, the most effective strategy is to disrupt membrane trafficking at discrete endocytic stages, despite the aforementioned caveats. Geographically, it does not seem likely that receptors in early endosomes and on the limiting membrane of the late endosome, would have access to different subsets of cytosolic effectors. However, the effectors may differentially associate with the various endocytic compartments either directly or through adaptor proteins. Together this analysis will generate a temporal and spatial map of EGFR:effector interactions that may be useful for anticipating how cell physiology is regulated.

In addition to delineating the receptor:effector interactions, another important question is whether the temporal/spatial regulation of EGFR:effector interaction is universal among all cell lines. This is a critical question because the EGFR mediates such a diverse array of physiological responses, endocytic regulation of EGFR signaling may provide important insight to explain the EGFR-dependent cell responses that are unique to a given cell line. This is particularly likely to be important in cancer cells that overexpress the EGFR. It is established that overexpression of the EGFR alters the endocytic trafficking of the EGFR and decreases the rate of receptor degradation. Since this effects both the duration and spatial placement of the activated receptor, it is reasonable to predict that there would be changes in signaling as well.

Ultimately, our goal for understanding the molecular basis of EGFR signaling is rooted in developing strategies for the pharmacological manipulation of signalling pathways. Knowing how the signaling pathways are regulated has a number of uses. First, understanding how each effector is activated will provide a better understanding of its contribution to a give cell physiology. Thus, the effector activity can be modulated downstream of the effector. Second, the endocytic pathway itself may be a useful target. Disrupting or accelerating endocytic trafficking may be sufficient to achieve desired changes in cell biology. Finally, an effort to study this regulation of signaling *in vivo* is necessary. Dissecting the *in vivo* regulation will not only help in develop anti-cancer therapeutics but also in other EGFR-mediated physiologies, such as wound healing.

8. Conclusion

Overexpression and hyperactivation of the EGFR as associated with many cancers. While inhibitors against the EGFR are effective for some EGFR-positive cancers, they are not effective in the treatment of breast cancers. In order to develop therapeutic agents to treat EGFR-positive breast cancers, a more thorough analysis of EGFR is needed, in particular, insight into how its signaling is regulated. Discussed here is the role of the endocytic pathway in controlling the duration and specificity of EGFR signaling. This field has made grade strides in understanding the relationship between the two processes. The basic science that underlies these studies has important implications in developing new tools for the detection, diagnosis, and treatment of breast cancers with elevated levels of the EGFR.

9. Acknowledgements

We apologize to our colleagues whose work was unable to be included due to space limitations. The author acknowledges support through NIH grant 1R01GM092874-01A1 and OCAST grant HR10-012.

10. References

Anderson, R.G., J.R. Falck, J.L. Goldstein, and M.S. Brown. 1984. Visualization of acidic organelles in intact cells by electron microscopy. *Proc Natl Acad Sci U S A*. 81:4838-4842.

Armstrong, D.K., S.H. Kaufmann, Y.L. Ottaviano, Y. Furuya, J.A. Buckley, J.T. Isaacs, and N.E. Davidson. 1994. Epidermal growth factor-mediated apoptosis of MDA-MB-468 human breast cancer cells. *Cancer Res*. 54:5280-5283.

Baselga, J., and C.L. Arteaga. 2005. Critical update and emerging trends in epidermal growth factor receptor targeting in cancer. *J Clin Oncol*. 23:2445-2459.

Cailleau, R., M. Olive, and Q.V. Cruciger. 1978. Long-term human breast carcinoma cell lines of metastatic origin: preliminary characterization. *In Vitro*. 14:911-915.

Cameron, D., M. Casey, C. Oliva, B. Newstat, B. Imwalle, and C.E. Geyer. 2010. Lapatinib plus capecitabine in women with HER-2-positive advanced breast cancer: final survival analysis of a phase III randomized trial. *Oncologist*. 15:924-934.

Ceresa, B.P. 2006. Regulation of EGFR endocytic trafficking by rab proteins. *Histol Histopathol*. 21:987-993.

Chen, G., Y. Ito, and Y. Imanishi. 1997. Photo-immobilization of epidermal growth factor enhances its mitogenic effect by artificial juxtacrine signaling. *Biochim Biophys Acta*. 1358:200-208.

Chen, P., J.E. Murphy-Ullrich, and A. Wells. 1996. A role for gelsolin in actuating epidermal growth factor receptor-mediated cell motility. *J Cell Biol*. 134:689-698.

Damke, H., T. Baba, D.E. Warnock, and S.L. Schmid. 1994. Induction of Mutant Dynamin Specifically Blocks Endocytic Coated Vesicle Formation. *J Cell Biol*. 127:915-934.

Dawson, J.P., M.B. Berger, C.C. Lin, J. Schlessinger, M.A. Lemmon, and K.M. Ferguson. 2005. Epidermal growth factor receptor dimerization and activation require ligand-induced conformational changes in the dimer interface. *Mol Cell Biol*. 25:7734-7742.

Dinneen, J.L., and B.P. Ceresa. 2004. Constitutive activation of rab5 results in a ligand independent redistribution of the EGFR and attenuates its ability to signal. *Traffic*. 5:606-615.

Feugaing, D.D., R. Tammi, F.G. Echtermeyer, H. Stenmark, H. Kresse, M. Smollich, E. Schonherr, L. Kiesel, and M. Gotte. 2007. Endocytosis of the dermatan sulfate proteoglycan decorin utilizes multiple pathways and is modulated by epidermal growth factor receptor signaling. *Biochimie*. 89:637-657.

Filmus, J., M.N. Pollak, R. Cailleau, and R.N. Buick. 1985. MDA-468, a human breast cancer cell line with a high number of epidermal growth factor (EGF) receptors, has an amplified EGF receptor gene and is growth inhibited by EGF. *Biochem Biophys Res Commun*. 128:898-905.

French, A.R., G.P. Sudlow, H.S. Wiley, and D.A. Lauffenburger. 1994. Postendocytic Trafficking of Epidermal Growth Factor-Receptor Complexes is Mediated through Saturable and Specific Endosomal Interactions. *J Biol Chem*. 269:15749-15755.

Gill, G.N., and C.S. Lazar. 1981. Increase phosphotyrosine content and inhibition of proliferation in EGF-treated A431 cells. *Nature*. 293:305-307.

Goh, L.K., F. Huang, W. Kim, S. Gygi, and A. Sorkin. 2010. Multiple mechanisms collectively regulate clathrin-mediated endocytosis of the epidermal growth factor receptor. *J Cell Biol*. 189:871-883.

Grandal, M.V., R. Zandi, M.W. Pedersen, B.M. Willumsen, B. van Deurs, and H.S. Poulsen. 2007. EGFRvIII escapes down-regulation due to impaired internalization and sorting to lysosomes. *Carcinogenesis*. 28:1408-1417.

Gruenberg, J., and F.R. Maxfield. 1995. Membrane Transport in the endocytic pathway. *Curr Opin Cell Biol*. 7:552-563.

Guerin, M., M. Barrois, M.J. Terrier, M. Spielmann, and G. Riou. 1988. Overexpression of either c-myc or c-erbB-2/neu proto-oncogenes in human breast carcinomas: correlation with poor prognosis. *Oncogene Res*. 3:21-31.

Harris, R.C., E. Chung, and R.J. Coffey. 2003. EGF Receptor ligands. *Exp Cell Res*. 284:2-13.

Haugh, J.M., A.C. Huang, H.S. Wiley, A. Wells, and D.A. Lauffenburger. 1999a. Internalized epidermal growth factor receptors participate in the activation of p21(ras) in fibroblasts. *J Biol Chem*. 274:34350-343560.

Haugh, J.M., K. Schooler, A. Wells, H.S. Wiley, and D.A. Lauffenburger. 1999b. Effect of epidermal growth factor receptor internalization on regulation of the phospholipase C-gamma1 signaling pathway. *J Biol Chem*. 274:8958-8965.

Herbst, J.J., L.K. Opresko, B.J. Walsh, D.A. Lauffenburger, and H.S. Wiley. 1994. Regulation of Postendocytic Trafficking of the Epidermal Growth Factor Receptor through Endosomal Retention. *J Biol Chem*. 269:12865-12873.

Hill, T.A., C.P. Gordon, A.B. McGeachie, B. Venn-Brown, L.R. Odell, N. Chau, A. Quan, A. Mariana, J.A. Sakoff, M. Chircop, P.J. Robinson, and A. McCluskey. 2009. Inhibition of dynamin mediated endocytosis by the dynoles--synthesis and functional activity of a family of indoles. *J Med Chem*. 52:3762-3773.

Huang, F., A. Khvorova, W. Marshall, and A. Sorkin. 2004. Analysis of clathrin-mediated endocytosis of epidermal growth factor receptor by RNA interfernce. *J Biol Chem*. 279:16657-16661.

Hyatt, D.C., and B.P. Ceresa. 2008. Cellular localization of the activated EGFR determines its effect on cell growth in MDA-MB-468 cells. *Exp Cell Res*. 314:3415-3425.

Hynes, N.E., and G. MacDonald. 2009. ErbB receptors and signaling pathways in cancer. *Curr Opin Cell Biol*. 21:177-184.

Johanessen, L.E., T. Ringerike, J. Molnes, and I.H. Madshus. 2000. Epidermal growth factor receptor efficiently activates mitogen-activated protein kinase in HeLa cells and HepG2 cells conditionally defective in clathrin-dependent endocytosis. *Exp Cell Res*. 260:136-145.

Jorissen, R.N., F. Walker, N. Pouliot, T.P.J. Garrett, C.W. Ward, and A.W. Burgess. 2003. Epidermal Growth Factor Receptor: Mechanisms of Activation and Signalling. *Exp Cell Res*. 284:31-53.

Kempiak, S.J., S.-C. Yip, J.M. Backer, and J.E. Segall. 2003. Local signaling by the EGF receptor. *J Cell Biol*. 162:781-787.

King, A.C. 1984. Monensin, like methylamine, prevents degradation of 125I-epidermal growth factor, causes intracellular accumulation of receptors and blocks the mitogenic response. *Biochem Biophys Res Commun*. 124:585-591.

Kottke, T.J., A.L. Blajeski, L.M. Martins, P.W. Mesner Jr., N.E. Davidson, W.C. Earnshaw, D.K. Armstrong, and S.H. Kaufmann. 1999. Comparison of Paclitaxel-, 5-Fluoro-2'-deoxyuridine-, and Epidermal Growth Factor (EGF)-induced Apoptosis. *J Biol Chem*. 274:15927-15936.

Larkin, J.M., M.S. Brown, J.L. Goldstein, and R.G. Anderson. 1983. Depletion of intracellular potassium arrests coated pit formation and receptor-mediated endocytosis in fibroblasts. *Cell*. 33:273-285.

Liao, H.J., and G. Carpenter. 2007. Role of the Sec61 translocon in EGF receptor trafficking to the nucleus and gene expression. *Mol Biol Cell*. 18:1064-1072.

Luetteke, N.C., T.H. Qiu, S.E. Fenton, K.L. Troyer, R.F. Riedel, A. Chang, and D.C. Lee. 1999. Targeted inactivation of the EGF and amphiregulin genes reveals distinct roles for

EGF receptor ligands in mouse mammary gland development. *Development*. 126:2739-2750.

Masui, H., L. Castro, and J. Mendelsohn. 1993. Consumption of EGF by A431 cells: evidence for receptor recycling. *J Cell Biol*. 120:85-93.

Matsui, Y., S.A. Halter, J.T. Holt, B.L. Hogan, and R.J. Coffey. 1990. Development of mammary hyperplasia and neoplasia in MMTV-TGF alpha transgenic mice. *Cell*. 61:1147-1155.

McClintock, J.L., and B.P. Ceresa. 2010. Transforming Growth Factor-α (TGF-α) Enhances Corneal Epithelial Cell Migration by Promoting EGFR Recycling. *Inv Opth Vis Sci*. doi:10.1167/iovs.09-4386.

Miettinen, P.J., J.E. Berger, J. Meneses, Y. Phung, R.A. Pedersen, Z. Werb, and R. Derynck. 1995. Epithelial immaturity and multi-organ failure in mice lacking epidermal growth factor receptor. *Nature*. 376:337-341.

Mosesson, Y., G.B. Mills, and Y. Yarden. 2008. Derailed endocytosis: an emerging feature of cancer. *Nat Rev Cancer*. 8:835-850.

Nicholson, R.I., J.M. Gee, and M.E. Harper. 2001. EGFR and cancer prognosis. *Eur J Cancer*. 37 Suppl 4:S9-15.

Offterdinger, M., and P.I. Bastiaens. 2008. Prolonged EGFR signaling by ERBB2-mediated sequestration at the plasma membrane. *Traffic*. 9:147-155.

Presly, J.F., S. Mayor, T.E. McGraw, K.W. Dunn, and F.R. Maxfield. 1997. Bafilomycin A1 treatment retards transferrin receptor recycling more than bulk membrane recycling. *J Biol Chem*. 272:13929-13936.

Ray, E., and A.K. Samanta. 1996. Dansyl Cadaverine regulates ligand induced endocytosis of interleukin-8 receptor in human polymorphonuclear neutrophils. *FEBS Lett*. 378:235-239.

Ringerike, T., E. Stang, L.E. Johanessen, D. Sandnes, F.O. Levy, and I.H. Madshus. 1998. High-affinity binding of epidermal growth factor (EGF) to EGF receptor is disrupted by overexpression of mutant dynamin (K44A). *J Biol Chem*. 273:16639-16642.

Roepstorff, K., M.V. Grandal, L. Henriksen, S.L. Knudsen, M. Lerdrup, L. Grovdal, B.M. Willumsen, and B. van Deurs. 2009. Differential Effects of EGFR Ligands on Endocytic Sorting of the Receptor. *Traffic*.

Rowinsky, E.K. 2004. The erbB Family: Targets for Therapeutic Develpment Against Cancer and Therapeutic strategies Using Monoclonal Antibodies and Tyrosine Kinase Inhibitors *Ann Rev of Med*. 55:433-457.

Rutten, M.J., P.J. Dempsey, C.A. Luttropp, M.A. Hawkey, B.C. Sheppard, R.A. Crass, C.W. Deveney, and R.J. Coffey, Jr. 1996. Identification of an EGF/TGF-alpha receptor in primary cultures of guinea pig gastric mucous epithelial cells. *Am J Physiol*. 270:G604-612.

Sandgren, E.P., N.C. Luetteke, T.H. Qiu, R.D. Palmiter, R.L. Brinster, and D.C. Lee. 1993. Transforming growth factor alpha dramatically enhances oncogene-induced carcinogenesis in transgenic mouse pancreas and liver. *Mol Cell Biol*. 13:320-330.

Sibilia, M., and E.F. Wagner. 1995. Strain-dependent epithelial defects in mice lacking the EGFR. *Science*. 269:234-238.

Stefonek, T.J., and K.S. Masters. 2007. Immobilized gradients of epidermal growth factor promote accelerated and directed keratinocyte migration. *Wound Repair Regen*. 15:847-855.

Stoscheck, C.M., and G. Carpenter. 1984. Down regulation of epidermal growth factor receptors: direct demonstration of receptor degradation in human fibroblasts. *J Cell Biol*. 98:1048-1053.

Threadgill, D.W., A.A. Dlugosz, L.A. Hansen, T. Tennenbaum, U. Lichti, D. Yee, C. LaMantia, T. Mourton, K. Herrup, R.C. Harris, and et al. 1995. Targeted disruption of mouse EGF receptor: effect of genetic background on mutant phenotype. *Science*. 269:230-234.

Tikhomirov, O., and G. Carpenter. 2004. Ligand-induced, p38-dependent Apoptosis in Cells Expressing High Levels of Epidermal Growth Factor Receptor and ErbB-2. *J Biol Chem*. 279:12988-12996.

Tullo, A.B., B. Esmaeli, P.I. Murray, E. Bristow, B.J. Forsythe, and K. Faulkner. 2005. Ocular findings in patients with solid tumour treated with the epidermal growth factor receptor tyrosine kinase inhibitor gefitinib ('Iressa', ZD1839) in Phase I and II clinical trials. *Eye*. 19:729-738.

Uberall, I., Z. Kolar, R. Trojanec, J. Berkovcova, and M. Hajduch. 2008. The status and role of ErbB receptors in human cancer. *Exp Mol Pathol*. 84:79-89.

Vanlandingham, P.A., and B.P. Ceresa. 2009. Rab7 regulates late endocytic trafficking downstream of multivesicular body biogenesis and cargo sequestration. *J Biol Chem*. 284:12110-12124.

Verveer, P.J., F.S. Wouters, A.R. Reynolds, and P.I.H. Bastiaens. 2000. Quantitative Imaging of Lateral ErbB1 Receptor Signal Propagation in the Plasma Membrane. *Science*. 290:1567-1570.

Vieira, A.V., C. Lamaze, and S.L. Schmid. 1996. Control of EGF Receptor Signaling by Clathrin-Mediated Endocytosis. *Science*. 274:2086-2089.

Wang, Y.N., H. Yamaguchi, J.M. Hsu, and M.C. Hung. 2010. Nuclear trafficking of the epidermal growth factor receptor family membrane proteins. *Oncogene*. 29:3997-4006.

Wells, A., J.B. Welsh, C.S. Lazar, H.S. Wiley, G.N. Gill, and M.G. Rosenfeld. 1990. Ligand-Induced Transformation by a Noninternalizing Epidermal Growth Factor Receptor. *Science*. 247:962-964.

Wikstrand, C.J., L.P. Hale, S.K. Batra, M.L. Hill, P.A. Humphrey, S.N. Kurpad, R.E. McLendon, D. Moscatello, C.N. Pegram, C.J. Reist, and et al. 1995. Monoclonal antibodies against EGFRvIII are tumor specific and react with breast and lung carcinomas and malignant gliomas. *Cancer Res*. 55:3140-3148.

Worthylake, R., L.K. Opresko, and H.S. Wiley. 1999. ErbB-2 amplification inhibits down-regulation and induces constitutive activation of both ErbB-2 and epidermal growth factor receptors. *J Biol Chem*. 274:8865-8874.

Zhang, G., S. Basti, and L.M. Jampol. 2007. Acquired trichomegaly and symptomatic external ocular changes in patients receiving epidermal growth factor inhibitors: case reports and a review of literature. *Cornea*. 26:858-860.

4

HER-2 Signaling in Human Breast Cancer

Kathleen M. Woods Ignatoski
University of Michigan,
USA

1. Introduction

1.1 *erb*B family

HER-2 is a member of the *erb*B family of receptor tyrosine kinases. Epidermal Growth Factor Receptor (EGFR) was first identified as the cellular homolog of the transduced oncogene of the avian retroviruses such as avian ERythroBlastosis virus, which causes erythroleukemia and fibrosarcoma and gives rise to the family name (erbB). EGFR, as its name implies, was shown by Stanley Cohen to induce the growth of epidermal cells (Todaro, DeLarco et al. 1976). The EGFR family consists of four members: *erb*B-1 (EGFR), *erb*B-2 (HER-2/neu), *erb*B-3 (HER-3), and *erb*B-4 (HER-4). Her-1, -2, and -3 have been associated with tumorigenesis (Suo, Emilsen et al. 1998). HER-4 has been implicated in development and tumor suppression, possibly by sequestration of the other *erb*B receptors in dimers. Ligand binding stabilizes dimer formation, leading to intracellular signaling. Each receptor consists of an extracellular domain that contains the ligand binding sites, an intracellular domain that contains the tyrosine kinase activity, and a cytoplasmic tail that is involved in cellular signaling. EGFR can be stimulated by an array of ligands, including EGF, transforming growth factor α (TGF-α), heparin-binding EGF (HB-EGF), and heregulins. HER-3 can bind heregulins (Holmes, Sliwkowski et al. 1992); although, it in and of itself does not have an active kinase domain. Heregulin binding to HER-3 facilitates dimerization with other *erb*B receptors which promote the phosphorylation of HER-3 and subsequent activation of downstream signals.

HER-2 does not have any known ligands; however, several intriguing papers have been published recently on this topic. The Calloway group has had a series of papers (Carraway, Carvajal et al. 1993; Carraway and Cantley 1994; Carraway, Sliwkowski et al. 1994; Carraway, Rossi et al. 1999; Komatsu, Jepson et al. 2001; Carraway and Carraway 2007; Kozloski, Carraway et al. 2010) showing that the extracellular domain of HER-2 can bind the intramembrane protein MUC4, suggesting that MUC4 was the ligand for HER-2. MUC4 appears to play a role in mammary gland development at the lactation step along with HER-2. In cancer, MUC 4 blocks apoptosis and stabilizes HER-2/HER-3 dimers. In normal epithelia, MUC 4 sequesters HER-2 to the apical surface, separating it from HER-3, which is on the lateral surface (Carraway and Carraway 2007). These data make a compelling argument for MUC4 as a ligand for HER-2.

More recently, Day, *et al.* (Najy, Day et al. 2008) showed that the extracellular domain of E-cadherin could activate HER-2 and EGFR. They have shown that the extracellular domain of E-cadherin is cleaved by the ADAM proteases. Since E-cadherin is normally present on epithelial cells and itself, or its sister protein N-cadherin, is present on cancer cells of epithelial origin, it is also a good candidate for a HER-2 ligand.

Pairings of the *erb*B receptors have been exquisitely elucidated by Josef Yarden and colleagues (Goldman, Benlevy et al. 1990; Karunagaran, Tzahar et al. 1996; Alroy and Yarden 1997). Yarden, *et al.* utilized the 32D cell line, an IL-3-independent murine myeloid cell line that does not express endogenous *erb*B receptors. They systematically expressed each family member separately and in pairs to determine which family members formed complexes. They found that each family member can homodimerize or heterodimerize with every other family member; although, certain heterodimers are preferred. Which dimer is present on the cell determines the biological phenotype of that cell. Although EGFR can homodimerize, it will pair with HER-2 when HER-2 is present and will only pair with itself when all of the HER-2 is paired or no HER-2 is present (Hendriks , Opresko et al. 2003).

EGFR dimerization results in the phosphorylation of tyrosine 1045 in the cytoplasmic domain. Phosphorylation of this tyrosine creates a docking site for the *cbl* protein (Yokouchi, Kondo et al. 1999). *Cbl* then recruits ubiquitin which targets the EGFR for degradation (Yokouchi, Kondo et al. 1999). Activation of HER-2 does not create a ubinquitin binding site, so HER-2 does not get degraded upon activation unless it is dimerized with EGFR. Over expression of HER-2 results in constitutive activation of both HER-2 and EGFR and in a decrease in degradation of both of the receptors.

Due to the fluidity of the plasma membrane, transient dimerization of the *erb*B receptors occurs. However, the transient dimers do not elicit a strong signal. Our model (*FIGURE 1*) (Woods Ignatoski, LaPointe et al. 1999) suggests that over expression of HER-2 leads to many transient homodimers. The transient homodimers lead to transphosphorylation of the receptor causing many small signals to be initiated. The overall effect is one of a strong, ligand-stabilized signal which results in constitutive activation of HER-2 and constitutive growth signals (*FIGURE 1C*). The type of HER-2 homo and heterodimerization, coupled with over expression, on mammary epithelial cells has consequences dealing with normal development, proliferation, and transformation.

2. HER-2 in development

HER-2 is expressed in almost all fetal tissues including the placenta, liver, kidney, mammary gland, brain, and lung (Kokai, Wada et al. 1988). On the basis of its expression pattern, HER-2 plays a role in general development. Although HER-2's role in tumorigenesis has been studied extensively, its role in normal mammary gland development has not. There are many articles about mammary gland development in HER-2 transgenic and knock-out mice, but since human and mouse mammary glands develop differently, the actual role of HER-2 in human mammary gland development is not fully understood. Mina Bissell and colleagues developed the three-dimensional *Matrigel* system to study mammary gland morphogenesis, discovering the role for integrins in anti-apoptotic signaling (Petersen, Ronnovjessen et al. 1992; Howlett, Bailey et al. 1995; Lochter, Galosy et al. 1997; Lochter, Navre et al. 1999). Joan Brugge and colleagues refined the *Matrigel* model to identify HER-2 as a modulator of the lumen compartment, by working through Bim-1 to regulate apoptosis of the pre-lumenal cells (Muthuswamy, Li et al. 2001). One caveat to the Brugge group's work is the use of a chimeric molecule that has an NGF extracellular domain and a HER-2 cytoplasmic domain that can be crosslinked to give a constitutive signal. While their work leads to important insight into the role of HER-2 in development, the system they use is not

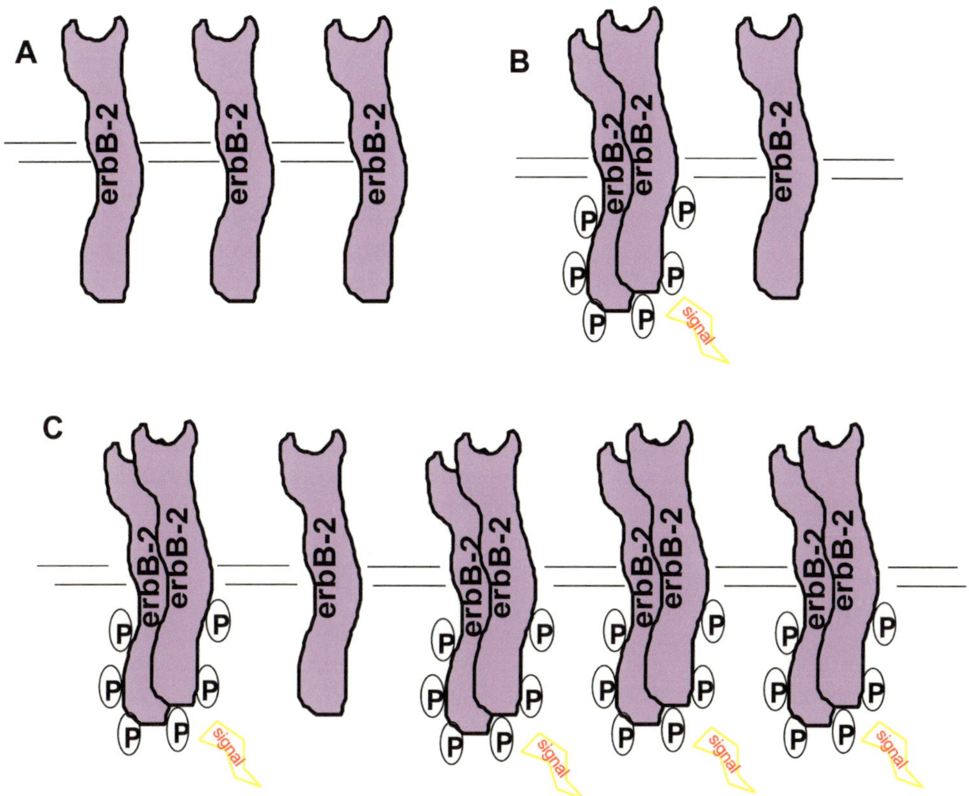

Fig. 1. Schematic of signaling from HER-2 during normal conditions and during over expression. (A) HER-2 is normally present as single molecules in the plasma membrane. (B) Due to the fluid nature of the membrane, random, transient dimers form producing weak signals that cannot elicit a response from the cell. (C) During over expression, many transient dimers produce a signal strong enough to elicit a response from the cell.

physiological, since HER-2 is not activated by a ligand but rather by the amount of protein, and constitutive HER-2 activation is not done by cross-linking the cytoplasmic domains.

Recently, we have developed a system that is more physiological than the one used by Brugge and colleagues (manuscript submitted). We used human mammary epithelial (HME) cells, obtained from reduction mammoplasties, plated in *Matrigel* to study the role of HER-2 in branching morphogenesis. We observed that HME cells form branching structures when plated in the 3D matrix *Matrigel* and determined that HER-2 is up-regulated at the time of branching. Using HER-2 over expressing HME cells (Woods Ignatoski, LaPointe et al. 1999) we showed that constitutive activation of HER-2 was necessary and sufficient to form the branches. By using genetic and chemical activators and inhibitors, we showed that AKT activation mediated the HER-2-facilitated branching morphogenesis. Our data imply that HER-2's role in mammary gland development is to facilitate ductal formation.

Korkaya, *et al.* (Korkaya, Paulson et al. 2008) and Magnifico, *et al.* (Magnifico, Albano et al. 2009) have shown that an increase in HER-2 in human mammary stem cells causes an increase in mammosphere formation and an increase in ductal structures when the cells are placed in animals. Both groups have also shown a reciprocal relationship between over expression of HER-2 and the expression of the developmental gene Notch. Their published data suggest that HER-2-mediated AKT activation is necessary for self-renewal leading to the ductal structures in their mouse models. Our data show that HER-2-mediated AKT activation is necessary for branching morphogenesis and is concordant with the data presented by Korkaya, *et al.* (Korkaya, Paulson et al. 2008) and Magnifico, *et al.* (Magnifico, Albano et al. 2009).

Since we have previously shown that HME cells in *Matrigel* and HER-2 over expressing cells have an increase in Focal Adhesion Kinase (FAK) phosphorylation (Woods Ignatoski and Ethier 1999), an implication of these data is that signaling from integrin binding to extracellular matrix may also play a role in this developmental phenotype. Indeed, Bissell, *et al.* (Petersen, Ronnovjessen et al. 1992; Howlett, Petersen et al. 1994; Howlett, Bailey et al. 1995; Gudjonsson, Ronnov-Jessen et al. 2002), has shown that β1 integrin is important in mammary cell morphology change. β1 integrins bind to and activate FAK (Zachary and Rozengurt 1992). FAK was shown to maintain the mammary gland stem cell pool (Nagy, Wei et al. 2007). Since HER-2 has recently been shown to play a role in human mammary stem cells (Korkaya, Paulson et al. 2008; Korkaya and Wicha 2009), the idea that FAK may be downstream of HER-2 to maintain the stem cell population is intriguing.

3. HER-2 signaling in transformation

HER-2 uses a variety of signaling pathways to elicit phenotypes associated with transformation and tumorigenesis. We and others used various *in vitro* methods in conjunction with constitutively active and dominantly negative mutants and chemical inhibitors to elucidate the multiple pathways HER-2 uses to transform cells (*FIGURE* 2).

Growth factor independence: One hallmark of a transformed cell is growth factor independence. Ram, *et al.* (Ram, Kokeny et al. 1995; Ram, Dilts et al. 1996) showed that human breast cancer (HBC) cells with increasing amounts of HER-2 had increasing degrees of growth factor independence. H16N2 cells, which are non-transformed, immortalized HME, have normal levels of HER-2 and required both insulin-like growth factor (IGF) and epidermal growth factor (EGF) to survive. 21MT-2 cells with an slight over expression of HER-2 still required EGF, but 21MT-1 cells with a clinically relevant HER-2 over expression did not require either IGF or EGF for growth. To determine the contribution of HER-2 over expression to growth factor independence without the other genetic abnormalities associated with HBC, we developed HME cell lines that over expressed HER-2 less than the HPV16-immortalized HME cell line (H16N2).

The MCF-10HER-2 cells were unable to grow in the absence of IGF, showing that a slight over expression resulted in IGF independence and that over expression to levels seen in amplified HBC cells conferred both IGF and EGF independence to the H16N2 cells (Woods Ignatoski, LaPointe et al. 1999). Over expression of HER-2 resulted in progressively increasing levels of tyrosine-phosphorylated HER-3, without any significant changes in HER-3 protein levels (Woods Ignatoski, LaPointe et al. 1999).

Our studies, while demonstrating a direct relationship between the level of expression, the activation of HER-2, and the requirements for IGF and EGF, suggest that genetic alterations present in breast cancer cells, or mediated by HPV-16-induced alterations, can influence the expression level and activation status of HER-2 and, in turn, their degree of growth factor independence. To this end, we were intrigued by the differences between

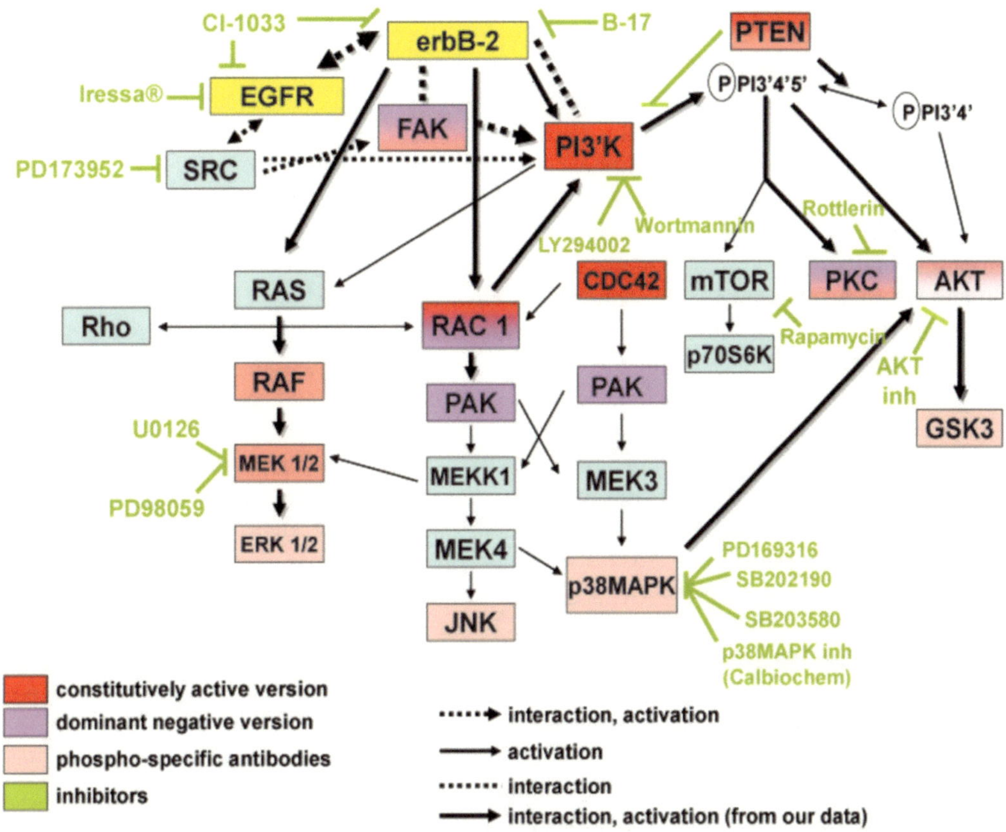

Fig. 2. The tools used to decipher HER-2 signaling. Various constitutively active and dominant negative constructs plus specific chemical inhibitors and phospho-specific antibodies were used to elucidate downstream signaling for HER-2 and associate them with transformed phenotypes.

the MCF-10A cell line and the H16N2 cell line in terms of their ability to over express HER-2 and their differences in growth factor independence. The biggest difference in the parental cell lines is the inclusion of the entire HPV16 genome in the H16N2 cells which is not in the MCF-10A cells. The HPV-16 genome produces the HPV E5, E6, and E7 oncogenes which have been shown to affect the tumor suppressors Rb and p53, among other proteins. To discern if the HPV genes played a role in HER-2-mediated transformation, we co-expressed E6, E7, or E6 and E7 with HER-2 in MCF-10A cells and tested for transformed phenotypes (Woods Ignatoski, Dziubinski et al. 2005). Co-expression of HER-2 with the HPV-16 oncoproteins E6 and E7 resulted in the emergence of fully EGF-independent cells that expressed very high levels of constitutively activated HER-2. Interestingly, co-expression of E7 with HER-2 resulted in cells that were EGF-independent for growth but which did not express HER-2 to higher levels than control MCF-10HER-2 cells. By contrast, co-expression of E6 with HER-2 resulted in cells expressing higher levels of HER-2 but which were still dependent on EGF for growth and survival. Examination of the expression and activation status of HER-1, -2 and -3 in the MCF-10HER-2 cells and their derivatives by immunoprecipitation/western blot analysis demonstrated that the EGF-independent MCF-10HER-2E7 cells and the HER-2/E6E7 cells exhibited constitutive EGF-independent activation of EGFR. Further, the constitutively active EGFR had a faster electrophoretic mobility than EGFR activated by exogenous growth factors. Exposure of MCF-10HER-2 cells and their derivatives as well as the HER-2 amplified SUM-225 breast cancer cell line to ZD1839 (IRESSA®) at concentrations specific for EGFR, eliminated EGFR tyrosine phosphorylation, blocked proliferation, but only modestly altered the levels of constitutively activated HER-2. By contrast, exposure of SUM-190 cells or MDA-351 cells, which have amplified HER-2 but express little or no EGFR, to these same concentrations of ZD1839 had little or no influence on cell proliferation. Our results showed that HER-2 over expression cooperates with EGFR and HPV-E7 to yield HME cells that are EGF-independent for growth. Together, HER-2, E6 and E7 cooperate with endogenous EGFR to yield fully transformed cells that express very high levels of HER-2 and that are growth factor autonomous for proliferation and survival.

Phophotidylinositol 3′ kinase (PI3′K) phosphorylates inositol in the plasma membrane at the 3′ position. Phosphorylation of inositol produces a docking site for the serine/threonine kinase AKT. Docking of AKT activates its kinase activity and elicits downstream signals. Activation of both HER-2 and HER-3 provide phosphotyrosines that can dock PI3′K and bring it to the membrane; therefore, activation of HER-2 mediates inositol phosphorylation and PI3′K signaling (Fedi, Pierce et al. 1994). Phospho-AKT remained detectable in HER-2 cells treated with the PI3′K inhibitor LY294002 or with expression of exogenous PTEN, a phosphatase that reverses the action of PI3′K, but was abolished by treatment with the p38 mitogen activated kinase (p38MAPK) inhibitor SB202190. Thus, both PI3K-dependent and p38MAPK-dependent pathways lead to activation of AKT. We also found that AKT was activated by p38MAPK in these cells, but this activation did not play a role in invasion (Woods Ignatoski, Livant et al. 2003). Since AKT has been shown in other systems to be a survival factor (Datta, Dudek et al. 1997; Brunet, Bonni et al. 1999; Hutchinson J, Jin J et al. 2001), we hypothesized that HER-2 mediated activation of AKT is necessary for growth factor independence. We found that, in the absence of EGF, p38MAPK-activated AKT is necessary for HER-2 over expressing cells to survive and to form colonies in soft agar (Woods Ignatoski, Livant et al. 2003). We showed that EGF works as a survival signal in the absence of p38MAPK-mediated activation of AKT and that HME cells expressing a constitutively active AKT did not require EGF for growth or colony formation in soft agar. Thus, our data indicate that AKT activation can compensate for EGF-mediated cell survival signals leading to growth factor-independence and anchorage-independent growth (Diehl, Grewal et al. 2007).

HER-2 in invasion: Using a model system for invasion that utilizes a naturally occurring membrane found in sea urchin embryos (Livant, Linn et al. 1995) in the configuration a cell would see upon extravasation (*FIGURE 3*), we determined that α5 integrin binding to the PHSRN sequence of fibronectin is necessary for invasion and that α4 integrin binding to the "LDV" sequence of fibronection abrogates invasion (Livant, Allen et al. 2000; Livant, Brabec et al. 2000; Woods Ignatoski, Maehama et al. 2000; Jia, Markwart et al. 2002) (*FIGURE 4*). Using this system, we showed that HER-2 requires PI3′K to drive invasion. With this same system we also showed that HER-2 mediates the down-regulation of α4 integrin from the cell surface to facilitate invasion via activation of p38MAPK (Woods Ignatoski, Maehama et al. 2000) (FIGURE 5).

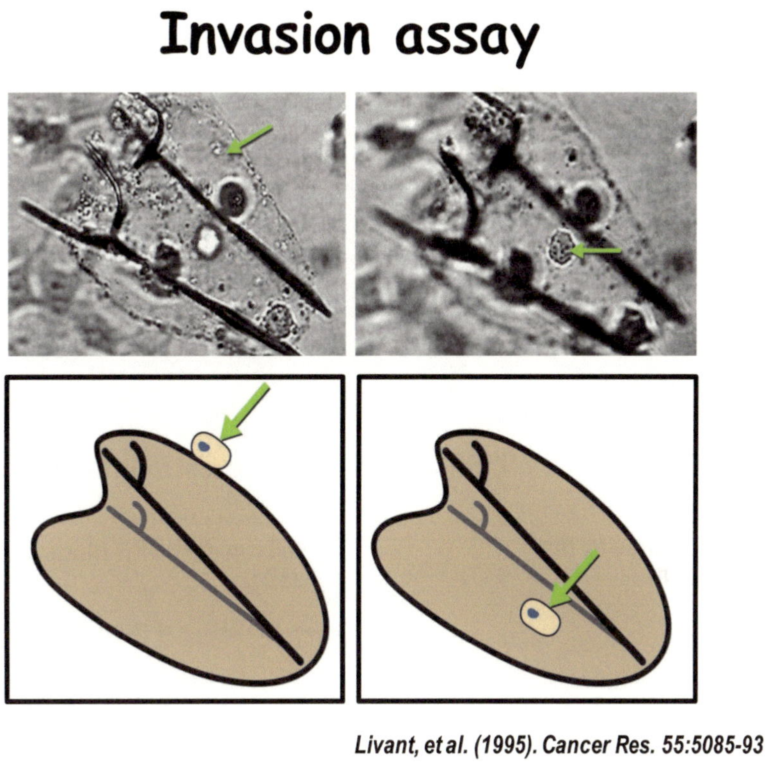

Fig. 3. Sea urchin embryo invasion assay. This assay utilizes the naturally occurring membrane found under a cell layer in sea urchin embryos. The outer cell layer is lysed and the cells are placed on top of the embryos. The number of cells that enter the embryo are blindly scored. Arrows point to cancer cells.

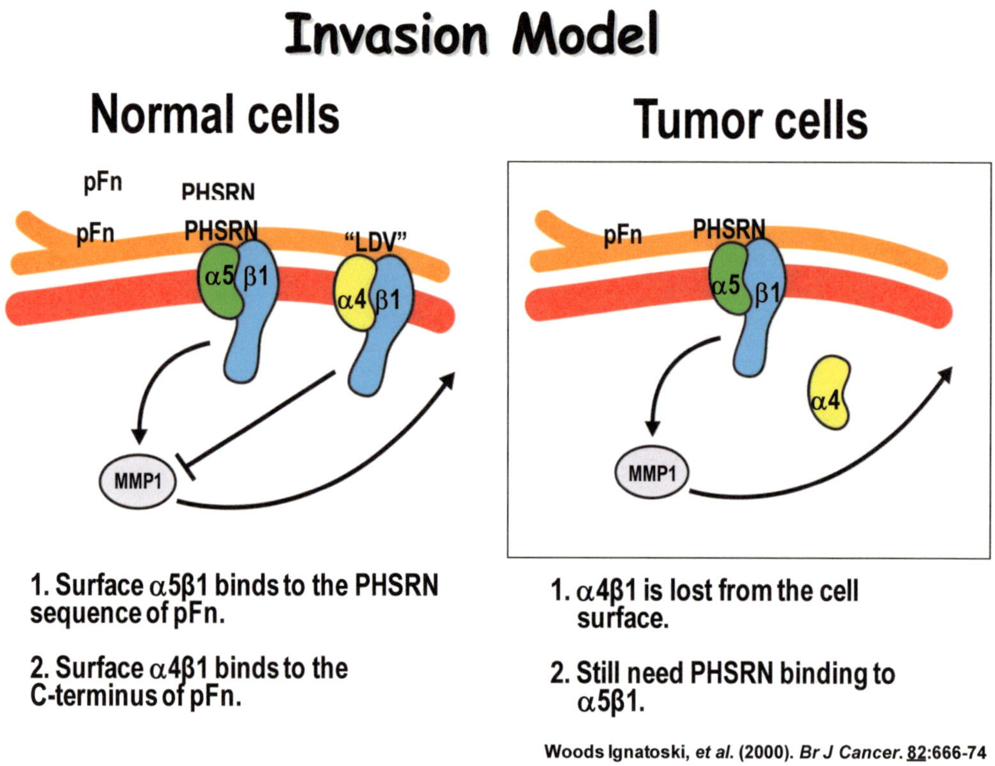

Fig. 4. Model of how cells are able to invade basement membranes. Fibronectin can bind α5 integrin through the PHSRN sequence. This binding drives the expression of MMP-1 and facilitates invasion. However, on normal cells, fibronectin binding to α4 integrin blocks MMP-1 release. On cancer cells, α4 integrin is not present on the cell surface, so invasion can proceed.

Utilizing a constitutively active form of PI3K, p110CAAX, we showed that PI3K can mediate most phenotypes observed in HER-2-overexpressing cells. PTEN expression blocked HER-2-mediated invasion. Down-regulated α4 integrin sequestered PTEN away from the surface, allowing PI3′K to activate PKCδ and facilitate the release of MMP-1 to drive invasion. These results led us to a model for HER-2-mediated invasion where the down-regulation of α4 integrin works in concert with the activation of PI3′K to facilitate the release of MMP-1 and drive invasion (*FIGURE 5*).

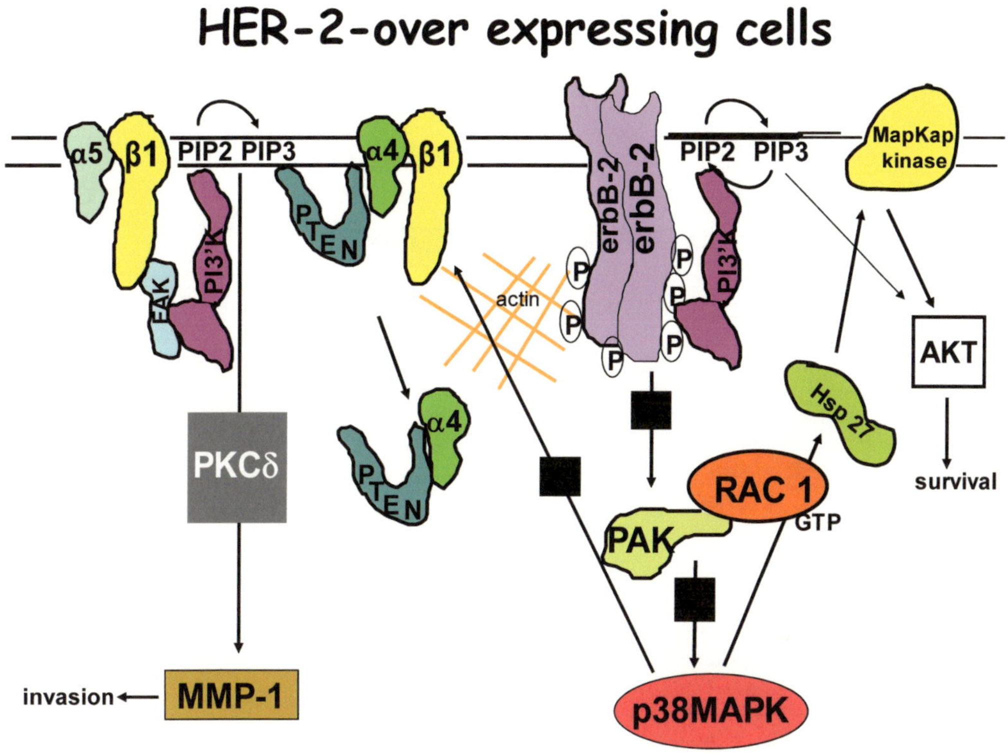

Fig. 5. Schematic of the signal pathways mediated by HER-2. HER-2 activates Rac 1 which activates p38MAPK. P38MAPK rearranges the actin cytoskeleton drawing α4 from the cell surface. It is hypothesized that PTEN is sequestered in the cytoplasm via its association with α4 (data not shown). Sequestration of PTEN allows PI3'K to activate PKCδ to release MMP-1 and facilitate invasion. P38MAPK also activates Hsp27 which activates MapKap kinase and, subsequently, AKT. AKT then facilitaes EGF-independent survival.

Using other *in vitro* transformation methods including anchorage-independent growth and cell motility assays, we were able to show that the PI3'K pathway can mediate most phenotypes observed when HER-2 is over expressed (Woods Ignatoski, Livant et al. 2003; Diehl, Woods Ignatoski et al. 2004). The HER-2-mediated signaling pathways are summarized in *FIGURE 6*.

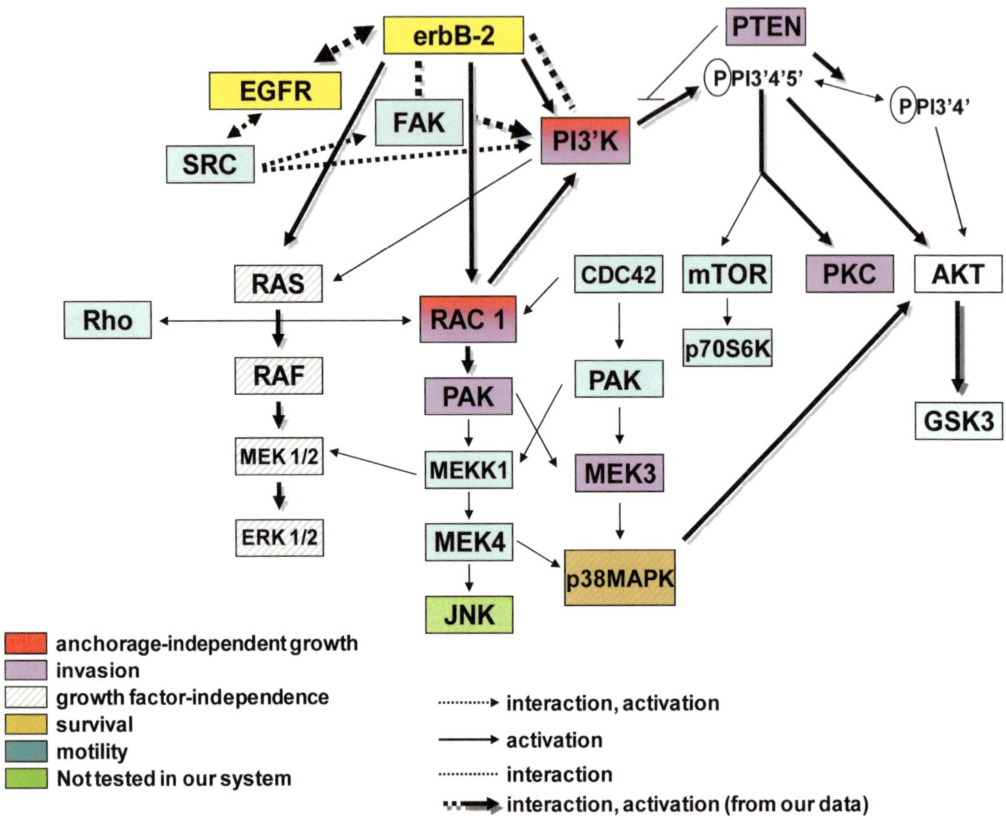

Fig. 6. Diagram of the HER-2-mediated signaling and designation of which pathways facilitate which transformed phenotypes.

Anti-HER-2 therapeutics: The presence of HER-2 over expression in HBC confers a poor prognosis (Slamon, Clark et al. 1987). Thus, the ultimate goal of the study of HER-2 is to offer women with HER-2 over expressing breast cancer an effective therapy. To this end, two relatively effective anti-HER-2 therapies have been FDA approved: trastuzumab (Herceptin®, *Genentech*) and lapatinib (Tykerb®, *Glaxo Smith-Kline*). Trastuzumab is a humanized anti-HER-2 antibody (Ewer, Gibbs et al. 1999; Palmieri, Powles et al. 2001; Rudlowski, Rath et al. 2001). The exact mode of action for trastuzumab is not known; however, trastuzumab is effective against 12-26% of HER-2-positive metastatic patients. Much of the resistance to trastuzumab has been shown to involve over activation of the PI3'K/ AKT pathway (O'Brien, Browne et al. 2010; Migliaccio I, Gutierrez et al. 2011). The survival advantage conferred upon a cell with an activated AKT overcomes the loss of HER-2 activity. Recently, Miller, *et al.* (Miller , Forbes et al. 2009) showed that trastuzumab in combination with rapamycin, which blocks the AKT pathway downstream of AKT at mTOR, could block HER-2 positive tumor growth in mice better than either treatment alone. Also, Zhang, *et al.* (Zhang, Huang et al. 2011) has shown that trastuzumab in combination with the *Src* inhibitor saracatinib can decrease HER-2 positive tumor growth in animals. *Src* is a non-receptor tyrosine kinase that has been shown to play a role in tumorigenesis. Zhang, *et al.* go on to show that *Src* activation is necessary for trastuzumab resistance and that all of the pathways that cause trastuzumab resistance, including different pathways that over activate AKT, originate from over active *Src*. Combination therapies, as the ones above, will be useful when using trastuzumab against HER-2 positive breast cancer.

Glaxo Smith-Kline has developed a small molecule EGFR/HER-2 dual inhibitor called lapatinib (Konecny, Pegram et al. 2006; Rusnak, Alligood et al. 2007; Molina, Kaufmann et al. 2008). Lapatinib has been shown to be a potent HER-2 inhibitor and a useful therapeutic against HER-2 positive breast cancer. Lapatinib, a 4-anilinoquinazoline kinase inhibitor of the intracellular tyrosine kinase domain of HER-2, is used with capecitabine for the treatment of advanced HER2-positive metastatic breast cancer (Molina, Kaufmann et al. 2008). Since response to lapatinib is predicted specifically by low levels of PTEN (Migliaccio I, Gutierrez et al. 2011) and resistance to trastuzumab is dependent on activation of the PI3'K pathway, studies showing the efficacy of a dual therapy using both lapatinib and trastuzumab will be very useful.

4. Conclusions

HER-2-mediated signaling is a convergence point that controls ductal development, the activity of the EGFR family of receptors, and many transformed phenotypes. Significantly abrogating the function of HER-2 is necessary to achieve prolonged survival for breast cancer patients.

5. References

Alroy, I. and Y. Yarden (1997). "The erbB signaling network in embryogenesis and oncogenesis: signal diversification through combinatorial ligand-receptor interactions." *FEBS Lett* 410: 83-86.

Brunet, A., A. Bonni, et al. (1999). "Akt promotes cell survival by phosphorylating and inhibiting a Forkhead transcription factor." *Cell* 96(6): 857-868.

Carraway, C. and K. Carraway (2007). "Sequestration and segregation of receptor kinases in epithelial cells: implications for ErbB2 oncogenesis." *Sci STKE* 2007(381): re3.

Carraway, C. A. C., M. E. Carvajal, et al. (1993). "Association of p185(neu) with Microfilaments via a Large Glycoprotein Complex in Mammary Carcinoma Microvilli - Evidence for a Microfilament-Associated Signal Transduction Particle." *J Biol Chem* 268(8): 5582-5587.

Carraway, K. L., 3rd, E. A. Rossi, et al. (1999). "An intramembrane modulator of the ErbB2 receptor tyrosine kinase that potentiates neuregulin signaling." *J Biol Chem* 274(9): 5263-5266.

Carraway, K. L. and L. C. Cantley (1994). "A neu acquaintance for ErbB3 and ErbB4: A role for receptor heterodimerization in growth signaling." *Cell* 78(1): 5-8.

Carraway, K. L., M. X. Sliwkowski, et al. (1994). "The erbB3 gene product is a receptor for heregulin." *J Biol Chem* 269(19): 14303-14306.

Datta, S. R., H. Dudek, et al. (1997). "Akt phosphorylation of BAD couples survival signals to the cell-intrinsic death machinery." *Cell* 91: 231-241.

Diehl, K. M., N. K. Grewal, et al. (2007). "p38MAPK-activated AKT in HER-2-over expressing human breast cancer cells acts as an EGF-independent survival signal." *Journal of Surgical Research* 142(1): 162-169.

Diehl, K. M., K. M. Woods Ignatoski, et al. (2004). "Signaling pathways in breast cancer cells influence the effects of the pan-erb-B kinase inhibitor CI-1033." *Proc. Am. Assoc. Cancer Res.* 45: 3683.

Ewer, M. S., H. R. Gibbs, et al. (1999). "Cardiotoxicity in patients receiving transtuzumab (Herceptin): primary toxicity, synergistic or sequential stress, or surveillance artifact? #1758." *Semin Oncol* 26(4 Suppl 12): 96-101.

Fedi, P., J. H. Pierce, et al. (1994). "Efficient Coupling with Phosphatidylinositol 3-Kinase, But Not Phospholipase C gamma or GTPase-Activating Protein, Distinguishes erbB-3 Signaling from That of Other erbB EGFr Family Members." *Mol Cell Biol* 14(1): 492-500.

Goldman, R., R. Benlevy, et al. (1990). "Heterodimerization of the erbB-1 and erbB-2 Receptors in Human Breast Carcinoma Cells - A Mechanism for Receptor Transregulation." *Biochemistry* 29(50): 11024-11028.

Gudjonsson, T., L. Ronnov-Jessen, et al. (2002). "Normal and tumor-derived myoepithelial cells differ in their ability to interact with luminal breast epithelial cells for polarity and basement membrane deposition." *J Cell Sci* 115(1): 39-50.

Hendriks , B. S., L. K. Opresko, et al. (2003). "Quantitative Analysis of HER2-mediated Effects on HER2 and Epidermal Growth Factor Receptor Endocytosis Distribution of Homo- AND Heterodimers Depends on Relative HER2 Levels." *J Biol Chem* 278(26): 23343-23351.

Holmes, W. E., M. X. Sliwkowski, et al. (1992). "Identification of heregulin, a specific activator of p185erb2 #636." *Science* 256: 1205-1210.

Howlett, A. R., N. Bailey, et al. (1995). "Cellular growth and survival are mediated by beta 1 integrins in normal human breast epithelium but not in breast carcinoma." *J Cell Sci* 108(Part 5): 1945-1957.

Howlett, A. R., O. W. Petersen, et al. (1994). "A novel function for the nm23-H1 gene: Overexpression in human breast carcinoma cells leads to the formation of basement membrane and growth arrest." *J Natl Cancer Inst* 86(24): 1838-1844.

Hutchinson J, Jin J, et al. (2001). "Activation of Akt (protein kinase B) in mammary epithelium provides a critical cell survival signal required for tumor progression." *Molecular and Cellular Biology* 21(6): 2203-2212.

Jia, Y., S. M. Markwart, et al. (2002). "Integrin receptors regulate MMP1 dependent invasion by breast cancer cells and by mammary epithelial cells." *Submitted to J Cell Biol.*

Karunagaran, D., E. Tzahar, et al. (1996). "ErbB-2 is a common auxiliary subunit of NDF and EGF receptors: Implications for breast cancer." *EMBO J* 15(2): 254-264.

Kokai, Y., T. Wada, et al. (1988). "The role of the neu oncogene product in cell transformation and normal development." *Princess Takamatsu Symp* 19: 45-57.

Komatsu, M., S. Jepson, et al. (2001). "Muc4/sialomucin complex, an intramembrane modulator of ErbB2/HER2/Neu, potentiates primary tumor growth and suppresses apoptosis in a xenotransplanted tumor." *Oncogene* 20(4): 461-470.

Konecny, G., M. Pegram, et al. (2006). "Activity of the dual kinase inhibitor lapatinib (GW572016) against HER-2-overexpressing and trastuzumab-treated breast cancer cells." *Cancer Research* 66(3): 1630-1639.

Korkaya, H., A. Paulson, et al. (2008). "HER2 regulates the mammary stem/progenitor cell population driving tumorigenesis and invasion." *Oncogene* 27(47): 6120-6130.

Korkaya, H. and M. Wicha (2009). "HER-2, notch, and breast cancer stem cells: targeting an axis of evil." *Clin Cancer Res* 15(6): 1845-1847.

Kozloski, G., C. Carraway, et al. (2010). "Mechanistic and signaling analysis of MUC4-ErbB2 signaling module: new insights into the mechanism of ligand-independent ErbB2 activity." *J Cell Physiol* 224(3): 649-657.

Livant, D. L., D. L. Allen, et al. (2000). "The PHSRN sequence induces extracellular matrix invasion and accelerates wound healing inobese diabetic mice." *J Clin Invest* 105(11): 1537-1545.

Livant, D. L., R. K. Brabec, et al. (2000). "Anti-invasive, antitumorigenic, and antimetastatic activities of the PHSCN sequence in prostate carcinoma." *Cancer Res* 60(2): 309-320.

Livant, D. L., S. Linn, et al. (1995). "Invasion of selectively permeable sea urchin embryo basement membranes by metastatic tumor cells, but not by their normal counterparts." *Cancer Res* 55: 5085-5093.

Lochter, A., S. Galosy, et al. (1997). "Matrix metalloproteinase stromelysin-1 triggers a cascade of molecular alterations that leads to stable epithelial-to-mesenchymal conversion and a premalignant phenotype in mammary epithelial cells." *J Cell Biol* 139(7): 1861-1872.

Lochter, A., M. Navre, et al. (1999). "alpha1 and alpha2 integrins mediate invasive activity of mouse mammary carcinoma cells through regulation of stromelysin-1 expression." *Mol Biol Cell* 10(2): 271-282.

Magnifico, A., L. Albano, et al. (2009). "Tumor-initiating cells of HER2-positive carcinoma cell lines express the highest oncoprotein levels and are sensitive to trastuzumab." *Clin Cancer Res* 15(6): 2010-2021.

Migliaccio I, D., M. Gutierrez, et al. (2011). "Loss of phosphatase and tensin homolog or phosphoinositol-3 kinase activation and response to trastuzumab or lapatinib in human epidermal growth factor receptor 2-overexpressing locally advanced breast cancers." *J Clin Oncol* 29(2): 166-173.

Miller , T., J. Forbes, et al. (2009). "Inhibition of mammalian target of rapamycin is required for optimal antitumor effect of HER2 inhibitors against HER2-overexpressing cancer cells." *Clin Cancer Res* 15(23): 7266-7276.

Molina, J., S. Kaufmann, et al. (2008). "Evaluation of Lapatinib andTopotecan CombinationTherapy:Tissue
Culture,Murine Xenograft, and Phase I ClinicalTrial Data." *Clin Cancer Res* 14(23): 7900-7908.

Muthuswamy, S., D. Li, et al. (2001). "ErbB2, but not ErbB1, reinitiates proliferation and induces luminal repopulation in epithelial acini." *Nat Cell Biol* 3(9): 785-792.

Nagy, T., H. Wei, et al. (2007). "Mammary epithelial-specific deletion of the focal adhesion kinase gene leads to severe lobulo-alveolar hypoplasia and secretory immaturity of the murine mammary gland." *J Biol Chem* 282(43): 1766-1776.

Najy, A., K. Day, et al. (2008). "The ectodomain shedding of E-cadherin by ADAM15 supports ErbB receptor activation." *J Biol Chem* 283(26): 18393-18401.

O'Brien, N., B. Browne, et al. (2010). "Activated phosphoinositide 3-kinase/AKT signaling confers resistance to trastuzumab but not to lapatinib." *Mol Cancer Ther* 9(6): 1489-1502.

Palmieri, C., T. Powles, et al. (2001). "Trastuzumab and breast cancer." *N Engl J Med* 345(13): 996-997.

Petersen, O. W., L. Ronnovjessen, et al. (1992). "Interaction with Basement Membrane Serves to Rapidly Distinguish Growth and Differentiation Pattern of Normal and Malignant Human Breast Epithelial Cells #713." *Proc Natl Acad Sci USA* 89(19): 9064-9068.

Ram, T. G., C. A. Dilts, et al. (1996). "Insulin-like growth factor and epidermal growth factor independence in human mammary carcinoma cells with c-erbB-2 gene amplification and progressively elevated levels of tyrosine phosphorylated erbB-2." *Mol. Carcinogen.* 15.: 227-238.

Ram, T. G., K. E. Kokeny, et al. (1995). "Mitogenic activity of neu differentiation factor/heregulin mimics that of epidermal growth factor and insulin-like growth factor-I in human mammary epithelial cells." *J. Cell. Physiol.* 163: 589-596.

Rudlowski, C., W. Rath, et al. (2001). "Trastuzumab and breast cancer." *N Engl J. Med* 345(13): 997-998.

Rusnak, D., K. Alligood, et al. (2007). "Assessment of epidermal growth factor receptor (EGFR, ErbB1) and HER2 (ErbB2) protein expression levels and response to lapatinib (Tykerb, GW572016) in an expanded panel of human normal and tumour cell lines." *Cell Prolif* 40(4): 580-594.

Slamon, D. J., G. M. Clark, et al. (1987). "Human breast cancer: Correlation of relapse and survival with amplification of the HER-2/neu oncogene." *Science* 235: 177-182.

Suo, Z., E. Emilsen, et al. (1998). "Type 1 protein tyrosine kinases in benign and malignant breast lesions #1767." *Histopathology* 33(6): 514-21.

Todaro, G. J., J. E. DeLarco, et al. (1976). "Transformation by murine and feline sarcoma viruses specifically blocks binding of epidermal growth factor to cells." *Nature* 264: 26-31.

Woods Ignatoski, K. and S. P. Ethier (1999). "Constitutive activation of pp 125fak in eleven newly isolated breast cancer cell lines." *Breast Cancer Res. and Treatment* 54: 173-182.

Woods Ignatoski, K. M., M. L. Dziubinski, et al. (2005). "Cooperative interactions of HER-2 and HPV-16 oncoproteins in the malignant transformation of human mammary epithelial cells." *Neoplasia* 7(8): 788-798.

Woods Ignatoski, K. M., A. J. LaPointe, et al. (1999). "ErbB-2 overexpression in human mammary epithelial cells confers growth factor independence." *Endocrinology* 140: 3615-3622.

Woods Ignatoski, K. M., D. L. Livant, et al. (2003). "The role of PI3'kinase and its downstream signals in erbB-2-mediated transformation." *Mol Cancer Res* 1(7): 551-560.

Woods Ignatoski, K. M., T. Maehama, et al. (2000). "ERBB-2 overexpression confers PI 3'-kinase-dependent invasion capacity on human mammary epithelial cells." *Br. J. Cancer* 82: 666-674.

Yokouchi, M., T. Kondo, et al. (1999). "Ligand-induced ubiquitination of the epidermal growth factor receptor involves the interaction of the c-Cbl RING finger and UbcH7." *J Biol Chem* 274(44): 31707-12.

Zachary, I. and E. Rozengurt (1992). "Focal Adhesion Kinase (p125(FAK)) - a Point of Convergence in the Action of Neuropeptides, Integrins, and Oncogenes." *Cell* 71(6): 891-894.

Zhang, S., W. Huang, et al. (2011). "Combating trastuzumab resistance by targeting SRC, a common node downstream of multiple resistance pathways." *Nat Med* 17(4): 461-469.

5

Brain Metastases Progression of Breast Cancer

Ala-Eddin Al Moustafa[1,2,3], Amber Yasmeen[2], Lina Ghabreau[4], Ali H. Mohamed[4] and Amal Achkhar[1,5]
[1]*Syrian Research Cancer Centre of the Syrian Society against Cancer, Aleppo*
[2]*Oncology Department, Faculty of Medicine, McGill University, Montréal*
[3]*Department of Mechanical Engineering, Concordia University, Montréal*
[4]*Deaptement of Pathology, Faculty of Medicine/University of Aleppo, Aleppo*
[5]*Faculty of Pharmacy, University of Aleppo, Aleppo*
[1,4,5]*Syria*
[2,3]*Canada*

1. Introduction

The development of brain metastases is one of the complications of breast cancer most feared by patients, having connotations of loss of identity and independence (Mayer, 2007). Clinically evident brain metastases occur in 20-30% of patients with metastatic breast cancer (Landis et al., 1999; Lin et al., 2004) and median survival of patients who develop breast cancer brain metastases (BCBMs) is generally poor, ranging from 2 to 9 months (Altundag et al., 2007; Lee et al., 2008; Ogawa et al., 2008). The treatment of metastasis to the brain is complicated by the unique characteristics of the brain. The blood-brain barrier (BBB), with its tight junctions and lack of lymphatic drainage, makes the delivery of chemotherapeutic agents difficult and represents a therapeutic haven from chemotherapy (Patchell, 2003; Ballabh et al., 2004; Nathoo et al., 2005). In addition, brain metastatic disease is the most poorly understood aspect of cancer progression. The potential of malignant cells to spread to distant organs including lung, bone and brain is the leading cause of death from breast cancer. Some breast cancer metastases display tissue-specific patterns to distant organs, such as the brain (Palmieri et al., 2006-2007; Sanna et al., 2007) and bone (Yang et al., 2007; Wang et al., 2007). The metastatic process is a complex phenomenon, and involves several genes. Recent studies recognize cell adhesion proteins especially E-cadherin and matrix metalloproteinases (MMPs), growth factor receptors such as EGF-R, ErbB-2, VEGF, and contributions from signal transduction pathways in addition to the activation of specific chemokines/cytokines, as major regulators of the metastatic process (Zeljko et al., 2011; Klein et al., 2009; Bos et al., 2009; Kennecke et al., 2010; Carotenuto et al., 2010; Hinton et al., 2010). Contrary to non-invasive breast cancer cells, malignant cells must display enhanced migratory behaviour and the ability to breach blood vessel walls and the dense collagenous matrix surrounding tumours. Additionally, metastatic cells must overcome the dynamics of a foreign microenvironment, to colonize and survive at a distant target site. Once metastasis has occurred, tumour growth is highly dependent on the ability of tumours to induce their own vascularization (Harlozinska, 2005; Hinton et al., 2008). There are key events to which malignant cells must adhere to complete their migration and angiogenesis: invasion of the surrounding stromal tissue, intravasation, evasion of programmed cell death and growth within a new microenvironment (Kaplan et al., 2006). These events are governed by several important genes that can regulate cell cancer invasion to a specific organ such as lung, bone and brain. In this chapter, we will discuss the contributions of E-cadherin, MMPs EGF-R, ErbB-2, VEGF and chemokine genes, to the induction and progression of metastasis of breast cancer especially to the brain.

2. MMPs and E-cadherin in brain metastasis

Ecadherin and MMPs family proteins are heavily involved in the metastases of the brain (VanMeter et al., 2001; Lewis-Tuffin et al., 2010). MMPs are a broad family of zinc-dependent proteinases that play a key role in extracellular matrix (ECM) degradation in metastasis (Kessenbrock et al., 2010); their expression is regulated via cytokines, and the ECM metalloprotease inducer is found on the surface of tumour cells. MMP activity is known to correlate with invasiveness, metastasis, and poor prognosis (Murphy, 2008; Kessenbrock et al., 2010). Earlier study found that MMP-2 is present in all metastatic brain tumours tested regardless of the site of origin and that the level of activity inversely correlated with survival (Jäälinojä et al., 2000; Deryugina and Quigley, 2006). Meanwhile, although MMP-9 was found to be up-regulated in all brain metastases and primary brain tumours, there was an inability to correlate up-regulation with survival (Arnold et al., 1999). Furthermore, previous studies showed that MMPs might be involved in the metastases of breast cancer to the brain (Cheng and Hung, 2007). A breast cancer brain metastases rat model was derived from injection of a carcinogen-induced mammary adenocarcinoma cell line in the left ventricle of rat (Mendes et al., 2005). The micro-metastasis in the brain showed a significantly higher expression of MMP-2, -3 and -9 and an increase in MMP-2 and MMP-3 activity compared to the normal brain tissue (Deryugina and Quigley, 2006). Furthermore, the development of brain metastasis was significantly decreased by the treatment with a selective synthetic MMP inhibitor (Mendes et al., 2005). This phenomenon was confirmed by another study in which human breast cancer cells over-expressed with MMP2 were inoculated into the left ventricle, a higher incidence of metastasis to brain was observed (Tester et al., 2004). Another study also showed that brain seeking breast cancer cells have a higher total and active amount MMP-1 and MMP-9 with higher migration and invasion capacity, which could be decreased by the application of MMP-1 and/or MMP-9 inhibitor (Stark et al., 2007).

On the other hand, E-cadherin/catenin complex is vital for the maintenance of both normal and tumour cytoarchitecture as well as a necessary mediator of cell-cell adhesion. β-catenin, as well as plakoglobin (γ-catenin), associate directly with the highly conserved cytoplasmic domain of E-cadherin in a mutually exclusive manner (Yasmeen et al., 2006; Al Moustafa et al., 2008). The E-cadherin/β-catenin complex is linked via α-catenin either directly or indirectly to the actin filament network via the actin-binding proteins α-actinin or vinculin (Yasmeen et al., 2006; Al Moustafa et al., 2008). The association of the E-cadherin/catenin complex with the cytoskeleton is essential for tight cell-cell adhesions. In the metastatic escape of a tumour, clone cells reduced intercellular adhesion and disrupted cytoarchitecture, and are thus prone to separation from the primary tumour mass (Al Moustafa et al., 2011). These clones are then free to invade both locally as well as to continue on to intravasation and further progress in the cascade (Nathoo et al., 2005).

Decreased expression of the E-cadherin/catenin complex has been correlated with invasion, metastasis, and unfavorable prognosis (Bremnes et al., 2002). Shabani et al. (2003) established a correlation between E-cadherin/catenin complex expression and an increased mindbomb homolog 1 (MIB1) index in metastatic adenocarcinomas. Further, E-cadherin is expressed in most meningiomas (Tohma et al., 1992; Figarella-Branger et al., 1994; Howng et al., 2002), and its loss may be associated with tumour progression (Schwechheimer et al., 1998). E-cadherin expression in glioblastoma multiforme or glioblastomas appears to be an exception to the epithelial-mesenchymal transition (EMT) rule, which is an important event in the progression cancer and metastasis (Lewis-Tuffin et al., 2010; Al Moustafa et al., 2011) (Figure 1). The molecular mechanisms underlying the contribution of E-cadherin to growth and/or invasiveness in glioblastomas are currently unknown. Although, the two main sources of brain metastasis - adenocarcinomas of the lung or the breast represent different models of the course of the disease (Bos et al., 2009); Zeljko et al. (2011) have showed that E-cadherin changes were frequent in metastases from both those malignancies. Moreover, Saad et al. (2008) demonstrated that loss of E-cadherin in patients with adenocarcinomas and squamous cell carcinomas of the lung is significantly associated to the increased risk of developing brain metastases. The results of other authors investigating E-cadherin involvement in brain metastasis (Arnold et al., 1999; Shabani et al., 2003; Prudkin et al., 2009) collectively demonstrate that Ecadherin is constantly expressed in metastatic deposits. Furthermore, our recent studies also demonstrated that E-cadherin-catenin complex is involved in cell migration and metastasis *in vivo* and *in vitro* (Yasmeen et al., 2007). In order to investigate the cooperation effect between ErbB-2 receptor and high-risk human papillomavirus (HPV) in breast carcinogenesis and metastasis, we generated double transgenic mice carrying ErbB-2 and E6/E7 of HPV type 16 under mouse mammary tumour virus (MMTV) and human keratin 14 (K14) promoters, respectively. Within six months, these double transgenic mice developed large and extensive invasive breast cancers to several vital organs including lung, bone and brain. Histological analysis of ErbB-2/E6/E7 transgenic mouse tumours revealed the presence of invasive breast carcinomas. However, breast tissues from ErbB-2 and E6/E7 singly transgenic mice showed only *in-situ* cancer and normal mammary phenotype, respectively (Yasmeen et al., 2007). In parallel, to assess the outcome of ErbB-2/E6/E7 cooperation in human breast carcinogenesis, we examined the effect of ErbB-2 and E6/E7 of HPV type 16 on the BT20 breast cancer cell lines. We found that ErbB-2/E6/E7 cooperate in the BT20 cell line to induce large colony formation and cell migration using soft agar and wound healing assays, respectively, in comparison with ErbB-2, E6/E7 and wild type cells. Moreover, we demonstrated that ErbB-2/E6/E7 cooperation induces a nuclear translocation of β-catenin in BT20 cells; regarding the mechanism of this translocation, we reported that ErbB-2/E6/E7 cooperation provokes a dissociation of E-cadherin/catenin complex by tyrosine phosphorylation of β-catenin through pp60(c-Src) kinase phosphorylation. Subsequently, the free β-catenin enters to the nucleus and modulates cell transcription via its association with the Tcf/Lef transcription factors (Yasmeen et al., 2007; Al Moustafa et al., 2008) (Figure 2). In conclusion, our *in vitro* and *in vivo* models demonstrated that the ErbB-2 tyrosine kinase receptor cooperates with E6/E7 of high-risk HPVs in breast tumorigenesis and metastasis via E-cadherin/catenin complex (Yasmeen et al., 2007; Al Moustafa et al., 2008). These studies provide evidence that MMPs and E-cadherin play an important role in brain metastases of breast cancer.

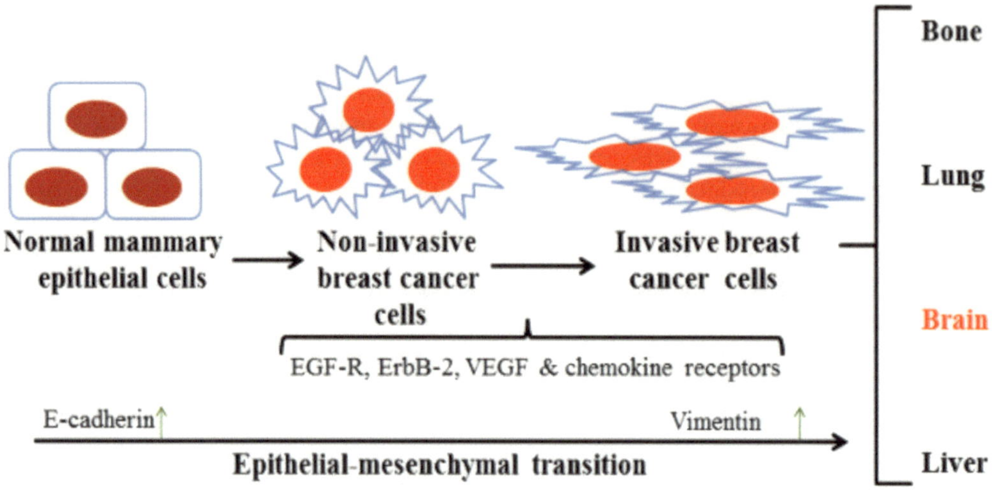

Fig. 1. Transformation of normal mammary epithelial to non-invasive and invasive cancer cells. Several oncogenes can transform normal epithelial cells to cancer ones; meanwhile, other genes such as, EGF-R, ErbB-2, VEGFs and chemokines, convert non-invasive cancer cells to invasive ones which can invade several vital organs including bone, lung, brain and liver. Invasion is a multi-step process which allows cell migration and invasion through dysfunctional cell–cell adhesive interactions, loss of cell–cell junctions and reorganization of the cytoskeleton; these procedures result in the loss of apical polarity and the acquisition of a more spindle-shaped morphology; this process is identified as the epithelial-mesenchymal transition (EMT). This event is accompanied by inhibition of epithelial markers such as E-cadherin and over-expression of mesenchymal markers such as vimentin.

3. EGF-R and ErbB-2 in brain metastasis

The epidermal growth factor receptor (EGFR) is a member of the ErbB family of receptor tyrosine kinases. This family includes four receptors: EGF-R/ErbB-1/HER-1, ErbB-2/HER-2/Neu, ErbB-3/HER-3, and ErbB-4/HER-4 (Carney et al., 2007; Lee-Hoeflich et al., 2008) that are structurally related. All HER members except HER-3 contain intracellular tyrosine kinase domain and all except HER-2, bind to extracellular ligands (Carpenter et al., 1990). Certain discrete genes, with several alternative splice variants, encode either the "Epidermal Growth Factor (EGF) receptor ligands" or the Neuregulins that bind to different ErbB receptors as a co-receptor. Different ligands bind to more than one receptor with high affinity; consequently ErbB-2 ligands readily activate ErbB-2 in combination with the appropriate high affinity co-receptor. The biological activity and affinity is often higher with the presence of ErbB2 complex than without it. The mammalian ligands that bind to the ErbB family include EGF, Transforming growth factor-α (TGF-α), heparin-binding EGF-like growth factor (HB-EGF), amphiregulin (AR), betacellulin (BTC), epiregulin (EPR), epigen, tomoregulin and neuregulins (NRG-1, NRG-2, NRG-3 and NRG-4) (Chang et al., 1997; Bublil and Yarden, 2007). The architecture of ErbB kinases, like most receptor tyrosine kinases (RTKs), is characterized by an extracellular ligand-binding domain, a transmembrane domain, a juxtamembrane (JM) segment, a kinase domain, and a COOH

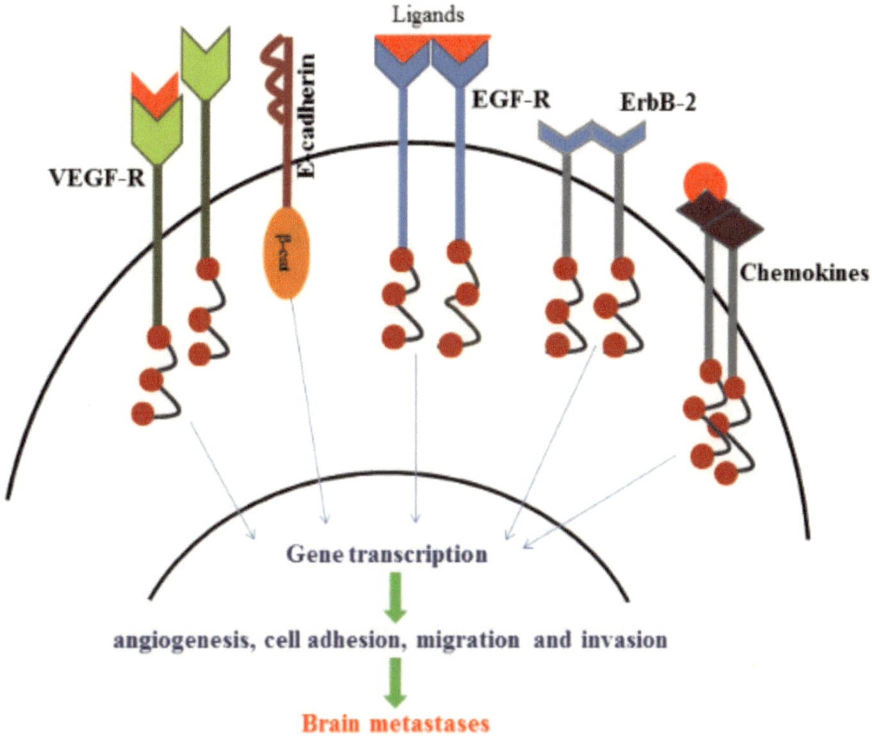

Fig. 2. VEGF-R, EGF-R, ErbB-2 and chemokines receptor signaling pathways in cancer cells. Ligands can activate downstream-signaling pathways of these receptors which also can interact with other protein complexes such E-cadherin/catenins. Therefore, these pathways alter the activity of multiple nuclear transcription factors which in turn can activate several genes implicated in diverse cellular procedures such as angiogenesis, cell adhesion, migration and invasion; after which cancer cells can migrate to several organs including brain.

terminal tail (C-terminal tail). The EGF-R is involved in many cellular processes including cell proliferation, motility, adhesion and angiogenesis via the activation of primarily two pathways: Phosphatidylinositol-3 Kinase (PI3K)/Akt pathway, and the External signal-Regulated Kinase (ERK) pathway (Yasmeen et al., 2006; Bublil and Yarden, 2007) (Figure 2). EGF-R is widely expressed in a variety of human cancers including non-small-cell lung cancer NSCLC, colorectal, pancreatic, breast, ovarian, prostate and gastric cancers (Raymond et al., 2000). It is thought that EGF-R plays an important role in the tumour development and progression (Grandis et al., 2004). In addition to their well established contributions to cell proliferation and survival, EGF-R and ErbB-2 are also linked with other characteristics of aggressive tumours such as local invasion and intravasation (Figure 2), independently of their effects on growth (Xue et al., 2006; Zhan et al., 2006). Gene expression profiling and immunohistochemical studies have indicated that 50–70% of basal-type breast tumours, which are ErbB-2 "triple-negative" carcinomas, exhibit EGF-R expression (Burness et al., 2010). This type of breast cancers is associated with large size, high tumour grade, increased frequency of distant metastases to several vital organs including brain (Da Silva et al., 2007).

ErbB-2/HER-2/Neu oncogene, located on the long arm of chromosome 17 (17q12-q21), is over-expressed or amplified in 18–35% of invasive breast cancers and in 60% of intraductal breast carcinomas but are not over-expressed relative to the normal breast epithelium (Pawlowski et al., 2000). Over-expression of ErbB-2 in breast carcinoma patients is associated with a shorter survival period and more frequent disease recurrence compared with patients without ErbB-2 over-expression (Slamon et al., 1987). Moreover, over-expression of ErbB-2 in breast cancer cell lines increases the portion of cells that present stem-like properties (Korkaya et al., 2008) and display intrinsic resistance to antiestrogen therapy (Jordan et al., 2007; Fan et al., 2009). ErbB-2 amplification/over-expression is a prognostic and predictive factor for the development of CNS metastases (Evans et al., 2004; Gabos et al., 2006). Autopsy data show that the incidence rate for CNS metastases in ErbB-2-positive breast cancer patients is higher (ie, 30% to 50%) than that in ErbB-2-negative breast cancer patients (approximately 30%) (Aragon-Ching et al., 2007). On the other hand, a retrospective study on 9524 women with early stage breast cancer identified ErbB-2 as a clear risk factor for the development of CNS relapse (Pestalozzi et al., 2006). However, the precise biological explanation for the tendency of ErbB-2-positive breast cancer cells to metastasize to CNS has not been completely elucidated; although it has been suggested that it may occur as a result of both the aggressiveness of this breast cancer subtype and of a particular affinity for CNS. Interestingly, the survival time after the diagnosis of brain metastasis is longer for patients with ErbB-2-positive disease than ErbB-2-negative. It is estimated that one-third of women receiving Herceptin for metastatic ErbB-2-positive breast cancer develop CNS metastases during the course of their illness (Bendell et al., 2003; Lai et al., 2004). Herceptin levels in cerebrospinal fluid are 300-fold lower than those in plasma (Pestalozzi et al., 2000; Rusnak et al., 2001), indicating that Herceptin cannot cross the BBB due to its large molecular weight. The inability of Herceptin to cross the BBB may also contribute to the increased incidence of brain metastases in patients with ErbB-2-over-expressing breast cancer. This is most likely because of the inherent aggressiveness of ErbB-2-positive disease, as well as the prolongation in survival and control of extracranial disease attributable to Herceptin therapy (Clayton et al., 2004). Interestingly, ErbB-3 expression was increased in breast cancer cells residing in the brain. Neuregulin-1, the ligand for this receptor, is abundantly expressed in the brain (Law et al., 2004; Da Silva et al., 2010). These findings suggest that neuregulin/ErbB-3 activation is an important mechanism for breast cancer cell colonization of the brain and imply that the inhibition of ErbB family receptors especially EGF-R and/or ErbB-2 may play a significant role in the treatment of patients with brain metastases from breast cancer.

4. VEGFs in brain metastasis

Vascular endothelial growth factor (VEGF) belongs to VEGF family that consists of five members: VEGF (or VEGF-A), VEGF-B, VEGF-C, VEGF-D, and placental growth factor (PlGF) (Li et al., 2001; Nagy et al., 2003; Yamazaki et al., 2003). There are three receptor protein-tyrosine kinases for the VEGF family ligands (VEGFR-1, VEGFR-2, and VEGFR-3), which are primarily expressed by the endothelium and are required for normal vascular development (Millauer et al., 1993; Peters et al., 1993; Terman et al., 1994). Each of these receptors consists of seven immunoglobulin-like loops in the extracellular domain, a single transmembrane domain, and an intracellular protein-tyrosine kinase segment that contains a kinase insert, and a carboxy-terminal tail (Fantl et al., 1993) (Figure 2). Several ligands of

VEGF family bind to two non-enzymatic receptors (neuropilin-1 and -2), and heparan sulfate proteoglycans that are found on the plasma membrane and in the extracellular matrix (Dougher et al., 1997; Gluzman-Poltorak et al., 2000). Binding of VEGF to its receptors induces proliferation and migration of cancer cells (Figure 1 and 2).

Although VEGF is considered potent mitogen for vascular endothehal cells, it is also considerably involved in the mitogenic activity of other cells. VEGF mRNA and protein are found in several tissues and organs (Berse et al., 1992; Ng et al., 2001; Maharaj et al., 2006). Also, VEGF gene expression and protein are found in many of human malignancies such as breast, non-small cell lung, colorectal, neuroblastoma, and prostate carcinomas (Fukuzawa et al., 2002; Hoeben et al., 2004; Xu et al., 2004). On the contrary, VEGF receptors are generally limited to endothelial cells in the cardiovascular and lymphatic systems (Kukk et al., 1996; Lymboussaki et al., 1999).

In the nervous tissue, VEGF is crucial for vascular growth during brain development (Breier et al., 1992; Ogunshola et al., 2000; Vates et al., 2005). However, in the intact adult CNS, the expression of VEGF becomes restricted to the choroid plexus, area postrema cerebellar granule cells (Monacci et al., 1993), and VEGF receptor expression becomes extremely low (Kremer et al., 1997; Soker et al., 1998). VEGF expression was demonstrated to be up-regulated in neurons and astroglia during pathological processes in the CNS that are associated with angiogenesis and increased BBB permeability, including tumours and ischemia (Pietsch et al., 1997; Issa et al., 1999; Lee et al., 1999; Plate et al., 1999; Jin et al., 2000; Graumann et al, 2003). VEGF direct application to fetal cortical and ventral mescencephalic explants has been shown to induce significant angiogenesis and astroglial proliferation (Silverman et al., 1999; Mani et al., 2005; Krum et al., 2008). Furthermore, continuous interstitial infusion of recombinant human VEGF165 protein administered to the cerebrum produced significant increases in the activity and, unexpectedly, in the astroglial proliferation within the adult CNS (Krum et al., 2002). VEGF, thus, was considered a direct astroglial mitogen (Krum et al., 2002).

It was postulated, forty years ago, by Folkman that tumours require to be vascularized to grow (Folkman, 1971). Tumour cells enter the vascular system after switching on the angiogenic process, and forming new ascites, leading to the initiation of metastasis. VEGF, among other various angiogenic factors, plays an essential role in tumour angiogenesis. VEGF is expressed and secreted by most solid tumours, but little occurs in endothelial cells (Ribatti et al., 1998; Shemirani and Crowe, 2000). In contrast, VEGF receptors (VEGFR-1 and VEGFR-2 mRNAs and proteins) are largely expressed in vessels lining and penetrating the tumours; where they are exclusively expressed in endothelial cells (Brown et al., 1995; Mentzel et al., 2001). These observations are consistent with the notion that VEGF acts in a paracrine manner, in which VEGF that is secreted from tumour cells influences nearby endothelial cells.

The finding that VEGF is highly expressed in metastatic cerebral tumours originating from angiosarcoma, renal cell carcinomas, melanomas, and adenocarcinomas provide further evidence that supports the significant role for VEGF in human metastases (Strugar et al., 1994). VEGF expression was associated with considerable staining of microvascular and the formation of vasogenic brain edema, revealing both the angiogenic and permeability properties of VEGF (Strugar et al., 1994). On the other hand, VEGF- mRNA is significantly correlated with vascularisation in both gliomas and meningiomas, indicating a pivotal role for VEGF in the vascularization of primary brain tumours (Samoto et al., 1995). It is currently well established that the formation of metastases correlates with the number of microvessels (the amount of vascularisation) that can be detected in a primary tumour.

A number of mechanisms account for tumour vascularisation, including sprouting angiogenesis, intussusceptions, recruitment of circulating endothelial precursors, cooption, mosaic vessels, and vascular mimicry. VEGF family members are considered the major players that control these mechanisms. Sprouting angiogenesis has been suggested as the mechanism that is used by the brain for vasculrization. In sprouting angiogenesis, VEGF-A produces vasodilatation of preexisting capillaries and increases permeability (Auguste et al., 2005). VEGF-A also induces endothelial cell proliferation (Auguste et al., 2005) and an increase in metalloproteases and plasminogen activators, which lead to the degradation of the extracellular matrix permitting endothelial cell migration (Pepper et al., 1991; Vu et al., 1998; Bergers et al., 2000). Vessel guidance mechanisms that direct host vessels into the tumour have been identified in the brain. VEGF and its receptors have been postulated as important guidance signal. It seems that cells located at the invading front of the blood vessels, huddle VEGFR-2 and follow a VEGF gradient (Gerhardt et al., 2003). Tumour cells injected into the brain were found to develop vascularization immediately by angiogenic sprouting with loss of the BBB. Tumour cells are speculated to be organized in cuffs of pseudopalisading cells around VEGFR-2 positive vessels, and to use these vessels to invade other brain areas. Vessels supply tumour cells with oxygen and nutriments.

A different mechanism of brain tumour vascularization that is distinct from the sprouting mechanism has been described. Accordingly, tumours in the brain can use a cooption mechanism for vascularization (Holash et al., 1999; Fischer et al., 2005). Vessels are surrounded by tumour cells, and cooped endothelial cells are induced to express angiopoietin-2. Binding of angiopoietin-2 to its receptors located at the endothelial cell surface leads to the dissociation of the mural cells from endothelial cells, and an increase in apoptosis. Angiopoietin-2 activity causes a significant decrease in tumour vessel number and an increase in vessel diameter. Accordingly, the scarcity of vessels leads to hypoxia which upregulates VEGF-A expression in tumour cells. As a consequence, strong angiogenesis develops mainly at the tumour periphery (Holash et al., 1999; Zagzag et al., 2000; Fischer et al, 2005). Rat mammary carcinomas was shown to be vascularized by cooption when cells are injected inside the brain. Metastases of Lewis lung carcinoma and melanoma cells into brain have been demonstrated to be partially vascularized by cooption (Holash et al., 1999; Kusters et al., 2002). Decreasing VEGF production, by antisense transfection, to 20–50% of original cell level was shown to be associated with inhibition of both angiogenesis and brain metastasis formation (Yano et al., 2000). In conclusion, VEGF is a key factor in the vascularization and metastasis of primary tumours into brain.

5. Chemokines and chemokine receptors

Chemotactic cytokines, or *chemo-kines*, are a large subfamily of cytokines that coordinate leukocyte recruitment and activation, two crucial elements in the pathogenesis of several immuno-mediated human diseases. Chemokines have been recognized in the last few years as important mediators in the pathogenesis of many human diseases and have assumed growing relevance in clinical pathology as markers of disease onset, progression, and remission (Hinton et al., 2010). Since the description of the first chemokine in 1977, over 40 related molecules have been discovered in humans and chemokines have been recognized as a family of functionally related small secreted molecules named "chemo-kine" because of leukocyte chemoattractant and cytokine-like activities (Luster, 1998; Locati and Murphy,

1999). Human chemokine family is currently known to include more than 40 chemokines and 20 chemokine receptors (Bonecchi et al., 2009). These receptors are defined by their ability to induce directional migration of cells toward a gradient of a chemotactic cytokine (a process known as chemotaxis) (Figure 2). Chemokine receptors are a family of seven transmembrane G protein-coupled cell surface receptors (GPCR) that are classified into four groups (CXC, CC, C, and CX3C) based on the position of the first two cysteines (Murphy et al., 2000; Zlotnik and Yoshie, 2000). While chemokine receptors have been found in many different cell types, these receptors were initially identified on leukocytes and were found to play an important role in the homing of such cells to sites of inflammation (Loetscher et al., 2000).

During the past several years, other types of non-hematopoietic cells have been found to express receptors for various chemokines found in their distinct tissue microenvironments. The interactions between such receptors and their respective chemokines are thought to help coordinate the trafficking and organization of cells within various tissue compartments (Baggiolini, 1998; Moser and Loetscher, 2001). CXCR4 is one of the best studied chemokine receptors, primarily due to its role as a co-receptor for HIV entry (Feng et al., 1996) and its ability to mediate the metastasis of a variety of cancers, including prostate cancer (Zlotnik, 2006a and b; Burger and Kipps, 2006; Sun et al., 2003). CXCR4 is a 352-amino acid rhodopsin-like GPCR that selectively binds the CXC chemokine stromal cell-derived factor 1 (SDF-1), also known as CXCL12 (Fredriksson et al., 2003; Burger and Kipps, 2006). On the other hand, lack of either SDF-1 or CXCR4 resulted in a phenotype almost identical to that of late gestational lethality with defects in B cell lymphopoiesis, bone marrow colonization, and cardiac septal formation (Nagasawa et al., 1996; Zou et al., 1998). These studies indicate that CXCR4 is essential for development, hematopoiesis, organogenesis, as well as vascularization (Tachibana et al., 1998; McGrath et al., 1999) and that it functions as a classical chemokine receptor in adults (Murphy, 1994; Baggiolini, 1998). A growing body of evidence now shows that CXCR4 has a role in both cancer metastasis and in cancer stem cells. The physiological mechanism of tissue-specific recruitment (i.e. a homing system for normal tissue replacement) also seems to be functional for cancer stem cells. The CXCR4-SDF-1 axis seems to have a large influence on the biology of tumours. High levels of SDF-1 in organs and tissue structures such as the lymph nodes, lungs, liver, brain and bones are believed to direct the metastasis of CXCR4-expressing tumour cells. In support of this hypothesis, several researchers have shown that multiple cancers expressing CXCR4 (e.g. breast, ovarian, and prostate cancers, as well as rhabdomyosarcomas and neuroblastomas) metastasize to the bones and the brain through the bloodstream in an SDF-1 (CXCL12)-dependent manner (Dontu et al., 3003; Porcile et al., 2004; Sun et al., 2003; Geminder et al., 2001; Hinton et al., 2010). The CXCR4-SDF-1-mediated trafficking/homing of tumour cells during metastasis seems to share some molecular mechanisms with normal stem cell processes. Additionally, the mobilization, trafficking and homing of both cancer and normal stem cells seem to be multistep processes, as described in several studies (Hattori et al., 2001; Lapidot et al., 2002; Hinton et al., 2010). Previous study by Muller et al. (2001) reported in breast cancer that CXCR4 and CXCL12 are central players in regulating metastasis by showing that normal breast tissues express little CXCR4, whereas breast neoplasms express high levels of CXCR4; CXCR4 signaling in response to CXCL12 mediates actin polymerization and pseudopodia formation, and subsequently induces chemotactic and invasive responses (Muller et al., 2001). These data formed the basis of the hypothesis that malignant cells may employ chemokine receptors to migrate toward chemokine ligands expressed at common metastatic sites, such as the lungs, bone marrow, brain and lymph nodes. Indeed, CXCR4 appears to be one of a limited number of genes that are enriched in a subpopulation of metastatic breast cancer cells, as over-expression of CXCR4 alone significantly increased the number of bone and brain metastases *in vivo* (Kang et al., 2003). Supporting evidence for the hypothesis was demonstrated by Liang et al. (2005) as blocking CXCR4 expression by siRNAs decreased breast cancer cell invasion *in vitro* and inhibited metastasis in animal models. Interestingly, the CXCR4 carboxy-terminal domain appears to play a major role in regulating receptor desensitization and down-regulation, whereas deletion of the C-terminal domain of CXCR4 leads to the down-regulation of cell-to-cell contact, enhanced motility, and proliferation in breast carcinoma cells (Ueda et al., 2006). Elucidation of the underlying mechanisms of breast cancer invasion and metastasis focusing on CXCR4 has resulted in several important observations. Ligand-binding studies indicate that the number and affinity of CXCR4 receptors are similar in nonmetastatic cells versus highly metastatic cells. In metastatic cells, CXCL12 binding to the Gαβγ/GDP protein complex leads to a GTP-for-GDP exchange, allowing Gαi to dissociate from the Gβγ subunit, leading to activation of ERK1/2, IκBα, JNK, Akt, p38 MAPK, and GSK-3αβ. In nonmetastatic cells, CXCR4 is able to independently form a complex with Gαi or Gβ subunits, but no Gαβγ heterotrimer could be associated with CXCR4 and, ultimately, Gβγ-dependent downstream signaling did not occur (Holland et al., 2006). Although the molecular basis for the difference in G-protein signaling in metastatic versus nonmetastatic cells remains to be elucidated, these studies have implications for clinical studies that are examining CXCR4 protein expression but not receptor function. As observed in breast cancer cell lines, detection of CXCR4 protein does not necessarily indicate CXCR4-mediated signaling (Fulton, 2009).

There is increasing evidence that CXCR4 interacts with several growth factor receptor tyrosine kinases. Upon activating IGF-1R, IGF-1 was shown to transactivate CXCR4 signal transduction in metastatic MDA-MB-231 cells but not in nonmetastatic MCF-7 cells, even though both cell lines are positive for IGF-1R and CXCR4 (Akekawatchai et al., 2005). Myofibroblasts associated with breast cancer, but not those in normal breast tissue, produce CXCL12 and enhance growth of tumours through mechanisms that include proliferation and survival of malignant cells and angiogenesis (Allinen et al., 2004; Orimo et al., 2005). Specific alleles of CXCL12 are associated with an increased risk of breast cancer (Razmkhah et al., 2005), and CXCL12 has been shown to transactivate ErbB-2 (Cabioglu et al., 2005). CXCR4 expression was also identified as a predictive factor of worse outcome in some metastatic tumours and in malignant gliomas (Scala et al., 2005; Ottaiano et al., 2006; Bian et al., 2007). CXCL12/CXCR4 axis is supposed to be crucial in brain metastases formation from breast cancer (Hinton et al., 2008). Recently, another CXCL12 receptor has been identified: the orphan G protein-coupled receptor (GPCR) RDC1, now called CXCR7 (Balabanian et al., 2005; Burns et al., 2006). This receptor does not mediate typical GPCR signaling through Gi or Ca2+ mobilization. Recent findings in zebrafish primordial germ cells showed a scavenger activity of CXCR7 generating a CXCL12 gradient that would lead to the formation of a guidance cue for CXCR4-positive cells (Thelen and Thelen, 2008). On the other hand, formation of CXCR4/CXCR7 heterodimers enhancing CXCL12 signaling in embryonic cells was observed, suggesting a potential interaction between the two receptors (Sierro et al., 2007). Nevertheless, CXCL12/CXCR4 relevance in brain metastasis establishment/progression needs more investigation especially on the molecular level.

6. Conclusions/Perspectives

Cancer cell migration and invasion are critical processes in the metastatic cascade. They can be induced and executed by various signalling pathways and regulatory networks. Many of these pathways seem to overlap with developmental processes and are being abused by invasive carcinomas cells and their microenvironment. Although we have made substantial progress in understanding the molecular mechanisms underlying cancer cell migration and invasion in experimental systems, we still lack sufficient insights into the actual processes at work in metastatic cancer patients especially brain metastatic disease. This divergence between clinicopathologic and experimental observations is mainly based on the lack of appropriate surrogate markers and the lack of complex *in vivo* models that appropriately recapitulate human stochastic carcinogenesis. However, it is expected that the ongoing cellular and molecular research on cell migration will provide the urgently needed tools for the development of improved diagnosis, prognosis and eventually for the design of innovative therapies.

There are few therapeutic approaches that are currently under development or in clinical trials specifically targeting metastatic breast cancer of the brain, such as interfering with specific pathways of some regulator genes of invasive cancer cells. However, by interfering with important signaling pathways that are known to modulate cell proliferation, survival, and differentiation, they may also affect cell migration and invasion. Examples are inhibitors against the activities of different receptor tyrosine kinases, such as EGF-R, ErbB-2, VEGF-Rs, fibroblast growth factor receptors, chemokine receptors, and c-Met, as well as various anti-angiogenesis regimen or even in combinations. Altogether, such multifaceted inhibitory approaches may provide efficient therapeutic measures that repress not only primary tumour outgrowth but also metastasis formation by interfering with cancer cell migration and invasion to the brain and other organs. However, the cellular and molecular variations to cancer cell migration discussed above raise the caveat that this endeavour will not be easy. We believe that using microarray technology and new *in vitro* and *in vivo* cancer metastatic models, including brain, should help us to understand the mechanism of cancer metastasis and consequently facilitate the design of more successful, personalized cancer therapies.

7. Acknowledgments

We are grateful to Mrs. A. Kassab and Mr. E Segal for their critical reading of the manuscript. The research works from Dr. Al Moustafa's laboratory has been supported by the Canadian Institutes for Health Research, the Cancer Research Society Inc. of Canada, the National Colorectal Cancer Campaign and the Fonds de la Recherche en Santé du Québec (FRSQ- Réseau du Cancer).

8. References

Akekawatchai C, Holland JD, Kochetkova M, Wallace JC, McColl SR. Transactivation of CXCR4 by the insulin-like growth factor-1 receptor (IGF-1R) in human MDA-MB-231 breast cancer epithelial cells. J Biol Chem. 2005 Dec 2;280(48):39701-8.

Al Moustafa A-E, Achkhar A, Yasmeen A. EGF-receptor signaling and epithelial-mesenchymal transition in human carcinomas. Frontiers in Bioscience journal, in press.

Al Moustafa AE, Kassab A, Darnel A, Yasmeen A. High-risk HPV/ErbB-2 interaction on E-cadherin/catenin regulation in human carcinogenesis. Curr Pharm Des. 2008;14(22):2159-72.

Allinen M, Beroukhim R, Cai L, Brennan C, Lahti-Domenici J, Huang H, Porter D, Hu M, Chin L, Richardson A, Schnitt S, Sellers WR, Polyak K. Molecular characterization of the tumor microenvironment in breast cancer. Cancer Cell. 2004 Jul;6(1):17-32.

Altundag K, Bondy ML, Mirza NQ, Kau SW, Broglio K, Hortobagyi GN, Rivera E. Clinicopathologic characteristics and prognostic factors in 420 metastatic breast cancer patients with central nervous system metastasis. Cancer. 2007 Dec 15;110(12):2640-7.

Aragon-Ching JB, Zujewski JA. (2007). CNS metastasis: an old problem in a new guise. Clin Cancer Res, vol.13, no.6, (mar 2007), pp. 1644-1647.

Arnold SM, Young AB, Munn RK, Patchell RA, Nanayakkara N, Markesbery WR. Expression of p53, bcl-2, E-cadherin, matrix metalloproteinase-9, and tissue inhibitor of metalloproteinases-1 in paired primary tumors and brain metastasis. Clin Cancer Res. 1999 Dec;5(12):4028-33.

Auguste P, Lemiere S, Larrieu-Lahargue F, Bikfalvi A. Molecular mechanisms of tumor vascularization. Crit Rev Oncol Hematol 2005;54:53–61.

Baggiolini M. Chemokines and leukocyte traffic. Nature 1998; 392: 565–8.

Balabanian K, Lagane B, Infantino S, Chow KY, Harriague J, Moepps B, Arenzana-Seisdedos F, Thelen M, Bachelerie F. The chemokine SDF-1/CXCL12 binds to and signals through the orphan receptor RDC1 in T lymphocytes. J Biol Chem. 2005 Oct 21;280(42):35760-6.

Ballabh P, Braun A, Nedergaard M.The blood-brain barrier: an overview: structure, regulation, and clinical implications. Neurobiol Dis. 2004 Jun;16(1):1-13.

Bartholdi, D., Rubin, B.P., Schwab, M.E., 1997. VEGF mRNA induction correlates with changes in the vascular architecture upon spinal cord damage in the rat. Eur. J. Neurosci. 9, 2549–2560.

Bendell JC, Domchek SM, Burstein HJ, et al. 2003. Central nervous system metastases in women who receive trastuzumab-based therapy for metastatic breast carcinoma. Cancer, vol. 97, no. 12, pp. 2972–2977.

Bergers G, Brekken R, McMahon G, et al. Matrix metalloproteinase- 9 triggers the angiogenic switch during carcinogenesis. Nat Cell Biol 2000;2:737–44.

Berse B, Brown LF, Van de Water L, Dvorak HF, Senger DR. Vascular permeability factor (vascular endothelial growth factor) gene is expressed differentially in normal tissues, macrophages, and tumors. Mol Biol Cell 1992;3:211–20.

Bian XW, Yang SX, Chen JH, Ping YF, Zhou XD, Wang QL, Jiang XF, Gong W, Xiao HL, Du LL, Chen ZQ, Zhao W, Shi JQ, Wang JM. Preferential expression of chemokine receptor CXCR4 by highly malignant human gliomas and its association with poor patient survival. Neurosurgery. 2007 Sep;61(3):570-8; discussion 578-9.

Bonecchi R, Galliera E, Borroni EM, Corsi MM, Locati M, Mantovani A. Chemokines and chemokine receptors: an overview. Front Biosci. 2009 Jan 1;14:540-51

Bos PD, Zhang XH, Nadal C, Shu W, Gomis RR, Nguyen DX, Minn AJ, van de Vijver MJ, Gerald WL, Foekens JA, Massagué J. Genes that mediate breast cancer metastasis to the brain. Nature. 2009 Jun 18;459(7249):1005-9.

Breier G, Albrecht U, Sterrer S, Risau W. Expression of vascular endothelial growth factor during embryonic angiogenesis and endothelial cell differentiation. Development 1992;114:521–32.

Bremnes RM, Veve R, Hirsch FR, Franklin WA. The E-cadherin cell-cell adhesion complex and lung cancer invasion, metastasis, and prognosis. Lung Cancer. 2002 May;36(2):115-24.

Brown, L. F., Berse, B., Jackman, R. W. Tognazzi, K. Guidi, A. J. Dvorak, H. F. Senger, D. R. Connolly, J. L. Schnitt, S. J. 1995. "Expression of vascular permeability factor (vascular endothelial growth factor) and its receptors in breast cancer." Hum Pathol 26(1): 86-91.

Bublil EM, Yarden Y. The EGF receptor family: spearheading a merger of signaling and therapeutics. Current opinion in cell biology 2007; 19:124-34.

Burger JA, Kipps TJ. CXCR4: A key receptor in the crosstalk between tumor cells and their microenvironment. Blood 2006; 107: 1761–7.

Burns JM, Summers BC, Wang Y, Melikian A, Berahovich R, Miao Z, Penfold ME, Sunshine MJ, Littman DR, Kuo CJ, Wei K, McMaster BE, Wright K, Howard MC, Schall TJ. A novel chemokine receptor for SDF-1 and I-TAC involved in cell survival, cell adhesion, and tumor development. J Exp Med. 2006 Sep 4;203(9):2201-13.

Burness ML, Grushko TA, Olopade OI. 2010. Epidermal growth factor receptor in triple-negative and basal-like breast cancer: promising clinical target or only a marker?. Cancer J, vol. 16, pp.23–32.

Cabioglu N, Summy J, Miller C, Parikh NU, Sahin AA, Tuzlali S, Pumiglia K, Gallick GE, Price JE. CXCL-12/stromal cell-derived factor-1alpha transactivates HER2-neu in breast cancer cells by a novel pathway involving Src kinase activation. Cancer Res. 2005 Aug 1;65(15):6493-7.

Carney W, Leitzel K, Ali S, Neumann R, Lipton A. 2007. HER-2 therapy. HER-2/neu diagnostics in breast cancer. Breast Cancer Res,. vol. 9:207.

Carotenuto P, Roma C, Rachiglio AM, Botti G, D'Alessio A, Normanno N. Triple negative breast cancer: from molecular portrait to therapeutic intervention. Crit Rev Eukaryot Gene Expr. 2010;20(1):17-34.

Carpenter G, Cohen S. Epidermal growth factor. 1990. J Biol Chem; vol. 265, pp.7709–7712.

Chang H, Riese DJ, 2nd, Gilbert W, Stern DF, McMahan UJ. Ligands for ErbB-family receptors encoded by a neuregulin-like gene. Nature 1997; 387:509-12.

Cheng X, Hung MC. Breast cancer brain metastases. Cancer Metastasis Rev. 2007 Dec;26(3-4):635-43.

Clayton AJ, Danson S, Jolly S, et al. 2004. Incidence of cerebral metastases in patients treated with trastuzumab for metastatic breast cancer. Br J Cancer, vol. 91, no. 4, pp. 639–643.

Da Silva L, Clarke C, Lakhani SR. 2007. Demystifying basal-like breast carcinomas. J Clin Pathol, vol. 60, no.12, pp 1328–1332.

Da Silva L, Simpson PT, Smart CE, Cocciardi S, Waddell N, et al. 2010. HER3 and downstream pathways are involved in colonization of brain metastases from breast cancer. Breast Cancer Research, vol. 12, no. 4, pp. 1–13.

Deryugina EI, Quigley JP. Matrix metalloproteinases and tumor metastasis. Cancer Metastasis Rev. 2006 Mar;25(1):9-34.

Dontu G, Al-Hajj M, Abdallah WM, Clarke MF, Wicha MS. Stem cells in normal breast development and breast cancer. Cell Prolif 2003; 36 (Suppl 1): 59–72.

Dougher, A. M., Wasserstrom, H., Torley, L. Shridaran, L. Westdock, P. Hileman, R. E. Fromm, J. R. Anderberg, R. Lyman, S. Linhardt, R. J. Kaplan, J. Terman, B. I. 1997. "Identification of a heparin binding peptide on the extracellular domain of the KDR VEGF receptor." Growth Factors 14(4): 257-68.

Evans AJ, James JJ, Cornford EJ, et al. Brain metastases from breast cancer: 2004.identification of a high-risk group. Clin Oncol (R Coll Radiol (Great Britain); vol. 16, no. 5, pp. 345–349.

Fan P, Yue W, Wang JP, Aiyar S, Li Y, Kim TH, et al. 2009. Mechanisms of resistance to structurally diverse antiestrogens differ under premenopausal and postmenopausal conditions: evidence from in vitro breast cancer cell models. Endocrinology, vol. 150, no.5, pp. 2036–2045.

Fantl WJ, Johnson DE, Williams LT. Signalling by receptor tyrosine kinases. Annu Rev Biochem 1993;62:453–81.

Feng Y, Broder CC, Kennedy PE, Berger EA. HIV-1 entry cofactor: Functional cDNA cloning of a seven-transmembrane, G protein-coupled receptor. Science 1996; 272: 872–7.

Figarella-Branger D, Pellissier JF, Bouillot P, Bianco N, Mayan M, Grisoli F, Rougon G.Expression of neural cell-adhesion molecule isoforms and epithelial cadherin adhesion molecules in 47 human meningiomas: correlation with clinical and morphological data. Mod Pathol. 1994 Sep;7(7):752-61.

Fischer, I., J. P. Gagner, Law, M. Newcomb, E. W. Zagzag, D. 2005. "Angiogenesis in gliomas: biology and molecular pathophysiology." Brain Pathol 15(4): 297-310.

Folkman J. (1971) Tumor angiogenesis: therapeutic implications. N Engl J Med; 285:1182-1186.

Fredriksson R, Lagerstrom MC, Lundin LG, Schioth HB. The G-protein-coupled receptors in the human genome form five main families. Phylogenetic analysis, paralogon groups, and fingerprints. Mol Pharmacol 2003; 63: 1256–72.

Fukuzawa, M., Sugiura, H., Koshinaga, T., Ikeda, T., Hagiwara, N., Sawada, T. (2002). "Expression of vascular endothelial growth factor and its receptor Flk-1 in human neuroblastoma using in situ hybridization." J Pediatr Surg 37(12): 1747-50.

Fulton AM. The chemokine receptors CXCR4 and CXCR3 in cancer. Curr Oncol Rep. 2009 Mar;11(2):125-31.

Furusato B, Mohamed A, Uhlén M, Rhim JS. CXCR4 and cancer. Pathol Int. 2010 Jul;60(7):497-505

Gabos Z, Sinha R, Hanson J, et al. 2006. Prognostic significance of human epidermal growth factor receptor positivity for the development of brain metastasis after newly diagnosed breast cancer. J Clin Oncol , vol. 24, no.36, pp. 5658–5663.

Geminder H, Sagi-Assif O, Goldberg L, Meshel T, Rechavi G, Witz IP, Ben-Baruch A. A possible role for CXCR4 and its ligand, the CXC chemokine stromal cell-derived factor-1, in the development of bone marrow metastases in neuroblastoma. J Immunol. 2001 Oct 15;167(8):4747-57.

Gerhardt H, Golding M, Fruttiger M, et al. VEGF guides angiogenic sprouting utilizing endothelial tip cell filopodia. J Cell Biol 2003;161:1163–77.

Gluzman-Poltorak, Z., Cohen, T., Herzog, Y. Neufeld, G. 2000. "Neuropilin-2 is a receptor for the vascular endothelial growth factor (VEGF) forms VEGF-145 and VEGF-165 [corrected]." J Biol Chem 275(24): 18040-5.

Grandis JR, Sok JC .(2004). Signaling through the epidermal growth factor receptor during the development of malignancy. Pharmacol Ther, vol 102, pp. 37- 46.

Graumann, U., R. Reynolds, Steck, A. J., Schaeren-Wiemers, N. 2003. "Molecular changes in normal appearing white matter in multiple sclerosis are characteristic of neuroprotective mechanisms against hypoxic insult." Brain Pathol 13(4): 554-73.

Harlozinska A. Progress in molecular mechanisms of tumor metastasis and angiogenesis. Anticancer Res. 2005; 25: 3327–33.

Hattori K, Heissig B, Tashiro K, Honjo T, Tateno M, Shieh JH, Hackett NR, Quitoriano MS, Crystal RG, Rafii S, Moore MA. Plasma elevation of stromal cell-derived factor-1 induces mobilization of mature and immature hematopoietic progenitor and stem cells. Blood. 2001 Jun 1;97(11):3354-60.

Hinton CV, Avraham S, Avraham HK. Contributions of integrin-linked kinase to breast cancer metastasis and tumourigenesis. J Cell Mol Med. 2008 Sep-Oct;12(5A):1517-26.

Hinton CV, Avraham S, Avraham HK. Role of the CXCR4/CXCL12 signaling axis in breast cancer metastasis to the brain. Clin Exp Metastasis. 2010 Feb;27(2):97-105.

Hoeben A, Landuyt B, Highley MS, Wildiers H, Van Oosterom AT, De Bruijn EA. Vascular endothelial growth factor and angiogenesis. Pharmacol Rev 2004;56:549–80.

Holash J, Maisonpierre PC, Compton D, et al. Vessel cooption, regression, and growth in tumors mediated by angiopoietins and VEGF. Science 1999;284:1994–8.

Holland JD, Kochetkova M, Akekawatchai C, Dottore M, Lopez A, McColl SR.Differential functional activation of chemokine receptor CXCR4 is mediated by G proteins in breast cancer cells. Cancer Res. 2006 Apr 15;66(8):4117-24.

Howng SL, Wu CH, Cheng TS, Sy WD, Lin PC, Wang C, Hong YR. Differential expression of Wnt genes, beta-catenin and E-cadherin in human brain tumors. Cancer Lett. 2002 Sep 8;183(1):95-101.

Issa, R., Krupinski, J., Bujny, T., Kumar, S., Kaluza, J., Kumar, P., 1999. Vascular endothelial growth factor and its receptor, KDR, in human brain tissue after ischemic stroke. Lab. Invest. 79, 417–425.

Jäälinojä J, Herva R, Korpela M, Höyhtyä M, Turpeenniemi-Hujanen T. Matrix metalloproteinase 2 (MMP-2) immunoreactive protein is associated with poor grade and survival in brain neoplasms. J Neurooncol. 2000;46(1):81-90.

Jin, K.L., Mao, X.O., Nagayama, T., Goldsmith, P.C., Greenberg, D.A., 2000. Induction of vascular endothelial growth factor and hypoxiainducible factor-1 alpha by global ischemia in rat brain. Neuroscience 99, 577–585.

Jordan VC, O'Malley BW. (2007). Selective estrogen-receptor modulators and antihormonal resistance in breast cancer. J Clin Oncol, vol. 25, no.36, pp. 5815–5824.

Kang Y, Siegel PM, Shu W, Drobnjak M, Kakonen SM, Cordón-Cardo C, Guise TA, Massagué J. A multigenic program mediating breast cancer metastasis to bone. Cancer Cell. 2003 Jun;3(6):537-49.

Kaplan RN, Rafii S, Lyden D. Preparing the "soil": the premetastatic niche. Cancer Res. 2006; 66: 11089–93.

Kennecke H, Yerushalmi R, Woods R, Cheang MC, Voduc D, Speers CH, Nielsen TO, Gelmon K. Metastatic behavior of breast cancer subtypes. J Clin Oncol. 2010 Jul 10;28(20):3271-7.

Kessenbrock K, Plaks V, Werb Z. Matrix metalloproteinases: regulators of the tumor microenvironment. Cell. 2010 Apr 2;141(1):52-67.

Klein A, Olendrowitz C, Schmutzler R, Hampl J, Schlag PM, Maass N, Arnold N, Wessel R, Ramser J, Meindl A, Scherneck S, Seitz S. Identification of brain- and bone-specific breast cancer metastasis genes. Cancer Lett. 2009 Apr 18;276(2):212-20

Korkaya H, Paulson A, Iovino F, Wicha MS. 2008. HER2 regulates the mammary stem/progenitor cell population driving tumorigenesis and invasion. Oncogene, vol. 27, pp. 6120–6130.

Kremer, C., Breier, G., Risau, W., Plate, K.H., 1997. Up-regulation of flk-1/vascular endothelial growth factor receptor 2 by its ligand in a cerebral slice culture system. Cancer Res. 57, 3852–3859.

Krum, J. M., Mani, N., Rosenstein, J. M. 2008. "Roles of the endogenous VEGF receptors flt-1 and flk-1 in astroglial and vascular remodeling after brain injury." Exp Neurol 212(1): 108-17.

Krum, J.M., Mani, N., Rosenstein, J.M., 2002. Angiogenic and astroglial responses to vascular endothelial growth factor administration in adult rat brain. Neuroscience 110, 589–604.

Krum, J.M., Rosenstein, J.M., 1999. Transient coexpression of nestin, GFAP, and vascular endothelial growth factor in mature reactive astroglia following neural grafting or brain wounds. Exp. Neurol. 160, 348–360.

Kukk E, Lymboussaki A, Taira S, et al. VEGF-C receptor binding and pattern of expression with VEGFR-3 suggests a role in lymphatic vascular development. Development 1996;122:3829–37.

Kunkel P, Ulbricht U, Bohlen P, et al. Inhibition of glioma angiogenesis and growth in vivo by systemic treatment with a monoclonal antibody against vascular endothelial growth factor receptor-2. Cancer Res 2001;61:6624–8.

Kusters B, Leenders WP, Wesseling P, et al. Vascular endothelial growth factor-A(165) induces progression of melanoma brain metastases without induction of sprouting angiogenesis. Cancer Res 2002;62:341–5.

Lai R, Dang CT, Malkin MG, Abrey LE. 2004. The risk of central nervous system metastases after trastuzumab therapy in patients with breast carcinoma. Cancer; vol. 101, pp. 810–6.

Landis SH, Murray T, Bolden S, Wingo PA. Cancer statistics, 1999. CA Cancer J Clin. 1999 Jan-Feb;49(1):8-31, 1.

Lapidot T, Petit I. Current understanding of stem cell mobilization: The roles of chemokines, proteolytic enzymes, adhesion molecules, cytokines, and stromal cells. Exp Hematol 2002; 30: 973–81.

Law AJ, Shannon Weickert C, Hyde TM, Kleinman JE, Harrison PJ. 2004. Neuregulin-1 (NRG-1) mRNA and protein in the adult human brain. Neuroscience, vol. 127, pp. 125-136.

Lee SS, Ahn JH, Kim MK, Sym SJ, Gong G, Ahn SD, Kim SB, Kim WK. Brain metastases in breast cancer: prognostic factors and management. Breast Cancer Res Treat. 2008 Oct;111(3):523-30.

Lee, M.Y., Ju, W.K., Cha, J.H., Son, B.C., Chun, M.H., Kang, J.K., Park, C.K., 1999. Expression of vascular endothelial growth factor mRNA following transient forebrain ischemia in rats. Neurosci. Lett. 265, 107–110.

Lee-Hoeflich ST, Crocker L, Yao E, Pham T, Munroe X, Hoeflich KP, et al. 2008. A central role for HER3 in HER2-amplified breast cancer: implications for targeted therapy. Cancer Res, vol. 68, pp. 5878–5887.

Lewis-Tuffin LJ, Rodriguez F, Giannini C, Scheithauer B, Necela BM, Sarkaria JN, Anastasiadis PZ. Misregulated E-cadherin expression associated with an aggressive brain tumor phenotype. PLoS One. 2010 Oct 27;5(10):e13665.

Li, X., U. Eriksson, Novel VEGF family members: VEGF-B, VEGF-C and VEGF-D, Int. J. Biochem. Cell Biol. 2001, 33, 421–426.

Liang Z, Yoon Y, Votaw J, Goodman MM, Williams L, Shim H. Silencing of CXCR4 blocks breast cancer metastasis. Cancer Res. 2005 Feb 1;65(3):967-71.

Lin NU, Bellon JR, Winer EP. CNS metastases in breast cancer. J Clin Oncol 2004;22:3608-3617.

Locati M, Murphy PM. Chemokines and chemokine receptors: biology and clinical relevance in inflammation and AIDS. Annu Rev Med. 1999;50:425-40.

Loetscher P, Moser B, Baggiolini M. Chemokines and their receptors in lymphocyte traffic and HIV infection. Adv Immunol 2000; 74: 127–80.

Luster AD. Chemokines--chemotactic cytokines that mediate inflammation. N Engl J Med. 1998 Feb 12;338(7):436-45

Lymboussaki, A., Olofsson, B., Eriksson, U., Alitalo, K., 1999. "Vascular endothelial growth factor (VEGF) and VEGF-C show overlapping binding sites in embryonic endothelia and distinct sites in differentiated adult endothelia." Circ Res 85(11): 992-9.

Maharaj AS, Saint-Geniez M, Maldonado AE, D'Amore PA. Vascular endothelial growth factor localization in the adult. Am J Pathol 2006;168:639–48.

Mani, N., Khaibullina, A., Krum, J. M., Rosenstein, J. M. 2005. "Astrocyte growth effects of vascular endothelial growth factor (VEGF) application to perinatal neocortical explants: receptor mediation and signal transduction pathways." Exp Neurol 192(2): 394-406.

Mayer M. A patient perspective on brain metastases in breast cancer. Clin Cancer Res 2007;13:1623-1624.

McGrath KE, Koniski AD, Maltby KM, McGann JK, Palis J. Embryonic expression and function of the chemokine SDF-1 and its receptor, CXCR4. Dev Biol 1999; 213: 442–56.

Mendes O, Kim HT, Stoica G. Expression of MMP2, MMP9 and MMP3 in breast cancer brain metastasis in a rat model. Clin Exp Metastasis. 2005;22(3):237-46.

Mentzel, T., L. F. Brown, Dvorak, H. F. Kuhnen, C. Stiller, K. J. Katenkamp, D. Fletcher, C. D. 2001. "The association between tumour progression and vascularity in myxofibrosarcoma and myxoid/round cell liposarcoma." Virchows Arch 438(1): 13-22.

Millauer, B., Wizigmann-Voos, S., Schnurch, H., Martinez, R., Moller, N.P., Risau, W., Ullrich, A., 1993. High affinity VEGF binding and developmental expression suggest Flk-1 as a major regulator of vasculogenesis and angiogenesis. Cell 72, 835–846.

Monacci, W.T., Merrill, M.J., Oldfield, E.H., 1993. Expression of vascular permeability factor/vascular endothelial growth factor in normal rat tissues. Am. J. Physiol. 264, 995-1002.

Moser B, Loetscher P. Lymphocyte traffic control by chemokines. Nat Immunol 2001; 2: 123-8.

Müller A, Homey B, Soto H, Ge N, Catron D, Buchanan ME, McClanahan T, Murphy E, Yuan W, Wagner SN, Barrera JL, Mohar A, Verástegui E, Zlotnik A. Involvement of chemokine receptors in breast cancer metastasis. Nature. 2001 Mar 1;410(6824):50-6.

Murphy G. The ADAMs: signalling scissors in the tumour microenvironment. Nat Rev Cancer. 2008 Dec;8(12):929-41.

Murphy PM, Baggiolini M, Charo IF, Hébert CA, Horuk R, Matsushima K, Miller LH, Oppenheim JJ, Power CA. International union of pharmacology. XXII. Nomenclature for chemokine receptors. Pharmacol Rev. 2000 Mar;52(1):145-76.

Murphy PM. The molecular biology of leukocyte chemoattractant receptors. Annu Rev Immunol 1994; 12: 593-633.

Nag, S., Takahashi, J.L., Kilty, D.W., 1997. Role of vascular endothelial growth factor in blood-brain barrier breakdown and angiogenesis in brain trauma. J. Neuropathol. Exp. Neurol. 56, 912-921.

Nagasawa T, Hirota S, Tachibana K, Takakura N, Nishikawa S, Kitamura Y, Yoshida N, Kikutani H, Kishimoto T. Defects of B-cell lymphopoiesis and bone-marrow myelopoiesis in mice lacking the CXC chemokine PBSF/SDF-1. Nature. 1996 Aug 15;382(6592):635-8.

Nagy, J.A., A.M. Dvorak, H.F. Dvorak, VEGF-A(164/165) and PlGF: roles in angiogenesis and arteriogenesis, Trends Cardiovasc. Med. 2003, 13, 169- 175.

Nathoo N, Chahlavi A, Barnett GH, Toms SA. Pathobiology of brain metastases. J Clin Pathol. 2005 Mar;58(3):237-42.

Ng YS, Rohan R, Sunday ME, Demello DE, D'Amore PA. Differential expression of VEGF isoforms in mouse during development and in the adult. Dev Dyn 2001;220:112-21.

Ogawa K, Yoshii Y, Nishimaki T, Tamaki N, Miyaguni T, Tsuchida Y, Kamada Y, Toita T, Kakinohana Y, Tamaki W, Iraha S, Adachi G, Hyodo A, Murayama S. Treatment and prognosis of brain metastases from breast cancer. J Neurooncol. 2008 Jan;86(2):231-8.

Ogunshola, O.O., Stewart, W.B., Mihalcik, V., Solli, T., Madri, J.A., Ment, L.R., 2000. Neuronal VEGF expression correlates with angiogenesis in postnatal developing rat brain. Brain Res. Dev. Brain Res. 119, 139- 153.

Orimo A, Gupta PB, Sgroi DC, Arenzana-Seisdedos F, Delaunay T, Naeem R, Carey VJ, Richardson AL, Weinberg RA. Stromal fibroblasts present in invasive human breast carcinomas promote tumor growth and angiogenesis through elevated SDF-1/CXCL12 secretion. Cell. 2005 May 6;121(3):335-48.

Ottaiano A, Franco R, Aiello Talamanca A, Liguori G, Tatangelo F, Delrio P, Nasti G, Barletta E, Facchini G, Daniele B, Di Blasi A, Napolitano M, Ieranò C, Calemma R, Leonardi E, Albino V, De Angelis V, Falanga M, Boccia V, Capuozzo M, Parisi V, Botti G, Castello G, Vincenzo Iaffaioli R, Scala S. Overexpression of both CXC chemokine receptor 4 and vascular endothelial growth factor proteins predicts early distant relapse in stage II-III colorectal cancer patients. Clin Cancer Res. 2006 May 1;12(9):2795-803.

Palmieri D, Smith QR, Lockman PR, Bronder J, Gril B, Chambers AF, Weil RJ, Steeg PS. Brain metastases of breast cancer. Breast Dis. 2006-2007; 26: 139–47.

Papavassiliou, E., Gogate, N., Proescholdt, M., Heiss, J.D., Walbridge, S., Edwards, N.A., Oldfield, E.H., Merrill, M.J., 1997. Vascular endothelial growth factor (vascular permeability factor) expression in injured rat brain. J. Neurosci. Res. 49, 451–460.

Patchell RA. The management of brain metastases. Cancer Treat Rev. 2003 Dec;29(6):533-40.

Pawlowski V, Revillion F, Hebbar M, Hornez L, Peyrat JP. 2000. Prognostic value of the type I growth factor receptors in a large series of human primary breast cancers quantified with a real-time reverse transcription-polymerase chain reaction assay. Clin Cancer Res, 6, pp. 4217–4225.

Pepper MS, Ferrara N, Orci L, Montesano R. Vascular endothelial growth factor (VEGF) induces plasminogen activators and plasminogen activator inhibitor-1 in microvascular endothelial cells. Biochem Biophys Res Commun 1991;181:902–6.

Pestalozzi BC, Brignoli S. 2000. Trastuzumab in CSF. J Clin Oncol, vol. 18, no.11, pp. 2349–2351.

Pestalozzi BC, Zahrieh D, Price KN, et al. 2006. Identifying breast cancer patients at risk for Central Nervous System (CNS) metastases in trials of the International Breast Cancer Study Group (IBCSG). Ann Oncol, vol. 17, no. 6, pp. 935–944.

Peters, K.G., De Vries, C., Williams, L.T., 1993. Vascular endothelial growth factor receptor expression during embryogenesis and tissue repair suggests a role in endothelial differentiation and blood vessel growth. Proc. Natl. Acad. Sci. USA 90, 8915–8919.

Pietsch, T., Valter, M.M., Wolf, H.K., von Deimling, A., Huang, H.J., Cavenee, W.K., Wiestler, O.D., 1997. Expression and distribution of vascular endothelial growth factor protein in human brain tumors. Acta Neuropathol. 93, 109–117.

Plate, K.H., Beck, H., Danner, S., Allegrini, P.R., Wiessner, C., 1999. Cell type specific upregulation of vascular endothelial growth factor in an MCA-occlusion model of cerebral infarct. J. Neuropathol. Exp. Neurol. 58, 654–666.

Porcile C, Bajetto A, Barbero S, Pirani P, Schettini G. CXCR4 activation induces epidermal growth factor receptor transactivation in an ovarian cancer cell line. Ann N Y Acad Sci 2004; 1030: 162–9.

Prudkin L, Liu DD, Ozburn NC, Sun M, Behrens C, Tang X, Brown KC, Bekele BN, Moran C, Wistuba II. Epithelial-to-mesenchymal transition in the development and progression of adenocarcinoma and squamous cell carcinoma of the lung. Mod Pathol. 2009 May;22(5):668-78.

Razmkhah M, Talei AR, Doroudchi M, Khalili-Azad T, Ghaderi A. Stromal cell-derived factor-1 (SDF-1) alleles and susceptibility to breast carcinoma. Cancer Lett. 2005 Jul 28;225(2):261-6.

Raymond E, Faivre S, Armand JP: Epidermal growth factor receptor tyrosine kinase as a target for anticancer therapy. Drugs 2000, 60 Suppl, no.1, pp. 15-23.

Ribatti, D., Alessandri, G., Vacca, A. Iurlaro, M., Ponzoni, M., (1998). "Human neuroblastoma cells produce extracellular matrix-degrading enzymes, induce endothelial cell proliferation and are angiogenic in vivo." Int J Cancer 77(3): 449-54.

Rusnak DW, Lackey K, Affleck K, et al. 2001. The effects of the novel, reversible epidermal growth factor receptor/ErbB-2 tyrosine kinase inhibitor,GW2016, on the growth of human normal and tumor-derived cell lines in vitro and in vivo. Mol Cancer Ther. 2001, vol. 1, no. 2, (Dec 2001), pp. 85–94.

Saad AG, Yeap BY, Thunnissen FB, Pinkus GS, Pinkus JL, Loda M, Sugarbaker DJ, Johnson BE, Chirieac LR. Immunohistochemical markers associated with brain metastases in patients with nonsmall cell lung carcinoma. Cancer. 2008 Oct 15;113(8):2129-38.

Samoto K, Ikezaki K, One M, Shone T, Kohno K, Kuwano M, Fukui M: Expression of vascular endothelial growth factor and its possible relation with ueovascularization in human brain tumours. *Cancer Res* 1995, 55:1189-1193.

Sanna G, Franceschelli L, Rotmensz N, Botteri E, Adamoli L, Marenghi C, Munzone E, Cossu Rocca M, Verri E, Minchella I, Medici M, Catania C, Magni E, Goldhirsch A, Nolè F. Brain metastases in patients with advanced breast cancer. Anticancer Res. 2007; 27: 2865–9.

Scala S, Ottaiano A, Ascierto PA, Cavalli M, Simeone E, Giuliano P, Napolitano M, Franco R, Botti G, Castello G. Expression of CXCR4 predicts poor prognosis in patients with malignant melanoma. Clin Cancer Res. 2005 Mar 1;11(5):1835-41.

Schwechheimer K, Zhou L, Birchmeier W. E-Cadherin in human brain tumours: loss of immunoreactivity in malignant meningiomas. Virchows Arch. 1998 Feb;432(2):163-7.

Shabani HK, Kitange G, Tsunoda K, Anda T, Tokunaga Y, Shibata S, Kaminogo M, Hayashi T, Ayabe H, Iseki M. Immunohistochemical expression of E-cadherin in metastatic brain tumors. Brain Tumor Pathol. 2003;20(1):7-12.

Shemirani, B. and D. L. Crowe. 2000. "Head and neck squamous cell carcinoma lines produce biologically active angiogenic factors." Oral Oncol 36(1): 61-6.

Sierro F, Biben C, Martínez-Muñoz L, Mellado M, Ransohoff RM, Li M, Woehl B, Leung H, Groom J, Batten M, Harvey RP, Martínez-A C, Mackay CR, Mackay F. Disrupted cardiac development but normal hematopoiesis in mice deficient in the second CXCL12/SDF-1 receptor, CXCR7. Proc Natl Acad Sci U S A. 2007 Sep 11;104(37):14759-64.

Silverman WF, Krum JM, Mani N, Rosenstein JM. Vascular, glial and neuronal effects of vascular endothelial growth factor in mesencephalic explant cultures. Neuroscience. 1999;90(4):1529-41.

Slamon DJ, Clark GM, Wong SG, et al. 1987. Human breast cancer: correlation of relapse and survival with amplification of the HER2/neu oncogene. Science, vol. 235, pp.177–182.

Soker, S., Takashima, S., Miao, H.Q., Neufeld, G., Klagsbrun, M., 1998. Neuropilin-1 is expressed by endothelial and tumor cells as an isoformspecific receptor for vascular endothelial growth factor. Cell 92, 735– 745.

Stark AM, Anuszkiewicz B, Mentlein R, Yoneda T, Mehdorn HM, Held-Feindt J. Differential expression of matrix metalloproteinases in brain- and bone-seeking clones of metastatic MDA-MB-231 breast cancer cells. J Neurooncol. 2007 Jan;81(1):39-48.

Strugar JS, Rothbart D, Harrington W, Criscuolo GR: Vascular permeability factor in brain metastases: correlation with vasogenic brain edema and tumour angiogenesis. *J Neurosurg* 1994, 81:560-566.

Sun YX, Wang J, Shelburne CE, Lopatin DE, Chinnaiyan AM, Rubin MA, Pienta KJ, Taichman RS. Expression of CXCR4 and CXCL12 (SDF-1) in human prostate cancers (PCa) in vivo. J Cell Biochem. 2003 Jun 1;89(3):462-73.

Tachibana K, Hirota S, Iizasa H, Yoshida H, Kawabata K, Kataoka Y, Kitamura Y, Matsushima K, Yoshida N, Nishikawa S, Kishimoto T, Nagasawa T. The chemokine receptor CXCR4 is essential for vascularization of the gastrointestinal tract. Nature. 1998 Jun 11;393(6685):591-4.

Terman B, Khandke L, Dougher-Vermazan M, Maglione D, Lassam NJ, Gospodarowicz D, Persico MG, Böhlen P, Eisinger M. VEGF receptor subtypes KDR and FLT1 show different sensitivities to heparin and placenta growth factor. Growth Factors. 1994;11(3):187-95.

Tester AM, Waltham M, Oh SJ, Bae SN, Bills MM, Walker EC, Kern FG, Stetler-Stevenson WG, Lippman ME, Thompson EW. Pro-matrix metalloproteinase-2 transfection increases orthotopic primary growth and experimental metastasis of MDA-MB-231 human breast cancer cells in nude mice. Cancer Res. 2004 Jan 15;64(2):652-8.

Thelen M, Thelen S. CXCR7, CXCR4 and CXCL12: an eccentric trio? J Neuroimmunol. 2008 Jul 31;198(1-2):9-13.

Tohma Y, Yamashima T, Yamashita J. Immunohistochemical localization of cell adhesion molecule epithelial cadherin in human arachnoid villi and meningiomas. Cancer Res. 1992 Apr 1;52(7):1981-7.

Tsao, M.N., Li, Y.Q., Lu, G., Xu, Y., Wong, C.S., 1999. Upregulation of vascular endothelial growth factor is associated with radiation-induced blood–spinal cord barrier breakdown. J. Neuropathol. Exp. Neurol. 58, 1051–1060.

Ueda Y, Neel NF, Schutyser E, Raman D, Richmond A. Deletion of the COOH-terminal domain of CXC chemokine receptor 4 leads to the down-regulation of cell-to-cell contact, enhanced motility and proliferation in breast carcinoma cells. Cancer Res. 2006 Jun 1;66(11):5665-75.

Vajkoczy P, Farhadi M, Gaumann A, et al. Microtumor growth initiates angiogenic sprouting with simultaneous expression of VEGF, VEGF receptor-2, and angiopoietin-2. J Clin Invest 2002;109:777–85.

VanMeter TE, Rooprai HK, Kibble MM, Fillmore HL, Broaddus WC, Pilkington GJ. The role of matrix metalloproteinase genes in glioma invasion: co-dependent and interactive proteolysis. J Neurooncol. 2001 Jun;53(2):213-35.

Vaquero, J., Zurita, M., de Oya, S., Coca, S., 1999. Vascular endothelial growth/permeability factor in spinal cord injury. J. Neurosurg. 90, 220–223.

Vates, G. E., Hashimoto, T., Young, W. L., Lawton, M. T. 2005. "Angiogenesis in the brain during development: the effects of vascular endothelial growth factor and angiopoietin-2 in an animal model." J Neurosurg 103(1): 136-45.

Vu TH, Shipley JM, Bergers G, et al. MMP-9/gelatinase B is a key regulator of growth plate angiogenesis and apoptosis of hypertrophic chondrocytes. Cell 1998;93:411–22.

Wang J, Jarrett J, Huang CC, Satcher RL Jr, Levenson AS. Identification of estrogen-responsive genes involved in breast cancer metastases to the bone. Clin Exp Metastasis. 2007; 24: 411–22.

Xu, T., Chen, D., Chen, J. 2004. "Expression of vascular endothelial growth factor C and its correlation with lymph node metastasis in colorectal carcinoma." J Huazhong Univ Sci Technolog Med Sci 24(6): 596-8.

Xue C, Liang F, Mahmood R, Vuolo M, Wyckoff J, et al. 2006. ErbB3-dependent motility and intravasation in breast cancer metastasis. Cancer Res, vol. 66, no.3, pp.1418–1426.

Yamazaki, Y. , K. Takani, H. Atoda, T. Morita, Snake venom vascular endothelial growth factors (VEGFs) exhibit potent activity through their specific recognition of KDR (VEGF receptor 2), J. Biol. Chem. 2003 278, 51985- 51988.

Yang W, Lam P, Kitching R, Kahn HJ, Yee A, Aubin JE, Seth A. Breast cancer metastasis in a human bone NOD/SCID mouse model. Cancer Biol Ther. 2007; 6: 1289–94.

Yang W, Lam P, Kitching R, Kahn HJ, Yee A, Aubin JE, Seth A. Breast cancer metastasis in a human bone NOD/SCID mouse model. Cancer Biol Ther. 2007; 6: 1289–94.

Yano, S., H. Shinohara, Herbst, R. S. Kuniyasu, H. Bucana, C. D. Ellis, L. M. Davis, D. W. McConkey, D. J. Fidler, I. J. 2000. "Expression of vascular endothelial growth factor is necessary but not sufficient for production and growth of brain metastasis." Cancer Res 60(17): 4959-67.

Yasmeen A, Bismar TA, Al Moustafa AE ErbB receptors and epithelial-cadherin-catenin complex in human carcinomas. Future Oncol. 2006 Dec;2(6):765-81.

Yasmeen A, Bismar TA, Dekhil H, Ricciardi R, Kassab A, Gambacorti-Passerini C, Al Moustafa AE. ErbB-2 receptor cooperates with E6/E7 oncoproteins of HPV type 16 in breast tumorigenesis. Cell Cycle. 2007 Dec 1;6(23):2939-43.

Zagzag D, Amirnovin R, Greco MA, et al. Vascular apoptosis and involution in gliomas precede neovascularization: a novel concept for glioma growth and angiogenesis. Lab Invest 2000;80: 837–49.

Zeljko M, Pecina-Slaus N, Martic TN, Kusec V, Beros V, Tomas D. Molecular alterations of E-cadherin and beta-catenin in brain metastases. Front Biosci (Elite Ed). 2011 Jan 1;3:616-24.

Zhan L, Xiang B, Muthuswamy SK. 2006. Controlled activation of ErbB1/ErbB2 heterodimerspromote invasion of three-dimensional organized epithelia in an ErbB1-dependent manner: implications for progression of ErbB2-overexpressing tumors. Cancer Res, 66, no. 3, pp. 5201–5208.

Zlotnik A, Yoshie O. Chemokines: a new classification system and their role in immunity. Immunity. 2000 Feb;12(2):121-7.

Zlotnik A. Chemokines and cancer. Int J Cancer 2006b; 119: 2026–9.

Zlotnik A. Involvement of chemokine receptors in organ-specific metastasis. Contrib Microbiol 2006a; 13: 191–9.

Zou YR, Kottmann AH, Kuroda M, Taniuchi I, Littman DR. Function of the chemokine receptor CXCR4 in haematopoiesis and in cerebellar development. Nature 1998; 393: 595–9.

6

Signal Transduction Pathways in Breast Cancer – Drug Targets and Challenges

Samar Azab[1] and Ayman Al-Hendy[2]
[1]*Pharmacology and Toxicology Department, Faculty of Pharmacy, Ain Shams University, Cairo,*
[2]*Center for Women Health Research, Department of Obstetrics and Gynecology, Meharry Medical College, Nashville, Tennessee,*
[1]*Egypt*
[2]*USA*

1. Introduction

Breast cancer is the most frequently diagnosed cancer and the leading cause of cancer death in females worldwide **[1].** Over 1.1 million cases of breast cancer are diagnosed across the world each year, compared with about 500,000 cases in 1975. This represents about 10% of all new cancer cases and 23% of all female cancers **[2-3]**. An annual prevalence of more than 4.4 million cases of breast cancer is expected worldwide by the year 2012 **[4]**.
In the past years, our knowledge of the genetic changes that contribute to breast cancer development & progression has tremendously changed **[5]**. Our knowledge of alterations in the cancer cell have allowed us to identify the signaling pathways that when disrupted allow a cancer cell to escape from normal control mechanisms **[6]**. On the other hand, these aberrant processes have also provided many therapeutic points for intervention, which is the major topic of this chapter. Following the successful introduction of trastuzumab, the first human epidermal growth factor receptor (HER) targeted therapy to become widely used in breast cancer patients, other agents have been developed **[7]**. Other potential hallmarks of malignancy that represent a new opportunity for therapeutic targeting include abrogation of apoptosis, lack of senescence, angiogenesis, tumor invasion and metastasis **[8]**. Therefore, new compounds are being developed that may interfere with these hallmarks and that may prove to be effective in monotherapy or in combination with cytotoxic therapy or other targeted therapies. Novel agents are needed because many of the current therapies have limitations. These include drug resistance, lack of target receptor expression in tumors and relatively small improvements in survival **[9-12]**.
Thus, this chapter provides an updated overview of the several signaling transduction pathways involved in development of breast cancer. In addition, it focuses on recent progress with the therapeutic strategies targeting these pathways contributing to their promising success in the clinical setting. Furthermore, molecular signals of its resistance phenotype and breast cancer stem cells & their therapeutic targeting are discussed briefly. Finally, the challenges facing the significant contribution of targeted therapeutics in breast cancer chemotherapy are also extensively discussed. Wherever possible, advances in drug analogs, accepted or controversial mechanisms described for their antitumor activity will be discussed within the framework of the current chapter.

Section A describes a reported panel of potential signal transduction pathways (STPs) that are altered in breast cancer and are undergoing research as targeted therapeutics. Some of these have yielded therapeutics that already had clinical success, while others are still in the experimental stages (**Fig. 1 & Tab.1**). Though many of the underlying mechanisms of the multi-drug resistance (MDR) phenotype are still not clearly identified, several potential molecular targets and pathways of activation have been suggested. The advances in this field provide an emerging picture of how MDR arises and how it could be therapeutically targeted. In **Section B**, we review the potential role of cancer stem cells molecular signaling in development of breast cancer & its resistance phenotype. It also discusses their putative modulation contributing to the success of targeted therapeutics in breast cancer chemotherapy.

	STP	STI	Mechanism
1	**Receptor tyrosine Kinase: I- HER2 receptor**	-Trastuzumab -Lapatinib, Erlotinib, Gefitinib and Neratinib	-Extracellular Targeted Therapeutic: Monoclonal Antibody inhibiting ligand binding to receptor -Intracellular Targeted Therapeutic: HER Receptor tyrosine kinase catalytic inhibitor
	Receptor tyrosine Kinase: II- Src receptor	Dasatinib	Intracellular Targeted Therapeutic: Src Receptor tyrosine kinase catalytic inhibitor
2	**MAPK Signaling Pathway**	Tipifarnib	Farnesyl transferase inhibitor
3	**PI3K/Akt/mTOR pathway**	-Perifosine -Temsirolimus and Everolimus -Octreotide	-Inhibitor of Akt phosphorylation -mTOR inhibitors -Inhibitor of IGF-1R signaling
4	**HSP90 signaling pathway**	Tanespimycin and Alvespimycin	Potent inhibitiors of HSP90 function
5	**PARP signaling pathway**	Olapraib Veliparib	PARP inhibitors
6	**Apoptosis & Autophagy pathways**		Inhibitors of the components of apoptotic & autophagic pathways
7	**Angiogenesis**	Bevacizumab	Extracellular Targeted Therapeutic: Monoclonal Antibody inhibiting ligand binding to receptor
8	**Multi-Target Therapeutics**	Sunitinib, Pazopanib, Sorafenib and Axitinib	Intracellular Targeted Therapeutic: Receptor tyrosine kinase catalytic inhibitors
9	**Estrogen signaling transduction**	-Tamoxifen -Letrozole	-Anti-estrogen -Aromatase inhibitor
10	**UPS signaling pathway**	Bortezomib	Proteasome inhibitor

Table 1. A list of the action site for signal transduction inhibitors (STIs) in breast cancer.

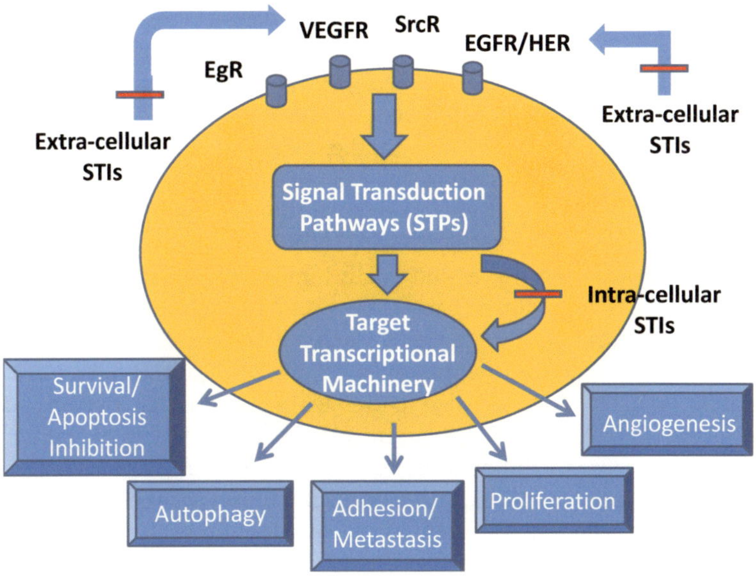

Fig. 1. Simplified schematic illustration of the multiple signal transduction pathways (STPs) in breast cancer.

2. Targeting signal transduction pathways in breast cancer

The mechanisms underlying the development of breast cancer are complex and vary among individual tumors **[13]**. Altered patterns of gene expression are associated with corresponding variations in growth rates, cellular composition and different prognoses **[14]**. Given the complex and varied factors that influence the development of breast cancer, and the use of increasingly sophisticated genetic analysis techniques, it is likely that more refined tumor subtypes and their associated prognoses will be identified**[13, 15]**. Advances in the understanding the etiology and biology of breast cancer have identified key targets among multiple signaling pathways involved in the development and survival of breast cancer cells. Thus, targeted therapies are among the most promising new agents for the treatment of breast cancer. Some of these reported breast cancer signaling transduction pathways (STPs) & their signal transduction inhibitors (STIs) are classified as follows:

2.1 STPs-1: Receptor Tyrosine Kinase (RTKs)

Altered patterns of gene expression can influence the activity of specific signaling pathways. For example, receptor tyrosine kinases (RTKs) are often aberrantly over-expressed or activated in human cancers. The epidermal growth factor receptor (EGFR) family is composed of cell surface tyrosine kinase receptors that are involved in the regulation of cellular proliferation and survival of epithelial cells. The EGFR (or also called HER) family includes four closely related receptors: EGFR/HER1/ErbB1, HER2 neu /ErbB2, HER3/ErbB3 and HER4/ErbB4 **[16]**.

2.1.1 HER2 receptor

Members of the HER family are encoded by genes on different chromosomes and regulate normal breast growth and development. The HER family couples to multiple signaling pathways that impact on all aspect of breast cancer biology. Through their interconnected cellular signaling network, the HER family regulates diverse biological processes, including cell proliferation, differentiation, and survival **[16-17].** Thus, they play a key role in the development and progression of breast cancer [16, 18-19].

Variations in the pathways associated with the HER family appear to be particularly important, not only in tumor development but also in treatment efficacy [20-21]**.** For example, in breast cancer, constitutive activation of the epidermal growth factor receptor (EGFR) and HER2 is found in approximately 16%-48% and 25%-30% of breast cancer tumors, respectively. Moreover, expression of HER family members in breast cancer tumors has a significant impact on tumor aggressiveness and patient survival. Importantly, their expression correlates with a more aggressive disease course, shorter survival time, and higher risk for resistance to endocrine therapies [10, 12, 22-27]. HER-3 expression, observed in approximately 18% of tumors, also correlates with shorter overall survival **[28].** Interestingly, expression of HER-4 (found in approximately 12% of tumors) has been associated with more favorable tumor characteristics and longer survival [27-28].

Each HER receptor has an extracellular domain (ECD) involved in ligand binding, a helical transmembrane segment, and an intracellular protein domain with tyrosine kinase activity. On ligand binding, the extracellular domains of the receptors undergo conformational changes, which allows them to form homodimers (consisting of two identical receptors) or heterodimers (consisting of two different receptors) of the HER family [16, 29]. Dimerization of HER receptors induces phosphorylation of their intracellular tyrosine kinase domains, which provide docking sites for adaptor proteins and signaling enzymes **[29]**.These molecules act as a link between membrane receptor kinases and "downstream" intracellular protein kinases, which results in the activation of multiple signaling pathways, of which the MAPK and PI3K pathways are probably the best studied **[29]**.

HER-2 is the preferred dimerization and signaling partner for all other members of the HER family, and it appears to function mainly as a co-receptor, increasing the affinity of ligand binding to dimerized receptor complexes [29-30]. With their multiple ligands, many dimerization combinations, and large number of downstream effectors, the HER family mediates an extensive range of signals, controlling a variety of cellular processes, including cellular proliferation, apoptosis, and angiogenesis [29, 31]. For example, HER2 receptor activation leads to the phosphorylation of the intracellular catalytic domains, and ultimately activation of signal transduction pathways that promote proliferation and survival, including the phosphatidylinositol 30-kinase (PI3K)/Akt/mTOR, the Erk1/2 mitogenactivated protein kinase (MAPK) and the Jak/Stat pathway **[32]**.

2.1.2 Src-family tyrosine kinases

The v-Src (Rous sarcoma virus) tyrosine kinase was the first oncogenic gene discovered **[33]**. The corresponding cellular gene, c-Src, is a non-receptor signaling kinase that functions as a hub of a vast array of signal transduction pathways that influence cellular proliferation, differentiation, motility and survival **[34]**. Several mechanisms lead to increased Src activity in tumors. Src is downstream in signaling from a number of growth factor receptors including PDGF receptor (PDGFR), epidermal growth factor receptor (EGFR) and insulin-like growth factor- 1 receptor (IGF-1R) **[35]**.

In many tumor types, over-expression of these receptors, their ligands or both is frequent **[36]**. For example, reported studies suggest an association between Src tyrosine kinase and the development, progression and metastasis of breast cancer [37-38]. In addition, it is described that mice over-expressing the HER2 oncogene develop highly metastatic mammary tumors with elevated Src activity **[37]**. Further supporting the role of Src in breast cancer, it has been demonstrated that Src activity is profoundly increased in human breast cancer tissues compared with benign breast tumors or adjacent normal breast tissues[38-39] and that elevated c-Src tyrosine kinase activity is correlated with early systemic relapse **[40]**. Taken together, these results strongly indicate that the Src may play an important role in the development and progression of breast cancer **[41]**.

2.2 STIs-1: Receptor Tyrosine Kinase Inhibitors (RTKIs)

2.2.1 HER2 receptor inhibitors

Numerous agents targeting individual members of the HER family have been developed for use in the treatment of breast cancer. Existing therapeutic approaches have largely focused on two classes of agents:

2.2.1.1 Extracellular targeted therapies

Monoclonal antibodies

The first comprises monoclonal antibodies that bind to extracellular regions of HER to interfere with receptor function (e.g., trastuzumab, pertuzumab, and a number of pan-HER inhibitors). Trastuzumab binds to the juxtamembrane region of HER-2 with high specificity, but it is not currently known how it specifically interferes with HER-2 function **[42]**. Pertuzumab is the first in a class of HER-2 dimerization inhibitors. Binding to HER-2 inhibits its dimerization with other HER receptors and this is thought to result in slowed tumor growth [43].

Trastuzumab, an HER2 specific humanized monoclonal antibody was one of the first biologicals to be approved for metastatic breast cancer treatment [44]. In patients, HER2 is over-expressed and/or amplified in one-fourth of breast tumors and confers a more aggressive clinical course and a worse survival [25, 45]. The outcome of these highly aggressive tumors has markedly improved with the development of anti-HER2 therapies. Trastuzumab (Herceptin®) is a recombinant humanised monoclonal antibody that binds with high affinity to the extracellular juxtamembrane domain of HER2 and inhibits the proliferation of human tumor cells that over-express HER2 in vitro and in vivo [46-48].

Trastuzumab. Trastuzumab, administered as an i.v. infusion, is approved in the U.S. and Europe for the treatment of HER-2–over-expressing metastatic breast cancer (MBC) [7]. It is standard-of-care treatment for MBC patients with HER-2–over-expressing tumors, both as first-line treatment in combination with chemotherapy and as a single agent in women who have HER-2–over-expressing breast cancer that has progressed after chemotherapy for metastatic disease[44, 49]. Trastuzumab is approved for the adjuvant treatment of HER-2+, node negative (ER-/progesterone receptor [PgR-]) or node-positive breast cancer, either in combination with chemotherapy or as a single agent following multi-modality anthracycline-based treatment.

In patients with HER2 amplified tumors, trastuzumab has single agent activity and improves survival in the first-line setting when combined with chemotherapy in patients with advanced disease [44, 50]. Recently, a number of well powered clinical trials have demonstrated that administration of trastuzumab in the adjuvant setting, in combination and/or sequentially after chemotherapy, results in an improvement in disease-free survival as well as overall survival **[51-54]**.

Trastuzumab efficacy in the metastatic setting has provided the rationale for several studies investigating the use of trastuzumab plus chemotherapy as adjuvant treatment for patients with earlystage HER-2+ breast cancer [52-53, 55-56]. Studies have evaluated a range of different trastuzumab-based combination regimens for the first-line treatment of MBC [50, 57]. Additionally, a number of trials are ongoing investigating trastuzumab in combination with hormonal therapy in MBC patients [58-59]. When administered as a single agent, trastuzumab has documented efficacy as a first-line therapy, with response rates typically in the range of 23%–33% [60-62]. Of those patients with MBC who do achieve an initial response, many experience disease progression within 12 months as a result of the high proportion of HER-2–over-expressing tumors that have intrinsic resistance to this agent **[63]**. Given the absence of known specific ligands for HER-2, thus there is no alternative approach to blocking this pathway except by trastuzumab. This has clinical implications as this may be related to the development of resistance to HER-2 blockade **[64]**.
On the other hand, changing the traditional treatment paradigm in patients progressing on trastuzumab and administering further trastuzumab-based therapy beyond disease progression may have clinical benefit [65-66].This "treatment beyond progression" approach is increasingly being studied in clinical trials by combining trastuzumab either with chemotherapy [67-68] or with another targeted agent, such as the RTKI lapatinib [69].
Trastuzumab-DM1 (T-DM1) is an anti–HER-2 antibody drug conjugate comprising trastuzumab linked to the maytansine derivative DM1. Combining these two agents facilitates anti–HER-2 activity as well as targeted intracellular delivery of a potent cytotoxic agent. Single-agent TDM1 as well tolerated, active and no dose-limiting cardiotoxicity was observed in a phase II study of 112 patients with pretreated MBC [7].

Limitations of Trastuzumab therapy

1. Trastuzumab is an effective treatment for patients with HER-2+ disease, yet its use is limited to this group (approximately 25%) [25]. Thus, accurate patient selection for treatment is important, using an appropriate method, such as immunohistochemistry or fluorescence in situ hybridization, to detect HER-2 over-expression.
2. Not all HER-2+ patients respond to treatment with trastuzumab, and the development of resistance is an issue. In the future, it may be possible to overcome resistance by combining trastuzumab with new therapies such as pertuzumab, by switching to an agent such as lapatinib that inhibits both HER-1 and HER-2 activity, or, if proven effective, the use of one of the pan-HER inhibitors currently in development.
3. Trastuzumab is unable to penetrate the blood– brain barrier (Guy et al., 1994) and over-expression of HER-2 is known to be associated with a greater risk for central nervous system (CNS) metastases [70]. Patients with HER-2+ MBC treated with trastuzumab appear to be at greater risk for developing CNS metastases than those who do not receive trastuzumab therapy [71]. However, HER-2+ patients with CNS metastases who are treated with trastuzumab appear to have a longer overall survival duration than those who are HER-2- or those unselected for HER-2 status. This may reflect greater control of extra-cranial disease as a result of trastuzumab therapy [72].
4. Treatment with trastuzumab is associated with a higher risk for cardiomyopathy (left ventricular dysfunction and congestive heart failure), particularly when used in combination with paclitaxel or anthracyclines [73]. However, these cardiotoxic effects appear to be reversible once trastuzumab treatment is discontinued or if they are managed with appropriate medical therapy [74-75]. The cellular mechanisms contributing to the cardiotoxicity observed with trastuzumab are still being explored. It

is known that HER-2 plays an important role in cardiomyocyte development and function, and trastuzumab- induced inhibition of HER-2 signaling in cardiomyocytes may be a central mechanism underlying the observed cardiomyopathy. However, the full explanation is likely to be more complex. Cardiotoxicity does not appear to be an issue with the RTKI lapatinib, which inhibits both HER-1 and HER- 2 [76]

5. Although cardiotoxicity is the primary safety concern with trastuzumab, potentially severe hypersensitivity reactions to infusion have also been reported [7].

Other example of novel anti-HER2 agents include antibodies that interfere with HER2 dimerisation. Pertuzumab is a recombinant, humanised MAb that targets an epitope within the HER2 dimerisation domain [77]. Once bound, pertuzumab inhibits ligand-activated HER dimerisation with HER2 and thereby inhibiting activation of intracellular signaling [78].

2.2.1.2 Intracellular targeted therapies

Receptor tyrosine kinase inhibitors (RKIs)

The second class of HER-targeted agents comprises the small molecule receptor tyrosine kinase inhibitors (RTKIs) that inhibit enzyme function of HER family members intracellularly. Oral RTKIs include lapatinib, neratinib (both inhibit HER-1 and HER-2), erlotinib and gefitinib that target the intracellular domain of HER-1, and the irreversible pan-HER inhibitors PF-00299804 and canertinib, which inhibit the kinase signaling of multiple HER family members [79].

Another strategy to target HER2 is with low molecular weight tyrosine kinase inhibitors. Lapatinib (Tykerb®) is a dual EGFR and HER2 inhibitor that has been studied extensively in multiple clinical settings. Lapatinib is approved in the U.S. (March 2007) and European Union (EU) (June 2008) for use (oral administration) in combination with capecitabine for the treatment of patients with advanced breast cancer or MBC whose tumors over-express HER-2 and who have received prior therapy including an anthracycline, a taxane, and trastuzumab [7].

Lapatinib increases survival in patients with advanced HER2-over-expressing breast cancer when given in combination with the chemotherapeutic agent capecitabine compared to capecitabine alone in patients that had previously failed anthracyclines and taxanes [80]. The incidences of adverse events (including those leading to treatment discontinuation) and symptomatic cardiac events were similar in both treatment groups. The observation that fewer patients in the lapatinib group developed central nervous system (CNS) metastases together with lapatinib's low molecular weight and capacity to cross the blood-brain barrier has led to a clinical trial to study the role of lapatinib in the treatment of brain metastasis in patients with HER2-over-expressing breast cancer [25, 28]. Thus, contrary to trastuzumab, lapatinib has a putative activity against CNS metastases in patients with HER-2+ breast cancer [81]. These data suggest that, as a small molecule RTKI, it may be able to cross the blood- brain barrier to provide effective therapeutic concentrations in cerebrospinal fluid (unlike monoclonal antibodies such as trastuzumab).

Lapatinib appears to be associated with less cardiotoxicity than trastuzumab [82]. However, as lapatinib development is extended to include the treatment of patients with lower-risk primary breast cancer, it will be increasingly important to monitor cardiotoxic effects. The most common adverse effects associated with lapatinib treatment are gastrointestinal; lapatinib-related diarrhea generally occurs early in the course of treatment, is mild to moderate, and does not require treatment, although monitoring is important to identify patients who may need intervention **[7]**.

Other examples of RTKIs include Erlotinib and Gefitinib. Recent clinical studies have not demonstrated any significant clinical benefit for erlotinib or gefitinib either as single agents or in combination with other agents in MBC [68, 83-85]. Given their lack of activity as monotherapy in MBC, studies continue to investigate the efficacy of erlotinib and gefitinib in combination with other targeted therapies, chemotherapy, or hormonal agents; however, tolerability issues may limit this approach.

Other anti-HER tyrosine kinase inhibitors in clinical development include HKI-272. Neratinib (HKI-272) is an orally administered, irreversible, pan-erbB kinase inhibitor [86] that covalently bind to the intracellular kinase domain. The observation that some patients with chronic myelogenous leukemia were developing resistance to the RTKI imatinib led to the development of neratinib. In preclinical models, neratinib has been shown to have promising antiproliferative activity in both HER-2–dependent cell lines and tumor xenografts.

Phase I/II data have confirmed that neratinib has antitumor activity in patients with HER-2+ MBC, either as a single agent in trastuzumab refractory patients or in combination with trastuzumab, and the safety profile of this agent has been manageable [87].

2.2.2 Src-family tyrosine kinases inhibitors

Currently, small-molecule Src inhibitors are in early phases of clinical development either as single agents, in combination with cytotoxic agents, biological therapies or in combination with hormonal treatment. Originally, dasatinib (BMS-354825) was selected as a synthetic small-molecule inhibitor of Src-family kinases; then, it was found to inhibit at least four other protein tyrosine kinases: bcr-abl, c-Kit, EphA2, PDGF-beta. Dasatinib is currently studied in clinical trials for the treatment of solid tumors, including breast cancer. Preclinical evidence suggests that dasatinib could be effective in breast cancer cell lines of basal-like subtype **[88]**. These findings provide scientific rationale for the clinical development of dasatinib in the treatment of patients with 'triple-negative' breast cancer, a tumor subtype that is categorised as being aggressive and lacking effective targeted treatments, such as endocrine therapies and anti- HER2 strategies. More recently, AZD-0530 a highly selective, dual-specific, orally available small-molecule inhibitor of Src kinase and Bcr-Abl has entered clinical trials **[89]**. In healthy volunteers, AZD-0530 has shown only mild adverse events.

Targeting downstream effector molecules

Targeting HER receptors with extracellular monoclonal antibodies and intracellular RTKIs has shown promising clinical activity. There is, however, a need for better treatment of MBC patients because many of these current therapies are restricted to a subset of the MBC patient population. Targeting cellular signaling pathways, such as the MAPK and PI3K pathways, downstream of HER receptors may be an attractive avenue for novel treatments. Additionally, there is some evidence that targeting heat shock proteins (Hsps) and the apoptotic pathway may be viable options for future therapeutic strategies in MBC. Recent developments in this field are briefly discussed in the following sections.

2.3 STPs-2: Targeting downstream MAPK signaling pathway

The MAPK pathway, also termed the extracellular signal-regulated kinase (ERK) pathway, contains downstream effectorsof the HER family and other tyrosine kinases, and is a central part of the signaling networks that control fundamental cellular processes, including cell proliferation, differentiation, and survival **[90]**.

2.4 STIs-2: Targeted therapies directed at the MAPK signaling pathway

The farnesyl transferase inhibitor tipifarnib (R115777) was evaluated in phase III trials for the treatment of breast cancer, although further development has now been terminated [91-93]. AZD6244 (ARRY-142886) is an inhibitor of the enzyme MEK, a component of the MAPK pathway. AZD6244 is currently in phase I clinical studies in several cancer types, including breast cancer.

2.5 STPs-3: Targeting downstream PI3K/Akt/mTOR pathway signaling pathway

The PI3K/Akt pathway plays a central role in diverse cellular functions including proliferation, growth, survival and metabolism. In addition to their physiological role, several isoforms of the PI3K family are implicated in tumor development, including cell proliferation, cell growth, cell motility, cell survival, and angiogenesis [29]. The relationship between dysregulated PI3K activity and the onset of cancer is well documented [94]. In particular, members of class 1A PI3Ks are often mutated in human cancer [95-100]. As a result of receptor tyrosine kinase RTK activation and phosphorylation, PI3K interacts with the intracellular domain of the receptors. Subsequent phosphorylation event by the mammalian target of rapamycin (mTOR)-complex is required for maximal Akt activity [101-102]. Akt is the central effector of the pathway. Akt reduces cell cycle inhibitors p27 and p21, and promotes cell cycle proteins c-Myc and cyclin D1, resulting in enhanced cellular proliferation. Its influence extends to a host of pro- and antiapoptotic proteins, such as the Bcl-2 family member Bad, limiting programmed cell death and boosting cellular survival. mTOR is a central regulator of cellular responses to multiple stimuli including amino acid availability and growth factor receptor signaling. In cells with sufficient nutrients, mTOR relays a signal to the translational machinery leading to an enhanced translation of mRNAs encoding proteins essential for cell growth and cell cycle progression [103-104].

There is growing evidence that uncontrolled activation of the phosphatidylinositol 3-kinase (PI3K)/Akt/mammalian target of rapamycin (mTOR) pathway, achieved via numerous genetic and epigenetic alterations, contributes to the development and progression of human cancers, including breast cancer [105]. In breast tumors, activating mutations in PIK3A, encoding the catalytic subunit of PI3K, or loss of PTEN, the negative regulator of PI3K activity, are very frequent and contribute to constitutive pathway activation and mTOR activity. Further, they may result in resistance to upstream anti-receptor agents. For example, trastuzumab depends on intact PTEN for its action in HER2-over-expressing breast cell lines, and PTEN loss predicts for trastuzumab resistance [106]. Therefore, this pathway is an attractive target for novel anticancer agents. Clinical trials are currently underway with mTOR, PI3K and Akt inhibitors.

2.6 STIs-3: Inhibitors of the PI3K/Akt/mTOR pathway

Therapies targeting the PI3K pathway include perifosine (KRX-0401), which inhibits Akt phosphorylation [107] and mTOR inhibitors are also further ahead in development within this class of agents. The rapamycin analogs that target mammalian target of rapamycin include temsirolimus (CCl-779) [108-109]. Rapamycin derivatives such as everolimus,

temsirolimus and deforolimus are potent inhibitors of mTOR and do not share the problems of poor solubility and chemical stability of rapamycin.
Recent data from two phase I trials suggest that everolimus can help overcome resistance to trastuzumab in women with HER-2+ MBC. Everolimus plus trastuzumab and weekly paclitaxel was shown to slow tumor growth in 77% of patients, and the combination of everolimus with trastuzumab and vinorelbine halted tumor growth in 62% of patients [110-111]. Although early indications suggest that targeting components of the PI3K pathway may have some activity in the treatment of MBC, additional data, including an understanding of combinations and patient selection, are required.
However, in unselected patients with breast cancer these agents have modest anti-tumor activity in the range of around 10% **[112]**. There is therefore a need to identify the subset of patients that may benefit from it, and PI3K/Akt/mTOR-dependency genetic signatures are being developed. In this direction, it has been recently observed that a majority of locally advanced and inflammatory breast cancers over-express the translation regulatory protein4E-BP1 and the initiation factor eIF4G, both of them are mTOR downstream targets. While additional studies are planned to further dissect this interaction, it does seem reasonable to explore the benefits of mTOR inhibitors in the treatment of locally advanced breast cancer [113].
Another potential explanation for the limited activity of mTOR inhibitors in breast cancer and other tumor types may be related to a 'collateral effect' of mTOR blockade. mTOR inhibition blocks the natural negative feed-back on IGF-1R signaling exerted on PI3K [114]. The result is an increase in PI3K and Akt activations which could potentially counteract the inhibition of mTOR. Thus, dual inhibition of both IGF-1 signaling, with either MAbs against the receptor or tyrosine kinase inhibitors, and mTOR results in superior anti-proliferative effect over each single strategy.
In the clinic there is indirect evidence that this approach may be fruitful as well. Octreotide has been shown to inhibit IGF-1R signaling. Although octreotide has limited activity in patients with refractory neuroendocrine tumors, it has been shown to that the combination of everolimus and octreotide has resulted in an impressive activity **[115]**.

2.7 STPs-4: HSP90 signaling pathway

Heat shock protein 90 (HSP90) is a molecular chaperone required for the stability and function of several conditionally activated and/or expressed signaling proteins ([116-117]. Many of these client proteins such as Akt, HER2, Bcr-Abl, c-Kit, EGFR and PDGFR-a are oncoproteins and important cell-signaling proteins [118-119]. As signal transducers and molecular switches, these client proteins are inherently unstable. HSP90 keeps unstable signaling proteins poised for activation until they are stabilised by conformational changes associated with the formation of signal transduction complexes. As such, it is a single molecular target that is a central integrator of multiple pathways important to cancer. Activation of HSP90-dependent client proteins proceeds through an ordered sequence of events linked to the ATPase activity of HSP90 and involves a variety of co-chaperone complexes **[120]**.
HER2 is among the most sensitive client proteins of HSP90, demonstrating degradation within 2 h of HSP90 inhibition in cell culture experiments **[121]**. Geldanamycin analogues (17-allylamino- 17-demethoxygeldanamycin [17-AAG] and 17-dimethylaminoethylamino-

17-demethoxygeldanamycin [17-DMAG]) have demonstrated potent inhibition of HSP90 function in HER2-over-expressing cell lines, demonstrating significant anti-tumor activity in both cell culture and animal studies [121-122].

2.8 STIs-4: HSP90 inhibitors

(HSP90) is an exciting new therapeutic target, inhibition of which delivers a combinatorial attack on multiple oncogenic targets and pathways and on all of the hallmark traits of malignancy **[123]**. In the clinic, initial studies with the HSP90 inhibitor have demonstrated safety and anti-tumor activity and tolerability in combination with trastuzumab in patients with trastuzumab-refractory HER2- positive metastatic breast cancer patients **[120]**. It will be important to determine whether HSP90 inhibitors will have clinical activity as single agents in breast cancer patients.

2.9 STPs-5: PARP signaling pathway

Poly (ADP-ribose) polymerase 1 (PARP-1) is the initial and best characterised member of a family of enzymes largely associated with the maintenance of genomic stability. Activation of PARP-1 is part of the immediate cellular response to DNA strand breaks, converting them into an intracellular signal via poly (ADP-ribosylation) of nuclear proteins [124-125]. This results in a highly negatively charged target, which in turn leads to the unwinding and repair of the damaged DNA through the base excision repair pathway. In addition, PARP-1 is also known to bind dsDNA breaks (DSB) preventing accidental recombination of homologous DNA [126]**.** Upon binding DNA breaks, the catalytic activity of PARP-1 is stimulated >500- fold [127]**.** Enhanced PARP-1 expression or activity has been also observed in a number of different tumor cell lines and could provide a greater level of resistance to both endogenous genotoxic stress and to DNA damage-inducing therapeutic agents.
Studies of PARP expression in various tumor types identified that breast cancers with negative estrogen receptor, progesterone receptor and HER2 expression were much more likely to over-express PARP [128]. Additionally, it has been recently shown that BRCA1 and BRCA2 dysfunction sensitises cells to the inhibition of PARP enzymatic activity, resulting in chromosomal instability, cell cycle arrest and subsequent apoptosis. This seems to develop because the inhibition of PARP leads to the persistence of DNA lesions normally repaired by homologous recombination **[128].**

2.10 STIs-5: PARP inhibitors

PARP inhibitors have been developed to investigate the role of PARP-1 in cell biology and to overcome DNA repair-mediated resistance of cancer cells to genotoxic agents [129]. These novel PARP inhibitors have been shown to enhance the anti-tumor activity of DNA-methylating agents, such as temozolomide, topoisomerase poisons and ionising radiation in preclinical studies [130], and to restore sensitivity of resistant tumors to methylating agents or topoisomerase I inhibitors, agents presently used for the treatment of breast cancer.

2.11 STPs-6: Apoptosis & autophagy signaling pathways

Apoptosis, the process of programmed cell death, is governed by complex, gene-directed pathways [131-133]. Dysregulation of apoptosis plays a key role in tumorigenesis and can allow tumor cells to become resistant to anticancer treatments [132-133]. Rationale for targeting apoptosis in the treatment of breast cancer includes the over-expression of the Bcl-2 protein in 40%–80% of human breast tumors, which is associated with both resistance to chemotherapy **[134]** and a better prognosis after chemotherapy **[135].** Additionally, the association of Bcl-2 with ER and/or PgR, loss of expression of the gene for the pro-apoptotic protein Bax, and differential expression of tumor necrosis factor-related apoptosis-inducing ligand-receptor 2 have all been correlated with prognosis in breast cancer patients [134-137].

On the other hand, autophagy is an evolutionarily conserved lysosomal pathway for degrading cytoplasmic proteins, macromolecules, and organelles [138]. Many studies have described the role of autophagy as a protective mechanism for cell survival that is initiated in response to metabolic or therapeutic stress. Furthermore, autophagy may delay apoptotic cell death caused by DNA damaging agents and hormonal therapies [139-141].

2.12 STIs-6: Targeted therapies directed at the apoptotic & autophagic pathways

Anticancer agents targeting the components of apoptotic pathways are in the early stages of development, and no agent specifically targeting apoptosis has yet been approved for use in cancer treatment. A range of approaches is being tested, including antisense DNA oligonucleotides and antibody and small molecule inhibitors of the components of apoptotic pathways. Few clinical data are currently available in breast cancer; however, preclinical studies show that such agents do have anticancer activity, suggesting that this may be a promising approach, particularly when used in combination with chemotherapy [7].

On the other hand, recent studies have demonstrated that the inhibition of autophagy in cancer cells may be therapeutically beneficial in some circumstances, as it can sensitize cancer cells to different therapies, including DNA-damaging agents, antihormone therapies (e.g., tamoxifen), and radiation therapy. This supports the hypothesis that inhibiting autophagy can increase cell death when combined with anticancer agents, providing a therapeutic advantage against cancer proliferation & drug resistance [139-141].

2.13 STPs-7: Targeting the angiogenesis pathway

It is increasingly being accepted that tumor cell proliferation alone is insufficient to result in a substantial tumor mass. Angiogenesis is essential for tumors to develop into detectable localized masses, and for metastasis to occur [142-143]. The process of angiogenesis (the formation of new blood vessels from a pre-existing vascular bed) is complex and dynamic, and it is regulated by a range of pro- and anti-angiogenic molecules **[144].** The VEGF and platelet-derived growth factor (PDGF) families of proteins and their receptors (VEGFR-1, VEGFR-2, VEGFR-3, PDGFR-α, and PDGFR-β) appear central to the process **[144].** Activation of VEGFRs and PDGFRs initiates signaling that results in numerous cellular responses, including survival, mitogenesis, migration, proliferation, and differentiation [144-145]. Activation of the VEGF pathway also increases vascular permeability and the movement of endothelial progenitor cells from the bone marrow into the peripheral circulation [144]. Primary breast tumors express a variety of different angiogenic factors, with VEGF being the most abundant.

High VEGF expression appears to be correlated with poor clinical prognosis and response **[146]**. Levels of VEGF in breast cancer tumors are a prognostic factor for relapse-free and overall survival in patients with both lymph node-negative and lymph node-positive disease [147-148], and they predict response to both tamoxifen and chemotherapy in advanced disease **[149]**. Similarly, a proportion of invasive breast cancers that over-express PDGFR-α have been associated with greater biological aggressiveness and a higher likelihood of lymph node metastasis [150].

Given their central roles in tumor angiogenesis and growth, the VEGF and PDGF signaling pathways are key targets for breast cancer therapy. However, with considerable redundancy in angiogenic signaling pathways, the inhibition of more than one receptor is likely necessary to block angiogenesis. It has been hypothesized that anti-VEGF agents may prevent the development of new tumor vasculature and induce normalization of existing, inefficient tumor vasculature (resulting from over-expression of VEGF) **[151]**. These agents, then, may allow better delivery of cytotoxic therapies to the tumor, suggesting a potential role for anti-VEGF therapy in conjunction with chemotherapy [151-152].

2.14 STIs-7: Targeted therapies directed at angiogenesis

Several therapies targeting angiogenesis are in development for breast cancer. These include monoclonal antibodies that act extracellularly by binding to receptors or their ligands, such as bevacizumab (Avastin®), and RTKIs that act intracellularly, such as sunitinib (Sutent®). Intracellular VEGF targeting therapeutics will be discussed later as they were proven to be targeting multiple sites.

Monoclonal antibodies: Bevacizumab

Bevacizumab is an anti-VEGF humanized monoclonal antibody administered as an i.v. infusion. It acts by binding to all VEGF isoforms, thus removing VEGF from the circulation and preventing activation of VEGFRs **[153]**. In 2008, the U.S. Food and Drug Administration (FDA) approved bevacizumab in combination with paclitaxel for the first-line treatment of locally recurrent breast cancer or MBC **[7]**.

Although bevacizumab has shown little activity as a single agent in MBC patients, combination therapy with chemotherapeutic agents has been associated with clinical activity in this patient population. Several phase III studies have investigated bevacizumab combined with chemotherapy [154-155]. These data suggest that VEGF inhibition combined with chemotherapy is a promising treatment strategy in this setting. Further studies are under way to explore the use of bevacizumab with different chemotherapeutic regimens, hormonal treatments, and other targeted therapies (including lapatinib and trastuzumab) in patients with MBC. Additionally, trials of bevacizumab are ongoing in the adjuvant and neoadjuvant settings, and preliminary reports suggest that this approach may be feasible.

Hypertension, bleeding, and thrombosis remain potential safety concerns with a number of anti-VEGF therapies, and this area requires further study. Future trials should focus on identifying those patients who will derive the most benefit from bevacizumab- based regimens and how best to combine bevacizumab with other cancer therapies (which therapies should be combined and whether sequential or concurrent administration is most effective). Overall, growing clinical experience with agents targeting angiogenic processes, such as bevacizumab, has provided proof of concept for the use of these treatments in MBC patients **[7]**.

2.15 STPs-8: Multi-target therapeutics

There appears to be extensive crosstalk between the pathways driving tumorigenic processes, and this provides a good rationale for inhibiting multiple pathways and processes with multi-targeted agents, either as single agents or in combination [7]. A number of single-agent RTKIs with multiple molecular targets have been developed as an alternative to combining multiple agents. These were developed based on previous studies showing that combining agents that target different pathways may have synergistic activity and delay or reverse resistance [156-158].

2.16 STIs-8: Multi-target inhibitors

A range of oral, antiangiogenic RTKIs with multiple targets is currently in development for MBC. These include sunitinib, pazopanib, sorafenib (Nexavar®) and axitinib.

Sunitinib selectively inhibits several receptor tyrosine kinases (VEGFR-1, VEGFR-2, VEGFR-3, PDGFR- α, PDGFR-β, Kit, FMS-like tyrosine kinase [FLT]-3, and colony-stimulating factor 1 receptor). It has both anti-angiogenic and anti-tumor activities. Sunitinib has been shown to have antitumor activity in breast cancer preclinical studies, both as a single agent and in combination with chemotherapy [159-163].

Data from a phase II study of sunitinib monotherapy in patients with refractory MBC reported single-agent activity in heavily pretreated patients, previously exposed to an anthracycline and a taxane [164]. The toxicities were manageable [164]. Studies and case series evaluating sunitinib given in combination with taxane therapy for MBC have reported antitumor activity and a manageable and tolerable safety profile [165-166]. Phase III trials of sunitinib in combination with a variety of cytotoxic agents are under way in first- and second-line MBC therapy [7].

Pazopanib targets VEGFR, PDGFR, and Kit and is currently in development in a number of tumor types, including breast cancer. Although originally developed as a Raf inhibitor, sorafenib also inhibits the activity of VEGFR-2 and VEGFR-3, PDGFR-β, FLT-3, and Kit; thus, it may inhibit tumor growth both directly (through Raf and Kit) and indirectly, through inhibition of angiogenesis [167-168].

Sorafenib inhibited MAPK activity in breast cancer cell lines expressing mutations of K-Ras or B-Raf, and showed antitumor and antiangiogenic activity in a human breast cancer xenograft model [168]. Significant and sustained increases in blood pressure were reported in a study of sorafenib monotherapy in patients with metastatic solid tumors **[169]**. Current data suggest little activity for sorafenib as a single agent in MBC patients; ongoing studies are exploring combination treatment with paclitaxel and with anastrozole in MBC.

Axitinib inhibits all known VEGFRs, in addition to PDGFR-β and the stem cell factor receptor Kit, and is currently being investigated in a range of tumor types, including breast cancer. In preclinical studies, axitinib was shown to selectively block VEGF-stimulated receptor phosphorylation in vitro, resulting in the inhibition of endothelial cell proliferation and survival. In a human breast cancer xenograft model, it significantly inhibited tumor growth and disrupted tumor microvasculature as assessed by dynamic contrast-enhanced magnetic resonance imaging **[170]**.

To date, the mult-itargeted RTKIs discussed have not been validated in phase III trials in MBC patients, although there is preliminary evidence of clinical activity. Of the four agents described above, three (pazopanib, sunitinib, and axitinib) appear to have the most clinical activity to date. Based on experience with other targeted agents in breast cancer, and with these RTKIs in other indications, combinations will hopefully show greater efficacy in the treatment of breast cancer [7].

2.17 STPs-9: Estrogen signaling transduction

Two of the genetic subtypes in breast cancer so far identified are those with gene expression characteristics typical of basal epithelial cells (which are predominantly estrogen receptor [ER-) and those with gene expression characteristics typical of luminal epithelial cells (which are predominantly ER+) [14, 171]. Typically, tumors of the ER-, basal subtype are associated with shorter relapse-free and overall survival times than those of the ER+, luminal subtype [171].

2.18 STIs-9: Estrogen signaling inhibitors

Endocrine therapy is widely used in the treatment of both early stage and recurrent/metastatic breast cancer. Tamoxifen and estrogen deprivation therapies such as aromatase inhibitors (AIs) and ovarian suppression have proved clinically effective and are generally well tolerated; they are the primary reason for the sustained improvement in survival for patients with early-stage [ER+] breast cancer [172]. Their long-term efficacy, however, is limited by relapse of disease and development of resistance following adjuvant endocrine therapy. This provides a strong rationale for using targeted agents against various growth factor and signaling pathways that are activated during endocrine resistance and for combining these targeted agents with ongoing endocrine therapy to either overcome endocrine resistance and enhance the efficacy of therapy for ER-positive breast cancer [173-174].

In this context, several selected targeted agents are being investigated in combination with endocrine therapy for patients with breast cancer in an attempt to overcome or prevent endocrine resistance. The role of EGFR/HER2 cross-talk with estrogen receptor (ER) signaling has been confirmed in preclinical studies [175] in which various inhibitors have yielded additive or synergistic effects when combined with endocrine agents. Recently, several results from clinical trials investigating this concept have been reported [59, 92].

2.19 STPs-10

Cancer progression is a multi-step process that enables tumor cells to invade through extracellular tissues and metastasize to distal organs **[8]**. Compelling recent evidence demonstrates that cooperation between signals from the extracellular matrix (ECM) and growth factors enhances malignant behaviors of aggressive cancer cells, such as proliferation, migration, survival, and invasion [176]. Examples of such cross talk signals include:

a. **The STATs** are a family of transcription factors that relay the interactions of cytokines and growth factors with their receptors at the cell surface to mediate changes in gene expression. In normal situations STATs are transiently activated; however, in many tumors tyrosine-phosphorylated STATs, mainly STAT3 and STAT5, can be detected, suggesting constitutive pathway activation [6].
b. **The NF-κB** pathway is triggered in response to microbial and viral infections and to pro-inflammatory cytokines. These agents activate the IκB kinase, which phosphoylates IκB allowing the liberated NF-κB family transcription factors to enter the nucleus. The pathway has an ever increasing interest for its role in human cancer [177]. The

association of NF-κB pathway activity with inflammation-associated tumor progression is well documented in mouse tumor models [178] and in human cancer cells [179].

c. **The Notch network** in mammals consists of four Notch receptors and five ligands. Once activated, the receptor undergoes intramembrane proteolysis leading to release and nuclear translocation of the intracellular domain, which has transcriptional activity. The Notch-4 gene is frequently rearranged in mammary glands by MMTV proviral integration. This rearrangement leads to expression of the intracellular domain under MMTV promoter control [180] an early demonstration of Notch's ability to induce mammary cancer.
d. **The UPS pathway**: The ubiquitin proteasome system (UPS) consists of several crucial enzymes contributing to most, if not all, cellular events. During the past decade, progress in endocrine therapy and the use of trastuzumab has significantly contributed to the decline in breast cancer mortality for hormone receptor-positive and HER2-positive cases, respectively. As a result of these advances, a breast cancer cluster with poor prognosis that is negative for the estrogen receptor (ER1), the progesterone receptor (PRGR) and HER2 (triple negative; basal like phenotype) has come to the forefront of medical therapeutic attention. DNA microarray analyses have revealed that this cluster is phenotypically most like the basal-like breast cancer that is caused by deficiencies in the **BRCA1 pathways**. BRCA1 acts as a hub protein that coordinates a diverse range of cellular pathways to maintain genomic stability [181]. Indeed, BRCA1 dysfunction in sporadic basal-like cancers has been reported [182]. Thus, investigating the BRCA1 pathway could be an important approach for the treatment of basal-like breast cancer.

2.20 STIs-10

To gain further improvements in breast cancer survival, new types of drugs might be required, and small molecules targeting the ubiquitin proteasome system have moved into the spotlight. The success of bortezomib in the treatment of multiple myeloma has sent encouraging signals that proteasome inhibitors could be used to treat other types of cancers [183]. In addition, ubiquitin enzymes involved in ER1, HER2 or BRCA1 pathways could be ideal targets for therapeutic intervention. The therapeutic effect of proteasome inhibitors on breast cancer remains to be determined but is greatly anticipated [184].

3. Targeting molecular signal in breast cancer stem cells responsible for development of multi-drug resistance (MDR)

Success in Breast cancer chemotherapy is challenged by the development of tumors having a multi-drug resistance (MDR) phenotype **[185]**. It is one of the major causes of failures to cancer chemotherapy. This phenotype is most prevalent in aggressive carcinomas as breast and ovarian carcinomas. By definition, MDR is a term used to describe the resistance developed by some tumors to protect themselves against a number of structurally and functionally unrelated chemotherapeutic agents. MDR is not only referred to the drug with which the patient has been treated but also to a wide range of other drugs used in cancer chemotherapy **[186]**.

Acquired drug resistance arises from exposure of tumor cells to chemotherapeutic agents. Random spontaneous mutations, acceleration of proliferation rate and alteration of cell sensitivity to growth factors can occur in tumor cells under the influence of cytotoxic drugs. On the other hand, MDR does not only develop as the result of treatment of tumor cells by a drug. It may be intrinsic, i.e. connected with the type of cell differentiation or genetic profile of tumor cells **[187]**.

Studies of resistance of tumor cells to cytotoxic drugs are necessary for understanding the mechanisms for restoring back their sensitivity. Although, MDR is a multi-factorial problem i.e. multiple mechanisms were hypothesized to account for this phenomenon, some of them were frequently observed and their clinical significance was determined. These mechanisms are acting either alone or in concert with each other for the development of the MDR phenotype in breast cancer cells **[188]**. Over-expression of ABC transporters, detoxification enzymes (aldehyde dehydrogenase), low cell turn over rate and the ability to activate the DNA check point response are possibly all involved and previously described with other mechanisms **[189]**. Innovative therapies, based on a better understanding of cancer stem cells, should lead to enhanced and long-term cure rates in breast cancer.

Given that tumor resistance to chemotherapy is believed to account for the majority of treatment failure in breast cancer, research attention in the last two decades focused on developing agents to reverse MDR and enhance the response of tumors to chemotherapeutic agents. Although hundreds of compounds have been found in-vitro to be able to modulate the MDR phenotype, their clinical application was limited owing to their high toxicity in-vivo [190-191]. Accordingly, searching for compounds able to modulate the MDR phenotype and have low toxicity continues to be an important challenge for optimizing cancer chemotherapy. The development of several therapeutics targeting the MDR phenotype in breast cancer cells have been previously reviewed **[189]**.

Recently, the possible roles of cancer stem cells in carcinogenesis have become more obvious. Numerous investigations have recently provided evidence that the genetic alterations occurring in the multi-potent tissue-specific adult stem cells and/or their early progenies may lead to their malignant transformation into cancer progenitor cells also designated as cancer stem cells or cancer-initiating cells **[192]**. A small population of undifferentiated- or poorly differentiated cancer progenitor cells, which possesses the stem cell-like properties including their self-renewal ability and capacity to give rise to the bulk mass of further differentiated malignant cells, appears to represent the principal cancer cells that are responsible for tumor formation [193]. Accumulating genetic alterations in tumorigenic cancer progenitor cells occurring during cancer progression may also confer to them the invasive and resistant properties that are essential for their remission and migration to distant metastatic sites [194-195].

The role of cancer stem cells in breast cancer chemoresistance was recently reviewed [196]. One characteristic of cancer stem cells that differentiates them from other normal cells in the tumor is that they have high levels of ABC transporter proteins, in particular ABCG2 [197]. The ABC transporter molecules are responsible for protecting cells from drug damage via efflux pumping mechanisms. Thus, cancer stem cells, as a result of these biological properties, are rendered resistant to drug treatment, including chemotherapeutic drugs [198].

Since all the stem cell-like properties attributed to cancer progenitor cells may provide them with a higher resistance to current cancer therapies, thus they constitute a substantial obstacle to the successful treatment of cancer patients [196]. This finding underlines the critical importance of targeting the cancer progenitor cells and their early progenies as well as their local microenvironment in the earlier stages of cancer treatment to counteract the rapid progression of certain cancer types and prevent the metastatic spread at distant sites. The simultaneous blockade of several oncogenic cascades activated in cancer progenitor cells during cancer progression may be essential for improving the current clinical treatments against high-risk, metastatic or relapsed breast cancers [189, 199].

Recent studies have revealed the possibility of using therapeutic agents targeting the EGFR, Wnt/β-catenin and/or Notch cascades to inhibit the ABC muli-drug efflux transporters and/or eliminate the cancer progenitor cells **[200]**. Moreover, one compound, salinomycin, reduces the proportion of cancer stem cells by >100-fold relative to paclitaxel, a commonly used breast cancer chemotherapeutic drug [201]. In addition, treatment of mice with salinomycin inhibits mammary tumor growth in vivo and induces increased epithelial differentiation of tumor cells **[199]**. What remains to be discovered is the extensive and in depth understanding of the molecular basis of cancer stem cell contribution to breast cancer development. Such extensive investigations enable the development of more effective and selective treatment strategies.

4. Concluding remarks and perspectives

Considerable progress has been made over the last several decades in understanding specific cellular, molecular and genetic mechanisms that contribute to cancer growth and progression **[202]**. In recent years, research efforts have focused on the signaling pathways involved in the growth and survival of breast cancer cells, leading to the development of a range of targeted agents with promising clinical activity. The encouraging success of trastuzumab, based on the identification of HER-2 as a molecular target, has provided the rationale for studying the array of targeted agents currently in clinical development for breast cancer **[7]**.

We have reviewed some of the most promising new targeted agents in breast cancer. This list, however, is far from complete. It should be pointed out that there are still many important additional classes of agents in clinical development in breast cancer. Examples include other tyrosine kinase inhibitors and also enhancers of apoptosis. We all hope that this list will keep developing. However, despite recent advances, there are still unanswered questions regarding the management of breast cancer with targeted agents.

With our knowledge of the molecular modifications in breast cancer and the increasing number of new targeted therapeutics, the current challenge is to select the best combinations of the so-called signal transduction inhibitors (STIs) for every patient [6]. The development of these targeted therapeutics will require a new set of challenging skills & investigations of unresolved issues **[120]**. These challenges are:

First, future studies are necessary to identify those patient subgroups likely to derive most benefit from a given therapy. Despite the temptation to use a targeted agent in all patients, identification of patient subgroups most likely to benefit must be a key goal and will be critical to the successful future use of these treatments **[7]**. These agents, unlike chemotherapy, will only work in the subset of tumors that show dependency on the target the therapy is being directed to.

If STI would have been developed in an unselected patient population, its anti-tumor activity would have been missed due to a dilutional effect brought in by the non-STPs-over-expressing population. This principle probably applies to the majority of classes of agents under study. The implication of this principle is that patient selection strategies will be of paramount importance in the development of these agents [120]. For example, accurate patient selection based on HER-2 over-expression is essential for trastuzumab-based treatment and is likely to be important for other agents in this class. However, identifying suitable patients may prove more difficult for RTKIs, because receptor over-expression alone does not seem to predict response to treatment [16].

Second, future studies are necessary to determine the optimal combinations, doses, and schedules required to maximize clinical activity while minimizing toxicity. Also, in early clinical studies with these agents in addition to establishing their safety and optimal doses and schedules, it may prove to be instrumental to also check for the presence of the target in the studied tumors and to seek for indications of target engagement with the study agent using careful analysis of [120]**2007**). The need to determine target engagement is currently being taken into account with the majority of clinical trials with novel agents that are moved into the clinic.

Third, Predictive markers are factors that are associated with upfront response or resistance to a particular therapy. Predictive markers are important in oncology as tumors of the same tissue of origin vary widely in their response to most available systemic therapies. Currently recommended oncological predictive markers include both estrogen and progesterone receptors for identifying patients with breast cancers likely to benefit from hormone therapy, HER-2 for the identification of breast cancer patients likely to benefit from trastuzumab [203]. Thus, the drive to identify new biomarkers of target engagement and sensitivity with these novel agents is also promoting the search for new clinical study designs in a minimally pre-treated population **[120]**.

Fourth, future studies will need to address how best to incorporate these agents into existing treatment regimens and to determine when and in which combinations targeted therapy should be administered **[7]**. Some of these agents will have limited activity by themselves and yet have the capacity to markedly enhance the anti-tumor activity of conventional agents like chemotherapy or even other biological agents. For example, anti angiogenesis MAb bevacizumab that has no activity as a single agent and yet is clinically active when combined with chemotherapy. Furthermore, HER-targeted agents may need to be used in combination with chemotherapy to provide clinically relevant activity.

Fifth, the therapy end-points with these agents also need to be revisited. Some of these agents are not expected to result in tumor shrinkage (or response), and therefore we cannot propose a unified definition of clinical benefit as it has been done with chemotherapy in the past. Furthermore, genetic assay techniques used to provide information on clinical outcomes, including the risk for tumor recurrence and individual benefit from a particular chemotherapy also needs further critical development **[204]**.

Sixth, Targeting HER-2 is associated with cardiac toxicity, which is an especially important consideration in the adjuvant setting and when combining anti–HER-2 agents with cardiotoxic chemotherapeutic drugs. Targeting HER-1 in combination with HER-2, as with the RTKIs lapatinib and neratinib, appears to reduce the risk for cardiotoxicity, although the exact mechanisms underlying this observation remain unclear **[7]**.

Finally, with the increase in the number of available lines of therapy in breast cancer, there is a danger that novel agents will be tested in a heavily pre-treated patient population. While there is little debate if patients with advanced disease receiving multiple lines of therapy may be appropriate study participants in early clinical studies. There is also a growing concern that patients with advanced disease may not be the ideal population to detect the anti-tumor activity of novel agents since their tumors may have become highly resistant to any type of therapy **[120]**.

In summary, the contribution of STIs in cancer chemotherapy continues to be encouraging, and clinical trials are currently addressing whether the promising preclinical activities of STIs will translate into benefits for patients. Hopefully, the previously mentioned suggestions and mechanisms will ultimately be put into practice. Moreover, cellular responses to cancer chemotherapeutic agents are complex and several mechanisms are commonly associated with the resistance of laboratory human breast cancer cell lines. Clinical testing of breast cancer STIs like other modern day targeted therapeutics must be rationally developed with a firm basis in the lessons learned in the laboratory and with proper selection of patient populations in which the predictive power and the potential for benefit is greatest.

5. References

[1] Jemal A., et al., *Global Cancer Statistics.* CANCER J CLIN, 2011. 61: p. 69–90.
[2] Jemal, A., et al., *Cancer statistics, 2009.* CA Cancer J Clin, 2009. 59(4): p. 225-49.
[3] Knutson, D. and E. Steiner, *Screening for breast cancer: current recommendations and future directions.* Am Fam Physician, 2007. 75(11): p. 1660-6.
[4] Gonzalez-Angulo, A.M., F. Morales-Vasquez, and G.N. Hortobagyi, *Overview of resistance to systemic therapy in patients with breast cancer.* Adv Exp Med Biol, 2007. 608: p. 1-22.
[5] Condeelis, J. and J.W. Pollard, *Macrophages: obligate partners for tumor cell migration, invasion, and metastasis.* Cell, 2006. 124(2): p. 263-6.
[6] Hynes, N.E. and W. Gullick, *Therapeutic targeting of signal transduction pathways and proteins in breast cancer.* J Mammary Gland Biol Neoplasia, 2006. 11(1): p. 1-2.
[7] Rosen, L.S., H.L. Ashurst, and L. Chap, *Targeting signal transduction pathways in metastatic breast cancer: a comprehensive review.* Oncologist, 2010. 15(3): p. 216-35.
[8] Hanahan, D. and R.A. Weinberg, *The hallmarks of cancer.* Cell, 2000. 100(1): p. 57-70.
[9] Bender, L.M. and R. Nahta, *Her2 cross talk and therapeutic resistance in breast cancer.* Front Biosci, 2008. 13: p. 3906-12.
[10] Menard, S., et al., *HER2 as a prognostic factor in breast cancer.* Oncology, 2001. 61 Suppl 2: p. 67-72.
[11] Milanezi, F., S. Carvalho, and F.C. Schmitt, *EGFR/HER2 in breast cancer: a biological approach for molecular diagnosis and therapy.* Expert Rev Mol Diagn, 2008. 8(4): p. 417-34.
[12] Slamon, D.J., et al., *Human breast cancer: correlation of relapse and survival with amplification of the HER-2/neu oncogene.* Science, 1987. 235(4785): p. 177-82.
[13] Gasparini, G., et al., *Therapy of breast cancer with molecular targeting agents.* Ann Oncol, 2005. 16 Suppl 4: p. iv28-36.
[14] Perou, C.M., et al., *Molecular portraits of human breast tumours.* Nature, 2000. 406(6797): p. 747-52.
[15] Martin, M., *Molecular biology of breast cancer.* Clin Transl Oncol, 2006. 8(1): p. 7-14.
[16] Lin, N.U. and E.P. Winer, *New targets for therapy in breast cancer: small molecule tyrosine kinase inhibitors.* Breast Cancer Res, 2004. 6(5): p. 204-10.
[17] Riese, D.J., 2nd and D.F. Stern, *Specificity within the EGF family/ErbB receptor family signaling network.* Bioessays, 1998. 20(1): p. 41-8.

[18] Mills, G.B., et al., *The role of genetic abnormalities of PTEN and the phosphatidylinositol 3-kinase pathway in breast and ovarian tumorigenesis, prognosis, and therapy.* Semin Oncol, 2001. 28(5 Suppl 16): p. 125-41.
[19] Salomon, D.S., et al., *Epidermal growth factor-related peptides and their receptors in human malignancies.* Crit Rev Oncol Hematol, 1995. 19(3): p. 183-232.
[20] Roskoski, R., Jr., *The ErbB/HER receptor protein-tyrosine kinases and cancer.* Biochem Biophys Res Commun, 2004. 319(1): p. 1-11.
[21] Stern, D.F., *Tyrosine kinase signalling in breast cancer: ErbB family receptor tyrosine kinases.* Breast Cancer Res, 2000. 2(3): p. 176-83.
[22] Barrett-Lee, P.J., *Growth factor signalling in clinical breast cancer and its impact on response to conventional therapies: a review of chemotherapy.* Endocr Relat Cancer, 2005. 12 Suppl 1: p. S125-33.
[23] Normanno, N., et al., *Mechanisms of endocrine resistance and novel therapeutic strategies in breast cancer.* Endocr Relat Cancer, 2005. 12(4): p. 721-47.
[24] Pawlowski, V., et al., *A real-time one-step reverse transcriptase-polymerase chain reaction method to quantify c-erbB-2 expression in human breast cancer.* Cancer Detect Prev, 2000. 24(3): p. 212-23.
[25] Slamon, D.J., et al., *Studies of the HER-2/neu proto-oncogene in human breast and ovarian cancer.* Science, 1989. 244(4905): p. 707-12.
[26] Tsutsui, S., et al., *Prognostic value of epidermal growth factor receptor (EGFR) and its relationship to the estrogen receptor status in 1029 patients with breast cancer.* Breast Cancer Res Treat, 2002. 71(1): p. 67-75.
[27] Vogt, U., et al., *Amplification of erbB-4 oncogene occurs less frequently than that of erbB-2 in primary human breast cancer.* Gene, 1998. 223(1-2): p. 375-80.
[28] Witton, C.J., *Structure of HER receptors and intracellular localisation of downstream effector elements gives insight into mechanism of tumour growth promotion.* Breast Cancer Res, 2003. 5(4): p. 206-7.
[29] Atalay, G., et al., *Novel therapeutic strategies targeting the epidermal growth factor receptor (EGFR) family and its downstream effectors in breast cancer.* Ann Oncol, 2003. 14(9): p. 1346-63.
[30] Graus-Porta, D., et al., *ErbB-2, the preferred heterodimerization partner of all ErbB receptors, is a mediator of lateral signaling.* EMBO J, 1997. 16(7): p. 1647-55.
[31] Prenzel, N., et al., *The epidermal growth factor receptor family as a central element for cellular signal transduction and diversification.* Endocr Relat Cancer, 2001. 8(1): p. 11-31.
[32] Schlessinger, J., *Common and distinct elements in cellular signaling via EGF and FGF receptors.* Science, 2004. 306(5701): p. 1506-7.
[33] Martin, G.S., *The hunting of the Src.* Nat Rev Mol Cell Biol, 2001. 2(6): p. 467-75.
[34] Thomas, S.M. and J.S. Brugge, *Cellular functions regulated by Src family kinases.* Annu Rev Cell Dev Biol, 1997. 13: p. 513-609.
[35] Bromann, P.A., H. Korkaya, and S.A. Courtneidge, *The interplay between Src family kinases and receptor tyrosine kinases.* Oncogene, 2004. 23(48): p. 7957-68.
[36] Blume-Jensen, P. and T. Hunter, *Oncogenic kinase signalling.* Nature, 2001. 411(6835): p. 355-65.
[37] Muthuswamy, S.K., et al., *Mammary tumors expressing the neu proto-oncogene possess elevated c-Src tyrosine kinase activity.* Mol Cell Biol, 1994. 14(1): p. 735-43.

[38] Verbeek, B.S., et al., *c-Src protein expression is increased in human breast cancer. An immunohistochemical and biochemical analysis.* J Pathol, 1996. 180(4): p. 383-8.

[39] Rosen, N., et al., *Analysis of pp60c-src protein kinase activity in human tumor cell lines and tissues.* J Biol Chem, 1986. 261(29): p. 13754-9.

[40] Ottenhoff-Kalff, A.E., et al., *Characterization of protein tyrosine kinases from human breast cancer: involvement of the c-src oncogene product.* Cancer Res, 1992. 52(17): p. 4773-8.

[41] Hiscox, S., et al., *Elevated Src activity promotes cellular invasion and motility in tamoxifen resistant breast cancer cells.* Breast Cancer Res Treat, 2006. 97(3): p. 263-74.

[42] Cho, H.S., et al., *Structure of the extracellular region of HER2 alone and in complex with the Herceptin Fab.* Nature, 2003. 421(6924): p. 756-60.

[43] Albanell, J., et al., *A phase I study of the safety and pharmacokinetics of the combination of pertuzumab (rhuMab 2C4) and capecitabine in patients with advanced solid tumors.* Clin Cancer Res, 2008. 14(9): p. 2726-31.

[44] Slamon, D.J., et al., *Use of chemotherapy plus a monoclonal antibody against HER2 for metastatic breast cancer that overexpresses HER2.* N Engl J Med, 2001. 344(11): p. 783-92.

[45] Yu, D. and M.C. Hung, *Overexpression of ErbB2 in cancer and ErbB2-targeting strategies.* Oncogene, 2000. 19(53): p. 6115-21.

[46] Baselga, J., et al., *Recombinant humanized anti-HER2 antibody (Herceptin) enhances the antitumor activity of paclitaxel and doxorubicin against HER2/neu overexpressing human breast cancer xenografts.* Cancer Res, 1998. 58(13): p. 2825-31.

[47] Carter, P., et al., *Humanization of an anti-p185HER2 antibody for human cancer therapy.* Proc Natl Acad Sci U S A, 1992. 89(10): p. 4285-9.

[48] Tokuda, Y., et al., *In vitro and in vivo anti-tumour effects of a humanised monoclonal antibody against c-erbB-2 product.* Br J Cancer, 1996. 73(11): p. 1362-5.

[49] Cobleigh, M.A., et al., *Multinational study of the efficacy and safety of humanized anti-HER2 monoclonal antibody in women who have HER2-overexpressing metastatic breast cancer that has progressed after chemotherapy for metastatic disease.* J Clin Oncol, 1999. 17(9): p. 2639-48.

[50] Marty, M., et al., *Randomized phase II trial of the efficacy and safety of trastuzumab combined with docetaxel in patients with human epidermal growth factor receptor 2-positive metastatic breast cancer administered as first-line treatment: the M77001 study group.* J Clin Oncol, 2005. 23(19): p. 4265-74.

[51] Joensuu, H., et al., *Adjuvant docetaxel or vinorelbine with or without trastuzumab for breast cancer.* N Engl J Med, 2006. 354(8): p. 809-20.

[52] Piccart-Gebhart, M.J., et al., *Trastuzumab after adjuvant chemotherapy in HER2-positive breast cancer.* N Engl J Med, 2005. 353(16): p. 1659-72.

[53] Romond, E.H., et al., *Trastuzumab plus adjuvant chemotherapy for operable HER2-positive breast cancer.* N Engl J Med, 2005. 353(16): p. 1673-84.

[54] Smith, I., et al., *2-year follow-up of trastuzumab after adjuvant chemotherapy in HER2-positive breast cancer: a randomised controlled trial.* Lancet, 2007. 369(9555): p. 29-36.

[55] Spielmann, M., et al., *Trastuzumab for patients with axillary-node-positive breast cancer: results of the FNCLCC-PACS 04 trial.* J Clin Oncol, 2009. 27(36): p. 6129-34.

[56] Untch, M. and C. Jackisch, *Optimal treatment strategies in hormone-responsive early breast cancer: the role of aromatase inhibitors.* Onkologie, 2007. 30(1-2): p. 55-64.

[57] Chia, S., et al., *Pegylated liposomal doxorubicin and trastuzumab in HER-2 overexpressing metastatic breast cancer: a multicenter phase II trial.* J Clin Oncol, 2006. 24(18): p. 2773-8.
[58] Kaufman, B., et al., *Trastuzumab plus anastrozole versus anastrozole alone for the treatment of postmenopausal women with human epidermal growth factor receptor 2-positive, hormone receptor-positive metastatic breast cancer: results from the randomized phase III TAnDEM study.* J Clin Oncol, 2009. 27(33): p. 5529-37.
[59] Marcom, P.K., et al., *The combination of letrozole and trastuzumab as first or second-line biological therapy produces durable responses in a subset of HER2 positive and ER positive advanced breast cancers.* Breast Cancer Res Treat, 2007. 102(1): p. 43-9.
[60] Burris, H., 3rd, et al., *Phase II trial of trastuzumab followed by weekly paclitaxel/carboplatin as first-line treatment for patients with metastatic breast cancer.* J Clin Oncol, 2004. 22(9): p. 1621-9.
[61] Sawaki, M., et al., *Efficacy and safety of trastuzumab as a single agent in heavily pretreated patients with HER-2/neu-overexpressing metastatic breast cancer.* Tumori, 2004. 90(1): p. 40-3.
[62] Vogel, C.L., et al., *Efficacy and safety of trastuzumab as a single agent in first-line treatment of HER2-overexpressing metastatic breast cancer.* J Clin Oncol, 2002. 20(3): p. 719-26.
[63] Nahta, R., et al., *Mechanisms of disease: understanding resistance to HER2-targeted therapy in human breast cancer.* Nat Clin Pract Oncol, 2006. 3(5): p. 269-80.
[64] Atalay, G., et al., *Clinical outcome of breast cancer patients with liver metastases alone in the anthracycline-taxane era: a retrospective analysis of two prospective, randomised metastatic breast cancer trials.* Eur J Cancer, 2003. 39(17): p. 2439-49.
[65] Bartsch, R., et al., *Analysis of trastuzumab and chemotherapy in advanced breast cancer after the failure of at least one earlier combination: an observational study.* BMC Cancer, 2006. 6: p. 63.
[66] Gelmon, K.A., et al., *Use of trastuzumab beyond disease progression: observations from a retrospective review of case histories.* Clin Breast Cancer, 2004. 5(1): p. 52-8; discussion 59-62.
[67] Bartsch, R., et al., *Capecitabine and trastuzumab in heavily pretreated metastatic breast cancer.* J Clin Oncol, 2007. 25(25): p. 3853-8.
[68] von Minckwitz, G., et al., *A multicentre phase II study on gefitinib in taxane- and anthracycline-pretreated metastatic breast cancer.* Breast Cancer Res Treat, 2005. 89(2): p. 165-72.
[69] Storniolo, A.M., et al., *Phase I dose escalation and pharmacokinetic study of lapatinib in combination with trastuzumab in patients with advanced ErbB2-positive breast cancer.* J Clin Oncol, 2008. 26(20): p. 3317-23.
[70] Kallioniemi, O.P., et al., *Association of c-erbB-2 protein over-expression with high rate of cell proliferation, increased risk of visceral metastasis and poor long-term survival in breast cancer.* Int J Cancer, 1991. 49(5): p. 650-5.
[71] Weil, R.J., et al., *Breast cancer metastasis to the central nervous system.* Am J Pathol, 2005. 167(4): p. 913-20.
[72] Gori, S., et al., *Central nervous system metastases in HER-2 positive metastatic breast cancer patients treated with trastuzumab: incidence, survival, and risk factors.* Oncologist, 2007. 12(7): p. 766-73.
[73] Ng, R., N. Better, and M.D. Green, *Anticancer agents and cardiotoxicity.* Semin Oncol, 2006. 33(1): p. 2-14.

[74] Ewer, M.S., et al., *Reversibility of trastuzumab-related cardiotoxicity: new insights based on clinical course and response to medical treatment.* J Clin Oncol, 2005. 23(31): p. 7820-6.
[75] Guarneri, V., et al., *Long-term cardiac tolerability of trastuzumab in metastatic breast cancer: the M.D. Anderson Cancer Center experience.* J Clin Oncol, 2006. 24(25): p. 4107-15.
[76] Force, T., D.S. Krause, and R.A. Van Etten, *Molecular mechanisms of cardiotoxicity of tyrosine kinase inhibition.* Nat Rev Cancer, 2007. 7(5): p. 332-44.
[77] Agus, D.B., et al., *Targeting ligand-activated ErbB2 signaling inhibits breast and prostate tumor growth.* Cancer Cell, 2002. 2(2): p. 127-37.
[78] Franklin, M.C., et al., *Insights into ErbB signaling from the structure of the ErbB2-pertuzumab complex.* Cancer Cell, 2004. 5(4): p. 317-28.
[79] Nemunaitis, J., et al., *Phase 1 clinical and pharmacokinetics evaluation of oral CI-1033 in patients with refractory cancer.* Clin Cancer Res, 2005. 11(10): p. 3846-53.
[80] Geyer, C.E., et al., *Lapatinib plus capecitabine for HER2-positive advanced breast cancer.* N Engl J Med, 2006. 355(26): p. 2733-43.
[81] Lin, N.U., et al., *Multicenter phase II study of lapatinib in patients with brain metastases from HER2-positive breast cancer.* Clin Cancer Res, 2009. 15(4): p. 1452-9.
[82] Perez, E.A., et al., *Cardiac safety of lapatinib: pooled analysis of 3689 patients enrolled in clinical trials.* Mayo Clin Proc, 2008. 83(6): p. 679-86.
[83] Arteaga, C.L., et al., *A phase I-II study of combined blockade of the ErbB receptor network with trastuzumab and gefitinib in patients with HER2 (ErbB2)-overexpressing metastatic breast cancer.* Clin Cancer Res, 2008. 14(19): p. 6277-83.
[84] Britten, C.D., et al., *A phase I/II trial of trastuzumab plus erlotinib in metastatic HER2-positive breast cancer: a dual ErbB targeted approach.* Clin Breast Cancer, 2009. 9(1): p. 16-22.
[85] Green, M.D., et al., *Gefitinib treatment in hormone-resistant and hormone receptor-negative advanced breast cancer.* Ann Oncol, 2009. 20(11): p. 1813-7.
[86] Bose, P. and H. Ozer, *Neratinib: an oral, irreversible dual EGFR/HER2 inhibitor for breast and non-small cell lung cancer.* Expert Opin Investig Drugs, 2009. 18(11): p. 1735-51.
[87] Chow, B.H., et al., *Increased expression of annexin I is associated with drug-resistance in nasopharyngeal carcinoma and other solid tumors.* Proteomics Clin Appl, 2009. 3(6): p. 654-62.
[88] Huang, F., et al., *Identification of candidate molecular markers predicting sensitivity in solid tumors to dasatinib: rationale for patient selection.* Cancer Res, 2007. 67(5): p. 2226-38.
[89] Hennequin, L.F., et al., *N-(5-chloro-1,3-benzodioxol-4-yl)-7-[2-(4-methylpiperazin-1-yl)ethoxy]-5- (tetrahydro-2H-pyran-4-yloxy)quinazolin-4-amine, a novel, highly selective, orally available, dual-specific c-Src/Abl kinase inhibitor.* J Med Chem, 2006. 49(22): p. 6465-88.
[90] Kolch, W., *Meaningful relationships: the regulation of the Ras/Raf/MEK/ERK pathway by protein interactions.* Biochem J, 2000. 351 Pt 2: p. 289-305.
[91] Johnston, S.R., et al., *Phase II study of the efficacy and tolerability of two dosing regimens of the farnesyl transferase inhibitor, R115777, in advanced breast cancer.* J Clin Oncol, 2003. 21(13): p. 2492-9.
[92] Johnston, S.R., et al., *A phase II, randomized, blinded study of the farnesyltransferase inhibitor tipifarnib combined with letrozole in the treatment of advanced breast cancer after antiestrogen therapy.* Breast Cancer Res Treat, 2008. 110(2): p. 327-35.

[93] Sparano, J.A., et al., *Targeted inhibition of farnesyltransferase in locally advanced breast cancer: a phase I and II trial of tipifarnib plus dose-dense doxorubicin and cyclophosphamide.* J Clin Oncol, 2006. 24(19): p. 3013-8.

[94] McCubrey, J.A., et al., *Roles of the Raf/MEK/ERK pathway in cell growth, malignant transformation and drug resistance.* Biochim Biophys Acta, 2007. 1773(8): p. 1263-84.

[95] Bachman, K.E., et al., *The PIK3CA gene is mutated with high frequency in human breast cancers.* Cancer Biol Ther, 2004. 3(8): p. 772-5.

[96] Campbell, I.G., et al., *Mutation of the PIK3CA gene in ovarian and breast cancer.* Cancer Res, 2004. 64(21): p. 7678-81.

[97] Lee, J.W., et al., *PIK3CA gene is frequently mutated in breast carcinomas and hepatocellular carcinomas.* Oncogene, 2005. 24(8): p. 1477-80.

[98] Levine, D.A., et al., *Frequent mutation of the PIK3CA gene in ovarian and breast cancers.* Clin Cancer Res, 2005. 11(8): p. 2875-8.

[99] Philp, A.J., et al., *The phosphatidylinositol 3'-kinase p85alpha gene is an oncogene in human ovarian and colon tumors.* Cancer Res, 2001. 61(20): p. 7426-9.

[100] Samuels, Y., et al., *High frequency of mutations of the PIK3CA gene in human cancers.* Science, 2004. 304(5670): p. 554.

[101] Cantley, L.C., *The phosphoinositide 3-kinase pathway.* Science, 2002. 296(5573): p. 1655-7.

[102] Sarbassov, D.D., et al., *Phosphorylation and regulation of Akt/PKB by the rictor-mTOR complex.* Science, 2005. 307(5712): p. 1098-101.

[103] Inoki, K., et al., *TSC2 is phosphorylated and inhibited by Akt and suppresses mTOR signalling.* Nat Cell Biol, 2002. 4(9): p. 648-57.

[104] Wullschleger, S., R. Loewith, and M.N. Hall, *TOR signaling in growth and metabolism.* Cell, 2006. 124(3): p. 471-84.

[105] Hennessy, B.T., et al., *Exploiting the PI3K/AKT pathway for cancer drug discovery.* Nat Rev Drug Discov, 2005. 4(12): p. 988-1004.

[106] Nagata, Y., et al., *PTEN activation contributes to tumor inhibition by trastuzumab, and loss of PTEN predicts trastuzumab resistance in patients.* Cancer Cell, 2004. 6(2): p. 117-27.

[107] Kondapaka, S.B., et al., *Perifosine, a novel alkylphospholipid, inhibits protein kinase B activation.* Mol Cancer Ther, 2003. 2(11): p. 1093-103.

[108] Baselga, J., et al., *Phase II and tumor pharmacodynamic study of gefitinib in patients with advanced breast cancer.* J Clin Oncol, 2005. 23(23): p. 5323-33.

[109] Chan, S., et al., *Phase II study of temsirolimus (CCI-779), a novel inhibitor of mTOR, in heavily pretreated patients with locally advanced or metastatic breast cancer.* J Clin Oncol, 2005. 23(23): p. 5314-22.

[110] Andre, F., et al., *Phase I study of everolimus plus weekly paclitaxel and trastuzumab in patients with metastatic breast cancer pretreated with trastuzumab.* J Clin Oncol, 2010. 28(34): p. 5110-5.

[111] Mariani, G., et al., *Trastuzumab as adjuvant systemic therapy for HER2-positive breast cancer.* Nat Clin Pract Oncol, 2009. 6(2): p. 93-104.

[112] Raymond, E., et al., *Safety and pharmacokinetics of escalated doses of weekly intravenous infusion of CCI-779, a novel mTOR inhibitor, in patients with cancer.* J Clin Oncol, 2004. 22(12): p. 2336-47.

[113] Braunstein, S., et al., *A hypoxia-controlled cap-dependent to cap-independent translation switch in breast cancer.* Mol Cell, 2007. 28(3): p. 501-12.

[114] O'Reilly, K.E., et al., *mTOR inhibition induces upstream receptor tyrosine kinase signaling and activates Akt.* Cancer Res, 2006. 66(3): p. 1500-8.
[115] Yao, J.C., et al., *Efficacy of RAD001 (everolimus) and octreotide LAR in advanced low- to intermediate-grade neuroendocrine tumors: results of a phase II study.* J Clin Oncol, 2008. 26(26): p. 4311-8.
[116] Neckers, L., A. Kern, and S. Tsutsumi, *Hsp90 inhibitors disrupt mitochondrial homeostasis in cancer cells.* Chem Biol, 2007. 14(11): p. 1204-6.
[117] Neckers, L., *Heat shock protein 90: the cancer chaperone.* J Biosci, 2007. 32(3): p. 517-30.
[118] Maloney, A. and P. Workman, *HSP90 as a new therapeutic target for cancer therapy: the story unfolds.* Expert Opin Biol Ther, 2002. 2(1): p. 3-24.
[119] Zhang, H. and F. Burrows, *Targeting multiple signal transduction pathways through inhibition of Hsp90.* J Mol Med, 2004. 82(8): p. 488-99.
[120] Di Cosimo, S. and J. Baselga, *Targeted therapies in breast cancer: where are we now?* Eur J Cancer, 2008. 44(18): p. 2781-90.
[121] Basso, A.D., et al., *Ansamycin antibiotics inhibit Akt activation and cyclin D expression in breast cancer cells that overexpress HER2.* Oncogene, 2002. 21(8): p. 1159-66.
[122] Neckers, L., *Effects of geldanamycin and other naturally occurring small molecule antagonists of heat shock protein 90 on HER2 protein expression.* Breast Dis, 2000. 11: p. 49-59.
[123] Powers, M.V. and P. Workman, *Targeting of multiple signalling pathways by heat shock protein 90 molecular chaperone inhibitors.* Endocr Relat Cancer, 2006. 13 Suppl 1: p. S125-35.
[124] Ame, J.C., et al., *PARP-2, A novel mammalian DNA damage-dependent poly(ADP-ribose) polymerase.* J Biol Chem, 1999. 274(25): p. 17860-8.
[125] Schreiber, V., et al., *Poly(ADP-ribose) polymerase-2 (PARP-2) is required for efficient base excision DNA repair in association with PARP-1 and XRCC1.* J Biol Chem, 2002. 277(25): p. 23028-36.
[126] Yang, Y.G., et al., *Ablation of PARP-1 does not interfere with the repair of DNA double-strand breaks, but compromises the reactivation of stalled replication forks.* Oncogene, 2004. 23(21): p. 3872-82.
[127] Schreiber, V., et al., *Poly(ADP-ribose): novel functions for an old molecule.* Nat Rev Mol Cell Biol, 2006. 7(7): p. 517-28.
[128] Farmer, H., et al., *Targeting the DNA repair defect in BRCA mutant cells as a therapeutic strategy.* Nature, 2005. 434(7035): p. 917-21.
[129] Ratnam, K. and J.A. Low, *Current development of clinical inhibitors of poly(ADP-ribose) polymerase in oncology.* Clin Cancer Res, 2007. 13(5): p. 1383-8.
[130] Graziani, G. and C. Szabo, *Clinical perspectives of PARP inhibitors.* Pharmacol Res, 2005. 52(1): p. 109-18.
[131] Lowe, S.W. and A.W. Lin, *Apoptosis in cancer.* Carcinogenesis, 2000. 21(3): p. 485-95.
[132] Reed, J.C., *Dysregulation of apoptosis in cancer.* J Clin Oncol, 1999. 17(9): p. 2941-53.
[133] Reed, J.C., *Apoptosis-targeted therapies for cancer.* Cancer Cell, 2003. 3(1): p. 17-22.
[134] Nahta, R. and F.J. Esteva, *Bcl-2 antisense oligonucleotides: a potential novel strategy for the treatment of breast cancer.* Semin Oncol, 2003. 30(5 Suppl 16): p. 143-9.
[135] Sjostrom, J., et al., *The predictive value of bcl-2, bax, bcl-xL, bag-1, fas, and fasL for chemotherapy response in advanced breast cancer.* Clin Cancer Res, 2002. 8(3): p. 811-6.

[136] Krajewski, S., et al., *Prognostic significance of apoptosis regulators in breast cancer.* Endocr Relat Cancer, 1999. 6(1): p. 29-40.
[137] McCarthy, M.M., et al., *Evaluating the expression and prognostic value of TRAIL-R1 and TRAIL-R2 in breast cancer.* Clin Cancer Res, 2005. 11(14): p. 5188-94.
[138] Dalby, K.N., et al., *Targeting the prodeath and prosurvival functions of autophagy as novel therapeutic strategies in cancer.* Autophagy, 2010. 6(3): p. 322-9.
[139] Abedin, M.J., et al., *Autophagy delays apoptotic death in breast cancer cells following DNA damage.* Cell Death Differ, 2007. 14(3): p. 500-10.
[140] Boya, P., et al., *Inhibition of macroautophagy triggers apoptosis.* Mol Cell Biol, 2005. 25(3): p. 1025-40.
[141] Qadir, M.A., et al., *Macroautophagy inhibition sensitizes tamoxifen-resistant breast cancer cells and enhances mitochondrial depolarization.* Breast Cancer Res Treat, 2008. 112(3): p. 389-403.
[142] Folkman, J., *Role of angiogenesis in tumor growth and metastasis.* Semin Oncol, 2002. 29(6 Suppl 16): p. 15-8.
[143] Folkman, J., *Angiogenesis.* Annu Rev Med, 2006. 57: p. 1-18.
[144] Board, R. and G.C. Jayson, *Platelet-derived growth factor receptor (PDGFR): a target for anticancer therapeutics.* Drug Resist Updat, 2005. 8(1-2): p. 75-83.
[145] Hicklin, D.J. and L.M. Ellis, *Role of the vascular endothelial growth factor pathway in tumor growth and angiogenesis.* J Clin Oncol, 2005. 23(5): p. 1011-27.
[146] Relf, M., et al., *Expression of the angiogenic factors vascular endothelial cell growth factor, acidic and basic fibroblast growth factor, tumor growth factor beta-1, platelet-derived endothelial cell growth factor, placenta growth factor, and pleiotrophin in human primary breast cancer and its relation to angiogenesis.* Cancer Res, 1997. 57(5): p. 963-9.
[147] Gasparini, G., et al., *Prognostic significance of vascular endothelial growth factor protein in node-negative breast carcinoma.* J Natl Cancer Inst, 1997. 89(2): p. 139-47.
[148] Gasparini, G., et al., *Clinical relevance of vascular endothelial growth factor and thymidine phosphorylase in patients with node-positive breast cancer treated with either adjuvant chemotherapy or hormone therapy.* Cancer J Sci Am, 1999. 5(2): p. 101-11.
[149] Foekens, J.A., et al., *High tumor levels of vascular endothelial growth factor predict poor response to systemic therapy in advanced breast cancer.* Cancer Res, 2001. 61(14): p. 5407-14.
[150] Carvalho, I., et al., *Overexpression of platelet-derived growth factor receptor alpha in breast cancer is associated with tumour progression.* Breast Cancer Res, 2005. 7(5): p. R788-95.
[151] Jain, R.K., *Normalization of tumor vasculature: an emerging concept in antiangiogenic therapy.* Science, 2005. 307(5706): p. 58-62.
[152] Rosen, L.S., *VEGF-targeted therapy: therapeutic potential and recent advances.* Oncologist, 2005. 10(6): p. 382-91.
[153] Presta, L.G., et al., *Humanization of an anti-vascular endothelial growth factor monoclonal antibody for the therapy of solid tumors and other disorders.* Cancer Res, 1997. 57(20): p. 4593-9.
[154] Miller, K., et al., *Paclitaxel plus bevacizumab versus paclitaxel alone for metastatic breast cancer.* N Engl J Med, 2007. 357(26): p. 2666-76.
[155] Miller, K.D., et al., *Randomized phase III trial of capecitabine compared with bevacizumab plus capecitabine in patients with previously treated metastatic breast cancer.* J Clin Oncol, 2005. 23(4): p. 792-9.

[156] Carraway, H. and M. Hidalgo, *New targets for therapy in breast cancer: mammalian target of rapamycin (mTOR) antagonists.* Breast Cancer Res, 2004. 6(5): p. 219-24.
[157] Chu, I., et al., *The dual ErbB1/ErbB2 inhibitor, lapatinib (GW572016), cooperates with tamoxifen to inhibit both cell proliferation- and estrogen-dependent gene expression in antiestrogen-resistant breast cancer.* Cancer Res, 2005. 65(1): p. 18-25.
[158] Konecny, G.E., et al., *Activity of the dual kinase inhibitor lapatinib (GW572016) against HER-2-overexpressing and trastuzumab-treated breast cancer cells.* Cancer Res, 2006. 66(3): p. 1630-9.
[159] Abrams, T.J., et al., *SU11248 inhibits KIT and platelet-derived growth factor receptor beta in preclinical models of human small cell lung cancer.* Mol Cancer Ther, 2003. 2(5): p. 471-8.
[160] Abrams, T.J., et al., *Preclinical evaluation of the tyrosine kinase inhibitor SU11248 as a single agent and in combination with "standard of care" therapeutic agents for the treatment of breast cancer.* Mol Cancer Ther, 2003. 2(10): p. 1011-21.
[161] Mendel, D.B., et al., *In vivo antitumor activity of SU11248, a novel tyrosine kinase inhibitor targeting vascular endothelial growth factor and platelet-derived growth factor receptors: determination of a pharmacokinetic/pharmacodynamic relationship.* Clin Cancer Res, 2003. 9(1): p. 327-37.
[162] Murray, L.J., et al., *SU11248 inhibits tumor growth and CSF-1R-dependent osteolysis in an experimental breast cancer bone metastasis model.* Clin Exp Metastasis, 2003. 20(8): p. 757-66.
[163] Sapi, E., *The role of CSF-1 in normal physiology of mammary gland and breast cancer: an update.* Exp Biol Med (Maywood), 2004. 229(1): p. 1-11.
[164] Burstein, H.J., et al., *Phase II study of sunitinib malate, an oral multitargeted tyrosine kinase inhibitor, in patients with metastatic breast cancer previously treated with an anthracycline and a taxane.* J Clin Oncol, 2008. 26(11): p. 1810-6.
[165] Kozloff, M., et al., *An exploratory study of sunitinib plus paclitaxel as first-line treatment for patients with advanced breast cancer.* Ann Oncol, 2010. 21(7): p. 1436-41.
[166] Liljegren, A., J. Bergh, and R. Castany, *Early experience with sunitinib, combined with docetaxel, in patients with metastatic breast cancer.* Breast, 2009. 18(4): p. 259-62.
[167] Adnane, L., et al., *Sorafenib (BAY 43-9006, Nexavar), a dual-action inhibitor that targets RAF/MEK/ERK pathway in tumor cells and tyrosine kinases VEGFR/PDGFR in tumor vasculature.* Methods Enzymol, 2006. 407: p. 597-612.
[168] Wilhelm, S.M., et al., *BAY 43-9006 exhibits broad spectrum oral antitumor activity and targets the RAF/MEK/ERK pathway and receptor tyrosine kinases involved in tumor progression and angiogenesis.* Cancer Res, 2004. 64(19): p. 7099-109.
[169] Veronese, M.L., et al., *Mechanisms of hypertension associated with BAY 43-9006.* J Clin Oncol, 2006. 24(9): p. 1363-9.
[170] Wilmes, L.J., et al., *AG-013736, a novel inhibitor of VEGF receptor tyrosine kinases, inhibits breast cancer growth and decreases vascular permeability as detected by dynamic contrast-enhanced magnetic resonance imaging.* Magn Reson Imaging, 2007. 25(3): p. 319-27.
[171] Sotiriou, C., et al., *Breast cancer classification and prognosis based on gene expression profiles from a population-based study.* Proc Natl Acad Sci U S A, 2003. 100(18): p. 10393-8.
[172] Sevelda, P., *[Tamoxifen in the treatment of patients with breast cancer: results of the latest meta-analysis of prospective randomized clinical trials].* Gynakol Geburtshilfliche Rundsch, 1998. 38(2): p. 81-4.

[173] Ali, S. and R.C. Coombes, *Endocrine-responsive breast cancer and strategies for combating resistance.* Nat Rev Cancer, 2002. 2(2): p. 101-12.

[174] Osborne, C.K. and R. Schiff, *Estrogen-receptor biology: continuing progress and therapeutic implications.* J Clin Oncol, 2005. 23(8): p. 1616-22.

[175] Shou, J., et al., *Mechanisms of tamoxifen resistance: increased estrogen receptor-HER2/neu cross-talk in ER/HER2-positive breast cancer.* J Natl Cancer Inst, 2004. 96(12): p. 926-35.

[176] Larsen, M., et al., *The matrix reorganized: extracellular matrix remodeling and integrin signaling.* Curr Opin Cell Biol, 2006. 18(5): p. 463-71.

[177] Karin, M., et al., *NF-kappaB in cancer: from innocent bystander to major culprit.* Nat Rev Cancer, 2002. 2(4): p. 301-10.

[178] Greten, F.R., et al., *IKKbeta links inflammation and tumorigenesis in a mouse model of colitis-associated cancer.* Cell, 2004. 118(3): p. 285-96.

[179] Wiener, Z., et al., *Synergistic induction of the Fas (CD95) ligand promoter by Max and NFkappaB in human non-small lung cancer cells.* Exp Cell Res, 2004. 299(1): p. 227-35.

[180] Robbins, J., et al., *Mouse mammary tumor gene int-3: a member of the notch gene family transforms mammary epithelial cells.* J Virol, 1992. 66(4): p. 2594-9.

[181] Zheng, L., et al., *Lessons learned from BRCA1 and BRCA2.* Oncogene, 2000. 19(53): p. 6159-75.

[182] Turner, N.C., et al., *BRCA1 dysfunction in sporadic basal-like breast cancer.* Oncogene, 2007. 26(14): p. 2126-32.

[183] Richardson, P.G., et al., *A phase 2 study of bortezomib in relapsed, refractory myeloma.* N Engl J Med, 2003. 348(26): p. 2609-17.

[184] Sato, K., E. Rajendra, and T. Ohta, *The UPS: a promising target for breast cancer treatment.* BMC Biochem, 2008. 9 Suppl 1: p. S2.

[185] Kuwano, M., et al., *Multidrug resistance-associated protein subfamily transporters and drug resistance.* Anticancer Drug Des, 1999. 14(2): p. 123-31.

[186] Dantzig, A.H., D.P. de Alwis, and M. Burgess, *Considerations in the design and development of transport inhibitors as adjuncts to drug therapy.* Adv Drug Deliv Rev, 2003. 55(1): p. 133-50.

[187] Nielsen, D., C. Maare, and T. Skovsgaard, *Cellular resistance to anthracyclines.* Gen Pharmacol, 1996. 27(2): p. 251-5.

[188] Stavrovskaya, A.A., *Cellular mechanisms of multidrug resistance of tumor cells.* Biochemistry (Mosc), 2000. 65(1): p. 95-106.

[189] Azab, S.S.E.-D., E. and Al-Hendy, A., *Multi-drug resistance as a problem challenging breast cancer chemotherapy* in *Aggressive Breast Cancer*, R.H.D. ed., Editor. 2010. p. pp. 53-100.

[190] Kerb, R., S. Hoffmeyer, and U. Brinkmann, *ABC drug transporters: hereditary polymorphisms and pharmacological impact in MDR1, MRP1 and MRP2.* Pharmacogenomics, 2001. 2(1): p. 51-64.

[191] Ling, V., *Multidrug resistance: molecular mechanisms and clinical relevance.* Cancer Chemother Pharmacol, 1997. 40 Suppl: p. S3-8.

[192] Mimeault, M. and S.K. Batra, *Recent advances on multiple tumorigenic cascades involved in prostatic cancer progression and targeting therapies.* Carcinogenesis, 2006. 27(1): p. 1-22.

[193] Rubin, L.L. and F.J. de Sauvage, *Targeting the Hedgehog pathway in cancer.* Nat Rev Drug Discov, 2006. 5(12): p. 1026-33.

[194] Mimeault, M., et al., *Recent advances in cancer stem/progenitor cell research: therapeutic implications for overcoming resistance to the most aggressive cancers.* J Cell Mol Med, 2007. 11(5): p. 981-1011.

[195] Nicolis, S.K., *Cancer stem cells and "stemness" genes in neuro-oncology.* Neurobiol Dis, 2007. 25(2): p. 217-29.

[196] Chuthapisith, S., et al., *Breast cancer chemoresistance: emerging importance of cancer stem cells.* Surg Oncol, 2010. 19(1): p. 27-32.

[197] Hirschmann-Jax, C., et al., *A distinct "side population" of cells with high drug efflux capacity in human tumor cells.* Proc Natl Acad Sci U S A, 2004. 101(39): p. 14228-33.

[198] Dean, M., T. Fojo, and S. Bates, *Tumour stem cells and drug resistance.* Nat Rev Cancer, 2005. 5(4): p. 275-84.

[199] Gupta, P.B., et al., *Identification of selective inhibitors of cancer stem cells by high-throughput screening.* Cell, 2009. 138(4): p. 645-59.

[200] Mimeault, M., R. Hauke, and S.K. Batra, *Recent advances on the molecular mechanisms involved in the drug resistance of cancer cells and novel targeting therapies.* Clin Pharmacol Ther, 2008. 83(5): p. 673-91.

[201] Al-Hajj, M., et al., *Prospective identification of tumorigenic breast cancer cells.* Proc Natl Acad Sci U S A, 2003. 100(7): p. 3983-8.

[202] Harari, P.M., *Epidermal growth factor receptor inhibition strategies in oncology.* Endocr Relat Cancer, 2004. 11(4): p. 689-708.

[203] Duffy, M.J., N. O'Donovan, and J. Crown, *Use of molecular markers for predicting therapy response in cancer patients.* Cancer Treat Rev, 2011. 37(2): p. 151-9.

[204] Paik, S., *Molecular profiling of breast cancer.* Curr Opin Obstet Gynecol, 2006. 18(1): p. 59-63.

7

ErbB2/HER2: Its Contribution to Basic Cancer Biology and the Development of Molecular Targeted Therapy

Tadashi Yamamoto et al.*
The Institute of Medical Science, The University of Tokyo, Japan

1. Introduction

ErbB2, one of the receptor tyrosine kinase superfamily has attracted the attention of cancer researchers since its discovery. Thirty years ago, *ErbB2* was discovered as an oncogene that transforms NIH3T3 cells. The first decade of ErbB2 research revealed that it is a member of the ErbB receptor family and is deregulated in various types of human cancer. In the second decade, one significant discovery came from the crystallography with the rational theory that explains why no ligands specific for ErbB2 have been identified so far, and the other breakthrough came from the clinical field with the appearance of ErbB-targeted therapeutics. Today, cancer researchers strive to describe the elaborate signaling network of ErbB receptors by proteomic analysis, and our knowledge of their function, which is far from complete, is being applied to develop more efficient ErbB-targeted therapeutics for cancer patients.

We will begin the story of *ErbB2* with its discovery as an oncogene called *neu*. In the dawn of oncogene research, this gene, derived from a rat tumor, was classified as one of the most pivotal genes in human cancer, along with the oncogenes Ras and Myc and the tumor suppressor gene p53. This is because *ErbB2* is frequently amplified and overexpressed in certain human cancers, such as breast carcinoma. Similar to other oncogenes, subsequent research demonstrated its indispensable role in development. Now, our interest is whether ErbB2 acts on the same target proteins in cancer and in normal development.

The signaling networks downstream of ErbB receptors are complex because there are various ligands for each receptor, except ErbB2, and the composition of the ErbB dimer seems to define downstream signaling targets. For example, EGFR (epidermal growth factor receptor)-containing heterodimers prefer to stimulate the mitogen-activated protein kinase (MAPK) cascade, while ErbB3-containing dimers preferably activate phosphatidylinositol 3-kinase (PI3K). This characteristic is reflected in the difficulty in choosing the best therapeutics corresponding to each case in the clinic.

---

* Makoto Saito[1], Kentaro Kumazawa[1], Ayano Doi[1], Atsuka Matsui[1], Shiori Takebe[1], Takuya Amari[1], Masaaki Oyama[2] and Kentaro Semba[1]
[1]*Department of Life Science and Medical Bioscience, Waseda University, Japan*
[2]*The Institute of Medical Science, The University of Tokyo, Japan*

Our passion for determining the function of ErbB2 in cancer has inspired us to develop experimental methods to reveal mechanisms of tumorigenesis in humans. One such method is the MCF10A morphogenesis assay, which will be useful for identifying new oncogenes.

2. Discovery of *ErbB2*

This section describes the history of the discovery of *ErbB2/HER2/neu*. The *ErbB2* gene was initially identified as an oncogene named *neu* in NIH3T3 cells. Soon after, several groups, including our laboratory revealed that this gene was the second member of the EGFR family. Initial studies showed that this gene was amplified in human cancer cell lines and tissues, indicating its importance in human cancer. This finding prompted the extensive studies of ErbB2 in human cancer. By the way, official NCBI gene symbol is ERBB2 (human), however, for simplicity, we will use one term "ErbB2" in this article.

2.1 *Neu*, an oncogene cloned from murine brain tumors

The origin of *ErbB2/HER2/neu* research can be traced back to the 1980s, when virtually all cancer researchers were hunting for novel oncogenes. Cancer researchers, using the tools for introducing foreign DNA into mammalian cells, were seeking genes that render normal cells cancerous, what we call "oncogenes." Scientists introduced genomic DNA that was isolated from mouse or human tumor cells into NIH3T3 mouse fibroblast cells (Shih et al., 1979) using the calcium-phosphate DNA precipitation technique (Graham & van der Eb, 1973) and examined their morphological changes, or their "transformation". This transformation assay described in detail in section 6 produced several fruitful discoveries. For us, the most significant was the discovery of *neu*.

The first report about *neu* came in 1981 when Shih et al. indicated that DNA prepared from rat neuro-/glioblastoma cell lines transformed NIH3T3 cells (Shih et al., 1981). In 1984, Schechter et al. demonstrated that several independently isolated transformed cells contained the same oncogene, based on resistance to inactivation by restriction enzyme cleavage, and thus named the oncogene "*neu*" (Schechter et al., 1984). They also showed that the *neu* gene encoded a protein of relative molecular mass 185,000 (p185), and it was related to EGFR serologically. This finding was consistent with the fact that *neu* showed significant similarity to v-*erbB*, a retroviral oncogene of avian erythroblastosis virus (Vennstrom & Bishop, 1982; Yamamoto et al., 1983), and was homologous with the cellular gene (c-*erbB*) encoding EGFR (Downward et al., 1984).

2.2 A second member of the ErbB family, *c-erbB2/HER2*

After the initial discoveries regarding *neu*, *neu* blossomed out into one of the most famous oncogenes. In 1985, Schechter et al. demonstrated that the homology between *neu* and *erbB* was limited to the region of the kinase domain of EGFR and that *neu* mapped to human chromosome 17, distinct from c-*erbB* on chromosome 7 (Schechter et al., 1985). Semba et al. identified the human v-*erbB*-related sequence as distinct from the EGFR gene and its amplification in the human adenocarcinoma of the salivary gland (Semba et al., 1985), and they named the gene c-*erbB2*, as a separate gene from c-*erbB1*, encoding EGFR. Soon after, several groups cloned this human version of the *neu* oncogene and designated it c-*erbB2* or *HER2* (Bargmann et al., 1986b; Coussens et al., 1985; Yamamoto et al., 1986), and cDNA clones of the *neu* oncogene itself were also isolated (Hung et al., 1986). Subsequent studies revealed that *ErbB2* encodes a 185-kDa transmembrane glycoprotein that is highly similar to

EGFR (Akiyama et al., 1986; Bargmann et al., 1986b). To date, there are four ErbB family receptors: EGFR (also ErbB1, HER1), ErbB2(HER2, Neu), ErbB3(HER3) (Kraus et al., 1989), and ErbB4(HER4) (Plowman et al., 1993). We will describe their structural similarities and differences in section 3.

In what ways does the *neu* oncogene cause murine neuro-/glioblastoma? In the case of the v-*erbB* oncogene, encoding the truncated form of EGFR, we could assume that its aberrant protein, which has no ligand binding domain, phosphorylates its substrates independently of ligand binding, resulting in hyperproliferation (Khazaie et al., 1988). The *neu* proto-oncogene, however, is activated by a single point mutation, V664E, in the transmembrane domain (Bargmann et al., 1986a), and not by gross rearrangements as seen in v-*erbB*. Does this single point mutation, which causes neuro-/glioblastoma in rats, also occur in humans? Interestingly, such a single point mutation of c-*erbB2* has never been observed in cancer patients. Instead, gene amplification and overexpression of its protein product are frequently observed in various types of human cancer, especially breast cancer (Slamon et al., 1989), as described in section 4.

3. Regulation of ErbB receptors and downstream signaling pathways

The ErbB receptors are closely related, single-chain glycoproteins. ErbB receptors are activated by binding to their specific ligands. Activated ErbB receptors then transmit signals to downstream signal transducers. In this section, we describe structural features of ErbB receptors and focus on recent observations of ErbB2 signal transduction pathways.

3.1 ErbB ligands

ErbB ligands act in a paracrine or autocrine fashion. Whereas paracrine ErbB ligands are derived from stromal cells, autocrine ErbB ligands are produced as transmembrane precursors that are subsequently cleaved by proteases to be released as soluble ligands when cells are stimulated (Hynes & Lane, 2005).

At least ten ErbB ligands are known (Figure 1) and are divided into three groups with respect to binding specificity. The first group includes EGF, amphiregulin (AR) and transforming growth factor-α (TGF-α), which bind specifically to ErbB1. The second group includes betacellulin (BTC), heparin-binding EGF (HB-EGF) and epiregulin (EPR), which show dual specificity, binding to both ErbB1 and ErbB4. The third group includes neuregulins (NRGs). They are composed of two subgroups. NRG1 and NRG2 bind specifically to both ErbB3 and ErbB4, whereas NRG3 and NRG4 bind specifically to only ErbB4 (Hynes & Lane, 2005).

None of these ErbB ligands bind and activate ErbB2. However, the mucin MUC4, a transmembrane glycoprotein, modulates the ErbB2 signaling pathway. MUC4 is composed of two subunits, ASGP-1, an O-glycosylated mucin subunit, and ASGP-2, an N-glycosylated transmembrane subunit. ASGP-2 possesses two EGF-like domains, EGF-1 and EGF-2, and interacts specifically with ErbB2, inducing its phosphorylation. MUC4 retains ErbB2 and ErbB3 on the cell membrane by suppressing their ligand-induced internalization. However, the mechanisms of ErbB2 signaling activation by MUC4 are largely unknown (Singh et al., 2007).

3.2 ErbB receptors

3.2.1 Structures of ErbB receptors and their conformational changes on ligand binding

Each ErbB receptor comprises five functional domains, the extracellular domain for ligand binding (~620 residues), the α-helical transmembrane segment (~23 residues), and

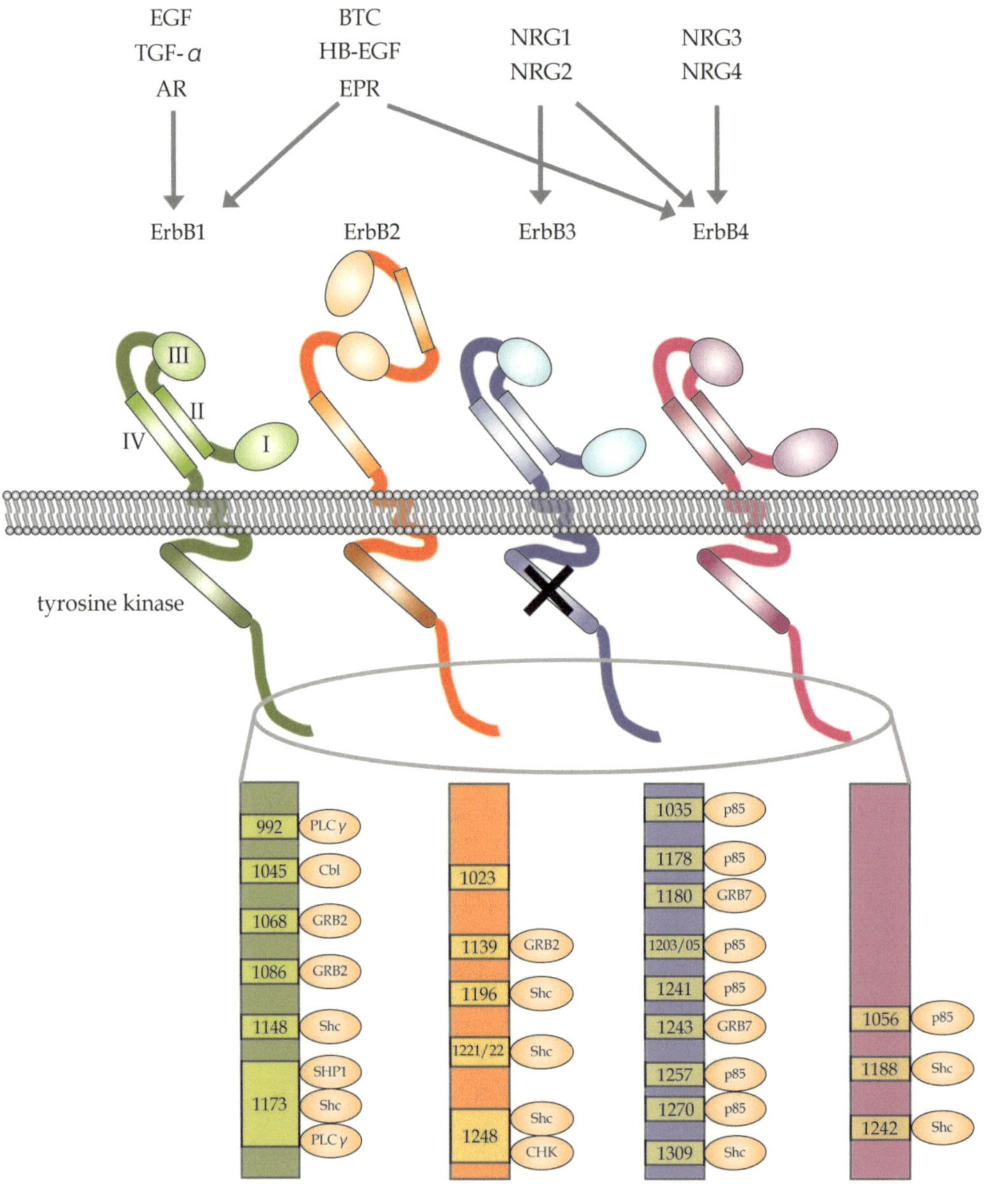

Fig. 1. ErbB ligands and receptors.
ErbB ligands, which act in an autocrine or paracrine fashion, are divided into three groups based on binding specificity. None of the ErbB ligands binds to ErbB2. However, MUC4 modulates ErbB2 signaling activity. Ligand binding to the extracellular domain of ErbB receptors changes the receptor's conformation and promotes homo- and heterodimerization. Its dimerization induces the tyrosine kinase activity of the intracellular domain, resulting in the cross-phosphorylation of specific tyrosine residues, which recruits and activates specific downstream signaling proteins. The intracellular domain of each ErbB receptor possesses unique docking sites for downstream signaling proteins, which consist of tyrosine residues and the surrounding amino acids (Baselga & Swain, 2009; Hynes & Lane, 2005; Olayioye et

al., 2000). ErbB1 has docking sites for growth factor receptor-bound 2 (GRB2) and Src homology 2-containing (Shc), which activate the MAPK and PI3K–Akt pathways though Ras activation, although it has no direct docking site for PI3K (Hynes & Lane, 2005). ErbB1 has a docking site for Cbl, an E3 ubiquitin ligase. ErbB1 dimerization induced by ligand binding induces receptor internalization into endosomes, which is followed by recycling. In the endosome, Cbl directly binds to tyrosine residues of ErbB1 and undergoes ubiquitylation, resulting in its degradation in lysosomes (Citri & Yarden, 2006). ErbB2 functions as the preferred partner of other ErbB receptors and possesses the strongest kinase activity. ErbB3 possesses six p85 docking sites, which effectively activate the PI3K–Akt pathway, although it lacks tyrosine kinase activity (Moasser, 2007). ErbB1, ErbB2 and ErbB3 are implicated in the progression of cancer. However, ErbB4 is associated with the inhibition of cell proliferation, although it has docking sites for p85 and Shc (Baselga & Swain, 2009).

a juxtamembranedomain (~40 residues), an intracellular tyrosine kinase domain (~260 residues), and a C-terminal regulatory region (~232residues) (Burgess et al., 2003). Intriguingly, the structures of ErbB2 and ErbB3 are unique among the ErbB family. ErbB2 is an orphan receptor, but it always has a ligand-activated conformation (Garrett et al., 2003), while ErbB3 has impaired intrinsic tyrosine kinase activity (P.M. Guy et al., 1994).

The ErbB family is conserved during evolution. Although we will not discuss the issue in detail, the biological significance of EGFR in the physiological state lies in its involvement in epithelial development in mammals (Miettinen et al., 1995; Sibilia & Wagner, 1995; Threadgill et al., 1995). EGFR has similar functions in invertebrates. For instance, both *Caenorhabditis elegans* and *Drosophila melanogaster* have a single EGFR homolog (Aroian et al., 1990; Livneh et al., 1985). EGFR regulates vulva development in *Caenorhabditis elegans* (Moghal & Sternberg, 2003) and the development of various organs in *Drosophila* (Shilo, 2003). In *Caenorhabditis elegans*, in parallel with the simplicity of the ErbB family of receptors, there are only one ligand for the receptors (Yarden & Sliwkowski, 2001), while humans have ten. The versatility of ErbB receptors and their ligands in mammals, which evolved from a simple cascade important for development in invertebrates, can endow signaling networks with not only robustness but also vulnerability, represented by tumorigenesis, a collapse of the regulatory circuit. The evolutional conservation of tumor-promoting ability of EGFR is well known, for instance, from the melanoma model of *Xiphophorus* (Gomez et al., 2004).

The extracellular domain consists of domains I–IV. Domain II promotes receptor dimerization. In the absence of ligand binding, ErbB exists in a tethered conformation in which intramolecular interaction between domains II and IV blocks the function of dimerization domain II. Ligand binding to ErbB receptors changes the tethered conformation into the extended conformation, which exposes domain II, allowing them to undergo homo- and heterodimerization (Hynes & Lane, 2005). However, ErbB3 lacks the ability to homodimerize (Baselga & Swain, 2009). ErbB2 has a unique structure of the ligand-activated conformation and is the most preferred partner for other ligand-bound ErbB receptors. This is because the structure of the ErbB2 extracellular domain originally resembles the extended conformation that exhibits no interaction between domain II and domain IV and exposes the dimerization domain II (Hynes & Lane, 2005). The intracellular domain possesses the protein tyrosine kinase activity and unique docking sites for specific downstream signaling proteins, which consist of tyrosine residues and surrounding amino acid side chains (Hynes & Lane, 2005). ErbB2 possesses the strongest tyrosine kinase activity among the ErbB receptors (Moasser, 2007). However, ErbB3 lacks the tyrosine kinase activity because it is unable to bind to ATP (Baselga & Swain, 2009).

3.2.2 HSP90–ErbB2 complex

Heat shock proteins (HSPs), a large family of highly conserved molecular chaperone proteins, mediate the conformational maturation and folding of target proteins. HSP90 protects the ErbB system from damage. Whereas other ErbB receptors are HSP90-independent, ErbB2 and several downstream signaling proteins are stabilized by HSP90. A ternary complex of HSP90, ErbB2 and a co-chaperone, CDC37, stabilizes ErbB2 at the cell membrane (Baselga & Swain, 2009; Citri & Yarden, 2006) . Inhibition of HSP90 function by specific drugs results in ubiquitylation and proteasomal degradation of ErbB2 and its downstream signaling proteins (Baselga & Swain, 2009). HSP90 also controls ErbB2 signaling activity. Binding of the complex of HSP90 and CDC37 to the tyrosine kinase domain of ErbB2 suppresses its tyrosine kinase activity and heterodimerization with other ligand-bound ErbB receptors.

3.3 Signaling pathways activated by ErbB receptors

Ligand-binding to the extracellular domain of ErbB receptors changes the tethered conformation into the extended conformation, inducing homo- and heterodimerization. Only ErbB2 is able to dimerize without ligand-binding. ErbB receptor dimerization results in phosphorylation on specific tyrosine residues of the intracellular domain. These phosphorylated tyrosine residues and surrounding amino acid side chains allow the recruitment and activation of downstream signaling proteins, which initiate multiple signaling pathways (Baselga & Swain, 2009).

The combination of ligands and heterodimer partners determines which downstream signaling proteins are recruited and which signaling pathways are activated. The heterodimer of ErbB2–ErbB3 is the most active in ErbB downstream signaling (Baselga & Swain, 2009).

Two main signaling pathways activated by ErbB receptors are the MAPK and the PI3K-Akt pathways. Other important ErbB signaling proteins are the signal transducers and activators of transcription (STATs) and the Src tyrosine kinase (Hynes & Lane, 2005). Although ErbB receptors are largely known as receptor tyrosine kinases (RTKs), recent studies indicate they can localize to the nucleus and act as transcription factors (S.-C. Wang et al., 2004).

3.3.1 MAPK pathway

GRB2, an adaptor protein, binds to ErbB receptors either indirectly through Shc or directly to the phosphorylated tyrosine residues. The GRB2–son of sevenless (Sos) complex, with or without Shc, recruits Ras and activates the MAPK pathway, inducing cell proliferation, migration, differentiation and angiogenesis (Baselga & Swain, 2009). Recent analysis using MCF10A cells showed that Shc is required for the inhibition of apoptosis and for paclitaxel resistance (see also section 6 for MCF10A system).

3.3.2 PI3K–Akt pathway

PI3K, a heterodimer composed of a p85 regulatory subunit and p110 catalytic subunit, is activated by at least two ErbB-related pathways. In the first pathway, p85 directly binds to phosphorylated tyrosine residues, triggering the activation of the p110 catalytic subunit. In the second pathway, GRB2 binds to ErbB either indirectly though Shc or directly to phosphorylated tyrosine residues and activates Ras, which also triggers the activation of p110 (Baselga & Swain, 2009; Cully et al., 2006). Activated PI3K phosphorylates phosphatidylinositol 4,5-bisphosphate (PIP2) into phosphatidylinositol 3,4,5-triphosphate (PIP3), which recruits Akt and phosphatidylinositol-dependent kinase 1 (PDK1) and activates PDK1. PDK1 phosphorylates and activates Akt. The tumor-suppressor phosphatase with tensin homology (PTEN) dephosphorylates PIP3 into PIP2 and inhibits PI3K–Akt pathway activation (Cully et al., 2006).

Activated Akt phosphorylates many target proteins associated with cell survival, proliferation (increased cell number), and growth (increased cell size). In addition, Akt promotes angiogenesis through vascular endothelial growth factor (VEGF) and hypoxia-inducible factor-1α (HIF-1α) (Vivanco & Sawyers, 2002).

3.3.2.1 Survival

Activated Akt directly phosphorylates several target proteins to suppress apoptosis. BAD, a pro-apoptotic member of the BCL2 family, antagonizes the survival protein BCL-X_L to promote cell death. Activated Akt phosphorylates BAD, which prevents it from interacting with BCL-X_L, allowing BCL-X_L to function as an anti-apoptotic protein. Caspase-9, a member of the cysteine-dependent aspartyl-specific protease family, cleaves and activates pro-caspase-3, resulting in apoptosis. Activated Akt phosphorylates caspase-9 and inhibits its catalytic activity. Forkhead box 1 (FOXO1), a member of the forkhead family of transcription factors, activates several pro-apoptotic proteins, including BIM and FAS ligand. Activated Akt phosphorylates FOXO1 and prevents its nuclear translocation. Nuclear factor κB (NF-κB), a transcription factor, is constantly inhibited by IκB. Activated Akt phosphorylates IκB kinase (IKK), which degrades IκB, allowing NF-κB to translocate to the nucleus and activate its target genes. Murine double minute (MDM2), a p53-binding protein, mediates proteasomal degradation of p53. Activated Akt phosphorylates and activates MDM2 (Vivanco & Sawyers, 2002).

3.3.2.2 Proliferation

Activated Akt directly phosphorylates several target proteins to regulate cell cycle control. Glycogen synthase kinase-3β (GSK-3β) phosphorylates cyclin D1 which mediates G1/S phase transition to induce its proteasomal degradation. Activated Akt directly phosphorylates and inhibits GSK-3β, which allows cyclin D1 to accumulate (Vivanco & Sawyers, 2002). Activated Akt phosphorylates and inhibits p27, a CDK inhibitor (CKI), promoting cell cycle entry. In addition, p27 expression is regulated by the transcription factor FOXO3A. FOXO3A activates p27 and BIM expression, and inhibit cyclin D1 expression. Activated Akt phosphorylates FOXO3A, which promotes its translocation from the nucleus. Activated Akt also modulates p21 activity by affecting its phosphorylation, presumably through other kinases (Cully et al., 2006).

3.3.2.3 Growth

Activated Akt directly phosphorylates tuberous sclerosis 2 (TSC2) to affect cell growth. TSC2 heterodimerizes with TSC1 to promote the GTPase activity of the Ras homolog enriched in brain (RHEB). Activated Akt phosphorylates TSC2 and inhibits the ability of the TSC1–TSC2 complex to act as RHEB-GTPase activating protein (RHEB-GAP), which allows GTP-bound RHEB to accumulate. Active GTP-bound RHEB promotes the kinase activity of the mammalian target of rapamycin (mTOR), a key regulator of cell growth. Activated mTOR, regulatory associated protein of TOR (raptor) and G-protein β-subunit-like (GβL) complex phosphorylates S6 kinase (S6K) and the eukaryotic translation-initiatin factor 4E (EIF4E)-inhibitory binding protein (4E-BP) to modulate the mRNA translation and protein synthesis (Cully et al., 2006).

3.3.3 ErB2–ErbB3 heterodimer and PI3K–Akt pathway

Several lines of evidence indicate that the heterodimer ErbB2–ErbB3 is the most important oncogenic signaling associated with the activation of the PI3K–Akt pathway. ErbB2, which lacks p85-binding sites, possesses strong kinase activity, and ErbB3, which lacks tyrosine kinase activity, possesses six p85-binding sites. Akt is frequently activated in ErbB2-overexpressing tumors, as well as in tumors generated in mouse mammary tumor virus (MMTV)-*neu* transgenic mice. Cell transformation by overexpressed ErbB2 *in vitro* is associated with increased ErbB3 phosphorylation and activation of the PI3K–Akt pathway. These results suggest the transactivation of ErbB3, and the PI3K–Akt pathway is strongly associated with the tumorigenic function of overexpressed ErbB2 (Moasser, 2007).

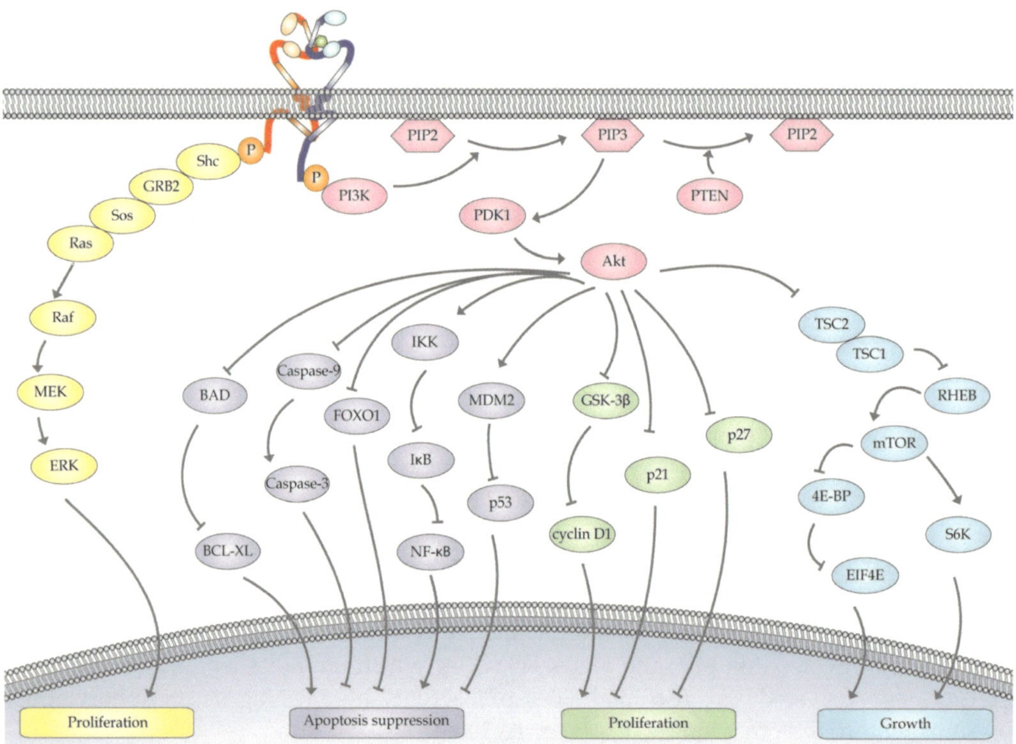

Fig. 2. Downstream signaling pathways of ErbB2–ErbB3 heterodimer.

The MAPK pathway and PI3K–Akt pathway are the two main pathways activated by ErbB receptors. GRB2–Sos complex, with or without Shc, recruits Ras and activates MAPK signaling, inducing cell proliferation, migration, differentiation and angiogenesis. PI3K is a heterodimer composed of a p85 regulatory subunit and a p110 catalytic subunit. p110 is activated by p85 directly binding to phosphorylated tyrosine residues or indirectly binding though the GRB2–Sos–Ras complex, with or without Shc, to phosphorylated tyrosine residues within RTKs. Activated PI3K phosphorylates PIP2 into PIP3, which recruits and activates PDK1. PDK1 phosphorylates and activates PI3K. PTEN dephosphorylates PIP3 into PIP2. Activated Akt phosphorylates many downstream proteins, inducing cell survival, proliferation, growth, and angiogenesis (Baselga & Swain, 2009; Cully et al., 2006; Vivanco & Sawyers, 2002). The heterodimer ErbB2–ErbB3 is the most oncogenic signaling activator of the PI3K–Akt pathway because ErbB2 possesses strong kinase activity, and ErbB3 possesses six p85-binding sites (Moasser, 2007).

3.3.4 Inhibition of PI3K–Akt signaling though PTEN by trastuzumab

Nagata et al. suggested the potency of trastuzumab (a humanized anti-ErbB2 monoclonal antibody, Herceptin®) is dependent on the ability to inhibit PI3K–Akt signaling pathway though activation of PTEN. PTEN dephosphorylates PIP3 into PIP2 and inhibits PI3K–Akt pathway activation. Overexpression of ErbB2 induces dimerization, resulting in phosphorylation on specific tyrosine residues of the intracellular domain. These phosphorylated tyrosine residues and surrounding amino acid side chains allow the recruitment and activation of downstream signaling proteins, including PI3K and Src. Activated PI3K activates PI3K–Akt pathway associated with cell survival, proliferation, growth and angiogenesis. Phosphorylated Src becomes activated and phosphorylates PTEN on tyrosine residues within the PTEN C2 domain, preventing PTEN from localizing to the cell membrane and dephosphorylating PI3K, and this also activates PI3K–Akt signaling. Treatment with trastuzumab keeps Src from binding ErbB2, leading to the dephosphorylation and inactivation of Src. PTEN is released from phosphorylation of Src and is localized to the cell membrane, which allows PTEN to antagonize PI3K function and negatively regulate the PI3K–Akt signaling pathway. However, Nagata et al. did not explore the mechanism that trastuzumab treatment rapidly keeps Src from ErbB2 (Crowder et al., 2004; Nagata et al., 2004).

3.3.5 The role of Src in the signaling pathway activated by ErbB2

Src, a non-receptor tyrosine kinase, is a critical component of multiple signaling pathways, leading to proliferation, survival, metastasis and angiogenesis. Several results indicate a functional and physical interaction between ErbB2 and Src. Src and ErbB receptors are overexpressed in ~70% of breast tumors (Ishizawar & Parsons, 2004). Src and Yes are activated in mammary tumors of MMTV-*neu* transgenic mice. Activation of Src is also observed in mammary epithelial cells transformed by ErbB2, but not by H-Ras, indicating that Src is a downstream signaling protein of ErbB2. Src directly interacts with the kinase domain of ErbB2. ErbB2 activates Src function by stabilizing Src and promoting increased Src expression or by directly phosphorylating Src in its SH2 domain. Src promotes ErbB2–ErbB3 dimerization, resulting in activation of their signaling activity. Src also phosphorylates the activation loop of the tyrosine kinase domain of ErbB2, which increases its kinase activity (Moasser, 2007).

3.3.6 The role of Cyclin D1 in ErbB2–induced tumorigenesis

Cyclin D1 is the key protein in ErbB2-induced tumorigenesis. ErbB2 overexpression in breast epithelial cells shows a short G1 phase and early S phase entry, mediated by the up-regulation of cyclin D1, cyclin E, and Cdk6 expression and enhanced degradation and relocalization of p21, leading to hyperproliferation (Timms et al., 2002). Cyclin D1-deficient mice show resistance to breast cancers induced by the *neu* oncogene, whereas they remain fully sensitive to other oncogenic pathways, such as c-myc or Wnt1 (Yu et al., 2001). Ectopic expression of *neu* or Wnt oncogene in the mammary glands of mice deficient in Cdk4, the partner of cyclin D1, shows Cdk4 expression is required for efficient *neu*-induced tumorigenesis, whereas it is not required for Wnt-induced tumorigenesis (Reddy, 2005). p16, a CKI, blocks Cdk4 and Cdk6 activity, and the MMTV-p16 transgene blocks ErbB2-induced tumorigenesis. These results suggest the importance of cyclin D1 in ErbB2-induced tumorigenesis and cell cycle control (Yang et al., 2004). Furthermore, cyclin D1 kinase activity is required for the self-renewal of mammary stem and progenitor cells that are targets of MMTV-ErbB2 tumorigenesis (Jeselsohn et al., 2010).

3.3.7 Cooperation of ErbB2 and α6β4 integrin to promote breast cancers

Integrins, heterodimeric cell surface proteins mediate adhesion between cells and the extracellular matrix (ECM) and also regulate signaling pathways. Guo et al. suggested β4 integrin amplifies ErbB2 signaling, promoting mammary tumorigenesis, by studying a targeted deletion of the β4 signaling domain in MMTV-*neu* mice. A complex of ErbB2, Src, and β4 integrin induces phosphorylation of the signaling domain of β4 integrin and the P loop kinase domain of ErbB2, which enhances ErbB2 kinase activity through activation of Src. Cooperative signaling by ErbB2 and α6β4 integrins activates Jun and STAT3. JNK-mediated phosphorylation of Jun promotes oncogenic hyperproliferation. STAT3 promotes the loss of epithelial adhesion and acquisition of an invasive phenotype (W. Guo et al., 2006; Muthuswamy, 2006).

3.3.8 The role of ErbB2 as a nuclear tyrosine kinase receptor

Although ErbB receptors have been considered strictly plasma membrane receptors, recent studies suggest that they can translocate to the nucleus and act as transcription factors. Full-length ErbB1 and ErbB3 translocate to the nucleus. Nuclear ErbB1 physically interacts with STAT3, leading to the transcriptional activation of inducible nitric oxide synthase (iNOS). An intracellular fragment of ErbB4 translocates to the nucleus. First, the extracellular domain of ErbB4 is cleaved by ADAM17/TACE. Second, the transmembrane domain is cleaved by γ-secretase, allowing the cytoplasmic fragment of ErbB4 to translocate to the nucleus (Citri & Yarden, 2006; S.-C. Wang et al., 2004). The study of Wang et al. suggested that ErbB2 acts as a nuclear tyrosine kinase receptor. Full-length ErbB2 is also localized in the nucleus in both cultured cells and primary tumor tissues, where it is recruited to several gene promoters. For example, ErbB2 is recruited to the cyclooxygenase-2 (COX-2) promoter and activates its transcription. The increased expression of COX-2 is associated with angiogenesis, invasiveness and anti-apoptotic effects (S.-C. Wang et al., 2004). Because it lacks a DNA-binding domain, however, ErbB2 may interact with other nuclear factors to indirectly bind to these promoters.

3.3.9 Mass spectrometry–based quantitative proteomics of ErbB2 signaling networks

Recent technological advances in mass spectrometry (MS) have enabled us to understand the whole signaling networks in combination of biological and mathematical analyses. Pioneering research investigated EGFR signaling with MS-based quantitative proteomics (Blagoev et al., 2004). In this report, three cell populations were labeled by stable isotopes using amino acids in a cell culture technique called SILAC, and each population was

stimulated by EGF for a variable length of time. Subsequently, tyrosine-phosphorylated proteins and associated proteins were purified by anti-phosphotyrosine antibodies and then quantified by MS. A large number of signaling proteins were identified, and the dynamics of their activation were revealed. Following this study, the ErbB2 signaling pathway was studied by similar methods (Bose, 2006). Three groups of cell lysates (ErbB2-overexpressing cells, cells transfected with empty vector, ErbB2-overexpressing cells with EGFR and the ErbB2 selective tyrosine kinase inhibitor PD168393) were affinity-purified. Phosphoproteins were separated by SDS-PAGE and subjected to liquid chromatography–tandem MS. In their study, 462 proteins were identified and quantified. There were four major patterns of dynamics in protein phosphorylation. For example, the adaptor protein Dok1 showed increased phosphorylation in ErbB2-overexpressing cells and decreased phosphorylation when treated with PD168393. Another adaptor protein, Fyn-binding protein (Fyb), showed increased phosphorylation in ErbB2-overexpressing cells, but under PD168393 treatment, there was no significant change in phosphorylation. Focal adhesion kinase (FAK) showed decreased phosphorylation in ErbB2-overexpressing cells, whereas Grb2 showed no significant changes in phosphorylation. Overall, 198 proteins showed remarkable (>1.5-fold) increases in phosphorylation, and 81 proteins showed remarkable (<0.66-fold) decreases.
Another report examined phosphorylation in the ErbB2 signaling pathway with MS (Wolf-Yadlin et al., 2006). In this report, ErbB2-overexpressing cells were stimulated by EGF or NRG. From this analysis, they identified 332 phosphorylated peptides from 175 proteins. Among these peptides, 289 were singly phosphorylated, 42 were doubly phosphorylated, and one was triply phosphorylated. Altogether, 20 phosphorylation sites were identified on EGFR, HER2, and HER3. These results show that EGF stimulation of ErbB2-overexpressing cells activates multiple signaling pathways to induce migration, while HRG stimulation of these cells leads to the amplification of a specific subset of proteins in the migratory signal pathway. Most of these novel phosphorylations have not been studied in detail, but these studies have definitely improved our understanding of ErbB2 signal transduction networks. Besides phosphorylation, EGF-induced ubiquitination network also has been studied (Argenzio et al., 2011).

4. ErbB2 in human cancer

ErbB2 amplification and overexpression have been reported in several human cancers, including breast, ovarian, lung and other cancers (Baselga & Swain, 2009; Santarius et al., 2010). In contrast, recent sequence analysis revealed that point mutation and internal deletion of *ErbB2* were rare (http://www.sanger.ac.uk/). ErbB2 overexpression is associated with poor prognosis in most cancers (Baselga & Swain, 2009; Santarius et al., 2010). ErbB2 is thus used as a tumor marker as well as a target for cancer therapy. ErbB2-targeted therapy uses the humanized monoclonal antibody trastuzumab or the ErbB kinase inhibitor lapatinib, pertuzumab, trastuzumab-DM1, or ertumaxomab (see section 5). However, resistance to trastuzumab is a critical issue for this therapy. As described above in section 3.3, PTEN and Src are the key modulators of trastuzumab resistance. PTEN function has been positively correlated with the clinical effect of trastuzumab (Baselga & Swain, 2009). A recent report showed that targeting Src in combination with trastuzumab sensitized trastuzumab-resistant cells to trastuzumab and eliminated trastuzumab-resistant tumors *in vivo* (Zhang et al., 2011). This section summarizes the current findings on *ErbB2* amplification and prognosis in each type of cancer (Table 1).

4.1 Breast cancer

In the initial study by Slamon et al., 28% of 189 breast tumors showed evidence of *ErbB2* gene amplification (Slamon et al., 1989). In other reports, amplification rates vary from 18 to 40% of breast cancers (Baselga & Swain, 2009; Santarius et al., 2010). ErbB2 is overexpressed in most amplified cases and in some non-amplified cases as well. *ErbB2* amplification and overexpression are associated with poor prognosis, namely overall survival and time to relapse (Baselga & Swain, 2009; Santarius et al., 2010; Sircoulomb et al., 2010). As described in section 6.2, various types of breast cancer models with enforced expression of ErbB2 have been developed. Intriguingly, the growth of both primary mammary tumors and pulmonary metastases depends on the continuous expression of ErbB2 (Moody et al., 2002).

Amplification of the *ErbB2* gene correlates with enhanced ErbB2 expression. One study of the transcriptional regulation of *ErbB2* demonstrated that the X-linked FOXP3, which is a member of the forkhead/winged helix transcription factor family, represses transcription of *ErbB2* (Zuo et al., 2007). X-linked tumor suppressor genes are relevant to tumorigenesis because several of such genes are subject to X inactivation, leading to the realization of Knudson's two-hit hypothesis. According to that report, FOXP3 binds to its consensus sequence in the 5′ promoter of the *ErbB2* gene and works as a transcriptional repressor. Moreover, somatic mutation of *FOXP3* was found in some breast cancer samples, and there was an inverse correlation between FOXP3 expression and that of ERBB2 among the samples, which is consistent with FOXP3's transcriptional activity. Finally, exogenous expression of FOXP3 inhibited the growth and tumorigenicity of various cancer cell lines. Recently, microRNAs (miRNAs) have attracted cancer researchers' attention because the relationships between deregulation of some miRNAs and tumorigenesis have been extensively reported. As expected, microarray analysis demonstrated that the expression level of each miRNA varied between types of cancer (Mattie et al., 2006). Interestingly, *miR-125b* and its homolog *miR-125a* were both downregulated in ErbB2-positive breast cancer. A subsequent study on the function of *miR-125* revealed that *miR-125* targeted the 3′-UTRs of *ErbB2* and *ErbB3*, and the overexpression of *miR-125* inhibited anchorage-dependent growth of SKBR3 and MCF10A cells. Interestingly, the migration and invasion of SKBR3 cells, which are derived from human ErbB2-positive breast cancer cells, was also inhibited by these miRNAs.

These results indicate that not only the amplification of the *ErbB2* gene but also regulation at the transcriptional level contributes to the overexpression of the gene, leading to human breast cancer.

4.2 Ovarian cancer

The initial study on ErbB2 in ovarian cancer was also conducted by Slamon et al., demonstrating that *ErbB2* is a reliable indicator of prognosis (Slamon et al., 1989). Among 73 ovarian cancers, 50 (68%) had staining similar to that of normal ovarian epithelium, while 23 (32%) showed strong staining (Berchuck et al., 1990). The prognosis of the 23 patients with ErbB2 overexpression was poorer than that of the 50 patients with normal ErbB2 expression (Berchuck et al., 1990). In ovarian cancer, therefore, ErbB2 is a predictor of prognosis. Recently, Zheng et al. showed that human immortalized ovarian epithelial cells with ErbB2 expression developed into papillary carcinoma in mice when injected intraperitoneally (Zheng et al., 2010).

cancer	amplification	mutation	prognosis	treatment	reference
breast cancer	18-40%	-	poor	trastuzumab, pertuzumab(phase III), trastuzumab-DM1(phase III), ertumaxomab(phase II), lapatinib	(Baselga & Swain, 2009; Santarius et al., 2010; Sircoulomb et al., 2010)
ovarian cancer	20%	-	poor	pertuzumab(phase II)	(Baselga & Swain, 2009; Berchuck et al., 1990; Santarius et al., 2010)
lung cancer	rare	10%	negative	lapatinib(phase II)	(Baselga & Swain, 2009; Hirsch et al., 2002; Santarius et al., 2010)
gastric cancer	10-30%	-	not clear	Trastuzumab(phase III), lapatinib(phase III)	(Baselga & Swain, 2009)
endometrial cancer	15-35%	-	poor	-	(Santarius et al., 2010)
oesophageal carcinoma	20%	-	poor	-	(Santarius et al., 2010)
bladder cancer	5-15%	-	poor	-	(Santarius et al., 2010)
medullo-blastoma	13%	-	poor	-	(Santarius et al., 2010)
glioma	-	-	poor	-	(Santarius et al., 2010)

Table 1. ErbB2 aberrations in human cancer.

4.3 Lung cancer

Ten percent of the adenocarcinoma subtype of lung cancer and a small proportion of non-small cell lung tumors show ErbB2-activating mutations in the kinase domain (Hirsch et al., 2002; Santarius et al., 2010). One important ErbB2 mutation is a G776 insertion in exon 20. *ErbB2* amplifications are rare in lung cancers (Hirsch et al., 2002). For example, among 238 non-small cell lung tumors, 39 (16%), including 35% of the adenocarcinomas, 20% of the large cell carcinomas and only 1% of the squamous cell carcinomas, were 2+ or 3+ overexpressed by immunohistochemistry using the HercepTest (S.E. Wang et al., 2006), whereas 3+ overexpression was rare (4%) (S.E. Wang et al., 2006). Inducible expression of ErbB2 mutations in lung epithelial cells causes invasive adenocarcinoma in mice (Perera et al., 2009). In contrast to EGFR, *ErbB2* mutations are not associated with prognosis (Tomizawa et al., 2011). In addition, one patient with the *ErbB2* mutation YVMA776-779ins responded to trastuzumab plus vinorelbine after failure of platinum-based chemotherapy and gefitinib.

4.4 Other cancers

10-30% of gastric cancers, 10–35% of endometrial cancers, 20% of Barrett's esophageal carcinomas, and 13% of medulloblastomas show *ErbB2* amplification and overexpression (Santarius et al., 2010). For example, in a panel of nine gastric cell lines, two of which showed *ErbB2* amplification and overexpression, were more sensitive to trastuzumab than cells without *ErbB2* amplification. In endometrial cancer and esophageal carcinomas, *ErbB2* amplifications are associated with poor prognosis.

5. ErbB2 as a therapeutic target

5.1 Antibody-based agents

Accumulating evidence demonstrating the significance of ErbB2 in human cancer has prompted researchers and pharmaceutical companies to develop ErbB2-targeting cancer therapies. Monoclonal antibody therapy has finally demonstrated significant benefits for patients with cancer and has been established as a standard of care. Antibodies can inhibit tumor growth by several mechanisms (Hansel et al., 2010). In contrast to other ErbB receptors, ErbB2 has no known ligand. Therefore, antibodies targeting ErbB2 suppress ErbB2 signaling by inhibiting receptor homo- or hetero-dimerization and/or internalization (Chen et al., 2003). Alternatively, tumor-bound antibodies can initiate an immunological assault against the cancer by activating antibody-dependent cellular cytotoxicity (ADCC) or complement-dependent cytotoxicity (CDC).

An important issue in the use of antibodies for therapy is the immunogenicity of the antibodies; antibodies derived from animals are easily recognized as foreign and cause strong immune responses (Khazaeli et al., 1994). This issue has been overcome by the generation of chimeric, humanized and fully human monoclonal antibodies, with a reduction in potentially immunogenic mouse components (Lonberg, 2005). The advances in antibody engineering have led to monoclonal antibodies with marked successes in the clinic (Adams & Weiner, 2005).

Trastuzumab, a humanized monoclonal antibody directed against the extracellular juxtamembrane (domain IV) of ErbB2, has had a major impact on the breast cancer therapy. In patients with breast cancer that overexpresses ErbB2, trastuzumab has anti-tumor activity and improves outcome and survival in combination with chemotherapy in patients with metastatic breast cancer (Slamon et al., 2001). Trastuzumab represents the standard of care in the adjuvant treatment of ErbB2-overexpressing breast cancers. The mechanisms through which trastuzumab exerts its effects are likely to include ADCC (Clynes et al., 2000), the inhibition of receptor dimerization and cleavage of the ErbB2 extracellular domain (Hudis, 2007).

However, the majority of patients with ErbB2-overexpressing tumors do not respond to trastuzumab or develop acquired resistance within a year. Several molecular mechanisms that could contribute to the development of trastuzumab resistance have been reported (Nahta & Esteva, 2006). In addition to alterations in ErbB2, other members of the ErbB family are thought to play roles in trastuzumab resistance by signaling downstream to the PI3K and MAPK pathways, bypassing trastuzumab's ErbB2-based inhibition of these pathways (Kruser & Wheeler, 2010). Loss of functionally of PTEN and mutations that activate PI3K are possible mechanisms of resistance to trastuzumab (see also 3.3.4 and Berns et al., 2007). Decreased interaction between trastuzumab and its target receptor ErbB2 due to steric hindrance of ErbB2 by MUC4 may prevent the actions of trastuzumab (Nagy et al., 2005). Because blocking ErbB2 to inhibit cancer cell growth can be circumvented through alternative signaling pathways, the combination of different agents that target molecules that contribute to anti-ErbB2 resistance may be a promising tool in the treatment of ErbB2-positive breast cancer.

Several other monoclonal antibodies that target ErbB2 are being tested in the clinic. Pertuzumab (developed by Genentech) is a humanized monoclonal antibody that binds to extracellular domain II of ErbB2, which is distinct from the binding site of trastuzumab. It sterically inhibits dimerization of ErbB2 with other ErbB proteins (Agus et al., 2002) and with IGF-1R (Nahta et al., 2005) and blocks the downstream signaling pathways of these dimers. The fact that pertuzumab and trastuzumab recognize different sites causes distinct downstream effects, and the combination of pertuzumab with trastuzumab synergistically inhibits the survival of breast tumor cells (Nahta et al., 2004).

Monoclonal antibodies are generally well tolerated in humans and are now established as targeted therapies. However, administration of mAbs carries the risk of immune and innate reactions (Presta, 2006). ErbB2-targeted therapies have been associated with cardiotoxicity because they can interrupt ErbB2 signaling, which is important for receptor signaling in the heart (Force et al., 2007). Fortunately, symptomatic cardiac toxicity frequently improves when trastuzumab therapy has been stopped (Romond et al., 2005).

The next generation of mAbs currently under development incorporates additional beneficial modifications, such as alterations in glycosylation and sequences that enhance ADCC (Lazar et al., 2006) or modifications in size and antigen-binding affinity that increase the ability of the mAb to penetrate solid tumors. Recombinant technology allows extensive modifications to be made to the structures of antibodies, including the production of recombinant antibody fragments. One advantage to this is that they are smaller and penetrate tissues and tumors more rapidly and deeply than whole antibodies (Jain, 1990). Bispecific and trispecific antibodies that target ErbB2 are also under investigation. These antibodies are designed to interact with other key proteins to facilitate, for example, the binding of a single antibody to all of the target antigens, to draw the immune cell into close proximity with the tumor cell that overexpresses ErbB2, with consequent recruitment of cytotoxic T cells to the T cell–antibody–tumor cell complex and immunological destruction of the tumor cell (Kiewe et al., 2006). Multifunctional mAbs will achieve more selective and effective cancer therapies.

5.2 Chemical compounds

In addition to antibodies targeting the extracellular domain of ErbR2, small-molecule tyrosine kinase inhibitors that directly inhibit the tyrosine kinase activity of ErbB2 have been developed. Among them, lapatinib (Tykerb®) is a dual tyrosine kinase inhibitor that targets both ErbB2 and EGFR. Lapatinib was developed as a safe and orally effective drug for the treatment of EGFR- or/and ErbB2-overexpressing breast cancer (Reid et al., 2007). It binds the ATP-binding pocket of the EGFR/ErbB2 protein kinase domain, preventing self-phosphorylation and the subsequent activation of the signaling cascade, leading to an increase in apoptosis and a decrease in cellular proliferation. In comparison to other tyrosine kinase inhibitors in clinical trials (for example, gefitinib and erlotinib), the interaction of lapatinib with EGFR and ErbB2 is reversible, but dissociation is much slower, allowing for prolonged downregulation of receptor tyrosine phosphorylation in tumor cells. Lapatinib in combination with trastuzumab exhibits a synergistic effect in ErbB2-overexpressing breast cancer cells, and it also has activity against trastuzumab-resistant cells (Konecny et al., 2006). Furthermore, due to the small size of lapatinib compared to antibodies, it can penetrate the blood-brain barrier and act against central nervous system (CNS) metastases. Moreover, clinical trials have demonstrated that lapatinib is a safe drug with no serious or symptomatic cardiotoxicity (Cameron & Stein, 2008).

5.3 Innovative materials for future drugs

Antibodies can also be used as a targeting device for other cytotoxic systems. The overexpression of ErbB2 on tumor cells and the accessibility of the extracellular domain of ErbB2 make it an ideal target for the targeted delivery of anti-tumor drugs as well as imaging agents (Colombo et al., 2010). Cytotoxic drugs, radioisotopes, toxins, enzymes or nano-scaled drug carriers can be conjugated with the antibody (Wu & Senter, 2005).

One successful application of such a complex is trastuzumab–DM1 (T–DM1), which consists of the trastuzumab antibody conjugated to the potent antimicrotubule drug DM1, a maytansine derivative. After binding to ErbB2, T–DM1 is internalized, and DM1 is subsequently released into the cell, thus delivering chemotherapy directly to cells that overexpress ErbB2. T-DM1 has antitumor activity in trastuzumab-sensitive and trastuzumab-resistant ErbB2-overexpressing breast cancer (Lewis Phillips et al., 2008).

Antibody-conjugated nano-scaled drug carriers offer major improvements in the therapeutic index of anticancer agents through the site-specific, efficient delivery of agents, which reduces side effects. Moreover, they can avoid multi-drug resistance (Peer et al., 2007). Many materials, such as liposomes, micelles, polymeric and metal nanoparticles, solid lipid particles, dendrimers and quantum dots, are used as nanocarriers. The material properties of each nanocarrier have been developed to enhance delivery to the tumor. These nano-scaled systems can be used to deliver small-molecule drugs as well as nucleic acid drugs. For example, anti-ErbB2 antibody fragment-conjugated, PEG-stabilized immunoliposomes display long-term circulation and selective delivery of the encapsulated drug into ErbB2-overexpressing cancer (Park et al., 2002). These anti-ErbB2 delivery systems greatly increase the therapeutic index by enhancing anti-tumor efficacy and reducing systemic toxicity. In part, this superior activity is attributed to the ability of the immunoliposomes to deliver their load inside the target cells via receptor-mediated endocytosis. The initial target accumulation could be achieved by passive targeting via the enhanced permeability and retention (EPR) effect (Maeda et al., 2009). Although antibody targeting is regarded as a promising strategy, some groups have reported that antibody targeting did not increase tumor localization but instead increased internalization (Kirpotin et al., 2006). Many pharmaceutical agents need to be delivered intracellularly to exert their therapeutic action in the cytoplasm or on individual organelles.

However, a problem with intracellular delivery is that any molecule/particle entering the cell via the endocytic pathway can become trapped in the endosome and eventually be degraded in the lysosome. As a result, only a small fraction of unaffected substance appears in the cytoplasm. Thus, even if efficient cellular uptake via endocytosis is observed, the delivery of intact agents is compromised by insufficient endosomal escape and subsequent lysosomal degradation (Lee et al., 2008). Improvement against lysosomal degradation is an important issue to be resolved.

6. Experimental methods to assesscellular transformation and tumorigenesis

This chapter focuses on representative experimental methods that have contributed to the studies of ErbB2 function, which include classical transformation assays using NIH3T3 cells, three-dimentional(3D) culture of MCF10A, transgenic and knock-in mice and recent techniques with non-germline genetically engineered mouse models.

6.1 Cell culture–based analysis

To analyze ErbB2 function, the transformation assay is the first choice because *ErbB2* was identified as an oncogene, as discussed above. We will review the classical transformation assay and introduce a novel, improved method we developed.

Transformation assays are usually carried out with NIH3T3 cells (Todaro & Green, 1963). The term "transformation assay" classically includes three representative assays: focus formation, colony formation, and tumor formation. Although they differ in detectable phenotype, the principle behind them is simple; if candidate genes introduced into NIH3T3 cells are oncogenic, they can confer cancerous phenotypes, such as the loss of contact inhibition, anchorage-independent growth, and tumorigenicity to the NIH3T3 cells.

The focus formation assay detects one of these oncogenic abilities, to cause the loss of contact inhibition. Contact inhibition is a phenotype usually present in NIH3T3 cells; NIH3T3 cells proliferate until they form a monolayer of cells. If oncogenes are introduced, then some of the cells might become transformed into cancer cells. Transformation can be quantified by the appearance of "foci" of transformants (Figure 3).

The colony formation assay detects another ability, to cause anchorage-independent growth. Anchorage-independent growth is a phenotype virtually all cancer cells have (Cifone & Fidler, 1980); cancer cells can multiply without attachment to the extracellular matrix or solid substrate, such as the bottom of the Petri dish. A transformant that can proliferate in soft agar in suspension forms a "colony", that is, amass of descendants from a single transformant. Thus, transformation activity can be quantified by the number of colonies formed.

The tumor formation assay detects the ability to generate tumors *in vivo*. In this assay, transformants are injected into a syngeneic host or immunocompromised mice, such as nude (*nu/nu*) mice, to examine whether they are able to grow and form tumors in their animal hosts.

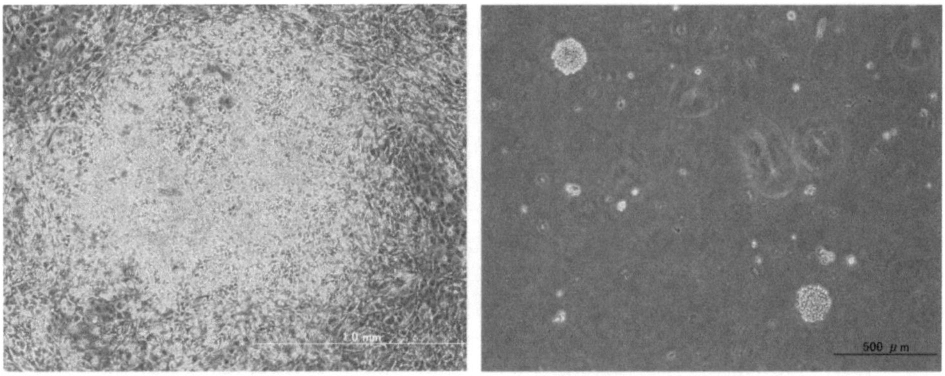

(a) ERBB2 V659E focus (b) H-RAS G12V colony

Fig. 3. Transformation assay with NIH3T3. (a)ERBB2 V659E has transformation activity. (b)H-RAS G12V, a mutant frequently observed in human cancer can also transform NIH3T3.

Rat *neu* transforms NIH3T3 cells, and the transformants are recognized as foci, which led to the discovery of *neu* itself (Schechter et al., 1984). Overexpression of wild-type ErbB2, as seen in human cancers, also transforms NIH3T3 cells (Di Fiore et al., 1987; Hudziak et al., 1987) by the colony formation and tumor formation assays. In contrast to human *ErbB2*, the rat *neu* proto-oncogene *ErbB2* does not transform cells when only expressed in NIH3T3 cells (Hung et al., 1986), but it transforms them when coexpressed with EGFR (Kokai et al., 1989). About ten years after its discovery, the *neu* oncogene was found not to transform the NIH3T3-7d cell line, which is devoid of detectable ErbB family members (Cohen et al., 1996). *ErbB2* itself probably does not have enough oncogenic activity to achieve the transformation of regular NIH3T3 cells but can transform them in the presence of EGFR. Our data also indicate that ErbB2 itself does not transform NIH3T3 cells (M.S., unpublished data), in contrast to DiFiore et al. (Di Fiore et al., 1987; Hudziak et al., 1987). This discrepancy probably results from the variations in the NIH3T3 cells used in these assays, as they have been passaged dozens of times since their early establishment. To detect a novel gene that transforms NIH3T3 cells in harmony with *ErbB2*, we established *ErbB2*-expressing NIH3T3 cells and introduced genes that are overexpressed in breast cancer using a retroviral expression vector. In fact, we demonstrated that one gene transforms NIH3T3 cells only in the presence of ErbB2 (M.S., unpublished data). This phenomenon seems to resemble the tumorigenesis of ErbB2-positive breast cancer *in vitro*.

Breast cancer can progress step by step along a continuum of changes from a normal phenotype to a malignant disease. The human mammary gland consists of multiple ducts and lobes (Vargo-Gogola & Rosen, 2007). Lobes are composed of multiple acinal structures with hollow lumens surrounded by layers of luminal epithelial cells, outer myoepithelial cells, and basement membranes. However, this well-organized structure is disrupted at early premalignant stages of breast cancer, such as ductal carcinoma *in situ* (DCIS). DCIS is the most common type of non-invasive breast cancer in women. DCIS can progress to malignant invasive breast cancer (IBC) and, subsequently, metastatic cancer (Espina & Liotta, 2010). The genetic events that cause progression to malignant stages are only partially understood.

A 3D culture of MCF10A cells within Matrigel, which are derived from the Englebreth-Holm Swarm (EHS) tumor (Kleinman et al., 1982), is an excellent *in vitro* model for understanding the biological processes and signaling pathways responsible for tissue morphogenesis *in vivo* and the disruption of epithelial architecture at early stages of tumorigenesis (Debnath & Brugge, 2005). MCF10A cells are a spontaneously immortalized but non-transformed human breast epithelial cell line (Soule et al., 1990). Following a reported method (Debnath, 2003b), MCF10A cells in Matrigel form acinar structures characterized by a hollow lumen surrounded by polarized, growth-arrested luminal epithelial cells, as shown in Figure 4. 3D cultures can provide a physiologically relevant context to the *in vivo* breast microenvironment, while monolayer cultures on plastic involve an environment that is considerably different from the *in vivo* environment (Vargo-Gogola & Rosen, 2007; Yamada & Cukierman, 2007). Certainly, both primary cultures of human tumor tissues and mouse models of cancer are practical to study carcinoma formation; however, they are relatively difficult to handle for understanding the biochemical and molecular biological pathways involved in the early stages of oncogenesis (Debnath, 2003b).

Madin-Darby canine kidney (MDCK) cells represent another widely used 3D culture model. When MDCK cells are embedded within collagen gels as single cells, they form polarized cysts with a central hollow lumen (Figure 5). During morphogenesis, intracellular vesicles containing apical membrane components are delivered to the cell surface between closely apposed cells, and membranes are separated, leading to the generation of several small lumens (Andrew & Ewald, 2010; Bryant & Mostov, 2008). Fusion of the lumens into a single large lumen subsequently occurs, and this phase requires apoptosis of luminal cells to clear

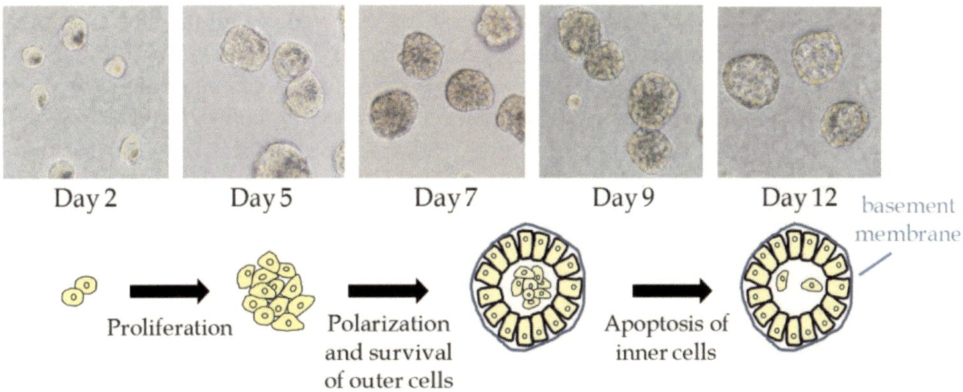

Fig. 4. MCF10A acinal structures constructed within Matrigel.
(1) Single cells embedded in Matrigel proliferate and form cell clusters. (2) At day 5–7, cells are distinguished between matrix-attached outer cells and matrix-deprived inner cells within each acinus. (3) After their fate has been determined, outer epithelial cells acquire apical-to-basal polarity and receive survival signals. (4) At day 8, however, non-polarized inner cells start to die via apoptosis. (5) Finally, replicated mammary acini with luminal spaces are constructed at day 14.

the lumen (Andrew & Ewald, 2010; Martin-Belmonte et al., 2008). Given that laminin is essential for initiating polarization mediated by the interaction between integrins and the ECM in the MDCK system, MDCK cells grown within the laminin-rich ECM, as within Matrigel, can polarize more efficiently than within collagen gels. The cells polarize and form clear lumens much faster, without the requirement of apoptosis (Martin-Belmonte et al., 2008).

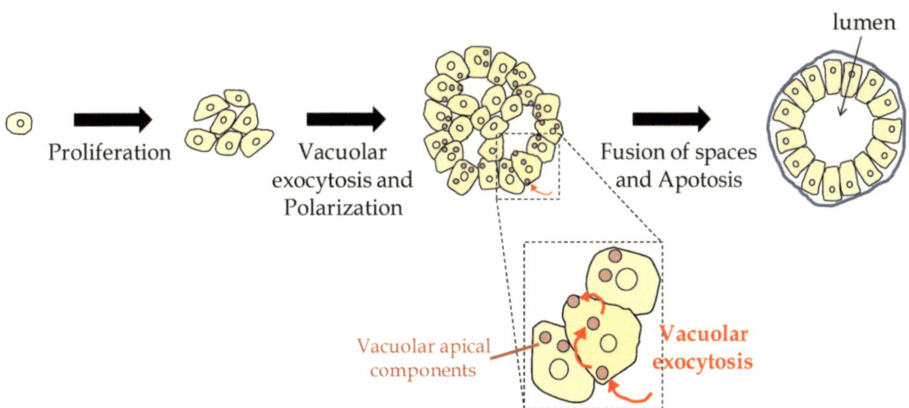

Fig. 5. Lumen formation by MDCK cells through vacuolar exocytosis of apical proteins.
(1) Single cells embedded in collagen gel or Matrigel proliferate to form groups of cells. (2) Intracellular vesicles containing apical membrane components are delivered to regions between cells and create luminal spaces via the fusion of vesicles and the plasma membrane. The surrounding cells now exhibit apical–basal polarity. (3) Several small lumens fuse with each other and generate one large lumen. Under the condition where cells are cultured within the laminin-lacking ECM, inner cell death by apoptosis is essential to clear the lumen (Andrew & Ewald, 2010; Bryant & Mostov, 2008).

Using the MCF10A 3D culture system, previous studies have revealed the effects of several oncogenes and viral oncoproteins on the process of acini formation (Debnath & Brugge, 2005; Shaw et al., 2004). For example, inactivation of the retinoblastoma protein (Rb) by HPV E7 facilitates proliferation (Debnath et al., 2002). Co-overexpression of CSF1-R and CSF1, both of which are elevated in mammary tumors, induces inner cell survival and loss of cell–cell adhesion, as well as hyperproliferation (Wrobel, 2004). Activated Akt leads to large, distorted, and filled-lumen structures (Debnath, 2003a). Each phenotype in these studies results from the biological activities of the introduced gene, suggesting that specific biological processes and pathways are modulated by the oncogene. Furthermore, these morphologies in 3D culture resemble the histological changes observed in human tumors *in vivo* (Debnath & Brugge, 2005).

Recently, the MCF10A 3D culture has been used to search for novel candidate oncogenes, such as the Yes kinase–associated protein (YAP) gene. *YAP* is included in the chromosome 11q22 amplicon that frequently appears in human tumors. Overexpression of YAP induces an anti-apoptotic and invasive morphology (Overholtzer, 2006). Further analysis has identified tumorigenic functions of generally non-tumorigenic proteins. For example, a study of MCF10A 3D structures suggested that not only oncogenes but also antioxidants could facilitate malignancy of carcinoma. In mammary acini, centrally located cells lack glucose transport and produce reactive oxygen species (ROS). Antioxidants could antagonize such metabolic stresses and promote the survival of cells detaching from the ECM by rescuing ATP production through fatty acid oxidation (FAO) (Schafer et al., 2009). Additionally, overexpression of a glycosyltransferase, N-acetylglucosaminyltransferase V (GnT-V) induces the disarrangement of mammary acinar morphogenesis, including increased cell proliferation, filled lumens, and disrupted polarity. Thus, altered expression of GnT-V, which catalyzes posttranslational modification, affects early stages of breast carcigenesis (H.B. Guo et al., 2010).

ERBB2 amplification in breast cancer is correlated with poor prognosis due to increased metastasis and resistance to chemotherapy. This gene is overexpressed in 50–60% of DCIS (Lu et al., 2009; Nofech-Mozes et al., 2005). Muthuswamy et al. showed that ErbB2-induced cells generate aberrant acini in 3D culture *in vitro*. To trigger homodimerization and activate ErbB2 signaling, they constructed chimeric receptors, as shown in Figure 6(a) (Muthuswamy et al., 1999; Muthuswamy et al., 2001). Treatment with AP1510 induced receptor homodimerization, leading to multi-acinar structures with filled lumens but no invasive phenotype. Therefore, additional genetic events as "second hits" may be required for invasion (Seton-Rogers, 2004). Those features are reminiscent of ErbB2-overexpressing DCIS *in vivo* (Muthuswamy et al., 2001). A recent analysis of ErbB2-mediated transformation indicated the significance of Tyr 1201 phosphorylation for the disruption of apical-basal polarity of MCF10A cells (Lucs et al., 2010).

Our laboratory uses a full-length *ErbB2* mutant, V659E, as a model of the constitutively activated ErbB2 receptor. It has higher intrinsic kinase activity and increased ability to induce transformation compared to wild-type ErbB2. This receptor can form a heterodimer with the other ErbB receptor family members as well as a homodimer, whereas chimeric receptors only form homodimers (Figure 6(b)). Thus our system may mimic physiological condition *in vivo* (A.D., unpublished data). We control the induction timing of ErbB2VE using the reverse tetracycline (Tet)-controlled transcriptional activator system, called "Tet-on". Induction of ErbB2VE leads to unregulated proliferation and filling of luminal spaces, whose structures are similar to "multi-acini" reported in a previous study (Muthuswamy et al., 2001).

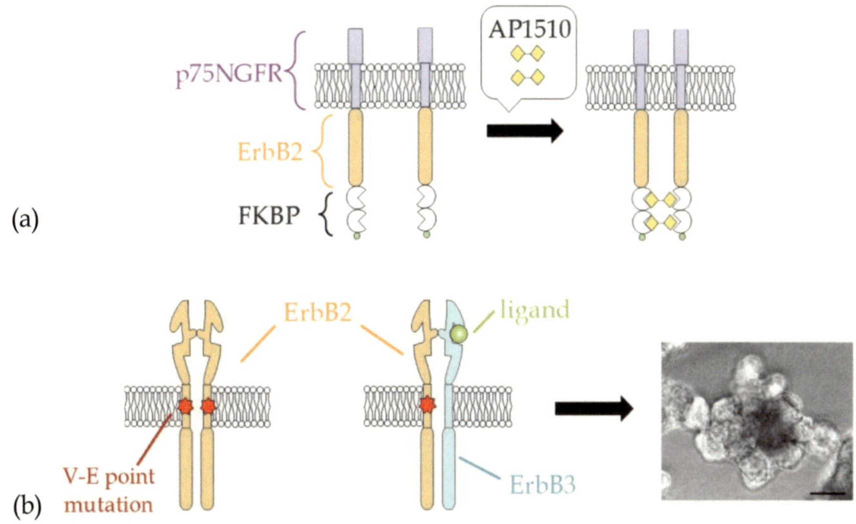

Fig. 6. Disruption of acinal structures due to ErbB2 signaling activation.
(a) Chimeric ErbB2 receptors induce homodimerization mediated by AP1510. MCF10A acini were treated with AP1510 at day 10 and cultured in Matrigel until day 20, resulting in the aberrant structure composed of multiple acini with filled lumens (Muthuswamy et al., 2001; Seton-Rogers, 2004). (b) In our laboratory, Tet-responsive ErbB2VE was expressed by treatment with Dox, forming both homo- and hetero-dimers. ErbB2VE activation from day 4 induces hyperproliferation and exhibits multi-acinar structures at day 12. This structure is similar to the phenotype previously reported (Muthuswamy et al., 2001). The scale bar represents 50 μm.

There is no evidence for how DCIS, which is a non-invasive and premalignant lesion, acquires invasive behavior. Given that DCIS with *ErbB2* amplification or overexpression frequently progresses to IBC, it is important to identify genes that collaborate with ErbB2 and induce tumor progression, including invasion and metastasis. Several investigators have been successful in detecting such factors using the MCF10A system. For example, either transforming growth factorβ (TGFβ) or prostate-derived Ets factor (PDEF) dramatically alters MCF10A spheroid-like acinal structures into protrusive cords invading the ECM in cooperation with ErbB2 (Gunawardane, 2005; Seton-Rogers, 2004). Additionally, co-overexpression of ErbB2 and 14-3-3γ, which shows increased expression in the early stages of breast cancer, results in larger acinar size, filled lumen, the gain of invasiveness, and disordered basal membrane protein laminin (Lu et al., 2009).

6.2 Animal models

Genetically engineered mouse (GEM) models have contributed broadly to the field of cancer research. First, we will review GEM models of breast cancer as a representative cancer related to the deregulation of ErbB2. The earliest model was generated by introducing *neu* oncogenes under the transcriptional control of the mouse mammary tumor virus (MMTV) LTR (Bouchard et al., 1989; C.T. Guy et al., 1992; Muller et al., 1988). MMTV LTR drives the expression of neu specifically in mammary gland intargeted mice. Tissue-specific expression is also achieved by using the whey acidic protein (WAP) promoter (Piechocki et al., 2003). The next useful development for GEM models was the Cre-loxP system (Wagner et al.,

1997). Cre-loxP models have genetic elements flanked by loxP sites that are processed by Cre recombinase, and its utility is widely known. Although *neu* under the strong viral LTR has questionable relevance to human breast cancers, mammary-specific expression of *neu* at endogenous levels had been desired. Thus, knock-in mice generated by interbreeding transgenic mice that have the *neu* promoter flanked by loxP sites with mice expressing Cre under the MMTV LTR (Andrechek et al., 2000) were developed, providing a valuable murine cancer model. *Neu* under the physiological promoter does not cause rapid tumor progression as seen in transgenic mice harboring MMTV-driven *neu*. However, they show amplification of the recombinant *neu* allele, as observed in human cancers (Andrechek et al., 2000). Furthermore, microarray profiling revealed that tumors arise in the knock-in mice, which demonstrated increased expression of GRB7 (Andrechek et al., 2003), as seen in human breast cancers.

More recently, several non-germline GEM models have been developed (Heyer et al., 2010). For example, generating chimeric mice is a novel way to increase the physiological relevance to human cancer, where cancer cells are surrounded by normal tissue, and it is also relatively cost-efficient. As in other models, chimeric mice carrying ErbB2 V659E in the lung, develop lung adenocarcinomas (Zhou et al., 2010). The necessity and desire to reproduce human cancers in mice will lead to more efficient translational research toward cancer therapies in the future.

7. Conclusion

We reviewed the history of the discovery of *ErbB2* with the recent progress on ErbB2 function. Thirty years have passed since the *neu* oncogene was discovered, and extensive research on ErbB proteins has been carried out since then. As long as tumor cell growth depends on ErbB2 expression, it is a rational target for therapy, and efforts will be made to develop more effective drugs than trastuzumab. In basic as well as clinical ErbB2 research, studies of cancer stem cells and the cells of origin (Visvader, 2011) of the ErbB2-induced tumors should be carried out. ErbB2 expression increases the population of stem/progenitor cells (Korkaya et al., 2008). Two distinct mammary progenitors have been identified, one of which is a target of MMTV-ErbB2 tumorigenesis and requires cyclin D1 kinase activity for its self-renewal (Jeselsohn et al., 2010). This suggests a combinational therapy with trastuzumab and cyclin D1 inhibitors may be more effective at treating ErbB2-mediated tumorigenesis than trastuzumab alone. The recent notion of non-oncogene addiction also needs to be considered (Luo et al., 2009). Identification of such genes will enable us to develop more effective targeted therapies as well as to understand the mechanism of ErbB2-mediated tumorigenesis itself.

8. Acknowledgement

We thank all the members of our laboratories, especially Jiro Fujimoto, Kosuke Ishikawa and Takaomi Ishida for valuable discussions.

9. References

Adams, G. P., & Weiner, L. M. (2005). Monoclonal antibody therapy of cancer. *Nat Biotechnol,* Vol.23, No.9, pp.1147-1157.

Agus, D. B., Akita, R. W., Fox, W. D., Lewis, G. D., Higgins, B., Pisacane, P. I., Lofgren, J. A., Tindell, C., Evans, D. P., Maiese, K., Scher, H. I., & Sliwkowski, M. X. (2002). Targeting ligand-activated ErbB2 signaling inhibits breast and prostate tumor growth. *Cancer Cell,* Vol.2, No.2, pp.127-137.

Akiyama, T., Sudo, C., Ogawara, H., Toyoshima, K., & Yamamoto, T. (1986). The product of the human c-erbB-2 gene: a 185-kilodalton glycoprotein with tyrosine kinase activity. *Science,* Vol.232, No.4758, pp.1644-1646.

Andrechek, E. R., Hardy, W. R., Siegel, P. M., Rudnicki, M. A., Cardiff, R. D., & Muller, W. J. (2000). Amplification of the neu/erbB-2 oncogene in a mouse model of mammary tumorigenesis. *Proc Natl Acad Sci USA,* Vol.97, No.7, pp.3444-3449.

Andrechek, E. R., Laing, M. A., Girgis-Gabardo, A. A., Siegel, P. M., Cardiff, R. D., & Muller, W. J. (2003). Gene expression profiling of neu-induced mammary tumors from transgenic mice reveals genetic and morphological similarities to ErbB2-expressing human breast cancers. *Cancer Res,* Vol.63, No.16, pp.4920-4926.

Andrew, D. J., & Ewald, A. J. (2010). Morphogenesis of epithelial tubes: Insights into tube formation, elongation, and elaboration. *Dev Biol,* Vol.341, No.1, pp.34-55.

Argenzio, E., Bange, T., Oldrini, B., Bianchi, F., Peesari, R., Mari, S., Di Fiore, P. P., Mann, M., Polo, S. (2011). Proteomic snapshot of the EGF-induced ubiquitin network. *Mol Syst Biol,* Vol.7.

Aroian, R. V., Koga, M., Mendel, J. E., Ohshima, Y., & Sternberg, P. W. (1990). The let-23 gene necessary for Caenorhabditis elegans vulval induction encodes a tyrosine kinase of the EGF receptor subfamily. *Nature,* Vol.348, No.6303, pp.693-699.

Bargmann, C. I., Hung, M. C., & Weinberg, R. A. (1986a). Multiple independent activations of the neu oncogene by a point mutation altering the transmembrane domain of p185. *Cell,* Vol.45, No.5, pp.649-657.

———. (1986b). The neu oncogene encodes an epidermal growth factor receptor-related protein. *Nature,* Vol.319, No.6050, pp.226-230.

Baselga, J., & Swain, S. M. (2009). Novel anticancer targets: revisiting ERBB2 and discovering ERBB3. *Nat Rev Cancer,* Vol.9, No.7, pp.463-475.

Berchuck, A., Kamel, A., Whitaker, R., Kerns, B., Olt, G., Kinney, R., Soper, J. T., Dodge, R., Clarke-Pearson, D. L., Marks, P., & et al. (1990). Overexpression of HER-2/neu is associated with poor survival in advanced epithelial ovarian cancer. *Cancer Res,* Vol.50, No.13, pp.4087-4091.

Berns, K., Horlings, H. M., Hennessy, B. T., Madiredjo, M., Hijmans, E. M., Beelen, K., Linn, S. C., Gonzalez-Angulo, A. M., Stemke-Hale, K., Hauptmann, M., Beijersbergen, R. L., Mills, G. B., van de Vijver, M. J., & Bernards, R. (2007). A functional genetic approach identifies the PI3K pathway as a major determinant of trastuzumab resistance in breast cancer. *Cancer Cell,* Vol.12, No.4, pp.395-402.

Blagoev, B., Ong, S-E., Kratchmarova, I., & Mann, M. (2004). Temporal analysis of phosphotyrosine-dependent signaling networks by quantitative proteomics. *Nat Biotechnol,* Vol.22, No.9, pp.1139-1145.

Bose, R. (2006). Phosphoproteomic analysis of Her2/neu signaling and inhibition. *Proc Natl Acad Sci USA,* Vol.103, No.26, pp.9773-9778.

Bouchard, L., Lamarre, L., Tremblay, P. J., & Jolicoeur, P. (1989). Stochastic appearance of mammary tumors in transgenic mice carrying the MMTV/c-neu oncogene. *Cell,* Vol.57, No.6, pp.931-936.

Bryant, D. M., & Mostov, K. E. (2008). From cells to organs: building polarized tissue. *Nat Rev Mol Cell Biol,* Vol.9, No.11, pp.887-901.

Burgess, A. W., Cho, H. S., Eigenbrot, C., Ferguson, K. M., Garrett, T. P., Leahy, D. J., Lemmon, M. A., Sliwkowski, M. X., Ward, C. W., & Yokoyama, S. (2003). An open-and-shut case? Recent insights into the activation of EGF/ErbB receptors. *Mol Cell,* Vol.12, No.3, pp.541-552.

Cameron, D. A., & Stein, S. (2008). Drug Insight: intracellular inhibitors of HER2--clinical development of lapatinib in breast cancer. *Nat Clin Pract Oncol,* Vol.5, No.9, pp.512-520.

Chen, J. S., Lan, K., & Hung, M. C. (2003). Strategies to target HER2/neu overexpression for cancer therapy. *Drug Resist Updat,* Vol.6, No.3, pp.129-136.

Cifone, M. A., & Fidler, I. J. (1980). Correlation of patterns of anchorage-independent growth with in vivo behavior of cells from a murine fibrosarcoma. *Proc Natl Acad Sci USA,* Vol.77, No.2, pp.1039-1043.

Citri, A., & Yarden, Y. (2006). EGF–ERBB signalling: towards the systems level. *Nat Rev Mol Cell Biol,* Vol.7, No.7, pp.505-516.

Clynes, R. A., Towers, T. L., Presta, L. G., & Ravetch, J. V. (2000). Inhibitory Fc receptors modulate in vivo cytoxicity against tumor targets. *Nat Med,* Vol.6, No.4, pp.443-446.

Cohen, B. D., Kiener, P. A., Green, J. M., Foy, L., Fell, H. P., & Zhang, K. (1996). The relationship between human epidermal growth-like factor receptor expression and cellular transformation in NIH3T3 cells. *J Biol Chem,* Vol.271, No.48, pp.30897-30903.

Colombo, M., Corsi, F., Foschi, D., Mazzantini, E., Mazzucchelli, S., Morasso, C., Occhipinti, E., Polito, L., Prosperi, D., Ronchi, S., & Verderio, P. (2010). HER2 targeting as a two-sided strategy for breast cancer diagnosis and treatment: Outlook and recent implications in nanomedical approaches. *Pharmacol Res,* Vol.62, No.2, pp.150-165.

Coussens, L., Yang-Feng, T. L., Liao, Y. C., Chen, E., Gray, A., McGrath, J., Seeburg, P. H., Libermann, T. A., Schlessinger, J., Francke, U., & et al. (1985). Tyrosine kinase receptor with extensive homology to EGF receptor shares chromosomal location with neu oncogene. *Science,* Vol.230, No.4730, pp.1132-1139.

Crowder, R. J., Lombardi, D. P., & Ellis, M. J. (2004). Successful targeting of ErbB2 receptors—is PTEN the key? *Cancer Cell,* Vol.6, No.2, pp.103-104.

Cully, M., You, H., Levine, A. J., & Mak, T. W. (2006). Beyond PTEN mutations: the PI3K pathway as an integrator of multiple inputs during tumorigenesis. *Nat Rev Cancer,* Vol.6, No.3, pp.184-192.

Debnath, J. (2003a). Akt activation disrupts mammary acinar architecture and enhances proliferation in an mTOR-dependent manner. *J Cell Biol,* Vol.163, No.2, pp.315-326.

———. (2003b). Morphogenesis and oncogenesis of MCF-10A mammary epithelial acini grown in three-dimensional basement membrane cultures. *Methods,* Vol.30, No.3, pp.256-268.

Debnath, J., Mills, K. R., Collins, N. L., Reginato, M. J., Muthuswamy, S. K., & Brugge, J. S. (2002). The role of apoptosis in creating and maintaining luminal space within normal and oncogene-expressing mammary acini. *Cell,* Vol.111, No.1, pp.29-40.

Debnath, J., & Brugge, J. S. (2005). Modelling glandular epithelial cancers in three-dimensional cultures. *Nat Rev Cancer,* Vol.5, No.9, pp.675-688.

Di Fiore, P. P., Pierce, J. H., Kraus, M. H., Segatto, O., King, C. R., & Aaronson, S. A. (1987). erbB-2 is a potent oncogene when overexpressed in NIH/3T3 cells. *Science,* Vol.237, No.4811, pp.178-182.

Downward, J., Yarden, Y., Mayes, E., Scrace, G., Totty, N., Stockwell, P., Ullrich, A., Schlessinger, J., & Waterfield, M. D. (1984). Close similarity of epidermal growth factor receptor and v-erb-B oncogene protein sequences. *Nature,* Vol.307, No.5951, pp.521-527.

Espina, V., & Liotta, L. A. (2010). What is the malignant nature of human ductal carcinoma in situ? *Nat Rev Cancer,* Vol.11, No.1, pp.68-75.

Force, T., Krause, D. S., & Van Etten, R. A. (2007). Molecular mechanisms of cardiotoxicity of tyrosine kinase inhibition. *Nat Rev Cancer,* Vol.7, No.5, pp.332-344.

Garrett, T. P., McKern, N. M., Lou, M., Elleman, T. C., Adams, T. E., Lovrecz, G. O., Kofler, M., Jorissen, R. N., Nice, E. C., Burgess, A. W., & Ward, C. W. (2003). The crystal structure of a truncated ErbB2 ectodomain reveals an active conformation, poised to interact with other ErbB receptors. *Mol Cell,* Vol.11, No.2, pp.495-505.

Gomez, A., Volff, J. N., Hornung, U., Schartl, M., & Wellbrock, C. (2004). Identification of a second egfr gene in Xiphophorus uncovers an expansion of the epidermal growth factor receptor family in fish. *Mol Biol Evol,* Vol.21, No.2, pp.266-275.

Graham, F. L., & van der Eb, A. J. (1973). A new technique for the assay of infectivity of human adenovirus 5 DNA. *Virology,* Vol.52, No.2, pp.456-467.

Gunawardane, R. N. (2005). Novel Role for PDEF in Epithelial Cell Migration and Invasion. *Cancer Res,* Vol.65, No.24, pp.11572-11580.

Guo, H. B., Johnson, H., Randolph, M., Nagy, T., Blalock, R., & Pierce, M. (2010). Specific posttranslational modification regulates early events in mammary carcinoma formation. *Proc Natl Acad Sci U S A,* Vol.107, No.49, pp.21116-21121.

Guo, W., Pylayeva, Y., Pepe, A., Yoshioka, T., Muller, W. J., Inghirami, G., & Giancotti, F. G. (2006). β4 Integrin Amplifies ErbB2 Signaling to Promote Mammary Tumorigenesis. *Cell,* Vol.126, No.3, pp.489-502.

Guy, C. T., Webster, M. A., Schaller, M., Parsons, T. J., Cardiff, R. D., & Muller, W. J. (1992). Expression of the neu protooncogene in the mammary epithelium of transgenic mice induces metastatic disease. *Proc Natl Acad Sci USA,* Vol.89, No.22, pp.10578-10582.

Guy, P. M., Platko, J. V., Cantley, L. C., Cerione, R. A., & Carraway, K. L., 3rd. (1994). Insect cell-expressed p180erbB3 possesses an impaired tyrosine kinase activity. *Proc Natl Acad Sci USA,* Vol.91, No.17, pp.8132-8136.

Hansel, T. T., Kropshofer, H., Singer, T., Mitchell, J. A., & George, A. J. (2010). The safety and side effects of monoclonal antibodies. *Nat Rev Drug Discov,* Vol.9, No.4, pp.325-338.

Heyer, J., Kwong, L. N., Lowe, S. W., & Chin, L. (2010). Non-germline genetically engineered mouse models for translational cancer research. *Nat Rev Cancer,* Vol.10, No.7, pp.470-480.

Hirsch, F. R., Varella-Garcia, M., Franklin, W. A., Veve, R., Chen, L., Helfrich, B., Zeng, C., Baron, A., & Bunn, P. A., Jr. (2002). Evaluation of HER-2/neu gene amplification and protein expression in non-small cell lung carcinomas. *Br J Cancer,* Vol.86, No.9, pp.1449-1456.

Hudis, C. A. (2007). Trastuzumab--mechanism of action and use in clinical practice. *N Engl J Med,* Vol.357, No.1, pp.39-51.

Hudziak, R. M., Schlessinger, J., & Ullrich, A. (1987). Increased expression of the putative growth factor receptor p185HER2 causes transformation and tumorigenesis of NIH 3T3 cells. *Proc Natl Acad Sci USA,* Vol.84, No.20, pp.7159-7163.

Hung, M. C., Schechter, A. L., Chevray, P. Y., Stern, D. F., & Weinberg, R. A. (1986). Molecular cloning of the neu gene: absence of gross structural alteration in oncogenic alleles. *Proc Natl Acad Sci USA,* Vol.83, No.2, pp.261-264.

Hynes, N. E., & Lane, H. A. (2005). ERBB receptors and cancer: the complexity of targeted inhibitors. *Nat Rev Cancer,* Vol.5, No.5, pp.341-354.

Ishizawar, R., & Parsons, S. J. (2004). c-Src and cooperating partners in human cancer. *Cancer Cell,* Vol.6, No.3, pp.209-214.

Jain, R. K. (1990). Physiological barriers to delivery of monoclonal antibodies and other macromolecules in tumors. *Cancer Res,* Vol.50, No.3 Suppl, pp.814s-819s.

Jeselsohn, R., Brown, N. E., Arendt, L., Klebba, I., Hu, M. G., Kuperwasser, C., & Hinds, P. W. (2010). Cyclin D1 kinase activity is required for the self-renewal of mammary stem and progenitor cells that are targets of MMTV-ErbB2 tumorigenesis. *Cancer Cell,* Vol.17, No.1, pp.65-76.

Khazaeli, M. B., Conry, R. M., & LoBuglio, A. F. (1994). Human immune response to monoclonal antibodies. *J Immunother Emphasis Tumor Immunol,* Vol.15, No.1, pp.42-52.

Khazaie, K., Dull, T. J., Graf, T., Schlessinger, J., Ullrich, A., Beug, H., & Vennstrom, B. (1988). Truncation of the human EGF receptor leads to differential transforming potentials in primary avian fibroblasts and erythroblasts. *EMBO J,* Vol.7, No.10, pp.3061-3071.

Kiewe, P., Hasmuller, S., Kahlert, S., Heinrigs, M., Rack, B., Marme, A., Korfel, A., Jager, M., Lindhofer, H., Sommer, H., Thiel, E., & Untch, M. (2006). Phase I trial of the trifunctional anti-HER2 x anti-CD3 antibody ertumaxomab in metastatic breast cancer. *Clin Cancer Res,* Vol.12, No.10, pp.3085-3091.

Kirpotin, D. B., Drummond, D. C., Shao, Y., Shalaby, M. R., Hong, K., Nielsen, U. B., Marks, J. D., Benz, C. C., & Park, J. W. (2006). Antibody targeting of long-circulating lipidic nanoparticles does not increase tumor localization but does increase internalization in animal models. *Cancer Res,* Vol.66, No.13, pp.6732-6740.

Kleinman, H. K., McGarvey, M. L., Liotta, L. A., Robey, P. G., Tryggvason, K., & Martin, G. R. (1982). Isolation and characterization of type IV procollagen, laminin, and heparan sulfate proteoglycan from the EHS sarcoma. *Biochemistry,* Vol.21, No.24, pp.6188-6193.

Kokai, Y., Myers, J. N., Wada, T., Brown, V. I., LeVea, C. M., Davis, J. G., Dobashi, K., & Greene, M. I. (1989). Synergistic interaction of p185c-neu and the EGF receptor leads to transformation of rodent fibroblasts. *Cell,* Vol.58, No.2, pp.287-292.

Konecny, G. E., Pegram, M. D., Venkatesan, N., Finn, R., Yang, G., Rahmeh, M., Untch, M., Rusnak, D. W., Spehar, G., Mullin, R. J., Keith, B. R., Gilmer, T. M., Berger, M., Podratz, K. C., & Slamon, D. J. (2006). Activity of the dual kinase inhibitor lapatinib (GW572016) against HER-2-overexpressing and trastuzumab-treated breast cancer cells. *Cancer Res,* Vol.66, No.3, pp.1630-1639.

Korkaya, H., Paulson, A., Iovino, F., & Wicha, M. S. (2008). HER2 regulates the mammary stem/progenitor cell population driving tumorigenesis and invasion. *Oncogene,* Vol.27, No.47, pp.6120-6130.

Kraus, M. H., Issing, W., Miki, T., Popescu, N. C., & Aaronson, S. A. (1989). Isolation and characterization of ERBB3, a third member of the ERBB/epidermal growth factor receptor family: evidence for overexpression in a subset of human mammary tumors. *Proc Natl Acad Sci USA,* Vol.86, No.23, pp.9193-9197.

Kruser, T. J., & Wheeler, D. L. (2010). Mechanisms of resistance to HER family targeting antibodies. *Exp Cell Res,* Vol.316, No.7, pp.1083-1100.

Lazar, G. A., Dang, W., Karki, S., Vafa, O., Peng, J. S., Hyun, L., Chan, C., Chung, H. S., Eivazi, A., Yoder, S. C., Vielmetter, J., Carmichael, D. F., Hayes, R. J., & Dahiyat, B. I. (2006). Engineered antibody Fc variants with enhanced effector function. *Proc Natl Acad Sci U S A,* Vol.103, No.11, pp.4005-4010.

Lee, E. S., Gao, Z., & Bae, Y. H. (2008). Recent progress in tumor pH targeting nanotechnology. *J Control Release,* Vol.132, No.3, pp.164-170.

Lewis Phillips, G. D., Li, G., Dugger, D. L., Crocker, L. M., Parsons, K. L., Mai, E., Blattler, W. A., Lambert, J. M., Chari, R. V., Lutz, R. J., Wong, W. L., Jacobson, F. S., Koeppen, H., Schwall, R. H., Kenkare-Mitra, S. R., Spencer, S. D., & Sliwkowski, M. X. (2008). Targeting HER2-positive breast cancer with trastuzumab-DM1, an antibody-cytotoxic drug conjugate. *Cancer Res,* Vol.68, No.22, pp.9280-9290.

Livneh, E., Glazer, L., Segal, D., Schlessinger, J., & Shilo, B. Z. (1985). The Drosophila EGF receptor gene homolog: conservation of both hormone binding and kinase domains. *Cell,* Vol.40, No.3, pp.599-607.

Lonberg, N. (2005). Human antibodies from transgenic animals. *Nat Biotechnol,* Vol.23, No.9, pp.1117-1125.

Lu, J., Guo, H., Treekitkarnmongkol, W., Li, P., Zhang, J., Shi, B., Ling, C., Zhou, X., Chen, T., Chiao, P. J., Feng, X., Seewaldt, V. L., Muller, W. J., Sahin, A., Hung, M. C., & Yu, D. (2009). 14-3-3ζ Cooperates with ErbB2 to Promote Ductal Carcinoma In Situ Progression to Invasive Breast Cancer by Inducing Epithelial-Mesenchymal Transition. *Cancer Cell,* Vol.16, No.3, pp.195-207.

Lucs, A. V., Muller, W. J., & Muthuswamy, S. K. (2010). Shc is required for ErbB2-induced inhibition of apoptosis but is dispensable for cell proliferation and disruption of cell polarity. *Oncogene,* Vol.29, No.2, pp.174-187.

Luo, J., Solimini, N. L., & Elledge, S. J. (2009). Principles of cancer therapy: oncogene and non-oncogene addiction. *Cell,* Vol.136, No.5, pp.823-837.

Maeda, H., Bharate, G. Y., & Daruwalla, J. (2009). Polymeric drugs for efficient tumor-targeted drug delivery based on EPR-effect. *Eur J Pharm Biopharm,* Vol.71, No.3, pp.409-419.

Martin-Belmonte, F., Yu, W., Rodriguez-Fraticelli, A. E., Ewald, A. J., Werb, Z., Alonso, M. A., & Mostov, K. (2008). Cell-polarity dynamics controls the mechanism of lumen formation in epithelial morphogenesis. *Curr Biol,* Vol.18, No.7, pp.507-513.

Mattie, M. D., Benz, C. C., Bowers, J., Sensinger, K., Wong, L., Scott, G. K., Fedele, V., Ginzinger, D., Getts, R., & Haqq, C. (2006). Optimized high-throughput microRNA expression profiling provides novel biomarker assessment of clinical prostate and breast cancer biopsies. *Mol Cancer,* Vol.5, p.24.

Miettinen, P. J., Berger, J. E., Meneses, J., Phung, Y., Pedersen, R. A., Werb, Z., & Derynck, R. (1995). Epithelial immaturity and multiorgan failure in mice lacking epidermal growth factor receptor. *Nature,* Vol.376, No.6538, pp.337-341.

Moasser, M. M. (2007). The oncogene HER2: its signaling and transforming functions and its role in human cancer pathogenesis. *Oncogene,* Vol.26, No.45, pp.6469-6487.

Moghal, N., & Sternberg, P. W. (2003). The epidermal growth factor system in Caenorhabditis elegans. *Exp Cell Res,* Vol.284, No.1, pp.150-159.

Moody, S. E., Sarkisian, C. J., Hahn, K. T., Gunther, E. J., Pickup, S., Dugan, K. D., Innocent, N., Cardiff, R. D., Schnall, M. D., & Chodosh, L. A. (2002). Conditional activation of Neu in the mammary epithelium of transgenic mice results in reversible pulmonary metastasis. *Cancer Cell,* Vol.2, No.6, pp.451-461.

Muller, W. J., Sinn, E., Pattengale, P. K., Wallace, R., & Leder, P. (1988). Single-step induction of mammary adenocarcinoma in transgenic mice bearing the activated c-neu oncogene. *Cell,* Vol.54, No.1, pp.105-115.

Muthuswamy, S. K., Gilman, M., & Brugge, J. S. (1999). Controlled dimerization of ErbB receptors provides evidence for differential signaling by homo- and heterodimers. *Mol Cell Biol,* Vol.19, No.10, pp.6845-6857.

Muthuswamy, S. K., Li, D., Lelievre, S., Bissell, M. J., & Brugge, J. S. (2001). ErbB2, but not ErbB1, reinitiates proliferation and induces luminal repopulation in epithelial acini. *Nat Cell Biol,* Vol.3, No.9, pp.785-792.

Muthuswamy, S. K. (2006). ErbB2 Makes β4 Integrin an Accomplice in Tumorigenesis. *Cell,* Vol.126, No.3, pp.443-445.

Nagata, Y., Lan, K.-H., Zhou, X., Tan, M., Esteva, F. J., Sahin, A. A., Klos, K. S., Li, P., Monia, B. P., Nguyen, N. T., Hortobagyi G. N., Hung, M. C., & Yu, D. (2004). PTEN activation contributes to tumor inhibition by trastuzumab, and loss of PTEN predicts trastuzumab resistance in patients. *Cancer Cell,* Vol.6, No.2, pp.117-127.

Nagy, P., Friedlander, E., Tanner, M., Kapanen, A. I., Carraway, K. L., Isola, J., & Jovin, T. M. (2005). Decreased accessibility and lack of activation of ErbB2 in JIMT-1, a herceptin-resistant, MUC4-expressing breast cancer cell line. *Cancer Res,* Vol.65, No.2, pp.473-482.

Nahta, R., & Esteva, F. J. (2006). Herceptin: mechanisms of action and resistance. *Cancer Lett,* Vol.232, No.2, pp.123-138.

Nahta, R., Hung, M. C., & Esteva, F. J. (2004). The HER-2-targeting antibodies trastuzumab and pertuzumab synergistically inhibit the survival of breast cancer cells. *Cancer Res,* Vol.64, No.7, pp.2343-2346.

Nahta, R., Yuan, L. X., Zhang, B., Kobayashi, R., & Esteva, F. J. (2005). Insulin-like growth factor-I receptor/human epidermal growth factor receptor 2 heterodimerization contributes to trastuzumab resistance of breast cancer cells. *Cancer Res,* Vol.65, No.23, pp.11118-11128.

Olayioye, M. A., Neve, R. M., Lane, H. A., & Hynes, N. E. (2000). The ErbB signaling network: receptor heterodimerization in development and cancer. *EMBO J,* Vol.19, No.13, pp.3159-3167.

Overholtzer, M. (2006). Transforming properties of YAP, a candidate oncogene on the chromosome 11q22 amplicon. *Proc Natl Acad Sci USA,* Vol.103, No.33, pp.12405-12410.

Park, J. W., Hong, K., Kirpotin, D. B., Colbern, G., Shalaby, R., Baselga, J., Shao, Y., Nielsen, U. B., Marks, J. D., Moore, D., Papahadjopoulos, D., & Benz, C. C. (2002). Anti-HER2 immunoliposomes: enhanced efficacy attributable to targeted delivery. *Clin Cancer Res,* Vol.8, No.4, pp.1172-1181.

Peer, D., Karp, J. M., Hong, S., Farokhzad, O. C., Margalit, R., & Langer, R. (2007). Nanocarriers as an emerging platform for cancer therapy. *Nat Nanotechnol,* Vol.2, No.12, pp.751-760.

Perera, S. A., Li, D., Shimamura, T., Raso, M. G., Ji, H., Chen, L., Borgman, C. L., Zaghlul, S., Brandstetter, K. A., Kubo, S., Takahashi, M., Chirieac, L. R., Padera, R. F., Bronson, R. T., Shapiro, G. I., Greulich, H., Meyerson, M., Guertler, U., Chesa, P. G., Solca, F., Wistuba, II, & Wong, K. K. (2009). HER2YVMA drives rapid development of adenosquamous lung tumors in mice that are sensitive to BIBW2992 and rapamycin combination therapy. *Proc Natl Acad Sci USA,* Vol.106, No.2, pp.474-479.

Piechocki, M. P., Ho, Y. S., Pilon, S., & Wei, W. Z. (2003). Human ErbB-2 (Her-2) transgenic mice: a model system for testing Her-2 based vaccines. *J Immunol,* Vol.171, No.11, pp.5787-5794.

Plowman, G. D., Culouscou, J. M., Whitney, G. S., Green, J. M., Carlton, G. W., Foy, L., Neubauer, M. G., & Shoyab, M. (1993). Ligand-specific activation of HER4/p180erbB4, a fourth member of the epidermal growth factor receptor family. *Proc Natl Acad Sci USA,* Vol.90, No.5, pp.1746-1750.

Presta, L. G. (2006). Engineering of therapeutic antibodies to minimize immunogenicity and optimize function. *Adv Drug Deliv Rev,* Vol.58, No.5-6, pp.640-656.

Reddy, H. K., Mettus, R. V., Rane, S. G., Graña., X., Litvin, J., Reddy, E. P. (2005). Cyclin-Dependent Kinase 4 Expression Is Essential for Neu-Induced Breast Tumorigenesis. *Cancer Res,* Vol.65, No.22, pp.10174-10178.

Reid, A., Vidal, L., Shaw, H., & de Bono, J. (2007). Dual inhibition of ErbB1 (EGFR/HER1) and ErbB2 (HER2/neu). *Eur J Cancer,* Vol.43, No.3, pp.481-489.

Romond, E. H., Perez, E. A., Bryant, J., Suman, V. J., Geyer, C. E., Jr., Davidson, N. E., Tan-Chiu, E., Martino, S., Paik, S., Kaufman, P. A., Swain, S. M., Pisansky, T. M., Fehrenbacher, L., Kutteh, L. A., Vogel, V. G., Visscher, D. W., Yothers, G., Jenkins, R. B., Brown, A. M., Dakhil, S. R., Mamounas, E. P., Lingle, W. L., Klein, P. M., Ingle, J. N., & Wolmark, N. (2005). Trastuzumab plus adjuvant chemotherapy for operable HER2-positive breast cancer. *N Engl J Med,* Vol.353, No.16, pp.1673-1684.

Santarius, T., Shipley, J., Brewer, D., Stratton, M. R., & Cooper, C. S. (2010). A census of amplified and overexpressed human cancer genes. *Nat Rev Cancer,* Vol.10, No.1, pp.59-64.

Schafer, Z. T., Grassian, A. R., Song, L., Jiang, Z., Gerhart-Hines, Z., Irie, H. Y., Gao, S., Puigserver, P., & Brugge, J. S. (2009). Antioxidant and oncogene rescue of metabolic defects caused by loss of matrix attachment. *Nature,* Vol.461, No.7260, pp.109-113.

Schechter, A. L., Hung, M. C., Vaidyanathan, L., Weinberg, R. A., Yang-Feng, T. L., Francke, U., Ullrich, A., & Coussens, L. (1985). The neu gene: an erbB-homologous gene distinct from and unlinked to the gene encoding the EGF receptor. *Science,* Vol.229, No.4717, pp.976-978.

Schechter, A. L., Stern, D. F., Vaidyanathan, L., Decker, S. J., Drebin, J. A., Greene, M. I., & Weinberg, R. A. (1984). The neu oncogene: an erb-B-related gene encoding a 185,000-Mr tumour antigen. *Nature,* Vol.312, No.5994, pp.513-516.

Scott, G. K., Goga, A., Bhaumik, D., Berger, C. E., Sullivan, C. S., & Benz, C. C. (2007). Coordinate suppression of ERBB2 and ERBB3 by enforced expression of micro-RNA miR-125a or miR-125b. *J Biol Chem,* Vol.282, No.2, pp.1479-1486.

Semba, K., Kamata, N., Toyoshima, K., & Yamamoto, T. (1985). A v-erbB-related protooncogene, c-erbB-2, is distinct from the c-erbB-1/epidermal growth factor-receptor gene and is amplified in a human salivary gland adenocarcinoma. *Proc Natl Acad Sci USA,* Vol.82, No.19, pp.6497-6501.

Seton-Rogers, S. E. (2004). Cooperation of the ErbB2 receptor and transforming growth factor in induction of migration and invasion in mammary epithelial cells. *Proc Natl Acad Sci USA,* Vol.101, No.5, pp.1257-1262.

Shaw, K. R. M., Wrobel, C. N., & Brugge, J. S. (2004). Use of Three-Dimensional Basement Membrane Cultures to Model Oncogene-Induced Changes in Mammary Epithelial Morphogenesis. *J Mammary Gland Biol Neoplasia,* Vol.9, No.4, pp.297-310.

Shih, C., Padhy, L. C., Murray, M., & Weinberg, R. A. (1981). Transforming genes of carcinomas and neuroblastomas introduced into mouse fibroblasts. *Nature,* Vol.290, No.5803, pp.261-264.

Shih, C., Shilo, B. Z., Goldfarb, M. P., Dannenberg, A., & Weinberg, R. A. (1979). Passage of phenotypes of chemically transformed cells via transfection of DNA and chromatin. *Proc Natl Acad Sci USA,* Vol.76, No.11, pp.5714-5718.

Shilo, B. Z. (2003). Signaling by the Drosophila epidermal growth factor receptor pathway during development. *Exp Cell Res,* Vol.284, No.1, pp.140-149.

Sibilia, M., & Wagner, E. F. (1995). Strain-dependent epithelial defects in mice lacking the EGF receptor. *Science,* Vol.269, No.5221, pp.234-238.

Singh, A. P., Chaturvedi, P., & Batra, S. K. (2007). Emerging Roles of MUC4 in Cancer: A Novel Target for Diagnosis and Therapy. *Cancer Res,* Vol.67, No.2, pp.433-436.

Sircoulomb, F., Bekhouche, I., Finetti, P., Adelaide, J., Ben Hamida, A., Bonansea, J., Raynaud, S., Innocenti, C., Charafe-Jauffret, E., Tarpin, C., Ben Ayed, F., Viens, P., Jacquemier, J., Bertucci, F., Birnbaum, D., & Chaffanet, M. (2010). Genome profiling of ERBB2-amplified breast cancers. *BMC cancer,* Vol.10, p.539.

Slamon, D. J., Godolphin, W., Jones, L. A., Holt, J. A., Wong, S. G., Keith, D. E., Levin, W. J., Stuart, S. G., Udove, J., Ullrich, A., & et al. (1989). Studies of the HER-2/neu proto-oncogene in human breast and ovarian cancer. *Science,* Vol.244, No.4905, pp.707-712.

Slamon, D. J., Leyland-Jones, B., Shak, S., Fuchs, H., Paton, V., Bajamonde, A., Fleming, T., Eiermann, W., Wolter, J., Pegram, M., Baselga, J., & Norton, L. (2001). Use of chemotherapy plus a monoclonal antibody against HER2 for metastatic breast cancer that overexpresses HER2. *N Engl J Med,* Vol.344, No.11, pp.783-792.

Soule, H. D., Maloney, T. M., Wolman, S. R., Peterson, W. D., Jr., Brenz, R., McGrath, C. M., Russo, J., Pauley, R. J., Jones, R. F., & Brooks, S. C. (1990). Isolation and characterization of a spontaneously immortalized human breast epithelial cell line, MCF-10. *Cancer Res,* Vol.50, No.18, pp.6075-6086.

Threadgill, D. W., Dlugosz, A. A., Hansen, L. A., Tennenbaum, T., Lichti, U., Yee, D., LaMantia, C., Mourton, T., Herrup, K., Harris, R. C., & et al. (1995). Targeted disruption of mouse EGF receptor: effect of genetic background on mutant phenotype. *Science,* Vol.269, No.5221, pp.230-234.

Timms, J. F., White, S. L., O'Hare, M. J., & Waterfield, M. D. (2002). Effects of ErbB-2 overexpression on mitogenic signalling and cell cycle progression in human breast luminal epithelial cells. *Oncogene,* Vol.21, No.43, pp.6573-6586.

Todaro, G. J., & Green, H. (1963). Quantitative studies of the growth of mouse embryo cells in culture and their development into established lines. *J Cell Biol,* Vol.17, pp.299-313.

Tomizawa, K., Suda, K., Onozato, R., Kosaka, T., Endoh, H., Sekido, Y., Shigematsu, H., Kuwano, H., Yatabe, Y., & Mitsudomi, T. (2011). Prognostic and predictive implications of HER2/ERBB2/neu gene mutations in lung cancers. *Lung Cancer.*

Vargo-Gogola, T., & Rosen, J. M. (2007). Modelling breast cancer: one size does not fit all. *Nat Rev Cancer,* Vol.7, No.9, pp.659-672.

Vennstrom, B., & Bishop, J. M. (1982). Isolation and characterization of chicken DNA homologous to the two putative oncogenes of avian erythroblastosis virus. *Cell,* Vol.28, No.1, pp.135-143.

Visvader, J. E. (2011). Cells of origin in cancer. *Nature,* Vol.469, No.7330, pp.314-322.

Vivanco, I., & Sawyers, C. L. (2002). The phosphatidylinositol 3-Kinase-AKT pathway in human cancer. *Nat Rev Cancer,* Vol.2, No.7, pp.489-501.

Wagner, K. U., Wall, R. J., St-Onge, L., Gruss, P., Wynshaw-Boris, A., Garrett, L., Li, M., Furth, P. A., & Hennighausen, L. (1997). Cre-mediated gene deletion in the mammary gland. *Nucleic Acids Res,* Vol.25, No.21, pp.4323-4330.

Wang, S. E., Narasanna, A., Perez-Torres, M., Xiang, B., Wu, F. Y., Yang, S., Carpenter, G., Gazdar, A. F., Muthuswamy, S. K., & Arteaga, C. L. (2006). HER2 kinase domain mutation results in constitutive phosphorylation and activation of HER2 and EGFR and resistance to EGFR tyrosine kinase inhibitors. *Cancer Cell,* Vol.10, No.1, pp.25-38.

Wang, S.-C., Lien, H.-C., Xia, W., Chen, I. F., Lo, H.-W., Wang, Z., Ali-Seyed, M., Lee, D.-F., Bartholomeusz, G., Ou-Yang, F., Giri, D. K., & Hung, M. C. (2004). Binding at and transactivation of the COX-2 promoter by nuclear tyrosine kinase receptor ErbB-2. *Cancer Cell,* Vol.6, No.3, pp.251-261.

Wolf-Yadlin, A., Kumar, N., Zhang, Y., Hautaniemi, S., Zaman, M., Kim, H.-D., Grantcharova, V., Lauffenburger, D. A., & White, F. M. (2006). Effects of HER2 overexpression on cell signaling networks governing proliferation and migration. *Mol Syst Biol,* Vol.2.

Wrobel, C. N. (2004). Autocrine CSF-1R activation promotes Src-dependent disruption of mammary epithelial architecture. *J Cell Biol,* Vol.165, No.2, pp.263-273.

Wu, A. M., & Senter, P. D. (2005). Arming antibodies: prospects and challenges for immunoconjugates. *Nat Biotechnol,* Vol.23, No.9, pp.1137-1146.

Yamada, K. M., & Cukierman, E. (2007). Modeling Tissue Morphogenesis and Cancer in 3D. *Cell,* Vol.130, No.4, pp.601-610.

Yamamoto, T., Ikawa, S., Akiyama, T., Semba, K., Nomura, N., Miyajima, N., Saito, T., & Toyoshima, K. (1986). Similarity of protein encoded by the human c-erb-B-2 gene to epidermal growth factor receptor. *Nature,* Vol.319, No.6050, pp.230-234.

Yamamoto, T., Nishida, T., Miyajima, N., Kawai, S., Ooi, T., & Toyoshima, K. (1983). The erbB gene of avian erythroblastosis virus is a member of the src gene family. *Cell,* Vol.35, No.1, pp.71-78.

Yang, C., Ionescu-Tiba, V., Burns, K., Gadd, M., Zukerberg, L., Louis, D. N., Sgroi, D., & Schmidt, E. V. (2004). The role of the cyclin D1-dependent kinases in ErbB2-mediated breast cancer. *Am J Pathol,* Vol.164, No.3, pp.1031-1038.

Yarden, Y., & Sliwkowski, M. X. (2001). Untangling the ErbB signalling network. *Nat Rev Mol Cell Biol,* Vol.2, No.2, pp.127-137.

Yu, Q., Geng, Y., & Sicinski, P. (2001). Specific protection against breast cancers by cyclin D1 ablation. *Nature,* Vol.411, No.6841, pp.1017-1021.

Zhang, S., Huang, W. C., Li, P., Guo, H., Poh, S. B., Brady, S. W., Xiong, Y., Tseng, L. M., Li, S. H., Ding, Z., Sahin, A. A., Esteva, F. J., Hortobagyi, G. N., Yu, D. (2011). Combating trastuzumab resistance by targeting SRC, a common node downstream of multiple resistance pathways. *Nat Med,* Vol.17, No.4, pp.461-469.

Zheng, J., Mercado-Uribe, I., Rosen, D. G., Chang, B., Liu, P., Yang, G., Malpica, A., Noara, H., Auersperg, N., Mills, G. B., Bast, R. C., & Liu, J. (2010). Induction of papillary carcinoma in human ovarian surface epithelial cells using combined genetic elements and peritoneal microenvironment. *Cell Cycle,* Vol.9, No.1, pp.140-146.

Zhou, Y., Rideout, W. M., 3rd, Zi, T., Bressel, A., Reddypalli, S., Rancourt, R., Woo, J. K., Horner, J. W., Chin, L., Chiu, M. I., Bosenberg, M., Jacks, T., Clark, S. C., Depinho, R. A., Robinson, M. O., & Heyer, J. (2010). Chimeric mouse tumor models reveal differences in pathway activation between ERBB family- and KRAS-dependent lung adenocarcinomas. *Nat Biotechnol,* Vol.28, No.1, pp.71-78.

Zuo, T., Liu, R., Zhang, H., Chang, X., Liu, Y., Wang, L., & Zheng, P. (2007). FOXP3 is a novel transcriptional repressor for the breast cancer oncogene SKP2. *J Clin Invest,* Vol.117, No.12, pp.3765-3773.

8

Trastuzumab-Resistance and Breast Cancer

Milos Dokmanovic and Wen Jin Wu*
Division of Monoclonal Antibodies, Office of Biotechnology Products, Office of Pharmaceutical Science, Center for Drug Evaluation and Research, U.S. Food and Drug Administration, Bethesda, Maryland, United States of America

1. Introduction

Evolution of therapeutic monoclonal antibodies significantly benefited from the recombinant DNA technologies that are used to generate chimeric, humanized, and human versions of monoclonal antibody to reduce the problem of immunogenicity and neutralization, as well as from understanding mechanisms of action mediated by monoclonal antibodies (Nelson et al., 2010; Reichert, 2009; Ranson & Sliwkowski , 2002). One of the significant advances in the application of monoclonal antibodies in oncology was the introduction and approval of trastuzumab, a humanized anti-HER2 antibody, for the treatment of HER2-positive breast cancer.

Despite initial successes and encouraging results, development of monoclonal antibody-based therapies faces several challenges (Yan et al., 2009). Among them are the selection of patients most likely to benefit from clinical trials and lack of understanding of mechanisms of resistance to monoclonal antibody-based therapies (Yan et al., 2009). Selection of patients most likely to benefit from clinical trials of monoclonal antibody-based therapies was initially based on the expression of the antigen targeted by the monoclonal antibody. The anti-HER-2 antibody trastuzumab was tested in patients whose breast tumors overexpress HER2 (Pegram et al., 1998) and the anti-epidermal growth factor receptor (EGFR) antibody cetuximab was used in patients with colorectal cancer and head and neck cancers that overexpress EGFR (Shin et al., 2001). Even with careful characterization of the antigen expression level in the patient population eligible for the clinical trials, primary resistance to monoclonal antibody-based therapies is a common problem. Up to 50% of EGFR-positive colorectal cancer patients are resistant to cetuximab (Saltz et al., 2004), and 74% of HER2-positive breast cancer patients are resistant to anti-HER2 antibody trastuzumab (Vogel et al., 2002).

It has emerged that the levels of antigen expression are not the only determinant of the patient response to monoclonal antibody therapies and that better understanding of the mechanisms of resistance to monoclonal antibodies in different patient subgroups has a potential to improve the effectiveness of the monoclonal antibody treatment. A retrospective analysis of the colorectal tumor samples from the patients that received cetuximab therapy indicated that EGFR-positive colorectal cancer patients with wild-type KRAS gene had increased overall

* Disclaimer: The information presented in this article reflects the views of the authors and does not represent the policy of the U.S. Food and Drug Administration.

survival, progression-free survival and improvement in the global health status compared to the patients whose tumors had KRAS mutations (Karapetis et al., 2008; Lievre et al., 2006). KRAS protein is a member of RAS super family of small GTP-binding proteins and a molecule downstream of the EGFR-mediated signaling cascade, and when aberrantly regulated, KRAS protein contributes to cancer development and progression (Karnoub & Weinberg, 2008). Cellular studies supported the role of KRAS mutations in the resistance to anti-EGFR antibody cetuximab (Benvenuti et al., 2007). Understanding of the role of the KRAS mutations in the resistance to the anti-EGFR antibody cetuximab has improved the selection of patients that are eligible for cetuximab treatment and as a consequence, cetuximab is currently approved for the treatment of EGFR-positive colorectal cancers that do not have KRAS mutations in codon 12 or 13. While KRAS mutations play a critical role in diminishing response to cetuximab in colorectal cancer patients, KRAS gene is infrequently mutated in breast cancer (Karnoub & Weinberg, 2008; Sanchez-Munoz et al., 2010), and it is therefore not likely to contribute to the resistance to anti-HER2 monoclonal antibody trastuzumab. The molecular basis for the resistance to anti-HER2 monoclonal antibody trastuzumab in breast cancer is still not well understood, and there are no clinically useful predictive biomarkers that can be used in conjunction with HER2 expression to predict the outcome of trastuzumab treatment in the HER2-positive breast cancer patients. Breast cancer is one of the most common cancers among women in the United States. It is the second leading cause of cancer death in women, after lung cancer. Women with HER2-overexpressing breast cancers have an increased risk of recurrence and shortened disease-free and overall survival rates (Press et al., 1993; Slamon et al., 1987; Slamon et al., 1989). Understanding the mechanism of resistance to trastuzumab and identifying the predictive biomarkers for the therapeutic resistance to trastuzumab could lead to important therapeutic advances.

Therapeutic monoclonal antibodies represent one of the most dynamic sectors in the biopharmaceutical industry (Reichert, 2009). Twelve monoclonal antibodies and antibodies-related products are licensed for the diagnosis and treatment of specific oncology indications in the U.S. (Table 1) (Note: gemtuzumab ozogamicin was withdrawn from the market in June 2010).

2. HER family of receptor tyrosine kinases

HER2 is a member of the HER family of receptor tyrosine kinases, which is composed of four type I receptors: EGFR/HER1/ErbB1, HER2/ErbB2, HER3/ErbB3, and HER4/ErbB4. All receptors share a similar structure composed of an extracellular ligand-binding region, a single transmembrane lipophilic segment and a cytoplasmic tyrosine kinase-containing domain (Zhang et al. 2007). The extracellular ligand-binding region of HER family receptors is composed of four domains (I-IV). Domains I and III are important for ligand binding. Domain II mediates receptor dimerization. Domain IV forms intramolecular interactions with the domain II and thus blocks dimerization (Garrett et al., 2003). Ligand binding to the extracellular domain of HER family members disrupts the autoinhibition conformation which results in the receptor homo- or hetero-dimerization, and transphosphorylation followed by the activation of the downstream signaling pathways which regulate cell growth and differentiation (Hudis, 2007; Hynes & Lane, 2005). The physiological ligand for HER2 has not been identified yet. HER3 function is particularly important due to its role in the development of resistance in HER2-overexpressing cancers. HER3 binds neuregulins via its extracellular region to mediate signals primarily by heterodimerization with HER2 in

Antibody name (USAN)	Antibody tradename	Therapeutic target	Antibody type	Clinical Indication	Year of approval
Ipilimumab	Yervoy	CTLA-4	IgG1/human	Advanced melanoma	2011
Ofatumumab	Arzerra	CD20	IgG1/human	Chronic lymphocytic leukemia	2009
Panitumumab	Vectibix	EGFR	IgG2/human	Colorectal cancer	2006
Cetuximab	Erbitux	EGFR	IgG1/chimeric	Colorectal cancer Head and Neck Squamous Cell Cancer	2004 2006
Bevacizumab	Avastin	VEGF-A	IgG1/humanized	Colorectal cancer	2004
I131-Tositumomab	Bexxar	CD20	IgG2/mouse	Non-Hodgkin lymphoma	2003
Y90 or I111-Ibritumomab-tiuxetan	Zevelin	CD20	IgG1/mouse	Non-Hodgkin lymphoma	2002
Alemtuzumab	Campath	CD52	IgG1/humanized	Chronic lymphocytic leukemia	2001
Gemtuzumab Ozogamicin	Mylotarg	CD33	IgG4/humanized linked to calichaemicin	Acute myeloid leukemia	2000 withdrawn in June 2010
Trastuzumab	Herceptin	HER2	IgG1/humanized	HER2-positive breast cancer	1998
Rituximab	Rituxan	CD20	IgG1/chimeric	Non-Hodgkin lymphoma	1997
Capromab pendetide	ProstaScint	PSMA	IgG1/murine	Prostate cancer imaging	1996

Table 1. FDA approved monoclonal antibodies used for diagnosis and treatment of different oncological indications.

tumors containing amplifications of HER2 (Baselga & Swain, 2009; Shi et al., 2010). In fact, HER3-HER2 is considered the most active HER signaling dimer (Tzahar et al., 1996). HER3 also plays a key role in the ability of HER2-overexpressing cells to escape the growth inhibition by the EGFR/HER2 dual-specific tyrosine kinase inhibitor (TKI) lapatinib (Sergina et al., 2007). Previously, the intracellular kinase domain of HER3 was thought to be an inactive pseudokinase, because it lacks several key conserved and catalytically important residues (Guy et al., 1994, Sierke et al., 1997). Recently however, HER3 was shown to have kinase activity and the ability to trans-autophosphorylate its intracellular region although it is substantially less active than EGFR (Shi et al., 2010). HER2 extracellular domain adopts a fixed conformation that resembles a ligand-activated state that permits it to form a dimer in the absence of a ligand (Cho at al., 2003; Garrett et al., 2003; Hynes & Lane, 2005). This likely explains why HER2 is the preferred dimerization partner for all of the other HER receptors (Graus-Porta et al., 1997). Moreover, although none of ligands for the HER family receptors directly binds to HER2, activation of EGFR, HER3, and HER4 can facilitate transactivation of HER2 through ligand-induced heterodimerization (Carraway et al., 1994; Wada et al., 1990).

Overexpression of HER2 has been reported in different types of cancer, including breast, gastric, ovarian and salivary gland (Baselga & Swain, 2009). Gene amplification is the most common mechanism resulting in HER2 overexpression in tumors. In addition, somatic mutations in the HER2 tyrosine kinase domain are reported in lung adenocarcinomas, epithelial ovarian cancer, hepatocellular carcinoma, gastric, colorectal and breast cancers, but the activating function for these mutations has not been clarified (Bekaii-Saab et al., 2006; Lee et al., 2006; Lin at al., 2011; Shigematsu et al., 2005). Recent studies also suggest that mutational inactivation in FOXP3 tumor suppressor may contribute to HER2 promoter activation in breast cancer tissues (Zuo et al., 2007). Regardless of the causative mechanisms resulting in HER2 overexpression in certain cancer, the number of HER2 molecules expressed on the surface of these cancer cells far exceeds the number expressed on normal cells, which facilitates the formation of HER2 heterodimers and the spontaneous formation of HER2 homodimers (Yarden & Sliwkowski, 2001). The consequence of this is an excess of HER2-mediated signaling, which drives oncogenic cell survival and proliferation (Yarden & Sliwkowski, 2001).

3. Trastuzumab and mechanisms of action of trastuzumab

For the past 20 years, the development of monoclonal antibodies and tyrosine kinase inhibitors (TKIs) targeting HER2 has been intensely pursued as important cancer therapeutic strategy. There are several reasons why HER2 is an attractive target in breast cancer treatment. First, the levels of HER2 in human cancer cells are higher than that in normal tissues and the elevated levels of HER2 correlate with the pathogenesis and prognosis in breast cancer (Natali et al., 1990; Slamon et al., 1987). Second, HER2 is overexpressed in approximately 20-30% of invasive breast cancer and is associated with poor disease-free survival and poor response to chemotherapy (Gusterson et al., 1992; Paik et al., 1990; Slamon et al., 1989). Third, HER2 is overexpressed in primary tumors and in metastatic sites suggesting that anti-HER2 therapy could be effective in all disease locations (Niehans et al., 1993). Trastuzumab is a recombinant humanized monoclonal antibody directed against the extracellular domain IV of HER2 and is approved for the treatment of HER2-positive breast cancer. In 2010, the European Medicines Agency approved trastuzumab for gastric cancer patients with high expression of HER2 (Okines et al., 2010). Subsequently, in October 2010, U.S. FDA approved trastuzumab in combination with chemotherapy for HER2-positive metastatic cancer of the stomach or the gastroesophageal junction.

Trastuzumab was engineered by inserting the antigen binding loops of a murine antibody (clone 4D5) into the framework of a consensus human IgG_1 using gene conversion mutagenesis strategy (Carter et al., 1992; Pegram et al., 1999). The humanized version of 4D5 (also known as rhuMabHER2; later named trastuzumab) showed significant effects in

HER2-overexpressing breast cancer cells and in HER2-overexpressing xenograft breast cancer models either alone or in combination with other chemotherapy agents (Pegram et al., 1999). While the mechanisms by which trastuzumab induces regression of HER2-positive breast cancers are still being investigated, it is currently believed that the binding of trastuzumab to HER2 contributes to its therapeutic effect by a) inducing HER2 endocytosis followed by receptor degradation; b) inhibiting either HER2 homodimerization or heterodimerization; c) preventing the cleavage of HER2 extracellular domain by the metalloprotease ADAM10 (Hudis, 2007). Taken together, binding of trastuzumab to the extracellular domain of HER2 reduces HER2-coupled mitogenic and pro-survival signaling pathways in tumor cells, leading to the inhibition of phosphatidylinositol 3-kinase (PI3K) and mitogen-activated protein kinase (MAPK) pathways, and the induction of the cyclin-dependent kinase inhibitor, p27 (Nahta & Esteva, 2006). Furthermore, trastuzumab is an IgG_1 subtype capable of inducing antibody-dependent cell mediated cytotoxicity (ADCC). Overexpression of HER2 in human tumor cells is closely associated with the increased angiogenesis and the expression of vascular endothelial growth factor (VEGF). Trastuzumab has also been shown to inhibit tumor angiogenesis, resulting in decreased microvessel density *in vivo* and reduced endothelial cell migration *in vitro* (Nahta & Esteva, 2006).

4. HER2-overexpression and clinical indications for trastuzumab

Trastuzumab is an anti-HER2 antibody indicated for the treatment of HER2-positive breast cancer and HER2-positive metastatic gastric or gastroesophageal (GE) junction adenocarcinoma. Three testing methodologies can be used to determine the HER2 status of the tumor samples: immunocytochemistry (IHC), fluorescence in situ hybridization (FISH), and chromogenic in situ hybridization (CISH) (Wolff et al., 2007). IHC detects the level of membrane bound HER2, whereas FISH and CISH detect the level of HER2 gene amplification. The American Society of Clinical Oncology/College of American Pathologists guideline was developed to define the status of HER2-positive breast cancer and recommended the use of a combination of IHC and FISH testing (Wolff et al., 2007). According to the guideline, a positive HER2 result is the IHC staining of 3+, and a FISH result of more than six HER2 gene copies per nucleus or a FISH ratio (HER2 gene signals to chromosome 17 signals) of more than 2.2 (Wolff et al., 2007). Trastuzumab was the first monoclonal antibody therapy to be approved with a companion diagnostic assay which was used to select the patients eligible for the trastuzumab treatment (Reichert, 2009).

Trastuzumab, when used as a single agent, produced an objective response rate up to 26% in the selected HER2-positive metastatic breast cancer patients (Vogel et al., 2002). Preclinical studies of the combinations of trastuzumab and different chemotherapy agents suggested the potential for additive and/or synergistic effects in the clinical settings (Baselga et al., 1998). Clinical studies then showed that trastuzumab in combination with chemotherapy in HER2-positive metastatic breast cancers significantly improved overall response rate, median overall survival, and time to disease progression (Burstein et al., 2001; Kaufman et al., 2009; Marty et al., 2005; O'Shaughnessy et al., 2004; Pegram et al., 1998; Perez et al., 2005; Slamon et al., 2001). Clinical benefit of trastuzumab treatment in HER2-positive metastatic breast cancer provided the rationale for testing the effects of trastuzumab treatment in the early stage HER2-positive breast cancer in the adjuvant and neoadjuvant setting. The adjuvant therapy is defined as any treatment given after the primary therapy, usually surgery, to increase the chance of long term survival, whereas neoadjuvant therapy refers to the treatment given before the primary therapy. While many clinical trials are still ongoing, there are promising results for the use of trastuzumab treatment in the adjuvant and neoadjuvant settings. It was reported that one year of trastuzumab treatment after adjuvant chemotherapy significantly improved disease free survival and that trastuzumab combined concurrently with the chemotherapy improved the outcomes among HER2-positive breast cancer patients (Piccart-Gebhart et al., 2005). In addition to the use of trastuzumab in adjuvant settings, some of the clinical studies addressed the potential benefit of offering trastuzumab in the neoadjuvant settings. Results from the GeparQuattro study suggested that neoadjuvant combination of trastuzumab and different chemotherapy agents induced a high pathological complete response (pCR) rate with the minimal toxicities (Untch et al., 2010). pCR is defined as the complete absence of intact tumor cells in the resected specimen. Trastuzumab is now a standard of care in combination with chemotherapy for patients with HER2-positive breast cancer (Banerjee & Smith, 2010).

5. Resistance to the EGFR-targeted therapies

Targeting the EGFR has been intensely pursued in the past decade as a cancer treatment strategy. Small molecule tyrosine kinase inhibitors (TKIs) and anti-EGFR monoclonal antibodies are the primary approaches to inhibit EGFR-coupled signaling pathways. To date, three tyrosine kinase inhibitors, erlotinib, gefitinib, and lapatinib, have been approved for oncology indications. Cetuximab, a chimeric IgG_1 directed against the extracellular domain of EGFR, was originally generated from a murine antibody, 225 (Goldstein et al., 1995). Preclinical studies showed that cetuximab was more effective than the murine antibody 225 in inhibiting tumor growth in A431 human tumor xenografts model. Based on the preclinical studies, cetuximab was found to inhibit EGFR activation by preventing ligand binding, which inhibits EGFR dimerization and induces the EGFR internalization and downregulation (Goldstein et al., 1995; Mendelsohn, 2002). Cetuximab was approved in 2004 by FDA for the treatment of EGFR expressing metastatic colorectal cancer. In 2006, FDA approved the use of cetuximab for the treatment of locally advanced or regionally advanced head and neck squamous cell carcinomas (HNSCC). In 2006, panitumumab, a human antibody directed against the EGFR was also approved for the treatment of EGFR expressing metastatic colorectal cancer (Giusti et al., 2008; Hecht et al., 2009; Van Cutsem et al., 2007).
Molecular mechanisms contributing to the resistance to EGFR kinase inhibitors have been extensively studied. Important findings suggest that there is a strong relationship between the resistance to EGFR TKIs and the absence of an activating mutation in the intracellular kinase domain of the receptor. These EGFR kinase domain mutations, such as the point mutation, L858R, and in-frame deletion in exon 19 around codons 746-750, enhance the ligand-dependent activation of EGFR, and simultaneously increase the sensitivity to the TKIs (Han et al., 2005; Mitsudomi et al., 2005; Morgillo et al., 2007). It has also been demonstrated that the patients with the EGFR mutation-positive tumors have an improved response rate and survival after treatment with TKIs compared to the patients with tumors that express wild-type EGFR (Han et al., 2005; Mitsudomi et al., 2005). Therefore, the lack of these mutations can be considered a predictor of the treatment resistance to TKI (Morgillo et al, 2007). Mechanisms contributing to the primary resistance to EGFR TKIs also include genetic alterations, for example, EGFR variant III (EGFRvIII) and activating KRAS mutations. EGFRvIII lacks the ligand binding domain and is a constitutively activated mutant. It has also been reported that a point mutation in the exon 20 (T790M) in the kinase

domain of the EGFR gene occurs in tumors with acquired resistance to EGFR kinase inhibitors, gefitinib and erlotinib (Pao et al., 2005). Because mutations within HER2 have not been commonly found in HER2-overexpressing breast tumors (Zito et al., 2008), the mechanisms of resistance to EGFR kinase inhibitors may not be relevant to trastuzumab.
Although EGFR tyrosine kinase domain mutations may predict response to the TKIs, no mutations in the EGFR have been associated with resistance to the antibody-based therapies, cetuximab and panitumumab (Mukohara et al., 2005; Kruser & Wheeler, 2010). While EGFR gene amplification may be both predictive and prognostic and associated with the objective tumor response to cetuximab therapy, IHC based assay measuring EGFR expression may not be an accurate predictive factor for response to cetuximab therapy in colorectal cancer (Chung et al., 2005; Lievre et al., 2006), indicating that different mechanisms may contribute to cetuximab-resistance. One of the most reliable predictive biomarkers to emerge in the clinic has been that of the KRAS mutation status in colorectal cancer (Kruser & Wheeler, 2010). Lievre et al. reported that KRAS mutation status was predictive of resistance to cetuximab therapy. In this report, 30 metastatic colorectal carcinoma patients treated with cetuximab were analyzed for KRAS mutations. The authors reported that KRAS mutation was found in 43% (13 tumors) and was significantly associated with resistance to cetuximab therapy (Lievre et al., 2006). A larger study was performed to measure the KRAS mutation status in 113 patients with refractory metastatic colorectal cancer treated with cetuximab. The authors found that KRAS wild-type is a strong predictor of significant increase in progression-free survival (PFS) and overall survival (OS) in this cohort of patients (De Roock et al., 2008). Many other clinical trials have confirmed these findings, leading to a Provisional Clinical Opinion from the American Society for Clinical Oncology (ASCO) stating that all patients with metastatic colorectal carcinoma who are candidates for anti-EGFR antibody therapy should have their tumor tested for KRAS mutations in a Clinical Laboratory Improvement Amendments (CLIA)-accredited laboratory (Allegra et al., 2009). If codon 12 or 13 of KRAS is found to be mutated then patients with metastatic colorectal cancer should not receive anti-EGFR antibody therapy as a part of their treatment (Allegra et al., 2009).

6. Therapeutic resistance to trastuzumab

6.1 Clinical evidence for trastuzumab-resistance

While trastuzumab has significantly changed the outcome for the treatment of HER2-positive breast cancer, mechanisms contributing to trastuzumab-resistance are less well understood. Both primary and acquired resistance to trastuzumab pose a significant hurdle in the breast cancer therapy (Nahta & Esteva, 2006). Primary trastuzumab resistance refers to the lack of response to trastuzumab treatment in the patients with HER2-positive breast tumors who were never treated with trastuzumab before, whereas acquired resistance indicates that the patients who achieve initial response to trastuzumab acquire resistance to this antibody. In the study which evaluated the efficacy and the safety of trastuzumab as a single agent, the reported rate of primary trastuzumab-resistance was 74%, indicating that the vast majority of HER2-positive metastatic breast cancer patients demonstrate intrinsic resistance to single-agent trastuzumab (Vogel et al., 2002). Moreover, while addition of trastuzumab to chemotherapy in the cohort of HER2-positive metastatic breast cancer patients results in the higher response rates, and the extension of time to disease progression, the durations of response to trastuzumab in either the single-agent setting or in the combination with chemotherapy has been reported to be 5-9 month (Kruser & Wheeler 2010; Nahta & Esteva, 2006; Slamon et al., 2001). Therefore, the majority of patients with HER2-positive breast cancer develops acquired resistance within one year. (Kruser & Wheeler 2010; Nahta & Esteva, 2006; Slamon et al., 2001). Understanding the mechanisms of trastuzumab-resistance and developing predictive biomarkers for therapeutic resistance to trastuzumab are critical to the discovery of novel agents that could overcome trastuzumab-resistance and potentially benefit HER2-positive breast cancer patients.

6.2 Preclinical studies

6.2.1 Cellular models used for the studies of trastuzumab-resistance

There are several preclinical cellular models developed to study the mechanisms of resistance to trastuzumab. HER2-positive breast cancer cell lines were chronically exposed to trastuzumab either *in vitro* (SKBR3 cell line) or in xenograft settings (BT474 cell line) in order to develop trastuzumab-resistant clones and populations (Nahta et al., 2004a; Ritter et al., 2007). In this approach, a comparison between parental trastuzumab-sensitive and derived trastuzumab-resistant clones was carried out in order to characterize the changes in the cell signaling pathways associated with trastuzumab-resistance. Recently, the JIMT-1 cell line was established from a breast cancer patient with HER2 gene amplification and primary resistance to trastuzumab and was used to study the mechanisms of resistance to trastuzumab (Tanner et al., 2004). These trastuzumab-resistant cell lines still overexpress HER2, suggesting that resistance to trastuzumab is not due to the loss of HER2 overexpression (Diermeier et al., 2005; Dokmanovic et al., 2009; Nagy et al., 2005; Ritter et al., 2007). Interestingly, it was reported recently that chronic exposure of BT-474 cells to trastuzumab gave rise to trastuzumab-resistant clones, which lost HER2 gene amplification and HER2 overexpression (Mittendorf et al., 2009). However, it is not clear whether trastuzumab eliminated HER2-overexpressing clones leaving only HER2-negative cancer clones or that the treatment with trastuzumab inhibited HER2 expression or induced downregulation of HER2, resulting in the loss of HER2 expression and resistance to trastuzumab.

6.2.2 Molecular mechanisms of trastuzumab-resistance

Trastuzumab-resistance may be broadly divided into two mechanistic categories. The first occurs at the cell membrane where aberrant regulation of HER2 results in deregulation of HER2 signaling pathways. The second results from changes to HER2-regulated intracellular signaling molecules that result in uncoupling signaling from their upstream regulation. Examples of the latter category include PTEN loss or expression of a constitutively activated PI3K mutant, PIK3CA.

Based on *in vitro* breast cancer cell models of trastuzumab-resistance, HER2 interactions with other membrane-associated proteins contribute to resistance. For example, in the JIMT-1 trastuzumab-resistant breast cancer cell line, binding of MUC4 glycoprotein to HER2 partially masks the trastuzumab binding site in HER2, resulting in reduced trastuzumab binding and contributing to trastuzumab-resistance (Nagy et al., 2005). Trastuzumab binding to HER2 in JIMT-1 cells was restored by downregulation of MUC4 protein (Nagy et al., 2005). Formation of homodimers, and heterodimers between EGFR, HER2, and HER3 due to overexpression of HER family ligands interferes with trastuzumab-mediated growth inhibition and contributes to trastuzumab-resistance (Diermeier et al., 2005; Motoyama 2002;

Ritter et al., 2007; Valabrega et al., 2005). *In vitro* models using breast cancer cells derived for resistance to trastuzumab found that Insulin-like growth factor-I receptor (IGF-IR) heterodimerizes with and phosphorylates ErbB2 suggesting that transactivation of ErbB2 by IGF1R may contribute to resistance (Nahta et al., 2005; Lu et al., 2004). Heterotrimerization of the growth factor receptors HER2, HER3 and IGF-IR in BT-474 breast cancer cells interferes with trastuzumab-associated p27 induction and therefore contributes to trastuzumab-resistance (Huang et al., 2010). Increased activity of small GTP-binding protein Rac1 interrupts with trastuzumab-induced HER2 endocytosis and degradation, resulting in the upregulated HER2-mediated signaling in SKBR3 breast cancer cells contributing to trastuzumab-resistance (Dokmanovic et al., 2009). The Met receptor tyrosine kinase, which is aberrantly expressed in breast cancer and predicts poor patient prognosis, is frequently expressed in HER2-overexpressing breast cancer cells, as well as in HER2-positive breast cancer, and Met activation protects cells against trastuzumab by abrogating p27 induction, thus contributing to trastuzumab resistance (Shattuck et al., 2008). Moreover, HER2-overexpressing breast cancer cells rapidly up-regulate Met expression after trastuzumab treatment, promoting their own resistance (Shattuck et al., 2008). As mentioned in the previous paragraph, loss of HER2 expression in HER2-overexpression breast cancer cells could be another mechanism contributing to trastuzumab resistance (Mittendorf et al., 2009). HER2 receptor initiated downstream signaling promotes cell proliferation and cell survival by the activation of RAS-MAPK and PI3K/Akt/mTOR pathways (Hudis, 2007; Zhou et al., 2004). Addition of trastuzumab to HER2-positive trastuzumab-sensitive cells results in the activation of PTEN, which acts as a tumor suppressor to induce inhibition of Akt phosphorylation and, therefore, antagonizes the PI3K/Akt survival pathway (Nagata et al., 2004). Nagata et al. reported that reducing PTEN in breast cancer cells by antisense oligonucleotides conferred trastuzumab-resistance and that inhibition of PI3K activity enhanced trastuzumab-mediated growth inhibition in a trastuzumab-resistant xenograft model (Nagata et al., 2004). PTEN knockdown in a large scale of RNA interference screening was found to be associated with selective isolation of cell clones resistant to trastuzumab (Berns et al., 2007). Constitutive activation of PI3K, such as PIK3CA mutant, can uncouple Akt signaling from the upstream regulation resulting in trastuzumab-resistance (Berns et al., 2007).

6.3 Clinical studies

Clinical studies have focused on characterization of the HER2 status and HER2-initiated downstream signaling pathways in the samples obtained from trastuzumab-sensitive patients and trastuzumab-resistant patients. A subtype of HER2-positive tumors with distinct biological and clinical features expresses a series of carboxyl terminal fragments of HER2 known as p95HER2. It is generally accepted that the p95HER2 can arise either by proteolytic shedding of the extracellular domain of the full-length HER2 by metalloproteinases ADAM10 at a site proximal to the transmembrane domain or by translation of the mRNA encoding truncated HER2 receptor from the internal initiation codons (Arribas et al., 2011). It is believed that trastuzumab has the ability to prevent proteolytic shedding of full-length HER2 on HER2-overexpressing breast cancer cells (Hudis, 2007). p95HER2 contains a hyperactive membrane anchored fragment that lacks the extracellular domain of HER2 and drives breast cancer progression *in vivo*. Of note, expression of p95HER2 fragments in transgenic mouse models leads to the generation of the breast tumors that were more aggressive and metastatic than those driven by full-length HER2 (Pedersen et al., 2009). Expression of the p95HER2 fragment is predictive of poor prognosis and correlates with resistance to trastuzumab treatment in breast cancer patients (Arribas et al., 2011; Carney et al., 2003). This is likely due to the absence of the extracellular domain (ECD) required for trastuzumab binding (Arribas et al., 2011). The ECD of HER2 can be released into the circulation after cleavage of HER2 by the metalloproteinases ADAM10. It was reported that the prevalence of increased levels of ECD in patient serum with primary breast cancer varied between 0% and 38%, whereas in metastatic breast cancer the range was from 23% to 80% (Carney et al., 2003). Moreover, Ali et al. reported that the decrease in serum levels of HER2 ECD was positively associated with trastuzumab-sensitivity (Ali et al., 2008). In particular, in an analysis of 307 patients with metastatic breast cancer, individuals who did not achieve a significant decline (defined as ≥ 20%) in serum level of serum HER2 ECD after receiving trastuzumab had decreased benefit from trastuzumab-based therapy (Ali et al., 2008).

The analysis of *HER2* gene amplification before and after trastuzumab therapy suggested that patients who had lost *HER2* gene amplification had a significantly decreased recurrence free survival (RFS) compared with patients whose tumors remained *HER2* amplified after trastuzumab treatment (Mittendorf et al., 2009). Nagata et al. revealed that patients with PTEN-deficient breast cancers had significantly reduced responses to trastuzumab-based therapy than those with normal PTEN, suggesting PTEN deficiency may be a predictor to trastuzumab resistance (Nagata et al., 2004). Analysis of the 137 patient samples with HER2-positive metastatic breast cancer who received trastuzumab therapy revealed that activation of PI3K either by PTEN loss and/or PIK3CA mutational activation was associated with a poor response to trastuzumab and a shorter patient survival time (Esteva et al., 2010). In a neoadjuvant clinical trial, which examined the association between response to trastuzumab therapy and the status of PTEN level and PIK3CA mutations, it was found that only 15.4% of subjects with low nuclear PTEN had pathological complete response (pCR) to trastuzumab compared to 44.4% of subjects with high nuclear PTEN levels. It was reported that 20% of patients with PIK3CA activating mutations achieved pCR compared to 38.1 % of patients with wild-type PIK3 status. When the two biomarkers (PTEN level and PIK3CA status) were combined together only 18.2% of patients with low PTEN or PIK3CA achieved pCR to trastuzumab compared to 66.7 % of patients who did not have low PTEN level or PI3KAC mutations (Dave et al., 2011). Taken together, loss of PTEN and PIK3CA activating mutations are associated with trastuzumab-resistance.

Cyclin E is a critical regulator of the cell cycle G1/S transition and cyclin E levels are regulated by HER2 signaling in breast cancer cells (Mittendorf et al., 2010). Trastuzumab treatment reduces cyclin E level and activity in breast cancer cells (Mittendorf et al., 2010).

It has been recently reported that in a cohort of 34 HER2-positive breast cancer patients treated with trastuzumab-based therapy, cyclin E amplification/overexpression was associated with a worse clinical benefit and a lower progression-free survival compared with non-overexpressing cyclin E tumors, suggesting that cyclin E amplification/overexpression may contribute to trastuzumab-resistance in HER-positive breast cancer patients (Scaltriti et al., 2011). Interestingly, in an analysis of 26 tumor samples (10 cyclin E positive and 16 cyclin E negative), cyclin E amplification only partially correlated with other clinically relevant trastuzumab-resistant markers, such as p95HER2 and PTEN loss (Scaltriti et al., 2011). This suggests that cyclin E amplification/overexpression might use a different mechanism to contribute to trastuzumab-resistance as compared to p95HER2 and PTEN loss.

7. Toxicity and trastuzumab-related cardiotoxicity

Trastuzumab is generally well tolerated with mild to moderate side effects and low incidence of chemotherapy associated adverse events (Brufsky, 2010). The side effects reported in different clinical trials include cardiomyopathy, infusion reactions, embryo-fetal toxicity, pulmonary toxicity, exacerbation of chemotherapy-induced neutropenia, diarrhea, burning sensation in the skin, rash, and nausea and vomiting, upper respiratory tract infection, increased cough. Among those side effects, the trastuzumab-related cardiotoxicity has drawn great attention for trastuzumab-based therapy.

Trastuzumab associated cardiac dysfunction was initially reported in a phase III trial, which tested the efficacy of combining chemotherapy with trastuzumab versus chemotherapy alone in metastatic breast cancer disease (Slamon et al., 2001). The addition of trastuzumab increased the incidence of chemotherapy-associated symptomatic and asymptomatic cardiac dysfunction. These manifested as severe congestive heart failure and as significant decrease in left ventricular ejection function (LVEF) (Slamon et al., 2001; Sutter et al., 2007). In the subgroup that received anthracyclines, cyclophosphamide and trastuzumab, the incidence of cardiac dysfunction was 27% compared to 8% for the subgroup that received anthracyclines and cyclophosphamide alone (Slamon et al., 2001). For the subgroup that received paclitaxel and trastuzumab the incidence of cardiac dysfunction was 13% compared to 1% for the subgroup that received paclitaxel alone (Slamon et al., 2001). Although the results of trastuzumab adjuvant trials indicate that the incidence of trastuzumab discontinuation due to cardiac disorder was low (4.3%) and that most patients with cardiac dysfunction recovered within 6 months period (Sutter et al., 2007), the finding of trastuzumab-induced cardiac dysfunction has influenced the design of subsequent trastuzumab adjuvant trials and implementation of cardiac screening prior to and during the trastuzumab adjuvant trial (Sutter et al., 2007). Meta analysis of adjuvant trastuzumab clinical trials have assessed the incidence of cardiac dysfunction and found a favorable benefit to risk ratio for trastuzumab treatment in the early breast cancer (Viani et al., 2007).

Cancer chemotherapy, in particular anthracycline therapy, was known to be associated with cardiac dysfunction, and trastuzumab treatment increased the incidence of chemotherapy-induced cardiac dysfunction in the early trials with metastatic breast cancer patients (Slamon et al., 20001). Subsequent analysis indicated that trastuzumab-associated cardiac toxicity was clinically different than cardiac dysfunction associated with anthracyclines treatment (Ewer et al., 2005). Currently, trastuzumab-associated cardiac dysfunction is recognized as type II chemotherapy related cardiac dysfunction (Ewer & Lipmann, 2005). Clinical studies indicate that the increase in patient plasma troponin I levels, which has been proposed as an early marker of high dose chemotherapy (HDCT)-induced cardiac dysfunction, is associated with a risk of trastuzumab-induced cardiac dysfunction and the lack of left ventricular ejection fraction (LVEF) recovery (Cardinale et al., 2010). The evidence from the clinical trials indicate that trastuzumab-induced cardiomyopathy is not dose dependent, and that it is increased when trastuzumab is administered concurrently with anthracyclines, and that it is at least partially reversible (Ewer et al., 2005).

HER2 signaling in heart is essential for cardiac development and function, as well as for the prevention of dilated cardiomyopathy (Negro et al., 2004). While the mechanisms contributing to trastuzumab-induced cardiac toxicity are still incompletely understood, it appears that blocking HER2 with anti-HER2 antibodies increases the production of reactive oxygen species and reduces human cardiomyocyte cell viability (Gordon et al., 2009). In other studies, treatment of rat cardiomyocytes with anti-HER2 antibodies increased mitochondria-dependent apoptosis by modulating the levels of Bcl-XL and Bcl-xS (Grazette et al., 2004). Consistent with the above studies, HER2 knockout mice have ventricular trabeculation deterioration, dilated cardiomyopathy, and increased sensitivity to anthracyclines toxicity (Lee et al., 1995; Negro et al., 2004). Molecular mechanisms by which trastuzumab induces cardiac dysfunction still remain elusive.

8. Strategies to overcome trastuzumab-resistance

Most examples of acquired therapeutic resistance to receptor tyrosine kinase inhibitors (TKIs) include development of mutations within the targeted receptors. For example, mutations in BCR/ABL in chronic myeloid leukemia and c-kit in gastrointestinal stromal tumors confer resistance to a specific BCR/ABL, c-kit kinase inhibitor Imatinib (Gleevec) (Litzow, 2006). Improvement of the binding of small molecules to their targets has been successfully used as a strategy to overcome resistance to imatinib (Guilhot et al.,2007; le Coutre et al.,2008).

While KRAS mutations have been found to be associated with primary resistance to cetuximab for the treatment of colorectal cancer, no predictive markers are currently used in the clinic to differentiate HER2-positive breast cancers that would respond favorably to trastuzumab from trastuzumab-resistant disease. Interestingly, KRAS, which signals downstream of both EGFR and HER2 receptors, is usually not mutated in HER2-positive breast cancer (Karnoub & Wenberg, 2008). Therefore, KRAS is not likely to contribute to therapeutic resistance to trastuzumab. Furthermore, mutations in HER2 have not been associated with resistance to trastuzumab. Based on these data, the strategies used to overcome therapeutic resistance to TKIs may not apply to trastuzumab-resistance.

8.1 Small molecule inhibitors used for the treatment of trastuzumab-resistant disease

Many new small molecule inhibitors are under clinical development to treat trastuzumab-resistant breast cancers. Early clinical studies suggest that TKIs that specifically target EGFR and HER2 have anti-tumor effects. Lapatinib, a reversible inhibitor targeting the ATP binding site of the tyrosine kinase domain of EGFR and HER2, has a mechanism of action distinct from trastuzumab. Based on the evidence obtained from preclinical and clinical studies, lapatinib activity is not dependent on the PTEN, p95HER2, and PI3K mutation status (Bartsch et al., 2007; Nahta & Esteva, 2006). Preclinical studies indicate that lapatinib is effective in inducing apoptosis in trastuzumab-resistant HER2-overexpressing breast cancer cells (Konecny et al, 2006; Nahta et al., 2007). Results from a phase I study of lapatinib in a cohort of EGFR and/or HER2 overexpressing breast cancer patients indicate that lapatinib was well tolerated and produced partial responses in patients with trastuzumab-resistant breast cancer (Burris et al., 2005). Taken together, these studies provided the rationale for clinical studies to evaluate the effect of lapatinib plus trastuzumab on duration of response. A randomized study of lapatinib alone versus the combination of lapatinib and trastuzumab in patients with trastuzumab-resistant HER2-positive metastatic breast cancer indicate that the combination of trastuzumab and lapatinib is superior to lapatinib alone for progression free survival (Blackwell et al., 2010).

Other TKIs in clinical development include neratinib which is a potent and irreversible TKI inhibitor of both EGFR and HER2. Neratinib showed promising results in clinical studies with HER2-positive breast cancer patients that were either heavily pretreated or not pretreated with trastuzumab (Burstein et al., 2010).

HER2 activates the PI3K/Akt/mammalian target of rapamycin pathway (mTOR), which represents a central signaling pathway that promotes proliferation, invasion, and survival of breast cancer cells (Zhou et al., 2004). Activation of the PI3K pathway either by loss of PTEN or by an activating mutation in PI3K, PIK3CA, is associated with lower response to anti-HER2 targeting agents, including trastuzumab (Berns et al., 2007; Nagata et al., 2004). Preclinical testing of combination of trastuzumab and PI3K, Akt or mTOR targeting agents showed that they have the potential to inhibit the growth of trastuzumab-resistant breast cancer cells and xenografts (Lu et al., 2007; Serra et al., 2008). These preclinical data are supported by recently published data of phase I trial where the oral mTOR inhibitor, everolimus, in combination with trastuzumab and vionorelbine had anti-tumor activity in HER2-positive metastatic breast cancer patients that progressed on trastuzumab (Jerusalem et al., 2011). Two additional mTOR inhibitors, rapamycin and temsirolimus, are also in clinical trials targeting trastuzumab-resistant breast cancers.

The chaperon Hsp90 has been implicated in the stabilization of a number of cellular proteins that play central roles in signaling transduction processes (Pratt & Toft, 2003). It has been reported that the intracellular domain of HER2 binds to Hsp90 and binding of Hsp90 to HER2 not only serves to maintain its physiological conformation, but also to restrain HER2 from forming active signaling dimer (Citri et al, 2004). Tanespimycin is a geldanamycin derivative that inhibits Hsp90 function in tumor cells, as well as in murine models (Zsebik et al., 2005). Cellular studies established that tanespimycin treatment either alone or in combination with trastuzumab inhibited cell growth and induced cell death in trastuzumab-sensitive and in trastuzumab-resistant cell lines (Zsebik et al., 2005). The inhibition of cell growth by tanespimycin was associated with decrease in membrane bound HER2 levels, most likely due to ubiquitination and lysosomal pathway dependent HER2 protein degradation (Raja et al., 2008). A phase I clinical testing of a combination of trastuzumab and tanespimycin showed safe and active in trastuzumab-resistant breast cancer and induced antitumor activity in HER2-positive metastatic breast cancers (Modi et al., 2007).

The following table provides information with regards to clinical trials testing multiple agents for the treatment of trastuzumab-resistant breast cancers. More detailed information can be found in the U.S. National Cancer Institute's website at http://www.cancer.gov/clinicaltrials.

8.2 Monoclonal antibodies indicated for the treatment of trastuzumab-resistant disease

Pertuzumab is an IgG_1 monoclonal antibody that binds to domain II of extracellular segment of HER2. Domain II mediates homo- and hetero-dimerization of HER2 with other members of the HER family. Therefore, binding of HER2 with pertuzumab prevents HER2-mediated dimerization and inhibits HER2-coupled signaling (Nahta et al., 2004b). Unlike pertuzumab, trastuzumab binds to domain IV of extracellular segment of HER2 receptor (Franklin et al., 2004). Cellular studies indicate that the combination of these two anti-HER2 antibodies exhibited synergistic effects in inhibiting breast cancer cell survival (Nahta et al., 2004b).

Clinical trial combination therapy for trastuzumab-resistant HER2 positive breast cancer	Molecular targets	Phase of clinical study
XL147/trastuzumab/paclitaxel	PI3K/HER2/microtubules	I,II
BKM120/trastuzumab	PI3K/HER2	I,II
AUY922/trastuzumab	Hsp90/HER2	I,II
GRN163L/trastuzumab	Telomerase/ErbB2	I
Everolimus/trastuzumab/vinorelbine	mTOR/HER2/tubulin	III
Rapamycin/trastuzumab	mTOR/HER2	II
Temsirolimus/neratinib	mTOR/EGFR, HER2	I,II
Panobinostat/trastuzumab	Histone deacetylase (HDAC)/HER2	I,II
BIBW2992/vinorelbine	EGFR, HER2/tubulin	III
BMS-754807/trastuzumab	Insulin-like growth factor-I receptor, insulin receptor/HER2	I,II

Table 2. Ongoing clinical trials testing multiple agents for trastuzumab-resistant breast cancer.

Addition of pertuzumab after progression to ongoing trastuzumab in xenografts synergistically increased tumor inhibition compared with trastuzumab alone (Friess et al., 2005). Taken together, these data suggest that trastuzumab and pertuzumab have complementary mechanisms of action and that the addition of pertuzumab to trastuzumab may improve clinical efficacy as a result of potentially broader blockade of the HER tumor cell proliferation and survival signaling (Friess et al., 2005). A Phase II trial of combination of pertuzumab and trastuzumab in HER2-positive patients that progressed on trastuzumab therapy indicated that the combination was active and well tolerated and adverse events were mild to moderate (Baselga et al., 2010). Data from this Phase II clinical trial indicated that objective response rate was 24.2%, the clinical benefit rate was 50%, and progression-free survival was 5.5 months in the cohort of patients (Baselga et al., 2010). Additionally, IMC-1121B (anti-VEGFR-2 monoclonal antibody) and IMC-18F1 (anti-VEGFR-1 monoclonal antibody) have been tested in clinical trials in combination with capecitabine, a chemotherapeutic agent that inhibits DNA synthesis and slows growth of tumor tissue, for the treatment of trastuzumab-resistant disease (National Cancer Institute, 2011; Schwartz et al., 2010; Spratin et al., 2010;).

8.3 Optimization of antibody structures

Advanced recombinant DNA technologies allow researchers to engineer therapeutic antibodies on a more rational basis. This can yield more homogeneous and stable molecules with additional properties such as increased cytotoxicity, dual-targeting, monovalent monoclonal antibodies, and enhanced penetration into solid tumors (Beck et al., 2010; Jin et al., 2008).

The variable region (Fv) of a monoclonal antibody is responsible for the binding of antibody to the antigens. Affinity maturation technology has been used to improve the binding affinity and specificity of Fv to the target. Targeting c-Met with antibodies had been difficult because most antibodies had intrinsic agonistic activity (Prat et al., 1998). A one-armed (OA) variant of the anti-c-Met antibody 5D5 was found to act as a pure antagonist and had the ability to inhibit the growth of cells dependent on SF/HGF-c-Met autocrine and paracrine signaling (Jin et al., 2008; Nguyen et al., 2003). Data have shown that monovalent 5D5 antibody potently inhibited glioma growth in an orthotopic *in vivo* model (Martens et al., 2006).

The constant region (Fc) of an antibody is essential for the interaction between antibody and Fc receptors presenting on immune cells (Bruhns et al., 2009). Fc functions can be modulated by altering glycosylation status and binding affinity to Fc receptors, resulting in changes in antibody-dependent cellular cytotoxicity (ADCC), serum half-life, anti-inflammatory properties, and complement activation. Musolino et al. reported that the response to trastuzumab in metastatic breast cancer correlates with expression of the high affinity allele of the activating FcγRIIIa (CD16a)-158V/V (Musolino et al., 2008). It was recently reported that MGAH22, an anti-HER2 monoclonal antibody, was engineered in the Fc domain to increase binding to both alleles of the CD16a (Nordstrom et al., 2010). It was also reported that MGAH22 had enhanced activity against HER2-expressing tumors in hCD16a-158F transgenic mice (Nordstrom et al., 2010). A preclinical study showed that MGAH22 conferred enhanced activity against HER2-positive breast tumor cells, including cells resistant to trastuzumab (Nordstrom et al., 2010). Furthermore, MGAH22 exhibited greater ADCC against HER2-expressing cancer cells with lower EC_{50} (Nordstrom et al., 2010). According to the information obtained from the website of the National Cancer Institute, MGAH22 is currently in phase I clinical trials for the treatment of the patients with the HER2-positive cancers, including breast cancer, that have not responded to the standard treatment (National Cancer Institute, 2011, http://www.cancer.gov/clinicaltrials).

Multiple signaling pathways contribute to cancer development and progression. Bispecific antibodies, which are directed against two antigens that drive cancer progression, might yield better therapeutic efficacy than inhibition of a single target (Chames & Baty, 2009). Bispecific antibodies can be obtained by combining the variable domains of two already characterized monoclonal antibodies (two V_L domains on the light chain and two V_H domains on the heavy chain) using the dual variable domain IgG (DVD-IgG) technology.

This technology enables the different specificities of two monoclonal antibodies to be engineered into a single functional, dual-specific, tetravalent IgG like molecule (Beck et al., 2010). A different approach consists of engineering an additional paratope, the antigen-binding site of an antibody, in the variable domain of an existing antibody, which results in simultaneous binding to two different antigens (Beck et al., 2010; Bostrom et al., 2009). The bispecific antibody (MM-111) was developed to target both ErbB2 and ErbB3. MM-111 was indicated to displace heregulin from ErbB3 and thereby prevents receptor phosphorylation, resulting in the inhibition of tumor growth. MM-111 in combination with trastuzumab is currently in a clinical trial to treat trastuzumab-resistant breast cancer (Arnett et al., 2011; National Cancer Institute, 2011, http://www.cancer.gov/clinicaltrials).

Polyclonal or oligoclonal antibodies refer to the recombinant polycolonal or oligoclonal antibodies directed against the same or different targets. For example, the Rhesus D blood group antigen-specific polyclonal antibody rozrolimupab (Sym001; Symphogen A/S), which is a mixture of 25 unique recombinant monoclonal antibodies, is currently in Phase II clinical trials for the treatment of chronic and acute idiopathic thrombocytopenic purpura (Beck et al, 2010; Swann, et al 2008;). Hopefully, in the near future we will see more optimized monoclonal antibodies entering the clinical trials to treat trastuzumab-resistant disease.

8.4 Antibody-drug conjugates (ADC)

An important approach to delivering a lethal quantity of cytotoxic agent to the cancer cells is to select an antibody that specifically binds to a cancer-specific antigen that can mediate a rapid rate of endocytosis of antibody conjugate and accumulate them at a high concentration in cancer cells, thus resulting in cancer cell-specific killing while minimizing damage to normal cells (Chen at al., 2005; Senter, 2009). Antibody-drug conjugates are monoclonal antibody-based products that are covalently attached to the cytotoxic agent by chemical linkers (Alley et al., 2010). It is now a common strategy to develop monoclonal antibody-cytotoxic drug conjugates to improve the efficacy of both the monoclonal antibody and the cytotoxic agent for cancer indications (Chen at al, 2005; Senter, 2009). Antibody-drug conjugates consist of three different elements: the monoclonal antibody, linker, and cytotoxic agent. Three different classes of cytotoxic agents, including calicheamicin-based, maytansinoid-based, and auristatin-based cytotoxic agents, are commonly used as drugs to be conjugated to antibodies. Calicheamicin is a natural product and has been the subject of extensive research for drug delivery, due to its ability to bind to DNA in the minor groove, resulting in DNA cleavage. Maytansinoid derivatives and auristatin represent other classes of highly potent drugs that have been widely utilized for antibody-drug conjugate development. Both cytotoxic agents, maytansinoid derivatives and auristatin, act by binding to tubulin to mediate inhibition of tubulin polymerization (Chari, 2008; Doronina et al, 2006; Doronina et al. 2003). Traditionally, the antibody in an antibody-drug conjugate functions as a vehicle to carry drugs to the tumor site and drugs with high systemic toxicity are selected as payload in the antibody-drug conjugate. Gemtuzumab ozogamicin (Mylotarg), an anti-CD33 antibody conjugated to calicheamicin, was granted marketing approval for the treatment of relapsed acute myeloid leukemia in 2000. It was withdrawn from the U.S. market in June 2010 when a clinical trial showed that the drug failed to demonstrate clinical benefit to the patients enrolled in clinical trials.

Trastuzumab-DM1 (T-DM1) is an antibody-drug conjugate that was generated by linking the maytansinoid derivative maytansin to trastuzumab via a thioether linker (Lewis Phillips et al., 2008). Testing of T-DM1 in a panel of HER2-positive trastuzumab-sensitive and trastuzumab-resistant cell lines indicated that T-DM1 was cytotoxic in both trastuzumab-sensitive and trastuzumab-resistant breast cancer cell lines (Lewis Phillips et al. 2008). T-DM1 also inhibited tumor growth and caused tumor regression in trastuzumab resistant animal xenograft models (Lewis Phillips et al. 2008). T-DM1 was reported to retain the mechanisms of action of trastuzumab and was also active against lapatinib-resistant cell lines and tumors (Junttila et al., 2010). A Phase I clinical trial testing of T-DM1 reported that T-DM1 was associated with clinical activity in HER2-positive patients who had progressed on trastuzumab-based therapy (Krop et al., 2010). A Phase II study recently reported that T-DM1 had robust single-agent activity in metastatic breast cancer patients who had progressed on the previous HER2-directed therapy (Burris III et al., 2011). These clinical studies provide the evidence that the HER2 pathway remains a valid therapeutic target following disease progression on trastuzumab and suggest that antibody-drug conjugates are a novel and effective approach that can be used to treat trastuzumab-resistant disease.

8.5 Development of novel therapeutic approaches: Mechanisms of resistance-based design of antibody drug conjugates

Significant effort has been made to understand the mechanisms of resistance to trastuzumab. Many different small molecules, for example PI3 kinase inhibitors and c-Src inhibitors have been shown to be able to revert trastuzumab-resistant phenotypes in preclinical settings (Junttila et al., 2009; Zhuang et al., 2010). Table 3 summarizes some of the novel proposed molecular targets involved in trastuzumab-resistance and small molecules that are able to override trastuzumab-resistant phenotypes based on the preclinical studies.

Molecular target implicated in trastuzumab resistance	Inhibitor for the target (preclinical studies)	Reference for the preclinical studies
Rac1	NSC23766	Dokmanovic et al., 2009
EGFR	Lapatinib Neratinib	Nahta et al.,2007 Burstein et al.,2010
PI3K	GDC-0941 LY294002 Wortmannin SF1126	Junttila et al., 2009 Clark et al., 2002 Nagata et al., 2004 Ozbay et al., 2010
Akt	Triciribine (API-2)	Lu et al.,2007
mTOR	RAD001(everolimus)	Lu et al.,2007
PI3K/mTOR	NVP-BEZ235	Serra et al., 2008
PDK-1/Akt	OSU-03012	Tseng et al., 2006
HSP90	SNX-2112 17-AAG	Chandarlapaty et al., 2010 Modi et al., 2007
TGF-β1	LY2109761	Wang et al., 2008
Src	Dasatinib	Zhuanget al., 2010
Proteasome	LLnL	Lu et al., 2004
Hyaluronan synthesis	4-MU (methylumbelliferon)	Palyi-Krekk et al., 2007
Fatty acid synthase	C-75	Vazquez-Martin et al., 2007

Table 3. Emerging molecular targets implicated in the trastuzumab-resistance and their respective inhibitors.

TGF-β is a secreted ligand that binds to type I and type II TGF-β receptors and induces the secretion of HER family ligands, such as TGF-α, amphiregulin, and heregulin. Secreted HER family ligands may enhance the association of p85 subunit of PI3K with HER3 and activate PI3K/Akt (Wang et al., 2008). Treatment with TGF-β or expression of TGF-β type I receptor in HER2-overexpressing cells reduced their sensitivity to the HER2 antibody trastuzumab. Inhibition of TGF-β type I receptor by LY2109761, a TGF-β receptor type I and type II dual inhibitor, restored sensitivity to trastuzumab (Wang et al., 2008). Rac1 is a Ras-like small GTPase which is believed to be associated with breast cancer progression and metastasis (Sahai & Marshall, 2002). Inhibition of Rac1 activity by Rac1 specific inhibitor, NSC23766, resulted in the restoration of the trastuzumab-mediated HER2 endocytic degradation and inhibition of the cell growth in trastuzumab-resistant cells (Dokmanovic et al., 2009). It has been reported that the inhibition of c-Src activity by dasatinib partially restored trastuzumab sensitivity in trastuzumab-resistant breast cancer cells (Zhuang et al., 2010). 4-MU inhibition of hyaluronan synthase enhanced trastuzumab-mediated growth inhibition in trastuzumab-resistant JIMT-1 xenografts (Palyi-Krekk et al., 2007). Inhibition of fatty acid syntheses (FASN) re-sensitized the trastuzumab-resistant SKBR3 cells to trastuzumab-mediated cell death (Vazquez-Martin et al., 2007).

Several other approaches were utilized to interfere with the molecular pathways associated with trastuzumab-resistance in the preclinical studies. It has been recently reported that the overexpression of FoxM1, an oncogenic transcription factor, confers resistance to the trastuzumab (Carr et al., 2010). Attenuation of FoxM1 expression either by small interfering RNA or by an alternate reading frame (ARF)-derived peptide inhibitor increased the sensitivity to trastuzumab (Carr et al., 2010). Damiano et al. report that a novel toll-like receptor 9 agonist, which is also referred as the immune modulatory oligonucleotide (IMO), exerts antiangiogenic effects by cooperating with anti-EGFR or anti-VEGF antobodies, (Damiano et al., 2009). It was also shown that IMO and trastuzumab exert a cooperative antiangiogenic effect on trastuzumab-resistant breast cancer xenografts and that combining IMO and trastuzumab may be a potential strategy for the treatment of trastuzumab-resistant breast cancers (Damiano et al., 2009). The Y-box binding protein-1 (YB-1) is an oncogenic transcription/translation factor mediating expression of growth promoting genes such as EGFR and HER2. YB-1 is activated by phosphorylation at Serine 102 residue, and a decoy cell permeable peptide (CPP) functions as interference peptide to prevent endogenous YB-1 phosphorylation and activation. This results in the down-regulation of both HER-2 and EGFR transcript level and protein expression (Law et al., 2010). Interestingly, treatment with CPP has been reported to enhance sensitivity and overcome resistance to trastuzumab in cells expressing amplified HER-2, suggesting that CPP may be a novel approach for the treatment of trastuzumab-resistant breast cancers (Law et al., 2010).

Even though there were multiple mechanisms of trastuzumab-resistance proposed from the preclinical studies, the question remains how the knowledge gained from these cellular and animal models can be translated into the next generation of monoclonal antibodies to overcome therapeutic resistance to trastuzumab. Based on literature and data from our laboratory (Dokmanovic et al., 2009), we propose a new approach by designing an antibody-drug conjugate (ADC) based on mechanisms of trastuzumab resistance. In this ADC, trastuzumab is conjugated by a small molecule that has ability to inhibit the cellular target(s) that has been demonstrated to contribute to trastuzumab-resistance. This proposed strategy may increase the magnitude and duration of the response to trastuzumab treatment.

9. Conclusions

Treatment with trastuzumab significantly improves outcomes for women with HER2-positive breast cancer. However, therapeutic resistance to trastuzumab poses a significant challenge in the treatment of human breast cancer. Pre-clinical studies conducted in the past few years have improved our understanding of molecular mechanisms contributing to the trastuzumab-resistance, and potential predictive biomarkers, such as the serum levels of extracellular cellular domain (ECD) of HER2, the status of p95HER2 and IGF-IR, and loss of PTEN, have been reported. However, no predictive markers are currently used in the clinic to differentiate HER2-positive breast cancers that would respond favorably to trastuzumab from trastuzumab-resistant disease. Validation of novel predictive biomarkers must be performed with clinical samples in the context of prospective clinical trial in which prognostic or predictive questions can be answered (Hirsch & Wu, 2007; Murphy et al., 2005). Resistance to monoclonal antibody therapeutics represents a common obstacle to the clinical efficacy for monoclonal antibody-based therapy. Understanding the molecular mechanisms of trastuzumab-resistance will lead to the discovery of new therapeutic targets, as well as more effective approaches. Innovative strategies to optimize antibody structures to develop next generation of monoclonal antibodies, such as antibody-drug conjugates, bispecific antibodies, and antibodies with either enhanced or silenced effector function, will also play a critical role in overcoming therapeutic resistance to monoclonal antibodies.

10. Acknowledgment

We thank Drs. Dianne S. Hirsch, David M. Frucht, and Patrick G. Swann for the critical review of this manuscript. Disclaimer: The information presented in this article reflects the views of the authors and does not represent the policy of the U.S. Food and Drug Administration.

11. References

Ali, SM., Carney, WP., Esteva, FJ., Fornier, M., Harris, L., Kostler, WJ., Lotz, J-P., Luftner, D., Pichon, MF., Lipton, A. & Serum HER-2/neu Study Group. Serum HER-2/neu and relative resistance to trastuzumab-based therapy in patients with metastatic breast cancer. (2008). *Cancer,* Vol.113, No.6, (September 2008), pp. (1294-1301).

Allegra, CJ., Jessup, JM., Somerfield, MR., Hamilton, SR., Hammond, EH., Hayes, DF., McAllister, PK., Morton RF. & Schilsky, RL. (2009). American Society of Clinical Oncology provisional clinical opinion: testing for KRAS gene mutations in patients with metastatic colorectal carcinoma to predict response to anti-epidermal growth factor receptor monoclonal antibody therapy. *Journal of Clinical Oncology,* Vol.27, No.12, (April 2009), pp. (2091–2096).

Alley, SC., Okeley, NM. & Senter, PD. (2010). Antibody-drug conjugates: targeted drug delivery for cancer. *Current Opinion in Chemical Biology,* Vol.14, No.4, (August 2010), pp. (529-537).

Arnett, SO., Teillaud, JL., Wurch, T., Reichert, JM., Dunlop, C. & Huber, M. (2011)..IBC's 21st

Annual Antibody Engineering and 8th Annual Antibody Therapeutics International Conferences and 2010 Annual Meeting of The Antibody Society December 5-9, 2010, San Diego, CA. *mAbs,*Vol. 3,No.2, (March 2011), pp. (133-152).

Arribas, J., Baselga, J., Pedersen, K. & Parra-Palau, JL. (2011). P95HER2 and Breast Cancer. *Cancer Research,* Vol.71, No.5, (March 2011), pp. (1515-1519).

Banerjee, S. & Smith, IE. (2010). Management of small HER2-positive breast cancers. *The Lancet Oncology,* Vol.11, No.12, (December 2010), pp. (1193-1199).

Bartsch, R., Wenzel, C., Zielinski, CC. & Steger, GG. (2007).HER-2-positive breast cancer: hope beyond trastuzumab. *BioDrugs,* Vol.21, No.2, pp.(69-77).

Baselga, J., Norton, L., Albanell, J., Kim YM. & Mendelsohn, J. (1998). Recombinant humanized anti-HER2 antibody (Herceptin) enhances the antitumor activity of paclitaxel and doxorubicine against HER2/neu overexpressing human breast cancer xenografts. *Cancer Research,* Vol.58, No.13, (July 1998), pp. (2825-2831).

Baselga, J. & Swain, SM. (2009). Novel anticancer targets: revisiting ERBB2 and discovering ERBB3. *Nature Reviews Cancer,* Vol. 9, No.7, (July2009), pp. (463-475).

Baselga, J., Gelmon, KA., Verma, S., Wardley, A., Conte, P., Miles, D., Bianchi, G., Cortes, J., McNally, VA., Ross, GA., Fumoleau, P. & Gianni, L. (2010). Phase II trial of pertuzumab and trastuzumab in patients with human epidermal growth factor receptor 2-positive metastatic breast cancer that progressed during prior trastuzumab therapy. *Journal of Clinical Oncology,* Vol.28, No.7, (March 2010), pp. (1138-1144).

Bekaii-Saab, T., Williams, N., Plass, C., Calero, MV. & Eng, C. (2006). A novel mutation in the tyrosine kinase domain of ERBB2 in hepatocellular carcinoma. *BMC Cancer,* Vol.6, (December 2006), pp.278.

Beck, A., Wurch, T., Bailly, C. & Corvaia, N. (2010). Strategies and challenges for the next generation of therapeutic antibodies. *Nature Reviews Immunology,*Vol.10, No.5, (May 2010), pp.(345-352).

Benvenuti, S., Sartore-Bianchi, A., Di Nicolantonio, F., Zanon, C., Moroni, M., Veronese, S., Siena, S. & Bardelli, A. (2007) .Oncogenic activation of the RAS/RAF signaling pathway impairs the response of metastatic colorectal cancers to anti-epidermal growth factor receptor antibody therapies. *Cancer Research,* Vol.67, No.6, (March 2007), pp. (2643-2648).

Berns, K., Horlings, HM., Hennessy, BT., Madiredjo, M., Hijmans, EM., Beelen, K., Linn, SC., Gonzalez-Angulo, AM., Stemke-Hale, K., Hauptmann, M., Beijersbergen, RL., Mills, GB., van de Vijver, MJ. & Bernards ,R. (2007). A functional genetic approach identifies the PI3K pathway as a major determinant of trastuzumab resistance in breast cancer. *Cancer Cell,* Vol.12, No.4, (October 2007), pp. (395-402).

Blackwell, KL., Burstein, HJ., Storniolo, AM., Rugo, H., Sledge, G., Koehler, M., Ellis, C., Casey, M., Vukelja, S., Bischoff, J., Baselga, J. & O'Shaughnessy, J. (2010). Randomized study of Lapatinib alone or in combination with trastuzumab in women with ErbB2-positive, trastuzumab-refractory metastatic breast cancer. *Journal of Clinical Oncology,* Vol.28, No.7, (March 2010), pp. (1124-1130).

Bostrom, J., Yu, SF., Kan, D., Appleton, BA., Lee, CV., Billeci, K., Man, W., Peale, F., Ross, S., Wiesmann, C. & Fuh, G.(2009). Variants of the antibody herceptin that interact with HER2 and VEGF at the antigen binding site. *Science,* Vol.323, No.5921, (March 2009), pp.(1610–1614).

Brufsky, A. (2010). Trastuzumab-based therapy for patients with HER2-positive breast Cancer: from early scientific development to foundation of care. *American Journal of Clinical Oncology,* Vol.33, No.2, (April 2010), pp. (186-195).

Bruhns, P., Iannascoli, B., England, P., Mancardi, DA., Fernandez, N., Jorieux, S. & Daëron, M. (2009).Specificity and affinity of human Fcgamma receptors and their polymorphic variants for human IgG subclasses. *Blood,* Vol.113, No.16, (April 2009), pp.(3716–3725).

Burris HA 3 rd., Rugo HS., Vukelja SJ., Vogel CL., Borson RA., Limentani S., Tan-Chiu E., Krop IE., Michaelson RA.,Girish S., Amler L., Zheng M., Chu YW., Klencke B.,& O'Shaughnessy, JA.(2011). Phase II study of the antibody-drug conjugate trastuzumab-DM1 for the treatment of human epidermal growth factor receptor 2(HER2)-positive breast cancer after prior HER2-directed therapy. *Journal of Clinical Oncology,* Vol.29, No.4, (February 2011), pp. (398-405).

Burris, HA 3rd., Hurwitz, HI., Dees, EC., Dowlati, A., Blackwell, KL., O'Neil, B., Marcom, PK., Ellis, MJ., Overmoyer, B., Jones, SJ., Harris, JL., Smith, DA., Koch, KM., Stead,

A., Mangum, S. & Spector, NL.(2005). Phase I safety, pharmacokinetics, and clinical activity study of lapatinib (GW572016), a reversible dual inhibitor of epidermal growth factor receptor tyrosine kinases, in heavily pretreated patients with metastatic carcinomas. *Journal of Clinical Oncology,* Vol.23, No.23, (August 2005), pp. (5305-5313).

Burstein, HJ., Kuter, I., Campos, SM., Gelman, RS., Tribou, L., Parker, LM., Manola, J., Younger, J., Matulonis, U., Bunnell, CA., Partridge, AH., Richardson, PG., Clarke, K., Shulman, LN. & Winer, EP. (2001). Clinical activity of trastuzumab and vinorelbine in women with HER2-overexpressing metastatic breast cancer. *Journal of Clinical Oncology,* Vol.19, No.10, (May 2001), pp. (2722-2730).

Burstein, HJ., Sun, Y., Dirix, LY., Jiang, Z., Paridaens, R., Tan, AR., Awada, A., Ranade, A., Jiao, S., Schwartz, G., Abbas, R., Powell, C., Turnbull, K., Vermette, J., Zacharchuk, C. & Badwe, R. (2010). Neratinib, an irreversible ErbB receptor tyrosine kinase inhibitor, in patients with advanced ErbB2-positive breast cancer. *Journal of Clinical Oncology,* Vol.28, No.8, (March 2010), pp. (1301-1307).

Cardinale, D., Colombo, A., Torrisi, R., Sandri, MT., Civelli, M., Salvatici, M., Lamantia, G., Colombo, N., Cortinovis, S., Dessanai, MA., Nole, F., Veglia, F. & Cipolla, CM. (2010). Trastuzumab-induced cardiotoxicity: clinical and prognostic implications of troponin I evaluation. *Journal of Clinical Oncology,* Vol.28, No.25, (September 2010), pp. (3910-3916).

Carney, WP. Neumann, R., Lipton, A., Leitzel K., Ali, S. & Price, CP. (2003).Potential clinical utility of serum HER2/neu oncoprotein concentrations in patients with breast cancer. *Clinical Chemistry,* Vol.49, No.10, (October 2003), pp. (1579-1598).

Carr, JR., Park, HJ. Wang, Z., Kiefer, MM. & Raychaudhuri, P. (2010). FoxM1 mediates resistance to herceptin and paclitaxel. *Cancer Research,* Vol.70, No.12, (June 2010), pp. (5054-5063).

Carraway, KL 3rd. & Cantley, LC. (1994). A neu acquaintance for erbB3 and erbB4: a role for receptor heterodimerization in growth signaling. *Cell,* Vol.78, No.1, (July 1994), pp.(5–8).

Carter, P., Presta, L., Gorman, CM., Ridgway, JB., Henner, D., Wong, WL., Rowland, AM., Kotts, C., Carver, ME.& Shepard, HM.(1992). Humanization of an anti-p185HER2 antibody for human cancer therapy. *Proceedings of the National Academy of Sciences of the United States of America,* Vol.89, No.10, (May 1992), pp.(4285-4289).

Chames, P. & Baty, D. (2009). Bispecific antibodies for cancer therapy: the light at the end of the tunnel? *mAbs,* Vol.1, No.6, (November-December 2009), pp.539–547.

Chandarlapaty, S., Scaltriti, M., Angelini, P., Ye, Q., Guzman, M., Hudis, CA., Norton, L., Solit, DB., Arribas, J., Baselga, J.& Rosen, N.(2010). Inhibitors of HSP90 block p95-HER2 signaling in Trastuzumab-resistant tumors and suppress their growth. *Oncogene,* Vol.29, No.3, (January 2010), pp.(325-334).

Chari, RV.(2008). Targeted cancer therapy: conferring specificity to cytotoxic drugs. *Accounts of Chemical Research,* Vol.41,No.1, (January 2008), pp.(98-107).

Chen, J., Jaracz, S., Zhao, X., Chen, S.& Ojima, I. (2005). Antibody-cytotoxic agent conjugates for cancer therapy. *Expert Opinion on Drug Delivery,* Vol.2, No.5, (September 2005),pp. (873-890).

Cho, HS., Mason, K., Ramyar, KX., Stanley, AM., Gabelli, SB., Denney, DW Jr. & Leahy, DJ. (2003). Structure of the extracellular region of HER2 alone and in complex with the Herceptin Fab. *Nature,* Vol.421, No.6924, (February 2003), pp. (756-760).

Chung, KY., Shia, J., Kemeny, NE., Shah, M., Schwartz, GK., Tse, A., Hamilton, A., Pan, D., Schrag, D., Schwartz, L., Klimstra, DS., Fridman, D., Kelsen, DP. & Saltz, LB. (2005). Cetuximab shows activity in colorectal cancer patients with tumors that do not express the epidermal growth factor receptor by immunohistochemistry. *Journal of Clinical Oncology,* Vol.23, No.9, (March 2005), pp. (1803–1810).

Citri, A., Gan, J., Mosesson, Y., Vereb, G., Sz¨oll″osi, J.& Yarden, Y. (2004). Hsp90 restrains ErbB2/HER2 signalling by limiting heterodimer formation. *EMBO Reports,* Vol.5, No.12, (December 2004), pp.(1165-1170).

Clark, AS., West, K., Streicher, S. & Dennis, PA. (2002). Constitutive and inducible Akt activity promotes resistance to chemotherapy, trastuzumab, or tamoxifen in breast cancer cells. *Molecular Cancer Therapeutics,* Vol.1, No.9, (July 2002), pp. (707-717).

Damiano, V., Garofalo, S., Rosa, R., Bianco, R., Caputo, R., Geraldi, T., Merola, G., Racioppi, L., Garbi, C., Kandimalla, ER., Agrawal S.& Tortora, G. (2009). A novel toll-like receptor 9 agonist cooperates with trastuzumab in trastuzumab-resistant breast tumors through multiple mechanisms of action. *Clinical Cancer Research,* Vol.15, No.22, (November 2009), pp. (6921-6930).

Dave, B., Migliaccio, I., Gutierrez, MC., Wu, MF., Chamness, GC., Wong, H., Narasanna, A., Chakrabarty, A., Hilsenbeck, SG., Huang, J., Rimawi, M., Schiff, R., Arteaga, C., Osborne, CK. & Chang, JC. Loss of phosphatase and tensin homolog or phosphoinositol-3 kinase activation and response to trastuzumab or lapatinib in human epidermal growth factor receptor 2-overexpressing locally advanced breast cancer. (2011). *Journal of Clinical Oncology,* Vol.29, No.2, (January 2011), pp.(166-173).

De Roock, W., Piessevaux, H., De Schutter, J., Janssens, M., De Hertogh, G., Personeni, N., Biesmans, B., Van Laethem, JL., Peeters, M., Humblet, Y., Van Cutsem, E. & Tejpar, S.(2008). KRAS wild-type state predicts survival and is associated to early radiological response in metastatic colorectal cancer treated with cetuximab. *Annals of Oncology,* Vol.19, No.3, (March 2008), pp. (508–515).

Diermeier, S., Horvath, G., Knuechel-Clarke, R., Hofstaedter, F., Szollosi, J. & Brockhoff, G. (2005). Epidermal growth factor receptor coexpression modulates susceptibility to Herceptin in HER2/neu overexpressing breast cancer cells via specific erbB-receptor interaction and activation. *Experimental Cell Research,* Vol.304, No.2, (April 2005), pp.(604–619).

Dokmanovic, M., Hirsch, DS., Shen, Y. & Wu, WJ. (2009). Rac1 contributes to trastuzumab resistance of breast cancer cells: Rac1 as a potential therapeutic target for the treatment of trastuzumab-resistant breast cancer. *Molecular Cancer Therapeutics,* Vol.8, No.6, (June 2009), pp. (1557-1569).

Doronina, SO., Mendelsohn, BA., Bovee, TD., Cerveny, CG., Alley, SC., Meyer, DL., Oflazoglu, E., Toki, BE., Sanderson, RJ., Zabinski, RF., Wahl, AF. & Senter, PD. (2006).Enhanced activity of monomethylauristatin F through monoclonal antibody delivery: effects of linker technology on efficacy and toxicity. *Bioconjugate Chemistry,* Vol.17,No.1, (January-February 2006), pp.(114-124).

Doronina, SO., Toki, BE., Torgov, MY., Mendelsohn, BA., Cerveny, CG., Chace, DF., DeBlanc, RL., Gearing, RP., Bovee, TD., Siegall, CB., Francisco, JA., Wahl, AF., Meyer, DL. & Senter, PD. (2003). Development of potent monoclonal antibody auristatin conjugates for cancer therapy. *Nature Biotechnology,* Vol.21, No.7, (July 2003), pp.(778-784).

Esteva, FJ., Guo, H., Zhang, S., Santa-Maria, C., Stone, S., Lanchbury, JS., Sahin, AA., Hortobagyi, GN.& Yu, D. (2010). PTEN, PIK3CA, p-AKT, and p-p70S6K status: association with trastuzumab response and survival in patients with HER2-positive metastatic breast cancer. *The American Journal of Pathology,* Vol. 177, No. 4, (October 2010), pp. (1647-1656).

Ewer, MS., Vooletich, MT., Durand, JB., Woods, ML., Davis, JR., Valero, V. & Lenihan, DJ. (2005).Reversibility of trastuzumab-related cardiotoxicity: new insights based on clinical course and response to medical treatment. *Journal of Clinical Oncology,* Vol.23, No.31, (November 2005), pp. (7820-7826).

Ewer, MS. & Lippman, SM. (2005). Type II chemotherapy-related cardiac dysfunction: time to recognize a new entity. *Journal of Clinical Oncology,* Vol.23, No.13, (May 2005), pp. (2900-2902).

Franklin, MC., Carey, KD., Vajdos FF., Leahy, DJ., de Vos, AM. & Sliwkowski, MX. (2004). Insights into ErbB signaling from the structure of the ErbB2-pertuzumab complex. *Cancer Cell,* Vol.5, No.4, (April 2004), pp. (317-328).

Friess, T., their, M., Scheuer, W. et al. (2005). Combination treatment with pertuzumab and trastuzumab against Calu-3 human NSCLC xenograft tumors is superior to monotherapy. *Presented at the 17th Annual Meeting of the American Association for Cancer Research–National Cancer Institute–European Organisation for Research and Treatment of Cancer,* Philadelphia, PA, November 14-18, 2005

Garrett, TP., McKern, NM., Lou, M., Elleman, TC., Adams, TE., Lovrecz, GO., Kofler, M., Jorissen, RN., Nice, EC., Burgess, AW. & Ward, CW. (2003). The crystal structure of truncated ErbB2 ectodomain reveals an active conformation, poised to interact with other ErbB receptors. *Molecular Cell,* Vol.11, No.2, (February 2003), pp. (495-505).

Giusti, RM., Shastri, K., Pilaro, AM., Fuchs, C., Cordoba-Rodriguez, R., Koti, K., Rothmann, M., Men, AY., Zhao, H., Hughes, M., Keegan, P., Weiss, KD. & Pazdur, R. (2008). U.S. Food and Drug Administration approval: panitumumab for epidermal growth factor receptor-expressing metastatic colorectal carcinoma with progression following fluoropyrimidine-, oxaliplatin-, and irinotecan-containing chemotherapy regimens. *Clinical Cancer Research,* Vol.14, No.5, (March 2008), pp.(1296–1302).

Goldstein, NI., Prewett, M., Zuklys, K., Rockwell, P.& Mendelsohn, J. (1995). Biological efficacy of a chimeric antibody to the epidermal growth factor receptor in a human tumor xenograft model. *Clinical Cancer Research,* Vol.1, No.11, (November 1995), pp. (1311–1318).

Gordon, LI., Burke, MA., Singh, A.T.., Prachand, S., Lieberman, ED., Sun, L., Naik, TJ., Prasad, SV. & Ardehali, H. (2009). Blockage of the erbB2 receptor induces cardiomyocyte death through mitochondrial and reactive oxygen species-dependent pathways. *The Journal of Biological Chemistry,* Vol.284, No.4, (January 2009), pp. (2080-2087).

Graus-Porta, D., Beerli, RR., Daly, JM. & Hynes, NE. (1997). ErbB-2, the preferred heterodimerization partner of all ErbB receptors, is a mediator of lateral signaling. *EMBO Journal*, Vol.16, No.7, (April 1997), pp.(1647-1655).

Grazette, LP., Boecker, W., Matsui, T., Semigran, M., Force, TL., Hajjar, RJ. & Rosenzweig, A.(2004). Inhibition of ErbB2 causes mitochondrial dysfunction in cardiomyocytes.: implications for Herceptin-induced cardiomyopathy. *Journal of American College of Cardiology*, Vol.44, No.11, (December 2004), pp. (2231-2238).

Guilhot, F., Apperley, J., Kim, DW., Bullorsky, EO., Baccarani, M., Roboz, GJ., Amadori, S., de Souza, CA., Lipton, JH., Hochhaus, A., Heim, D., Larson, RA., Branford, S., Muller, MC., Agarwal, P., Gollerkeri, A. & Talpaz, M. (2007). Dasatinib induces significant hematologic and cytogenetic responses in patients with imatinib-resistant or -intolerant chronic myeloid leukemia in accelerated phase. *Blood*, Vol.109, No.10, (May 2007), pp.(4143-4150).

Gusterson, BA., Gelber, RD., Goldhirsch, A., Price, KN., Save-Soderborgh, J., Anbazhagan, R., Styles, J., Rudenstam, CM., Golouh, R., Reed, R., Martinez-Tello, F., Tiltman, A., Torhorst, J., Grigolato, P., Bettelheim, R., Neville, AM., Burki, K., Castiglione, M., Collins, J., Lindtner, J. & Senn, HJ for the International (Ludwig)Breast Cancer Study Group. (1992). Prognostic importance of c-erbB-2 expression in breast cancer. International (Ludwig) Breast Cancer Study Group. *Journal of Clinical Oncology*, Vol.10, No.7, (July 1992), pp.(1049-1056).

Guy, PM., Platko, JV., Cantley, LC., Cerione, RA. & Carraway, KL 3rd. (1994). Insect cell-expressed p180erbB3 possesses an impaired tyrosine kinase activity. *Proceedings of the National Academy of Sciences of the United States of America*, Vol.91, No.17, (August 1994), pp.(8132–8136).

Han, SW., Kim, TY., Hwang, PG., Jeong, S., Kim, J., Choi, IS., Oh, DY., Kim, JH., Kim, DW., Chung, DH., Im, SA., Kim,YT., Lee, JS., Heo, DS., Bang, YJ. & Kim, NK. (2005). Predictive and prognostic impact of epidermal growth factor receptor mutation in non-small-cell lung cancer patients treated with gefitinib. *Journal of Clinical Oncology*, Vol.23, No.11, (April 2005), pp.(2493–2501).

Hecht, JR., Mitchell, E., Chidiac, T., Scroggin, C., Hagenstad, C., Spigel, D., Marshall, J., Cohn, A., McCollum, D., Stella, P., Deeter, R., Shahin, S. & Amado, RG. (2009). A randomized phase IIIB trial of chemotherapy, bevacizumab, and panitumumab compared with chemotherapy and bevacizumab alone for metastatic colorectal cancer. *Journal of Clinical Oncology*, Vol.27, No.5, (February 2009), pp. (672–680).

Hirsch, DS. & Wu, WJ.(2007). Cdc42: an effector and regulator of ErbB1 as a strategic target in breast cancer therapy. *Expert Review of Anticancer Therapy*, Vol.7,No.2, (February 2007), pp.(147-157).

Huang, X., Gao, L., Wang, S., McManaman, JL., Thor, AD., Yang, X., Esteva, FJ. & Liu, B. (2010). Heterotrimerization of the growth factor receptors erbB2, erbB3 and insulin-like growth factor-i receptor in breast cancer cells resistant to herceptin. *Cancer Research*, Vol.70, No.3, (February 2010), pp.(1204-1214).

Hudis, CA. (2007). Trastuzumab-mechanism of action and use in clinical practice. *The New England Journal of Medicine*, Vol.357, No.1, (July 2007), pp. (39-51).

Hynes, NE. & Lane, HA. (2005). ERBB receptors and cancer: the complexity of targeted inhibitors. *Nature Reviews Cancer*, Vol.5, No.5, (May 2005), pp.(341-354).

Jerusalem, G., Fasolo, A., Dieras, V., Cardoso, F., Bergh, J., Vittori, L., Zhang, Y., Massacesi, C., Sahmoud, T. & Gianni, L. (2011). Phase I trial of oral mTOR inhibitor everolimus in combination with trastuzumab and vinoirelbine in pre-treated patients with HER2-overexpressing metastatic breast cancer. *Breast Cancer Research and Treatment,* Vol.125, No.2, (January 2011), pp. (447-455).

Jin, H., Yang, R., Zheng, Z., Romero, M., Ross, J., Bou-Reslan, H., Carano, RA., Kasman, I., Mai, E., Young, J., Zha, J., Zhang, Z., Ross, S., Schwall, R., Colbern, G. & Merchant, M. (2008). MetMAb, the one-armed 5D5 anti-c-Met antibody, inhibits orthotopic pancreatic tumor growth and improves survival. *Cancer Res.earch,* Vol.68, No.11 (Jun 2008), pp. (4360-4368).

Junttila, TT., Li, G., Parsons, K., Phillips, GL. & Sliwkowski, MX. (2010). Trastuzumab-DM1 (T-DM1) retains all the mechanisms of action of trastuzumab and efficiently inhibits growth of lapatinib insensitive breast cancer. *Breast Cancer Research and Treatment,* (August 2010).

Junttila, TT., Akita, RW., Parsons, K., Fields, C., Lewis Phillips, GD., Friedman, LS., Sampath, D. & Sliwkowski, MX. (2009). Ligand-independent HER2/HER3/PI3K complex is disrupted by trastuzumab and is effectively inhibited by the PI3K inhibitor GDC-0941. *Cancer Cell,* Vol.15, No.5, (May 2009), pp. (429-440)

Karapetis, CS., Khambata-Ford, S., Jonker, DJ., O'Callaghan, CJ., Tu, D., Tebbutt, NC., Simes, RJ., Chalchal, H., Shapiro, JD., Robitaille, S., Price, TJ., Shepherd, L., Au, HJ., Langer, C., Moore, MJ. & Zalcberg, JR. (2008). K-ras mutations and benefit from cetuximab in advanced colorectal cancer. *The New England Journal of Medicine,* Vol.359, No.17, (October 2008), pp. (1757-1765).

Karnoub, AE. & Weinberg, RA. (2008). Ras oncogenes: split personalities. *Nature Reviews Molecular Cell Biology,* Vol. 9, No.7, (July 2008), pp. (517-531).

Kaufman B., Mackey, JR., Clemens, MR., Bapsy, PP., Vaid, A., Wardley, A., Tjulandin, S., Jahn, M., Lehle, M., Feyereislova, A., Revil, C.,& Jones, A. (2009). Trastuzumab plus anastrozole versus anastrozole alone for the treatment of postmenopausal women with human epidermal growth factor receptor 2-positive, hormone receptor-positive metastatic breast cancer: results from the randomized phase III TAnDEM study. (2009). *Journal of Clinical Oncology,* Vol.27, No.33, (November 2009), pp. (5529-5537).

Konecny, GE., Pegram, MD., Venkatesan, N., Finn, R., Yang, G., Rahmeh, M., Untch, M., Rusnak, DW., Spehar, G., Mullin, RJ., Keith, BR., Gilmer, TM., Berger, M., Podratz, KC. & Slamon DJ. (2006). Activity of the dual kinase inhibitor lapatinib (GW572016) against HER-2-overexpressing and trastuzumab-treated BC cells. *Cancer Research,* Vol.66, No.3, (February 2006), pp. (1630-1639).

Krop, IE., Beeram, M., Modi, S., Jones, SF., Holden, SN., Yu, W., Girish, S., Tibbitts, J., Yi, J H., Sliwkowski, MX., Jacobson, F., Lutzker, SG. & Burris, HA. (2010). Phase I study of trastuzumab-DM1, an HER2 antibody-drug conjugate, given every 3 weeks to patients with HER2-positive metastatic breast cancer. *Journal of Clinical Oncology,* Vol.28, No.16, (June 2010), pp. (2698-2704).

Kruser, TJ. & Wheeler,DL. (2010). Mechanisms of resistance to HER family targeting antibodies. *Experimental Cell Research,* Vol.316, No.7, (April 2010), pp.(1083-1100).

Law, JH., Li, Y., To, K., Wang, M., Astanehe, A., Lambie, K., Dhillon, J., Jones, SJ., Gleave, ME., Eaves, CJ. & Dunn, SE. (2010). Molecular decoy to the Y-box binding protein-1 suppresses the growth of breast and prostate cancer cells whilst sparing normal cell viability. *PLOS One,* Vol.5, No.9, (September 2010), pp. e12661.

le Coutre, P., Ottmann, OG., Giles, F., Kim, DW., Cortes, J., Gattermann, N., Apperley, JF., Larson, RA., Abruzzese, E., O'Brien, SG., Kuliczkowski, K., Hochhaus, A., Mahon, FX., Saglio, G., Gobbi, M., Kwong, YL., Baccarani, M., Hughes, T., Martinelli, G., Radich, JP., Zheng, M., Shou, Y. & Kantarjian, H. (2008). Nilotinib (formerly AMN107), a highly selective BCR-ABL tyrosine kinase inhibitor, is active in patients with imatinib-resistant or -intolerant accelerated-phase chronic myelogenous leukemia. *Blood,* Vol.111, No.4, (February 2008), pp.(1834-1839).

Lee, KF., Simon, H., Chen, H., Bates, B., Hung, MC. & Hauser, C. (1995). Requirement for neuregulin receptor erbB2 in neural and cardiac development. *Nature,* Vol.378, No.6555, (November 1995), pp. (394-398).

Lee, JW., Soung, YH., Seo, SH., Kim, SY., Park, CH., Wang, YP., Park, K., Nam, SW., Park, WS., Kim, SH., Lee, JY., Yoo, NJ.& Lee, SH. (2006). Somatic mutations of ERBB2 kinase domain in gastric, colorectal, and breast carcinomas. *Clinical Cancer Research,* Vol.12, No.1, (January 2006), pp. (57–61).

Lewis Phillips, GD., Li, G., Dugger, DL., Crocker, LM., Parsons, KL., Mai, E., Blattler, WA., Lambert, JM., Chari, RV., Lutz, RJ., Wong, WL., Jacobson, FS., Koeppen, H., Schwall ,RH., Kenkare-Mitra, SR., Spencer, SD. & Sliwkowski, MX. (2008). Targeting HER2-positive breast cancer with trastuzumab-DM1, an antibody-cytotoxic drug conjugate. *Cancer Research,* Vol.68, No.22, (November 2008), pp. (9280-9290).

Lievre, A., Bachet, JB., Le Corre, D., Boige, V., Landi, B., Emile, JF., Cote, JF., Tomasic, G., Penna, C., Ducreux, M., Rougier, P., Penault-Llorca, F. & Laurent-Puig, P. (2006). KRAS mutation status is predictive of response to cetuximab therapy in colorectal cancer. *Cancer Research,* Vol.66, No.8, (April 2006), pp. (3992-3995).

Lin, WL., Kuo, WH., Chen FL., Lee, MY., Ruan, A., Tyan, YS., Hsu, JD., Chiang, H. & Han, CP. (2011). Identification of the Coexisting HER2 Gene Amplification and Novel Mutations in the HER2 Protein-Overexpressed Mucinous Epithelial Ovarian Cancer. *Annals of Surgical Oncology,* (February 2011).

Litzow, MR. (2006). Imatinib resistance: obstacles and opportunities. *Archives of Pathology and Laboratory Medicine,* Vol.130, No.5, (May 2006), pp.(669-689).

Lu, CH., Wyszomierski, SL., Tseng, LM., Sun, MH., Lan, KH., Neal, CL., Mills, GB., Hortobagyi, GN., Esteva, FJ. & Yu, D. (2007). Preclinical testing of clinically applicable strategies for overcoming trastuzumab resistance caused by PTEN deficiency. *Clinical Cancer Research,* Vol.13, No.19, (October 2007), pp. (5883-5888).

Lu, Y., Zi, X. & Pollak, M. (2004). Molecular mechanisms underlying IGF-I-induced attenuation of the growth-inhibitory activity of trastuzumab (Herceptin) on SKBR3 breast cancer cells. *International Journal of Cancer,* Vol.108, No.3, (January 2004), pp. (334-341).

Martens, T., Schmidt, NO., Eckerich, C., Fillbrandt, R., Merchant, M., Schwall, R., Westphal, M., Lamszus, K. (2006). A novel one-armed anti-c-Met antibody inhibits glioblastoma growth in vivo. *Clinical Cancer Research,* Vol.12, No.20 Pt1, (October 2006) pp. (6144-6152).

Marty, M., Cognetti, F., Maraninchi, D., Snyder, R., Mauriac, L., Tubiana-Hulin, M., Chan, S., Grimes, D., Anton, A., Lluch, A., Kennedy, J., O'Byrne, K., Conte, P., Green, M.,

Ward, C., Mayne, K., & Extra, JM. (2005). Randomized phase II trial of the efficacy and safety of trastuzumab combined with docetaxel in patients with human epidermal growth factor receptor 2-positive metastatic breast cancer administered as first-line treatment: the M77001 study group. *Journal of Clinical Oncology,* Vol.23, No.19, (July 2005), pp. (4265-4274).

Mendelsohn, J. (2002). Targeting the epidermal growth factor receptor for cancer therapy. *Journal of Clinical Oncology,* Vol.20, No.18 Suppl, (September 2002), pp. (1S–13S).

Mittendorf, EA., Wu, Y., Scaltriti, M., Meric-Bernstam, F., Hunt, KK., Dawood, S., Esteva, FJ., Buzdar, AU., Chen, H., Eksambi, S., Hortobagyi, GN., Baselga, J. & Gonzalez-Angulo, AM.(2009). Loss of HER2 amplification following trastuzumab-based neoadjuvant systemic therapy and survival outcomes. *Clinical Cancer Research,* Vol.15, No.23, (December 2009), pp. (7381-7388).

Mittendorf, EA., Liu, Y., Tucker, SL., Mckenzie, T., Qiao, N., Akli, S., Biernacka, A., Liu, Y., Meijer, L., Keyomarsi, K. & Hunt, KK. (2010). A novel interaction between HER2/neu and cyclin E in breast cancer. *Oncogene,*Vol. 29, No.27, (July 2010), pp. (3896-3907).

Mitsudomi, T., Kosaka, T., Endoh, H., Horio, Y., Hida, T., Mori, S., Hatooka, S., Shinoda, M., Takahashi, T. & Yatabe, Y. (2005). Mutations of the epidermal growth factor receptor gene predict prolonged survival after gefitinib treatment in patients with non-small-cell lung cancer with postoperative recurrence. *Journal of Clinical Oncology,* Vol.23, No.11, (April 2005), pp. (2513–2520).

Modi, S., Stopeck, AT., Gordon, MS., Mendelson, D., Solit, DB., Bagatell, R., Ma, W., Wheler, J., Rosen, N., Norton, L., Cropp, GF., Johnson, RG., Hannah, AL. & Hudis, CA. (2007). Combination of trastuzumab and tanespimycin (17-AAG, KOS-953) is safe and active in trastuzumab-refractory HER-2 overexpressing breast cancer: a phase I dose-escalation study. *Journal of Clinical Oncology,* Vol. 25, No.34, (December 2007), pp. (5410-5417).

Morgillo, F., Bareschino, MA., Bianco, R., Tortora, G. & Ciardiello, F. (2007). Primary and acquired resistance to anti-EGFR targeted drugs in cancer therapy. *Differentiation,* Vol.75, No.9, (November 2007), pp. (788–799).

Motoyama, AB., Hynes, NE. & Lane, HA. (2002).The efficacy of ErbB receptor-targeted anticancer therapeutics is influenced by the availability of epidermal growth factor-related peptides. *Cancer Research,* Vol.62, No.11, (June 2002), pp. (3151–3158).

Mukohara, T., Engelman, JA., Hanna, NH., Yeap, BY., Kobayashi, S., Lindeman, N., Halmos, B., Pearlberg, J., Tsuchihashi, Z., Cantley, LC., Tenen, DG., Johnson, BE. & Jänne, PA. (2005). Differential effects of gefitinib and cetuximab on non - small-cell lung cancers bearing epidermal growth factor receptor mutations. *Journal of the National Cancer Institute,* Vol.97, No.16, (August 2005), pp. (1185-1194).

Murphy, N., Millar, E. & Lee, CS. (2005).Gene expression profiling in breast cancer: towards individualizing patient management. Pathology, Vol.37, No.4, (August 2005), pp.(271-277).

Musolino, A., Naldi, N., Bortesi, B., Pezzuolo, D., Capelletti, M., Missale, G., Laccabue, D., Zerbini, A., Camisa, R., Bisagni, G., Neri, TM. & Ardizzoni, A. (2008). Immunoglobulin G fragment C receptor polymorphisms and clinical efficacy of trastuzumab-based therapy in patients with HER-2/neu-positive metastatic breast cancer. *Journal of Clinical Oncology,* Vol.26, No.11, (April 2008), pp. (1789-1796)

Nagata, Y., Lan, KH., Zhou, X., Tan, M., Esteva, FJ., Sahin, AA., Klos, KS., Li, P., Monia, BP., Nguyen, NT., Hortobagyi, GN., Hung, MC. & Yu, D. (2004). PTEN activation contributes to tumor inhibition by trastuzumab, and loss of PTEN predicts trastuzumab resistance in patients. *Cancer Cell,* Vol.6, No.2, (August 2004), pp. (117-127).

Nagy, P., Friedlander, E., Tanner, M., Kapanen, AI., Carraway, KL., Isola, J. & Jovin, TM.(2005). Decreased accessibility and lack of activation of ErbB2 in JIMT-1, a herceptin-resistant, MUC4-expressing breast cancer cell line. *Cancer Research,* Vol.65, No.2, (January 2005), pp. (473-482).

Nahta, R., Takahashi, T., Ueno, NT., Hung, MC. & Esteva, FJ. (2004a). $P27^{kip1}$ down-regulation is associated with trastuzumab resistance in breast cancer cells. *Cancer Research,* Vol.64, No.11, (June 2004), pp. (3981-3986).

Nahta, R., Hung, MC. & Esteva, FJ. (2004b). The HER-2 targeting antibodies trastuzumab and pertuzumab synergistically inhibit the survival of breast cancer cells. *Cancer Research,* Vol.64, No.7, (April 2004), pp. (2343-2346).

Nahta, R., Yuan, LX., Zhang, B., Kobayashi, R. & Esteva, FJ. (2005). Insulin-like growth factor I receptor/human epidermal growth factor receptor 2 heterodimerization contributes to trastuzumab resistance of breast cancer cells. *Cancer Research,* Vol. 65, No. 23, (December 2005), pp.(11118-11128).

Nahta, R. & Esteva, FJ. (2006). Herceptin: mechanisms of action and resistance. *Cancer Letters,* Vol.232, No.2, (February 2006), pp. (123-138).

Nahta, R., Yuan, LX., Du, Y. & Esteva, FJ. (2007). Lapatinib induces apoptosis in trastuzumab-resistant breast cancer cells: effects on insulin-like growth factor I signaling. *Molecular Cancer Therapeutics,* Vol.6, No.2, (February 2007), pp. (667-674).

Natali, PG., Nicotra, MR., Bigotti, A., Venturo, I., Slamon, DJ., Fendly, BM. & Ullrich, A. (1990). Expression of the p185 encoded by HER2 oncogene in normal and transformed human tissues. *International Journal of Cancer,* Vol.45, No.3, (March 1990), pp. (457-461).

Negro, A., Brar, BK. & Lee, KF. (2004). Essential roles of Her2/erbB2 in cardiac development and function. *Recent Progress in Hormone Research,* Vol.59, pp. (1-12).

Nelson, AL., Dhimolea, E. & Reichert, JM. (2010). Development trends for human monoclonal antibody therapeutics. *Nature Reviews Drug Discovery,* Vol.9, No.10, (October 2010), pp. (767-774).

Nguyen, TH., Loux, N., Dagher, I., Vons, C., Carey, K., Briand, P., Hadchouel, M., Franco, D., Jouanneau, J., Schwall, R. & Weber, A. (2003). Improved gene transfer selectivity to hepatocarcinoma cells by retrovirus vector displaying single-chain variable fragment antibody against c-Met. *Cancer Gene Therapy,* Vol. 10, No.11, (November 2003), pp.(840-849).

Niehans, GA., Singleton, TP., Dykosk,i D., & Kiang, DT. (1993). Stability of HER-2/neu expression over time and at multiple metastatic sites. *Journal of the National Cancer Institute,* Vol.85, No.15, (August 1993), pp. (1230-1235).

Nordstrom, JL., Huang, L., Yang, Y., Tuaillon, N., Stavenhagen, JB., Stewart, S., Moore, PA., Johnson, S., Koenig, S., Bonvini; E.(2010). Preclinical antitumor activity of an Fc domain-optimized HER2 monoclonal antibody (mAb). Abstract (e13135) of 2010 American Society of Clinical Oncology Annual Meeting, Chicago, IL June 2010.

O'Shaughnessy, JA., Vukelja, S., Marsland, T., Kimmel, G., Ratnam, S. & Pippen, JE. (2004). Phase II study of trastuzumab plus gemcitabine in chemotherapy-pretreated patients with metastatic breast cancer. *Clinical Breast Cancer*, Vol.5, No.2, (June 2004), pp. (142-147).

Ohashi K., Marion PL., Nakai H., Meuse L., Cullen JM., Bordier BB., Schwall R., Greenberg HB., Glenn JS. & Kay MA. (2000) .Sustained survival of human hepatocytes in mice: A model for in vivo infection with human hepatitis B and hepatitis delta viruses. *Nature Medicine*, Vol. 6, No.3, (Mar 2000), pp.(327-331).

Okines, AF. & Cunningham, D. (2010).Trastuzumab in gastric cancer. *European Journal of Cancer*, Vol.46, No.11, (July 2010), pp. (1949–1959).

Ozbay, T., Durden, DL., Liu, T., O'Regan, RM. & Nahta, R. (2010). In vitro evaluation of pan-PI3-kinase inhibitor SF1126 in trastuzumab-sensitive and trastuzumab-resistant HER2-over-expressing breast cancer cells. *Cancer Chemotherapy and Pharmacology*, Vol.65, No.4, (March 2010), pp. (697-706).

Paik, S., Hazan, R., Fisher, ER., Sass, RE., Fisher, B., Redmond, C., Schlessinger, J., Lippman, ME., & King, CR. (1990). Pathologic findings from the National Surgical Adjuvant Breast and Bowel Project: prognostic significance of erbB-2 protein overexpression in primary breast cancer. *Journal of Clinical Oncology*, Vol.8, No.1, (January 1990), pp. (103-112).

Palyi-Krekk, Z., Barok, M., Isola, J., Tammi, M., Szollosi, J. & Nagy, P. (2007). Hyaluronan-induced masking of ErbB2 and CD44-enhanced trastuzumab internalization in trastuzumab resistant breast cancer. *European Journal of Cancer*, Vol.43, No.16, (November 2007), pp. (2423-2433).

Pao, W., Miller, VA., Politi, KA., Riely, GJ., Somwar, R., Zakowski, MF., Kris, MG. & Varmus, H. (2005). Acquired resistance of lung adenocarcinomas to gefitinib or erlotinib is associated with a second mutation in the EGFR kinase domain. *PLoS Med*, Vol.2, No.3, (March 2005), pp. e73.

Prat, M., Crepaldi, T., Pennacchietti, S., Bussolino, F.& Comoglio, PM. (1998). Agonistic monoclonal antibodies against the Met receptor dissect the biological responses to HGF. *Journal of Cell Science*, Vol. 111, No. Pt2, (January 1998), pp. (237-247).

Pedersen, K., Angelini, PD., Laos, S., Bach-Faig, A., Cunningham, MP., Ferrer-Ramon, C., Luque-Garcia, A., Garcia-Castillo, J., Parra-Palau, JL., Scaltriti, M., Ramon y Cajal, S., Baselga, J. & Arribas, J. (2009). A naturally occurring HER2 carboxy-terminal fragment promotes mammary tumor growth and metastasis. *Molecular and Cellular Biology*, Vol.29, No.12, (June 2009), pp. (3319-3331).

Pegram, MD., Lipton, A., Hayes, DF., Weber, BL., Baselga, JM., Tripathy, D., Baly, D., Baughman, SA., Twaddell, T., Glaspy, JA.& Slamon, DJ.(1998). Phase II study of receptor-enhanced chemosensitivity using recombinant humanized anti-p185 $^{HER2/neu}$ monoclonal antibody plus cisplatin in patients with HER2/neu-overexpressing metastatic breast cancer refractory to chemotherapy treatment. *Journal of Clinical Oncology*, Vol.16, No.8, (August 1998), pp. (2659-2671).

Pegram, M., Hsu, S., Lewis, G., Pietras, R., Beryt, M., Sliwkowski, M., Coombs, D., Baly, D., Kabbinavar, F. & Slamon, D. (1999). Inhibitory effects of combinations of HER-2/neu antibody and chemotherapeutic agents used for treatment of human breast cancer. *Oncogene*, Vol.18, No.13, (April 1999), pp. (2241-2251).

Perez, EA., Suman, VJ., Rowland, KM., Ingle, JN., Salim, M., Loprinzi, CL., Flynn, PJ., Mailliard,JA., Kardinal, CG., Krook, JE., Thrower, AR., Visscher, DW. & Jenkins, RB. (2005). Two concurrent phase II trials of paclitaxel/carboplatin/trastuzumab (weekly or every-3-week schedule) as first-line therapy in women with HER2-overexpressing metastatic breast cancer: NCCTG study 983252.*Clinical Breast Cancer,* Vol.6, No.5, (December 2005), pp. (425-432).

Piccart-Gebhart, MJ., Procter, M., Leyland-Jones, B., Goldhirsch, A., Untch, M., Smith, I., Gianni, L., Baselga, J., Bell, R., Jackisch, C., Cameron, D., Dowsett, M., Barrios, CH., Steger, G., Huang, CS., Andersson, M., Inbar, M., Lichinitser, M., Lang, I., Nitz, U., Iwata, H., Thomssen, C., Lohrisch, C., Suter, TM., Ruschoff, J., Suto, T.,Greatorex, V., Ward, C., Straehle, C., McFadden, E., Dolci, MS., & Gelber, RD. for the Herceptin Adjuvant (HERA) Trial Study Team. (2005). Trastuzumab after adjuvant chemotherapy in HER2 -positive breast cancer. *The New England Journal of Medicine,* Vol.353, No.16, (October 2005), pp. (1659-1672).

Pratt, WB.& Toft, DO. (2003). Regulation of signaling protein function and trafficking by the hsp90/hsp70-based chaperone machinery. *Experimental Biology and Medicine (Maywood),* Vol.228 ,No.2, (February 2003) pp.(111–133).

Press, MF., Pike, MC., Chazin, VR., Hung, G., Udove, JA., Markowicz, M., Danyluk, J., Godolphin, W., Sliwkowski, M., Akita, R., Paterson, MC. & Slamon, DJ. (1993). Her-2/neu expression in node-negative breast cancer: direct tissue quantitation by computerized image analysis and association of overexpression with increased risk of recurrent disease. *Cancer Research,* Vol.53, No.20, (October 1993), pp. (4960-4970) .

Raja, SM., Clubb, RJ., Bhattacharyya, M., Dimri, M.,Cheng, H., Pan, W.,Ortega-Cava, C., Lakku-Reddi, A., Naramura, M., Band, V. & Band, H. A combination of Trastuzumab and 17-AAG induces enhanced ubiquitination and lysosomal pathway-dependent ErbB2 degradation and cytotoxicity in ErbB2-overexpressing breast cancer cells. *Cancer Biology& Therapy,* Vol.7, No.10, (October 2008), pp. (1630-1640)

Ranson, M. & Sliwkowski, MX. (2002). Perspectives on anti-HER antibodies. *Oncology,* Vol. 63,Suppl 1, (November 2002), pp. (17-24).

Reichert, JM. (2009). Global antibody development trends. *mABs,* Vol.1, No.1, (January/February 2009), pp. (86-87).

Ritter, CA., Perez-Torres, M., Rinehart, C., Guix, M., Dugger, T., Engelman, JA. & Arteaga, CL. (2007). Human breast cancer cells selected for resistance to trastuzumab *in vivo* overexpress epidermal growth factor receptor and ErbB ligands and remain dependent on the ErbB receptor network. *Clinical Cancer Research,* Vol.13, No.16, (August 2007), pp. (4909-4919).

Sahai E.& Marshall, CJ. (2002). RHO-GTPases and cancer. *Nature Reviews Cancer.,* Vol. 2, No.2, (February 2002), pp. (133-142).

Saltz, LB., Meropol, NJ., Loehrer, PJ Sr., Needle, MN., Kopit, J. & Mayer, RJ. (2004). Phase II trial of cetuximab in patients with refractory colorectal cancer that expresses the epidermal growth factor receptor. *Journal of Clinical Oncology,* Vol.22, No.7, (April 2004), pp. (1201-1208).

Sanchez-Munoz, A., Gallego, E., de Luque, V., Perez-Rivas, LG., Vicioso, L., Ribelles, N., Lozano, J. & Alba, E. (2010). Lack of evidence for KRAS oncogenic mutations in triple-negative breast cancer. *BMC Cancer,* Vol.10, (April 2010), pp. 136.

Scaltriti, M., Eichhorn, PJ., Cortes, J., Prudkin, L., Aura, C., Jimenez, J., Chandarlapaty, S., Serra, V., Prat, A., Ibrahim, YH., Guzman, M., Gili, M., Rodriguez, O., Rodriguez, S., Perez, J., Green, SR., Mai, S., Rosen, N., Hudis, C. & Baselga, J. (2011).Cyclin E amplification/overexpression is a mechanism of trastuzumab resistance in HER2+ breast cancer patients. *Proceedings of the National Academy of Sciences of the Unites States of America,* Vol.108, No.9, (March 2011), pp. (3761-3766).

Schwartz, JD., Rowinsky, EK., Youssoufian, H., Pytowki, B. & Wu, Y. (2010). Vascular endothelial growth factor receptor-1 in human cancer: concise review and rationale for development of IMC-18F1 (Human antibody targeting vascular endothelial growth factor receptor-1). *Cancer,* Vol.116, No.4Suppl, (February 2010), pp. (1027-1032).

Senter, PD. (2009). Potent antibody drug conjugates for cancer therapy. *Current opinion in chemical biology,* Vol.13, No.3, (June 2009), pp. (235-244).

Sergina, NV., Rausch, M., Wang, D., Blair, J., Hann, B., Shokat, KM. & Moasser, MM. (2007). Escape from HER-family tyrosine kinase inhibitor therapy by the kinase-inactive HER3. *Nature,* Vol.445, No.7126, (January 2007), pp. (437–441).

Serra, V., Markman, B., Scaltriti, M., Eichhorn, PJ., Valero, V., Guzman, M., Botero, ML., Llonch, E., Atzori, F., Di Cosimo, S., Maira, M., Garcia-Echeverria, C., Parra, JL., Arribas, J. & Baselga, J. (2008). NVP-BEZ235, a dual PI3K/mTOR inhibitor, prevents PI3K signaling and inhibits the growth of cancer cells with activating PI3K mutations. *Cancer Research,* Vol.68, No. 19, (October 2008), pp. (8022-8030).

Shattuck, DL., Miller, JK., Carraway, KL 3rd.& Sweeney, C. (2008). Met receptor contributes to trastuzumab resistance of Her2-overexpressing breast cancer cells. *Cancer Research,* Vol. 68, No. 5 (March 2008), pp.(1471-1477).

Shi, F., Telesco, SE., Liu, Y., Radhakrishnan, R. & Lemmon, MA. (2010). ErbB3/HER3 intracellular domain is competent to bind ATP and catalyze autophosphorylation. *Proceedings of the National Academy of Sciences of the United States of America,* Vol.107, No.17, (April 2010), pp. (7692-7697).

Shigematsu, H., Takahashi, T., Nomura, M., Majmudar, K., Suzuki, M., Lee, H., Wistuba, II., Fong, KM., Toyooka, S., Shimizu, N., Fujisawa, T., Minna, JD. & Gazdar, AF. (2005). Somatic mutations of the HER2 kinase domain in lung adenocarcinoma. *Cancer Research,* Vol.65, No.5, (March 2005), pp. (1642-1646).

Shin, DM., Donato, NJ., Perez-Soler, R., Shin, HJ., Wu, JY., Zhang, P., Lawhorn, K., Khuri, FR., Glisson, BS., Myers, J., Clayman, G., Pfister, D., Falcey, J., Waksal, H., Mendelsohn, J. & Hong, WK. (2001). Epidermal growth factor receptor-targeted therapy with C225 and cisplatin in patients with head and neck cancer. *Clinical Cancer Research,* Vol.7, No.5, (May 2001), pp. (1204-1213).

Sierke, SL., Cheng, K., Kim, HH. & Koland, JG. (1997). Biochemical characterization of the protein tyrosine kinase homology domain of the ErbB3 (HER3) receptor protein. *Biochemistry Journal,* Vol.322, No.Pt 3, (March 1997), pp. (757–763).

Slamon, DJ., Clark, GM., Wong, SG., Levin, WJ., Ullrich, A. &McGuire, WL. (1987). Human breast cancer: correlation of relapse and survival with amplification of the HER-2/neu oncogene. *Science,* Vol.235, No.4785, (January 1987), pp. (177-182).

Slamon, DJ., Godolphin, W., Jones, LA., Holt, JA., Wong, SG., Keith, DE., Levin, WJ., Stuart, SG., Udove, J., Ullrich, A. & Press, MF. (1989). Studies of the HER-2/neu proto-oncogene in human breast and ovarian cancer. *Science,* Vol.244, No.4905, (May 1989), pp. (707-712).

Slamon, DJ., Leyland-Jones, B., Shak, S., Fuchs, H., Paton, V., Bajamonde, A., Fleming, T., Eiermann, W., Wolter, J., Pegram, M., Baselga, J. & Norton, L. (2001). Use of chemotherapy plus a monoclonal antibody against HER2 for metastatic breast cancer that overexpresses HER2. *The New England Journal of Medicine,* Vol.344, No.11, (March 2001), pp. (783-792).

Spratlin, JL., Cohen, RB., Eadens, M., Gore, L., Camidge, DR., Diab, S., Leong, S., O'Bryant, C., Chow, LQ., Serkova, NJ., Meropol, NJ., Lewis, NL., Chiorean, EG., Fox, F., Youssoufian, H., Rowinsky, EK.& Eckhardt, SG. (2010). Phase I pharmacological and biological study of ramucirumab (IMC-1121B), a fully human immunoglobulin G1 monoclonal antibody targeting the vascular endothelial growth factor receptor-2. *Journal of Clinical Oncology,* Vol.28, No.5, (February 2010), pp. (780-787).

Sutter, TM., Procter, M., van Veldhuisen, DJ., Muscholl, M., Bergh, J., Carlomagno, C., Perren, T., Passalacqua, R., Bighin, C., Klijn, J.G.M., Ageev, FT., Hitre, E., Groetz, J., Iwata, H., Knap, M., Gnant, M., Muehlbauer, S.,Spence, A., Gelber, RD. & Piccart-Gebhart ,MJ. (2007). Trastuzumab-associated cardiac adverse effects in the herceptin adjuvant trial. *Journal of Clinical Oncology,* Vol.25, No.26, (September 2007), pp. (3859-3865).

Swann, PG., Tolnay, M., Muthukkumar, S., Shapiro, MA., Rellahan, BL. & Clouse, KA. (2008). Considerations for the development of therapeutic monoclonal antibodies. *Current Opinion in Immunology,* Vol.20, No.4, (August 2008), pp. (493–499).

Tanner, M., Kapanen, AI., Junttila, T., Raheem, O., Grenman, S., Elo, J., Elenius, K. & Isola, J. (2004). Characterization of a novel cell line established from a patient with Herceptin-resistant breast cancer. *Molecular Cancer Therapeutics,* Vol.3, No.12, (December 2004), pp. (1585-1592).

Tseng, PH., Wang, YC., Weng, SC., Weng, JR., Chen, CS., Brueggemeier, RW., Shapiro, CL., Chen, CY., Dunn, SE., Pollak, M. & Chen, CS. (2006). Overcoming trastuzumab resistance in HER2-overexpressing breast cancer cells by using a novel celecoxib-derived phosphoinositide-dependent kinase-1 inhibitor. *Molecular Pharmacology,* Vol.70, No.5, (November 2006), pp. (1534-1541).

Tzahar, E., Waterman, H., Chen, X., Levkowitz, G., Karunagaran, D., Lavi, S., Ratzkin, BJ. & Yarden, Y. (1996). A hierarchical network of interreceptor interactions determines signal transduction by Neu differentiation factor/neuregulin and epidermal growth factor. *Molecular and Cellular Biology,* Vol.16, No.10, (October 1996), pp. (5276–5287).

Untch, M., Rezai, M., Loibl, S., Fasching, PA., Huober, J., Tesch, H., Bauerfeind, I., Hilfrich, J., Eidtmann, H., Gerber, B., Hanusch, C., Kuhn, T., du Bois, A., Blohmer, JU., Thomssen, C., Dan Costa, S., Jackisch, C., Kaufmann, M., Mehta, K., & von Minckwitz, G. (2010). Neoadjuvant treatment with trastuzumab in HER2-positive breast cancer: results from the GeparQuattro study. *Journal of Clinical Oncology,* Vol.28, No.12, (April 2010), pp. (2024-2031).

Valabrega, G., Montemurro, F., Sarotto, I., Petrelli, A., Rubini, P., Tacchetti, C., Aglietta, M., Comoglio, PM. & Giordano, S. (2005). TGF alpha expression impairs Trastuzumab-induced HER2 downregulation. *Oncogene,* Vol.24, No.18, (April 2005), pp. (3002-3010).

Van Cutsem, E., Peeters, M., Siena, S., Humblet, Y., Hendlisz, A., Neyns, B., Canon, JL., Van Laethem, JL., Maurel, J., Richardson, G., Wolf, M. & Amado, RG. (2007). Open-label phase III , trial of panitumumab plus best supportive care compared with best supportive care alone in patients with chemotherapy-refractory metastatic colorectal cancer. *Journal of Clinical Oncology*, Vol.25, No.13, (May 2007), pp. (1658–1664).

Vazquez-Martin, A., Colomer, R., Brunet, J. & Menendez, JA. (2007). Pharmacological blockage of fatty acid synthase (FASN) reverses acquired autoresistance to trastuzumab (Herceptin) by transcriptionally inhibiting "HER2 super-expression" occurring in high-dose trastuzumab-conditioned SKBR3/Tzb100 breast cancer cells. *International Journal of Oncology*, Vol.31, No.4, (October 2007), pp. (769-776).

Viani, GA., Afonso, SL., Stefano, EJ., De Fendi, LI. & Soares, FV. (2007). Adjuvant trastuzumab in the treatment of her-2-positive early breast cancer: a meta-analysis of published randomized trials. *BMC Cancer*, Vol.7, (August 2007), pp.153.

Vogel, CL., Cobleigh, MA., Tripathy, D., Gutheil, JC., Harris, LN., Fehrenbacher, L., Slamon, DJ., Murphy, M., Novotny, WF., Burchmore, M., Shak, S., Stewart, SJ. & Press, M. (2002). Efficacy and safety of trastuzumab as a single agent in first-line treatment of HER2-overexpressing metastatic breast cancer. *Journal of Clinical Oncology*, Vol.20, No.3, (February 2002), pp. (719-726).

Wada, T., Qian, XL. & Greene, MI. (1990). Intermolecular association of the p185neu protein and EGF receptor modulates EGF receptor function. *Cell*, Vol.61, No.7, (June 1990), pp. (1339–1347).

Wang, SE., Xiang, B., Guix, M., Olivares, MG., Parker, J., Chung, CH., Pandiella, A. & Arteaga, CL. (2008). Transforming growth factor beta engages TACE and ErbB3 to activate phosphatidylinositol-3 kinase/Akt in ErbB2-overexpressing breast cancer and desensitizes cells to trastuzumab. *Molecular and Cellular Biology*, Vol.28, No.18, (September 2008), pp. (5605-5620).

Wolff, AC., Hammond, ME., Schwartz, JN., Hagerty, KL., Allred, DC., Cote, RJ., Dowsett, M., Fitzgibbons, PL., Hanna, WM., Langer, A., McShane, LM., Paik, S., Pegram, MD., Perez, EA., Press, MF., Rhodes, A., Sturgeon, C., Taube, SE., Tubbs, R., Vance, GH., van de Vijver, M., Wheeler, TM. & Hayes, DF. (2007). American Society of Clinical Oncology/College of American Pathologist guideline recommendations for human epidermal growth factor receptor 2 testing in breast cancer. *Journal of Clinical Oncology*, Vol.25, No.1, (January 2007), pp. (118-145).

Yan, L., Ehrlich, PJ. , Gibson, R., Pickett, C. & Beckman, RA. (2009).How can we improve antibody-based cancer therapy? *mAbs*, Vol.*1, No. 1*, (January/February 2009), pp. (67-70).

Yarden, Y. & Sliwkowski, M.X. (2001).Untangling the ErbB signalling network. *Nature Reviews Molecular Cell Biology*, Vol.2, No.2, (February 2001), pp. (127–137).

Zhang, H., Berezov, A., Wang, Q., Zhang, G., Drebin, J., Mural,i R.& Greene, MI. (2007). ErbB receptors: from oncogenes to targeted cancer therapies. *The Journal of Clinical Investigation*, Vol.117, No.8, (August 2007), pp. (2051-2058).

Zhou, X., Tan, M., Stone Hawthorne, V., Klos, KS., Lan, KH., Yang, Y., Yang, W., Smith, TL., Shi, D. & Yu, D.(2004). Activation of the Akt/mammalian target of rapamycin/4E-BP1 pathway by ErbB2 overexpression predicts tumor progression in breast cancers. *Clinical Cancer Research*, Vol.10, No.20, (October 2004), pp. (6779-6788).

Zhuang, G., Brantley-Sieders, DM., Vaught, D., Yu, J., Xie, L., Wells, S., Jackson, D., Muraoka-Cook, R., Arteaga, C. & Chen, J. (2010). Elevation of receptor tyrosine kinase ephA2 mediates resistance to trastuzumab therapy. *Cancer Research,* Vol.70, No.1, (January 2010), pp. (299-308).

Zito, CI., Riches, D., Kolmakova, J., Simons, J., Egholm, M. & Stern, DF.(2008). Direct resequencing of the complete ERBB2 coding sequence reveals an absence of activating mutations in ERBB2 amplified breast cancer. *Genes, Chromosomes and Cancer* , Vol.47, No.7, (July 2008), pp. (633- 638).

Zuo, T., Wang, L., Morrison, C., Chang, X., Zhang, H., Li, W., Liu, Y., Wang, Y., Liu, X., Chan, MW., Liu, JQ., Love, R., Liu, CG., Godfrey, V., Shen, R., Huang, T.H.., Yang, T., Park, BK., Wang, CY., Zheng, P. & Liu, Y. (2007). FOXP3 is an X-linked breast cancer suppressor gene and an important repressor of the HER-2/ErbB2 oncogene. *Cell,* Vol.129, No.7, (June 2007), pp. (1275-1286).

Zsebik, B., Citri, A., Isola, J., Yarden, Y., Szollosi, J. & Vereb, G. (2006). Hsp90 inhibitor 17-AAG reduces ErbB2 levels and inhibits proliferation of the trastuzumab resistant breast tumor cell line JIMT-1. *Immunology Letters,* Vol.104, No.1-2, (April 2006), pp. (146-155).

9

Targeting HER-2 Signaling Network: Implication in Radiation Response

In Ah Kim
Department of Radiation Oncology, Seoul National University, Republic of Korea

1. Introduction

The Human Epidermal Growth Factor Receptor 2 (HER2) oncogene encodes a 185 kDa type I tyrosine kinase receptor that is a member of the epidermal growth factor receptor (EGFR) family including HER1, HER2, HER3 and HER4 (Yarden & Sliwkowski, 2001). Overexpression of HER2 is observed in 25-30% of human breast cancers and is associated with poor prognosis (Slamon et al., 1989; Cooke et al., 2001).

HER2 overexpression activates multiple signaling pathways and promotes tumor growth, proliferation, and survival. The underlying mechanism for this action was elucidated by several studies involving critical components of the HER2 regulated pathway including phosphatidylinositol 3-kinase (PI3K) and mitogen-activated protein kinase (MAPK) cascades (Huang & Lau, 1999). The most widely used anti-HER2 therapy is the recombinant humanized antibody trastuzumab, which represented the proof of principle for the targeting of tyrosine kinase receptors in breast cancer. Trastuzumab exerts its antitumor activity by induction of receptor degradation (Klapper et al., 2000), prevention of HER2 ectodomain cleavage (Molina et al., 2001), inhibition of HER2 kinase signal transduction via antibody-dependent cellular cytotoxicity (Clynes et al., 2000) and inhibition of angiogenesis (Izumi et al., 2002). Trastuzumab has been approved as a front-line therapy for HER2-positive breast cancer patients in both adjuvant and metastatic settings (Hudis, 2007), however, trastuzumab fails in 50-70% of HER2-positive patients (Vogel et al., 2002; Slamon et al., 2001).

Radiotherapy is employed as an integral part of the current comprehensive breast cancer treatment regimen, and may be used to eradicate remaining cancer cells in the breast, chest wall, or axilla after surgery or to reduce the size of an advanced tumor before surgery. A series of studies have shown the evidences regarding the potential value of targeting HER-2 signaling to enhance the anti-tumor activity of ionizing radiation. However, therapeutic resistance, resulting from several factors including activation of downstream pathway or alternative survival pathways, as well as molecular resistance mechanisms, has been emerged as an important issue in clinic.

We have been trying to identify the component(s) implicated in radiation response in HER-2 signaling network and also screening the useful approaches to overcome therapeutic resistance such as targeting downstream effectors, ligand-independent modulation via heat shock protein 90 (HSP90) inhibition and epigenetic modulation of HER-2 signaling via inhibition of histone deacetylases (HDACs). The efficacy and clinical relevance of each strategy and the diverse mechanisms of radiosensitization will be discussed.

2. Targeting downstream signaling

Overamplification of the HER2 gene results in formation of a ligand-independent HER2 homodimer that is able to initiate downstream signaling cascades such as the PI3K and MAPK pathways (Pinkas-Kramarski et al., 1996). While the inhibition of MEK-ERK signaling did not increase the radiosensitivity of SKBR3 breast cancer cells exhibiting over-amplification of HER2, selective inhibition of PI3K-Akt-mTOR pathway components radiosensitized SKBR3 cells (No et al., 2009). Loss of PTEN (phosphatase and tensin homolog deleted one chromosome ten) expression results in trastuzumab resistance, and PI3K inhibitors restore trastuzumab sensitivity in PTEN-deficient cells (Nagata et al., 2004). Berns et al. recently provided strong confirmatory evidence that activation of the PI3K pathway through loss of the tumor suppressor PTEN or through oncogenic stimulation of PI3K can mediate trastuzumab resistance (Berns et al., 2007).

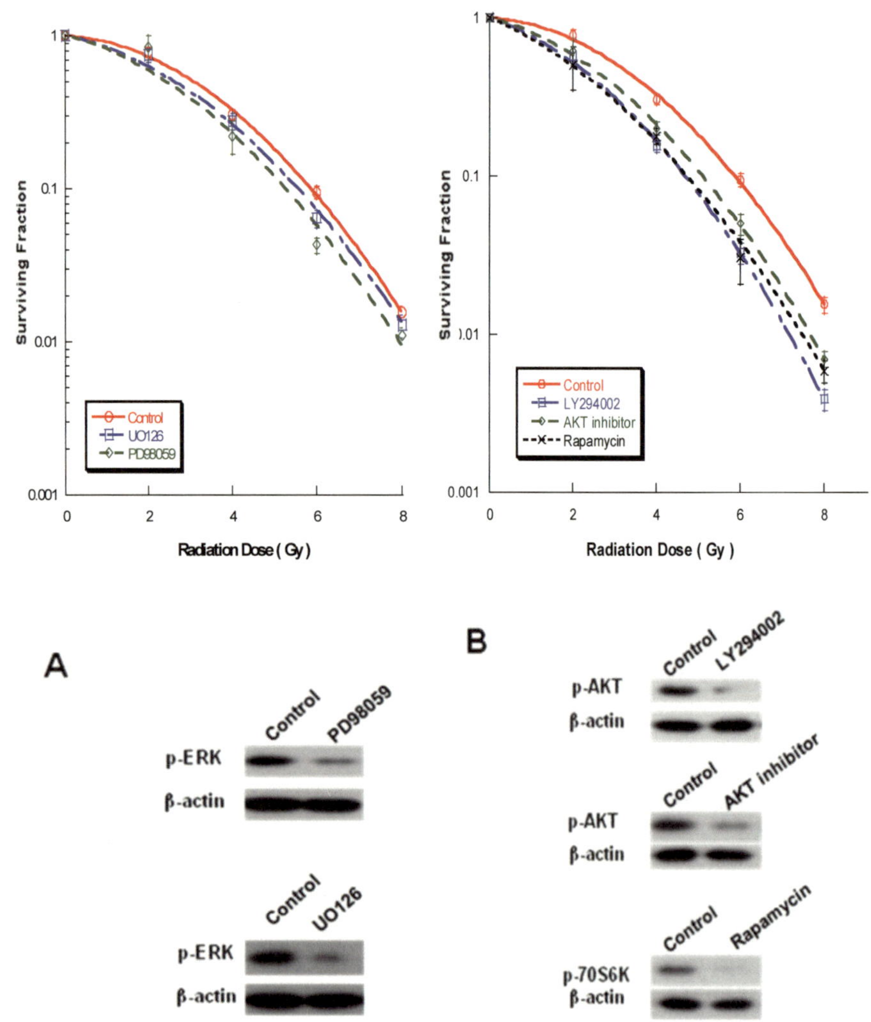

Fig. 1. Targeting downstream of HER-2 signaling (No et al, 2009).

2.1 Targeting PI3K-AKT-mTOR pathway

2.1.1 Targeting PI3K

PI3K, a heterodimer consisting of p85 regulatory subunit and a 110 catalytic subunit, plays a central role in growth regulation and tumorigenesis. It generates specific inositol lipids (PIP2, PIP3) that have been implicated in the regulation of cell proliferation, differentiation, survival, and angiogenesis (Engelman et al., 2006). Recently, several groups reported that 18-40% of human breast cancers harbor somatic mutations of PI3K (Levin et al, 2005), resulting in constitutive activation of PI3K signaling. PTEN inhibits PI3K by dephosphorylation of the second messenger PIP3. PTEN appears to be controlled by down-regulation of gene expression and genetic alterations of this tumor suppressor are found in a moderate proportion of breast cancers.

2.1.2 Targeting AKT

AKT/PKB is a serine/threonine kinase that plays an important role in cancer progression and cell survival and is activated in a PI3K-dependent manner by a variety of stimuli through growth factor receptors. Among the specific AKT family members, increased AKT1 activity was reported in 40% of breast cancers (Manning et al., 2007). We previously showed that inhibition of AKT1 using RNAi increased radiosensitivity of EGFR- or Ras-activated cell lines (Kim et al., 2005) and the other study showed that AKT inhibitor (API) or AKT1 siRNA inhibited repair of DNA double strand breaks (DSBs) in EGFR-activated lung cancer cell lines as measured by the γH2AX foci assay (Toulany et al., 2008). SKBR3 breast cancer cells having activated HER-2 signaling also showed similar findings (Figure 3, No et al., 2009).

2.1.3 Targeting m-TOR

The mammalian target of rapamycin (mTOR) is an important downstream component of the PI3K-AKT signaling pathway. mTOR inhibitors can effectively block the pro-growth, pro-proliferative, and pro-survival actions of mTOR by inactivating its downstream effectors such as p70S6 kinase and 4E-binding protein1 and decreasing protein synthesis (Shaw et al., 2006; Guertin & Sabatini, 2007). mTOR presents an attractive target in the pathway because its inhibition could avoid possible side effects associated with inhibition of upstream PI3K/AKT signaling molecules with broader function. We previously showed that the radiosensitizing effect of Rapamycin is related to inhibition of DNA damage repair, as demonstrated by the γH2AX foci assay using SKBR3 cells (Fig. 2, No et al., 2009). Recent report showed that RAD001 attenuated prosurvival AKT/mTOR signaling and increased radiation sensitivity of MDA-MB-231 breast cancer cells (Albert et al., 2006).

2.1.4 Targeting class I PI3K and m-TOR

One of the reasonable approaches would be the targeting more than one component of tumor specific signaling that less affect normal cell survival. Inhibition of PI3K using LY294002 lacks specificity and has shown unacceptable toxicities in preclinical studies. Previous study showed that specific inhibition of class I PI3K using RNAi enhanced the radiosensitivity of tumor cells having activated PI3K signaling resulting from overexpression of EGFR or mutation of RAS oncogene (Kim et al., 2005). The PI103 is known as a dual inhibitor which targets class I PI3K and mTOR signaling which reduce radiation survival of tumor cells with AKT activation. (Prevo et al., 2008). PI103 effectively radiosensitized SKBR3 cells with activated HER2 signaling and this sensitizing effect

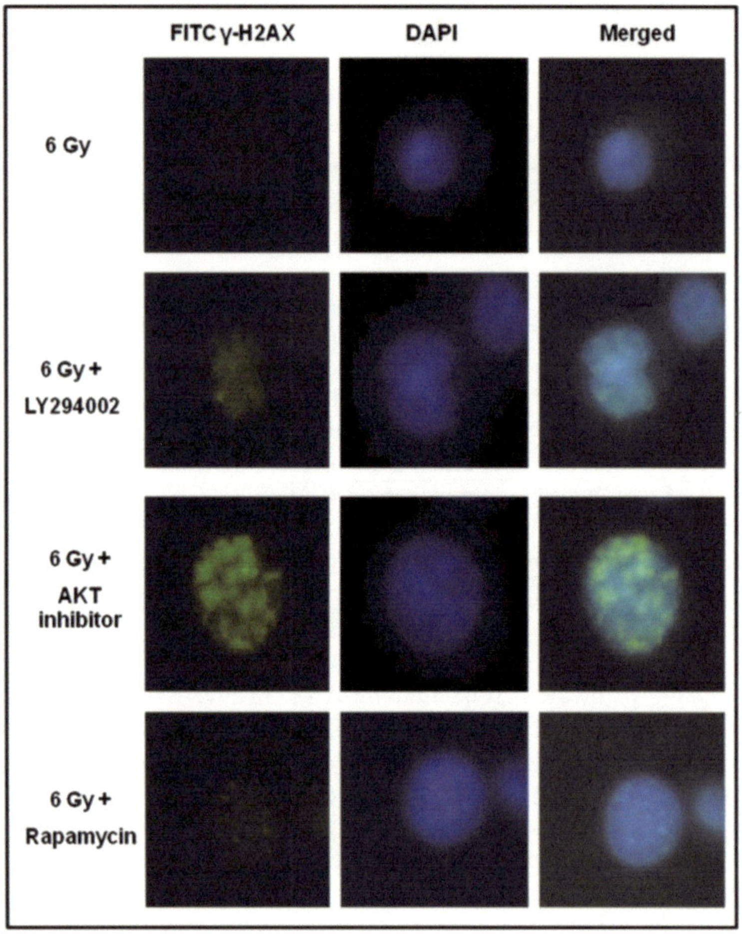

Fig. 2. Persistent γH2AX foci following orradiation by selective inhibition of PI3K-AKT-mTOR signalling (No et al., 2009).

was associated with prolongation of γH2AX foci following irradiation. Decreased phosphorylation of DNA-PKs by pretreatment of inhibitors targeting PI3K-AKT indicated that the functional requirement of PI3K-AKT pathway in regulation of DNA repair following radiation (Fig.3 & 4, No et al., 2009). While apoptosis was the major mode of cell death when the cells were pretreated with LY294002 or AKT inhibitor VIII, cells were pretreated by Rapamycin or PI103 showed the mixed mode of cell death including autophagy (Fig. 5, No et al., 2009).

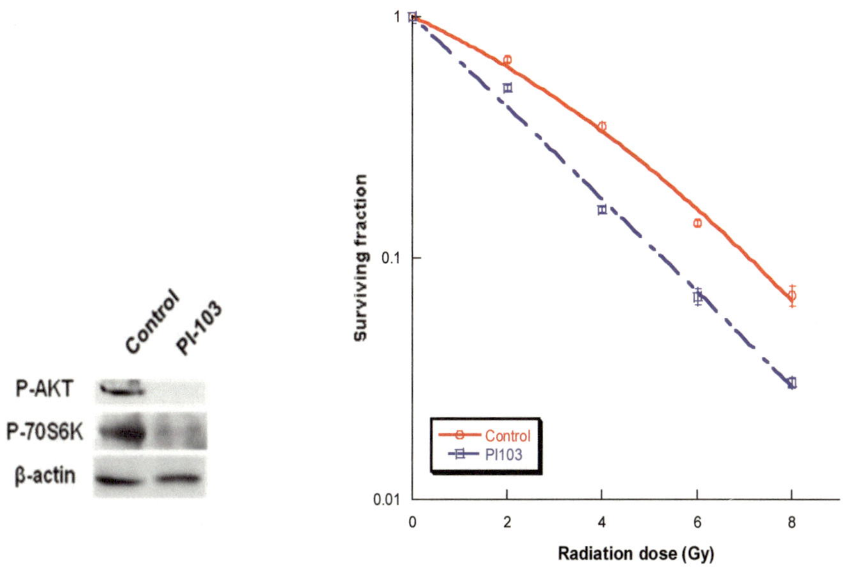

Fig. 3. Targeting Class I PI3K and m-TOR using dual inhibitor (No et al., 2009).

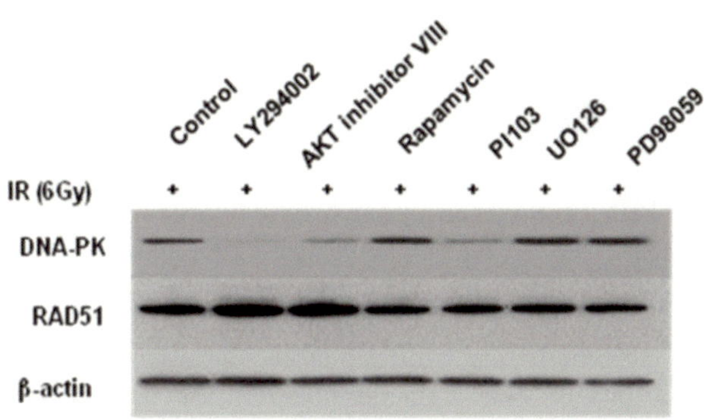

Fig. 4. Targeting Class I PI3K-Akt down-regulated DNA-PK expression (No et al., 2009).

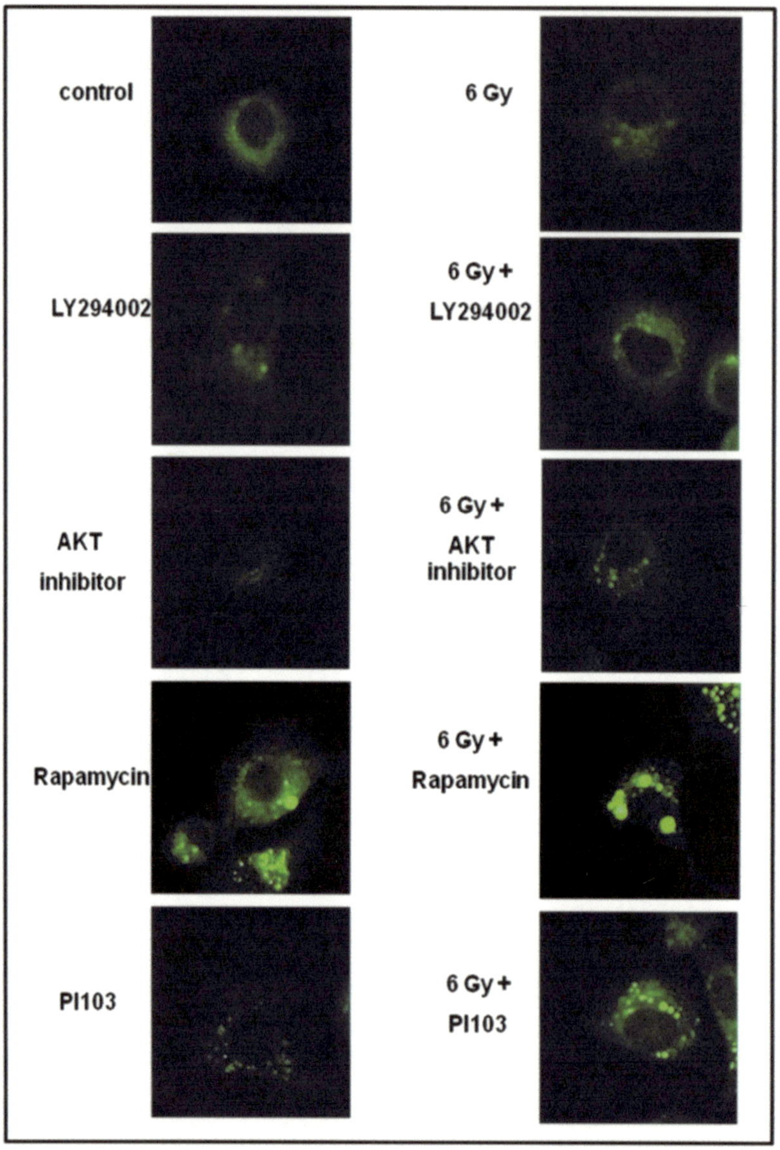

Fig. 5. Rapamycin and PI103 induced autophagy following irradiation. (No et al., 2009).

3. Ligand-independent modulation of HER-2 signaling: HSP90 inhibition

The majority of breast cancers involve multiple molecular abnormalities that are likely to be involved in malignant progression. It is possible that several different molecules from diverse pathways have synergistic properties that promote malignant relapse or metastasis. In that situation, HSP90 could be a pivotal key molecule, as its chaperone function ensures the correct conformation, activity, intracellular localization, and proteolytic turnover of a range of proteins involved in cell growth, differentiation, and survival (Neckers et al., 2003). This molecular chaperon is essential for the stability and function of many oncogenic client proteins, which contributes to the hallmark trait of cancers such as ER, HER-2, and AKT (Powers & Workman, 2006). The inhibition of multiple targets through the abrogation of HSP90 could be more effective in the management of breast cancers, since its inhibition counteracts multiple oncogenic molecules and prosurvival signaling pathways at the same time.

Additional data supports the identification of HSP90 as an important molecular target relevant to breast cancers. HER2, which is associated with poor prognosis in breast cancer, is one of the most important client proteins of HSP90, and HSP90 inhibitors have shown antitumor activity in a HER2-driven xenograft model (Kamal et al, 2003). Additionally, HSP90 inhibitors bind selectively to HSP90 in cancerous cells versus normal cells (Munster et al, 2001). Breast cancer cells resistant to conventional chemotherapy, radiation therapy, and trastuzumab, are known to involve the PI3K signaling pathway. The key molecule of this pathway, AKT, is also an important client protein of HSP90.

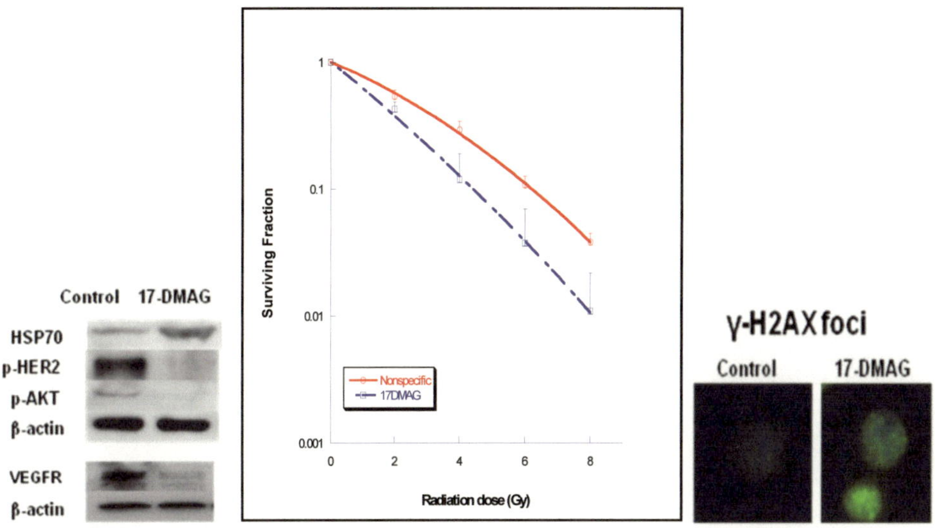

Fig. 6. 17-DMAG, a HSP90 inhibitor radiosensitized SKBR-3 cells with HER-2 overexpression.

A HSP90 inhibitor, 17-(allylamino)-17-demethoxy-geldanamycin (17-AAG) downregulated HER2 in trastuzumab-resistant breast cancer cells (Zsebik et al., 2006). We also have observed that 17-DMAG, led to downregulation of HER-2 and p-AKT, and radiosensitized HER-2 activated breast cancer cells. This radiosensitizing effect was associated with persistence of γH2AX foci following irradiation (Figure 6, unpublished data).

Our previous immunihistochemical study using tissue samples from 212 patients who underwent surgical resection for primary invasive breast cancer, have shown that expression of HSP90 from invasive breast cancer was associated with an increased risk of early recurrence (Fig. 7, Song et al., 2010). Co-expression of HSP90 and PI3K or expression of HSP90 in combination with the loss of PTEN was significantly associated with RFS especially in the patient group having HER-2 overexpression (Fig.8, Song et al., 2010). This study provides direct evidence that the expression of HSP90 predicts early relapse in patients with invasive breast cancers and validates the significance of HSP90 as a clinically significant therapeutic target.

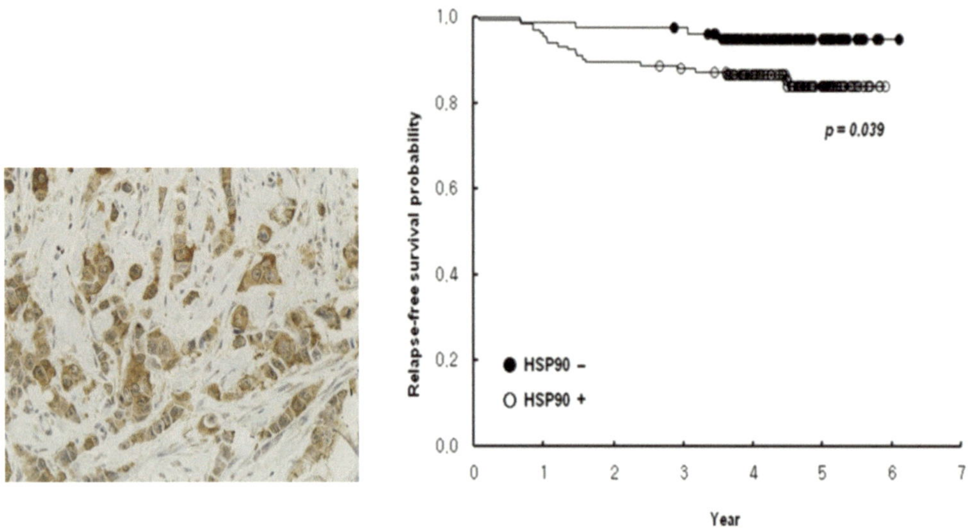

Fig. 7. Relapse free survival of patients according to HSP90 overexpression (Song et al., 2010).

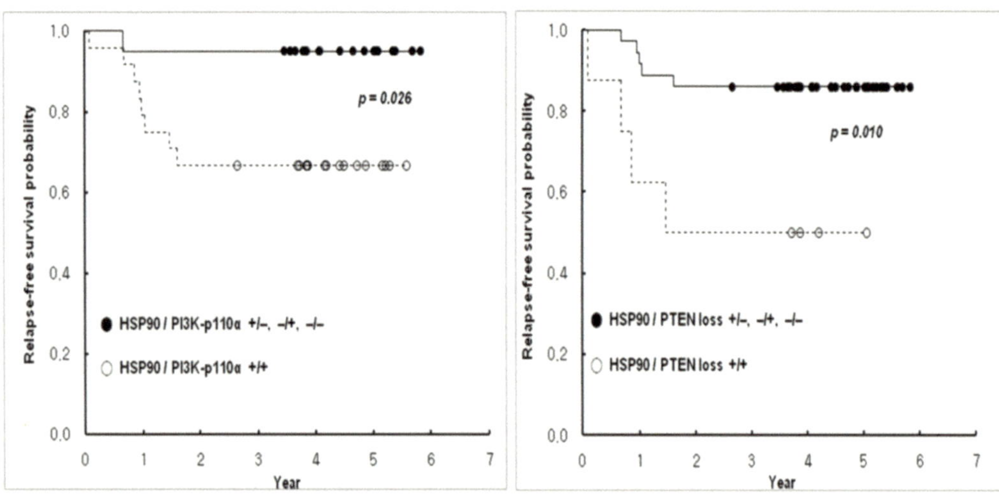

Fig. 8. Relapse free survival of patients with HER-2 overexpression (Song et al., 2010).

4. Epigenetic modulation of HER-2 signlaing: Histone deacetylase inhibition

Histone deacetylase inhibitiors (HDIs) are capable of modifying gene expression without directly interacting with DNA by affecting the acetylation state of DNA-associated proteins, as well as other proteins.

We previously reported that HER-2 activated cells were preferentially radiosensitized by LBH589, the cinnamyl hydroxamic acid analogue panHDAC inhibitor compared to the effect of TSA or SK7041 at iso-effective concentrations and that this was associated with down-regulation of HER-2 signaling of SKBR-3 cells (Fig.9, Kim et al., 2009).

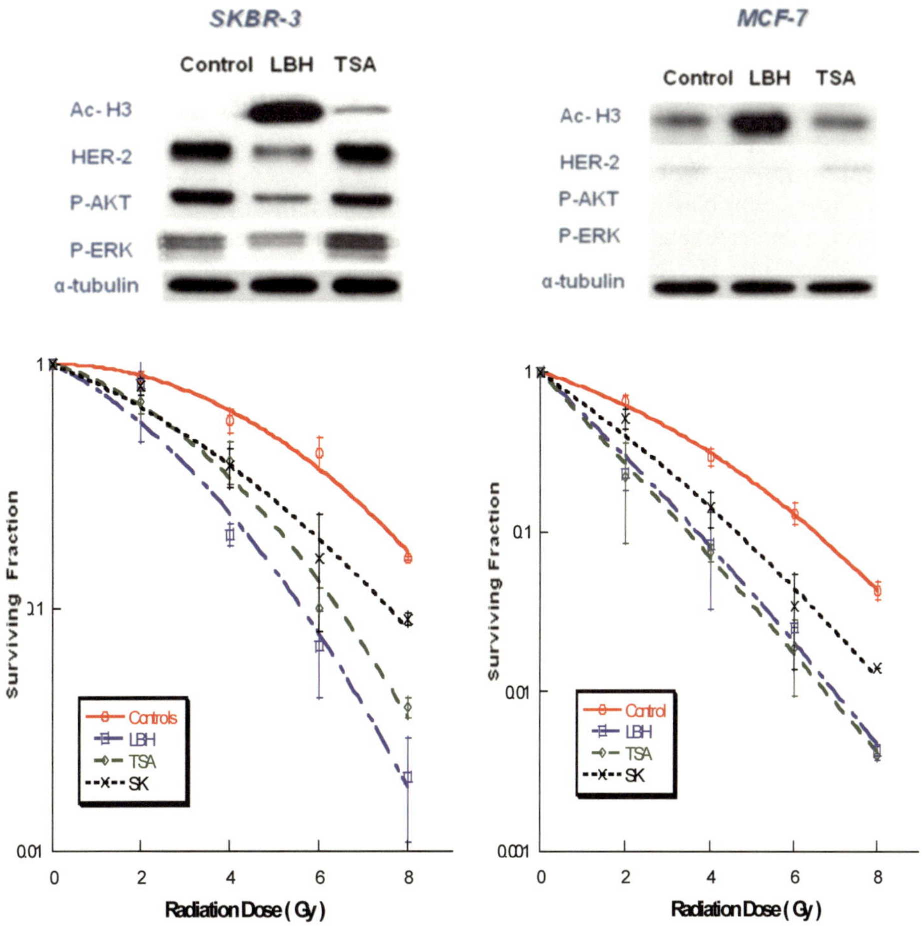

Fig. 9. LBH589 preferentially radiosensitizes breast cancer cells with HER-2 amplification (Kim et al., 2009).

The acetylation level of HSP90 and the relative inhibition of HDAC6 by the three different HDIs at iso-effective concentrations provided a mechanistic clue to explain this preferential radiosensitization by LBH589. Selective inhibition of HDAC6 led to acetylation of HSP90 resulting in ubiquitination and depletion of pro-survival client proteins including HER-2 and its downstream effectors. Specific inhibition of HDAC6 using RNAi increased acetylation of HSP 90 and attenuated the expression level of its client proteins such as p-AKT and p-ERK. This was associated with increased radiosensitivity of SKBR-3 cells (Fig.10, unpublished data).

The first evidence of non-nuclear and non-histone associated activity for a HDAC member came from the characterization of HDAC 6, one of the class IIB members. It possesses two deacetylase domains and zinc finger motif. The central part of this motif is similar to region found in BRAP (BRCA1-associated protein 2) and several ubiquitin-specific proteases. This motif is also known as PAZ (polyubiquitin-associated zinc finger) due to its ubiquitin-binding ability. It has been implicated as a critical link between proteasome degradation and autophagy (Kawaguchi et al., 2003; Boyault et al., 200; Pandei et al., 2007). HDAC6 has been implicated in modulating receptor tyrosine kinase signaling. Increased acetylation of heat shock protein such as HSP90 by HDAC 6 inhibition may lead to mis-folding and degradation of survival associated client proteins such as oncogenic tyrosine kinases, RAF, and AKT (Bali et al., 2005). Stable knockdown of HDAC6 expression also causes a decrease platelet-derived growth factor receptor α (Kamera et al., 2008). Lee et al. recently found that HDAC6 deficient fibroblasts were more resistant to oncogenic Ras and HER2-dependent transformation, indicating a critical role of HDAC6 in oncogene-induced transformation (Lee et al., 2008). Thus, HDAC6 could be a good therapeutic target regulating critical cancer-relevant biologic functions. These reports and the current study suggest that HDAC 6 may be a useful target for overcoming therapeutic resistance to available HER2 inhibitors combined with radiation.

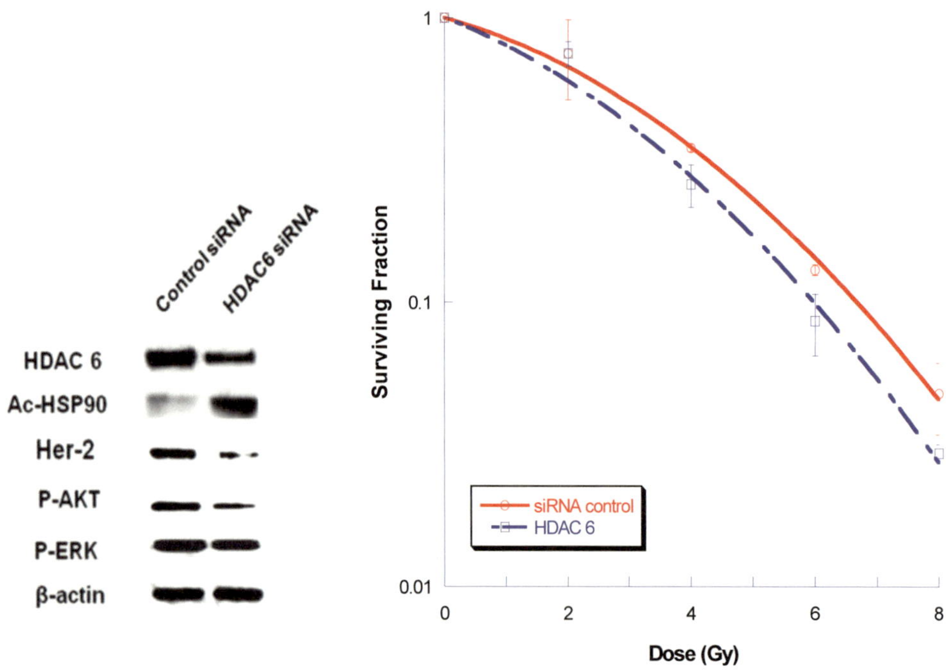

Fig. 10. Selective inhibition of HDAC6 radiosensitized SKBR-3 cells.

5. Conclusion

Identification of the prognostic significance of HER2 and its targeted therapy are the best examples of proof of concept (Hassa et al., 2005). A series of studies have shown solid preclinical and clinical evidences regarding the potential value of targeting HER-2 signaling to enhance the anti-tumor activity of ionizing radiation (Sartor et al., 2003; Sambade et al.,

2010). However, therapeutic resistance resulting from several factors including activation of downstream pathway or alternative survival pathways, as well as molecular resistance mechanisms, have emerged as an important issue in the clinic. Based on previous studies and our data, we propose that targeting downstream, ligand-inependent modulation via HSP90 inhibitor, and epigentic modulation via HDAC inhibiton could be an alternative approaches to tackle factors such as these that limit the therapeutic benefit of HER-2 targeted therapy combined with radiation.

6. Acknowledgment

This work was supported by the National Research Foundation grants (Nuclear R&D Program, BAERI #2007-2001193, #313-2007-2-E00381 and #531-2006-1-E00061) from Korean Ministry of Education, Science & Technology to Kim IA and Cancer Control Program(#0820010) from Korean Ministry of Health & Welfare

7. References

Yarden Y, Sliwkowski M. (2001) Untangling the ErbB signalling network. *Nature Rev Mol Cell Biol* 2:127-37.

Slamon DJ, Godolphin W, Jones LA, Holt JA, Wong SG, Keith DE, et al. (1989). Studies of HER2/neu proto-oncogene in human breast and ovarian cancer. *Science*; 244: 707-712.

Cooke T, Reeves J, Lanigan A, Stanton P. (2001). HER2 as a prognostic and predictive marker for breast cancer. *Ann Oncol*; 12: S23-S28.

Huang MC, Lau YK: Basic science of HER2/neu. a review (1999). *Semin Oncol* 26:51-59.

Klapper L, Waterman H, Sela M, Yarden Y. (2000) Tumor-inhibitory antibodies to HER2/ErbB2 may act by recruiting c-Cbl and enhancing ubiquitination of HER2. *Cancer Res* 60:3384-8.

Molina MA, Codony-Servat J, Albanell J, Rojo F, Arribas J, Balselga J. (2001). Trastuzumab, a humanized anti-her2 receptor monoclonal antibody inhibits basal and activated HER2 ectodomain cleavage in breast cancer cells. *Cancer Res* 61: 4744-9.

Clynes RA, Towers TL, Presta LG, Ravetch JV. (2000). Inhibitory Fc receptors modulate in vivo cytotoxicity against tumor targets. *Nat Med* 6: 443-6.

Izumi Y, Xu L, di Tomaso E, Fukumura D, Jain RK. (2002) Tumour biology: Herceptin acts as an anti-angiogenic cocktail. *Nature* 416:279-80.

Hudis CA. Trastuzumab - mechanism of action and use in clinical practice. (2007) *N Engl J Med* 357:39-51.

Vogel CL, Cobleigh MA, Tripathy D, Gutheil JC, Harris LN, Fehrenbacher L,et al. (2002). Efficacy and safety of trastuzumab as a single agent in first-line treatment of HER2 overexpressing metastatic breast cancer. *J Clin Oncol* 20:719-26.

Slamon DJ, Leyland-Jones B, Shak S, Fuchs H, Paton V, Bajamonde A, et al. (2001). Use of chemotherapy plus monoclonal antibody against HER2 for metastatic breast cancer that overexpress HER2. *N Engl J Med* 344:783-792.

Kim IA, Bae SS, Fernandes A, Wu J, Muschel RJ, McKenna WG, et al. (2005). Selective inhibition of Ras, Phosphoinositide 3 kinase, and Akt isoforms increases the radiosensitivity of human carcinoma cell lines. *Cancer Res* 1: 65(17):7902-10.

Berns K, Horlings HM, Hennessy BT, Madiredjo M, Hijmans EM, Beelen K, et al. (2007). A functional Genetic Approach identifies the PI3K pathway as a major determinant of tratuzumab resistance in breast cancer. *Cancer Cell* 12: 395-402.

Nagata Y, Lan KH, Zhou X, Tan M, Esteva FJ, Sahin AA, et al. (2004). PTEN activation contributes to tumor inhibition by tratuzumab, and loss of PTEN predicts trastuzumab resistance in patients. *Cancer Cell* 6:117-27.

Pinkas-Kramarski R, Soussan L, Waterman H, Levkowitz G, Alroy I, Klapper L, Lavi S, et al. (1996). Diversification of Neu differentiation factor and epidermal growth factor signaling by combinatorial receptor interactions. *EMBO J* 15:2452-67.

Engelman JA, Luo J, Catley LC. (2006). The evolution of phosphatidylinositol 3-kinases as regulators of growth and metabolism. *Nat Rev Genetics* 7: 606-619.

Lee JY, Engelman JA, Catley LC. (2007). PI3K charges ahead. *Science* 317: 206-207.

Levine DA, Bogomolniy F, Yee CJ, Lash A, Barakat RR, Borgen PI et al. (2005). Frequent mutation of PI3KA gene in ovarian and breast cancers. *Clin Can Res* 11:2875-8.

Manning BD, Catley LC. AKT/PKB Signaling: Navigating Downstream. (2007). *Cell* 129:1261-1274.

Toulany M, Kehlbach R, Florczak U, Sak A, Wang S, Chen J, et al. (2008). Targeting of AKT1 enhances radiation toxicity of human tumor cells by inhibiting DNA-PKs-dependent DNA double-strand break repair. *Mol Can Ther* 7(7):1772-1781.

Bozulic L, Surucu B, Hynx D, Hemmings BA. (2008). PKBα/AKT1 acts downstream of DNA-PK in DNA double-stand break response and promotes survival. *Mol Cell* 30:203-213

Shaw RJ, Cantley LC. (2006). Ras, PI3K and mTOR signalling controls tumour cell growth. *Nature* 441:424-430.

Guertin DA, Sabatini DM (2007). Defining the role of mTOR in Cancer. *Cancer Cell* 12:9-22.

Albert JM, Kim KW, Cao C, Lu B. (2006). Targeting the Akt/mammalian target of rapamycin pathway for radiosensitization of breast cancer. *Mol Cancer Ther* 5: 1183-42.

Prevo R, Deutsch E, Sampson O, Diplexcito J, Cengel K, Harper J, et al. (2008). Class I PI3 kinase inhibition by the pyridinylfuranopyrimidine inhibitor PI-103 enhances tumor radiosensitivity. *Cancer Res* 15:68(14):5915-23.

Neckers L, Ivy SP. (2003). Heat shock protein 90. *Curr Opin Oncol* 15:419-424.

Powers M, Workman P. Targeting multiple signalling pathways by heat shock protein 90 molecular chaperone inhibiotrs. *Endocrine -Related Cancer* 2006, 13:S125-35

Kamal A, Thao L, Sensintaffar J, Zhang L, Boehm MF, Fritz LC, Burrows FJ. (2003). A high-affinity conformation of HSP90 confers tumour selectivity on HSP90 inhibitors. *Nature* 425:407-410.

Munster PN, Basso A, Solit D, Norton L, Rosen N. Modulation of HSP90 function by ansamycin sensitize breast cancer cells to chemotherapy-induced apoptosis in a RB- and schedule-dependent manner. *Clin Cancer Res* 2001, 7:2228-36

Zsebik B, Citri A, Isola J, Yarden Y, Szöllosi J, Vereb G. HSP90 inhibitor 17-AAG reduces ErbB2 levels and inhibits proliferation of the trastuzumab resistant breast tumor cell line JIMT-1. *Immunol Lett* 2006, 104:146-155.

McKee JA, Yao TP. Histone deacetylases in the response to misfolded proteins p167-169 in *Histone Deacetylases: transcriptional regulation and other cellular functions.* edited by Verdin E. Humania pres. 2006

Kawaguchi Y, Kovacs JJ, McLaurin A, Vance JM, Ito A, Yao P. The Deacetylase HDAC6 regulates aggresome formation and cell viability in response to misfolded protein stress. *Cell* 2003;115:727-738

Boyault C, Sadoul K, Pabion M, Khochbin S. (2007). HDAC6, at the crossroad between cytoskelecton and cell signaling by acetylation and ubiquitination. *Oncogene* 26:5468-5476

Pandey UB, Nie Z, Batlevi Y, McCray BA, Ritson GP, Nedelsky NB, Schwartz SL, DiProspero NA, Knight MA, Schuldiner O, Padmanabhan R, Hild M, Berry DL, Garza D, Hubbert CC, Yao TP, Baehrecke EH, Taylor JP. (2007). HDAC6 rescues neurodegeneration and provides an essential link between autophagy and the UPS. *Nature* 14:447(7146):859-63.

Bali P, Pranpat M, Bradner J, Balasis M, Fiskus W, Guo F, Bhalla K. (2005). Inhibition of Histone Deacetylase 6 acetylates and disrupts the chaperone function of Heat Shock Protein 90. *J Biol Chem* 29:26729-26734

Kamemura K, Ito A, Shimazu T, Matsuyama A, Maeda S, Yao TP, Horinouchi S, Khochbin S, Yoshida M. (2008). Effects of downregulated HDAC6 expression on the proliferation of lung cancer cells. *Biochem Biophys Res Commun* 12:374 (1):84-89

Lee YS, Lim KH, Guo X, Kawaguchi Y, Gao Y, Barrientos T, Ordentlich P, *et al.* (2008). The cytoplasmic deacetylase HDAC6 is required for efficient oncogenic tumorigenesis. *Can Res* 68:7561- 7569

Huang SM, Bock JM, Harari PM. (1999). Epidermal growth factor recetor blockade with C225 modulates proliferation, apoptosis and radiosensitivity in squmous cell carcinomas of head and neck. *Cancer Res* 59:1935-1940

Bonner JA, Harari PM, Giralt J, Azarnia N, ShinDM, Cohen RB, Jones CU, *et al.* (2006). Radiotherapy plus Cetuximab for squamous-cell carcinoma of head and neck. *N Engl J Med* 9: 354 (6):567-78

Sartor CI. Epidermal growth factor family receptors and inhibitors: radiation response modulators.(2003). *Semin Radiat Oncol* 13(1): 22-30

Sambade MJ, Kimple RJ, Camp JT, *et al.* (2010). Lapatinib in combination with radiation diminishes tumor regrowth in HER2+ and basal-like/EGFR+ breast tumor xenografts. *Int J Radiat Oncol Biol Phys* 77:575-581.

No M, Choi EJ, Kim IA. (2009). Targeting HER2 signaling pathway for radiosensitization: Alternative strategy for therapeutic resistance. *Cancer Biology & Therapy* 8(24):2351-2361

Kim IA, No M, Lee JM *et al.* (2009). Epigenetic modulation of radiation response in human cancer cells with activated EGFR or HER-2 signaling: Potential role of histone deacetylase 6. *Radiotherapy & Oncology*: 92:125-132

Song CH, Park SY, Eom KY, Kim JH, Kim SW, Kim JS, Kim IA. (2010). Potential prognostic value of heat-shock protein 90 in the presence of phosphatidylinositol-3-kinase overexpression or loss of PTEN, in invasive breast cancers. *Breast Cancer Res.* 12(2):R20.

Part 2

Estrogen Receptors

10

The Importance of ERα/ERβ Ratio in Breast Cancer: Mitochondrial Function and Oxidative Stress

Pilar Roca, Jordi Oliver, Jorge Sastre-Serra and Mercedes Nadal-Serrano
Universitat de les Illes Balears
Spain

1. Introduction

Breast cancer is the most commonly diagnosed malignancy within the female population of developed countries and is the first leading cause of cancer deaths in women. In the European Union (EU27) every year there are an estimated 319.000 new cases diagnosed, and approximately 131.000 deaths, which comprises 16.7% of all cancer caused deaths in women (Ferlay et al., 2007).
The causes of breast cancer are not fully understood, but the epidemiology of the disease clearly shows that hormonal factors play a key role. Estrogen production appears as one potential risk factor among women worldwide because it stimulates the proliferation of breast epithelial cells (Ekbom et al., 1997; Ferlay et al., 2007). Coincident with this proliferation, breast cancer risk increases in early menarche, late menopause and with obesity in postmenopausal women (situations where there is a direct association between estrogen and breast cancer risk). In general, breast cancer risk decreases around 5% with each year that menarche is delayed. Breast cancer incidence rates also increase more slowly after menopause; therefore a woman with a natural menopause at age 45 years has half the risk of developing this type of cancer that a woman with menopause at age 55 (Kelsey et al., 1993; Key et al., 2001).
Childbearing seems to have a dual effect on risk of breast cancer (Key et al., 2001). On one hand the immediate effect is to temporarily increase the risk after a birth, yet on the other, this risk diminishes in the long term and the overall effect of a pregnancy is to reduce the overall risk of developing this disease. It appears that the negative short term effect is due to the increase in estradiol levels in early pregnancy. However, has been seen that premenopausal parous women have lower global levels of circulating estradiol than in nulliparous premenopausal women. This effect is observed among postmenopausal women, suggesting that this diminution is stable (Ewertz et al., 1990). Women who have had at least one child have around a 25% reduction in breast cancer risk compared to nulliparous women (Layde et al., 1989; Ewertz et al., 1990).
Moreover, the use of menopausal hormonal therapy increases the risk of breast cancer; in fact, the use of these estrogen preparations over a period of 10 years, increases cancer risk by 35%(Key et al., 2001). Other risk factor associated with breast cancer is family history and genetic predisposition. Women with a first-degree relative have about a two-fold risk of

developing breast cancer. However the risk is lower when only second-degree relatives are affected (Pharoah et al., 1997). Several germline mutations that have a predisposition for the development of breast cancer have been identified: BRCA1, BRCA2, P53, PTEN, ATM, NBS1, RAD50, BRIP1, PALB2 and CHEK2 (Walsh and King, 2007). In addition, the International Agency for Research on Cancer (IARC) estimates that 25% of all cancers are associated with overweight and obesity. This increase in cancer risk is approximately linear with increasing body-mass index, yet is reduced in the more physically active, equivalent population (McTiernan, 2003). In the European Union, 13.000 cases of breast cancer could be avoided annually by maintaining a normal body weight (Devenish et al., 1979). The increased risk in obese postmenopausal women may be due to higher levels of circulating estrogens (Lahmann et al., 2004). For many years this risk has been linked to higher estrogenic synthesis by the aromatase process in the adipose tissue and recent studies showed that the hormones secreted for this tissue have the capacity to induce tumour cell proliferation and survival (Catalano et al., 2003; Lahmann et al., 2004; Garofalo and Surmacz, 2006).

The most common type of breast cancer is invasive ductal carcinoma (IDC), and about 80% of all breast cancers are of this histological type. The second most common type is invasive lobular carcinoma (ILC), represents approximately 10%. Tubular carcinoma of the breast is a rare subtype of invasive ductal carcinoma, and accounts for only 1-2% of all breast cancer cases (Novelli et al., 2008).

2. Estrogen receptors

2.1 History of estrogen

Estrogen is term derived from Greek *oistros*¸ a word which refers to oestrus, the phase in which females are sexually receptive. In women with active menstrual cycles, daily ovary estrogen production is between 70 and 500 micrograms, with 17β-estradiol (E_2) the most important one. Studies report that the production E_2 of increases under the influence of gonadotropins secreted by the pituitary gland and by the maturation of ovarian follicles. Follicular estrogens induce the growth and development of female sex organs and to maintain sexual characteristics, as well as influence female behaviour (Morani et al., 2008). Studies of action of E_2 on the uterus, directed by Jensen, led to the conclusion that the biological effects of estrogen occur through the activation of estrogen receptor (ER) (Jensen et al., 1972). In the classical scheme of reproductive organ development, estrogens were considered as "female hormones", while testosterone was thought to be the "male hormone". In the 1980's the studies began to analyse effects of estrogen in non-target organs for the action of this hormone, i.e. in organs that are not associated with reproduction. The importance of estrogens in the bone homeostasis was recognised because of the observed increased risk of osteoporosis in postmenopausal women. However, it was a publication in 1994 of a case report of male with an ER mutation who had abnormal bone density and impaired glucose tolerance that finally confirmed the importance of estrogens in both males and females (Smith et al., 1994).

It was only until 1985, 23 years after the discovery of ER by Jensen, that this receptor was identified as a member of nuclear receptor superfamily (Greene et al., 1980; Walter et al., 1985; Green et al., 1986). Ten years later, in 1995, Gustafsson's laboratory discovered a second ER. The "Jensen" receptor was than named ERα and the new receptor ERβ (Kuiper et al., 1996). ERα and ERβ have distinct tissue expression patterns (Kuiper et al., 1997). In fact, many tissues previously thought to be "estrogen-insensitive tissue" were found to be ERβ positive and estrogen sensitive, with ERβ highly expressed and is almost the exclusive ER in ovarian granulose cells. ERα is the main ER subtype in the liver, breast and ovaries, while ERβ is predominantly in the prostate, colon and lung (Gustafsson, 1999; Pearce and Jordan, 2004). Thus, the proliferative actions of estrogens mediated via ERα can be opposed by ERβ (Pearce and Jordan, 2004; Chang et al., 2008; Jensen et al., 2010).

2.2 Estrogen receptors structure

ERα and ERβ have the typical structure of the nuclear receptor family (figure 1): a highly variable N-terminal region (A/B domain, involved in protein-protein interactions with transcriptional machinery and cofactors), a highly conserved DNA-binding domain (C), a hinge domain (D), a ligand-binding domain (E) and a C-terminal domain (F) (Giguere et al., 1986; Kumar et al., 1987).

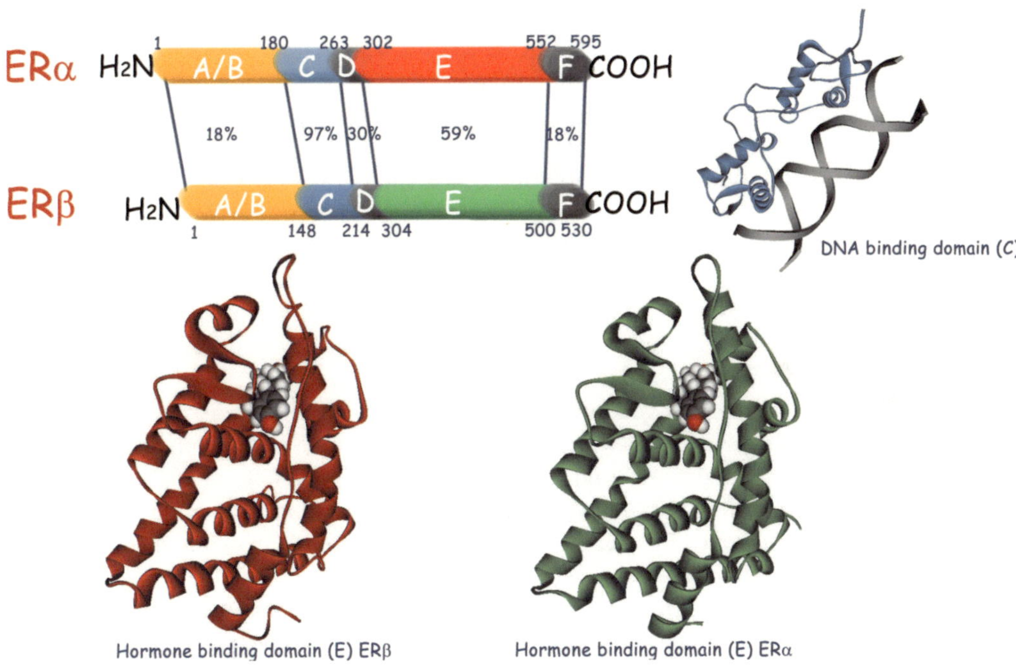

Fig. 1. ERα and ERβ structures. Schematic representation of the structure ERα and ERβ, structure DNA binding domain and structure of the hormone binding domain of both estrogen receptors.

ERα (595 aa) and ERβ (530 aa) receptors are codified by two different genes with less than 18% homology between them in A/B domain, although there is a 97% of homology between their respective DNA-binding domains (the most conserved). This domain (C) contains two zinc fingers and has a short motif, called a P-box, which is responsible for DNA specificity and is also involved in dimerization (Nilsson et al., 2001; Morani et al., 2008). Consequently both receptors ERα and ERβ bind to DNA in a similar manner, but the association with different cofactors enables them to modulate transcription genes (Giguere et al., 1986; Kumar et al., 1987). The D domain has nuclear localization signals and could provide malleability between the C and E domains. The E domain has the property for ligand binding, with its ligand-binding pocket formed by 12 alpha-helixes, and which is 60% conserved between the two estrogen receptors (Spithill et al., 1979; Morani et al., 2008). Moreover this domain is also involved in other functions such as receptor dimerization, nuclear localization and cofactor interaction. Finally, the F domain is extremely variable and contributes gene transactivation capacity (Morani et al., 2008).

2.3 Mechanisms of ER activation

Estrogens can act through different mechanisms and pathways to cause their biological effects (Gonzalez et al., 1993; Nilsson et al., 2001). There is a typical nuclear receptor superfamily mechanism to modulate the expression of several genes. Estrogen activates ER by ligand binding to the receptor, but this unity can occur in to forms. The first can occur when E_2-ER complex has formed in the cytoplasm and then is transported to the nucleus through cytoskeleton regulated mechanisms. The second form has the same final product, but occurs by a direct E_2 binding to the ER in the nucleus, with this union allowing for eventual ER dissociation of the chaperon proteins and the restoration of the ER to the inactive state. After this dissociation, ER can form either heterodimers or homodimers and bind directly to estrogen response element (ERE) through the DNA-binding domain as well as by association with different gene regulation co activators (Nilsson et al., 2001; Morani et al., 2008).

Another mechanism includes the involvement of the SP1 protein in the formation of the bridge between the activated estrogen receptor dimer and ERE (Kushner et al., 2000; Saville et al., 2000). This mechanism forms an indirect activation/inhibition of E_2 regulated genes and some authors have found differences dependant on the ERα and ERβ union to ERE (Sidhu and Tauro, 1979; Morani et al., 2008).

Another action of ERs, in a non-genomic process, involves the interaction of activated ERs with secondary messenger proteins (SM) with rapid, concomitant effects in many tissues, although this process is still not well understood (Heldring et al., 2007).

Furthermore, ERs have a ligand-independent activation mechanism, involving kinases that phosphorylate and activate ERs and this mechanism could explain the hormone-independent growth of some tumours.

Other factors have an important role in the activation mechanisms of ERs and serve as corregulators (or cofactors) recruited by the ERs to activate (coactivator) or to repress (corepressor) the transcriptional activity of ERs. These corregulators can modify the affinity of the ERs to EREs and can be in the form of acetylases/deacetylases, kinases/phosphatases and methylases/demethylases. It must be emphasized, however, that the pool of corregulators can differ according to the type of tissue, and it is the fact that has been proposed as an explanation for the differential tissue effects of estrogen and selective estrogen receptor modulator (SERMS).

Moreover, not only do corregulators differ according to tissue, the distribution of ERα and ERβ has also been reported to vary. In the tissues when both ERα and ERβ coexist, their effects seem to counteract each other. Thus, in the uterus, mammary glands and the immune systems, ERα promotes cell proliferation while ERβ has proapoptotic and cell differentiation functions (Morani et al., 2008).

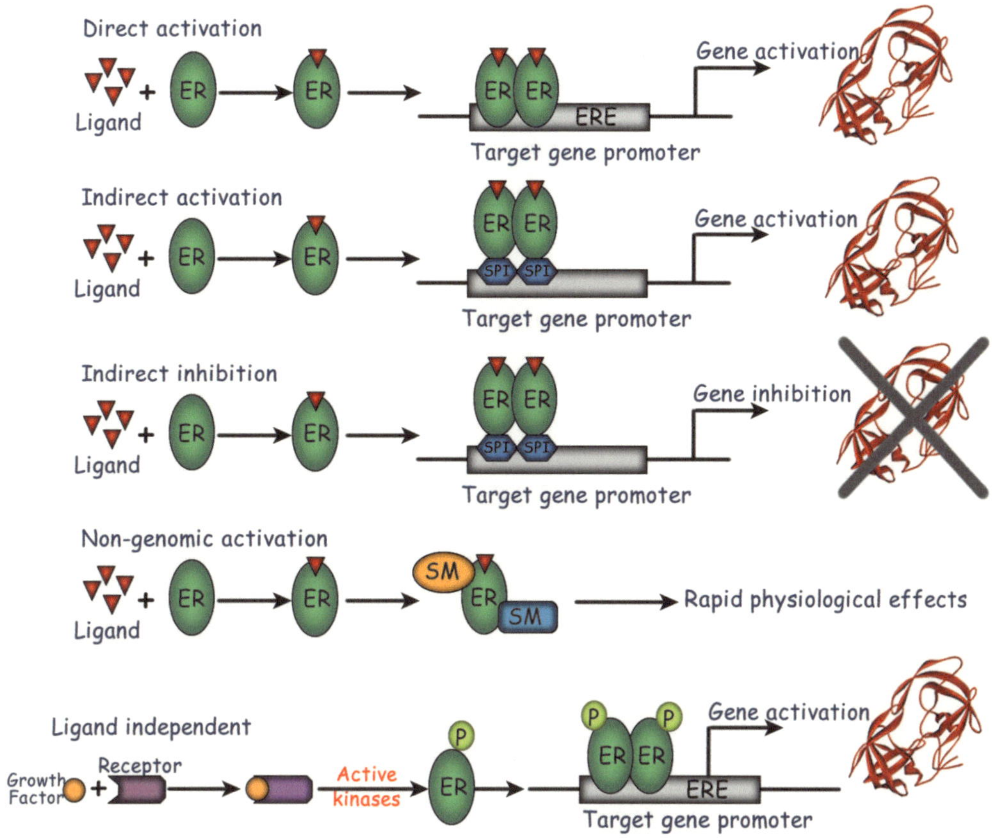

Fig. 2. Mechanisms ER activation.

3. Breast cancer and estrogens

3.1 Mammary gland and estrogens

Development and physiology of the mammary gland are under estrogen control and suffers important changes during a women's lifespan and estrogens have an active role in these changes. During puberty the glands undergoes an increased cellular division and in adult life there is a proliferation/involution cycle according to menstrual cycle (Russo et al., 1999). The role of estrogen in mammary epithelial proliferation has been unclear, because the proliferation markers in ductal epithelial cells never co localize with ERα (Saji et al., 2000). For a long time, estrogens were believed to induce proliferation through indirect effects, such as growth factor secretion to the stroma. However, recent studies suggest that when ERα is activated by estrogen it is quickly lost in the beginning of the G1 phase of the cell cycle. This fact could be explain the non-colocalisation of ERα with proliferation markers, such as cyclin A or PCNA, tipycal from the S phase (Morani et al., 2008).
Ductal cells in the mammary gland appear to be one example of cells where ERα and ERβ counteract each other in estrogen-stimulated proliferation. The proliferative response to E_2 seems to be determined by the ratio of ERα / ERβ. The functions of ERβ in the breast are probably related to its antiproliferative as well as its prodifferentiative functions (Strom et al., 2004).

In studies with MCF7 cells, a breast cancer cell line expressing ERα but not ERβ, showed that E_2 increases proliferation, and when ERβ was artificially introduced into these cells, E_2-induced proliferation was inhibited (Schatz, 1979).

3.2 Breast cancer estrogen induction

Estrogens are a major risk factor for breast cancer initiation and progression, as they affect epithelial mammary cell growth and these cells are more susceptible to make DNA replication errors. Another point of view is that estrogens produce oxidant species for their metabolism (quinine metabolites) that can form adducts in DNA and generate reactive oxygen species (ROS) through a redox cycle (Russo et al., 2003; Yager and Davidson, 2006).

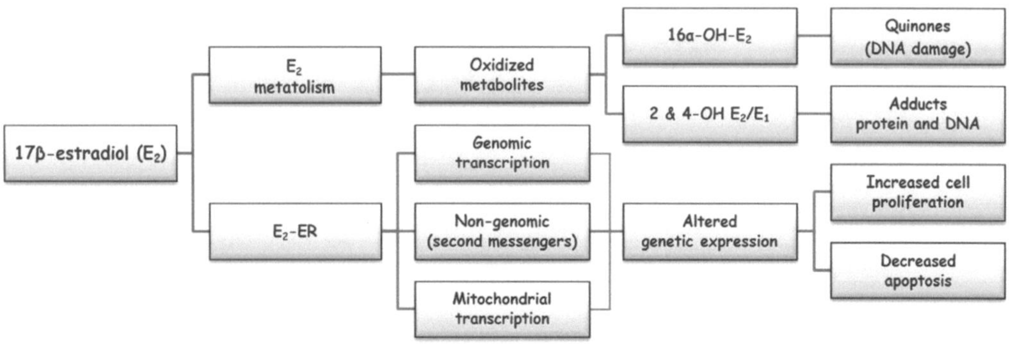

Fig. 3. Estrogen carcinogenesis mechanisms: E_2: 17β-estradiol. ER: estrogen receptor. 16α-OH-E_2: 16α-hydroxyE_2. 2-OH-E_2: 2-hydroxyE_2. 4-OH-E_2: 4-hydroxyE_2. 2-OH-E_1 2-hydroxyestrone. 4-OH-E_1 4-hydroxyestrone.

In recent years, EREs have been found in mitochondrial DNA, suggesting that the carcinogenic role of estrogen could be mediated by the action of these molecules in the mitochondria (Gonzalez et al., 1993; Sogl et al., 2000). Moreover, as mentioned earlier, the two subtypes of estrogen receptors have different actions in several tissues and therefore it is entirely possible that the effects will differ in mitochondria as well. Other papers have studied the localization of ERα and ERβ in the mitochondria and the regulation of mitochondrial genes (Gonzalez et al., 1993; Sogl et al., 2000; Chen et al., 2004; Pedram et al., 2006; Amutha et al., 2009; Usmanova et al., 2011). Furthermore, apoptotic pathways and the presence of estrogen receptor in the mitochondria could be important for carcinogenic processes (Gonzalez et al., 1993; Sogl et al., 2000).

The majority of ER-positive breast tumours contain both ERα and ERβ subtypes, although some tumours have only ERβ and may have distinct clinical behaviours and responses. In contrast to ERα, studies suggest that ERβ expression declines during breast tumourigenesis (Roger et al., 2001; Skliris et al., 2003; Bardin et al., 2004; Hartman et al., 2009). The mechanism by which ERβ is downregulated is not fully understood, but epigenetic changes could play an important role (Zhao et al., 2003). This downregulation of ERβ in breast cancers indicates a role for ERβ as a tumour suppressor (Novelli et al., 2008; Fox et al., 2008). Characterization of the role of ERβ in ERα negative tumors is basically unexplored, but available data suggest that the role of ERβ may differ depending if it is co-expressed with ERα or expressed alone (Fox et al., 2008; Skliris et al., 2008; Hartman et al., 2009). Classically, the ERα negative tumors are considered endocrine resistant since they lack a receptor to mediate the estrogenic response. However, it has been observed that approximately 50% of this subgroup expresses ERβ (Skliris et al., 2006). Several studies have been published different conclusions for correlations with ERβ, prognostic markers and clinical outcome. Reports have shown that tumours that co-expressed ERβ and ERα have a good prognosis and good clinical outcome with adjuvant therapy. Additional studies have considered the addition of ERβ to ERα as clinical tumor marker as beneficial (Murphy and Watson, 2006; Skliris et al., 2006; Gruvberger-Saal et al., 2007; Skliris et al., 2008; Hartman et al., 2009). Conversely, very few studies have focused on ERβ expression in ERα negative breast tumors; where ERβ has been described as a marker for poor prognosis and endocrine resistance (Leygue et al., 1998; Speirs et al., 1999; O'Neill et al., 2004; Skliris et al., 2006; Fox et al., 2008; Skliris et al., 2008; Hartman et al., 2009) (table 1).

ERα and ERβ status	Clinical outcome
ERα+/ ERβ+	Increased overall survival and disease-free survival correlated ERβ+
ERα+/ ERβ-	Worst prognosis
ERα-/ ERβ+	Less favorable prognosis, ERβ seems to correlate with the proliferation

Table 1. Clinical correlation between ERα/ ERβ expression and evaluation response to endocrine therapy in breast cancer.

An increased ERα/ERβ ratio respect to non tumoral breast tissue is an important factor for the development of the cancerous phenotype (Stossi et al., 2004; Strom et al., 2004; Adam et al., 2006; Garcia-Roves et al., 2007; Morani et al., 2008). On the contrary, a decrease in this ratio (due to ERβ increase) is indicative of a poor prognosis and problems with antiestrogen treatment (Power and Thompson, 2003). This evidence could also explain the different action of estrogens and phytoestrogens through varing ERα and ERβ levels (Sotoca et al., 2008).

Another difference between ERα and ERβ is estrogen activation, because estrogen stimulates both ERα and ERβ receptors, although it is 10 times more selective for ERα than ERβ (Kuiper et al., 1998; Quaedackers et al., 2001). Furthermore, several authors shave shown that estrogen regulation of ERα and ERβ expression, causing a decrease in ERα and an increase in ERβ in ERα-positive cell lines such as MCF-7 and T47D (Power and Thompson, 2003; Lee et al., 2005). In addition to this important fact, oxidative stress also regulates ERα and ERβ levels, and in the same manner, causes downregulation of ERα and upregulation of ERβ (Tamir et al., 2002).

4. Estrogens, mitochondria and oxidative stress

Classically, it has been suggested that estrogens induce growth in mammary gland epithelial cells. This high cell proliferation can increase susceptibility to the acquirement of error-induced mutations during DNA replication, which if not corrected can establish a malignant phenotype (Gonzalez et al., 1993). Another mechanism to explain this association is that estrogens can produce genotoxic metabolites during their metabolism (cathecol estrogens), that can make DNA adducts and create ROS through redox cycle (Russo et al., 2003; Yager and Davidson, 2006), but for these compounds to have a relevant impact, the estrogen concentration must be higher than physiological levels.

Recently, ERs have been found in the mitochondria, and in mitochondrial DNA there are EREs. Moreover, mitochondrial biogenesis and ROS production are under estrogen influence. For this reason, some authors give estrogens a new role in the carcinogenesis process, in the modulation of mitochondrial function (Addison and McCormick, 1978; Sogl et al., 2000). The changes in mitochondrial function cause an increase in ROS production, which alters the control that mitochondria exerts in cellular proliferation and apoptosis, and which could explain the action of estrogen in cancer development (Addison and McCormick, 1978; Gonzalez et al., 1993).

4.1 Mitochondria

Mitochondria are important organelles in eukaryotic cells. The structure of the mitochondrion is delimited by an outer and inner membrane. The former is wrinkled and completely surrounds the organelle. The later has infolding called cristae where the mitochondrial respiratory chain (MRC) resides. The inner compartment of mitochondria, the matrix, is a concentrated aqueous solution of many enzymes and chemical intermediates involved in energy-yielding metabolism. The outer membrane is a relatively simple phospholipid bilayer, containing protein structures called porins which render it permeable to molecules of about 10 kDA or less (the size of the smallest proteins). Ions, nutrient molecules, ATP, ADP, etc. can pass through the outer membrane with ease. The inner membrane is only freely permeable to oxygen, carbon dioxide, and water. Its structure is highly complex, including all of the complexes of the electron transport system, the ATP synthase complex and transport proteins.

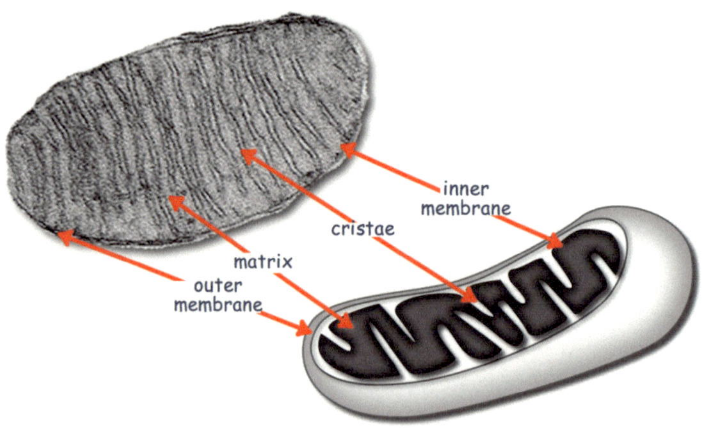

Fig. 4. Mitochondrial structure.

Mitochondria are the intracellular organelles responsible for the supply of ATP (generation of more than 90% of the cell's energy requirements) and are also the main intracellular source and target of reactive oxygen species (ROS). Mitochondria also participate in the regulation of intracellular calcium homeostasis by controlling various ion channels and transporters and participation in heme and steroid biosynthesis. In addition, mitochondria play a role in the regulation of cellular proliferation and apoptosis (Gonzalez et al., 1993).
The primary role of mitochondria is the generation of ATP through a complex process of controlled substrate degradation and oxygen consumption known as oxidative phosphorylation (OXPHOS) (Korb and Neupert, 1978). The inner membrane mitochondrial contains the large protein complexes that are necessary for energy transduction and ATP synthesis. Briefly, oxidation of reduced nutrient molecules, such as carbohydrates, lipids,

and proteins, through cellular metabolism yields electrons in the form of the reduced hydrogen carriers $NADH^+$ and $FADH_2$. These reduced cofactors donate electrons to a series of protein complexes of the electron transport chain embedded in the inner mitochondrial membrane. These complexes (complex I, III and IV) use the energy released from electron transport for the active pumping of protons across the inner membrane, thereby generating an electrochemical gradient. The ultimate destiny of these electrons is the reduction of molecular oxygen at complex IV to yield a molecule of water, whereas the energy, conserved as a proton gradient, is used by the F_0F_1 ATP synthase (or complex V) to phosphorylate ADP through the return of protons into the mitochondrial matrix (Devenish et al., 1978).

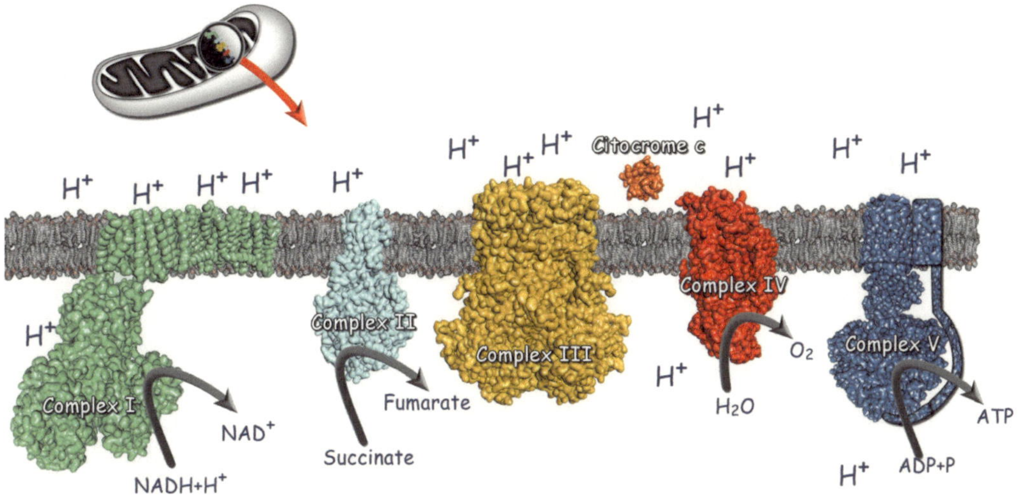

Fig. 5. The mitochondrial oxidative phosphorylation system.

Although mitochondria have their own genome, most of the proteins and enzymes that reside in the mitochondrial membranes are nuclear gene products. Each mammalian cell contains several hundred to more than a thousand mitochondria, and each organelle harbours 2–10 copies of mitochondrial DNA (mtDNA) (Amutha et al., 2008). The double-strand circular mtDNA consists of 16,500 base pairs (bp). This DNA encodes 13 protein coding genes (or polypeptides), 22 transfer RNA (or tRNA) and 2 ribosomal RNA (or rRNA) necessary for the translation. The 13 polypeptides including seven subunits of complex I-NADH dehydrogenase (ND1, ND2, ND3, ND4, ND4L, ND5, and ND6), three subunits of complex III-cytochrome c oxidase (COI, COII, and COIII), two subunits of complex V-F_0F_1ATPase (ATPase 6 and ATPase 8), and cytochrome b are encoded by mtDNA and synthesized in the organelle (Molina-Navarro et al., 2006). A single major noncoding region, referred to as the displacement loop (D-loop), contains the primary regulatory sequences for transcription and imitation of replication (Menassa et al., 1997). mtDNA is first transcribed to a larger mitochondrial transcript precursor, from which the 13 mRNAs, 22 tRNAs and 2 rRNAs are derived (Menassa et al., 1997).

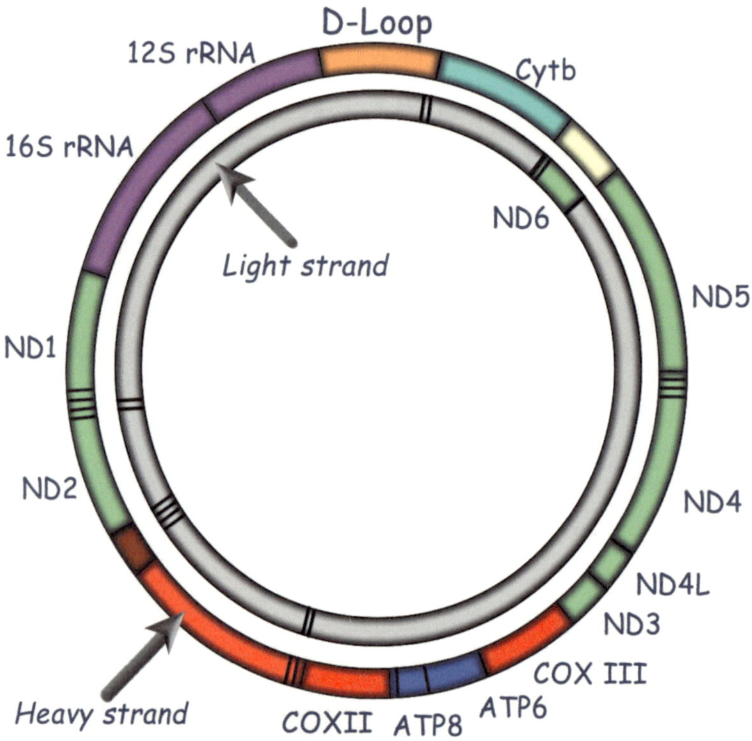

Fig. 6. The mitochondrial genome. The mammalian mitochondrial genome is a circular double stranded molecule, composed of one heavy and one light strand.

The assembly and functioning of the respiratory enzyme complexes in mammalian cells require coordinated expression and interaction between gene products of the mitochondrial and nuclear genomes (Menassa et al., 1997). Correct mitochondrial biogenesis relies on the spatiotemporally coordinated synthesis and import of ~1000 proteins encoded by the nuclear genome, of which some are assembled with proteins encoded by mitochondrial DNA within the newly synthesized phospholipid membranes of the inner and outer mitochondrial membranes. (Klingenspor et al., 1996).

	Complex I	Complex II	Complex III	Complex IV	Complex V
mtDNA	7	0	1	3	2
nDNA	39	4	9	10	10

Table 2. Nuclear and mitochondrial respiratory subunits.

Transcription and replication of mitochondrial DNA is driven by the nuclear-encoded mitochondrial transcription factor A (TFAM), which binds to a common upstream enhancer of the promoter sites of the two mitochondrial DNA strands. (Klingenspor et al., 1996) Additionally, two proteins that interact with the mammalian mitochondrial RNA polymerase and TFAM, TFB1M and TFB2M, can support promoter-specific mtDNA transcription (Addya et al., 1997). Nuclear respiratory factors 1 and 2 control (NRF1 and NRF2) play an important role in the regulation of mitochondrial respiratory function, as they on one hand control nuclear transcription of the subunits of the respiratory chain complexes (Schuster, 1994) as well as activate the expression of factors involved in the initiation of transcription of the mitochondrial genome, such as TFAM, and TFB2M TFB1M (Addya et al., 1997).

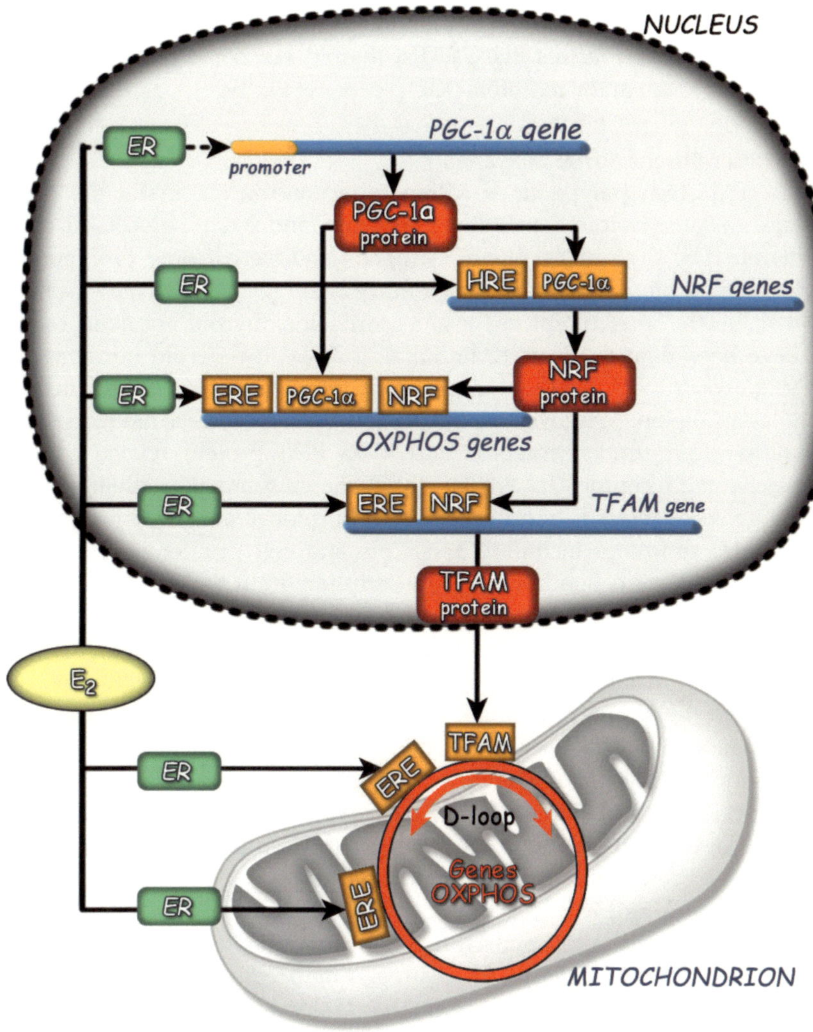

Fig. 7. Coordination of transcription of nuclear and mitochondrial genes encoding OXPHOS by steroid hormones.

The TFAM promoter contains recognition sites for NRF1 and/or NRF2, thus allowing coordination between mitochondrial and nuclear activation during mitochondrial biogenesis. However, there is a subset of genes that does not appear to be regulated by NRFs. For example, fatty acid transport proteins and oxidation enzyme genes are mainly regulated by the peroxisome proliferator-activated receptor alpha PPARα (Klingenspor et al., 1996).

Peroxisome proliferator-activated receptor gamma co-activator (PGC-1α) lacks DNA-binding activity but interacts with and co-activates numerous transcription factors including NRFs on the promoter of TFAM. Mitochondrial biogenesis and respiration are stimulated by PGC-1α through a powerful induction of NRF1 and NRF2 gene expression (Giege et al., 2008). Data are accumulating that show PGC-1α to be a master regulator of mitochondrial biogenesis in mammals (Klingenspor et al., 1996). In addition to NRFs, PGC-1α also interacts with and co-activates other transcription factors like PPARs, thyroid hormone, glucocorticoid, estrogen, and estrogen-related ERRα and γ receptors (Klingenspor et al., 1996).

4.2 Estrogen and mitochondrial biogenesis

The synthesis of thirteen polypeptides within mitochondria are under the regulation of hormones and other factors, including cortisol, androgen, glucocorticoids, 1,25α-dihydroxyvitamin D3, thyroid hormone, estrogens and peroxisome proliferators, which have profound effects on mitochondrial respiratory chain (MRC) activities (Gonzalez et al., 1993; Sogl et al., 2000). Thus, receptors for glucocorticoids, thyroid hormone, estrogens and androgens have been detected in mitochondrial and specific steroid hormone responsive elements for glucocorticoids, thyroid hormone and estrogen are found in the human mtDNA regulatory region. Moreover the ligand-activated glucocorticoid receptor, a variant form of the thyroid hormone receptor and a 45 kDa protein related to peroxisome proliferation-activated receptor γ2, have each been shown to mediate stimulatory effects on mitochondrial gene expression. In addition, these hormones and their receptors control a number of cellular processes including apoptosis and cell proliferation. It is likely that hormonal regulation of mitochondrial gene transcription occur through mechanisms similar to those that control nuclear gene transcription. These insights have extended our understanding of hormone action at the cellular level (Gonzalez et al., 1993).

In the last years, there has been increasing evidence pointing to the MRC as a novel and important target for the actions of E_2 and ERs in a number of cell types and tissues that have high demand for mitochondrial energy metabolism for their biological activities. This novel E2-mediated mitochondrial pathway involves the cooperation of the nuclear ERα and ERβ with mitochondrial localized ERs and their co-activators on the coordinate regulation of both-encoded genes and mtDNA-encoded genes for MRC proteins (Sogl et al., 2000).

ERα and ERβ have been detected in the mitochondria of several human cells, including breast cancer cells such as MCF7 (Chen et al., 2004; Pedram et al., 2006). Thus estrogens regulate the biogenesis and mitochondrial function through cross-talk between the nucleus and the mitochondria to control the estrogen-induced signaling involved in the proliferation, apoptosis and differentiation cellular (Felty and Roy, 2005). E_2 stimulates the expression of TFAM and possibly TFB1M and TFB2M via the activation of NRF-1 and NRF-2, and it is likely that E_2 and ERs stimulate the transcription via activation of the expression of these mitochondrial transcriptional factors (Sogl et al., 2000). Moreover, it has been found that E_2 significantly enhanced the amounts of mitochondrial ERα and ERβ in a time- and concentration-dependent manner and that these effects are accompanied by a significant increase in the transcript levels of mtDNA-encoded genes (Chen et al., 2004).

4.3 Estrogen and mitochondrial ROS production

Mitochondrial ROS production is under estrogen influence and the consequences of this production in the control that mitochondria exerts in cellular proliferation and apoptosis could be explain the action of estrogen in cancer development (Gonzalez et al., 1993; Sogl et al., 2000).

Mitochondria are the most important source of ROS production in mammalian cells, as under normal physiological conditions about 1% of electrons during transfer along the respiratory chain, escape and form a single electron reduction of molecular oxygen to form a superoxide anion ($O2^{\bullet-}$), which in turn is the precursor of other ROS (Fariss et al., 2005; Murphy, 2009). Aerobic respiration involves the complete reduction of oxygen to water, which is catalyzed by complex IV (or cytochrome c oxidase). Superoxide is rapidly converted to hydrogen peroxide (H_2O_2), either spontaneously or is enzymatically catalyzed by superoxide dismutase (SOD). H_2O_2, although not an oxygen free radical, can lead to the production, in the presence of ferrous iron via the Fenton reaction, of the highly reactive hydroxyl radical ($^{\bullet}OH$). ROS production can be significantly enhanced with a high mitochondrial potential membrane that can occur with abundant fuel supply (high NADH production) or with the functional impairment of complexes I or III of respiratory chain, while ROS production decreased with reduced energy demand (Lenaz, 2001; Chen et al., 2003; Fariss et al., 2005).

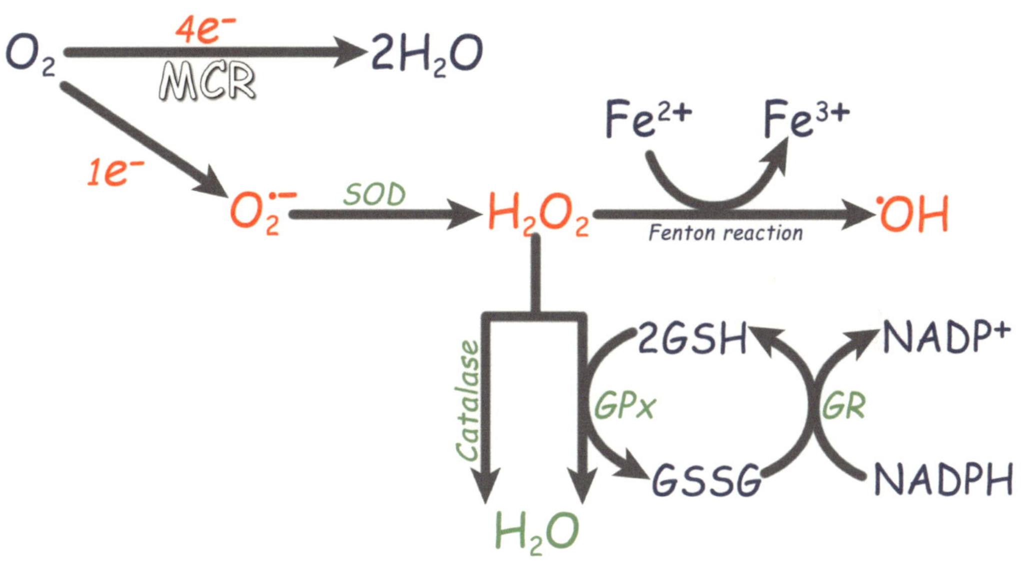

Fig. 8. ROS detoxification mechanisms.

ROS can be dissipated by the action of several enzymes, as SOD, glutation peroxidase (GPx) and glutation reductase (GR). SOD transforms $O2^{\bullet-}$ in H_2O_2, which is detoxified by the action of two enzymes, catalase and GPx yielding H_2O. Glutathione (GSH) is regenerated from glutathione disulfide (GSSG) by the action of GR, using NADPH as a reducing equivalent. Non-enzymatic antioxidants (as vitamins C and E) provide alternative targets to ROS reactivity, thus avoiding the deleterious effects on cell components (Fariss et al., 2005; Murphy, 2009).

Another mechanism to be included within the systems that can protect against oxidative damage are the uncoupling proteins or UCPs (Addison and McCormick, 1978; Echtay, 2007).

UCPs are a family of inner mitochondrial membrane proteins whose function is to allow the re-entry of protons into the mitochondrial matrix dissipate the proton gradient and, subsequently, decrease the membrane potential and ROS production (Addison and McCormick, 1978; Echtay, 2007).

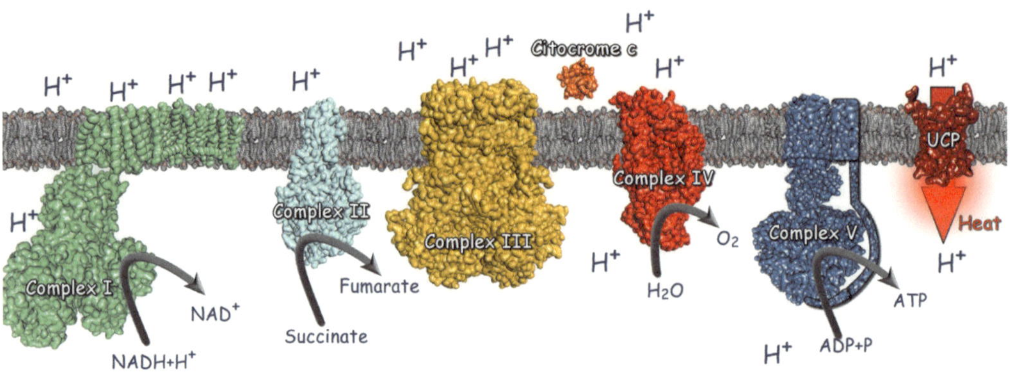

Fig. 9. Mitochondrial oxidative phosphorylation system and uncoupling protein.

When cellular production of ROS overwhelms the overall antioxidant defenses, free radicals may escape and exert their deleterious effects. This situation is oxidative stress, and is supposed to be responsible for the accrual of cellular damage during its lifetime, thereby playing a role in the etiogenesis and course of numerous pathologies and in the aging process (Addison and McCormick, 1978; Lenaz, 2001). Macromolecules within the mitochondria are more prone to ROS-induced damage due to their physical proximity to ROS sources. In addition, mitochondrial DNA, which lacks protective histone shields and also has limited DNA-repair systems, is especially vulnerable to such damage. It is worth noting that the damage exerted by ROS on mitochondrial DNA may lead to a higher degree of mitochondrial dysfunction and in turn, to a higher ROS production, leading to a vicious cycle of ROS amplification (Fariss et al., 2005).

Nevertheless, ROS should not be seen only in a negative light or as just damaging to molecules. It is worth noting that the rapidly-produced, short-lived, and highly diffusible ROS also perfectly fits the characteristics of a second messenger molecule. In fact, although ROS do cause damage, low levels of ROS are thought to participate in cell signaling processes such as cell proliferation, inflammation, apoptosis and phagocytosis (Obbink et al., 1977). Thus, it is well established by many studies that ROS may act as second messengers in cellular signaling transduction cascade pathways, including stress-activated protein kinases (SAPK) with both p38MAPK and c-Jun N-terminal kinase (JNK), p53 (universal sensor of genotoxic stress) through PI3K/PKB and NF-κB pathways (Harkness et al., 1994; Sauer et al., 2001; Martindale and Holbrook, 2002; Sanders et al., 2004; Murphy, 2009). In this complex context, low levels of ROS stimulate cellular proliferation, while high levels induce apoptosis. In summary, many cellular signal pathways are sensible to ROS levels and the final cellular response depends on the final cell interpretation, which is the result of equilibrium between apoptotic signals and proliferative and survival signals (Addison and McCormick, 1978).

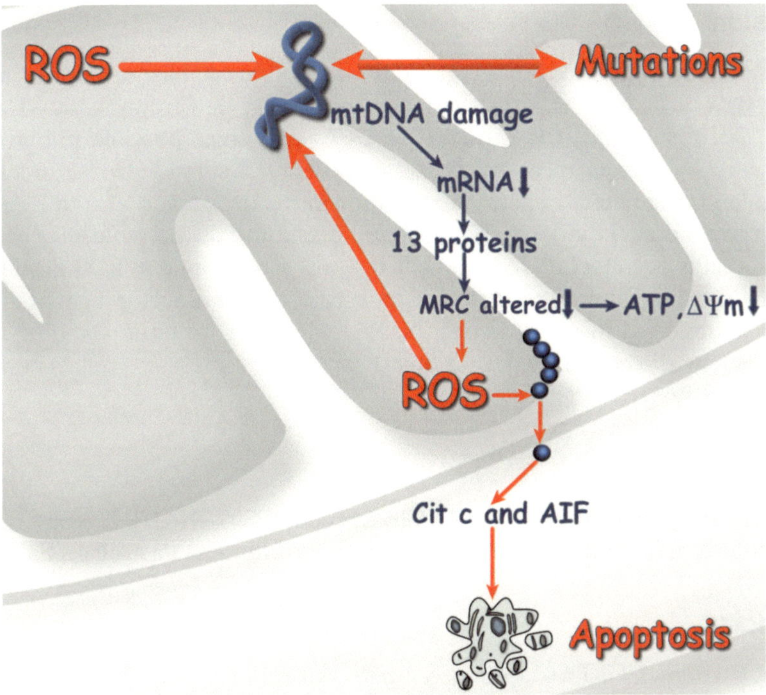

Fig. 10. Mitochondrial DNA and oxidative stress and apoptosis.

Estrogens can mediate in the complex process of ROS cellular level control. Thus, estrogens control mitochondrial biogenesis and maintenance, which are induced by signal pathways related to cellular proliferation, differentiation and apoptosis (Gonzalez et al., 1993). Moreover, mitochondrial ROS production can be regulated by estrogens through both nuclear and mitochondrial ER, with regulation by these via mitochondrial structure and function (Vic et al., 1982; Tam and Wong, 1991). Additionally estrogen controls the ROS dissipation, since expression of antioxidant enzymes and UCPs are induced by ERE (Chen et al., 2004). However, the literature is contradictory in this aspect, as the effect depends on tissue studied, estrogen concentration and *in vitro* or *in vivo* studies. For example, while oxidative stress induction in breast and prostate cancer cell lines has been described, in liver, brain, skeletal and cardiac muscle as well as adipose tissue, a protector role has been described to estrogen for the avoidance of oxidative stress (Valle et al., 2005; Colom et al., 2007a; Colom et al., 2007b; Valle et al., 2007a; Valle et al., 2007b; Guevara et al., 2008; Valle et al., 2008). This controversy could be attributed to the different ERα and ERβ ratios in different tissues. Thus in MCF7 breast cancer cell lines (with a high ratio of ERα/ERβ) estrogen induces oxidative stress either by or in combination with mitochondrial dysfunction, decrease in antioxidant enzymes and/or UCPs. On the contrary, in MDA-MB-231 breast cancer cell lines (with only ERα) no effects have been detected in the same conditions (Garcia-Roves et al., 2007). In addition it has been described , for prostrate cell lines which had the greatest levels of ERβ and the lowest ERα/ERβ ratio, that E_2 treatment caused the up-regulation of antioxidant enzymes and UCPs with a look-up decrease in ROS production. These effects were reversed when the cells were treated with E_2 in the presence of an ERβ antagonist (Houstek et al., 1990).

5. Conclusion

ERα and ERβ endowment can be of great importance in the establishment of oxidative stress in mitochondria, and may explain the opposite effects of estrogens found in different tissues. On the other hand, the presence of UCPs and their possible implication in the oxidative balance of breast cancer cell lines is notable and it should also be underscored that UCP expression is regulated, or sensible to, estrogen regulation and also to ERα/ERβ ratio. For the above mentioned evidence, a better understanding of the molecular action of ERα and ERβ, especially at mitochondrial level, is needed, as their role in ROS production could explain both the implication of estrogen in breast cancer development and its cancer protective role observed in other tissues. Additionally, a better understanding at this level could provide new dietary strategies for breast cancer prevention as well as new anticancer therapeutic procedures.

6. Acknowledgment

This work was supported by the Spanish Government (PS09/01637). J. Sastre-Serra and M. Nadal-Serrano were funded by grants of Comunidad Autónoma de las Islas Baleares.

7. References

Adam, A.C., Bornhovd, C., Prokisch, H., Neupert, W., & Hell, K. (2006). The Nfs1 interacting protein Isd11 has an essential role in Fe/S cluster biogenesis in mitochondria. *EMBO Journal,* Vol.25. No.1, (Jan 11). pp. 174-183, ISSN 0261-4189.

Addison, R., & McCormick, D.B. (1978). Biogenesis of flavoprotein and cytochrome components in hepatic mitochondria from riboflavin-deficient rats. *Biochemical and Biophysical Research Communications,* Vol.81. No.1, (Mar 15). pp. 133-138, ISSN 0006-291X.

Addya, S., Anandatheerthavarada, H.K., Biswas, G., Bhagwat, S.V., Mullick, J., & Avadhani, N.G. (1997). Targeting of NH2-terminal-processed microsomal protein to mitochondria: a novel pathway for the biogenesis of hepatic mitochondrial P450MT2. *Journal of Cell Biology,* Vol.139. No.3, (Nov 3). pp. 589-599, ISSN 0021-9525.

Amutha, B., Gordon, D.M., Dancis, A., & Pain, D. (2009). Chapter 14 Nucleotide-dependent iron-sulfur cluster biogenesis of endogenous and imported apoproteins in isolated intact mitochondria. *Methods in Enzymology,* Vol.456. pp. 247-266, ISSN 1557-7988.

Amutha, B., Gordon, D.M., Gu, Y., Lyver, E.R., Dancis, A., & Pain, D. (2008). GTP is required for iron-sulfur cluster biogenesis in mitochondria. *Journal of Biological Chemistry,* Vol.283. No.3, (Jan 18). pp. 1362-1371, ISSN 0021-9258.

Bardin, A., Boulle, N., Lazennec, G., Vignon, F., & Pujol, P. (2004). Loss of ERbeta expression as a common step in estrogen-dependent tumor progression. *Endocrine-Related Cancer,* Vol.11. No.3, (Sep). pp. 537-551, ISSN 1351-0088.

Catalano, S., Marsico, S., Giordano, C., Mauro, L., Rizza, P., Panno, M.L., & Ando, S. (2003). Leptin enhances, via AP-1, expression of aromatase in the MCF-7 cell line. *Journal of Biological Chemistry,* Vol.278. No.31, (Aug 1). pp. 28668-28676, ISSN 0021-9258.

Colom, B., Alcolea, M.P., Valle, A., Oliver, J., Roca, P., & Garcia-Palmer, F.J. (2007). Skeletal muscle of female rats exhibit higher mitochondrial mass and oxidativephosphorylative capacities compared to males. *Cellular Physiology and Biochemistry,* Vol.19. No.1-4, pp. 205-212, ISSN 1015-8987.

Colom, B., Oliver, J., Roca, P., & Garcia-Palmer, F.J. (2007). Caloric restriction and gender modulate cardiac muscle mitochondrial H2O2 production and oxidative damage. *Cardiovascular Research,* Vol.74. No.3, (Jun 1). pp. 456-465, ISSN 0008-6363.

Chang, E.C., Charn, T.H., Park, S.H., Helferich, W.G., Komm, B., Katzenellenbogen, J.A., & Katzenellenbogen, B.S. (2008). Estrogen Receptors alpha and beta as determinants of gene expression: influence of ligand, dose, and chromatin binding. *Molecular Endocrinology,* Vol.22. No.5, (May). pp. 1032-1043, ISSN 0888-8809.

Chen, J.Q., Delannoy, M., Cooke, C., & Yager, J.D. (2004). Mitochondrial localization of ERalpha and ERbeta in human MCF7 cells. *American Journal of Physiology Endocrinology and Metabolism,* Vol.286. No.6, (Jun). pp. E1011-1022, ISSN 0193-1849.

Chen, Q., Vazquez, E.J., Moghaddas, S., Hoppel, C.L., & Lesnefsky, E.J. (2003). Production of reactive oxygen species by mitochondria: central role of complex III. *Journal of Biological Chemistry,* Vol.278. No.38, (Sep 19). pp. 36027-36031, ISSN 0021-9258.

Devenish, R.J., Englisn, K.J., Hall, R.M., Linnase, A.W., & Lukins, H.B. (1978). Biogenesis of mitochondria 49 identification and mapping of a new mitochondrial locus (tsr1) which maps within polar region of yeast mitochondrial genome. *Molecular and General Genetics,* Vol.161. No.3, (May 31). pp. 251-259, ISSN 0026-8925.

Devenish, R.J., Hall, R.M., Linnane, A.W., & Lukins, H.B. (1979). Biogenesis of mitochondria. 52. Deletions in petite strains occurring in the mitochondrial gene for the 21 S ribosomal RNA, that affect the properties of mitochondrial recombination. *Molecular and General Genetics,* Vol.174. No.3, (Jul 24). pp. 297-305, ISSN 0026-8925.

Echtay, K.S. (2007). Mitochondrial uncoupling proteins--what is their physiological role? *Free Radical Biology and Medicine,* Vol.43. No.10, (Nov 15). pp. 1351-1371, ISSN 0891-5849.

Ekbom, A., Hsieh, C.C., Lipworth, L., Adami, H.Q., & Trichopoulos, D. (1997). Intrauterine environment and breast cancer risk in women: a population-based study. *Journal of the National Cancer Institute,* Vol.89. No.1, (Jan 1). pp. 71-76, ISSN 0027-8874.

Ewertz, M., Duffy, S.W., Adami, H.O., Kvale, G., Lund, E., Meirik, O., Mellemgaard, A., Soini, I., & Tulinius, H. (1990). Age at first birth, parity and risk of breast cancer: a meta-analysis of 8 studies from the Nordic countries. *International Journal of Cancer,* Vol.46. No.4, (Oct 15). pp. 597-603, ISSN 0020-7136.

Fariss, M.W., Chan, C.B., Patel, M., Van Houten, B., & Orrenius, S. (2005). Role of mitochondria in toxic oxidative stress. *Molecular Interventions,* Vol.5. No.2, (Apr). pp. 94-111, ISSN 1534-0384.

Felty, Q., & Roy, D. (2005). Estrogen, mitochondria, and growth of cancer and non-cancer cells. *Journal of Carcinogenesis,* Vol.4. No.1, (Jan 15). pp. 1, ISSN 1477-316.

Ferlay, J., Autier, P., Boniol, M., Heanue, M., Colombet, M., & Boyle, P. (2007). Estimates of the cancer incidence and mortality in Europe in 2006. *Annals of Oncology,* Vol.18. No.3, (Mar). pp. 581-592, ISSN 0923-7534.

Fox, E.M., Davis, R.J., & Shupnik, M.A. (2008). ERbeta in breast cancer--onlooker, passive player, or active protector? *Steroids,* Vol.73. No.11, (Oct). pp. 1039-1051, ISSN 0039-128X.

Garcia-Roves, P., Huss, J.M., Han, D.H., Hancock, C.R., Iglesias-Gutierrez, E., Chen, M., & Holloszy, J.O. (2007). Raising plasma fatty acid concentration induces increased biogenesis of mitochondria in skeletal muscle. *Proceedings of the National Academy of Sciences of the United States of America,* Vol.104. No.25, (Jun 19). pp. 10709-10713, ISSN 0027-8424.

Garofalo, C., & Surmacz, E. (2006). Leptin and cancer. *Journal of Cellular Physiology,* Vol.207. No.1, (Apr). pp. 12-22, ISSN 0021-9541.

Giege, P., Grienenberger, J.M., & Bonnard, G. (2008). Cytochrome c biogenesis in mitochondria. *Mitochondrion,* Vol.8. No.1, (Jan). pp. 61-73, ISSN 1567-7249.

Giguere, V., Hollenberg, S.M., Rosenfeld, M.G., & Evans, R.M. (1986). Functional domains of the human glucocorticoid receptor. *Cell,* Vol.46. No.5, (Aug 29). pp. 645-652, ISSN 0092-8674.

Gonzalez, D.H., Bonnard, G., & Grienenberger, J.M. (1993). A gene involved in the biogenesis of c-type cytochromes is co-transcribed with a ribosomal protein gene in wheat mitochondria [corrected]. *Current Genetics,* Vol.24. No.3, (Sep). pp. 248-255, ISSN 0172-8083.

Green, S., Walter, P., Greene, G., Krust, A., Goffin, C., Jensen, E., Scrace, G., Waterfield, M., & Chambon, P. (1986). Cloning of the human oestrogen receptor cDNA. *Journal of Steroid Biochemistry and Molecular Biology,* Vol.24. No.1, (Jan). pp. 77-83, ISSN 0022-4731.

Greene, G.L., Nolan, C., Engler, J.P., & Jensen, E.V. (1980). Monoclonal antibodies to human estrogen receptor. *Proceedings of the National Academy of Sciences of the United States of America,* Vol.77. No.9, (Sep). pp. 5115-5119, ISSN 0027-8424.

Gruvberger-Saal, S.K., Bendahl, P.O., Saal, L.H., Laakso, M., Hegardt, C., Eden, P., Peterson, C., Malmstrom, P., Isola, J., Borg, A., & Ferno, M. (2007). Estrogen receptor beta expression is associated with tamoxifen response in ERalpha-negative breast carcinoma. *Clinical Cancer Research,* Vol.13. No.7, (Apr 1). pp. 1987-1994, ISSN 1078-0432.

Guevara, R., Santandreu, F.M., Valle, A., Gianotti, M., Oliver, J., & Roca, P. (2008). Sex-dependent differences in aged rat brain mitochondrial function and oxidative stress. *Free Radical Biology and Medicine.* (Oct 17). ISSN 0891-5849.

Gustafsson, J.A. (1999). Estrogen receptor beta--a new dimension in estrogen mechanism of action. *Journal of Endocrinology,* Vol.163. No.3, (Dec). pp. 379-383, ISSN 0022-0795.

Harkness, T.A., Nargang, F.E., van der Klei, I., Neupert, W., & Lill, R. (1994). A crucial role of the mitochondrial protein import receptor MOM19 for the biogenesis of mitochondria. *Journal of Cell Biology,* Vol.124. No.5, (Mar). pp. 637-648, ISSN 0021-9525.

Hartman, J., Strom, A., & Gustafsson, J.A. (2009). Estrogen receptor beta in breast cancer--diagnostic and therapeutic implications. *Steroids,* Vol.74. No.8, (Aug). pp. 635-641, ISSN 1878-5867.

Heldring, N., Pike, A., Andersson, S., Matthews, J., Cheng, G., Hartman, J., Tujague, M., Strom, A., Treuter, E., Warner, M., & Gustafsson, J.A. (2007). Estrogen receptors: how do they signal and what are their targets. *Physiological Reviews,* Vol.87. No.3, (Jul). pp. 905-931, ISSN 0031-9333.

Houstek, J., Kopecky, J., Baudysova, M., Janikova, D., Pavelka, S., & Klement, P. (1990). Differentiation of brown adipose tissue and biogenesis of thermogenic mitochondria in situ and in cell culture. *Biochimica et Biophysica Acta,* Vol.1018. No.2-3, (Jul 25). pp. 243-247, ISSN 0006-3002.

Jensen, E.V., Jacobson, H.I., Smith, S., Jungblut, P.W., & De Sombre, E.R. (1972). The use of estrogen antagonists in hormone receptor studies. *Gynecologic Investigation,* Vol.3. No.1, pp. 108-123, ISSN 0017-5986.

Jensen, E.V., Jacobson, H.I., Walf, A.A., & Frye, C.A. (2010). Estrogen action: a historic perspective on the implications of considering alternative approaches. *Physiology & Behavior,* Vol.99. No.2, (Feb 9). pp. 151-162, ISSN 1873-507X.

Kelsey, J.L., Gammon, M.D., & John, E.M. (1993). Reproductive factors and breast cancer. *Epidemiologic Reviews,* Vol.15. No.1, pp. 36-47, ISSN 0193-936X.

Key, T.J., Verkasalo, P.K., & Banks, E. (2001). Epidemiology of breast cancer. *The Lancet Oncology,* Vol.2. No.3, (Mar). pp. 133-140, ISSN 1470-2045.

Klingenspor, M., Ivemeyer, M., Wiesinger, H., Haas, K., Heldmaier, G., & Wiesner, R.J. (1996). Biogenesis of thermogenic mitochondria in brown adipose tissue of Djungarian hamsters during cold adaptation. *Biochemical Journal,* Vol.316 (Pt 2). (Jun 1). pp. 607-613, ISSN 0264-6021.

Korb, H., & Neupert, W. (1978). Biogenesis of cytochrome c in Neurospora crassa. Synthesis of apocytochrome c, transfer to mitochondria and conversion to Holocytochrome c. *European Journal of Biochemistry,* Vol.91. No.2, (Nov 15). pp. 609-620, ISSN 0014-2956.

Kuiper, G.G., Carlsson, B., Grandien, K., Enmark, E., Haggblad, J., Nilsson, S., & Gustafsson, J.A. (1997). Comparison of the ligand binding specificity and transcript tissue distribution of estrogen receptors alpha and beta. *Endocrinology,* Vol.138. No.3, (Mar). pp. 863-870, ISSN 0013-7227.

Kuiper, G.G., Enmark, E., Pelto-Huikko, M., Nilsson, S., & Gustafsson, J.A. (1996). Cloning of a novel receptor expressed in rat prostate and ovary. *Proceedings of the National Academy of Sciences of the United States of America,* Vol.93. No.12, (Jun 11). pp. 5925-5930, ISSN 0027-8424.

Kuiper, G.G., Lemmen, J.G., Carlsson, B., Corton, J.C., Safe, S.H., van der Saag, P.T., van der Burg, B., & Gustafsson, J.A. (1998). Interaction of estrogenic chemicals and phytoestrogens with estrogen receptor beta. *Endocrinology,* Vol.139. No.10, (Oct). pp. 4252-4263, ISSN 0013-7227.

Kumar, V., Green, S., Stack, G., Berry, M., Jin, J.R., & Chambon, P. (1987). Functional domains of the human estrogen receptor. *Cell,* Vol.51. No.6, (Dec 24). pp. 941-951, ISSN 0092-8674.

Kushner, P.J., Agard, D.A., Greene, G.L., Scanlan, T.S., Shiau, A.K., Uht, R.M., & Webb, P. (2000). Estrogen receptor pathways to AP-1. *Journal of Steroid Biochemistry and Molecular Biology,* Vol.74. No.5, (Nov 30). pp. 311-317, ISSN 0960-0760.

Lahmann, P.H., Hoffmann, K., Allen, N., van Gils, C.H., Khaw, K.T., Tehard, B., Berrino, F., Tjonneland, A., Bigaard, J., Olsen, A., Overvad, K., Clavel-Chapelon, F., Nagel, G., Boeing, H., Trichopoulos, D., Economou, G., Bellos, G., Palli, D., Tumino, R., Panico, S., Sacerdote, C., Krogh, V., Peeters, P.H., Bueno-de-Mesquita, H.B., Lund, E., Ardanaz, E., Amiano, P., Pera, G., Quiros, J.R., Martinez, C., Tormo, M.J., Wirfalt, E., Berglund, G., Hallmans, G., Key, T.J., Reeves, G., Bingham, S., Norat, T., Biessy, C., Kaaks, R., & Riboli, E. (2004). Body size and breast cancer risk: findings from the European Prospective Investigation into Cancer And Nutrition (EPIC). *International Journal of Cancer,* Vol.111. No.5, (Sep 20). pp. 762-771, ISSN 0020-7136.

Layde, P.M., Webster, L.A., Baughman, A.L., Wingo, P.A., Rubin, G.L., & Ory, H.W. (1989). The independent associations of parity, age at first full term pregnancy, and duration of breastfeeding with the risk of breast cancer. Cancer and Steroid Hormone Study Group. *Journal of Clinical Epidemiology,* Vol.42. No.10, pp. 963-973, ISSN 0895-4356.

Lee, Y.R., Park, J., Yu, H.N., Kim, J.S., Youn, H.J., & Jung, S.H. (2005). Up-regulation of PI3K/Akt signaling by 17beta-estradiol through activation of estrogen receptor-alpha, but not estrogen receptor-beta, and stimulates cell growth in breast cancer cells. *Biochemical and Biophysical Research Communications,* Vol.336. No.4, (Nov 4). pp. 1221-1226, ISSN 0006-291X.

Lenaz, G. (2001). The mitochondrial production of reactive oxygen species: mechanisms and implications in human pathology. *IUBMB Life,* Vol.52. No.3-5, (Sep-Nov). pp. 159-164, ISSN 1521-6543.

Leygue, E., Dotzlaw, H., Watson, P.H., & Murphy, L.C. (1998). Altered estrogen receptor alpha and beta messenger RNA expression during human breast tumorigenesis. *Cancer Research,* Vol.58. No.15, (Aug 1). pp. 3197-3201, ISSN 0008-5472.

Martindale, J.L., & Holbrook, N.J. (2002). Cellular response to oxidative stress: signaling for suicide and survival. *Journal of Cellular Physiology,* Vol.192. No.1, (Jul). pp. 1-15, ISSN 0021-9541.

McTiernan, A. (2003). Behavioral risk factors in breast cancer: can risk be modified? *Oncologist,* Vol.8. No.4, pp. 326-334, ISSN 1083-7159.

Menassa, R., El-Rouby, N., & Brown, G.G. (1997). An open reading frame for a protein involved in cytochrome c biogenesis is split into two parts in Brassica mitochondria. *Current Genetics,* Vol.31. No.1, (Jan). pp. 70-79, ISSN 0172-8083.

Molina-Navarro, M.M., Casas, C., Piedrafita, L., Belli, G., & Herrero, E. (2006). Prokaryotic and eukaryotic monothiol glutaredoxins are able to perform the functions of Grx5 in the biogenesis of Fe/S clusters in yeast mitochondria. *FEBS Letters,* Vol.580. No.9, (Apr 17). pp. 2273-2280, ISSN 0014-5793.

Morani, A., Warner, M., & Gustafsson, J.A. (2008). Biological functions and clinical implications of oestrogen receptors alfa and beta in epithelial tissues. *Journal of Internal Medicine,* Vol.264. No.2, (Aug). pp. 128-142, ISSN 1365-2796.

Murphy, L.C., & Watson, P.H. (2006). Is oestrogen receptor-beta a predictor of endocrine therapy responsiveness in human breast cancer? *Endocrine-Related Cancer,* Vol.13. No.2, (Jun). pp. 327-334, ISSN 1351-0088.

Murphy, M.P. (2009). How mitochondria produce reactive oxygen species. *Biochemical Journal,* Vol.417. No.1, (Jan 1). pp. 1-13, ISSN 1470-8728.

Nilsson, S., Makela, S., Treuter, E., Tujague, M., Thomsen, J., Andersson, G., Enmark, E., Pettersson, K., Warner, M., & Gustafsson, J.A. (2001). Mechanisms of estrogen action. *Physiological Reviews,* Vol.81. No.4, (Oct). pp. 1535-1565, ISSN 0031-9333.

Novelli, F., Milella, M., Melucci, E., Di Benedetto, A., Sperduti, I., Perrone-Donnorso, R., Perracchio, L., Venturo, I., Nistico, C., Fabi, A., Buglioni, S., Natali, P.G., & Mottolese, M. (2008). A divergent role for estrogen receptor-beta in node-positive and node-negative breast cancer classified according to molecular subtypes: an observational prospective study. *Breast Cancer Research,* Vol.10. No.5, pp. R74, ISSN 1465-5411.

O'Neill, P.A., Davies, M.P., Shaaban, A.M., Innes, H., Torevell, A., Sibson, D.R., & Foster, C.S. (2004). Wild-type oestrogen receptor beta (ERbeta1) mRNA and protein expression in Tamoxifen-treated post-menopausal breast cancers. *British Journal of Cancer,* Vol.91. No.9, (Nov 1). pp. 1694-1702, ISSN 0007-0920.

Obbink, D.J., Spithill, T.W., Maxwell, R.J., & Linnane, A.W. (1977). Biogenesis of mitochondria 48: mikamycin resistance in Saccharomyces cerevisiae--a mitochondrial mutation conferring resistance to an antimycin A-like contaminant in mikamycin. *Molecular and General Genetics,* Vol.151. No.2, (Mar 7). pp. 127-136, ISSN 0026-8925.

Pearce, S.T., & Jordan, V.C. (2004). The biological role of estrogen receptors alpha and beta in cancer. *Critical Reviews in Oncology/Hematology,* Vol.50. No.1, (Apr). pp. 3-22, ISSN 1040-8428.

Pedram, A., Razandi, M., Wallace, D.C., & Levin, E.R. (2006). Functional estrogen receptors in the mitochondria of breast cancer cells. *Molecular Biology of the Cell,* Vol.17. No.5, (May). pp. 2125-2137, ISSN 1059-1524.

Pharoah, P.D., Day, N.E., Duffy, S., Easton, D.F., & Ponder, B.A. (1997). Family history and the risk of breast cancer: a systematic review and meta-analysis. *International Journal of Cancer,* Vol.71. No.5, (May 29). pp. 800-809, ISSN 0020-7136.

Power, K.A., & Thompson, L.U. (2003). Ligand-induced regulation of ERalpha and ERbeta is indicative of human breast cancer cell proliferation. *Breast Cancer Research and Treatment,* Vol.81. No.3, (Oct). pp. 209-221, ISSN 0167-6806.

Quaedackers, M.E., Van Den Brink, C.E., Wissink, S., Schreurs, R.H., Gustafsson, J.A., Van Der Saag, P.T., & Van Der Burg, B.B. (2001). 4-hydroxytamoxifen trans-represses nuclear factor-kappa B activity in human osteoblastic U2-OS cells through estrogen receptor (ER)alpha, and not through ER beta. *Endocrinology,* Vol.142. No.3, (Mar). pp. 1156-1166, ISSN 0013-7227.

Roger, P., Sahla, M.E., Makela, S., Gustafsson, J.A., Baldet, P., & Rochefort, H. (2001). Decreased expression of estrogen receptor beta protein in proliferative preinvasive mammary tumors. *Cancer Research,* Vol.61. No.6, (Mar 15). pp. 2537-2541, ISSN 0008-5472.

Russo, J., Ao, X., Grill, C., & Russo, I.H. (1999). Pattern of distribution of cells positive for estrogen receptor alpha and progesterone receptor in relation to proliferating cells in the mammary gland. *Breast Cancer Research and Treatment,* Vol.53. No.3, (Feb). pp. 217-227, ISSN 0167-6806.

Russo, J., Hasan Lareef, M., Balogh, G., Guo, S., & Russo, I.H. (2003). Estrogen and its metabolites are carcinogenic agents in human breast epithelial cells. *Journal of Steroid Biochemistry and Molecular Biology,* Vol.87. No.1, (Oct). pp. 1-25, ISSN 0960-0760.

Saji, S., Jensen, E.V., Nilsson, S., Rylander, T., Warner, M., & Gustafsson, J.A. (2000). Estrogen receptors alpha and beta in the rodent mammary gland. *Proceedings of the National Academy of Sciences of the United States of America,* Vol.97. No.1, (Jan 4). pp. 337-342, ISSN 0027-8424.

Sanders, L.M., Henderson, C.E., Hong, M.Y., Barhoumi, R., Burghardt, R.C., Wang, N., Spinka, C.M., Carroll, R.J., Turner, N.D., Chapkin, R.S., & Lupton, J.R. (2004). An increase in reactive oxygen species by dietary fish oil coupled with the attenuation of antioxidant defenses by dietary pectin enhances rat colonocyte apoptosis. *The Journal of Nutrition,* Vol.134. No.12, (Dec). pp. 3233-3238, ISSN 0022-3166.

Sauer, H., Wartenberg, M., & Hescheler, J. (2001). Reactive oxygen species as intracellular messengers during cell growth and differentiation. *Cellular Physiology and Biochemistry,* Vol.11. No.4, pp. 173-186, ISSN 1015-8987.

Saville, B., Wormke, M., Wang, F., Nguyen, T., Enmark, E., Kuiper, G., Gustafsson, J.A., & Safe, S. (2000). Ligand-, cell-, and estrogen receptor subtype (alpha/beta)-dependent activation at GC-rich (Sp1) promoter elements. *Journal of Biological Chemistry,* Vol.275. No.8, (Feb 25). pp. 5379-5387, ISSN 0021-9258.

Schatz, G. (1979). Biogenesis of yeast mitochondria: synthesis of cytochrome c oxidase and cytochrome c. *Methods in Enzymology,* Vol.56. pp. 40-50, ISSN 0076-6879.

Schuster, W. (1994). The highly edited orf206 in Oenothera mitochondria may encode a component of a heme transporter involved in cytochrome c biogenesis. *Plant Molecular Biology,* Vol.25. No.1, (Apr). pp. 33-42, ISSN 0167-4412.

Sidhu, R.S., & Tauro, P. (1979). Biogenesis of mitochondria in yeast Saccharomyces cerevisiae: Part I--Nuclear control of mitochondria biogenesis. *Indian Journal of Experimental Biology,* Vol.17. No.1, (Jan). pp. 19-23, ISSN 0019-5189.

Skliris, G.P., Leygue, E., Curtis-Snell, L., Watson, P.H., & Murphy, L.C. (2006). Expression of oestrogen receptor-beta in oestrogen receptor-alpha negative human breast tumours. *British Journal of Cancer,* Vol.95. No.5, (Sep 4). pp. 616-626, ISSN 0007-0920.

Skliris, G.P., Leygue, E., Watson, P.H., & Murphy, L.C. (2008). Estrogen receptor alpha negative breast cancer patients: estrogen receptor beta as a therapeutic target. *Journal of Steroid Biochemistry and Molecular Biology,* Vol.109. No.1-2, (Mar). pp. 1-10, ISSN 0960-0760.

Skliris, G.P., Munot, K., Bell, S.M., Carder, P.J., Lane, S., Horgan, K., Lansdown, M.R., Parkes, A.T., Hanby, A.M., Markham, A.F., & Speirs, V. (2003). Reduced expression of oestrogen receptor beta in invasive breast cancer and its re-expression using DNA methyl transferase inhibitors in a cell line model. *The Journal of Pathology,* Vol.201. No.2, (Oct). pp. 213-220, ISSN 0022-3417.

Smith, E.P., Boyd, J., Frank, G.R., Takahashi, H., Cohen, R.M., Specker, B., Williams, T.C., Lubahn, D.B., & Korach, K.S. (1994). Estrogen resistance caused by a mutation in the estrogen-receptor gene in a man. *New England Journal of Medicine,* Vol.331. No.16, (Oct 20). pp. 1056-1061, ISSN 0028-4793.

Sogl, B., Gellissen, G., & Wiesner, R.J. (2000). Biogenesis of giant mitochondria during insect flight muscle development in the locust, Locusta migratoria (L.). Transcription, translation and copy number of mitochondrial DNA. *European Journal of Biochemistry,* Vol.267. No.1, (Jan). pp. 11-17, ISSN 0014-2956.

Sotoca, A.M., Ratman, D., van der Saag, P., Strom, A., Gustafsson, J.A., Vervoort, J., Rietjens, I.M., & Murk, A.J. (2008). Phytoestrogen-mediated inhibition of proliferation of the human T47D breast cancer cells depends on the ERalpha/ERbeta ratio. *Journal of Steroid Biochemistry and Molecular Biology,* Vol.112. No.4-5, (Dec). pp. 171-178, ISSN 0960-0760.

Speirs, V., Malone, C., Walton, D.S., Kerin, M.J., & Atkin, S.L. (1999). Increased expression of estrogen receptor beta mRNA in tamoxifen-resistant breast cancer patients. *Cancer Research,* Vol.59. No.21, (Nov 1). pp. 5421-5424, ISSN 0008-5472.

Spithill, T.W., Nagley, P., & Linnane, A.W. (1979). Biogenesis of mitochondria 51: biochemical characterization of a mitochondrial mutation in Saccharomyces cerevisiae affecting the mitochondrial ribosome by conferring resistance to aminoglycoside antibiotics. *Molecular and General Genetics,* Vol.173. No.2, (Jun 7). pp. 159-170, ISSN 0026-8925.

Stossi, F., Barnett, D.H., Frasor, J., Komm, B., Lyttle, C.R., & Katzenellenbogen, B.S. (2004). Transcriptional profiling of estrogen-regulated gene expression via estrogen receptor (ER) alpha or ERbeta in human osteosarcoma cells: distinct and common target genes for these receptors. *Endocrinology,* Vol.145. No.7, (Jul). pp. 3473-3486, ISSN 0013-7227.

Strom, A., Hartman, J., Foster, J.S., Kietz, S., Wimalasena, J., & Gustafsson, J.A. (2004). Estrogen receptor beta inhibits 17beta-estradiol-stimulated proliferation of the breast cancer cell line T47D. *Proceedings of the National Academy of Sciences of the United States of America,* Vol.101. No.6, (Feb 10). pp. 1566-1571, ISSN 0027-8424.

Tam, C.C., & Wong, Y.C. (1991). Ultrastructural study of the effects of 17 beta-oestradiol on the lateral prostate and seminal vesicle of the castrated guinea pig. *Acta Anatomica (Basel),* Vol.141. No.1, pp. 51-62, ISSN 0001-5180.

Tamir, S., Izrael, S., & Vaya, J. (2002). The effect of oxidative stress on ERalpha and ERbeta expression. *Journal of Steroid Biochemistry and Molecular Biology,* Vol.81. No.4-5, (Aug). pp. 327-332, ISSN 0960-0760.

Usmanova, N., Tomilin, N., Zhivotovsky, B., & Kropotov, A. (2011). Transcription factor GABP/NRF-2 controlling biogenesis of mitochondria regulates basal expression of peroxiredoxin V but the mitochondrial function of peroxiredoxin V is dispensable in the dog. *Biochimie,* Vol.93. No.2, (Feb). pp. 306-313, ISSN 1638-6183.

Valle, A., Catala-Niell, A., Colom, B., Garcia-Palmer, F.J., Oliver, J., & Roca, P. (2005). Sex-related differences in energy balance in response to caloric restriction. *American Journal of Physiology Endocrinology and Metabolism,* Vol.289. No.1, (Jul). pp. E15-22, ISSN 0193-1849.

Valle, A., Garcia-Palmer, F.J., Oliver, J., & Roca, P. (2007). Sex differences in brown adipose tissue thermogenic features during caloric restriction. *Cellular Physiology and Biochemistry,* Vol.19. No.1-4, pp. 195-204, ISSN 1015-8987.

Valle, A., Guevara, R., Garcia-Palmer, F.J., Roca, P., & Oliver, J. (2007). Sexual dimorphism in liver mitochondrial oxidative capacity is conserved under caloric restriction conditions. *American Journal of Physiology. Cell Physiology,* Vol.293. No.4, (Oct). pp. C1302-1308, ISSN 0363-6143.

Valle, A., Guevara, R., Garcia-Palmer, F.J., Roca, P., & Oliver, J. (2008). Caloric restriction retards the age-related decline in mitochondrial function of brown adipose tissue. *Rejuvenation Research,* Vol.11. No.3, (Jun). pp. 597-604, ISSN 1549-1684.

Vic, P., Vignon, F., Derocq, D., & Rochefort, H. (1982). Effect of estradiol on the ultrastructure of the MCF7 human breast cancer cells in culture. *Cancer Research,* Vol.42. No.2, (Feb). pp. 667-673, ISSN 0008-5472.

Walsh, T., & King, M.C. (2007). Ten genes for inherited breast cancer. *Cancer Cell,* Vol.11. No.2, (Feb). pp. 103-105, ISSN 1535-6108.

Walter, P., Green, S., Greene, G., Krust, A., Bornert, J.M., Jeltsch, J.M., Staub, A., Jensen, E., Scrace, G., Waterfield, M., & et al. (1985). Cloning of the human estrogen receptor cDNA. *Proceedings of the National Academy of Sciences of the United States of America,* Vol.82. No.23, (Dec). pp. 7889-7893, ISSN 0027-8424.

Yager, J.D., & Davidson, N.E. (2006). Estrogen carcinogenesis in breast cancer. *New England Journal of Medicine,* Vol.354. No.3, (Jan 19). pp. 270-282, ISSN 1533-4406.

Zhao, C., Lam, E.W., Sunters, A., Enmark, E., De Bella, M.T., Coombes, R.C., Gustafsson, J.A., & Dahlman-Wright, K. (2003). Expression of estrogen receptor beta isoforms in normal breast epithelial cells and breast cancer: regulation by methylation. *Oncogene*, Vol.22. No.48, (Oct 23). pp. 7600-7606, ISSN 0950-9232.

11

Heterogeneity of Phenotype in Breast Cancer Cell Lines

Bruce C. Baguley and Euphemia Leung
Auckland Cancer Society Research Centre, University of Auckland, New Zealand

1. Introduction

Breast cancer is a major challenge to current medicine; it is the disease with highest death rate in the female population and is even of significance to the male population. Although breast cancer is effectively treated by surgery at early stages, patients who present with breast cancer metastases at diagnosis or who subsequently develop metastatic disease have a much poorer prognosis. A feature of the normal breast endothelium is its regulation by the endocrine system; steroid hormones such as oestrogen are released predominantly by the ovary and control both proliferation and differentiation of epithelial cells. The proliferation of corresponding carcinoma cells that arise in early breast cancer has a similar dependence on endocrine hormones. Thus, one of the main methods for treating early breast cancer, apart from surgery, is to block the growth promoting action of oestrogen, either by blocking the downstream action with antioestrogens such as tamoxifen or by reducing the concentration of circulating oestrogen through oophorectomy or treatment with aromatase inhibitors. While such treatment is generally effective, the consequent emergence of aggressive tumours is common and poses a major barrier to successful disease management. Heterogeneity has been postulated to be a key property of both breast cancer and epithelial subtypes of normal breast tissue (Visvader, 2009). MCF-7, a commonly used breast cancer cell line, has been propagated for many years by multiple groups and it might be expected that such propagation would select a single phenotype that had the highest growth rate. However, the finding of extensive heterogeneity among MCF-7 lines used by different groups (Nugoli et al., 2003) suggests that mechanisms may be operating within proliferating MCF-7 populations to generate phenotypic diversity continuously. The aim of this chapter is to discuss the evidence of the way that the MCF-7 breast cancer cell line is heterogeneous with respect to both the expression of hormone receptors and to the utilization of the signalling pathways linked to these receptors. Such heterogeneity may be reflected by the presence of multiple phenotypes within a tumour population that differ markedly in their relative expression of receptors such as progesterone receptor (PR), oestrogen receptor (ER), epidermal growth factor receptor (EGFR) and epidermal growth factor receptor-2 (HER2; also known as ErbB2).

2. Detection of cellular heterogeneity in the MCF-7 breast cancer cell line

Several approaches have been employed to investigate phenotypic heterogeneity in MCF-7 cell lines. Cassanelli et al. (1995) isolated a series of individual MCF-7 clones and measured their expression of PR, finding that two thirds were PR-negative and that the remainder showed various degrees of PR expression. They also showed that PR expression was related to proliferation rate in culture. Coser et al. (2009) isolated multiple MCF-7 clones using two different culture conditions. Firstly, they picked individual colonies from low density MCF-7 cultures to establish antioestrogen-sensitive MCF-7 sub-lines. Secondly, they picked individual antioestrogen-resistant colonies from MCF-7 cultures that had previously been grown to high density and exposed to either 4-hydroxytamoxifen (1 μM) or to fulvestrant (10–100 nM) for 21 days. The surviving cells (less than 0.001% of the population) were allowed to recover in drug-free growth medium for 7 days before isolation of the colonies, and all sub-lines subsequently characterized within a 20 population doubling period of culture. The isolated sub-lines could be distinguished by morphology, gene expression profile, gene copy number variations and the presence of individual genetic changes. The results indicated that all of the antioestrogen-resistant MCF-7 sub-lines were derived from a common ancestor.

In a somewhat different approach, Leung et al. (2010) set out to mimic, *in vitro*, the conditions that lead to the development clinical resistance to antioestrogens (Leung et al., 2010). Three different conditions were used to generate sub-lines. Firstly, MCF-7 cells were grown continuously in standard growth medium in the presence of increasing amounts of tamoxifen to produce the TamR7 sub-line. Oestrogen (which is present in foetal bovine serum) was not specifically excluded, thus mimicking clinical antioestrogen therapy. Secondly, cells were grown continuously in culture medium in the absence of both oestrogen and phenol red (which has oestrogenic properties) to produce the TamC3 and TamC6 sub-lines. The foetal bovine serum, used as a source of growth factors, had been previously absorbed with charcoal to remove oestrogen, thus mimicking the clinical effects of either oophorectomy or treatment with aromatase inhibitors such as letrozole. Thirdly, cells were grown continuously as above in the absence of oestrogen but with the addition of tamoxifen to produce the TamR3 and TamR6 sub-lines, thus mimicking the effect of combined therapy with antioestrogens plus aromatase inhibitors. Independent studies were undertaken using different batches of foetal calf serum, one batch giving the "3-series" (TamC3 and TamR3) and another giving the "6-series" (TamC6 and TamR6). Each condition resulted initially in the death of a high proportion of the cell population, followed over a period of at least 6 months by the emergence of resistant cells; however, the sub-lines were not clonally derived. Some of the properties of these sub-lines are shown in Table 1; all were shown by microsatellite analysis to be related to the parental MCF-7 cell line (Leung et al., 2010).

	Parental	TamR7	TamC3	TamR3	TamC6	TamR6
DNA content (ploidy)	1.5	1.9	1.4	1.4	2.0	2.1
Modal cell volume (pL)	2.4	2.6	1.6	1.7	2.2	2.0
Cell cycle time (hours)	31	31	27	27	36	37

Table 1. Characteristics of the MCF-7 line and of its sub-lines. From previously published data (Leung et al., 2010).

The above sub-lines were each found to be resistant to tamoxifen and were initially characterized by DNA content, cell cycle time and cell size. Flow cytometry was utilized to measure DNA content following staining of DNA with propidium bromide; cell size was determined by forward scatter in a flow cytometer; cell cycle time was measured by a stathmokinetic method involving the arrest of cell division by the mitotic poison paclitaxel and subsequent measurement of the reduction in the incorporation of ^{3}H-thymidine by the S-phase (Baguley et al., 1995). Surprisingly, DNA content alone distinguished four of the five sub-lines (Fig. 1). The parental MCF-7 line was aneuploid with a DNA content of 1.5x diploid, while the ploidy of derived sub-lines ranged from 1.4x diploid to 2.1x diploid. Changes in ploidy arise as a consequence of chromosomal instability, which in turn is related to the presence of extra centrosomes (Ganem et al., 2009). Control of centrosome number is in turn influenced by the expression of oncogenic and tumour suppressor proteins (Fukasawa, 2007). Changes in ploidy of a tumour population appear to occur gradually as a function of cell division, providing an effective measure of divergence of individual cells in a population.

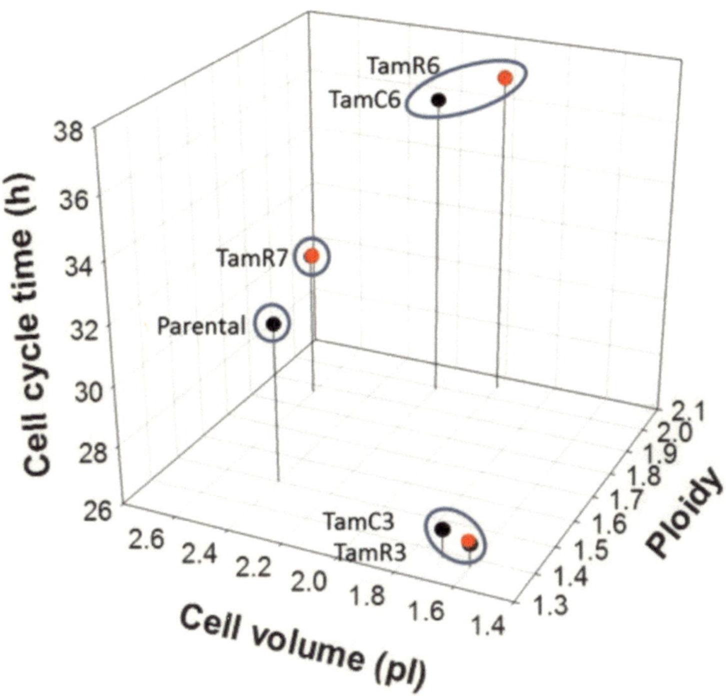

Fig. 1. Relationship between DNA ploidy, modal cell volume and cell cycle time of MCF-7 sub-lines. Figure reproduced from previously published data (Leung et al., 2010).

Mean cell cycle time and modal cell volume were also used to distinguish the sub-lines. Surprisingly, cell volume did not appear to be related to DNA content (Fig. 1). It was of interest that two lines, TamC6 and TamR6, which were derived under very different growth conditions (one in the presence of tamoxifen and one in its absence) showed very similar DNA content, cell cycle time and modal cell volume; the same situation applied to TamC3 and TamR3, which are very similar to each other although differing substantially from TamC6 and TamR6 (Fig. 1). Although it is likely that the constituent cell lines in each of these pairs are not identical, their similar properties suggest they are closely related. Such hierarchies might be expected on the basis of molecular signatures derived from gene expression arrays (Coser et al., 2009).

3. Steroid hormone receptor expression

The results in the previous section demonstrate the presence of heterogeneity in the MCF-7 cell lines and imply that small sub-populations existing in the parental line can be expanded under appropriate selective conditions. The time scale of the *in vitro* selection process (6 months or more) is consistent with the long period of time that occurs clinically in the development of resistance to antioestrogens or aromatase inhibitors in breast cancer patients. However, a critical question with regard to therapy is whether the emerging sub-lines express altered receptors and associated signalling pathways. This question was addressed using the sub-lines in Table 1. Expression of ER is shown in Fig. 2 and that of PR is shown in Fig. 3. MCF-7 is an ER+ tumour but as can be seen from Fig. 2, ER expression was weak when compared to that of the tamoxifen-resistant sub-lines with the exception of TamC6, which also expressed ER weakly. On the other hand, expression of PR was strong in the parental line, weak in TamC6 and virtually absent in the remaining sub-lines.

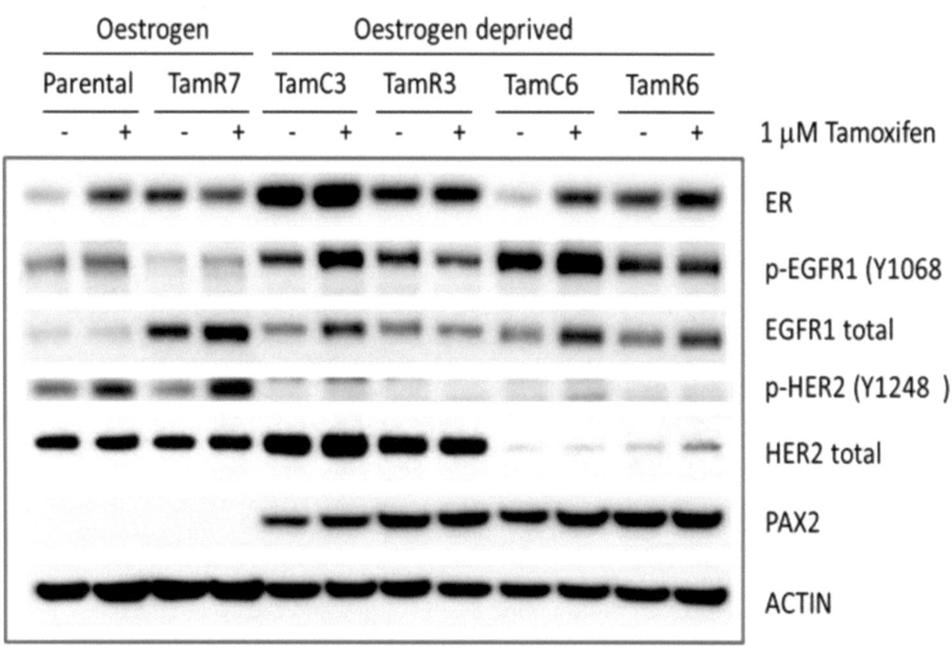

Fig. 2. Relative expression of ER, EGFR and HER2 by MCF-7 and its sub-lines in the absence (-) and presence (+) of tamoxifen (1 μM). Reproduced from previously published data (Leung et al., 2010).

None of the tamoxifen-resistant lines showed complete absence of ER expression but this may have been a result of the selection method. Tamoxifen is a partial ER agonist, probably acting on ER associated with the plasma membrane and selection in the presence of tamoxifen may favour cells expressing ER. An alternative approach was carried out by Liu et al. (2006), who used fulvestrant as a "pure" antioestrogen for cell line selection. This resulted in the generation of a MCF-7 sub-line (MCF-7/F) that did not express ER and that grew independently of either oestrogen or antioestrogens (Liu et al., 2006).

4. Growth factor receptor expression

The growth of breast cancer cells is controlled not only by ER and PR but also by plasma membrane-associated growth factor receptors. Two particularly important members of this large family are EGFR, which is activated by epidermal growth factor (EGF), and HER2. The expression of the two receptors was compared in MCF-7 cells and in their tamoxifen-resistant sub-lines. EGFR was expressed very weakly in parental MCF-7 cells but was upregulated in the sub-lines with strongest expression in the TamR7 sub-line (Leung et al., 2010). It was also upregulated in an MCF-7 sub-line (MCF-7/F) that does not express ER (Liu et al., 2006). Since EGFR is activated by phosphorylation, expression of the phosphorylated form of EGFR is more indicative of activity. As shown in Fig. 2, the parental and TamR7 cell lines show weak phosphorylation and TamC6 strong phosphorylation, while the other lines show intermediate phosphorylation (Leung et al., 2010). For most of the sub-lines, addition of tamoxifen increased EGFR phosphorylation, suggesting a relationship between ER and EGFR pathway utilization, in keeping with other studies implicating cross-talk between these pathways in breast cancer (Johnston, 2010).

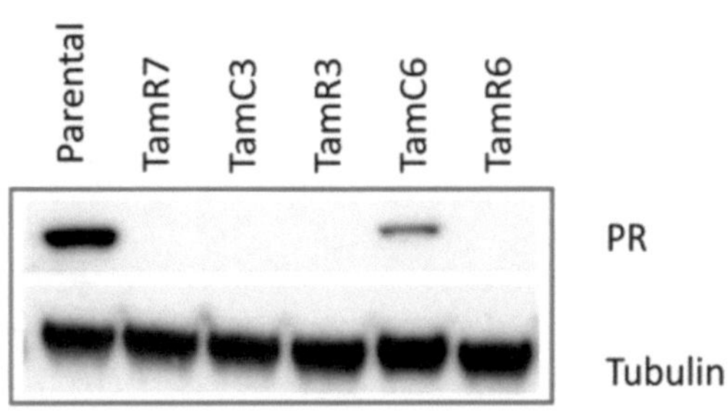

Fig. 3. Relative expression of PR by MCF-7 and its sub-lines.

Expression of the HER2 also varied across the cell lines. It was moderate in the parental MCF-7 line and TamR7, increased in TamC3 and TamR3, and low or absent in the TamC6 and Tam R6 sub-lines (Fig. 2). Previously, it was reported that PAX2 played an important role in the HER2 expression (Hurtado et al., 2008) and that of two MCF-7 phenotypes identified in this study, one expressed HER2 but not PAX2, while the other expressing PAX2 but not HER2. PAX2 is a paired box protein involved in lineage determination that is expressed during development and is commonly expressed in breast cancers (Muratovska et al., 2003). Hurtado et al. (2008) suggested that this inverse relationship arises because PAX2 competes with ER and its co-activator SRC-3 for binding sites on the *HER2* promoter, so that expression of PAX2 leads to repression of HER2 expression. While these two phenotypes are each evident in Fig. 2, a third phenotype expressing both HER2 and PAX2 proteins is also apparent as represented by TamC3 and TamR3. This suggests that the regulation of HER2 expression is more complex and that HER2 can sometimes be co-expressed with PAX2.

As discussed in the previous two sections, MCF-7 sub-lines demonstrate a wide divergence in the relative expression of ER, PR and HER2. It would be interesting to determine whether a sub-line of MCF-7 exhibiting "triple negative" properties could be isolated using appropriate selection procedures; this might form a useful model for understanding triple negative breast cancers that are encountered in clinical practice. Thus, the generation of variants of a single cancer cell line might be able to recapitulate the development of multiple phenotypes in clinical cancer.

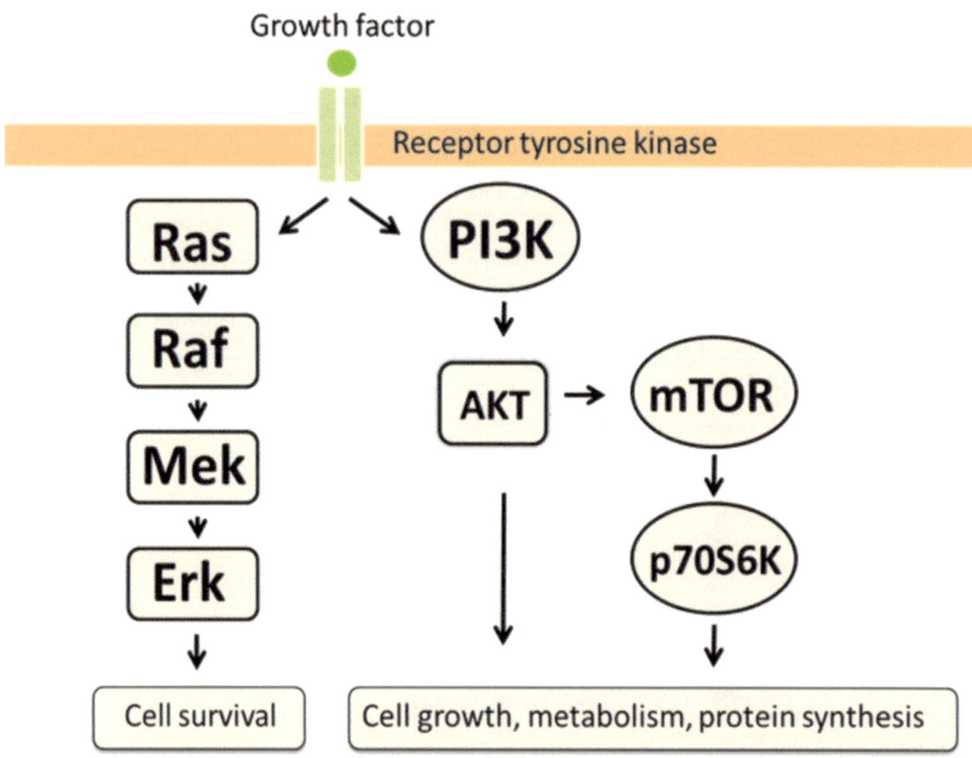

Fig. 4. Simplified diagram of the main pathways involving ERK, AKT (PKB) and mTOR.

5. Growth factor receptor pathways

Growth factor receptors such as EGFR and HER2 largely signal through a common pathway; self-association of adjacent receptors leads through tyrosine kinase phosphorylation to the activation of the receptor complex and recruitment of a series of associated signalling proteins that include RAS, phosphoinositide-3-kinase (PI3K) and RAF, ultimately contributing to the control of proliferation and survival; a simplified summary of these pathways is shown in Fig. 4. Members of the GTPase RAS family of proteins activate both the PI3K and RAF proteins, which in turn activate three key pathways: AKT (PKB; protein kinase B), ERK (extracellular related kinase) and mTOR (mammalian target of rapamycin). RAF activates ERK through the intermediate kinase MEK (mitogen-activated protein kinase kinase), while mTOR activates p70S6K, which is involved in the regulation of protein synthesis. Some measure of the crucial significance of these pathways to cancer growth is indicated by the incidence of mutations of the genes which control these signalling proteins; in particular, mutations of PIK3*CA*, the gene specifying PI3K, are found in 15-40% of patients with breast cancer (Isakoff et al., 2005) and a *PIK3CA* mutation is also found in MCF-7 cells. The impact of these mutations is to provide a decreased dependence on external stimulation of the pathways by growth factors such as EGF. Measurement of the utilization of the above pathways demonstrated considerable variation among the different MCF-7 sub-lines (Leung et al., 2010) and the results are summarized in Fig. 5. Utilization of the PI3K pathway can be assessed by phosphorylation of AKT; since the PIK3CA mutation and the gain of *PIK3CA* copy number in the MCF-7 cell line (Wu et al., 2005) lead to constitutive activation of PI3K, one might expect a high degree of AKT phosphorylation.

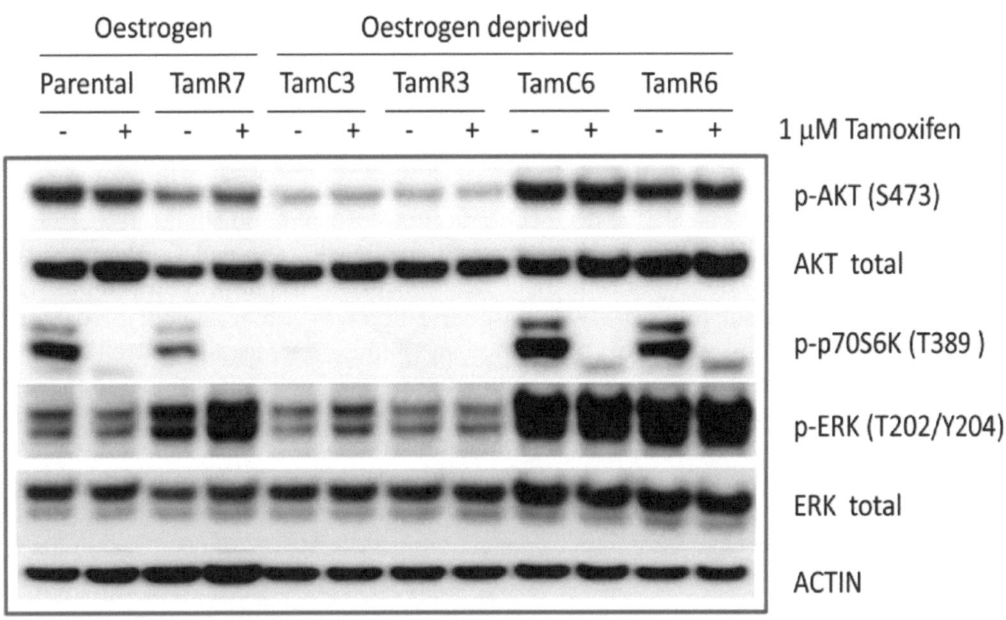

Fig. 5. Relative expression of AKT and its phosphorylated form p-AKT, phosphorylated p-p70S6K, ERK and phosphorylated form p-ERK. Data are shown for MCF-7 and its sub-lines in the absence (-) and presence (+) of tamoxifen (1 μM). Reproduced from previously published data (Leung et al., 2010).

Surprisingly, two of resistant MCF-7 sub-lines, TamC3 and TamR3, show low levels of phosphorylation of AKT, suggesting a comparatively low level of utilization. Utilization of the RAF pathway was assessed by measurement of ERK phosphorylation and here the parental line, as well as the TamC3 and TamR3 sub-lines, exhibited low phosphorylation while TamC6 and TamR6 exhibited high utilization and TamR7 showed intermediate phosphorylation. Utilization of the mTOR pathway was assessed by measurement of phosphorylation of the downstream signalling molecules p70S6K. Here the parental line, as well as the TamC3, TamR3 and TamR7 sub-lines, exhibited low phosphorylation levels while the TamC6 and TamR6 show higher utilization. The wide divergence in pathway utilization among the different sub-lines, as well as a lack of correlation between pathway utilization and expression of ER, PR, EGFR and HER2, was a surprising aspect of this study.

6. Response of MCF-7 sub-lines to therapeutic agents

It is clear from the previous section that the MCF-7 sub-lines vary considerably in their utilization of the AKT (PKB), ERK and mTOR signalling pathways. An important question arising from this observation is whether a high level of utilization of a particular pathway is related to sensitivity to inhibitors of this pathway. For instance, based on the data in Fig. 4, are the parental and TamC6 cell lines, which show higher phosphorylation of AKT than the other sub-lines, differentially susceptible to inhibitors of PI3K? Furthermore, do PI3K inhibitors differentially inhibit AKT phosphorylation in cell lines showing increased phosphorylation? It should be noted that MCF-7 cells have a PIK3CA mutation and the consequently activated PI3K activity makes them generally more sensitive to inhibitors of PI3K than other cell lines containing the wild type enzyme (Serra et al., 2008).

Since there are currently no PI3K inhibitors in routine clinical use, the question of differential sensitivity to PI3K inhibition was addressed using NVP-BEZ235 and GSK2126458 (Leung et al., 2011). NVP-BEZ235 is currently being tested in phase I/II clinical trials in breast cancer patients with advanced disease while GSK2126458 is being evaluated in a phase I trial in patients with solid tumours or lymphoma[1]. Examination of drug inhibitory properties showed that at drug concentrations of 1 μM and 50 nM, respectively, the parental and TamR7 lines were the most sensitive while TamC6 and TamR6 were the most resistant (Fig. 6). Thus, drug sensitivity was not related to pathway utilization. The question of differential inhibition of AKT phosphorylation was also examined; the parental and TamR7 were the most sensitive while TamC6 and TamR6 were least sensitive (Leung et al., 2011). This correlated well with inhibition of cell proliferation. A subsequent commentary on this work emphasises the importance of understanding the principles underlying sensitivity and resistance to inhibitors of this pathway (Butt, 2011).

A second example is provided by the mTOR pathway. Rapamycin is the classical inhibitor of this pathway and mTOR inhibitors such as everolimus and temsorolimus are in clinical trial. Moreover, treatment of mice with rapamycin sensitizes MCF-7 tumour xenografts to inhibition by tamoxifen (deGraffenried et al., 2004). Are MCF-7 sub-lines that highly phosphorylate the mTOR substrate p70S6K differentially sensitive to rapamycin? As measured by growth inhibition assays, the parental line and TamR7 were the most sensitive (Leung et al., 2010) while TamC6 and TamR6, where p70S6K are also highly phosphorylated, are resistant (Fig. 5). A third example is provided by the ERK pathway. No inhibitors of MEK, the enzyme that phosphorylates ERK, are yet in clinical use but CI-1040 has undergone clinical trial. Are MCF-7 sub-lines that show high phosphorylation of ERK, the MEK substrate, differentially sensitive to CI-1040? This does not appear to be the case because TamC3 was the most sensitive to CI-1040 despite showing only moderate phosphorylation of the ERK protein (Fig. 5).

Taken together, these results indicate a lack of a clear relationship between the degree of utilization of a particular pathway and the degree of dependence of cell growth on that pathway. While this may at first seem counter-intuitive, it should be kept in mind that phosphorylation pathways are utilized by the cell not only to promote proliferation but also to promote survival. Growth in culture in the presence of the multiple growth factors and antioxidants provided by foetal bovine serum is very different from growth *in vivo*, where

---

[1] http://clinicaltrials.gov/ct2/show/NCT00620594 and http://clinicaltrials.gov/ct2/show/NCT00972686.

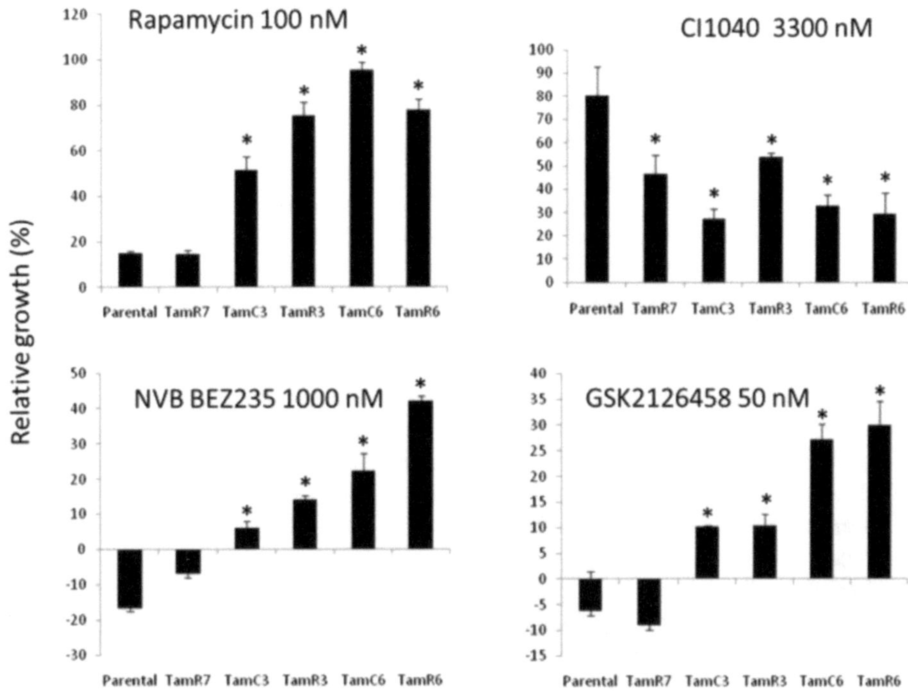

Fig. 6. Relative effects of inhibitors of mTOR (rapamycin), MEK (CI-1040) and PI3K (NVP BEZ235 and GSK2126458). Asterisks represent significant increases ($p < 0.05$) and negative values indicate evidence of cell killing. The two lower graphs are reproduced from previously published data (Leung et al., 2011).

the microenvironment is much more hostile. It is of interest in the case of the inhibitors of PI3K that the induction of apoptosis, if observed at all, was seen only at the highest drug concentrations tested, and that the main basis for inhibition of culture growth, particularly in the determination of IC_{50} values, was the induction of cell cycle arrest (Leung et al., 2011). It can thus be hypothesized that there are many alternative pathways that can be accentuated to promote cell survival and that different sub-lines have developed individual combinations of survival mechanisms. Only a small proportion of the overall signalling may be required to maintain cells in a proliferating state.

7. Conclusion

The hypothesis that emerges from these studies is that the human breast MCF-7 line, although often treated as a single entity, comprises a large number of individual phenotypes, most of which constitute only small proportions of the total population. These phenotypes differ in gene expression profile, receptor expression and signalling pathway usage. Despite differences in proliferation rate of individual phenotypes, a balance of multiple phenotypes is somehow maintained during progressive culturing of the line, perhaps by some type of signalling co-operation. The proportion of the dominant phenotype may be maintained by the growth conditions; in the case of MCF-7 the predominance of the ER+ phenotype could maintained by the presence of small amounts of oestrogen in the foetal bovine serum. However, extended growth in the absence of oestrogen would select for variants that rely on EGFR, HER2 and other stimulators of signalling pathways.

If the above hypothesis is correct, it raises three important questions. The first is whether such heterogeneity is a feature of all human breast cancer cell lines. Based on current literature, this is likely to be the case. Multiple antigenic phenotypes have been identified in several breast cancer cell lines (Edwards et al., 1985). Studies with T47D breast cancer cells using multidimensional flow cytometry have shown the presence of different phenotypes that differ not only in the expression of PR but also in DNA content (Graham et al., 1992). Further research is needed to explore the generality of these observations.

The second question is whether human breast cancers growing *in vivo* show similar levels of heterogeneity to those of the derived cell lines. This question is difficult to answer unless individual cells can be identified, but evidence of heterogeneity of *EGFR* copy number has been detected in fine needle biopsies from 29 breast cancer patients, as well as in samples of the MCF-7, SKBR3, and T47D cell lines (Sauer et al., 2005). An answer to this question is critical because it could imply a common ancestry not only for breast cancer cells that differ in receptor status but also in histological status and growth rate.

The third question is whether the mechanisms responsible for generating the heterogeneity of breast cancer cell types also apply to normal mammary tissue. There is increasing evidence for the existence of a differentiation hierarchy in the adult mammary epithelium, where precursor cells at various levels of the hierarchy are able to switch expression of proteins involved in differentiation; such switching includes the epidermal-mesenchymal transition (Visvader, 2009). The mechanism of such phenotype switching is not yet understood but is thought to involve epigenetic changes mediated by changes in DNA methylation, histone modification and concentrations of non-coding RNA (Huang & Esteller, 2010). These studies imply that the mechanism for generation of multiple phenotypes in breast cancer cells could be based on existing mechanisms that occur in the normal breast epithelium, with additional tumour-specific mechanisms arising from genetic alteration, chromosomal instability and possibly the presence of a mutated PI3K enzyme (Meyer et al. 2011).

8. Acknowledgements

The authors thank the Auckland Cancer Society, the New Zealand Breast Cancer Foundation, the New Zealand Lottery Commission, the Maurice and Phyllis Paykel trust and the Genesis Oncology Trust for their support of these studies.

9. References

Baguley, B C, Marshall, E. S., Whittaker, J. R., Dotchin, M. C., Nixon, J., McCrystal, M. R., Finlay, G. J., Matthews, J. H. L., Holdaway, K. M. & van Zijl, P. (1995). Resistance mechanisms determining the *in vitro* sensitivity to paclitaxel of tumour cells cultured from patients with ovarian cancer. *European Journal of Cancer*, 31A, 230-237.

Butt, A J (2011). Overcoming resistance: Targeting the PI3K/mTOR pathway in endocrine refractory breast cancer. *Cancer Biology and Therapy*, 11, 947-949

Cassanelli, S, Louis, J. & Seigneurin, D. (1995). Progesterone receptor heterogeneity in MCF-7 cell subclones is related to clonal origin and kinetics data. *Tumour Biology*, 16, 222-229.

Coser, K R, Wittner, B. S., Rosenthal, N. F., Collins, S. C., Melas, A., Smith, S. L., Mahoney, C. J., Shioda, K., Isselbacher, K. J., Ramaswamy, S. & Shioda, T. (2009). Antiestrogen-resistant subclones of MCF-7 human breast cancer cells are derived from a common monoclonal drug-resistant progenitor. *Proceedings of the National Academy of Sciences U S A*, 106, 14536-14541.

deGraffenried, L A, Friedrichs, W. E., Russell, D. H., Donzis, E. J., Middleton, A. K., Silva, J. M., Roth, R. A. & Hidalgo, M. (2004). Inhibition of mTOR activity restores tamoxifen response in breast cancer cells with aberrant Akt Activity. *Clinical Cancer Research*, 10, 8059-8067.

Edwards, P A, Skilton, R. A., Payne, A. W. & Ormerod, M. G. (1985). Antigenic heterogeneity of breast cell lines detected by monoclonal antibodies and its relationship with the cell cycle. *Journal of Cell Science*, 73, 321-333.

Fukasawa, K (2007). Oncogenes and tumour suppressors take on centrosomes. *Nature Reviews Cancer*, 7, 911-924.

Ganem, N J, Godinho, S. A. & Pellman, D. (2009). A mechanism linking extra centrosomes to chromosomal instability. *Nature*, 460, 278-282.

Graham, M L, Smith, J. A., Jewett, P. B. & Horwitz, K. B. (1992). Heterogeneity of progesterone receptor content and remodeling by tamoxifen characterize subpopulations of cultured human breast cancer cells: analysis by quantitative dual parameter flow cytometry. *Cancer Research*, 52, 593-602.

Huang, T H & Esteller, M. (2010) Chromatin remodeling in mammary gland differentiation and breast tumorigenesis. *Cold Spring Harbor Perspectives in Biology*, 2, a004515.

Hurtado, A, Holmes, K. A., Geistlinger, T. R., Hutcheson, I. R., Nicholson, R. I., Brown, M., Jiang, J., Howat, W. J., Ali, S. & Carroll, J. S. (2008). Regulation of ERBB2 by oestrogen receptor-PAX2 determines response to tamoxifen. *Nature*, 456, 663-666.

Isakoff, S J, Engelman, J. A., Irie, H. Y., Luo, J., Brachmann, S. M., Pearline, R. V., Cantley, L. C. & Brugge, J. S. (2005). Breast cancer-associated PIK3CA mutations are oncogenic in mammary epithelial cells. *Cancer Research*, 65, 10992-11000.

Johnston, S R (2010). New strategies in estrogen receptor-positive breast cancer. *Clinical Cancer Res*, 16, 1979-1987.

Leung, E, Kannan, N., Krissansen, G. W., Findlay, M. P. & Baguley, B. C. (2010). MCF-7 breast cancer cells selected for tamoxifen resistance acquire new phenotypes differing in DNA content, phospho-HER2 and PAX2 expression, and rapamycin sensitivity. *Cancer Biology and Therapy*, 9, 717-724.

Leung, E, Kim, J. E., Rewcastle, G. W., Finlay, G. J. & Baguley, B. C. (2011). Comparison of the effects of the PI3K/mTOR inhibitors NVP-BEZ235 and GSK2126458 on tamoxifen-resistant breast cancer cells. *Cancer Biology and Therapy*, 11, 938-946.

Liu, H, Cheng, D., Weichel, A. K., Osipo, C., Wing, L. K., Chen, B., Louis, T. E. & Jordan, V. C. (2006). Cooperative effect of gefitinib and fumitremorgin c on cell growth and chemosensitivity in estrogen receptor negative fulvestrant-resistant MCF-7 cells. *International Journal of Cancer*, 129, 1237-1246.

Meyer, D. S., Brinkhaus, H., Müller, U., Müller, M, Cardiff, R. D. Alj, M. B. (2011). Luminal expression of PIK3CA mutant H1047R in the mammary gland induces heterogeneous tumors. *Cancer Research*, in press.

Muratovska, A, Zhou, C., He, S., Goodyer, P. & Eccles, M. R. (2003). Paired-Box genes are frequently expressed in cancer and often required for cancer cell survival. *Oncogene*, 22, 7989-7997.

Nugoli, M, Chuchana, P., Vendrell, J., Orsetti, B., Ursule, L., Nguyen, C., Birnbaum, D., Douzery, E. J., Cohen, P. & Theillet, C. (2003). Genetic variability in MCF-7 sublines: evidence of rapid genomic and RNA expression profile modifications. *BMC Cancer*, 3, 13:1-12.

Sauer, T, Beraki, K., Noren, T., Garred, O. & Naess, O. (2005). EGFR gene copy number heterogeneity in fine-needle aspiration cytology from breast carcinomas determined by chromogenic in situ hybridization. *Diagnostic Cytopathology*, 33, 228-232.

Serra, V, Markman, B., Scaltriti, M., Eichhorn, P. J., Valero, V., Guzman, M., Botero, M. L., Llonch, E., Atzori, F., Di Cosimo, S., Maira, M., Garcia-Echeverria, C., Parra, J. L., Arribas, J. & Baselga, J. (2008). NVP-BEZ235, a dual PI3K/mTOR inhibitor, prevents PI3K signaling and inhibits the growth of cancer cells with activating PI3K mutations. *Cancer Research*, 68, 19, 8022-8030

Visvader, J. E. (2009). Keeping abreast of the mammary epithelial hierarchy and breast tumorigenesis. *Genes and Development*, 23, 2563-2577.

Wu, G., Xing, M., Mambo, E., Huang, X., Liu, J., Guo, Z.,Chatterjee, A., Goldenberg, D., Gollin, S. M., Sukumar, S., Trink, B., Sidransky, D. (2005). Somatic mutation and gain of copy number of PIK3CA in human breast cancer. *Breast Cancer Research*, 7, R609 - R16.

12

Metabolomics and Transcriptional Responses in Estrogen Receptor Positive Breast Cancer Cells

Soma Mandal, Protiti Khan, Lin Li and James R. Davie
Manitoba Institute of Cell Biology, University of Manitoba, Winnipeg, Manitoba, Canada

1. Introduction

Estrogen exposure is well recognized as a high risk factor of breast cancer, despite the fact that the hormone transcriptionally regulates the expression of tumor suppressor genes, like BRCA1 (Hockings *et al.*, 2008). Estrogen acts through the estrogen receptor α (ERα) in target cells (Ali and Coombes, 2000). ERα overexpression occurs in about 70% of breast cancers, referred as "ER positive" (ER+) (Dickson and Lippman, 1988). ERα is a primary target for chemoprevention as well as other therapeutic interventions for breast cancer with the ER+ phenotype. Clinically, in pathological lesions such as women with benign breast tumors, who underwent surgery, presented with a high proportion of ER positivity than the control group. In such cases, logistic regression yielded an adjusted odds ratio of 6.5 for risk of development of breast cancer compared to 0.3 odds ratio for PR (progesterone receptor); there was an increased proportion of cells expressing ERα by immunohistochemical staining, thereby demonstrating the importance of ERα as a breast cancer risk marker (Khan *et al.*, 1994). Estrogen or E2 mostly exerts its mitogenic effects by the modulation of metabolic responses and through the transcriptional induction of genes regulating crucial cellular processes like the cell cycle (Prall *et al.*, 1998). Microarray and RNA interference studies suggest that the transcriptional regulation of about 60% of estrogen responsive genes (induced or repressed) is dependent upon ERα and Sp1/3 transcription factors (Bazley and Gullick, 2005). The basal expression of ERα, in turn, is regulated by Sp1 in ER+ breast cancer cells (deGraffenried *et al.*, 2002). Sp1 and Sp3 are ubiquitously expressed in mammalian cells and are abnormally expressed in various cancers, including breast (Li and Davie, 2010). Sp1 and Sp3 bind to the same DNA sequence defined as Sp1/3 sites, with similar affinity. Sp1 and Sp3 play important roles in regulating genes critical to the initiation and progression of breast cancers (Hirokawa, 1984; Lu and Archer, 2010). Targeting these proteins is a promising cancer therapeutic approach (Jia *et al.*, 2010).

In most cases, ER+ breast cancers present a better clinical prognosis than the ER- breast cancers. Moreover, it is an encouraging fact that the leading antiestrogenic drugs such as tamoxifen have effectively improved the overall survival of pre and postmenopausal women by the reduction of cancer incidence and formation of new tumors (Ferguson and Davidson, 1997; Muss, 2001). However, a major obstacle to breast cancer treatment is the development of drug resistance. Resistance is commonly associated with an increased expression of Erb proteins including EGFR (epidermal growth factor receptor); in addition, there is evidence of non-hormonal role of ERα in hormone sensitive MCF-7 cells to maintain basal proliferation (Salazar *et al.*, 2011). Interestingly, there was no expression of Erb2 and 3, but ERα supported a population of basal fraction of actively dividing S phase cells which were unaffected by hormone depletion or hydroxy tamoxifen treatment (Salazar *et al.*, 2011). Like breast tumors, breast cancer cell lines can also yield clonal populations of tamoxifen resistant cells that have variable ER dependence (Coser *et al.*, 2009). This *in vitro* evidence supports the fact that the basal population of hormone sensitive cells may be a prerequisite condition for eventual occurrence of hormone insensitive tumors where current therapies such as tamoxifen are no more effective (Salazar *et al.*, 2011). Development of resistance to tamoxifen or aromatase inhibitors (AIs) is a result of adaptive changes which lead to the activation of alternate signaling pathways. ER+ tumors unresponsive to front line therapy drugs such as tamoxifen or AIs will eventually become resistant; as seen in xenograft or cell line models, there is an eventual constitutive activation of the RAS-MAPK (RAS-mitogen activated protein kinase) signaling pathway and dependency on growth factor receptor (EGFR/HER1 and HER2/neu) signaling. Constitutive RAS-MAPK activation by EGFR or HER2 overexpression in ER- breast cancers results in the downstream activation of mitogen and stress activated kinase 1 and 2 (MSK1 and MSK2) as well as several MSK substrates that are implicated in oncogenic programming. Given these detrimental adaptive cellular changes, there is a lot of attention given to breast cancers during the ER+ stage, such that alternative strategies can be used to circumvent the problem of drug resistance. One such approach is the use of synthetic peptides with sequences of natural biological molecules, such as ERα. A peptide analog, ERα17p with a 17 amino acid motif (PLMIKRSKKNSLALSLT; P295-T311 of ERα) was synthesized which contained the third nuclear localization signal of ERα, a proteolysis site, as well as a binding site for calmodulin. This 17 amino acid motif of ERα is responsible for a number of post-transcriptional modifications as well as of the recruitment of co-regulators. It was reported to elicit (pseudo)-estrogenic responses in ER+ MCF-7 cells (Gallo *et al.*, 2007). Further studies showed that the ERα17p peptide induced apoptosis in the ER+ MCF-7 and T47D cells and also in the ER- MDA-MB-231 and SKBr-3 cells through ERα independent mechanisms. This peptide also caused regression of ER- breast cancer tumor xenografts without apparent toxicity. This suggested a potentially new attractive tool for the development of promising therapeutic approaches, and also provided an insight to the cellular fate of ERα (Pelekanou *et al.*, 2011).

The differences of the ER+ or ER- breast cancer not only relate to their morphology, but are also largely due to the differential metabolomics and differences in their transcriptional responses, which overall is a reflection of the selectivity of gene usage. Differences between these two wide phenotypes are reflected in the metabolism of sugars, fatty acids, proteins or even drugs that accelerate or decelerate proliferation. In the ER+ breast cancer cells, E2 is pivotal in controlling diverse energy metabolic pathways such as glucose transport, glycolysis, TCA (tricarboxylic acid) cycle, mitochondrial respiratory chain, adenosine nucleotide translocator and fatty acid β-oxidation and synthesis respectively. Estrogen has positive effects on carbohydrate and lipid metabolism. Absence of ERα causes hyperplasia and hypertrophy of the adipose tissue, insulin resistance, and reduced energy expenditure respectively [(Chen *et al.*, 2009) and references therein]. Hence disturbances in the E2/ER metabolic pathways are likely to cause metabolic diseases such as heart disease, obesity and also cancer. Thus breast cancer progression and unresponsiveness to therapy are interrelated.

MCF-7 is a model cell line of the ER+ phenotype and the highly metastatic MDA-MB-231 is a model cell line of ER- phenotype. Both these cell lines have been widely used for *in vitro* cell culture and *in vivo* xenograft studies. We used microarray expression data obtained from public repositories for MCF-7 (non-stimulated) and MDA-MB-231 to compare interrelated factors that regulate the transition of breast cancer towards the more aggressive phenotype (Mandal *et al.*, 2007b; Mandal and Davie, 2007). In this chapter, we review, discuss, and compare some salient features and experimental findings of major energy metabolic pathways, the importance of pathways that are constitutively activated and transcriptional responses with particular emphasis on ER+ breast cancers.

2. Glucose metabolism

The binding of estrogen to its receptor induces crucial metabolic changes through the activation of various estrogen responsive genes. Estrogen stimulates glucose metabolism, including glycolysis and glycogen synthesis, in target organs such as the uterus, which is a classic estrogen target organ (Shinkarenko *et al.*, 1994; Smith and Gorski, 1968). It has been shown in many studies that estrogen stimulates the incorporation of labeled glucose (^{14}C-labeled glucose) into lipid, RNA, and protein (Bitman *et al.*, 1965; Nicolette and Gorski, 1964; Swigart *et al.*, 1961). The influence of estrogen in glucose metabolism is also well studied in another estrogen target tissue, the breast. Several studies in breast cancer cell lines have that the incorporation of the glucose analogue, [^{18}F]-fluoro-2-deoxy-D-glucose (^{18}F-FDG) varies with the ERα status, the acquisition of drug resistance, or alterations in the expression of ERα. Clinically, ^{18}F-FDG is used for non-invasive detection of breast cancer and staging of axillary lymph node metastases by PET (positron emission tomography) scan (Utech *et al.*, 1996). PET technology utilizes the metabolic characteristic of enhanced glucose utilization by tumor cells (Moreno-Sanchez *et al.*, 2007). Hence this advanced technology can be effectively used to study metabolic characteristics in drug resistance or hormone related metabolic changes.

Tumors refractory to chemotherapy are prone to the acquisition of drug resistance. One of the mechanisms of acquired resistance is through alterations of glucose metabolism and the differential expression of GLUT (glucose transporter) expression. The higher gene and protein expression of GLUTs in tumors is well documented (Macheda *et al.*, 2005; Medina and Owen, 2002; Wood and Trayhurn, 2003). This phenomenon provides an advantage to tumors to harness increased glucose utilization through the glycolysis pathway. Glucose transporters such as GLUT12, initially identified in MCF-7 cells, have been shown to have deregulated and increased expression in breast tumors (Rogers *et al.*, 2003). Facilitated transport of polar glucose molecules across the plasma membrane is dependent on GLUT proteins. GLUT proteins 1-5 have been identified in mammalian cells. These transporter proteins impart unique metabolic properties to cells (Rogers *et al.*, 2003). There is evidence that in both the ER+ MCF-7 cells and the ER- MDA-MB-231 cells, there is an increased expression of GLUT1 under hypoxic conditions (Rivenzon-Segal *et al.*, 2003). MCF-7 cells rendered resistant to the drug 5-fluorouracil by long term exposure (the drug-sensitive parental cell line in medium with increasing concentrations for a period of two years), had a decreased ^{18}F-FDG incorporation. Microarray data showed that the expression of GLUTs 8 and 10 was decreased in resistant cells, while GLUT1 was only increased in cells resistant to the lowest concentration of 5-fluorouracil. There were no alterations in the hexokinase activity, but there was a increase in glucose transport (Smith *et al.*, 2007). On the other hand, estrogen produces an positive increase in the ^{18}F-FDG uptake which has been demonstrated in ER+ cells. A comparative study between the ER+ T47D cells and the ER- cell lines, MDA-MB-231 and MDA-MB-468 demonstrated the dependence of estrogen in mediating the glucose uptake. In the ER- breast cancer cells, the ^{18}F-FDG uptake was totally absent; this correlated positively with the fact that these cells are totally unresponsive to the estrogen dependent effect on glucose uptake. To further demonstrate this estrogen dependence, it was seen that when the ER+ T47D cells were pretreated with the pure antiestrogen ICI182,780 (fulvestrant), the glucose uptake was totally abrogated. Unlike fulvestrant, the partial antiestrogen tamoxifen was incapable of blocking this estrogen response (Ko *et al.*, 2010).

Comparison of metabolic and morphological differences between normal breast and ER+ breast cancer cells gave insights into the adaptive responses adaptive responses which enable cancer cells to better utilize cellular energy resources. Glucose metabolism was studied in the finite lifespan normal human mammary epithelial cell line (HMECs) as well as the classical ER+ the classical ER+ MCF-7 cancer cell line. Cells were induced to grow rapidly under routine tissue culture conditions in nutrient rich media containing ^{13}C-labeled glucose and the isotopic enrichment of cellular metabolites was quantified to calculate metabolic fluxes in key pathways. Cells grown in culture dishes of various sizes (with different surface areas) exhibited very different metabolic and morphological profiles. MCF-7 cells have about an 80% smaller exposed surface area and contain 26% less protein per cell than the HMECs. The per-cell glucose consumption, lactate production, and glutamine consumption rate was 225-250% higher per cell relative to the cancer cells. However, the calculated flux per the exposed area for glucose, lactate, and glutamine was much higher in MCF-7 cells; MCF-7 cells also consumed amino acids at rates much higher than that required for protein synthesis demonstrating a greater efficacy of transport mechanisms (Meadows *et al.*, 2008). In addition, the energy efficiency was much higher in MCF-7 cells which also had a higher dependence on the TCA cycle. These observations form the basis of rational drug design for metabolic drugs (Meadows *et al.*, 2008).

2.1 Glucose metabolism – A comparative analysis in ER+ and ER- breast cancer cells

Glycolysis is the metabolic pathway where glucose is oxidized to pyruvate under aerobic conditions to yield ATP; however, under anaerobic conditions, pyruvate is converted to lactic acid. This biochemical pathway is regulated by the enzymes hexokinase, phosphofructokinase, and pyruvate kinase respectively, which are also potential sites of control and in most organisms these steps are irreversible. The opposite action of glycolysis is gluconeogenesis, which occurs when the blood sugar level falls, thus aiding in the replenishment of blood sugar levels. The gene expression in glycolysis and gluconeogenesis pathways is depicted in Fig. 1A in the ER+ MCF-7 cells and the ER- MDA-MB-231 cells. Some of the key patterns of gene expression are seen between the ER+ and ER- phenotypes:

a. In both cases, the expression of genes and proteins coding for facilitated transmembrane GLUTs (SLCs, solute carrier family of proteins) is either absent or down-regulated. Interestingly, the protein encoded by the gene, *GPI* (phosphoglucose isomerase) catalyzing the irreversible isomerization of G-6-PO_4 (glucose-6-phosphate) to F-6-PO_4 (fructose-6-phosphate), is key in energy pathways and is down-regulated in MDA-MB-231 cells whereas, it is up-regulated in MCF-7 cells. This agrees with our previous studies where we had shown that the more aggressive ER+ cells have a reduced utilization of genes involved in the energy production and expenditure pathways similar to the ER- breast cancer phenotype (Mandal and Davie, 2007).

b. Of the three isozymes of PFK (phosphofructokinase) which catalyze the conversion of fructose 6-phosphate (F-6-PO_4) to the 1, 6-diphosphate form, PFKM is highly expressed in MCF-7 cells and is down-regulated in MDA-MB-231 cells; PFKM is responsible for the phosphorylation of F 6-PO_4 to F 1, 6-bisPO_4. On the other hand, expression of PFKP is quite high in MDA-MB-231 cells and this isoform is responsible for the catalytic conversion of F 6-PO_4 to F 1, 6-bisPO_4 and PFKP is a key regulatory enzyme of glycolysis. Mutations in this key enzyme can cause glycogen storage disease.
c. A crucial difference is the down-regulated expression of the isozymes of lactate dehydrogenase (LDH) in MCF-7 (LDHA, LDHC) versus their up-regulation in MDA-MB-231 cells. The proteins encoded by both these genes catalyze the conversion of L-lactate and NAD to pyruvate and NADH as the final step of anaerobic glycolysis, a feature of the metastatic phenotype.
d. Genes encoding for glycolytic enzymes like phosphoglycerate kinases (*PGK1/2*) are either down-regulated (*PGK1* in MCF-7), or have low expression (*PGK1* in MDA-MB-231), or are absent (*PGK2,* in MCF7 and MDA-MB-231).
e. Aldolases catalyzing the reversible aldol cleavage of fructose 1, 6-biphosphate and fructose 1-phosphate to dihydroxyacetone phosphate and either glyceraldehyde-3-phosphate or glyceraldehyde respectively are either absent (*ALDOA, B*) or are highly expressed in MCF-7 cells, but down-regulated in MDA-MB-231 cells. The same pattern of opposite gene expression is also seen with *TPI1* (triosephosphate isomerase 1), which catalyzes the isomerization of glyceraldehydes 3-phosphate (G3P) and dihydroxy-acetone phosphate (DHAP) in glycolysis and gluconeogenesis.

Glycogenesis is the glycogen synthesis process, in which glucose molecules are added to chains of glycogen for storage. We compared the gene expression analysis between MCF-7 and MDA-MB-231 cells where in general, there was a down-regulation or absence of genes involved in critical steps [such as debranching (AGL), phosphate transfer to glucose molecules (*PGM1*)] within the pathway (Fig. 1B). Notably, mutations of most of the genes involved in the glycogenesis pathway are associated with glycogen storage disease. Interestingly, there was a selective up-regulation of genes *(PPP2R3A, PPP2CA, PPP2R5A, PPP2R5B, PPP2R2C)* in MDA-MB-231 cells encoding for protein phosphatases; the proteins of these genes are involved in the negative control of cell division and growth.

3. Fatty acid (FA) metabolism

The first step to the biosynthesis of fatty acids is the transport of citrate from the mitochondria to the cytoplasm. Lipogenesis is controlled by the enzyme fatty acid synthase or FASN, which is highly expressed in breast carcinomas and is thus an important cancer therapeutic target. The breakdown of fatty acids is regulated by carnitine palmitoyltransferase-1 or CPT-I. The preferential expression of FASN in cancer cells including breast cancer, in particular in ER+ breast cancer cells, is of importance because the production and levels of palmitate substantially differ in cancer cells. Blocking FASN has antiproliferative effects on breast cancer cells. A natural antibiotic, known as cerulenin derived from the fungus, *C. ceruleans,* caused apoptosis in cancer cells; C75 is a natural derivative of cerulenin. C75 has antitumor effects and its action is postulated to be on CPT-1 and production of high levels of malonyl CoA respectively. In a comparative study between C75 and EGCG (epigallocatechin-3-gallate), a main constituent of green tea, it was seen that EGCG caused induction of apoptosis uncoupled to the effects of CPT-1 in breast cancer cells through the targeted inhibition of FASN (Puig *et al.*, 2008). (Information source of individual genes: www.ncbi.nlm.nih.gov).

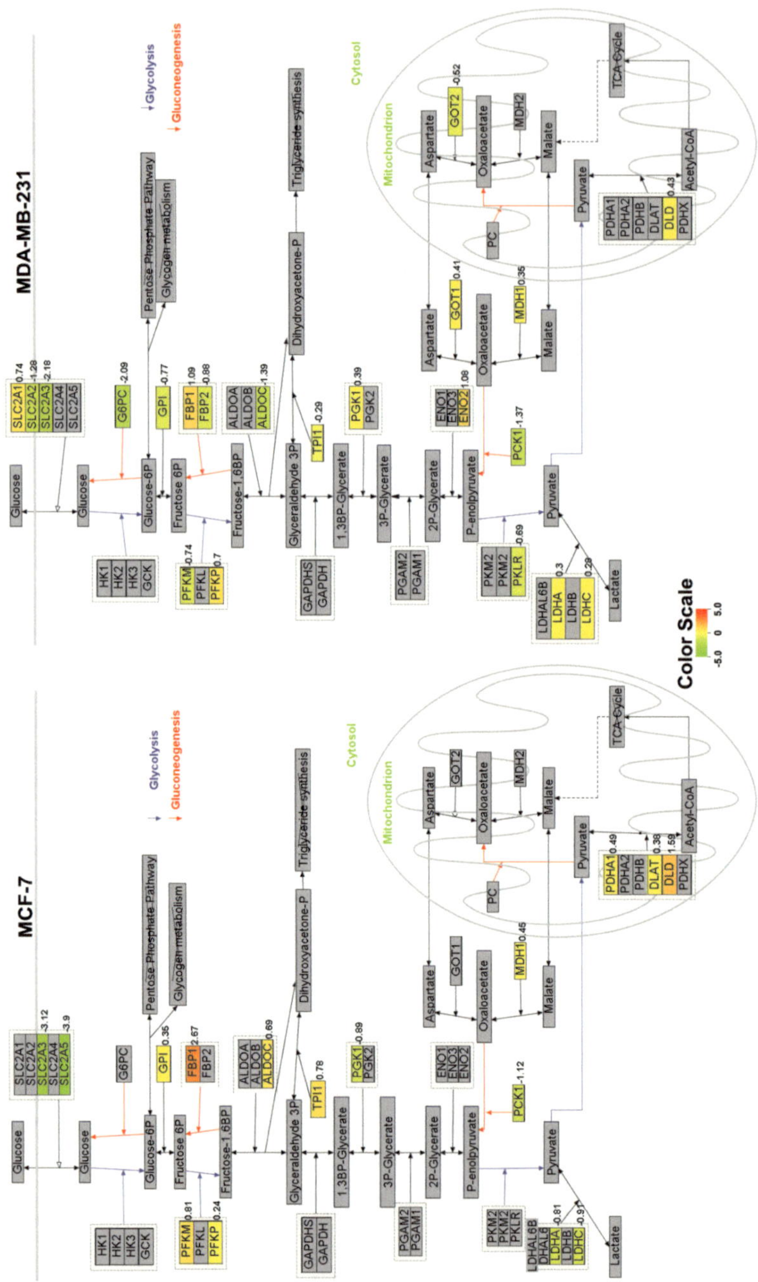

Fig. 1A. A comparative view of the glycolysis and gluconeogenesis pathways operating in the ER+ MCF-7 and ER- MDA-MB-231 cells is shown. The pathway maps were generated using the pathway visualization tool, PathVisio (Version 2). The software generated a color scale for the visualization of expression (red is up-regulation and green is down-regulation of gene expression). Expression values (SLR, signal log ratio) with a cutoff value of ≥ 0.2 or ≤- 0.2 was used and in case of duplicate SLR values, an average SLR was taken. **Note**: Only the controlled irreversible steps of each pathway are colored.

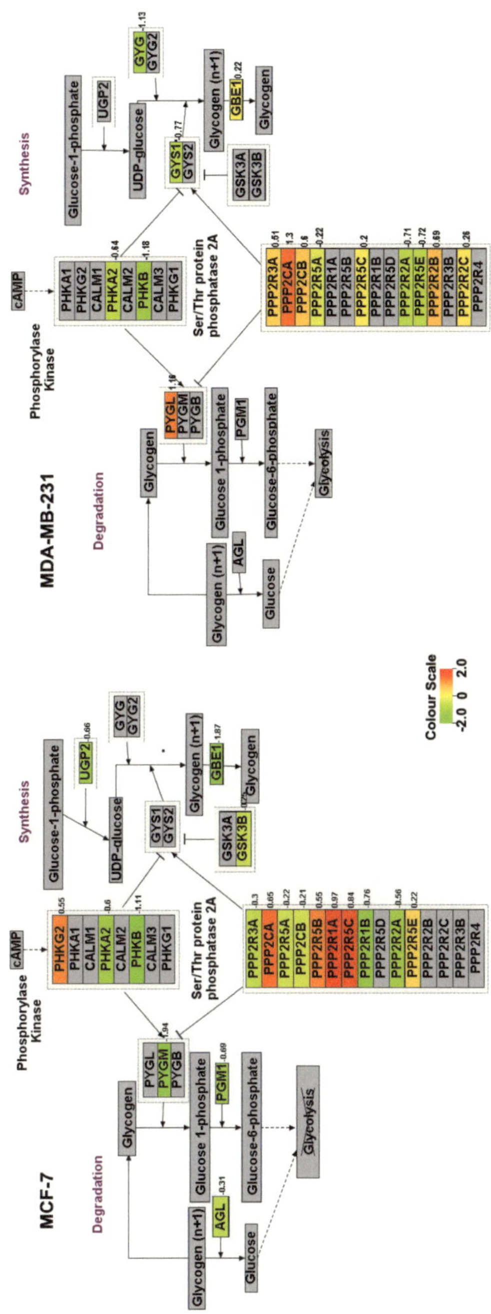

Fig. 1B. A comparative view of the glycogenesis pathway operating in MCF-7 and MDA-MB-231 cells is shown. The pathway maps were generated using the pathway visualization tool, PathVisio (Version 2). The software generated a color scale for the visualization of expression (red is up-regulation and green is down-regulation of gene expression). Expression values (SLR, signal log ratio) with a cutoff value of ≥ 0.2 or ≤ -0.2 was used and in case of duplicate SLR values, an average SLR was taken.

The n-3 PUFAs (n-3 polyunsaturated fatty acids) have beneficial effects as chemopreventive and chemotherapeutic agents in the treatment of cancer. It is of particular interest that in recent years several *in vitro* and *in vivo* xenograft studies and clinical trials have presented evidence that there are beneficial effects of n-3 PUFAs when administered with conventional antineoplastic drugs and radiotherapy against many different types of cancers including breast cancer. Combination of drugs such as doxorubicin/epirubicin/paclitaxel with the n-3 PUFA, DHA (docosahexaenoic acid) had antiproliferative effects such as apoptosis induction, inhibition of neo-angiogenesis, or inhibition of invasiveness in MCF-7 and MDA-MB-231 cells [(Calviello *et al.*, 2009) and references therein]. The cellular antiproliferative actions of n-3 PUFAs include modulation of metabolism, expression of cell cycle and apoptosis factors including caspases, and the ability of fatty acids to sensitize tumor cells to anticancer drugs by increasing membrane permeability. Such beneficial properties have been exploited to develop an interesting strategy of drug delivery, which is the design of liposomes for the targeted delivery of anticancer drugs. This system utilizes the fact that conventional drugs like doxorubicin and cisplatin in liposomal formulations are activated by secretory phospholipase A_2 or $sPLA_2$ which is overexpressed in inflammatory and tumor tissues (Andresen *et al.*, 2005; Laye and Gill, 2003). However, such an approach has not been successful in ER+ (MCF-7) or ER- (MDA-MB-231) cells (Rasmussen *et al.*, 2010). The metabolic modulatory effects of PUFAs leading to antiproliferation include alterations in arachidonic acid (AA) oxidative metabolism and metabolic conversion of n-3 PUFAs to bioactive derivatives. The cellular production of some AA-derived eicosanoids such as prostaglandin E_2 is high in cancer and their formation is inhibited by n-3 PUFAs. Moreover, n-3 PUFAs also competitively inhibit the COX2 enzyme (a very potent oncogene) to produce the less biologically effective n-3 PUFA derived eicosanoids (Chell *et al.*, 2006). A promising finding is the ability of n-3 PUFA to overcome resistance of breast cancer cells treated with tamoxifen. As the n-3 PUFAs are known to inhibit the Akt activity, it was found that EPA (eicosapentaenoic acid) cotreatment of breast cancer cells overexpressing Akt made cells more responsive to tamoxifen. Conjugated preparations of novel anticancer agent, propofol with n-3 PUFAs, DHA and EPA caused significant induction of apoptosis, induction of caspase 3 activity, inhibition of cell adhesion and migration in MDA-MB-231 cells. The drug alone or in combination with the n-3 PUFAs was minimally effective to cause these effects (Siddiqui *et al.*, 2005).

3.1 FA metabolism – A comparative analysis in ER+ and ER- breast cancer cells

In general, the ER+ MCF-7 cells show a greater number of up-regulated genes for proteins catalyzing the FA biosynthesis in comparison to the ER- MDA-MB-231 cells (Fig. 2A). The key features of gene expression are as follows:

a. Notably, the gene expressing the primary enzyme for FA biosynthesis is *FASN*, which is up-regulated in MCF-7 cells in contrast to a down-regulated expression in MDA-MB-231 cells. Genes encoding for enzymes catalyzing the production of FA acetyl Co-A esters from the TCA cycle intermediate, citrate and acetyl CoA (*ACYL, FASN*), or via its intermediate malonyl CoA (ACACB), were up-regulated in MCF-7 cells, but were down-regulated or absent in MDA-MB-231 cells (*ACYL, FASN, ACACA, ACACB*).
b. Interestingly, in both cell types, genes for the enzymes catalyzing the production of triglycerides from FA CoA (*ACSL1, 3, ACAS2*) were down-regulated. These ligases play a key role not only in biosynthesis, but also in FA degradation. Thus, while it is evident that MCF-7 cells differ from ER- cells in the production of palmitate, the synthesis of triglycerides seems to be restricted in both cell types and may be a predominant adaptive response of cancer cells (Fig. 2A).

Similar to FA biosynthesis, genes encoding for enzymes of FA degradation and cholesterol biosynthesis (Fig. 2B) are also mostly up-regulated in MCF-7 cells in contrast to MDA-MB-231 cells.

a. Genes regulating cholesterol biosynthesis may be favored in a hormone responsive environment, cholesterol being the building block of all steroid hormones, including estradiol. Notably among them, is *SQLE* (squalene epoxidase), the protein product of which is a key enzyme in cholesterol key enzyme of cholesterol biosynthesis. MCF-7 cells have an up-regulated expression of the gene, while it is down-regulated in MDA-MB-231 cells. Clinical studies have shown that higher expression of *SQLE* is inversely correlated with distant metastasis-free survival in ER+ stage 1/II breast cancer patients (Helms *et al.*, 2008).
b. Other notable differences include the up-regulated expression of genes of enzymes (*MVK, PMVK*) producing the phosphorylated forms of mevalonic acid, which is a key intermediate of steroid biosynthesis, in MCF-7 cells.
c. Gene of the enzyme catalyzing the dimerization of 2 farnesyl diphosphate molecules to form squalene, is down-regulated, but forms an important step in cholesterol synthesis. It may be assumed that this step of cholesterol biosynthesis, and hence the synthesis of squalene is tightly controlled with respect to the need of steroid hormone synthesis.
d. Notably, in both cell lines, the NAD(P) dependent steroid dehydrogenase-like (NSDHL) enzyme is slightly up-regulated; this may be indicative of an advantage of cancer cells to produce cholesterol depending on its cellular needs.
e. Two other genes whose proteins (*SC4MOL, CYP51A1*) are involved in the synthesis of the cholesterol intermediate, lathosterol are either absent (MDA-MB-231) or down-regulated (MCF-7). Notably, among these, the *CYP51A1* gene encodes for a member of the cytochrome P450 superfamily of monooxygenase enzymes which catalyze many reactions involved in drug metabolism and synthesis of cholesterol, steroids and other lipids. The absence or down-regulation of this enzyme allows cancer cells to metabolize therapeutic drugs aimed to arrest or cause death and thus aid in their overall survival.

4. Retinoic acid (RA) metabolism

The retinoids comprise of RA (vitamin A, all-*trans* retinoic acid) and related signaling molecules which are essential in the differentiation of various types of stem cells. A compromised retinoid signaling is often seen early in carcinogenesis including in breast carcinogenesis, where retinoids interact with the estrogen signaling pathways. These molecules are used for cancer therapeutics because they can induce differentiation and growth arrest. Efficacy of retinoid treatment is often challenged by the fact that these molecules are rapidly metabolized. Moreover, compromised responses, including resistance, to pharmacological doses of retinoids to cancer cells are also the result of epigenetic changes, such as the expression of various transcriptional coactivators and corepressors, the hypermethylation of CpGs in specific promoters in cancer cells, and the activities of other signaling pathways respectively. A combination therapy of retinoids with epigenetic drugs such as histone deacetylase or DNA methytransferase inhibitors or with other classical chemotherapeutic drugs may be a potential alternative route of treatment (Tang and Gudas, 2011). Moreover, another reason limiting the potent anticarcinogenic activities of RA is the fact that it exhibits a paradoxical behavior in that in some cancers it facilitates proliferation rather than inhibition of growth (Schug *et al.*, 2008). (Information source of individual genes: www.ncbi.nlm.nih.gov)

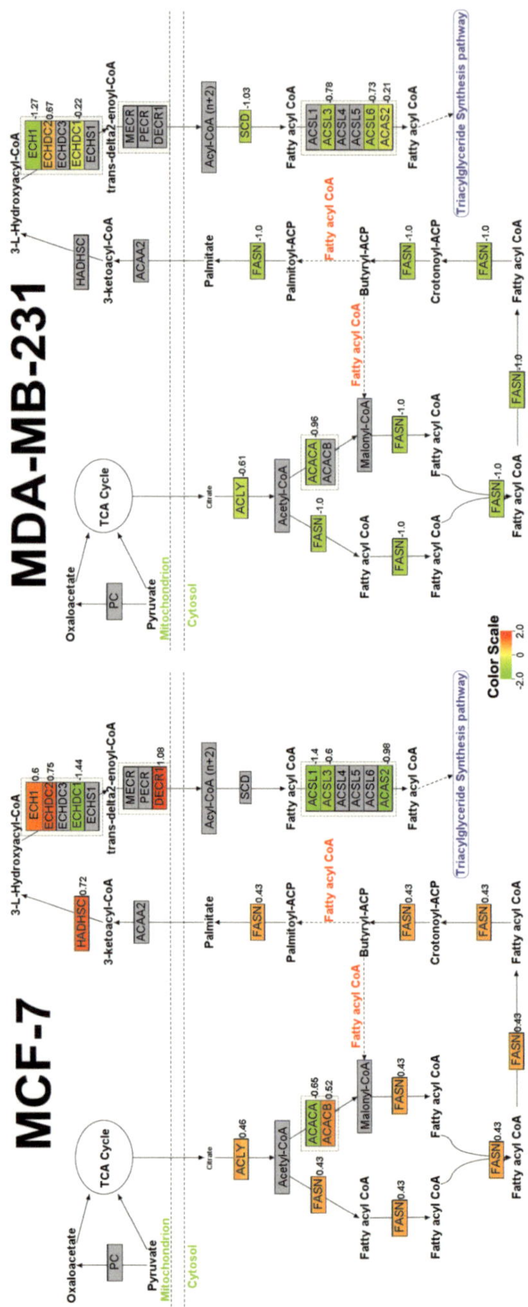

Fig. 2A. A comparative view of fatty acid biosynthesis pathways operating in MCF-7 and MDA-MB-231 cells is shown. The pathway maps were generated using the pathway visualization tool, PathVisio (Version 2). The software generated a color scale for the visualization of expression (red is up-regulation and green is down-regulation of gene expression). Expression values (SLR, signal log ratio) with a cutoff value of ≥ 0.2 or ≤- 0.2 was used and in case of duplicate SLR values, an average SLR was taken.

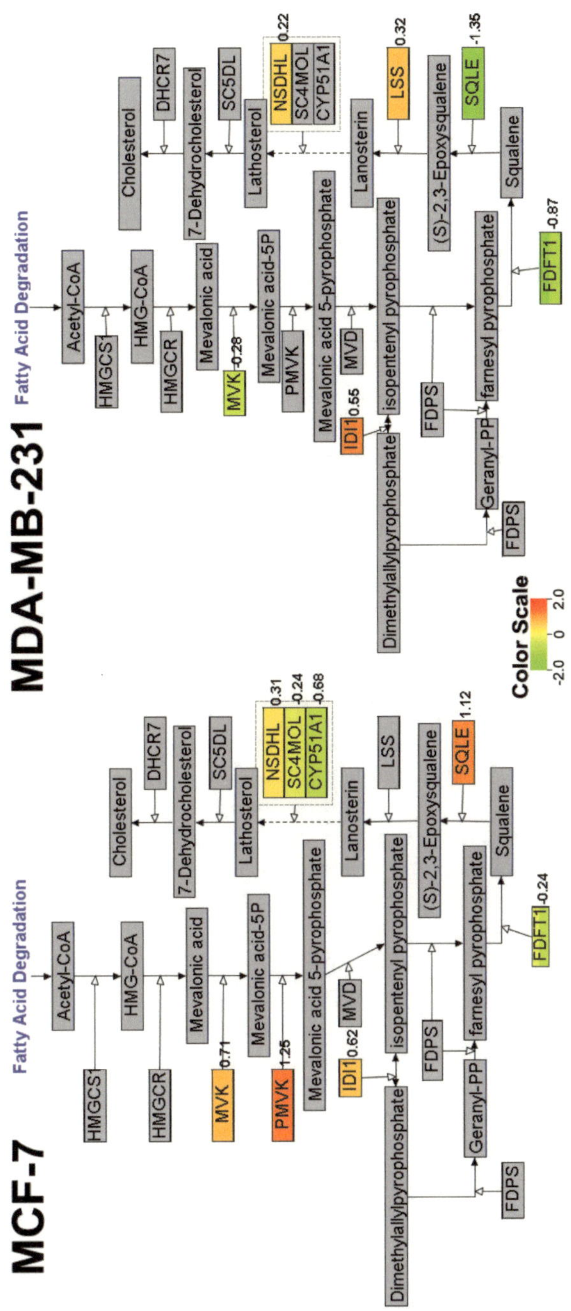

Fig. 2B. A comparative view of fatty acid degradation pathway operating in MCF-7 and MDA-MB-231 cells is shown. The pathway maps were generated using the pathway visualization tool, PathVisio (Version 2). The software generated a color scale for the visualization of expression (red is up-regulation and green is down-regulation of gene expression). Expression values (SLR, signal log ratio) with a cutoff value of ≥ 0.2 or ≤- 0.2 was used and in case of duplicate SLR values, an average SLR was taken.

The intracellular concentrations of various forms of retinoids are under the control of several metabolic enzymes (Duester, 2008). Within the RA generating tissue, retinol or vitamin A (retinol) is first converted to the aldehyde form (retinaldehyde) and then to the carboxylic acid (retinoic acid, RA). The expression of several alcohol and retinol dehydrogenases is widespread and overlapping in a variety of tissues. However, during mouse embryogenesis, the expression of the enzymes (retinaldehyde dehydrogenases) responsible for the second step which leads to RA generation, is tissue specific and non-overlapping (Mic *et al.*, 2002). Oxidation of RA leads to its degradation to more polar metabolites such as 4-oxo-RA (and other more polar RA metabolites); this oxidative degradation is catalyzed by three cytochrome P450 (CYP) enzymes, CYP26A1, B1, and C1 respectively (bu-Abed *et al.*, 1998). Enzymes controlling the synthesis of RA are expressed in very low levels in breast cancers relative to normal breast cells. The ability of normal HMECs from reduction mammoplasty has been shown to be competent in RA synthesis and the ability is still retained by immortal, non-tumorigenic breast epithelial cells, such as MCF10A. However, in the ER+ MCF-7 and T47D cells, the impaired RA activity appeared due to the impaired biosynthesis of RA; treatment with the CYP26 inhibitor, liarozole did not affect the low and undetectable levels of RA (Mira *et al.*, 2000). Likewise, a defect found in human primary breast tumors is the aberrantly high expression of the degradation enzyme, CYP26A1. The ducts and lobules of normal breast tissues demonstrated weak staining which was in contrast to distinct strong cytoplasmic staining in 46% of breast carcinomas (primary and metastatic breast carcinomas) examined within a tissue microarray. Kaplan-Meier analysis of these breast cancer cases suggested an association of high expression of CYP26A1 with a lower disease free and overall survival period. While overexpression of CYP26A1 in transfected AC2M2 (a breast metastatic ER- variant cell line) caused a decreased sensitivity to apoptosis, CYP26A1 siRNA silencing partially abrogated cells from the apoptosis sensitivity. In RA sensitive ER+ T47D cells, the induction of this enzyme was also more rapid than the ER- MDA-MB-231 cells. The growth inhibitory properties of RA were increased by the effect of treatment of an RA metabolism inhibitor, liarozole. Thus both *in vivo* and *in vitro* evidence suggested the potential oncogenic capacity (decreased apoptosis and increased cell survival) of RA degradation enzymes (Osanai *et al.*, 2010; Sonneveld *et al.*, 1998).
Studies show that two critical steps in RA metabolism responsible for synthesis and degradation of RA are sometimes impaired in breast cancers. Thus, defects in RA metabolism influences its effectiveness as a cancer antiproliferative drug in the ER+/ER- breast cells. RA inhibited cell growth and induced apoptosis in ER+ breast cancer cell lines, MCF-7 and T47D, but not in ER- MDA-MB-231 and MDA-MB-453 cells. The differences were due to the ability of ER+ cells to uptake RA rapidly (by hour 2) and by hour 24 there was a disappearance of RA uptake from the medium and cells leaving oxidation products in the culture medium. In sharp contrast, ER- cells showed lower accumulation without any sharp increase and subsequent steep decline; the result was the presence of more RA in these cells and the culture medium (Okamoto *et al.*, 2000). Interestingly, the ER- cell line MDA-MB-468 cells still retain the ability to synthesize RA (Mira *et al.*, 2000). Though a triple negative ER- cell line with EGFR amplification, the MDA-MB-468 cells are responsive to novel drugs along with the nuclear localization of a pseudo wild-type p53 and delocalization of mutant p53 (Mandal *et al.*, 2007a).

4.1 Comparative analysis of RA metabolism between ER+ and ER- cells

RA acts through its binding to the RA receptor (RAR), which in turn is bound to DNA as a heterodimer with the retinoid X receptor (RXR) in the RA response elements (RAREs).

Binding of RA ligand to RAR alters the conformation of the RAR resulting in the transcriptional induction or repression of RA target genes. As discussed in the previous paragraphs, the genes of proteins catalyzing the metabolism of RA has profound effects on breast cancer and hence also on its antiproliferative actions. Here we discuss the pattern of expression of genes encoding for proteins involved in RA metabolism in the ER+ and ER- breast cancer cells (Fig. 3). Essentially, there is a generalized down-regulation of genes encoding proteins involved in the production of various RA metabolites. Major differences are seen in RAR, RA binding proteins, and sulfotransferase enzymes (SULT) respectively. The key differences and similarities are discussed below:

a. The protein encoded by SCARB1 is a plasma membrane receptor for HDL (high density lipoprotein) cholesterol. SCARB1 protein mediates cholesterol transfer to and from HDL. This gene is down-regulated in both cell lines. Among the metabolic genes, there is retinol saturase, (*RETSAT*); the protein of this gene catalyzes the conversion of all-trans retinol to all-trans-13, 14-dihydroretinol, an intermediate of 13, 14-dehydroRA. All-trans-13, 14-dihydroretinol binds to the RARs in the nucleus and it is selectively up-regulated in MCF-7, but is absent in MDA-MB-231 cells. Also, in the ER+ MCF-7 we see a selective up-regulation of CYP2E1, a RA degradation enzyme, which is highly up-regulated in aggressive breast tumors as discussed above. The first step of RAR activation is mediated by the delivery of RA from the cytosol to the receptor in the nucleus, a step which involves the cellular retinoic acid-binding protein 2 (*CRABP2*); this gene is highly up-regulated in MCF-7 cells (Schug *et al.*, 2008).
b. In MCF-7 cells the expression of genes encoding for SULT enzymes, *SULT2A1* and *B1*, are highly up-regulated. These enzymes catalyze the sulfate conjugation of many hormones, neurotransmitters, drugs, and xenobiotic compounds. In particular, the enzyme SULT2B1 sulfates dehydroepiandrosterone, but not 4-nitrophenol, a typical substrate for the phenol and estrogen sulfotransferase subfamilies. MDA-MB-231 cells did not show expression of these genes. In support of this, we found that the GO term molecular functions are associated with sulfotransferase activity within the RA network in E2 stimulated MCF-7 cells; genes of the RA network are associated with biological processes such as the cell cycle and its regulation, protein metabolic processes amino acid methylation and alkylation and sulphur compound biosynthetic process respectively.
c. *RARa/RXRa*-these RARs are selectively up-regulated in MCF-7, but are low in expression and absent in MDA-MB-231 cells. This selective expression can be correlated to the fact that RARa protein is involved with functions such as apoptosis and differentiation and together as hetero/homodimers mediate the biological effects by RA-mediated gene activation.
d. *RARb/RXRb-RARb* binds to RA and mediates cellular signaling in embryonic morphogenesis, cell growth and differentiation. This protein has antiproliferative effects in many cell types. This gene is down-regulated in both cell types; however, its heterodimeric counterpart, RXRb gene lies within the MHC class II region on chromosome 6a, is selectively up-regulated in MDA-MB-231 cells. The significance of this discrepancy is unknown, but may be a feature of de-regulated immune responses present in ER- breast cancer cells (Mandal *et al.*, 2007b).

RARg/RXRG-these nuclear hormone receptors are ligand-dependent transcriptional regulators. RXRg, the counterpart of RARg, mediates the antiproliferative effects of RA. RXRg is expressed at significantly lower levels in non-small cell lung cancer cells. This receptor pair is down-regulated in MDA-MB-231 cells, but RARg is selectively up-regulated in MCF-7 cells. (Information source of individual genes: www.ncbi.nlm.nih.gov)

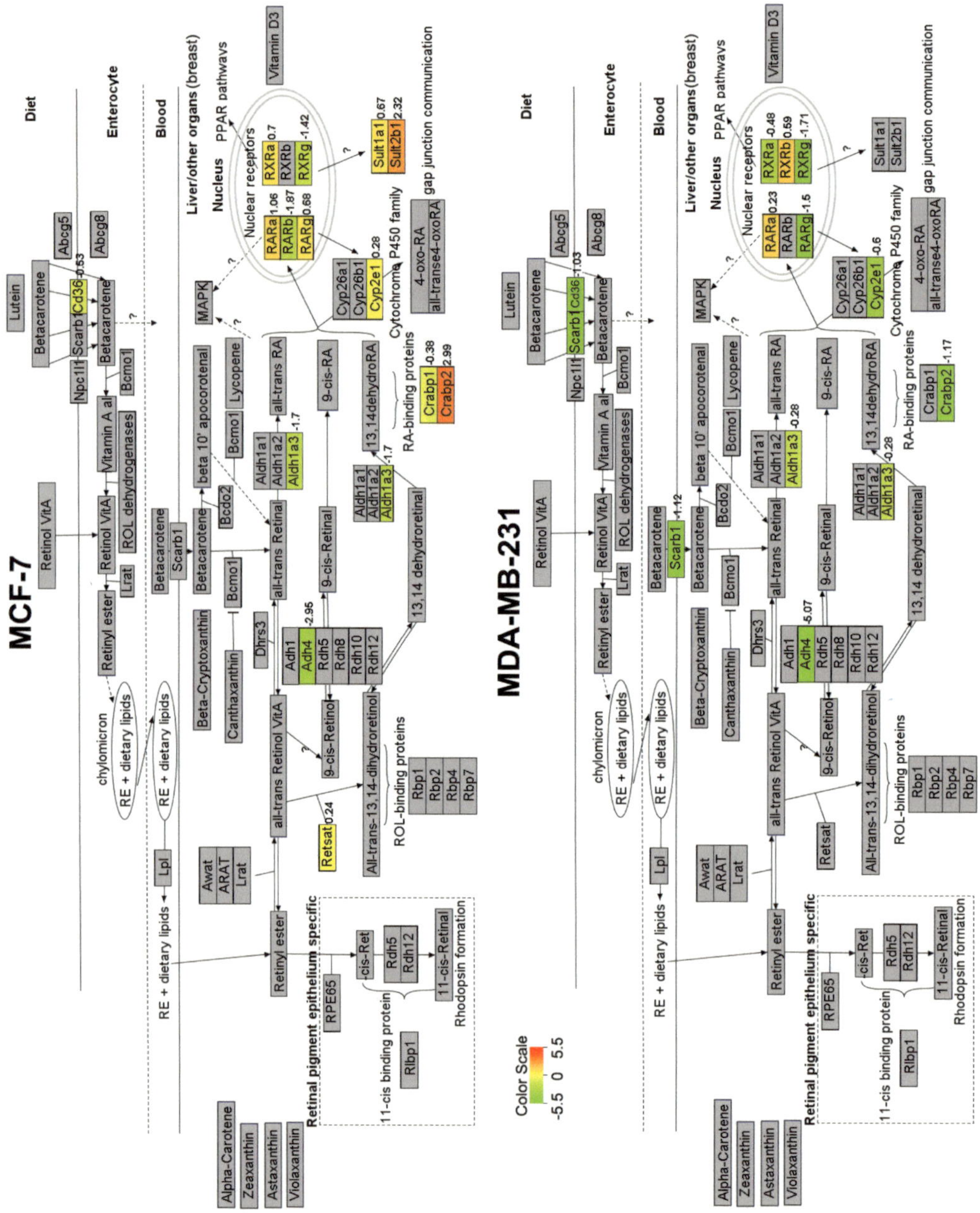

Fig. 3. A comparative view of retinoic acid metabolic pathways operating in MCF-7 and MDA-MB-231 cells is shown. The pathway maps were generated using the pathway visualization tool, PathVisio (Version 2). The software generated a color scale for the visualization of expression (red is up-regulation and green is down-regulation of gene expression). Expression values (SLR, signal log ratio) with a cutoff value of ≥ 0.2 or ≤- 0.2 was used and in case of duplicate SLR values, an average SLR was taken. Abbreviations used: ROL=retinol; RAL=retinaldehyde; RA=retinoic acid; RE=retinyl ester; RPE=retinal pigment epithelium.

5. The role of mitogen and stress activated kinase (MSK) in breast cancer

Mitogen and stress activated kinases 1 and 2 (MSK1/RPS6KA5, MSK2/RPS6KA4) are serine-threonine kinases that are activated by the p38 or RAS-MAPK signaling pathway. In breast cancer, there is overexpression of the growth factor receptors EGFR/HER1 and HER2/neu; in 25-30% of breast tumors HER2 is overexpressed and 45% of breast tumors test positive for EGFR (Klijn *et al.*, 1992; Slamon *et al.*, 1989). The overexpression of these receptors leads to the constitutive activation of the RAS-MAPK signaling pathway and the subsequent phosphorylation and activation of MSK1 and MSK2. Once activated, MSK1 and 2 can act on several substrates that are relevant to cancer signaling pathways. Importantly, MSKs can phosphorylate the serine residues S10 and S28 on the N-terminal tail of the histone protein H3 (Soloaga *et al.*, 2003). MSK1/2 mediated H3 modification is an event that can lead to chromatin remodeling and the expression of immediate-early (IE) genes such as *FOS*, *COX2*, and *JUN*, which are often up-regulated during oncogenesis (Drobic *et al.*, 2010; Dunn *et al.*, 2005). MSK proteins can also phosphorylate and activate various transcription factors such as CREB, ATF1, ER81, and the p65 subunit of NFκB, which activate the transcription of genes involved in tumorigenic and metastatic progression (Arthur and Cohen, 2000; Vermeulen *et al.*, 2003; Wiggin *et al.*, 2002).

The role of MSKs in cancer progression spans from their contribution to the process of anchorage-independent growth to a potential role in epithelial mesenchymal transition (EMT). MSK has been implied in the anchorage independent growth of mouse epidermal cells, *H-ras* transformed mouse fibroblasts and v-Src transformed mouse Balb3T3 cells (Kim *et al.*, 2008; Perez-Cadahia *et al.*, 2011; Tange *et al.*, 2009). Inhibition of MSK by the small molecule inhibitor H89 implicates MSK in the EMT process in *H-RAS* overexpressing Caco-H human colon cancer cells (Pelaez *et al.*, 2010). In the ER+ breast cancer cell line MCF-7, stimulation with the phorbol ester 12-O-tetradecanoylphorbol-13-acetate (TPA) causes the activation of the RAS-MAPK pathway and hence H3S10 phosphorylation and the induction of the E2 response gene, *TFF1* (trefoil factor 1), which has been implicated in breast cancer progression (Espino *et al.*, 2006). Interestingly, MSK activation by TPA in MCF-7 cells induces H3S10 phosphorylation but not H3S28 phosphorylation by an unknown mechanism (Espino *et al.*, 2006). However, a recent study has called into question the value of using *TFF1* as a prognostic marker in breast cancer, as it demonstrates that knockdown of *TFF1* in MCF-7 cells leads to enhanced colony formation in soft agar, and that *TFF1* knock-out mice have a higher tumor incidence in mammary glands (Buache *et al.*, 2011).

In the ER- MDA-MB-231 and SKBR-3 cells, MSK is implicated in the expression of the pro-inflammatory cytokine IL-6, whereby IL-6 is constitutively expressed and MSK is recruited to the IL-6 promoter following TNF-α signaling. The MSK-mediated expression of IL-6 involves MSK-mediated phosphorylation of $NF\kappa Bp65^{S276}$, recruitment of MSK and phosphorylation of H3S10 on the IL-6 promoter, followed by subsequent chromatin remodeling of the promoter via the recruitment of the BRG1 subunit of the SWI/SNF chromatin remodeling complex (Ndlovu *et al.*, 2009). Similarly, MSK mediated H3S10 phosphorylation can induce the chromatin remodeling of the mouse mammary tumor virus (MMTV) promoter in MTVL breast cancer cells that have a stably integrated luciferase reporter gene driven by the MMTV promoter (Vicent *et al.*, 2008). In this system, progestin treatment leads to the formation of a ternary complex comprised of the PR and phosphorylated ERK (pERK) and MSK1 (pMSK1). The PR/pERK/pMSK1 complex is recruited to the MMTV promoter followed by phosphorylation of H3S10 by pMSK, leading to the displacement of the HP1γ repressor complex and the subsequent activation of gene transcription in these cells (Vicent *et al.*, 2008; Vicent *et al.*, 2009). In the ER- cells (eg., MDA-MB-231) MSK has been implicated in the migration and invasion of cells to lymphatic endothelial cells *in vitro* as well as in *in vivo* mouse xenograft model through the possible NFκB binding to the chemokine receptor CCR7 (Pan *et al.*, 2009). MSK has also been implicated in cancer-related inflammation through *COX2* expression. It has been observed that MSK-mediated *COX2* expression in mouse epidermal cells induces neoplastic transformation (Yan *et al.*, 2006). MSK recruitment and H3S10 and H3S28 phosphorylation occur at the upstream regulatory promoter region of *COX2* in mouse fibroblasts in addition to the recruitment of chromatin remodeling factors and transcriptional activation histone marks at these sites (Drobic *et al.*, 2010). In MCF-7, TPA selectively induces *COX2* expression (Degner *et al.*, 2006). From these data it can be speculated that MSK may be involved in *COX2* expression/regulation in breast cancer cells, although this has yet to be experimentally reported. MSKs contribute to breast cancer progression through a variety of mechanisms including the induction of genes involved in transformation or inflammation, and priming gene promoters for chromatin remodeling and activation.

5.1 A comparative analysis of the MAPK pathway in ER+ and ER- breast cancer

As discussed in the previous paragraphs, genes of the MAPK pathway have profound effects on the progression of breast cancer. An overall comparison between MCF-7 and MDA-MB-231 shows that all the caspases are either absent or down-regulated in both cell lines, *EGFR* is up-regulated in the MDA-MB-231. cells, and the early responsive genes, *FOS* and *JUN* are oppositely expressed, and the p50/p105 (NFκB1) subunit of NFκB is up-regulated. *BDNF* (brain-derived neurotrophic factor) is highly expressed in MDA-MB-231 cells, but is totally absent in MCF-7 cells. The high expression of *BDNF* is of speculative importance because the gene encoding for this protein of the nerve growth factor family is responsible for the survival of striatal neurons and also responds to stress. Different members of MAP kinases are differntially up/down-regulated in the two cell lines, which may be a reflection of aggressiveness. The key differences and similarities are discussed below (Fig. 4):

a. *DUSP*- dual specificity protein phosphatase enzymes play important roles in regulating cellular response to environmental stress are also negative regulators of cell proliferation. They negatively regulate members of the mitogen-activated protein (MAP) kinase superfamily, which are associated with cellular proliferation and differentiation. Different members of this family of phosphatases have distinct substrate specificities for various MAP kinases, different tissue distribution and subcellular localization, and different modes of inducibility of their expression by extracellular stimuli. Interestingly, genes encoding for these phosphatases are down-regulated in MCF-7 and are up-regulated in MDA-MB-231 cells.
b. *PRKC (B, Z, H, G, D)*-Protein kinase C (PKC) is a family of serine- and threonine-specific protein kinases that can be activated by calcium and second messenger DAG (diacylglycerol). PKC family members phosphorylate a wide variety of protein targets and participate in diverse cellular signaling pathways. PKCs are major receptors for phorbol esters; in the comparative gene analysis, we find that most of the PKCs are down-regulated or absent with the exception of a few, but we have shown that the ER+ MCF-7 cells activate the MAPK pathway in response to TPA (Espino *et al.*, 2006). (Information source of individual genes: www.ncbi.nlm.nih.gov)

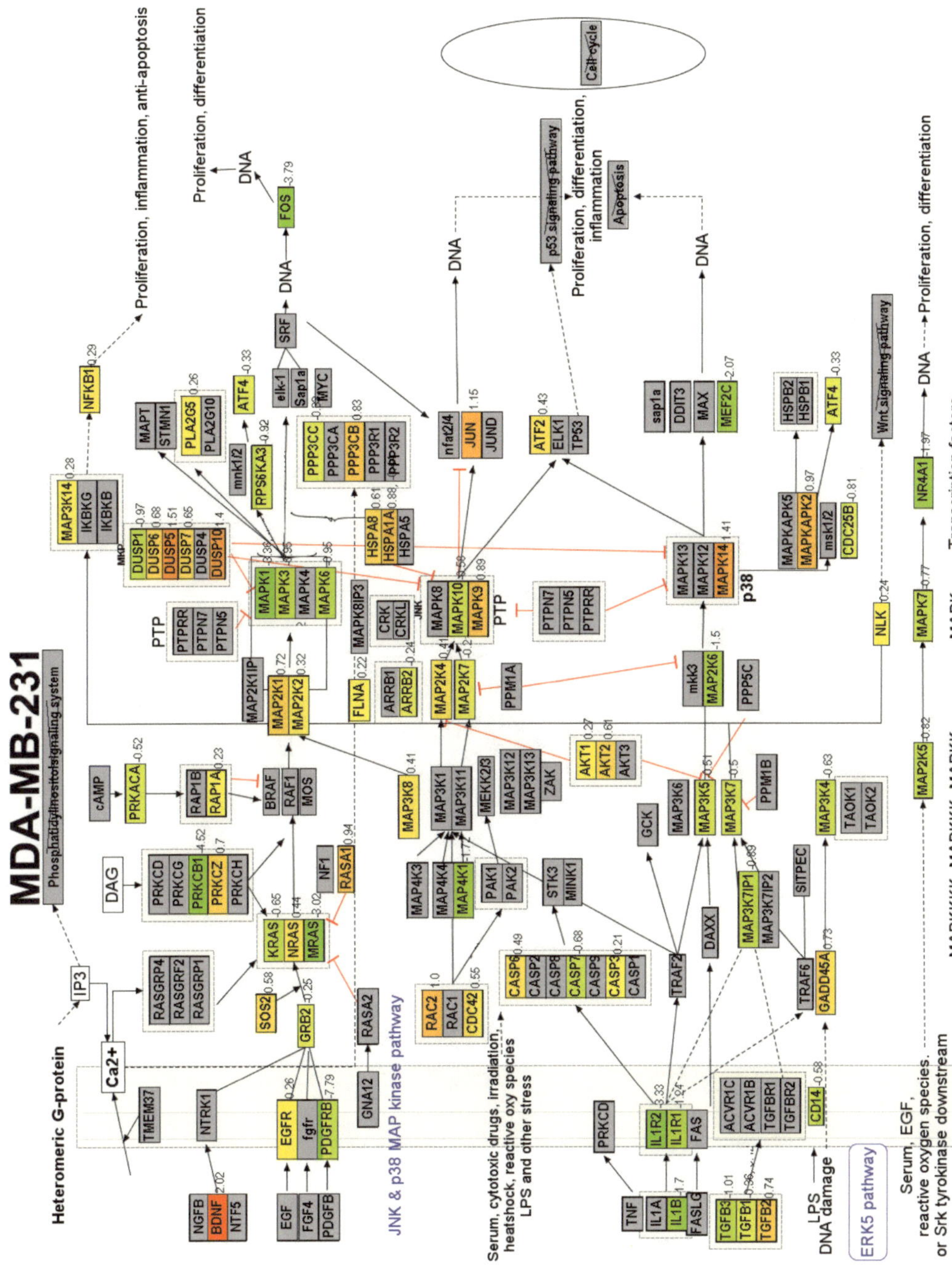

Fig. 4. (Continued)

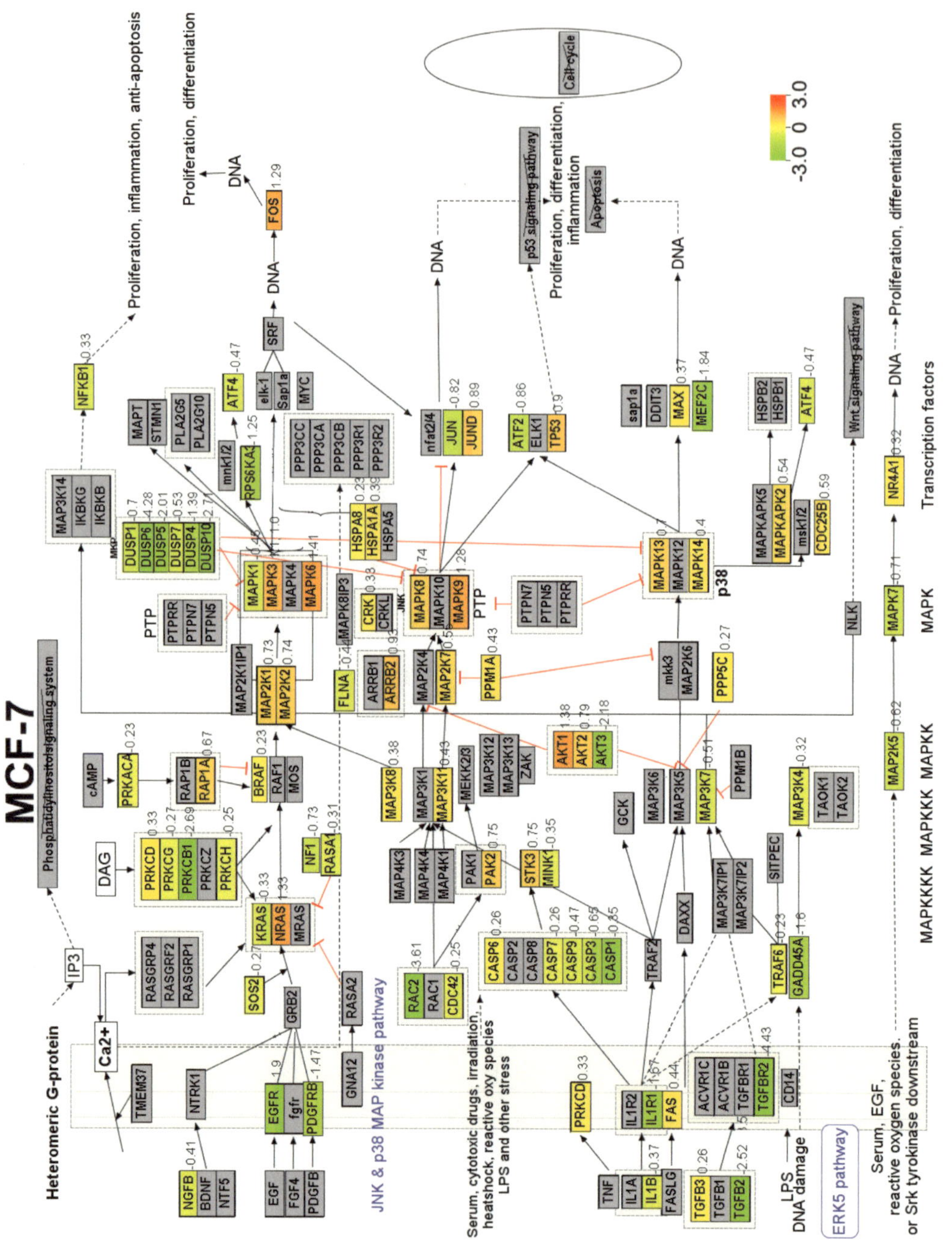

Fig. 4. A comparative view of the MAPK pathway operating in MCF-7 and MDA-MB-231 cells is shown. The pathway maps were generated using the pathway visualization tool, PathVisio (Version 2). The software generated a color scale for the visualization of expression (red is up-regulation and green is down-regulation of gene expression). Expression values (SLR, signal log ratio) with a cutoff value of ≥ 0.2 or ≤- 0.2 was used and in case of duplicate values, an average SLR was taken.

6. Role of transcription factors, Sp1 and Sp3 in breast cancer

Sp1 and Sp3 proteins are overexpressed in breast tumors and contribute to the proliferative and angiogenic phenotype, characteristics which correlate to poor prognosis (Li *et al.*, 2004; Mertens-Talcott *et al.*, 2007). There are an estimated 12000 Sp1 and Sp3 binding sites in human genome (Cawley *et al.*, 2004). Inhibition of Sp1 binding to DNA by mithramycin A or knocking down Sp1 to the normal expression level, decreased tumor formation, growth and metastasis (Lou *et al.*, 2005; Yuan *et al.*, 2007). Likewise, antiproliferative agents such as, betulinic acid and curcumin reduced the expression of Sp1 and Sp3 and their target genes (*EGFR, CCND1, VEGF, SREBF2, CD151*), which have roles in metastasis (Chadalapaka *et al.*, 2010; Kang and Chen, 2009). Knocking out Sp1/Sp3 was lethal and caused the death of knockout mice at different developmental stages. Compounded Sp1 and Sp3 knockout mice were not viable suggesting that both these transcription factors are required to maintain appropriate gene expression programs (Bouwman *et al.*, 2000; Kruger *et al.*, 2007; Marin *et al.*, 1997; Van Loo *et al.*, 2003). This agrees with the fact that Sp1 and Sp3 are autoregulated genes with Sp1 and Sp3 binding sites in their proximal promoter regions (Nicolas *et al.*, 2001).

In the estrogen and breast cancer context, it is known that many estrogen responsive genes have Sp1/3(s) sites in the estrogen response elements of their promoters (Castro-Rivera *et al.*, 2001; Higgins *et al.*, 2006; Mandal and Davie, 2010; Sun *et al.*, 2002; Sun *et al.*, 2005). *TFF1* is a highly expressed estrogen responsive gene in malignant breast epithelial cells but not normal mammary cells (Rio *et al.*, 1987). In our studies, we predicted and validated a Sp1/3 site 6 bp upstream of the imperfect ERE site and the dynamic association of ERα, Sp protein, KATs and HDACs on the *TFF1* proximal promoter in response to E2 using TFSEARCH, ChIP (chromatin immunoprecipitation) assay and promoter analysis. We found Sp3, but not Sp1, to be the major Sp protein activating the *TFF1* upstream promoter region in response to E2 (Sun *et al.*, 2005). This was supported by other studies where it was shown that Sp3 plays a major role in ERα/Sp-mediated gene expression in MCF-7 cells (Khan *et al.*, 2007). In general, Sp1 usually activates transcription and Sp3 represses or most weakly activates transcription (Higgins *et al.*, 2006; Jaiswal *et al.*, 2006; Noe *et al.*, 2001). Though in some studies it was shown that Sp1 and Sp3 synergistically enhanced gene promoter function, we have shown that Sp1 and Sp3 did not exist in the same protein complexes in the *TFF1* promoter in MCF-7 cells (Hantusch *et al.*, 2007; He *et al.*, 2005; Lee *et al.*, 2009; Li and Davie, 2008).

6.1 Regulation of transcriptional responses of Sp1 and Sp3

Sp1 and Sp3 have multiple isoforms, of which Sp1 has two and Sp3 has four isoforms (Li and Davie, 2010). Four Sp3 isoforms have been reported. The two long forms of Sp3 and Sp1 contain two trans-activation domains A and B, one serine / threonine rich domain for post-translational modifications (PTMs) and the DNA binding domain C. Sp1 has domain D at the C-terminus which is critical for its synergistic activation. As the Sp family signature, the DNA binding domain C features the three Cys2His2 zinc 'fingers' required for sequence-specific DNA association. The consensus Sp1 and Sp3 binding DNA sequence is GGGGCGGGG. Although recognizing the same DNA binding sequence, Sp1 and Sp3 differ structurally in the location of their inhibitory domains; it is at the N-terminus for Sp1 and for Sp3 this domain lies immediately in front of the DNA binding domain (Suske, 1999).

PTMs such as sumoylation and acetylation of Sp1 and Sp3 regulate their functional roles (Li *et al.*, 2004; Li and Davie, 2010). Sumoylated Sp1 was deficient in proteolytic processing; it was proposed that Sp1 sumoylation preserves the integrity of a negative regulatory domain and inhibits the Sp1-dependent transcription (Spengler and Brattain, 2006). In another study however, sumoylation was found to aid in Sp1 interaction with the proteosome (Wang *et al.*, 2008). The major sumoylation of Sp3 long and short forms occurs at K551, which is a single lysine in its inhibitory domain and a minor sumoylation site (K120) is in the long form. The K551 modification silenced or significantly decreased Sp3 activity and mutation of this site converted the short Sp3 isoforms into potent transactivators of the SRC 1A gene promoter, but did not affect the transcriptional properties of Sp3 long forms (Ellis *et al.*, 2006; Ross *et al.*, 2002; Sapetschnig *et al.*, 2002; Spengler *et al.*, 2008). Interestingly, acetylation of K551 by KAT p300 converts Sp3 to a transcriptional activator; thus the activity of Sp3 can be repressing or activating depending on PTM of K551 (Ammanamanchi *et al.*, 2003). Sp1 can also be acetylated by p300, but the exact role of acetylation is unclear (Song *et al.*, 2003). Another PTM is methylation within or around Sp1/3 site(s), which regulates Sp1 and Sp3 association with DNA to regulate gene expression (Mudduluru and Allgayer, 2008). Whereas methylation within the consensus Sp1/3 site did not influence binding of Sp1/Sp3 to the $p21^{Waf1/Cip1}$ promoter, this modification outside the GC boxes reduced Sp1/Sp3 binding to $p21^{Waf1/Cip1}$ and mouse *Abcc6* promoter with repression of gene expression (Zhu *et al.*, 2003). Thus these Sp1/Sp3 PTMs likely influence the functional roles of these transcription factors for gene activation and repression.

6.2 A comparative analysis of Sp1-Sp3 interactions in ER+ and ER- breast cancer – The Sp1 and Sp3 target genes

Sp1 and Sp3 participate in the regulation of tissue-specific, viral, and inducible genes (Davie *et al.*, 2008; Lu and Archer, 2010). Genes include regulators of cell cycle progression and arrest (eg. cyclins), pro- and anti-angiogenic factors involved in invasion and metastasis, pro- and anti-apoptotic factors involved in genomic stability, proto-oncogenes (eg. *MYC*), tumor suppressors (eg. *p53*), enhancers of cell proliferation and oncogenesis (Abdelrahim *et al.*, 2002; DesJardins and Hay, 1993; Feng *et al.*, 2000; Kavurma *et al.*, 2001; Lagger *et al.*, 2003; Olofsson *et al.*, 2007; Yuan *et al.*, 2007). Analysis by Ingenuity Pathway Analysis (IPA) tool showed that in MCF-7 and MDA-MB-231 cells, Sp1 and Sp3 share a network of interconnected genes inclusive of all categories discussed above (Fig. 5A, 5B). Fig. 5C is a snapshot cluster view of the Sp1-Sp3 gene network. Comparison showed that in the ER+ MCF-7 cells Sp1 was up-regulated and Sp3 was expressed at lower levels, while Sp3 was highly expressed in the MDA-MB-231 cells. In case of the $p21^{Waf1/Cip1}$ promoter, we also observed a lower Sp3 association in response to estrogen stimulation in MCF-7 cells (Mandal and Davie, 2007). We demonstrated that both Sp1 and Sp3 associated with *TFF1*, but Sp3, not Sp1, plays a major role in the estrogen activated ERα/Sp-mediated gene expression in MCF-7 cells (Khan *et al.*, 2007; Li and Davie, 2008). Therefore, in the context of estrogen stimulation, Sp1 and Sp3 play dual roles in regulating gene expression.

7. Conclusions

The evidence presented here show that metabolic patterns, transcriptional responses and gene expression in pathways in ER+ cells considerably differ from the ER- breast cancer counterpart. Generally, gene expression of energy metabolic pathways is low to absent for the more metastatic ER- cancer cells. Estrogen is a major mitogen which drives metabolic processes related to glucose and fatty acid metabolism and the hormone is also responsible

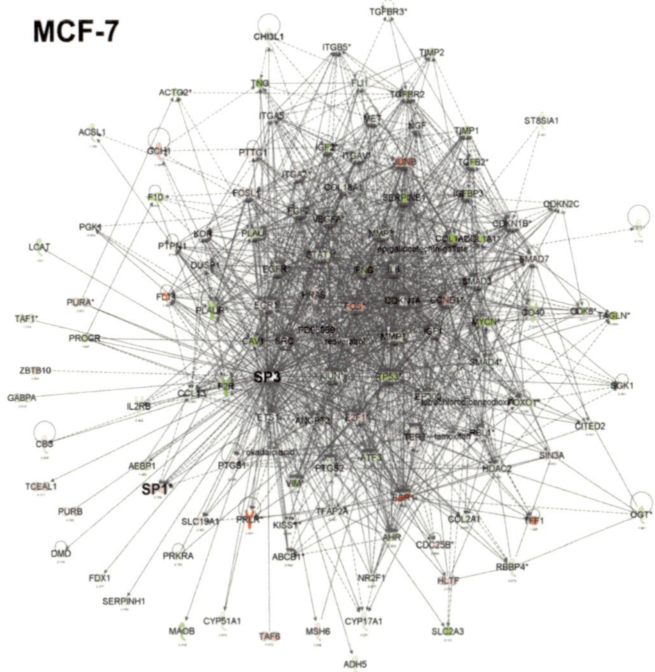

5A

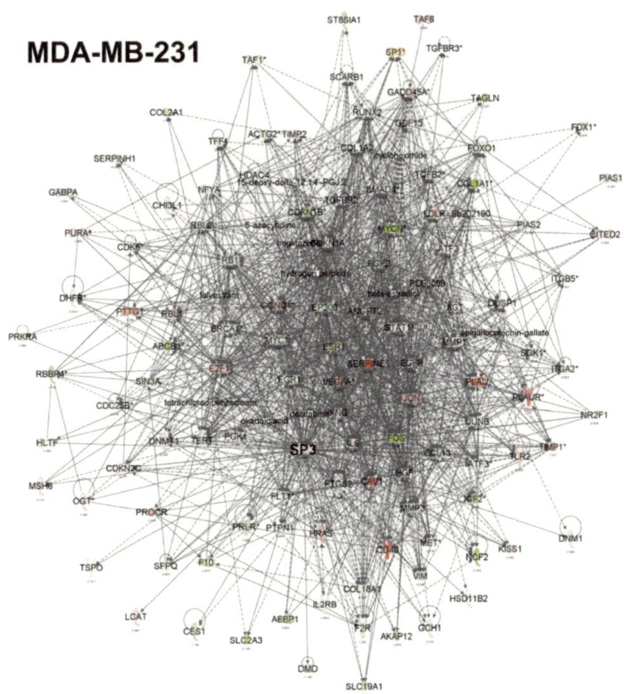

5B

Fig. 5. (Continued)

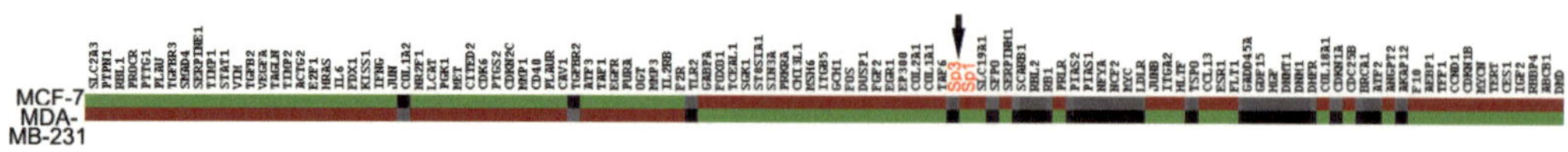

5C

Fig. 5. A network of genes connected to the transcription factors Sp1 and Sp3 in (A) in the ER+ MCF-7 and the (B) ER- MDA-MB-231 cells. This network was generated using IPA (Ingenuity Pathway Analysis) tool. Red indicates positive and green indicates negative expression. (C) A cluster view of the genes in the network (Cluster Tree view; red is positive, green is negative, grey is total absence of expression); cluster analysis was done as described previously (Eisen *et al.*, 1998). Expression values (SLR, signal log ratio) with a cutoff value of ≥ 0.2 or ≤- 0.2 was used and in case of duplicate values, an average SLR was taken.

for the Sp1 and Sp3 transcriptionally driven expression of many estrogen responsive genes. The functional role of Sp1 and Sp3 in estrogen stimulated breast cancer cells is determined by the type of PTM, protein interaction, promoter context, collectively all of which contribute to the progression of the disease. The contribution of MSK to breast cancer progression is manifold. Importantly, MSK proteins can be inhibited by small molecules (e.g. H89) which reverse the epigenetic effects of MSK on gene transcription, and thereby make MSK an attractive target for cancer therapy. Moreover, it has been shown that treatment with MEK1/2 inhibitors such as PD98059, can cause radio-sensitization of MCF-7 cells in clonogenic survival assay. The MAPK pathway can also be proapoptotic in breast cancer cells. In the ER+ T47D cells, p38 kinase inhibitors (SB202190, SB203580, PD169316) abolished activin-mediated growth arrest, suggesting that this pathway can be utilized by a growth factor for growth inhibitory effects (Cocolakis *et al.*, 2001). Further studies are required to determine the mechanisms by which MEK1/2 inhibitors commit cells to killing via apoptotic and non-apoptotic mechanisms (Qiao *et al.*, 2002). On the other hand, targeting these major transcription factors is also a promising therapeutic approach. Most of the current studies have focused on Sp1 mRNA/protein expression and more studies on Sp3 isoforms are required to develop better Sp protein targeting cancer therapies. Several approaches to the development and delivery of metabolic drugs also hold promise to the treatment of hormone responsive tumors.

8. Acknowledgments

Research support has been provided by a grant from the Canadian Breast Cancer Foundation to JRD and a Canada Research Chair to JRD. Lin Li was a recipient of the U.S. Army Medical and Materiel Command Breast Cancer Research Program Foundation Studentship grant W81XWH-05-1-0284.

9. References

Abdelrahim, M. *et al.* (2002). Small inhibitory RNA duplexes for Sp1 mRNA block basal and estrogen-induced gene expression and cell cycle progression in MCF-7 breast cancer cells. *J Biol Chem* 277, 28815-28822.

Ali, S., Coombes, R. C. (2000). Estrogen receptor alpha in human breast cancer: occurrence and significance. *J Mammary Gland Biol Neoplasia* 5, 271-281.

Ammanamanchi, S. *et al.* (2003). Acetylated sp3 is a transcriptional activator. *J Biol Chem* 278, 35775-35780.

Andresen, T. L. *et al.* (2005). Advanced strategies in liposomal cancer therapy: problems and prospects of active and tumor specific drug release. *Prog Lipid Res* 44, 68-97.

Arthur, J. S., Cohen, P. (2000). MSK1 is required for CREB phosphorylation in response to mitogens in mouse embryonic stem cells. *FEBS Lett* 482, 44-48.

Bazley, L. A., Gullick, W. J. (2005). The epidermal growth factor receptor family. *Endocr Relat Cancer* 12 Suppl 1, S17-S27.

Bitman, J. *et al.* (1965). Kinetics of in vivo glycogen synthesis in the estrogen-stimulated rat uterus. *Endocrinology* 76, 63-69.

Bouwman, P. *et al.* (2000). Transcription factor Sp3 is essential for post-natal survival and late tooth development. *EMBO J* 19, 655-661.

bu-Abed, S. S. *et al.* (1998). Mouse P450RAI (CYP26) expression and retinoic acid-inducible retinoic acid metabolism in F9 cells are regulated by retinoic acid receptor gamma and retinoid X receptor alpha. *J Biol Chem* 273, 2409-2415.

Buache, E. *et al.* (2011). Deficiency in trefoil factor 1 (TFF1) increases tumorigenicity of human breast cancer cells and mammary tumor development in TFF1-knockout mice. *Oncogene*.

Calviello, G. *et al.* (2009). Antineoplastic effects of n-3 polyunsaturated fatty acids in combination with drugs and radiotherapy: preventive and therapeutic strategies. *Nutr Cancer* 61, 287-301.

Castro-Rivera, E. *et al.* (2001). Estrogen regulation of cyclin D1 gene expression in ZR-75 breast cancer cells involves multiple enhancer elements. *J Biol Chem* 276, 30853-30861.

Cawley, S. *et al.* (2004). Unbiased mapping of transcription factor binding sites along human chromosomes 21 and 22 points to widespread regulation of noncoding RNAs. *Cell* 116, 499-509.

Chadalapaka, G. *et al.* (2010). Drugs that target specificity proteins downregulate epidermal growth factor receptor in bladder cancer cells. *Mol Cancer Res* 8, 739-750.

Chell, S. *et al.* (2006). Mediators of PGE2 synthesis and signalling downstream of COX-2 represent potential targets for the prevention/treatment of colorectal cancer. *Biochim Biophys Acta* 1766, 104-119.

Chen, J. Q. *et al.* (2009). Regulation of energy metabolism pathways by estrogens and estrogenic chemicals and potential implications in obesity associated with increased exposure to endocrine disruptors. *Biochim Biophys Acta* 1793, 1128-1143.

Cocolakis, E. *et al.* (2001). The p38 MAPK pathway is required for cell growth inhibition of human breast cancer cells in response to activin. *J Biol Chem* 276, 18430-18436.

Coser, K. R. *et al.* (2009). Antiestrogen-resistant subclones of MCF-7 human breast cancer cells are derived from a common monoclonal drug-resistant progenitor. *Proc Natl Acad Sci U S A* 106, 14536-14541.

Davie, J. R. *et al.* (2008). Nuclear organization and chromatin dynamics--Sp1, Sp3 and histone deacetylases. *Adv Enzyme Regul* 48, 189-208.

Degner, S. C. *et al.* (2006). Conjugated linoleic acid attenuates cyclooxygenase-2 transcriptional activity via an anti-AP-1 mechanism in MCF-7 breast cancer cells. *J Nutr* 136, 421-427.

deGraffenried, L. A. *et al.* (2002). Sp1 is essential for estrogen receptor alpha gene transcription. *J Steroid Biochem Mol Biol* 82, 7-18.

DesJardins, E., Hay, N. (1993). Repeated CT elements bound by zinc finger proteins control the absolute and relative activities of the two principal human c-myc promoters. *Mol Cell Biol* 13, 5710-5724.

Dickson, R. B., Lippman, M. E. (1988). Control of human breast cancer by estrogen, growth factors, and oncogenes. *Cancer Treat Res* 40, 119-165.

Drobic, B. *et al.* (2010). Promoter chromatin remodeling of immediate-early genes is mediated through H3 phosphorylation at either serine 28 or 10 by the MSK1 multi-protein complex. *Nucleic Acids Res* 38, 3196-3208.

Duester, G. (2008). Retinoic acid synthesis and signaling during early organogenesis. *Cell* 134, 921-931.

Dunn, K. L. *et al.* (2005). The Ras-MAPK signal transduction pathway, cancer and chromatin remodeling. *Biochem Cell Biol* 83, 1-14.

Eisen, M. B. *et al.* (1998). Cluster analysis and display of genome-wide expression patterns. *Proc Natl Acad Sci U S A* 95, 14863-14868.

Ellis, D. J. *et al.* (2006). The modification of Sp3 isoforms by Sumoylation has differential effects on the SRC1A promoter. *Gene* 379, 68-78.

Espino, P. S. *et al.* (2006). Chromatin modification of the trefoil factor 1 gene in human breast cancer cells by the Ras/mitogen-activated protein kinase pathway. *Cancer Res* 66, 4610-4616.

Feng, X. H. *et al.* (2000). Smad2, Smad3 and Smad4 cooperate with Sp1 to induce p15(Ink4B) transcription in response to TGF-beta. *EMBO J* 19, 5178-5193.

Ferguson, A. T., Davidson, N. E. (1997). Regulation of estrogen receptor alpha function in breast cancer. *Crit Rev Oncog* 8, 29-46.

Gallo, D. *et al.* (2007). Calmodulin-independent, agonistic properties of a peptide containing the calmodulin binding site of estrogen receptor alpha. *Mol Cell Endocrinol* 268, 37-49.

Hantusch, B. *et al.* (2007). Sp1/Sp3 and DNA-methylation contribute to basal transcriptional activation of human podoplanin in MG63 versus Saos-2 osteoblastic cells. *BMC Mol Biol* 8, 20.

He, S. *et al.* (2005). Differential intranuclear organization of transcription factors Sp1 and Sp3. *Mol Biol Cell* 16, 4073-4083.

Helms, M. W. *et al.* (2008). Squalene epoxidase, located on chromosome 8q24.1, is upregulated in 8q+ breast cancer and indicates poor clinical outcome in stage I and II disease. *Br J Cancer* 99, 774-780.

Higgins, K. J. *et al.* (2006). Vascular endothelial growth factor receptor-2 expression is induced by 17beta-estradiol in ZR-75 breast cancer cells by estrogen receptor alpha/Sp proteins. *Endocrinology* 147, 3285-3295.

Hirokawa, T. (1984). [Experimental chemotherapy using a transplanted head and neck cancer model in athymic nude mice]. *Nippon Jibiinkoka Gakkai Kaiho* 87, 182-194.

Hockings, J. K. *et al.* (2008). Involvement of a specificity proteins-binding element in regulation of basal and estrogen-induced transcription activity of the BRCA1 gene. *Breast Cancer Res* 10, R29.

Jaiswal, A. S. *et al.* (2006). 7,12-Dimethylbenzanthracene-dependent transcriptional regulation of adenomatous polyposis coli (APC) gene expression in normal breast epithelial cells is mediated by GC-box binding protein Sp3. *Carcinogenesis* 27, 252-261.

Jia, Z. *et al.* (2010). Combined treatment of pancreatic cancer with mithramycin A and tolfenamic acid promotes Sp1 degradation and synergistic antitumor activity. *Cancer Res* 70, 1111-1119.

Kang, Q., Chen, A. (2009). Curcumin inhibits srebp-2 expression in activated hepatic stellate cells in vitro by reducing the activity of specificity protein-1. *Endocrinology* 150, 5384-5394.

Kavurma, M. M. *et al.* (2001). Sp1 phosphorylation regulates apoptosis via extracellular FasL-Fas engagement. *J Biol Chem* 276, 4964-4971.

Khan, S. *et al.* (2007). Role of specificity protein transcription factors in estrogen-induced gene expression in MCF-7 breast cancer cells. *J Mol Endocrinol* 39, 289-304.

Khan, S. A. *et al.* (1994). Estrogen receptor expression of benign breast epithelium and its association with breast cancer. *Cancer Res* 54, 993-997.

Kim, H. G. *et al.* (2008). Mitogen- and stress-activated kinase 1-mediated histone H3 phosphorylation is crucial for cell transformation. *Cancer Res* 68, 2538-2547.

Klijn, J. G. *et al.* (1992). The clinical significance of epidermal growth factor receptor (EGF-R) in human breast cancer: a review on 5232 patients. *Endocr Rev* 13, 3-17.

Ko, B. H. *et al.* (2010). 17beta-estradiol augments 18F-FDG uptake and glycolysis of T47D breast cancer cells via membrane-initiated rapid PI3K-Akt activation. *J Nucl Med* 51, 1740-1747.

Kruger, I. *et al.* (2007). Sp1/Sp3 compound heterozygous mice are not viable: impaired erythropoiesis and severe placental defects. *Dev Dyn* 236, 2235-2244.

Lagger, G. *et al.* (2003). The tumor suppressor p53 and histone deacetylase 1 are antagonistic regulators of the cyclin-dependent kinase inhibitor p21/WAF1/CIP1 gene. *Mol Cell Biol* 23, 2669-2679.

Laye, J. P., Gill, J. H. (2003). Phospholipase A2 expression in tumours: a target for therapeutic intervention? *Drug Discov Today* 8, 710-716.

Lee, V. H. *et al.* (2009). Regulation of RASSF1A in nasopharyngeal cells and its response to UV irradiation. *Gene* 443, 55-63.

Li, L., Davie, J. R. (2008). Association of Sp3 and estrogen receptor alpha with the transcriptionally active trefoil factor 1 promoter in MCF-7 breast cancer cells. *J Cell Biochem* 105, 365-369.

Li, L., Davie, J. R. (2010). The role of Sp1 and Sp3 in normal and cancer cell biology. *Ann Anat* 192, 275-283.

Li, L. *et al.* (2004). Gene regulation by Sp1 and Sp3. *Biochem Cell Biol* 82, 460-471.

Li, Y. *et al.* (2011). The histone modifications governing TFF1 transcription mediated by estrogen receptor. *J Biol Chem.*

Lou, Z. *et al.* (2005). Down-regulation of overexpressed sp1 protein in human fibrosarcoma cell lines inhibits tumor formation. *Cancer Res* 65, 1007-1017.

Lu, S., Archer, M. C. (2010). Sp1 coordinately regulates de novo lipogenesis and proliferation in cancer cells. *Int J Cancer* 126, 416-425.

Macheda, M. L. *et al.* (2005). Molecular and cellular regulation of glucose transporter (GLUT) proteins in cancer. *J Cell Physiol* 202, 654-662.

Mandal, S. *et al.* (2007a). A novel series of potent cytotoxic agents targeting G2/M phase of the cell cycle and demonstrating cell killing by apoptosis in human breast cancer cells. *Bioorg Med Chem Lett* 17, 4955-4960.

Mandal, S. *et al.* (2007b). S100A7 (psoriasin) influences immune response genes in human breast cancer. *Exp Cell Res* 313, 3016-3025.

Mandal, S., Davie, J. R. (2007). An integrated analysis of genes and pathways exhibiting metabolic differences between estrogen receptor positive breast cancer cells. *BMC Cancer* 7, 181.

Mandal, S., Davie, J. R. (2010). Estrogen regulated expression of the p21(Waf1/Cip1) gene in estrogen receptor positive human breast cancer cells. *J Cell Physiol* 224, 28-32.

Marin, M. *et al.* (1997). Transcription factor Sp1 is essential for early embryonic development but dispensable for cell growth and differentiation. *Cell* 89, 619-628.

Meadows, A. L. *et al.* (2008). Metabolic and morphological differences between rapidly proliferating cancerous and normal breast epithelial cells. *Biotechnol Prog* 24, 334-341.

Medina, R. A., Owen, G. I. (2002). Glucose transporters: expression, regulation and cancer. *Biol Res* 35, 9-26.

Mertens-Talcott, S. U. *et al.* (2007). The oncogenic microRNA-27a targets genes that regulate specificity protein transcription factors and the G2-M checkpoint in MDA-MB-231 breast cancer cells. *Cancer Res* 67, 11001-11011.

Mic, F. A. *et al.* (2002). Novel retinoic acid generating activities in the neural tube and heart identified by conditional rescue of Raldh2 null mutant mice. *Development* 129, 2271-2282.

Mira, Y. L. *et al.* (2000). Retinol conversion to retinoic acid is impaired in breast cancer cell lines relative to normal cells. *J Cell Physiol* 185, 302-309.

Moreno-Sanchez, R. *et al.* (2007). Energy metabolism in tumor cells. *FEBS J* 274, 1393-1418.

Mudduluru, G., Allgayer, H. (2008). The human receptor tyrosine kinase Axl gene--promoter characterization and regulation of constitutive expression by Sp1, Sp3 and CpG methylation. *Biosci Rep* 28, 161-176.

Muss, H. B. (2001). Role of adjuvant endocrine therapy in early-stage breast cancer. *Semin Oncol* 28, 313-321.

Ndlovu, N. *et al.* (2009). Hyperactivated NF-{kappa}B and AP-1 transcription factors promote highly accessible chromatin and constitutive transcription across the interleukin-6 gene promoter in metastatic breast cancer cells. *Mol Cell Biol* 29, 5488-5504.

Nicolas, M. *et al.* (2001). Cloning and characterization of the 5'-flanking region of the human transcription factor Sp1 gene. *J Biol Chem* 276, 22126-22132.

Nicolette, J. A., Gorski, J. (1964). Effect of estradiol on glucose-u-c-14 metabolism in the rat uterus. *Arch Biochem Biophys* 107, 279-283.

Noe, V. *et al.* (2001). Sp1 involvement in the 4beta-phorbol 12-myristate 13-acetate (TPA)-mediated increase in resistance to methotrexate in Chinese hamster ovary cells. *Eur J Biochem* 268, 3163-3173.

Okamoto, K. *et al.* (2000). Differences in uptake and metabolism of retinoic acid between estrogen receptor-positive and -negative human breast cancer cells. *Cancer Chemother Pharmacol* 46, 128-134.

Olofsson, B. A. *et al.* (2007). Phosphorylation of Sp1 in response to DNA damage by ataxia telangiectasia-mutated kinase. *Mol Cancer Res* 5, 1319-1330.

Osanai, M. *et al.* (2010). Oncogenic and cell survival properties of the retinoic acid metabolizing enzyme, CYP26A1. *Oncogene* 29, 1135-1144.

Pan, M. R. *et al.* (2009). Tubocapsanolide A inhibits transforming growth factor-beta-activating kinase 1 to suppress NF-kappaB-induced CCR7. *J Biol Chem* 284, 2746-2754.

Pelaez, I. M. *et al.* (2010). Oncogenic RAS alters the global and gene-specific histone modification pattern during epithelial-mesenchymal transition in colorectal carcinoma cells. *Int J Biochem Cell Biol* 42, 911-920.

Pelekanou, V. *et al.* (2011). The estrogen receptor alpha-derived peptide ERalpha17p (P(295)-T(311)) exerts pro-apoptotic actions in breast cancer cells in vitro and in vivo, independently from their ERalpha status. *Mol Oncol* 5, 36-47.

Perez-Cadahia, B. *et al.* (2011). Role of MSK1 in the malignant phenotype of Ras-transformed mouse fibroblasts. *J Biol Chem* 286, 42-49.

Prall, O. W. *et al.* (1998). Estrogen regulation of cell cycle progression in breast cancer cells. *J Steroid Biochem Mol Biol* 65, 169-174.

Puig, T. *et al.* (2008). Fatty acid metabolism in breast cancer cells: differential inhibitory effects of epigallocatechin gallate (EGCG) and C75. *Breast Cancer Res Treat* 109, 471-479.

Qiao, L. *et al.* (2002). Pharmocologic inhibitors of the mitogen activated protein kinase cascade have the potential to interact with ionizing radiation exposure to induce cell death in carcinoma cells by multiple mechanisms. *Cancer Biol Ther* 1, 168-176.

Rasmussen, N. *et al.* (2010). Effect of free fatty acids and lysolipids on cellular uptake of doxorubicin in human breast cancer cell lines. *Anticancer Drugs* 21, 674-677.

Rio, M. C. *et al.* (1987). Specific expression of the pS2 gene in subclasses of breast cancers in comparison with expression of the estrogen and progesterone receptors and the oncogene ERBB2. *Proc Natl Acad Sci U S A* 84, 9243-9247.

Rivenzon-Segal, D. *et al.* (2003). Glycolysis and glucose transporter 1 as markers of response to hormonal therapy in breast cancer. *Int J Cancer* 107, 177-182.

Rogers, S. *et al.* (2003). Differential expression of GLUT12 in breast cancer and normal breast tissue. *Cancer Lett* 193, 225-233.

Ross, S. *et al.* (2002). SUMO-1 modification represses Sp3 transcriptional activation and modulates its subnuclear localization. *Mol Cell* 10, 831-842.

Salazar, M. D. *et al.* (2011). During hormone depletion or tamoxifen treatment of breast cancer cells the estrogen receptor apoprotein supports cell cycling through the retinoic acid receptor alpha1 apoprotein. *Breast Cancer Res* 13, R18.

Sapetschnig, A. *et al.* (2002). Transcription factor Sp3 is silenced through SUMO modification by PIAS1. *EMBO J* 21, 5206-5215.

Schug, T. T. *et al.* (2008). Overcoming retinoic acid-resistance of mammary carcinomas by diverting retinoic acid from PPARbeta/delta to RAR. *Proc Natl Acad Sci U S A* 105, 7546-7551.

Shinkarenko, L. *et al.* (1994). 13C NMR kinetic studies of the rapid stimulation of glucose metabolism by estrogen in immature rat uterus. *NMR Biomed* 7, 209-217.

Siddiqui, R. A. *et al.* (2005). Anticancer properties of propofol-docosahexaenoate and propofol-eicosapentaenoate on breast cancer cells. *Breast Cancer Res* 7, R645-R654.

Slamon, D. J. *et al.* (1989). Studies of the HER-2/neu proto-oncogene in human breast and ovarian cancer. *Science* 244, 707-712.

Smith, D. E., Gorski, J. (1968). Extrogen control of uterine glucose metabolism. An analysis based on the transport and phosphorylation of 2-deoxyglucose. *J Biol Chem* 243, 4169-4174.

Smith, T. A. *et al.* (2007). Decreased [18F]fluoro-2-deoxy-d-glucose incorporation and increased glucose transport are associated with resistance to 5FU in MCF7 cells in vitro. *Nucl Med Biol* 34, 955-960.

Soloaga, A. *et al.* (2003). MSK2 and MSK1 mediate the mitogen- and stress-induced phosphorylation of histone H3 and HMG-14. *EMBO J* 22, 2788-2797.

Song, C. Z. *et al.* (2003). Functional interplay between CBP and PCAF in acetylation and regulation of transcription factor KLF13 activity. *J Mol Biol* 329, 207-215.

Sonneveld, E. *et al.* (1998). Human retinoic acid (RA) 4-hydroxylase (CYP26) is highly specific for all-trans-RA and can be induced through RA receptors in human breast and colon carcinoma cells. *Cell Growth Differ* 9, 629-637.

Spengler, M. L., Brattain, M. G. (2006). Sumoylation inhibits cleavage of Sp1 N-terminal negative regulatory domain and inhibits Sp1-dependent transcription. *J Biol Chem* 281, 5567-5574.

Spengler, M. L. *et al.* (2008). Phosphorylation mediates Sp1 coupled activities of proteolytic processing, desumoylation and degradation. *Cell Cycle* 7, 623-630.

Sun, J. M. *et al.* (2002). The transcriptional repressor Sp3 is associated with CK2-phosphorylated histone deacetylase 2. *J Biol Chem* 277, 35783-35786.

Sun, J. M. *et al.* (2005). Estrogen regulation of trefoil factor 1 expression by estrogen receptor alpha and Sp proteins. *Exp Cell Res* 302, 96-107.

Suske, G. (1999). The Sp-family of transcription factors. *Gene* 238, 291-300.

Swigart, R. H. *et al.* (1961). Glycogen in the uterus of alloxan-diabetic rats. *Endocrinology* 68, 643-646.

Tang, X. H., Gudas, L. J. (2011). Retinoids, retinoic acid receptors, and cancer. *Annu Rev Pathol* 6, 345-364.

Tange, S. *et al.* (2009). Phosphorylation of histone H3 at Ser10: its role in cell transformation by v-Src. *Biochem Biophys Res Commun* 386, 588-592.

Utech, C. I. *et al.* (1996). Prospective evaluation of fluorine-18 fluorodeoxyclucose positron emission tomography in breast cancer for staging of the axilla related to surgery and immunocytochemistry. *Eur J Nucl Med* 23, 1588-1593.

Van Loo, P. F. *et al.* (2003). Impaired hematopoiesis in mice lacking the transcription factor Sp3. *Blood* 102, 858-866.

Vermeulen, L. *et al.* (2003). Transcriptional activation of the NF-kappaB p65 subunit by mitogen- and stress-activated protein kinase-1 (MSK1). *EMBO J* 22, 1313-1324.

Vicent, G. P. *et al.* (2008). Convergence on chromatin of non-genomic and genomic pathways of hormone signaling. *J Steroid Biochem Mol Biol* 109, 344-349.

Vicent, G. P. *et al.* (2009). Erk signaling and chromatin remodeling in MMTV promoter activation by progestins. *Nucl Recept Signal* 7, e008.

Wang, Y. T. *et al.* (2008). Sumoylation of specificity protein 1 augments its degradation by changing the localization and increasing the specificity protein 1 proteolytic process. *J Mol Biol* 380, 869-885.

Wiggin, G. R. *et al.* (2002). MSK1 and MSK2 are required for the mitogen- and stress-induced phosphorylation of CREB and ATF1 in fibroblasts. *Mol Cell Biol* 22, 2871-2881.

Wood, I. S., Trayhurn, P. (2003). Glucose transporters (GLUT and SGLT): expanded families of sugar transport proteins. *Br J Nutr* 89, 3-9.

Yan, Y. *et al.* (2006). NFAT3 is specifically required for TNF-alpha-induced cyclooxygenase-2 (COX-2) expression and transformation of Cl41 cells. *J Cell Sci* 119, 2985-2994.

Yuan, P. *et al.* (2007). Therapeutic inhibition of Sp1 expression in growing tumors by mithramycin a correlates directly with potent antiangiogenic effects on human pancreatic cancer. *Cancer* 110, 2682-2690.

Zhu, W. G. *et al.* (2003). Methylation of adjacent CpG sites affects Sp1/Sp3 binding and activity in the p21(Cip1) promoter. *Mol Cell Biol* 23, 4056-4065.

13

ER-Alpha36 Mediates Non-Genomic Estrogen and Anti-Estrogen Signaling in Breast Cancer Cells

ZhaoYi Wang, XianTian Zhang and LianGuo Kang
Department of Medical Microbiology & Immunology, Creighton University Medical School, Omaha, NE, USA

1. Introduction

Estrogen signaling is essential in the initiation and development of neoplasia in mammary gland. In the past several decades, extensive efforts have been dedicated to understand the underlying mechanisms of this important signaling pathway in mammary carcinogenesis, which have facilitated the development of anti-estrogen therapy, the first targeted therapy for human cancer.

It has been well documented that the diverse activities of estrogens and anti-estrogens are mediated by specific receptors designated as estrogen receptors (ERs). Currently, there are two identified ERs, ER-α and ER-β, both of which are ligand-activated transcription factors that stimulate target gene transcription. Compelling evidence indicates that estrogens, especially 17β-estradiol (E2β), up-regulate the expression and function of c-Myc and cyclin D1, activate cyclin E-Cdk2 complexes and promotes cell cycle progression from G1 to S phase in mammary epithelial cells. Thus, stimulation of target gene expression by ERs in response to estrogens is prevailingly thought to be responsible for estrogen-stimulated mammary carcinoma initiation and progression.

Despite the clarity with which ERs have been shown to act as ligand-dependent transcription factors, it became apparent now that not all of the activities mediated by ERs are accomplished through a direct effect on gene transcription. Another signaling pathway (also known as a non-classic, non-genomic, extra-nuclear or membrane-initiated signaling pathway) exists that involves cytoplasmic signaling proteins, growth factor receptors and other membrane-initiated signaling pathways. Several intracellular signaling pathways have been shown cross-talking with the membrane-initiated estrogen signaling: the adenylate cyclase pathway, the phospholipase C pathway, the G-protein-coupled receptor-activated pathways, the PI3K/AKT and the MAPK pathways.

Currently, the identity of the membrane-based estrogen receptor that mediates non-genomic estrogen effects has not been fully established. ER-β, two forms of ER-α, full-length (66-kDa) and short form (46-kDa) have been found on or near the plasma membrane and mediates membrane-initiated estrogen signaling. In addition, there is also evidence indicating that GPR30, an orphan G-protein-coupled-receptor, mediates the rapid, non-genomic responses to estrogens. In 2005, our laboratory identified and cloned a novel variant of ER-α, which has a molecular weight of 36-kDa and thus we have termed it ER-α36. This ER-α variant differs from the original 66 kDa ER-α (ER-α66) by lacking both transcriptional activation domains (AF-1 and AF-2) but retaining the DNA-binding domain and partial dimerization and ligand-binding domains. ER-α36 is predominantly expressed on the plasma membrane of both ER-positive and –negative breast cancer cells, mediates membrane-initiated estrogen and anti-estrogen signaling such as activation of the MAPK/ERK and PI3K/AKT signaling pathways and stimulation of cell proliferation. Thus, ER-α36 is a novel membrane-associated estrogen receptor that mediates membrane-initiated estrogen and anti-estrogen signaling in both ER-positive and -negative breast cancer cells.

In this chapter, we highlight the historical understanding of non-genomic estrogen signaling and its role in cell survival and proliferation, and specifically illustrate the biological function and the possible underlying mechanisms of ER-α36 in non-genomic estrogen and anti-estrogen signaling in both ER-positive and –negative breast cancer cells. We also discuss the integral roles of EGFR, Src and STAT5 in the non-genomic estrogen signaling mediated by ER-α36 and the complex regulatory network among ER-α66, 46 and 36. In addition, the novel biology of non-genomic estrogen signaling mediated by ER-α36 also has significance for understanding the physiology of bone remodeling. Thus, ER-α36-mediated signaling has a broad appeal in physiology of non-classical estrogen targeting tissues and general cancer research.

2. Estrogen receptors and genomic estrogen signaling

Estrogen signaling is pivotal in the establishment and maintenance of reproductive function in men and women. It is also involved in normal development and physiology of bone, liver, cardiovascular and neuronal systems. Inappropriate estrogen signaling is involved in osteoporosis, atherosclerosis and Alzheimer's disease and is essential in the initiation and development of neoplasia in breast and endometrial cancers (Nilsson et al., 2001). Hence, it is important to understand the molecular mechanisms by which this important signaling pathway functions, so its participation in a wide variety of different biological processes can be clarified, including how its dysregulation contributes to different diseases and even neoplastic transformation.

The diverse physiological and pathological functions of estrogens are mediated by specific receptors designated as estrogen receptors (ERs). In 1986, the cloning of the estrogen receptor (ER) was first reported (Green et al., 1986; Greene et al., 1986). Until 1996, it was assumed that there was only one ER responsible for all of the physiological and pharmacological effects of natural and synthetic estrogens and anti-estrogens. However, in 1996, a second ER was cloned (Kuiper et al., 1996). Currently, the first ER discovered is referred to as ER-α, while the second is called ER-β.

ER-α and ER-β share a common structural architecture (Reviewed by Kong et al., 2003; Zheng et al., 2003). Both are composed of three independent but interacting functional domains: the N-terminal A/B domain, the C or DNA-binding domain, and the D/E/F or ligand-binding domain. The N-terminal domain of ERs encodes a ligand-independent activation function (AF-1), a region involved in interaction with co-activators, and transcriptional activation of target genes. The DNA-binding domain or C domain contains a two zinc-finger structure, which is involved in receptor dimerization and binding to specific DNA sequences. The C-terminal E/F domain is a ligand-binding domain that mediates ligand binding, receptor dimerization, nuclear translocation, and a ligand-dependent transactivation function (AF-2). The relative contributions that both AF-1 and AF-2 exert on transcriptional control vary in a cell-specific and DNA promoter-specific manner (Berry et al., 1990; Tzukerman et al., 1994).

It is well established that estrogen receptors are members of the nuclear receptor superfamily of ligand-activated transcription factors that control various physiological processes. It is prevailingly thought that this control often occurs through the regulation of gene transcription (Reviewed by Katzenellenbogen & Katzenellenbogen, 2000; McDonnell & Norris, 2002). The estrogen receptor utilizes multiple mechanisms to either activate or repress transcription of its target genes. These mechanisms include: (a) direct interaction of the ligand-occupied receptor with DNA at a consensus estrogen response elements (ERE, GGTCAnnnTGACC) followed by recruitment of transcriptional coregulator or mediator complexes (Reviewed by Klinge, 2001), (b) interaction of the ligand-occupied ER with other transcription factors such as AP-1 (Kushner at al., 2000), Sp1 (Safe, 2001) or NF-κB (McKay & Cidlowski, 1999), or (c) indirect modulation of gene transcription via sequestration of general/common transcriptional components (Harnish et al., 2000; Speir et al., 2000). In addition, the ability of an estrogen receptor to regulate transcription through these mechanisms appears to be cell-type specific, perhaps due to differences in the complement of transcriptional co-regulatory factors available in each cell type (Cerillo et al., 1998; Evans et al., 2001; Maret et al., 1999). Also, transcriptional regulation is dependent upon the nature of the ligand, with various natural and synthetic selective estrogen receptor modulators (SERM) acting as either estrogen receptor agonists or antagonists through these various mechanisms (Shang & Brown, 2002; Katzenellenbogen & Katzenellenbogen, 2002; Margeat et al., 2003).

3. Estrogen signaling and breast cancer

Experimental and clinical evidence for the role of endogenous estrogens in normal development of mammary glands and breast cancer etiology has been well documented (Reviewed by Feigelson & Henderson, 1996). Estrogen signaling is involved in mammary epithelial cell proliferation and differentiation. Dysregulated estrogen signaling increases the rate of cell proliferation and thus the risk for development of breast cancer.

ER-α is expressed in approximately 15-30% of luminal epithelial cells and not at all in any other cell types in the normal human breast (Clarke *et. al.*, 1997). However, dual label immunofluorescent technique revealed that ER-α expressing cells are separate from those labeled with proliferation markers such as Ki67 and cyclin A in both normal human and rodent mammary glands (Clarke et al., 1997; Zeps et al., 1999). This is in direct contrast to estrogen action in breast cancer cells, where estrogens, especially 17β-estradiol (E2β), functions as potent mitogens through promoting cell cycle progression from G1 to S phase (Prall et al., 1998; Altucci et al., 1996 & 1997). Thus, it is thought that estrogens directly interact with ERs in ER-positive human breast cancer cells, where they induce transcriptional activation of "immediate early" and cyclin genes, and promote cell cycle progression. Consistent with its role in mammary carcinogenesis, ER-α expression is increased at the earliest stages of ductal hyperplasia and increases even more with increasing atypia, such that most cells in atypical ductal hyperplasias and in ductal cancer in situ of low and intermediate grade contain ER-α (Khan et. al., 1994). As ER-α expression increases during breast cancer development, the inverse relationship between ER-α expression and cell proliferation become dysregulated (Shoker *et. al.*, 1999 a and b).

Approximately 70% of invasive breast carcinomas express the ER-α and most of these tumors contain ER-α positive proliferating cells (Clarke *et. al.*, 1997).
Currently, ER-α is the most widely used marker in diagnosis of human breast cancer. Breast cancers are diagnosed either as ER-positive or -negative depending on the existence or absence of ER-α. At the onset, 46%-77% of breast cancers are ER-positive (Robertson *et. al.*, 1996). The ER-positive tumors are histologically well differentiated and diploid, and patients with ER-positive tumors generally have a better prognosis since they respond well to anti-estrogen treatment (Clark *et. al.*, 1984; Osborne *et. al.*, 1980). ER-negative breast cancers that account for about one third of breast cancers diagnosed, however, are more malignant and aggressive through a still unknown mechanism (Sheikh *et. al.*, 1994), and they generally respond poorly to anti-estrogen treatment.
ER-negative breast cancers are often considered to be the result of tumor progression from ER-positive premalignant lesions or ER-positive breast cancers by epigenetic alterations such as promoter methylation (Ferguson et. al., 1995) or ER-α protein degradation by the proteasome system after hypoxia in non-vascularized tumors (Stoner et. al., 2002). However, immunohistochemical studies in human breast cancers showed that some proliferative ductal lesions and many high-grade ductal carcinomas in situ (DCIS) are ER-α-negative (Roger et. al., 2000), suggesting some ER-negative breast cancers may be progressed directly from ER-negative premalignant lesions.

4. Non-genomic estrogen signaling

It become clear now that estrogens elicit two signaling pathways; the first requires hours to days to result in transcriptional changes of target genes and is known as genomic, classic or nuclear signaling pathway while the second occurs in seconds to minutes after estrogen treatment and usually initiates at the plasma membrane. Thus, the second signaling pathway is also known as a non-classic, non-genomic, extra-nuclear or membrane-initiated signaling pathway which is mediated by estrogen binding proteins associated with the plasma membrane and employs various cytoplasmic signaling proteins, growth factor receptors and G-protein-coupled-receptor signaling pathways (Segars & Driggers, 2002; Driggers & Segars, 2002; Kelly & Levin, 2001; Levin, 2002; Hammes & Levin, 2007).
Pietras and Szego first described the rapid estrogen signaling more than 30 years ago (Pietras & Szego, 1975 &1977), noting immediate calcium fluxes in endometrial cells induced by estrogen and specific binding sites at the outer surfaces of isolated endometrial cells. Quick estrogen responses were also recorded in neuroendocrine tissue such as a rapid rise of intracellular calcium in pituitary cells, which leads to cell depolarization within 1 min (Dufy et al., 1979). Rapid estrogen signaling also induces prolactin secretion from pituitary tumor cells (Watson et al., 1999). Such signaling of estrogens has also been described in uterine (Aronica et al., 1994) and ovarian cells (Morley et al., 1992; Tesarik & Mendoza, 1997) as well as bone (Endoh et al., 1997; Longo et al., 2004; Sylvia et al., 2001), vascular endothelial (Russell et al., 2000; Lu et al., 2004) and neuronal cells (Kelly et al., 1977; Mermelstein et al., 1996), indicating that the rapid, non-genomic estrogen signaling is involved in various physiological and pathological estrogen activities.
Non-genomic estrogen signaling has been also documented in breast cancer cells for cell proliferation and survival (Song et al., 2002; Migliaccio et al., 1996; Ahmad et al., 1999; Lobenhofer et al., 2000; Castoria et al., 1999 & 2001). These findings strongly suggest that the

rapid, non-genomic estrogen signaling is involved in estrogen-induced proliferation in breast cancer cells.

5. Nature of membrane-based estrogen receptor

While it is clear that membrane-initiated estrogen signaling exists, the identity of the membrane-based estrogen receptor that mediates these rapid estrogen effects, especially the effects in mammary epithelial cell proliferation and survival, has not been fully established. Laboratory evidence indicated that both ER-α and ER-β are involved in the rapid, non-genomic estrogen signaling (Razandi et al., 1999). However, evidence also suggests that more than one membrane-initiated signaling pathway is associated with estrogen action. Data from several laboratories using the membrane-impermeable compound 17β-estradiol-bovine serum albumin (E2β-BSA) indicates the existence of two functionally distinct membrane-associated pathways: one sensitive to anti-estrogens and one resistant (Chen et al., 1999; Russell et al., 2000; Watters et al., 1997). For example, ER-α/knockout mice retained rapid estrogen-stimulated membrane effects in neurons, which were not blocked by anti-estrogen ICI-182, 780 (Gu, et. al., 1999). These findings suggest that another membrane-based ER may exist since all known ERs are sensitive to anti-estrogen inhibition. As a consequence, an orphan G-protein coupled receptor, GPCR30, and some other unknown proteins have been reported to mediate this anti-estrogen resistant non-genomic estrogen signaling.

6. ER-α

A large body of experimental evidence indicated that ER-α is involved in both genomic and non-genomic estrogen signaling. Immunofluorescent staining of non-permeabilized pituitary tumor cells with anti-ER-α antibodies revealed a punctuated staining pattern on cell surface although most ER-α were localized in cell nuclei (Watson et al., 1999). ER-α associated with the plasma membrane is also detected by a panel of antibodies targeting different domains of ER-α in intact breast cancer cells and in breast cancer specimens (Pietras et al., 2005; Kim et al., 2006). The findings that transfection of the nuclear ER-α cDNA into ER-"null" Chinese hamster ovary (CHO) cells leads to expression of both membrane and nuclear ER-α further support the notion that membrane-associated ER-α is derived from the same transcript as nuclear ER-α (Razandi et al., 1999). However, recent evidence indicates that the CHO-K1, Rat2-fibroblasts and COS7 cells previously considered as ER "null' cells and extensively used to transfect ER cDNAs in order to demonstrate rapid estrogen signaling actually exhibit strong non-genomic estrogen signaling such as activation of the MAPK/ERK before transfection (Nethrapalli et al., 2005), suggesting these cells already posses some unknown proteins other than classical ERs that mediate the rapid estrogen signaling.

It is widely accepted that estrogen signaling promotes cell proliferation in target cells. However, the explanation of this effect of estrogen signaling simply by the function of ER-α is confounding. When ER-α was expressed in ER-"null" CHO cells (Kushner *et. al.*, 1990), and human cervical cancer HeLa cells (Touitou *et. al.*, 1990), E2β failed to stimulate cell growth. On the contrary, E2β inhibited cell proliferation and even induced cell apoptosis. Likewise, the ER-negative immortal MCF10A breast epithelial cells (Pilat *et. al.*, 1996), and MDA-MB-231 breast cancer cells (Jiang & Jordan, 1992) were both growth inhibited by estrogen when stably transfected with ER-α cDNA. These experimental results argue against a positive function of the well-known ER-α alone in mitogenic estrogen signaling.

7. ER-β

ER-β acts as a classical ligand-induced transcription factor. Like ER-α, ligand-bound ER-β functions by regulating downstream target genes. ER-β also heterodimerizes with ER-α and modulates ER-α function (Reviewed by Harris, 2007; Deroo & Buensuceso, 2010). ER-β has been shown to be S-palmitoylated, which facilitates the localization of ER-β at the plasma membrane to mediate the rapid, non-genomic estrogen effects (Marino & Ascenzi, 2008). Indeed, the involvement of ER-β in rapid, non-genomic estrogen signaling has been documented when ER-β cDNA was introduced into CHO cells (Razandi et al., 1999). In colon cancer, pro-apoptotic activities of ER-β have been reported to be mediated by membrane-initiated signaling; induction of ER-β via the MAPK/p38 signaling pathway, which in turn leads to downstream apoptotic events (Caiazza et al., 2007), indicating a potential role of ER-β as a tumor suppressor. In addition, inhibition of ER-β palmitoylation in colon cancer cells abrogated the pro-apoptotic activity of ER-β (Galluzzo et al., 2007), suggesting that non-genomic effects mediated by membrane–associated ER-β is important for its pro-apoptotic function.

The biological significance of ER-β in breast cancer has not been well established. Approximately 70% of breast tumor express ER-β and most tumor co-express both ER-α and -β (Dotzlaw et al., 1997; Fuqua et al., 1999 & 2003). Studies indicated that ER-β expression in human breast cancer is associated with a poorer prognosis, compared with tumors that only express ER-α (Speirs et al., 1999). ER-β expression is associated with elevated levels of proliferation markers, Ki67 and cyclin A, in human breast cancer (Jensen et al., 2001) These studies suggested that ER-β may promote cell proliferation and breast cancer progression.

In contrast, accumulating evidence indicated that ER-β acts as a tumor suppressor in breast cancer. ER-β is expressed in both normal and malignant mammary glands (Warner et al., 2000; Speirs et al., 2002). In the rodent mammary gland, ER-β expressing cells can proliferate but the majority cells that express proliferation markers do not express either ER (Saji et al., 2001). The levels of ER-β expression are highest in normal mammary gland and are decreased as tumors progress from pre-invasive to invasive (Leygue et al., 1998; Iwao et al., 2000; Roger et al., 2001). The presence of ER-β in breast cancer confers a more favorable prognosis and is associated with node-negative, low-grade tumors (Jarvinen et al., 2000) as well as a greater disease-free survival rate (Omoto et al., 2001). Several laboratory studies demonstrated that ER-β inhibited angiogenesis and malignant growth of T47D breast tumor xenograft and malignant growth of MCF7 breast cancer cells *in vitro* and in nude mice (Hartman et al., 2006; Paruthiyil et al., 2004). Intriguingly, ER-β also inhibited proliferation of ER-negative breast cancer MDA-MB-231 cells in a ligand-independent manner whereas ER-α inhibition of MDA-MB-231 cell proliferation is estrogen-dependent (Lazennec et al., 2001). These results indicate that ER-β negatively regulates mitogenic estrogen signaling.

8. ER-α46

Previously, it was reported that a 46-kDa antigen is tightly associated with ER-α in human breast cancer samples (Diaz-Chico *et. al.*, 1988). This 46-kDa antigen is enriched in the cell cytosol and could be recognized by an isolated monoclonal antibody, E476, raised against the human ER-α (Diaz-Chico *et. al.,* 1988). Similarly, Jozan (1991) later reported that there are two species of ER with different molecular weight (65 and 47 kDa), and three species of tumors (36% containing the highest form of ER alone, 49% bearing the two forms in variable amounts, and 15% bearing only the minor form). These results strongly suggest that two different forms of ER-α exist at different ratios in human breast cancer.

In 2000, Flouriot *et. al.* cloned a 46-kDa isoform of ER-α and demonstrated that the 46-kDa isoform lacks the first 173 amino acids (A/B or AF-1 domain) and is derived from alternative splicing of the ER-α gene by skipping exon 1. This alternative splicing event generates an mRNA that has an AUG in a favorable Kozak sequence for translation initiation in frame with the remainder of the open reading frame of ER-α (Flouriot et. al., 2000). This new isoform of ER-α is named as ER-α46 and the original one as ER-α66. ER-α46 forms homo-dimers and binds to an ERE, and it can also form heterodimers with ER-α66 (Flouriot et. al., 2000). Furthermore, the ER-α46/66 heterodimers form preferentially over the ER-α66 homodimers and ER-α46 acts competitively to inhibit transactivation mediated by AF-1 domain of ER-α66 but without effect on AF-2-dependent transactivation (Floutiot et. al., 2000). Therefore, ER-α46 is a naturally occurring isoform of ER-α that regulates genomic estrogen signaling mediated by the AF-1 domain of ER-α66.

Previously, two forms of ER-α, full-length (66-kDa) and short form (46-kDa) were co-purified with 5' nucleotidase, a plasma membrane-marker enzyme (Marquez & Pietras, 2001), suggesting a possible role of ER-α46 in the rapid, non-genomic estrogen signaling. Recently, ER-α46 was localized on the plasma membrane, in the cytosol, and nucleus of endothelial cells and mediated rapid estrogen signaling such as activation of the Src/PI3K/AKT signaling and stimulation of NO synthesis (Kim & Bender, 2005; Li *et. al.,* 2003; Reviewed by Moriarty et al., 2006), further confirming that the ER-α46 isoform functions as a membrane-associated estrogen receptor.

Although it is clear now that ER-α46 is involved in both genomic and non-genomic estrogen signaling, its function in breast cancer has been less investigated. Forced expression of ER-α46 inhibited proliferation of MCF-7 breast cancer cells and cyclin D1 promoter activity (Penot et al., 2005). Overexpression of both ER-α46 and ER-α66 in ER-negative MDA-MB-231 cells revealed that ER-α46 inhibited basal transcription of the estrogen responsive gene pS2 while estrogen treatment released this inhibition (Metivier et al., 2004). Recently, expression levels of ER-α46 was found to be down-regulated in tamoxifen-resistant breast cancer cells and re-introduction of ER-α46 into these cells inhibited cell proliferation and ER-α66-regulated gene transcription (Klinge et al., 2010). Thus, these results suggest that ER-α46 may function as a negative-regulator of mitogenic estrogen signaling in ER-positive breast cancer cells.

9. ER-α36

In 2005, our laboratory identified a 5.4 kb cDNA clone from a normal human edometrium cDNA library (RZPD clone number: DKFZp686N23123) and later cloned this cDNA from a human placenta cDNA library (Wang et al., 2005). This cDNA clone harbors a 310 amino acid open-reading frame that can produce a protein with a predicted molecular weight of 35.7 kDa. To differentiate it from ER-α66 and 46, and apply consistent nomenclature, this novel isoform of ER-α was named as ER-α36.

The cDNA sequence of the open-reading frame matches 100% to the DNA sequence of the exons 2 to 6 of the ER-α66 gene. The 5′untraslated region (5′UTR) of the cDNA showed 100% homology to the DNA sequence of the first intron of the ER-α66 gene. Thus, the transcript of this ER-α isoform is initiated from a previously unidentified promoter in the first intron of the ER-α66 gene (Figure 1, Zou et al., 2009). A small, non-coding novel exon in the first intron of the ER-α66 gene was designated as exon 1′. The exon 1′ is then spliced directly into the exon 2 of the ER-α66 gene and continues from exon 2 to exon 6 of the ER-α66 gene. Exon 6 is then spliced to an exon located 64,141 bp downstream of the ER-α66 gene (Figure 1). The cDNA sequence encoding the last 27 amino acids and the 4,293 bp 3′untranslated region (3′UTR) was matched 100% to a continuous sequence from the genomic sequence of clone RP1-1304 on chromosome 6q24.2-25.3 (GeneBank accession number AL78582), indicating the remaining cDNA sequence of this novel ER-α isoform is transcribed from one big exon of 4,374 bp located downstream of the ER-α66 gene. This exon is thus designated as exon 9 to reflect the extra exon beyond the previous reported eight exons for ER-α66 gene (Figure 1). All of these splicing events are supported by the identification of perfect splice donors and acceptors at the splice juncture. The protein ER-α36 can be produced from a perfect Kozak sequence located in the second exon, the same initiation codon used to produce ER-α46 (Flouriot *et. al.,* 2000). ER-α36 differs from the ER-α66 by lacking both transcriptional activation domains (AF-1 and AF-2) but retaining the DNA-binding and dimerization domains, and partial ligand-binding domains. It also possesses an extra, unique 27 amino acid domain to replace the last 138 amino acids encoded by exon 7 and 8 of the ER-α66 (Figure 2). Thus, ER-α36 is another naturally occurring novel isoform of ER-α that may play an important role in both genomic and non-genomic estrogen signaling. Currently, there are three major ER-α isoforms observed in ER-positive breast cancer MCF7 cells that correspond to three mRNA variants generated from different promoter usage and alternative splicing (Figure 2).

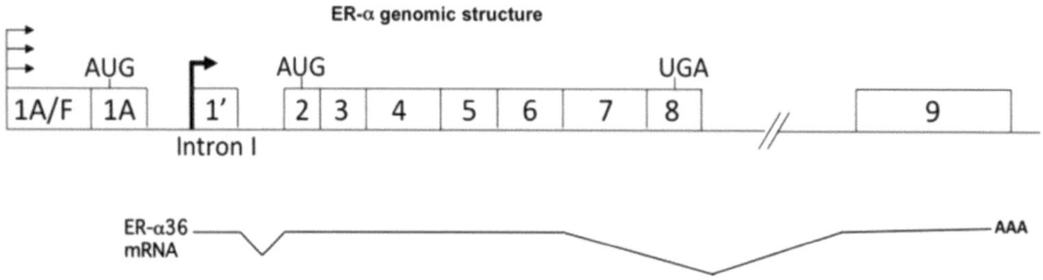

Fig. 1. Genomic organization of the human ER-α36 gene. The locations of multiple promoters of human ER-α66 gene are shown as arrows. The translation start and stop codons are indicated as AUG and UGA. The common exons are shown as numbered open boxes. The extra exon that is beyond the 8 exons of the human ER-α66 gene is numbered as 9 in the open box. The intron 1 is also shown with the exon 1′ in the open box. The lower panel shows mRNA structure of human ER-α36 isoform.

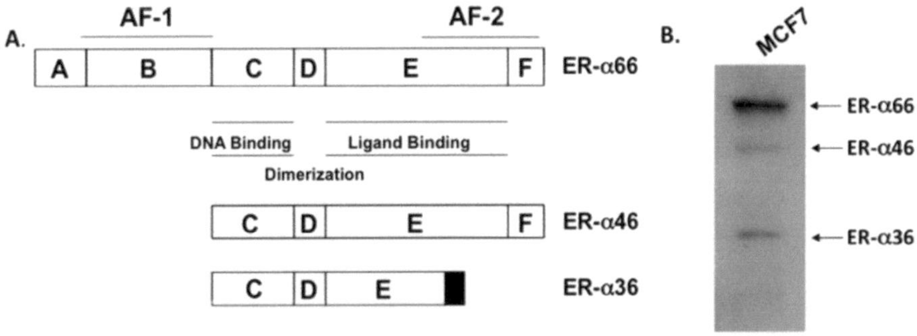

Fig. 2. Domain structure and expression of human estrogen receptor-α variants in ER-positive breast cancer MCF7 cells. (A). Domain structure representation of human ER-α isoforms. Domains (labeled A–F), and activation function domains (AF-1 and -2) are shown. The function of each domain is indicated. The last 27 amino acids of human ER-α36 are indicated as a filled box. (B). Western blot analysis of three human ER-α isoforms in MCF7 cells with an anti-ER-α66 antibody (H222).

10. GPR30

Previously, different laboratories demonstrated the existence of two distinct membrane-associated pathways: one sensitive to anti-estrogens and one resistant (Chen et al., 1999; Russell et al., 2000; Watters et al., 1997). These results suggest that another membrane-associated estrogen receptor may exist since both ER-α and -β are sensitive to anti-estrogen inhibition.

An orphan G protein-coupled receptor, GPR30 was reported to mediate the rapid, non-genomic estrogen signaling that was insensitive to ICI 182,780; estrogen stimulates changes of Ca^{2+} currents and cAMP signaling in cells expressing GPR30 (Revankar et al., 2005) and activates the MAPK/ERK phosphorylation and the PI3K/Akt signalling pathways via transactivation of the EGFR pathway in ER-negative but GPR30-positive breast cancer cells (Filardo et al., 2000 & 2007). Thus, GPR30 was considered as a novel type of membrane-associated estrogen receptor that mediates the rapid, non-genomic estrogen signaling.

There are also reports that challenge the role of GPR30 as a novel estrogen receptor. A study showed that introduction of GPR30 anti-sense oligonucleotides failed to block the MAPK/ERK activation and cell growth induced by estrogen in ER-positive breast cancer cells (Ahola et al., 2002). Pedram *et al.* (2006) failed to observe the cAMP or ERK activation in GPR30-positive, ER-negative breast cancer cells. Another study demonstrated that the GPR30 selective agonist G1 failed to exert estrogenic effect in two classical estrogen target organs, the uterus and the mammary gland (Otto et al., 2008). Recently, Otto *et al.* generated GPR30-deficient mice and demonstrated that the development of reproductive organs was unimpaired in these mice and the estrogenic responses in the uterus and the mammary gland were completely maintained in GPR30-deficient animals (Otto et al., 2009).

Recently, our group reported that knockdown of GPR30 expression in ER-negative breast cancer SK-BR-3 cells down-regulated the expression levels of ER-α36 (Kang et al., 2010b). Introduction of a GPR30 expression vector into GPR30 non-expressing cells induced endogenous ER-α36 expression and GPR30 activated the promoter activity of ER-α36 via an AP-1 binding site located in the 5′-flanking region of ER-α36 (Kang et al., 2010b). Thus, ERα36 is a downstream target gene of GPR30-mediated signaling and the previously reported activities of GPR30 as a membrane-based estrogen receptor are through its ability to induce ER-α36 expression.

11. Other putative estrogen receptors

Other unknown proteins that may be involved in the rapid, non-genomic estrogen signaling have been also reported. For an example, a report that E2β activated the MAPK/ERK signaling in un-trasnfected CHO-K1, COS7 and Rat2-fibroblasts (Nethrapalli et al., 2005) suggested the existence of an unidentified membrane-associated mER. Recently, we reported that un-transfected COS7 cells express high levels of endogenous ER-α36 (Kang et al., 2010b) and found that CHO-K1 cells also express ER-α36 (Kang et al., unpublished observations), suggesting that ER-α36 may mediates the rapid, non-genomic estrogen signaling observed in these cells.

Another unique membrane-associated ER with an estimated molecular weight of 63-65 kDa, referred to as ER-X, is developmentally regulated differently from both ER-α and -β. Its pharmacological profile was also different from ER-α and -β, even with some features opposite to those shown for these two receptors (Toran-Allerand et al., 2002). For examples, ER-X mediated rapid estrogen signaling was not sensitive to anti-estrogen, and the association of Hsp90 is required for the inactive state of ER-α while ER-X requires to be associated with hsp90 for its activity (Toran-Allerand et al., 2002). Whereas ER-X shares limited similarities with ER-α36, such as reaction with antibodies to the ligand-binding domain of ER-α66 and responding equally to 17α- and β-estradiol, the molecular similarity of these two receptors awaits for the cloning and sequencing of ER-X.

Additionally, a heterodimeric estrogen-binding protein, referred to as the putative ER (pER), was reported to bind to E2β at a sub-nanomolar affinity but was unable to bind other estrogens or anti-estrogens. Depending on cell types, pER is expressed on the plasma and/or nuclear membranes or in the cytoplasm and nucleus (Rao et al., 1998). Since the polyclonal anti-pER antibody failed to react with estrogen receptors and was unable to detect pER expression in reproductive organs (Rao et al., 1998), the role of this putative estrogen receptor in non-genomic estrogen signaling of breast cancer cells remains elusive.

12. Negative regulation of genomic estrogen signaling by ER-α36

Comparison of protein structures of ER-α66 and ER-α36 indicated that ER-α36 lacks both AF-1 and -2 transcription activation domains but retains the DNA-binding domain and dimerization domain. Transient co-transfection assays using a luciferase-expressing reporter construct that contains two Estrogen Response Element (ERE) placed upstream of the thymidine kinase promoter (2 X ERE-tk-Luc) revealed that ER-α36 has no intrinsic transcriptional activity in the presence and absence of E2β (Wang et al., 2006). However, ER-α36 strongly inhibited the transactivation activities mediated by the AF-1 and -2 domains of both ER-α66 and ER-β (Wang et al., 2006). These data indicate that ER-α36 itself is unable to mediate genomic estrogen signaling by regulate target gene expression. However, ER-α36 acts as a naturally occurring dominant-negative regulator of the genomic estrogen signaling mediated by the AF1 and AF2 domains of ER-α66 and ER-β.

13. Membrane-association and mitogenic signaling of ER-α36

The fact that ER-α36 posses no intrinsic transcription regulatory activity suggests that ER-α36 may be a membrane-associated estrogen receptor. The sub-cellular fractionation assay in ER-α36 transfected HEK293 cells revealed that a high percentage of ER-α36 (~50%) is localized on or near the plasma membrane and a low percentage of it in cytosol (~40%) and nucleus (~10%) (Wang *et al.*, 2006). Immuno-fluorescence staining of intact breast cancer MCF7 cells and endometrial cancer Hec1A cells using the ER-α36 specific antibody recognizing the last 20 amino acids that are unique to ER-α36 exhibits a membrane expression pattern that is co-localized with caviolin-1, a typical cell-surface protein (Lin et al., 2010). Immunohistochemistry analysis of specimens from breast cancer patients also demonstrated an expression pattern of ER-α36 predominantly on the breast cancer cell surface (Lee et al., 2008; Vranic et al., 2011). This anti-ER-α36 specific antibody also blocked ER-α36-mediated non-genomic estrogen signaling such as activation of the MAPK/ERK signaling in breast cancer cells presumably through steric hindrance of estrogen accesses to its binding pocket (Kang *et. al.*, 2010b), indicating that the antibody is accessible to the C-terminal region of the plasma membrane-associated ER-α36 in intact cells. These results thus demonstrated that ER-α36 is expressed on or near the plasma membrane and suggested that ER-α36 may be also shuttled to the cell cytoplasm and nucleus depending on cell context and extracellular signals.

Both 17β-estradiol (E2β) and BSA-conjugated E2β elicit the rapid, membrane-initiated estrogen signaling such as activation of the MAPK/ERK signaling pathway and stimulation of cell proliferation in ER-α36 transfected HEK293 cells, which is not blocked by anti-estrogens such as tamoxifen, 4-hydroxy-tamoxifen and ICI 182, 780 (Wang et al., 2006). In addition, other estrogens including estrone (E1), 17α-estradiol (E2α), estriol (E3) and estetrol (E4) all activate the ERK1/2 phosphorylation at a very similar level (Wang et al., 2006). Recently, it was reported that ER-α36 even mediated testosterone-stimulated activation of the MAPK/ERK and PI3K/Akt signaling pathways in endometrial cancer Hec1A cells (Lin et al., 2009). ER-α36 also mediates estrogen activation of the PKCδ/ERK signaling pathway (Tong et al., 2010). The finding that the non-genomic estrogen signaling mediated by ER-α36 was insensitive to anti-estrogens suggests that ER-α36 may be a receptor involved in the anti-estrogen-insensitive estrogen signaling described in different systems before. Taken together, ER-α36 is a membrane-associated estrogen receptor that mediates rapid and mitogenic estrogen signaling.

14. ER-α36 in anti-estrogen signaling and anti-estrogen resistance

Since mitogenic estrogen signaling plays a pivotal role in development and maintenance of ER-positive breast cancer, treatment with anti-estrogens such as tamoxifen (TAM) has become a first-line therapy for advanced ER-positive breast cancer. However, laboratory and clinical evidence indicated that TAM and its metabolites such as 4-hydroxytamoxifen (4-OHT) have mixed agonist/antagonist or estrogenic/anti-estrogenic actions depending on cell and tissue context, and the agonist activity of tamoxifen may contribute to tamoxifen resistance observed in almost all patients treated with tamoxifen. As a consequence, a more potent and "pure" anti-estrogen, ICI 182, 780 (Fulvestrant, Faslodex) has been developed (Reviewed by Howell et al., 2000).

TAM and 4-OHT are thought to function as antagonists by competing with E2β and other estrogens for binding to ERs. Further structural studies revealed that TAM induces an ER-α conformation that does not recruit coactivators to trans-activate target genes but recruits co-repressors (Shang *et. al.*, 2000), suggesting that TAM- and 4-OHT-bounded ER-α66 is unable to effectively activate genes involved in cell growth and breast cancer development. On the other hand, ICI 182, 780, a 'pure' antiestrogen without estrogenic activity, works in a different mechanism. ICI 182, 780 binds to ERs, impairs receptor dimerization and inhibits nuclear localization of receptor (Fawell, *et. al.*, 1990; Dauvois *et. al.*, 1992). Furthermore, ICI 182, 780 also accelerates degradation of the ER-α66 protein without a reduction of ER-α66 mRNA (Nicholson *et. al.*, 1995). Thus, ICI 182, 780 binds ER-α66 and accelerates degradation of ER-α66 protein, resulting in a complete inhibition of estrogen signaling mediated by ER-α66.

Although ICI 182, 780 has been depicted as a non-agonist or 'full' or 'pure' anti-estrogen, different laboratories documented estrogenic agonist activities of ICI 182, 780 in different systems. Estrogenic agonist activity of ICI 182, 780 has been found in hippocampal neurons and in bone cells where ICI 182, 780 promoted bone growth (Zhao et al., 2006; Sibonga et al., 1998). Agonist-like activities of ICI 182, 780 have also been reported in tamoxifen-resistant KPL-1 breast cancer cells (Kurebayashi et al., 1998) and Yeast (Dudley et al., 2000). Both tamoxifen and ICI 182, 780 were also reported to induce phosphorylation of the adhesion molecules p130Cas/BCR1, FAK and Src in ER-positive breast cancer MCF7 cells (Cowell et al., 2006). The molecular mechanisms by which ICI 182, 780 acts as an estrogenic agonist have never been elucidated. Studies from a number of laboratories suggested that a membrane associated estrogen-binding receptor mediates the agonist actions of ICI 182, 780 in neurons (Reviewed by Brinton 2001; Zhao et al., 2005; McEwen, 2002).

As described above, ER-α36 mediated non-genomic estrogen signaling is insensitive to anti-estrogens such as TAM and ICI 182, 780 (Wang et al., 2006). ER-α36 also mediates agonist activities of tamoxifen and ICI 182, 780 such as activation of the MAPK/ERK and the PI3K/AKT signaling pathways in breast and endometrial cancer cells (Wang *et. al.*, 2006; Lin *et. al.*, 2010). ICI 182, 780 failed to induce degradation of ER-α36 (Kang et al., 2010a) presumably because ER-α36 has a truncated ligand-binding domain that lacks the last 4 helixes (helix 9–12) of ER-α66 (Wang et al., 2005). The helix-12 domain is critical in protein degradation induced by ICI 182, 780 and different positioning of the helix 12 and the F domain of ER-α66 regulates functional differences between agonists and antagonists (Mahfoudi et al., 1995; Pearce et al., 2003). Thus, it is possible that ER-α36 is a receptor that mediates agonist activities of TAM and ICI 182, 780 recorded in different systems.

Despite the significant anti-neoplastic activities of anti-estrogens, most breast tumors are eventually resistant to anti-estrogen therapy. Essentially, two forms of anti-estrogen resistance occur: *de novo* and acquired resistance (Reviewed by Clarke *et. al.*, 2001 & 2003; Ring & Dowestt, 2004). Although absence of ER-α66 expression is the most common *de novo* resistance mechanism, about 40-50% ER-positive tumors are already resistant to anti-estrogens by the time of diagnosis; this *de novo* resistance mechanism in these ER-positive tumors is largely unknown (Reviewed by Clarke *et. al.*, 2001 & 2003; Ring & Dowestt, 2004). Furthermore, most initially responsive breast tumors gradually acquire anti-estrogen resistance by loss of anti-estrogen responsiveness. The underlying mechanism of breast tumors loss their anti-estrogen responsiveness remains unknown. Breast tumors with acquired TAM resistance frequently but not always retain levels of ER-α66 expression that would still define them as ER-positive tumors (Reviewed by Clarke *et. al.*, 2001 & 2003). Therefore, a loss of ER-α66 expression is not the major mechanism driving acquired anti-estrogen resistance. Up-regulation of Erb-B2 (Her2/Neu) and activation of the MAPK signaling pathways are usually associated with development of anti-estrogen resistance (Reviewed by Clarke *et. al.*, 2001 & 2003; Ring & Dowsett, 2004).

A recent retrospective study of 896 cases of breast cancer patients revealed that about 40% cases of human breast cancer patients were positive for ER-α36; about 40% cases ER-positive breast cancer co-expressed ER-α66 and ER-α36 and about 40% cases of ER-negative breast cancer that lacked ER-α66 expression were positive for ER-α36 (Shi et al., 2009). The breast cancer patients with tumors expressing high levels of ER-α36 were less benefited from tamoxifen therapy than those with low levels of ER-α36 expression did, and ER-α36 expression is significantly associated with Her2/Neu expression (Shi *et. al.*, 2009). These data suggest that high levels of ER-α36 expression in breast cancer cells is one of the underlying mechanisms of *de novo* tamoxifen resistance found in ER-positive breast cancer patients.

The aromatase inhibitors (AIs), on the other hand, inhibit the action of the enzyme aromatase, which converts testosterone to E2 (estradiol) and androstenedione to E1 (estrone). The third generation AIs exemplified by anastrazole and letrozole, provides a second line therapeutic strategy in advanced ER-positive patients (Reviewed by Santen, 2003). However, breast cancer cells that express high levels of ER-α36 are super sensitive to estrogen; activation of the MAPK/ERK in response to an extreme low concentration of estrogen, 1 X 10^{-16} M/L (Zhang et al., 2011). The anastrozole usually suppresses a plasma level of E2β to a mean of 2.6 pmol/L and letrozole to a mean of 2.1 pmol/L (Geisler et al., 2002). These data suggest that breast cancer patients with tumors expressing high levels of ER-α36 may also be refractory to the third generation of AIs.

15. ER-α36 in ER-negative breast cancer

Because of the lack of ER-α66 expression, it is prevailingly thought that estrogen signaling is not involved in development and progression of ER-negative breast cancer. However, early study showed that ovariectomy prevents formation of both ER-positive and –negative breast cancers (Nissen-Meyer, 1964). In addition, BRCA1 mutation related tumors, the vast majority of which are ER-negative, are also effectively prevented by prophylactic ovariectomy (Rebbeck et al., 1999). The increased risk developing breast cancer following pregnancy is assumed due to the ability of pregnancy-associated hormones such as estrogen to stimulate mammary epithelial cell proliferation. Surprisingly, however, the majority of breast cancers that develop following pregnancy are negative for either estrogen and progesterone receptors. To explain this contradictory findings, Gupta et al., (2007) proposed that estrogen may promote the growth of ER-negative breast cancer via a systemic increase in host angiogenesis.

Rapid activation of the PI3K/Akt pathway in ER-negative breast cancer MDA-MB-231 cells that could not be blocked by estrogen antagonists was reported (Tsai *et. al.*, 2001), which was explained as estrogen signaling through an ER-independent pathway. Taken together, these data suggest that subsets of ER-negative breast cancer cells may retain non-genomic estrogen signaling, which may contribute to development and progression of ER-negative breast cancers. Several studies demonstrated that ER-α36 variant is expressed in established

ER-negative breast cancer cell lines such as MDA-MB-231 and MDA-MB-436 and about 40% specimens from ER-negative breast cancer patients (Wang et al., 2006; Lee et al., 2008; Shi et al., 2009). Our group recently reported that E2β treatment activated the MAPK/ERK signaling pathway, induced expression of growth-promoting genes, c-Myc and cyclin D1, stimulated cell proliferation and accelerated tumor growth *in vivo* in ER-negative breast cancer MDA-MB-231 and MDA-MB-436 cells, all of which could be abrogated by knock-down of ER-α36 expression using ER-α36 specific shRNA (Zhang et al., 2011). Thus, ER-α36-mediated mitogenic estrogen signaling contributes malignant growth of ER-negative breast cancer cells.

16. Underlying mechanism of mitogenic estrogen signaling mediated by ER-α36

Compelling evidence demonstrated that estrogens up-regulate the expression and function of c-Myc and cyclin D1, and activate cyclin E-Cdk2 complexes, all of which are rate limiting factors for cell cycle progression from G1 to S phase (Prall *et. al.*, 1998; Altucci *et. al.*, 1996 & 1997). Based on these findings, it is believed that estrogens directly interact with ERs in ER-positive human breast cancer cells, where they induce transcriptional activation of "immediate early" and cyclin genes and promote cell cycle progression. However, membrane-initiated estrogen signaling, including rapid changes of the signal transduction cascades, has been proposed to be also essential for the mitogenic action of estrogen signaling. Castoria *et. al.*, (1999) reported that NIH3T3 fibroblasts are made equally E2β-responsive in terms of DNA synthesis by transient transfection with either the wild-type or the transcriptionally inactive ER-α66 mutant. Castoria *et. al.*, (2001) later demonstrated that the PI3K/Akt signaling pathway and Src together mediates activation of cyclin D1 promoter activity and promotion of the S-phase entry in estrogen–stimulated ER-positive breast cancer MCF7 cells. These findings together with other reports (Song et al., 2002; Migliaccio et al., 1996; Ahmad et al., 1999; Lobenhofer et al., 2000) highlight the importance of the non-genomic action of estrogen signaling in estrogen-stimulated cell proliferation and mammary tumorigenesis.

The epidermal growth factor receptor (EGFR) is essential for ductal morphogenesis during normal mammary gland development and its overexpression either at the gene or protein levels is well documented in human breast cancer (Reviewed by Troyer & Lee, 2001). Overexpression of EGFR alone usually does not constitute efficient transformation and tumorigenesis in breast cancer models. However, co-expression with the non-receptor kinase c-Src dramatically increases tumorigenesis (Maa et al., 1995; Tice et al., 1999; Biscardi et al., 1998). Co-expression of EGFR and c-Src in breast cancer cell lines results in their association and c-Src-mediated phosphorylation of the EGFR at tyrosine 845 (Tyr845) within its catalytic domain, which contributes to enhanced proliferation *in vitro* and tumor formation *in vivo* (Biscardi et al., 1998; Maa et al., 1995; Tice et al., 1999; Biscardi et al., 2000). Accumulating evidence indicated that c-Src is involved in non-genomic estrogen signaling by interacting with ER-α66 in ER-positive breast cancer cells (Shupnik, 2004). In ER-negative breast cancer cells, E2β induced the MAPK/ERK activation through a mechanism that involves the interaction between ER-α36 and the EGFR/Src/Shc complex (Zhang et al, 2011). Intriguingly, ER-α36 interacts strongly with EGFR in the absence of estrogen and is progressively dissociated from EGFR after estrogen treatment (Zhang et al., 2011), which is in contradictory to the finding that estrogen stimulates recruitment of ER-α66 to the EGFR complex (Reviewed by Levin, 2003). Like ER-α66 (Song et al., 2002), interaction between ER-α36 and the Src/Shc was estrogen-dependent (Zhang et al., 2011), which results in Src-Tyr-416 phosphorylation and phosphorylation of the EGFR-Tyr-845 but not the major auto-phosphorylation sites of EGFR such as Tyr-992, -1068 and -1073. Tyr-845 in the EGFR is not an auto-phosphorylation site and is not required for EGFR kinase activity but is phosphorylated by Src (Biscardi et al., 1998).

Signal transducer and activator of transcription 5b (STAT5b), c-Src and EGFR play important roles in estrogen-stimulated proliferation of ER-positive breast cancer cells (Fox et al., 2008). Estrogen-induced Src activation and Src-dependent phosphorylation of EGFR-Tyr-845 recruit STAT5b as a downstream effector of phosphorylated EGFR-Tyr-845 to induce c-Myc and cyclin D1 expression (Fox et al., 2008). Introduction of a dominant-negative STAT5a into ER-positive T47D breast cancer cells inhibits E2β-stimulated cell proliferation and induces apoptosis (Yamashita et al., 2003). The involvement of STAT5 in ER-α36-mediated estrogen activation of the cyclin D1 promoter activity has been established (Zhang et al., unpublished data). Thus, it is possible that ER-α36 mediates mitogenic estrogen signaling through the EGFR/Src/STAT5 pathway in breast cancer cells.

17. Transcriptional regulation of ER-α36

Transcription of ER-α36 is initiated from a previously unidentified promoter in the first intron of the ER-α66 gene (Figure 1). The putative 5′-flanking region of the ER-α36 has been cloned and sequenced (Zou et al., 2009). Computer analysis revealed a TATA binding protein (TBP) recognition sequence upstream of the cDNA start site and several Sp1, NF-κB and Ap1 binding sites in the 5′-flanking region of ER-α36. A perfect half ERE site was identified at the promoter region of ER-α36 that is involved in suppression of ER-α36 promoter activity by ER-α66, indicating that ER-α36 expression is subjected to negative regulation of ER-α66 (Zou et al., 2009). This is consistent with the finding that ER-positive breast cancer cells tend to express lower levels of ER-α36 compared to ER-negative breast cancer cells (Wang et al., 2006; Zou et al., 2009). ER-α46 that lacks the AF-1 domain, however, had no effect on ER-α36 promoter activity while ER-α46 released the suppression activity of ER-α66 when co-expressed with ER-α66 (Zou et al., 2009). Thus ER-α66 suppresses the promoter activity of ER-α36 presumably through ligand-independent activity mediated by its AF1 domain, which can be blocked by ER-α46. In addition, co-expression of ER-α36 also released the suppression activity mediated by ER-α66 (Zou et al., 2009), suggesting that ER-α36 may be regulated by a positive-feedback mechanism.

BRCA1 mutations and downregulation are found in familial and sporadic breast cancers and BRCA1-related tumors are more likely to be ER-negative than are non-BRCA1 related breast cancers. It is still unknown why dysfunctional BRCA1 only predispose to cancers of estrogen responsive tissues and why these BRCA1-related breast tumors are often ER-negative. BRCA1 mediates the ligand-independent transcriptional repression activity of the ER-α66 through its AF-1 domain (Zheng *et. al.,* 2003). Since ER-α66 represses the promoter activity of ER-α36 through its AF-1 domain, it is reasonable to postulate that loss of BRCA1 function either by mutations or downregulation may activate ER-α36 expression, which then activates ER-α36-mediated mitogenic estrogen signaling that eventually leads to development of breast cancers characterized as ER-negative since they lack ER-α66 expression.

The analysis of ER-α36 promoter revealed several important features of transcriptional regulation of this potentially important player in estrogen signaling. The finding of several NF-κB binding sites indicates that ER-α36 is subject to regulation by the NF-κB signaling pathway and by different cytokines that activate the NF-κB signaling pathway. The existence of Ap-1 binding sites in the ER-α36 promoter region raised the possibility that growth factor signaling may regulate ER-α36 expression, which was confirmed by our recent report that EGFR-mediated signaling induces ER-α36 expression via one of the Ap-1 binding sites (Zhang et al., 2011). Thus, further study of the transcription regulation of ER-α36 will provide more information about the mechanisms underlying regulation of ER-α36 mediated non-genomic estrogen signaling in cells and tissues other than mammary gland.

18. Cross-regulation of ER-α36 and members of the EGFR family

In ER-positive breast cancer cells, it has been well documented that the cross-communication between EGFR and ER-α66 leads to serine phosphorylation of ER-α66 and ligand-independent activation of the ER-α66-mediated transcription (Kato et al., 1995; Bunone et al., 1996). Conversely, EGF signaling is strongly enhanced by the ER-α66 in ER-positive MCF7 cells and anti-estrogen ICI 182, 780 was able to block the EGF signaling (Migliaccio et al., 2006). In addition, our group has reported another level of cross-talk mechanism by which EGFR and ER-α36 positively regulate each other's expression in triple-negative breast cancer cells (Zhang et al., 2011); EGFR signaling activates the promoter activity of ER-α36 and ER-α36 stabilizes the steady state levels of EGFR protein. This positive feedback loop provides a molecular explanation to the aggressiveness of triple-negative breast cancer. A similar cross-regulation between Her2/Neu and ER-α36 was also found (Kang et al., unpublished observations). However, unlike EGFR, ER-α36-mediated estrogen signaling up-regulates the promoter activity of Her2/Neu gene, suggesting that ER-α36 positively regulates Her2/Neu expression. This data is consistent with the finding that ER-α36 expression is significantly correlated with Her-2/Neu expression in specimens from breast cancer patients (Shi et al., 2009). Thus, the interplay between growth factor receptors and ER-α36 may play an important role in development and progression of subsets of breast cancer that highly express ER-α36.

19. ER-α36 in osteoporosis

Non-genomic estrogen signaling plays an important role in bone protection; estrogen is able to protect the adult skeleton against bone loss by maintaining a focal balance between bone formation and resorption, which mainly results from the opposite effects of osteoblasts (OBs) and osteoclasts (OCs). Estrogen has anti-apoptotic effects on OBs and pro-apoptotic effects on OCs through an extra-nuclear signaling that leads to activation of the MAPK/ERK signaling pathway and kinase-dependent changes in transcription activities (Reviewed by Manolagas, 2000; Manolagas et al., 2004). However, the underlying mechanisms of this opposite effects of estrogen signaling have not been established. Xie et al., (2011) recently reported that the postmenopausal level of E2β induces mitogenic, anti-apoptotic and anti-osteogenic effects in postmenopausal OBs and pro-apoptotic effects in postmenopausal OCs, respectively. ER-α36 mediates the effects of post-menopausal-level E2β on proliferation, apoptosis, and differentiation of OBs through transient activation of the MAPK/ERK pathway, whereas ER-α36 mediates post-menopausal-level E2β induced apoptosis of OCs through prolonged or sustained activation of the MAPK/ERK pathway. The levels of ER-α36 expression in bone are positively associated with bone mineral density in post-menopausal women. Thus, the high levels of ER-α36 expression are required for preserving bone mass in post-menopausal and menopausal women.

20. Conclusions

Most previous studies of estrogen signaling in human breast cancer were focused on the ER-α66, the only known estrogen receptor for many years. The discovery of ER-α36 in our laboratory, combined with the previous reports of membrane-based ER-α46, raised the intriguing possibility that ER-α36 and ER-α46 are also involved in estrogen signaling. Net estrogen response in a specific target cell thus depends on absolute and relative levels of the regulated expression of full-length and alternatively processed estrogen receptor-α isoforms.

It is well established that estrogen stimulates mammary epithelial cell proliferation. However, the function of ER-α66, ER-β and ER-α46 in mitogenic estrogen signaling is confounding. A plethora of experimental evidence indicates that ER-α66, ER-α46, and ER-β negatively regulate mitogenic estrogen signaling in transfected cells, which argue against the positive role of these receptors in estrogen-stimulated cell proliferation. Thus far, ER-α36 is the only reported estrogen receptor that mediates mitogenic estrogen signaling and stimulates cell proliferation in transfected cells and in ER-negative breast cancer cells that lack expression of ER-α66, ER-α46 and ER-β but express high level of endogenous ER-α36. In addition, the finding that ER-α36 functions as a potent dominant-negative regulator of the genomic estrogen signaling mediated by ER-α66 and ER-β implicates that when ER-α36 mediates mitogenic estrogen signalling, it may require the silence of genomic estrogen signaling. This again challenges the well-known role of genomic estrogen signaling in estrogen-stimulated cell proliferation.

Accumulating evidence highlights the importance of ER-α36-mediated non-genomic estrogen signaling in malignant growth of breast cancer and endometrial cancer cells. The expression of ER-α36 has also been detected in other types of human cancer such as human colon cancer and liver cancer (Jiang et al., 2008; Miceli et al., 2011), suggesting that ER-α36 may also involved in initiation and development of human malignancy in non-classical estrogen targeting organs. Elucidating the functions of ER-α36-mediated non-genomic estrogen signaling in different types of human malignancy could provide more informed approaches to better understand the underlying mechanisms of mitogenic estrogen signaling in mammary carcinogenesis. We hope that further investigation of the function and underlying mechanisms of this ER variant in different subtypes of human breast cancer and even in the putative breast cancer stem/progenitor cells will lead to development of high efficacy, less toxic therapeutic agents for patients affected with mammary malignancies.

21. Acknowledgments

We regret the inability to cite many fine papers that contribute to this field due to space limitations. This work was supported by grants from the National Institute of Health, Susan G. Komen for the Cure and the Nebraska Tobacco Settlement Biomedical Research Program.

22. References

Ahmad, S., Singh, N. & Glazer, RI. (1999). Role of AKT1 in 17beta-estradiol- and insulin-like growth factor I (IGF-I)-dependent proliferation and prevention of apoptosis in MCF-7 breast carcinoma cells. *Biochem Pharmacol* 58:425-430.

Ahola, TM., Alkio, N., Manninen, T. & Ylikomi, T. (2002). Progestin and G protein-coupled receptor 30 inhibit mitogen-activated protein kinase activity in MCF-7 breast cancer cells. *Endocrinology.* 143:4620-4626.

Altucci, L., Addeo, R., Cicatiello, L., Dauvois, S., Parker, MG., Truss, M., Beato, M., Sica, V., Bresciani, F. & Weisz, A. (1996). 17beta-Estradiol induces cyclin D1 gene transcription, p36D1-p34cdk4 complex activation and p105Rb phosphorylation during mitogenic stimulation of G1-arrested human breast cancer cells. *Oncogene.* 12:2315-2324.

Altucci, L., Addeo, R., Cicatiello, L., Germano, D., Pacilio, C., Battista, T., Cancemi, M., Petrizzi, VB., Bresciani, F. & Weisz, A. (1997). Estrogen induces early and timed activation of cyclin-dependent kinases 4, 5, and 6 and increases cyclin messenger ribonucleic acid expression in rat uterus. *Endocrinology.* 138:978-984.

Aronica, SM., Kraus, WL. & Katzenellenbogen, BS. (1994). Estrogen action via the cAMP signaling pathway: stimulation of adenylate cyclase and cAMP-regulated gene transcription. *Proc Natl Acad Sci U S A.* 91:8517-8521.

Berry, M., Metzger, D. & Chambon, P. (1990). Role of the two activating domains of the oestrogen receptor in the cell-type and promoter-context dependent agonistic activity of the anti-oestrogen 4-hydroxytamoxifen. *EMBO J.* 9:2811-2818.

Biscardi, JS., Belsches, AP. & Parsons, SJ. (1998). Characterization of human epidermal growth factor receptor and c-Src interactions in human breast tumor cells. *Mol. Carcinog.* 21:261-272.

Biscardi, JS., Ishizawar, RC., Silva, CM. & Parsons, SJ. (2000). Tyrosine kinase signalling in breast cancer: epidermal growth factor receptor and c-Src interactions in breast cancer. *Breast Cancer. Res.* 2:203-210.

Brinton, RD. (2001). Cellular and molecular mechanisms of estrogen regulation of memory function and neuroprotection against Alzheimer's disease: recent insights and remaining challenges. *Learn Mem.* 8:121-133.

Bunone, G., Briand, PA., Miksicek, RJ. & Picard, D. (1996). Activation of the unliganded estrogen receptor by EGF involves the MAP kinase pathway and direct phosphorylation. *EMBO J.* 15:2174-2183.

Caiazza F, Galluzzo P, Lorenzetti S, Marino M (2007) 17Beta-estradiol induces ERbeta up-regulation via p38/MAPK activation in colon cancer cells. *Biochem Biophys Res Commun* 359:102-107.

Castoria, G., Barone, M.V, Di Domenico, M., Bilancio, A., Ametrano, D., Migliaccio, A. & Auricchio, F. (1999). Non-transcriptional action of oestradiol and progestin triggers DNA synthesis. *EMBO J.* 18:2500-2510.

Castoria, G., Migliaccio, A., Bilancio, A., Di Domenico, M., de Falco, A., Lombardi, M., Fiorentino, R., Varricchio, L., Barone, MV. & Auricchio, F. (2001). PI3-kinase in concert with Src promotes the S-phase entry of oestradiol-stimulated MCF-7 cells. *EMBO J.* 20:6050-6059.

Cerillo, G., Rees, A., Manchanda, N., Reilly, C., Brogan, I., White, A. & Needham, M. (1998). The oestrogen receptor regulates NFkappaB and AP-1 activity in a cell-specific manner. *J Steroid Biochem. Mol. Biol.* 67:79-88.

Chen, Z., Yuhanna, IS., Galcheva-Gargova, Z., Karas, RH., Mendelsohn, ME. & Shaul, PW. (1999.) Estrogen receptor alpha mediates the nongenomic activation of endothelial nitric oxide synthase by estrogen. *J Clin. Invest.* 103:401-406.

Clark, GM., Osborne, CK. & McGuire, WL. (1984). Correlations between estrogen receptor, progesterone receptor, and patient characteristics in human breast cancer. *J Clin Oncol.* 2:1102-1109.

Clark, GM. (2000). Prognostic and predictive factors. *Diseases of the breast*, Lippincott Williams & Wilkins, Vol. 2:489-514.

Clarke, R., Leonessa, F., Welch, JN. & Skaar, TC. (2001). Cellular and molecular pharmacology of antiestrogen action and resistance. *Pharmacol. Rev.* 53:25-71.

Clarke, R., Liu, MC., Bouker, KB., Gu, Z., Lee, RY., Zhu, Y., Skaar, TC., Gomez, B., O'Brien, K., Wang, Y. & Hilakivi-Clarke, LA. (2003). Antiestrogen resistance in breast cancer and the role of estrogen receptor signaling. *Oncogene.* 22:7316-7339.

Clarke, R., Howell, A., Potten, CS. & Anderson, E. (1997). Dissociation between steroid receptor expression and cell proliferation in the human breast. *Cancer Res.* 57:4987-4991.

Cowell, LN., Graham, JD., Bouton, AH., Clarke, CL. & O'Neill, GM. (2006). Tamoxifen treatment promotes phosphorylation of the adhesion molecules, p130Cas/BCAR1, FAK and Src, via an adhesion-dependent pathway. *Oncogene.* 25:7597-7607.

Dauvois, S., Danielian, PS., White, R. & Parker, MG. (1992.) Antiestrogen ICI 164,384 reduces cellular estrogen receptor content by increasing its turnover. *Proc Natl Acad Sci U S A.* 89:4037-4041.

Deroo, BJ. & Buensuceso, AV. (2010.) Minireview: Estrogen receptor-beta: mechanistic insights from recent studies. *Mol. Endocrinol.* 24:1703-1714.

Diaz-Chico, BN., Ogasawara, Y., Chamness, GC., Salman, M. & McGuire, WL. (1988). A 46-kDa antigen associated with estrogen receptor in human breast cancer. *J Steroid Biochem.* 30:315-320.

Dotzlaw, H., Leygue, E., Watson, PH. & Murphy, LC. (1997). Expression of estrogen receptor-beta in human breast tumors. *J Clin. Endocrino.l Metab.* 82:2371-2374.

Driggers, PH. & Segars, JH. (2002). Estrogen action and cytoplasmic signaling pathways. Part II: the role of growth factors and phosphorylation in estrogen signaling. *Trends Endocrinol. Metab.* 13:422-427.

Dudley, MW., Sheeler, CQ., Wang, H. & Khan, S. (2000). Activation of the human estrogen receptor by the antiestrogens ICI 182,780 and tamoxifen in yeast genetic systems: implications for their mechanism of action. *Proc Natl Acad Sci U S A.* 97:3696-3701.

Dufy, B., Vincent, JD., Fleury, H., Du Pasquier, P., Gourdji, D & Tixier-Vidal, A. (1979). Membrane effects of thyrotropin-releasing hormone and estrogen shown by intracellular recording from pituitary cells. *Science.* 204:509-511.

Endoh, H., Sasaki, H., Maruyama, K., Takeyama, K., Waga, I., Shimizu, T., Kato, S. & Kawashima, H. (1997). Rapid activation of MAP kinase by estrogen in the bone cell line. *Biochem. Biophys. Res. Commun.* 235:99-102.

Evans, MJ., Eckert, A., Lai, K., Adelman, SJ. & Harnish, DC. (2001). Reciprocal antagonism between estrogen receptor and NF-kappaB activity in vivo. *Circ. Res.* 89:823-830.

Fawell, SE., White, R., Hoare, S., Sydenham, M., Page, M. & Parker, MG. (1990). Inhibition of estrogen receptor-DNA binding by the "pure" antiestrogen ICI 164,384 appears to be mediated by impaired receptor dimerization. *Proc Natl Acad Sci U S A.* 87:6883-6887.

Feigelson, HS. & Henderson, BE. (1996). Estrogens and breast cancer. *Carcinogenesis.* 17:2279-2284.

Ferguson, AT., Lapidus, RG., Baylin, SB. & Davidson, NE. (1995). Demethylation of the estrogen receptor gene in estrogen receptor-negative breast cancer cells can reactivate estrogen receptor gene expression. *Cancer Res.* 55:2279-2283.

Filardo, EJ., Quinn, JA., Bland, KI. & Frackelton, AR. Jr. (2000). Estrogen-induced activation of Erk-1 and Erk-2 requires the G protein-coupled receptor homolog, GPR30, and occurs via trans-activation of the epidermal growth factor receptor through release of HB-EGF. *Mol. Endocrinol.* 14:1649-1660.

Filardo, E., Quinn, J., Pang, Y., Graeber, C., Shaw, S., Dong, J. & Thomas, P. (2007). Activation of the novel estrogen receptor G protein-coupled receptor 30 (GPR30) at the plasma membrane. *Endocrinology* 148:3236-3245.

Flouriot, G, Brand, H., Denger, S., Metivier, R., Kos, M., Reid, G., Sonntag-Buck, V. & Gannon, F. (2000). Identification of a new isoform of the human estrogen receptor-alpha (hER-alpha) that is encoded by distinct transcripts and that is able to repress hER-alpha activation function 1. *EMBO J.* 19:4688-4700.

Fox, EM., Bernaciak, TM., Wen, J., Weaver, AM., Shupnik, MA. & Silva, CM. (2008). Signal transducer and activator of transcription 5b, c-Src, and epidermal growth factor receptor signaling play integral roles in estrogen-stimulated proliferation of estrogen receptor-positive breast cancer cells. *Mol. Endocrinol.* 22:1781-1796.

Fuqua, SA., Schiff, R., Parra, I., Friedrichs, WE., Su, JL., McKee, DD., Slentz-Kesler, K., Moore, LB., Willson, TM. & Moore, JT. (1999). Expression of wild-type estrogen receptor beta and variant isoforms in human breast cancer. *Cancer Res.* 59:5425-5428.

Fuqua, SA., Schiff, R., Parra, I., Moore, JT., Mohsin, SK., Osborne, CK., Clark, GM & Allred, DC. (2003). Estrogen receptor beta protein in human breast cancer: correlation with clinical tumor parameters. *Cancer Res.* 63:2434-2439.

Galluzzo, P., Caiazza, F., Moreno, S. & Marino, M. (2007). Role of ER-beta palmitoylation in the inhibition of human colon cancer cell proliferation. *Endocr. Relat. Cancer.* 14:153-167.

Geisler, J., Haynes, B., Anker, G., Dowsett, M. & Lonning, PE. (2002). Influence of letrozole and anastrozole on total body aromatization and plasma estrogen levels in postmenopausal breast cancer patients evaluated in a randomized, cross-over study. *J Clin. Oncol.* 20:751-757.

Green, S., Walter, P., Kumar, V., Krust, A., Bornert, JM., Argos, P. & Chambon, P. (1986). Human oestrogen receptor cDNA: sequence, expression and homology to v-erb-A. *Nature.* 320:134-139.

Greene, GL., Gilna, P., Waterfield, M., Baker, A, Hort, Y. & Shine, J. (1986). Sequence and expression of human estrogen receptor complementary DNA. *Science.* 231:1150-1154.

Gu, Q., Korach, KS. & Moss, RL. (1999). Rapid action of 17beta-estradiol on kainate-induced currents in hippocampal neurons lacking intracellular estrogen receptors. *Endocrinology.* 140:660-666.

Gupta, PB., Proia, D., Cingoz, O., Weremowicz, J., Naber, SP., Weinberg, RA. & Kuperwasser, C. (2007). Systemic stromal effects of estrogen promote the growth of estrogen receptor-negative cancers. *Cancer Res.* 67:2062-2071.

Hammes, SR. & Levin, ER. (2007). Extranuclear steroid receptors: nature and actions. *Endocr. Rev.* 28:726-741.

Harnish, DC., Scicchitano, MS., Adelman, SJ., Lyttle, CR. & Karathanasis, SK. (2000). The role of CBP in estrogen receptor cross-talk with nuclear factor-kappaB in HepG2 cells. *Endocrinology.* 141:3403-3411.

Harris, HA. (2007). Estrogen receptor-beta: recent lessons from in vivo studies. *Mol. Endocrinol* .21:1-13.

Hartman, J., Lindberg, K., Morani, A., Inzunza, J., Strom, A & Gustafsson, JA. (2006). Estrogen receptor beta inhibits angiogenesis and growth of T47D breast cancer xenografts. *Cancer Res.* 66:11207-11213.

Howell, A., Osborne, CK., Morris, C. & Wakeling, AE. (2000). ICI 182,780 (Faslodex): development of a novel, "pure" antiestrogen. *Cancer.* 89:817-825.

Iwao, K., Miyoshi, Y., Egawa, C., Ikeda, N. & Noguchi, S. (2000). Quantitative analysis of estrogen receptor-beta mRNA and its variants in human breast cancers. *Int. J Cancer.* 88:733-736.

Jarvinen, TA., Pelto-Huikko, M., Holli, K. & Isola, J. (2000). Estrogen receptor beta is coexpressed with ER-alpha and PR and associated with nodal status, grade, and proliferation rate in breast cancer. *Am. J Pathol.* 156:29-35.

Jensen, EV., Cheng, G., Palmieri, C., Saji, S., Makela, S., Van Noorden, S., Wahlstrom, T., Warner, M., Coombes, RC & Gustafsson, JA. (2001). Estrogen receptors and proliferation markers in primary and recurrent breast cancer. *Proc Natl Acad Sci U S A.* 98:15197-15202.

Jiang, H., Teng, R., Wang, Q., Zhang, XT., Wang, H., Wang, ZY., Cao, J. & Teng, L. (2008). Transcriptional analysis of estrogen receptor alpha variant mRNAs in colorectal cancers and their matched normal colorectal tissues. *J Steroid Biochem. Mol. Biol.* 112:20-24.

Jiang, SY. & Jordan, VC. (1992). Growth regulation of estrogen receptor-negative breast cancer cells transfected with complementary DNAs for estrogen receptor. *J Natl. Cancer Inst.* 84:580-591.

Jozan, S., Julia, AM., Carretie, A., Eche, N., Maisongrosse, V., Fouet, B., Marques, B. & David, JF. (1991). 65 and 47 kDa forms of estrogen receptor in human breast cancer: relation with estrogen responsiveness. *Breast Cancer Res. Treat.* 19:103-109.

Kang, LG. & Wang, ZY. (2010a). Breast cancer cell growth inhibition by phenethyl isothiocyanate is associated with down-regulation of oestrogen receptor-alpha36. *J Cell Mol. Med.* 14:1485-1493.

Kang, LG., Zhang, XT., Xie, Y., Tu, YP., Wang, D., Liu, ZM. & Wang, ZY. (2010b). Involvement of estrogen receptor variant ER-alpha36, not GPR30, in nongenomic estrogen signaling. *Mol. Endocrinol.* 24:709-721.

Kato, S., Endoh, H., Masuhiro, Y., Kitamoto, T., Uchiyama, S., Sasaki, H., Masushige, S., Gotoh, Y., Nishida, E., Kawashima, H., Metzger, D. & Chambon, P. (1995). Activation of the estrogen receptor through phosphorylation by mitogen-activated protein kinase. *Science.* 270:1491-1494.

Katzenellenbogen, BS. & Katzenellenbogen, JA. (2000). Estrogen receptor transcription and transactivation: Estrogen receptor alpha and estrogen receptor beta: regulation by selective estrogen receptor modulators and importance in breast cancer. *Breast Cancer Res.* 2:335-344.

Katzenellenbogen, BS. & Katzenellenbogen, JA. (2002). Biomedicine. Defining the "S" in SERMs. *Science.* 295:2380-2381.

Kelly, MJ. & Levin, ER. (2001). Rapid actions of plasma membrane estrogen receptors. *Trends Endocrinol. Metab.* 12:152-156.

Kelly, MJ., Moss, RL., & Dudley, CA. (1976) Differential sensitivity of preoptic-septal neurons to microelectrophoresed estrogen during the estrous cycle. *Brain Res* 114:152-157.

Kelly, MJ., Moss, RL., Dudley, CA. & Fawcett, CP. (1977). The specificity of the response of preoptic-septal area neurons to estrogen: 17alpha-estradiol versus 17beta-estradiol and the response of extrahypothalamic neurons. *Exp. Brain Res.* 30:43-52.

Khan, SA., Rogers, MA., Obando, JA. & Tamsen, A. (1994). Estrogen receptor expression of benign breast epithelium and its association with breast cancer. *Cancer Res.* 54:993-997.

Kim, KH. & Bender, JR. (2005). Rapid, estrogen receptor-mediated signaling: why is the endothelium so special? *Sci. STKE.* 2005:pe28.

Kim, R., Kaneko, M., Arihiro, K., Emi, M., Tanabe, K., Murakami, S., Osaki, A. & Inai, K. (2006). Extranuclear expression of hormone receptors in primary breast cancer. *Ann Oncol* 17:1213-1220.

Klinge, CM. (2001). Estrogen receptor interaction with estrogen response elements. *Nucleic Acids Res.* 29:2905-2919.

Klinge, CM., Riggs, KA., Wickramasinghe, NS., Emberts, CG., McConda, DB., Barry, PN. &, Magnusen, JE. (2010). Estrogen receptor alpha 46 is reduced in tamoxifen resistant breast cancer cells and re-expression inhibits cell proliferation and estrogen receptor alpha 66-regulated target gene transcription. *Mol. Cell Endocrinol.* 323:268-276.

Kong, EH., Pike, AC. & Hubbard, RE. (2003). Structure and mechanism of the oestrogen receptor. *Biochem. Soc. Trans.* 31:56-59.

Kuiper, GG., Enmark, E., Pelto-Huikko, M., Nilsson, S. & Gustafsson, J.A. (1996). Cloning of a novelreceptor expressed in rat prostate and ovary. *Proc. Natl. Acad. Sci. USA.* 93: 5925-5930.

Kurebayashi J, Otsuki T, Yamamoto S, Kurosumi M, Nakata T, Akinaga S, Sonoo H (1998) A pure antiestrogen, ICI 182,780, stimulates the growth of tamoxifen-resistant KPL-1 human breast cancer cells in vivo but not in vitro. *Oncology* 55 Suppl 1:23-34.

Kushner, PJ., Agard, DA., Greene, GL., Scanlan, TS., Shiau, AK., Uht, RM. & Webb, P. (2000). Estrogen receptor pathways to AP-1. *J Steroid Biochem. Mol. Biol.* 74:311-317.

Kushner, PJ., Hort, E., Shine, J., Baxter, JD. & Greene, GL. (1990). Construction of cell lines that express high levels of the human estrogen receptor and are killed by estrogens. *Mol. Endocrinol.* 4:1465-1473.

Lazennec, G., Bresson, D., Lucas, A., Chauveau, C. & Vignon, F. (2001). ER beta inhibits proliferation and invasion of breast cancer cells. *Endocrinology.* 142:4120-4130.

Lee, LM., Cao, J., Deng, H., Chen, P., Gatalica, Z. & Wang, ZY. (2008). ER-alpha36, a novel variant of ER-alpha, is expressed in ER-positive and -negative human breast carcinomas. *Anticancer Res.* 28:479-483.

Levin, ER. (2002). Cellular functions of plasma membrane estrogen receptors. *Steroids.* 67:471-475.

Levin, ER. (2003). Bidirectional signaling between the estrogen receptor and the epidermal growth factor receptor. *Mol. Endocrinol.* 17:309-317.

Leygue, E., Dotzlaw, H., Watson, PH. & Murphy, LC. (1998). Altered estrogen receptor alpha and beta messenger RNA expression during human breast tumorigenesis. *Cancer Res.* 58:3197-3201.

Li, L., Haynes, MP. & Bender, JR. (2003.) Plasma membrane localization and function of the estrogen receptor alpha variant (ER46) in human endothelial cells. *Proc Natl Acad Sci U S A.* 100:4807-4812.

Lin, SL., Yan, LY., Liang, XW., Wang, ZB., Wang, ZY., Qiao, J., Schatten, H. & Sun, QY. (2009). A novel variant of ER-alpha, ER-alpha36 mediates testosterone-stimulated ERK and Akt activation in endometrial cancer Hec1A cells. *Reprod. Biol. Endocrinol.* 7:102.

Lin, SL., Yan, LY., Zhang, XT., Yuan, J., Li, M., Qiao, J., Wang, ZY. & Sun, QY. (2010). ER-alpha36, a variant of ER-alpha, promotes tamoxifen agonist action in endometrial cancer cells via the MAPK/ERK and PI3K/Akt pathways. *PLoS One.* 5:e9013.

Lobenhofer, EK., Huper, G., Iglehart, JD. & Marks, JR. (2000). Inhibition of mitogen-activated protein kinase and phosphatidylinositol 3-kinase activity in MCF-7 cells prevents estrogen-induced mitogenesis. *Cell Growth Differ.* 11:99-110.

Longo, M., Brama, M., Marino, M., Bernardini, S., Korach, KS., Wetsel, WC., Scandurra, R., Faraggiana, T., Spera, G., Baron, R., Teti, A. & Migliaccio, S. (2004). Interaction of estrogen receptor alpha with protein kinase C alpha and c-Src in osteoblasts during differentiation. *Bone.* 34:100-111.

Lu Q, Pallas DC, Surks HK, Baur WE, Mendelsohn ME, Karas RH (2004) Striatin assembles a membrane signaling complex necessary for rapid, nongenomic activation of endothelial NO synthase by estrogen receptor alpha. *Proc Natl Acad Sci U S A* 101:17126-17131.

Maa, MC., Leu, TH., McCarley, DJ., Schatzman, RC. & Parsons, SJ. (1995). Potentiation of epidermal growth factor receptor-mediated oncogenesis by c-Src: implications for the etiology of multiple human cancers. *Proc Natl Acad Sci U S A.* 92:6981-6985.

Mahfoudi, A., Roulet, E., Dauvois, S., Parker, MG. & Wahli, W. (1995). Specific mutations in the estrogen receptor change the properties of antiestrogens to full agonists. *Proc Natl Acad Sci U S A.* 92:4206-4210.

Manolagas, SC. (2000). Birth and death of bone cells: basic regulatory mechanisms and implications for the pathogenesis and treatment of osteoporosis. *Endocr. Rev.* 21:115-137.

Manolagas, SC., Kousteni, S., Chen, JR., Schuller, M., Plotkin, L. & Bellido, T. (2004). Kinase-mediated transcription, activators of nongenotropic estrogen-like signaling (ANGELS), and osteoporosis: a different perspective on the HRT dilemma. *Kidney Int. Suppl*: S41-49.

Maret, A., Clamens, S., Delrieu, I., Elhage, R., Arnal, JF. & Bayard, F. (1999). Expression of the interleukin-6 gene is constitutive and not regulated by estrogen in rat vascular smooth muscle cells in culture. *Endocrinology.* 140:2876-2882.

Margeat, E., Bourdoncle, A., Margueron, R., Poujol, N., Cavailles, V. & Royer, C. (2003). Ligands differentially modulate the protein interactions of the human estrogen receptors alpha and beta. *J Mol. Biol.* 326:77-92.

Marino, M. & Ascenzi, P. (2008). Membrane association of estrogen receptor alpha and beta influences 17beta-estradiol-mediated cancer cell proliferation. *Steroids.* 73:853-858.

Marquez, DC. & Pietras, RJ. (2001). Membrane-associated binding sites for estrogen contribute to growth regulation of human breast cancer cells. *Oncogene.* 20:5420-5430.

McDonnell, DP. & Norris, JD. (2002). Connections and regulation of the human estrogen receptor. *Science.* 296:1642-1644.

McEwen, B. (2002). Estrogen actions throughout the brain. *Recent Prog. Horm. Res.* 57:357-384.

McKay LI, Cidlowski JA (1999) Molecular control of immune/inflammatory responses: interactions between nuclear factor-kappa B and steroid receptor-signaling pathways. *Endocr Rev* 20:435-459.

Mermelstein, PG., Becker, JB. & Surmeier, DJ. (1996). Estradiol reduces calcium currents in rat neostriatal neurons via a membrane receptor. *J Neurosci.* 16:595-604.

Metivier, R., Penot, G., Carmouche, RP., Hubner, MR., Reid, G., Denger, S., Manu, D., Brand, H., Kos, M., Benes, V. & Gannon, F. (2004). Transcriptional complexes engaged by apo-estrogen receptor-alpha isoforms have divergent outcomes. *EMBO J.* 23:3653-3666.

Miceli, V., Cocciadiferro, L., Fregapane, M., Zarcone, M., Montalto, G., Polito, LM., Agostara, B., Granata, OM. & Carruba, G. (2011). Expression of Wild-Type and Variant Estrogen Receptor Alpha in Liver Carcinogenesis and Tumor Progression. *OMICS.* [Epub ahead of print].

Migliaccio, A., Castoria, G., Di Domenico, M., Ciociola, A., Lombardi, M., De Falco, A., Nanayakkara, M., Bottero, D., De Stasio, R., Varricchio, L. & Auricchio, F (2006). Crosstalk between EGFR and extranuclear steroid receptors. *Ann N Y Acad Sci* 1089:194-200.

Migliaccio, A., Di Domenico, M., Castoria, G., de Falco, A., Bontempo, P., Nola, E. & Auricchio, F. (1996). Tyrosine kinase/p21ras/MAP-kinase pathway activation by estradiol-receptor complex in MCF-7 cells. *EMBO J* 15:1292-1300.

Moriarty, K., Kim, KH. & Bender, JR (2006). Minireview: estrogen receptor-mediated rapid signaling. *Endocrinology.* 147:5557-5563.

Morley, P., Whitfield, JF., Vanderhyden, BC., Tsang, BK. & Schwartz, JL. (1992). A new, nongenomic estrogen action: the rapid release of intracellular calcium. *Endocrinology.* 131:1305-1312.

Nethrapalli, IS., Tinnikov, AA., Krishnan, V., Lei, CD. & Toran-Allerand, CD. (2005). Estrogen activates mitogen-activated protein kinase in native, nontransfected CHO-K1, COS-7, and RAT2 fibroblast cell lines. *Endocrinology.* 146:56-63.

Nicholson, RI., Gee, JM., Manning, DL., Wakeling, AE., Montano, MM. & Katzenellenbogen, BS. (1995). Responses to pure antiestrogens (ICI 164384, ICI 182780) in estrogen-sensitive and -resistant experimental and clinical breast cancer. *Ann. N Y Acad. Sci.* 761:148-163.

Nilsson, S., Makela, S., Treuter, E., Tujague, M., Thomsen, J., Andersson, G., Enmark, E., Pettersson, K., Warner, M. & Gustafsson, JA. (2001). Mechanisms of estrogen action. *Physiol. Rev.* 81:1535-1565.

Nissen-Meyer, R. (1964). "Prophylactic" ovariectomy and ovarian irradiation in breast cancer. *Acta. Unio. Int. Contra. Cancrum.* 20:527-530.

Omoto, Y., Inoue, S., Ogawa, S., Toyama, T., Yamashita, H., Muramatsu, M., Kobayashi, S. & Iwase, H. (2001). Clinical value of the wild-type estrogen receptor beta expression in breast cancer. *Cancer Lett.* 163:207-212.

Osborne, CK., Yochmowitz, MG., Knight, WA., 3rd. & McGuire, WL. (1980). The value of estrogen and progesterone receptors in the treatment of breast cancer. *Cancer.* 46:2884-2888.

Otto, C, Fuchs, I., Kauselmann, G., Kern, H., Zevnik, B., Andreasen, P., Schwarz, G., Altmann, H., Klewer, M.,, Schoor M., Vonk, R. & Fritzemeier, KH. (2009). GPR30 does not mediate estrogenic responses in reproductive organs in mice. *Biol. Reprod.* 80:34-41.

Otto, C., Rohde-Schulz, B, Schwarz, G., Fuchs, I., Klewer, M., Brittain, D., Langer, G., Bader, B., Prelle, K., Nubbemeyer, R. & Fritzemeier, KH. (2008). G protein-coupled receptor 30 localizes to the endoplasmic reticulum and is not activated by estradiol. *Endocrinology.* 149:4846-4856.

Paruthiyil, S., Parmar, H., Kerekatte, V., Cunha, GR., Firestone, GL. & Leitman, DC. (2004). Estrogen receptor beta inhibits human breast cancer cell proliferation and tumor formation by causing a G2 cell cycle arrest. *Cancer Res.* 64:423-428.

Pearce, ST., Liu, H. & Jordan, VC. (2003). Modulation of estrogen receptor alpha function and stability by tamoxifen and a critical amino acid (Asp-538) in helix 12. *J Biol. Chem.* 278:7630-7638.

Pedram, A., Razandi, M. & Levin, ER. (2006). Nature of functional estrogen receptors at the plasma membrane. *Mol. Endocrinol.* 20:1996-2009.

Penot, G., Le Peron, C., Merot, Y., Grimaud-Fanouillere, E., Ferriere, F., Boujrad, N., Kah, O., Saligaut, C., Ducouret, B., Metivier, R. & Flouriot, G. (2005). The human estrogen receptor-alpha isoform hERalpha46 antagonizes the proliferative influence of hERalpha66 in MCF7 breast cancer cells. *Endocrinology.* 146:5474-5484.

Pietras, RJ., Marquez, DC., Chen, HW., Tsai, E., Weinberg, O. & Fishbein, M. (2005). Estrogen and growth factor receptor interactions in human breast and non-small cell lung cancer cells. *Steroids.* 70:372-381.

Pietras, RJ. & Szego, CM. (1975). Endometrial cell calcium and oestrogen action. *Nature.* 253:357-359.

Pietras, RJ. & Szego, CM. (1977). Specific binding sites for oestrogen at the outer surfaces of isolated endometrial cells. *Nature.* 265:69-72.

Pilat, MJ., Christman, JK. & Brooks, SC. (1996). Characterization of the estrogen receptor transfected MCF10A breast cell line 139B6. *Breast Cancer Res. Treat.* 37:253-266.

Prall, OW., Rogan, EM. & Sutherland, RL. (1998). Estrogen regulation of cell cycle progression in breast cancer cells. *J Steroid Biochem. Mol. Biol.* 65:169-174.

Rao, BR. (1998). Isolation and characterization of an estrogen binding protein which may integrate the plethora of estrogenic actions in non-reproductive organs. *J Steroid Biochem, Mol Biol.* 65:3-41.

Razandi, M., Pedram, A., Greene GL & Levin, ER. (1999). Cell membrane and nuclear estrogen receptors (ERs) originate from a single transcript: studies of ER-alpha and ER-beta expressed in Chinese hamster ovary cells. *Mol Endocrinol.* 13:307-319.

Rebbeck, TR., Levin, AM., Eisen, A., Snyder, C., Watson, P., Cannon-Albright, L., Isaacs, C., Olopade, O., Garber, JE., Godwin, AK., Daly, MB., Narod, SA., Neuhausen, SL., Lynch, HT & Weber, BL. (1999). Breast cancer risk after bilateral prophylactic oophorectomy in BRCA1 mutation carriers. *J Natl. Cancer Inst.* 91:1475-1479.

Revankar, CM., Cimino, DF., Sklar, LA., Arterburn, JB. & Prossnitz, ER. (2005). A transmembrane intracellular estrogen receptor mediates rapid cell signaling. *Science.* 307:1625-1630.

Ring, A. & Dowsett, M. (2004.) Mechanisms of tamoxifen resistance. *Endocr. Relat. Cancer.* 11:643-658.

Robertson, JF. (1996). Oestrogen receptor: a stable phenotype in breast cancer. *Br. J Cancer.* 73: 5-12.

Rochefort, H. (1995). Oestrogen- and anti-oestrogen-regulated genes in human breast cancer. *Ciba. Found. Symp.* 191:254-265.

Roger, P., Daures, JP., Maudelonde, T., Pignodel, C., Gleizes, M., Chapelle, J., Marty-Double, C., Baldet, P., Mares, P., Laffargue, F. & Rochefort, H. (2000). Dissociated overexpression of cathepsin D and estrogen receptor alpha in preinvasive mammary tumors. *Hum. Pathol.* 31:593-600.

Roger, P., Sahla, ME, Makela, S., Gustafsson, JA, Baldet, P. & Rochefort, H. (2001). Decreased expression of estrogen receptor beta protein in proliferative preinvasive mammary tumors. *Cancer Res.* 61:2537-2541.

Russell, KS., Haynes, MP., Sinha D., Clerisme, E. & Bender, JR. (2000). Human vascular endothelial cells contain membrane binding sites for estradiol, which mediate rapid intracellular signaling. *Proc Natl Acad Sci U S A.* 97:5930-5935.

Safe, S. (2001). Transcriptional activation of genes by 17 beta-estradiol through estrogen receptor-Sp1 interactions. *Vitam. Horm.* 62:231-252.

Saji,. S, Sakaguchi, H., Andersson, S., Warne,r M. & Gustafsson, J (2001). Quantitative analysis of estrogen receptor proteins in rat mammary gland. *Endocrinology.* 142:3177-3186.

Santen, RJ. (2003). Inhibition of aromatase: insights from recent studies. *Steroids.* 68:559-567.

Segars, JH. & Driggers, PH. (2002). Estrogen action and cytoplasmic signaling cascades. Part I: membrane-associated signaling complexes. *Trends Endocrinol. Metab.* 13:349-354.

Shang, YF. & Brown, M. (2002). Molecular determinants for the tissue specificity of SERMs. *Science.* 295:2465-2468.

Shang, YF., Hu, X., DiRenzo, J., Lazar, MA. & Brown, M. (2000). Cofactor dynamics and sufficiency in estrogen receptor-regulated transcription. *Cell.* 103:843-852.

Sheikh, MS., Garcia, M., Pujol, P., Fontana, JA. & Rochefort, H. (1994). Why are estrogen-receptor-negative breast cancers more aggressive than the estrogen-receptor-positive breast cancers? *Invasion Metastasis.* 14:329-336.

Shi, .L, Dong, B., Li, Z., Lu, Y., Ouyang, T., Li, J., Wang, T., Fan, Z., Fan, T., Lin, B., Wang, ZY. & Xie, YT. (2009). Expression of ER-{alpha}36, a novel variant of estrogen receptor {alpha}, and resistance to tamoxifen treatment in breast cancer. *J Clin. Oncol.* 27:3423-3429.

Shoker, BS., Jarvis, C., Clarke, RB., Anderson, E., Hewlett, J., Davies, MP., Sibson, DR. & Sloane, JP (1999a). Estrogen receptor-positive proliferating cells in the normal and precancerous breast. *Am. J Pathol.* 155:1811-1815.

Shoker, BS., Jarvis, C., Sibson, DR., Walker, C. & Sloane, JP. (1999b). Oestrogen receptor expression in the normal and pre-cancerous breast. *J Pathol.* 188:237-244.

Shupnik, MA. (2004) Crosstalk between steroid receptors and the c-Src-receptor tyrosine kinase pathways: implications for cell proliferation. *Oncogene.* 23:7979-7989.

Sibonga, JD., Dobnig, H., Harden, RM. & Turner, RT. (1998). Effect of the high-affinity estrogen receptor ligand ICI 182,780 on the rat tibia. *Endocrinology.* 139:3736-3742.

Song, RX., McPherson, RA., Adam, L., Bao, Y., Shupnik, MA., Kumar, R. & Santen, RJ. (2002). Linkage of rapid estrogen action to MAPK activation by ERalpha-Shc association and Shc pathway activation. *Mol. Endocrinol.* 16:116-127.

Speir, E., Yu, ZX., Takeda, K., Ferrans, VJ. & Cannon, RO., 3rd. (2000). Competition for p300 regulates transcription by estrogen receptors and nuclear factor-kappaB in human coronary smooth muscle cells. *Circ. Res.* 87:1006-1011.

Speirs, V., Parkes, AT., Kerin, MJ., Walton, DS., Carleton, PJ., Fox, JN. & Atkin, SL. (1999). Coexpression of estrogen receptor alpha and beta: poor prognostic factors in human breast cancer? *Cancer Res.* 59:525-528.

Speirs, V., Skliris, GP., Burdall, SE. & Carder, PJ. (2002). Distinct expression patterns of ER alpha and ER beta in normal human mammary gland. *J Clin. Pathol.* 55:371-374.

Stoner, M., Saville, B., Wormke, M., Dean, D., Burghardt, R. & Safe, S. (2002). Hypoxia induces proteasome-dependent degradation of estrogen receptor alpha in ZR-75 breast cancer cells. *Mol. Endocrinol.* 16:2231-2242.

Sylvia, VL., Walton, J., Lopez, D., Dean, DD., Boyan, BD. & Schwartz, Z. (2001). 17 beta-estradiol-BSA conjugates and 17 beta-estradiol regulate growth plate chondrocytes by common membrane associated mechanisms involving PKC dependent and independent signal transduction. *J Cell Biochem.* 81:413-429.

Tesarik, J. & Mendoza, C. (1997). Direct non-genomic effects of follicular steroids on maturing human oocytes: oestrogen versus androgen antagonism. *Hum. Reprod. Update.* 3:95-100.

Tice, DA., Biscardi, JS., Nickles, AL. & Parsons, SJ. (1999). Mechanism of biological synergy between cellular Src and epidermal growth factor receptor. *Proc Natl Acad Sci U S A.* 96:1415-1420.

Tong, JS., Zhang, QH., Wang, ZB., Li, S., Yang, CR., Fu, XQ., Hou, Y., Wang, ZY., Sheng, J. & Sun, QY. (2010), ER-alpha36, a novel variant of ER-alpha, mediates estrogen-stimulated proliferation of endometrial carcinoma cells via the PKCdelta/ERK pathway. *PLoS One.* 5:e15408.

Toran-Allerand, CD., Guan, X., MacLusky, NJ., Horvath, TL., Diano, S., Singh, M., Connolly, ES., Jr., Nethrapalli, IS. & Tinnikov, A. (2002). ER-X: a novel, plasma membrane-associated, putative estrogen receptor that is regulated during development and after ischemic brain injury. *J Neurosci.* 22:8391-8401.

Touitou, I., Mathieu, M,. & Rochefort, H. (1990). Stable transfection of the estrogen receptor cDNA into Hela cells induces estrogen responsiveness of endogenous cathepsin D gene but not of cell growth. *Biochem. Biophys. Res. Commun.* 169:109-115.

Troyer, KL. & Lee, DC. (2001.) Regulation of mouse mammary gland development and tumorigenesis by the ERBB signaling network. *J Mammary Gland Biol. Neoplasia.* 6:7-21.

Tsai, EM., Wang, SC., Lee, JN. & Hung, MC. (2001). Akt activation by estrogen in estrogen receptor-negative breast cancer cells. *Cancer Res.* 61:8390-8392.

Tzukerman, MT., Esty, A., Santiso-Mere, D., Danielian, P., Parker, MG., Stein, RB., Pike, JW. & McDonnell, DP. (1994). Human estrogen receptor transactivational capacity is determined by both cellular and promoter context and mediated by two functionally distinct intramolecular regions. *Mol. Endocrinol.* 8:21-30.

Vranic, S., Gatalica, Z., Deng, H., Frkovic-Grazio, S., Lee, MJ., Olga Gurjeva, O. & Wang, Z-Y. (2011). ER-α36, a novel isoform of ER-α66, is commonly over-expressed in apocrine and adenoid cystic carcinomas of the breast". *J. of Clinical Pathology.* 64: 54-57.

Wang, ZY., Zhang, XT., Shen, P., Loggie, BW., Chang, Y. & Deuel, TF. (2005). Identification, cloning, and expression of human estrogen receptor-alpha36, a novel variant of human estrogen receptor-alpha66. *Biochem. Biophys. Res. Commun.* 336:1023-1027.

Wang, ZY., Zhang, XT., Shen, P., Loggie, BW., Chang, Y. & Deuel, TF. (2006). A variant of estrogen receptor-{alpha}, hER-{alpha}36: transduction of estrogen- and antiestrogen-dependent membrane-initiated mitogenic signaling. *Proc Natl Acad Sci U S A.* 103:9063-9068.

Warner, M., Saji, S. & Gustafsson, JA. (2000.) The normal and malignant mammary gland: a fresh look with ER-beta onboard. *J Mammary Gland Biol. Neoplasia.* 5:289-294.

Watson, C., Norfleet, A., Pappas, T. & Gametchu, B. (1999). Rapid actions of estrogens in GH3/B6 pituitary tumor cells via a plasma membrane version of estrogen receptor-α. *Steroids.* 64:5–13

Watters, JJ., Campbell, JS., Cunningham, MJ., Krebs, EG. & Dorsa, DM. (1997). Rapid membrane effects of steroids in neuroblastoma cells: effects of estrogen on mitogen activated protein kinase signaling cascade and c-fos immediate early gene transcription. *Endocrinology.* 138:4030-4033.

Xie, H., Sun, M., Liao, XB., Yuan, LQ., Sheng, Z.F, Meng, JC., Wang, D., Yu, ZY., Zhang, LY, Zhou, HD., Luo, XH., Li, H., Wu, XP., Wei, QY., Tang, SY., Wang, ZY. & Liao, EY. (2011). Estrogen receptor alpha36 mediates a bone-sparing effect of 17beta-estrodiol in postmenopausal women. *J Bone Miner. Res.* 26:156-168.

Yamashita, H., Iwase, H., Toyama, T. & Fujii, Y. (2003). Naturally occurring dominant-negative Stat5 suppresses transcriptional activity of estrogen receptors and induces apoptosis in T47D breast cancer cells. *Oncogene.* 22:1638-1652.

Zeps, N., Bentel, JM., Papadimitriou, JM., Dawkins, HJ. (1999). Murine progesterone receptor expression in proliferating mammary epithelial cells during normal pubertal development and adult estrous cycle. Association with eralpha and erbeta status. *J Histochem. Cytochem.* 47:1323-1330.

Zhang, XT., Kang, LG., Ding, L., Vranic, S., Gatalica, Z. & Wang, ZY. (2011). A positive feedback loop of ER-alpha36/EGFR promotes malignant growth of ER-negative breast cancer cells. *Oncogene.* 30:770-780.

Zhao, L., O'Neill, K. & Brinton, RD. (2006). Estrogenic agonist activity of ICI 182,780 (Faslodex) in hippocampal neurons: implications for basic science understanding of estrogen signaling and development of estrogen modulators with a dual therapeutic profile. *J Pharmacol. Exp. Ther.* 319:1124-1132.

Zhao, L., O'Neill, K., Diaz Brinton, R. (2005,) Selective estrogen receptor modulators (SERMs) for the brain: current status and remaining challenges for developing Neuro-SERMs. *Brain Res. Rev.* 49:472-493.

Zheng, WH., Andersson, S., Cheng, G., Simpson, ER., Warner, M. & Gustafsson, JA. (2003). Update on estrogen signaling. *FEBS Lett.* 546:17-24.

Zou, Y., Ding, L., Coleman, M. & Wang, ZY. (2009). Estrogen receptor-alpha (ER-alpha) suppresses expression of its variant ER-alpha 36. *FEBS Lett.* 583:1368-1374.

14

Estrogen-Related Receptors and Breast Cancer: A Mini Review

Christina T. Teng[1] and Peggy R. Teng[2]
[1]*Division of National Toxicology Program, National Institute of Environmental Health Sciences, National Institutes of Health, Durham*
[2]*Department of Experimental Pathology and Laboratory Medicine, Anderson School of Management, UCLA Alumnus, Los Angeles*
United States of America

1. Introduction

The estrogen-related receptors (ERRs) α, β and γ comprise the NR3B orphan subgroup within the nuclear receptor superfamily. Although the ERRs were identified based on their sequence homology to estrogen receptor alpha (ERα), they do not bind estrogen or any other natural hormones. Recent studies have defined the roles of ERRs in the regulation of target genes at the transcriptional level as well as their participation in a broad range of physiological functions such as energy metabolism and growth progression. The expression of ERRs has been shown to be up-regulated in advanced breast cancer cells and is considered to be a negative prognostic marker for the diagnosis of the disease. This review will cover what is currently known in regards to the gene structure of ERRs in addition to their regulation, function and relationship to breast cancer.

Breast cancer is a complicated disease with 200,000 women diagnosed in the United States each year. There are many factors that influence breast cancer development and progression with hormone and nuclear receptors playing critical roles. Several reviews have been written on the emerging roles of estrogen and nuclear receptors in breast cancer (reviews (Conzen 2008; Hayashi, Niwa et al. 2009; Riggins, Mazzotta et al. 2010)). In this review we will focus on the estrogen-related receptor alpha, beta and gamma (ERRα, β and γ). ERRα and ERRβ were the first orphan nuclear receptors to be cloned in the late 1980's (Giguere, Yang et al. 1988) with ERRγ following 10 years later (Eudy, Yao et al. 1998; Hong, Yang et al. 1999; Heard, Norby et al. 2000). Although these receptors were cloned many years ago based on their sequence homology at the DNA binding domain to estrogen receptor alpha (ERα), their biological relevance (s) has only recently been uncovered (Giguere 2008; Villena and Kralli 2008) along with potential roles in cancer, and more specifically breast cancer.

1.1 Background of nuclear receptor family

ERRs belong to the orphan nuclear receptor NR3B subfamily which do not bind to any known natural ligands and are constitutively active in transcription (Benoit, Cooney et al. 2006). Crystal structure analyses of the ERRs revealed that the AF-2 containing helix 12, essential for coactivator interaction (Nettles and Greene 2005), is in an active conformation while the ligand-binding pocket (LBP) remains empty (Greschik, Wurtz et al. 2002; Kallen, Schlaeppi et al. 2004). ERRs bind to TCAA/GGTCA elements called SFRE/ERRE and continually transactivate the target gene (Yang, Shigeta et al. 1996; Sladek, Beatty et al. 1997). While there are three members in this subfamily, both ERRβ (Zhou, Liu et al. 2006; Bombail, Collins et al. 2010) and ERRγ (Heard, Norby et al. 2000) have multiple variants that are expressed in a tissue-specific manner whereas there are no reports on variants of ERRα.

Although ERRs have high amino acid sequence homology, they are located on different chromosomes and cover a wide range of genomic space. The ESRRA gene is located at chromosome 11q13.1 (Shi, Shigeta et al. 1997) with a processed pseudogene present at 13q12.1 (Sladek, Beatty et al. 1997). It contains 7 exons and spans approximately 11 kbp genomic-space. The ESRRB gene is located at chromosome 14q24.3, has 12 exons and at least 5 variants from alternative splicing. It covers 130 kbp genomic-space ((Zhou, Liu et al. 2006; Collin, Kalay et al. 2008); Ensembl genome browser 61). The ESRRG gene spans 635 kbp genomic space, is located at chromosome 1q41 with 9 exons and 5 variants ((Eudy, Yao et al. 1998; Hong, Yang et al. 1999; Heard, Norby et al. 2000); Ensembl genome browser). A diagrammatic presentation of the relationship between ERRs and the ERs protein demonstrated that the highly conserved DNA binding domain (DBD) among the ERRs is closely related to the ERs DBD (Fig. 1). As indicated above, the ERR genes are located on different chromosomes which suggests that the gene and/or genome duplication event occurred over a long period of evolutionary time. Additionally, some of the coding exons are separated by large introns while others are clustered together.

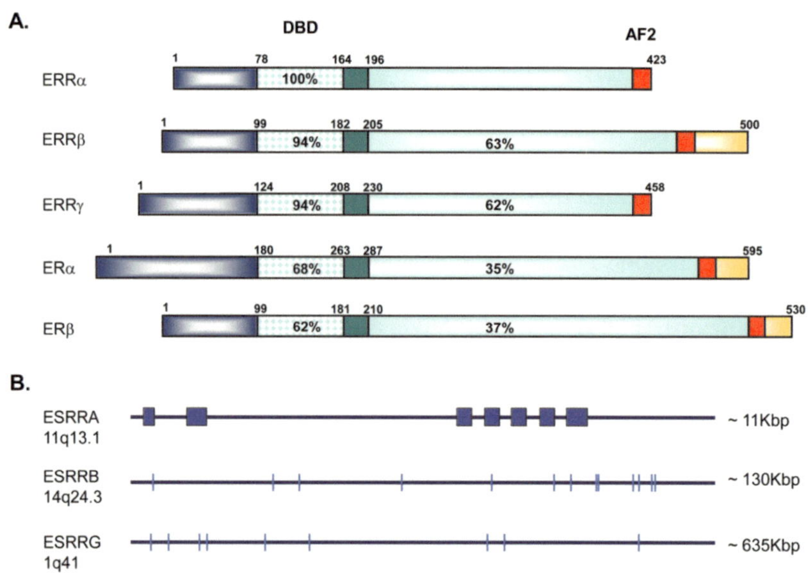

Fig. 1. A. Protein structures of the ERRs and ERs. DBD, DNA binding domain; AF2, activation function 2. Number on top indicates the amino acid position of the modular domains for the nuclear receptor. % in the box indicates the amino acid sequence homology to ERRα within the same domain. B: Gene structures of the ERRs. The size of the gene and the locations of the exons (vertical bar or box) are in approximation. Chromosome locations and the approximate gene sizes are indicated.

1.2 Expression of ERRs

Surveying the expression of all 49 nuclear receptors from 39 mouse tissues uncovered the coordination of several nuclear receptor groups with the transcriptional programs necessary to affect distinct physiologic pathways (Bookout, Jeong et al. 2006). Indeed expression of some of the nuclear receptors including the ERRs is linked to the circadian clock in key metabolic tissues suggesting their role in regulation of nutrient and energy metabolism (Horard, Castet et al. 2004; Yang, Downes et al. 2006; Giguere 2008; Villena and Kralli 2008). These studies underscore the importance of regulation and expression of nuclear receptors in normal and abnormal physiological conditions. ERRα is ubiquitously expressed in all tissues examined and is especially abundant in those with high metabolic needs such as heart, skeletal muscle and kidney (Giguere 2008). In addition, ERRα is expressed in both human and mouse embryonic stem cells (Xie, Jeong et al. 2009), during adipocyte differentiation (Fu, Sun et al. 2005) and bone morphogenesis (Bonnelye and Aubin 2002; Bonnelye, Kung et al. 2002) suggesting its roles in differentiation and development. Although expression of ERRγ is more restricted and not detectable in every tissue examined with levels that are lower than ERRα, it is still highly expressed in metabolically active tissues such as brain, skeletal muscle, heart and kidney (Zhang and Teng 2007; Giguere 2008). It was thought that ERRβ was mainly expressed in embryo (Giguere, Yang et al. 1988; Luo, Sladek et al. 1997), however as detection methods improved, ERRβ expression was found to be present in eye, brain, thyroid, kidney and the heart of adult tissues (Bookout, Jeong et al. 2006). Although ERRβ is present at lower levels as compared to ERRα and ERRγ, it also exhibited a distinct diurnal rhythmic expression much like the other two in white fat (WAT), brown fat (BAT), liver and skeletal muscle. This suggests a potential role in the coordination of oxidative metabolism in these tissues (Yang, Downes et al. 2006). The expression of ERRs in these metabolically active tissues under circadian rhythm hints to potential overlapping functions in energy metabolism.

As stated earlier, the expression level of the receptors could be closely linked to their biological function in a cell-type specific manner. This is particularly relevant for a constitutive activator since they are not regulated by the addition of ligands. Therefore the function of ERRs could be controlled by their expression level; however information regarding the mechanisms and signals that regulate their expression is limited.

1.3 Regulation of ERRs

1.3.1 Estrogen regulation of ERRs

ERRα was demonstrated to be the target gene for estrogen in the mouse uterus (Shigeta, Zuo et al. 1997) 15 years ago. Later, a combinatorial estrogen response element which can bind several nuclear receptors termed multiple hormone response element (MHRE) was identified in the human ERRα gene promoter (Liu, Zhang et al. 2003). Under the influence of estrogen, the estrogen receptor alpha (ERα), (but not the estrogen receptor beta (ERβ)) was recruited to the chromatin of the human ERRα promoter which interacted with the MHRE in an indirect tethering manner and transactivated the promoter (Liu, Zhang et al. 2003; Hu, Kinyamu et al. 2008). Surprisingly, in a similar experiment conducted with ER negative SKBR3 cells, estrogen treatment also induced chromatin modification around the MHRE region and recruited the coregulators and RNA polymerase II to the ERRα promoter (Li, Birnbaumer et al. 2010). This suggests that the ERRα gene can be regulated by estrogen in a non-ER dependent manner. Indeed, the MHRE (a 57 bp region in human and a 34 bp region) in mouse of the ERRα gene is a pleiopropic response element for multiple nuclear receptors

(Liu, Zhang et al. 2005) and also serves as the binding site for ERRα and ERRγ (Laganiere, Tremblay et al. 2004; Mootha, Handschin et al. 2004; Liu, Zhang et al. 2005). ERRγ was recently found to be responsive to estrogen, its expression able to be stimulated in a dose dependent manner. Furthermore, this response can be blocked by the pure estrogen antagonist ICI 182,780 (Ijichi, Shigekawa et al. 2011). By using chromatin immunoprecipitation (ChIP)-on chip analysis with MCF-cells, a number of potential EREs in the second intron of the human ERRγ gene were previously identified (Carroll, Meyer et al. 2006). These studies demonstrated a functional cross-talk between ERs and ERRs in the estrogen signaling pathway.

1.3.2 PCG-1α regulation of ERRα

While nuclear receptor binding to its target gene is important for transcriptional activation, it requires specific interactions with coregulatory proteins (Glass, Rose et al. 1997; McKenna, Lanz et al. 1999). One of the key regulators in energy metabolism is peroxisome proliferator-activated receptor γ coactivator -1α (PGC-1α). PGC-1α not only interacts with and stimulates ERRα transcriptional activity, it also enhances its expression in an autoregulatory loop mechanism (Schreiber, Knutti et al. 2003; Laganiere, Tremblay et al. 2004; Mootha, Handschin et al. 2004; Zhang and Teng 2007; Wang, Li et al. 2008). By combining PGC-1α induced genome-wide transcriptional profiles with a computational strategy to detect cis-regulatory motifs approach, ERRα was discovered to be a key transcription factor that is involved in cross-talk with PGC-1α in regulating the oxidative phosphorylation pathway (Mootha, Handschin et al. 2004). PGC-1α is capable of co-activating nearly all known nuclear receptors and many other transcription factors (Puigserver and Spiegelman 2003), yet it possesses a unique protein interaction surface that is dedicated specifically to the ERRs (see review and references therein (Villena and Kralli 2008)). With this unique relationship, ERRα expression is co-regulated with PGC-1α under various physiological stimuli such as during fasting (Ichida, Nemoto et al. 2002), under cold exposure (Schreiber, Knutti et al. 2003) and exercise (Cartoni, Leger et al. 2005). Therefore, induction of PGC-1α expression by physiological stimuli also induces ERRα expression in a positive feed-forward mechanism. The expression level of ERRα is also affected by ERRγ (Liu, Zhang et al. 2005; Zhang and Teng 2007) and cAMP (Liu, Benlhabib et al. 2009). These studies showed that multiple mechanisms are involved in the regulation of ERRs expression and function.

1.4 Function of the ERRs

1.4.1 ERRs interactions with ERs and other nuclear receptors

Understanding the role of ERRs in ER-mediated function starts with their cloning. ERRα and ERRβ were identified based on a search for genes with sequence homology at the DNA binding domain to ERα (Giguere, Yang et al. 1988). Eight years later, ERRα was re-cloned as a specific binding protein to an extended hormone response element (HRE) half-site, the TCAAGGTCATC region of the human lactoferrin gene promoter (Yang, Shigeta et al. 1996). This finding revealed that ERRα binds to the steroidogenic factor 1 (SF-1) binding element termed SFRE and later renamed this element to ERRE as estrogen-related receptor response element whenever addressing the ERRs binding (Sladek, Bader et al. 1997). It was demonstrated that binding of ERRα to this ERRE enhances the ER-mediated estrogen response of the lactoferrin gene (Yang, Shigeta et al. 1996). ERRα was later shown to bind a variety of EREs as a monomer or homodimer (Johnston, Liu et al. 1997; Vanacker, Pettersson et al. 1999; Zhang and Teng 2000; Zhang and Teng 2001) and genes possessing such ERE or

ERRE or both were subject to ERRα regulation (Sladek, Beatty et al. 1997; Vega and Kelly 1997; Vanacker, Bonnelye et al. 1998; Vanacker, Delmarre et al. 1998; Sumi and Ignarro 2003). Other than the binding elements, ERRs and ERs recognize similar co-activators and co-repressors (Xie, Hong et al. 1999; Zhang and Teng 2000). Therefore, an extensive cross-talk between the ERRα and ERα occurs at the multiple steps of the transcriptional process ((Giguere 2002) and references therein). Depending on the EREs and the surrounding elements, ERRα could either enhance or inhibit the estrogen responsiveness of the target genes (Yang, Shigeta et al. 1996; Kraus, Ariazi et al. 2002; Zhang, Chen et al. 2006).

ERRβ represses glucocorticoid receptor (GR) activity (Trapp and Holsboer 1996) and inhibits the function of NF-E2 Related Factor 2 (Nrf2) on antioxidant response element mediated gene expression (Zhou, Lo et al. 2007) in a cell-specific manner. Recently, variant isoforms (Long and Short) of ERRβ were found in the human endometrium. Increasing the expression of the Long form enhanced the ERα-mediated stimulation of c-myc expression and cell proliferation in Ishikawa cells whereas the Short form had no effect (Bombail, Collins et al. 2010). Interestingly, ERRγ (but not ERRα or ERRβ) was shown to activate the orphan nuclear receptor small heterodimer partner (SHP; NR0B2) (Sanyal, Kim et al. 2002) and the dosage-sensitive sex reversal (DAX-1) promoter (Park, Ahn et al. 2005). ERRs could bind to the promoter of other nuclear receptors such as thyroid hormone receptor (TR) (Vanacker, Bonnelye et al. 1998; Castet, Herledan et al. 2006), PPARα (Huss, Torra et al. 2004), RXRα and RXRβ (Sonoda, Laganiere et al. 2007) thus potentially regulating their expression. These nuclear receptors are also involved in a wide range of physiological functions. Therefore, the cross-talk of ERRs with other nuclear receptors expands their functional roles and points to the importance of their expression in normal and diseased conditions.

1.4.2 The role of ERRs in homeostasis

A major advance in understanding the role of ERRα in energy homeostasis comes from the observation that the medium-chain acyl-coenzyme A dehydrogenase (MCAD) is an ERRα target (Sladek, Bader et al. 1997; Vega and Kelly 1997). The MCAD is an enzyme that mediates the first step in the mitochondrial β-oxidation of fatty acids (Schulz 1991). This was followed by the discovery of a close relationship between ERRα and PGC-1α in transcriptional regulation (Huss, Kopp et al. 2002; Ichida, Nemoto et al. 2002; Schreiber, Knutti et al. 2003). Evidence indicates that PGC-1α serves as a key regulator of mitochondrial biogenesis in mammals. This includes the activation of the transcription of mitochondrial uncoupling protein -1 (UCP-1) and the induction of the expression of NRF-1, NRF-2 and Tfam, all critical factors for mitochondrial function and maintenance. Furthermore, PGC-1α up-regulates the expression of genes involved in mitochondrial fatty acid oxidation and triggers mitochondrial proliferation (see review (Kelly and Scarpulla 2004)). The regulatory roles of PGC-1α in these key metabolic processes were mediated by ERRα (see review and references therein (Giguere 2008; Villena and Kralli 2008)). In microarray studies, over expression of PGC-1α in culture cells induced hundred of genes encoding mitochondrial proteins involved in fatty acid oxidation (FAO), the tricarboxylic acid cycle (TCA), oxidative phosphorylation (OXPHOS), mitochondrial membrane and carbohydrate metabolism. Interestingly, these PGC-1α effects can be blocked by siRNA against ERRα or be induced by over expression of constitutively active ERRα (Mootha, Handschin et al. 2004; Schreiber, Emter et al. 2004). Taken together, ERRα plays a major role in the regulation of sets of genes involved in a wide range of energy balance activities such as lipid transport, fatty acid oxidation, TCA cycle, oxidative phosphorylation, and mitochondrial biogenesis to name a few.

2. ERRs in breast cancer

Searching for therapeutic targets in cancer biology is an important endeavor and the nuclear receptor has been shown to be one such target. Recently, the expression profile of 48 nuclear receptors in 51 human cancer cell lines derived from nine different tissues from the NC160 collection was investigated (Holbeck, Chang et al. 2010). The results uncovered a number of potential receptor-drug interactions and demonstrated that the individual receptor levels may predict a response to therapeutic intervention. Like all cancers, breast cancer is a complicated disease and many factors, estrogen in particular, contributes to its development and progression (Kelsey and Bernstein 1996). Although estrogen action is mediated through two receptors (ERα (Greene, Gilna et al. 1986) and ERβ (Kuiper, Enmark et al. 1996)), 70% of breast cancers express ERα which serves as the mediator for estrogen action (Russo, Hu et al. 2000; Conzen 2008; Hayashi, Niwa et al. 2009). In view of the structural similarity and functional cross-talk of the ERs and ERRs, it is possible that ERRs are also involved in breast cancer biology (review and references therein (Ariazi and Jordan 2006; Riggins, Mazzotta et al. 2010)).

2.1 ERRs as potential biomarkers

Using qPCR to measure the mRNA levels of ERs, epidermal growth factor receptor, ErbB family members, and ERR mRNA levels in 38 unselected primary breast tumors and 9 normal mammary gland epithelial cells from breast reduction surgery revealed that ERRα is highly expressed in a subset of tumors with elevated levels of ErbB2, an indicator of aggressive tumor behavior and nonfunctional ERα. Unlike ERRα, expression of ERRγ in breast tumors correlates with ER-positive status and ErbB4 expression which is a preferred clinical marker. These studies suggest that ERRα can be used as an unfavorable whereas ERRγ can serve as a favorable marker for diagnosis of clinical outcome. The mRNA level of ERRβ in the above mentioned breast tumor samples is very low and the potential as a biomarker unclear (Ariazi, Clark et al. 2002). Despite the proposed use of ERRγ as a favorable marker, over expression of ERRγ contributed to the development of tamoxifen (TAM)- resistance in cell lines derived from invasive lobular carcinoma (Riggins, Lan et al. 2008). Additional studies using an immunohistochemistry approach combined with RT-PCR supports the earlier findings that ERRα expression in breast carcinoma is associated with an increased risk of recurrence and an adverse clinical outcome (Suzuki, Miki et al. 2004).

2.2 ERRα and breast cancer cell growth

ERRα has been extensively studied in the context of breast cancer (Ariazi, Clark et al. 2002; Suzuki, Miki et al. 2004; Barry and Giguere 2005; Ariazi and Jordan 2006; Ariazi, Kraus et al. 2007; Stein, Chang et al. 2008; Chisamore, Wilkinson et al. 2009; Deblois, Hall et al. 2009; Stein, Gaillard et al. 2009; Dwyer, Joseph et al. 2010). Correlation between the expression of ERRs and disease outcome presents a first glimpse of the potential role of ERRs in breast cancer. Further studies using an unbiased microarray approach to understand the cross-talk between ERs and ERRs in MCF-7 cells yielded unexpected results (Stein, Chang et al. 2008). Despite the functional cross-talk between ERs and ERRs presented earlier, ERRα was found to regulate a smaller set of genes that overlapped with ERα despite regulating many more genes not involved in estrogen signaling. Analysis of the microarray data from ER-regulated and ERR-regulated genes in MCF-7 cells by gene ontology (GO) showed that the majority of genes regulated by ERRα are involved in energy metabolism, oxidative stress and detoxification as expected. Interestingly, ERRα also induces vascular endothelial growth factor (VEGF), a highly angiogenic factor. Importantly, knockdown ERRα expression in MDA-MB-231 cells reduced tumor cell migration *in vitro* and tumor growth as xenografts *in vivo* (Stein, Chang et al. 2008). Further studies demonstrated that ERRα-dependent activation of VEGF mRNA expression occurs in several different breast cancer cell lines (Stein, Gaillard et al. 2009). This suggests that ERRα promotes tumor cell growth by stimulating VEGF expression. These studies together with the finding that ERRα also induces the pro-migratory factor, WNT11 (Dwyer, Joseph et al. 2010) provides a basis for highly expressed ERRα to be considered an overall negative phenotype of breast cancers.

2.3 ERRα and aromatase

As indicated above, there is much evidence that points to potential mechanisms of how ERRα influences breast cancer biology. ERRα plays a role in the local production of estrogen in breast cancer cells with levels in tumor tissue being several-fold higher than in normal circulating estrogen (Thorsen, Tangen et al. 1982; van Landeghem, Poortman et al. 1985) and aromatase, a key enzyme in converting androgens to estrogens, is also up-regulated in tumor cells (Miller and O'Neill 1987; Sasano and Harada 1998; Chen, Zhou et al. 1999). The presence of aromatase mRNA in the intra-tumoral location of 19 breast carcinoma tissues was detected using laser capture microdissection (LCM) and quantitative reverse transcription-PCR (q-PCR) while aromatase protein was verified by immunohistochemistry (Miki, Suzuki et al. 2007). Furthermore, microarray expression profiling of aromatase and ERRα mRNA in isolated carcinoma cells demonstrated a significant positive correlation (Miki, Suzuki et al. 2007). Although regulation of aromatase expression is tissue- and promoter-specific, its activity in breast carcinoma is higher than in normal tissue of the same patients (Silva, Rowlands et al. 1989; Miller, Anderson et al. 1990; Lipton, Santen et al. 1992). This suggests that the regulation of aromatase expression in breast cancer cells of the patient has been changed. Indeed, promoter switching in breast cancer tissue has been reported (Chen, Zhou et al. 1999; Chen, Reierstad et al. 2009) and ERRα plays a positive role (Yang, Zhou et al. 1998; Miao, Shi et al. 2010). Taken together, ERRα functions as a key modulator of intratumoral estrogen production in human breast carcinoma by stimulating the expression of the androgen-estrogen key converting enzyme, aromatase via tumor specific promoter usage.

2.4 ERRα and EGFR

ERRα has a close relationship with the ErbB2/epidermal growth factor receptor (EGFR) signaling pathway. ErbB2 is a receptor tyrosine kinase and in combination with EGFR, activates a complex array of downstream signaling pathways which leads to phosphorylation of multiple transcription factors including ERRα. Phosphorylation of these transcription factors promotes growth and proliferation (reviewed in ref. (Yarden and Sliwkowski 2001)). Upon EGF treatment, ERRα in MCF-7 cells was phosphorylated and preferentially recruited to the pS2 promoter. Furthermore, phosphorylated ERRα showed enhanced DNA binding capability in an *in vitro* study (Barry and Giguere 2005). Additionally, mitogen-activated protein kinases (MAPK) and Akts (components of the

ErbB2 pathway) are involved in ERRα phorphorylation and transactivation since inhibitors to MAPK and Akt also block ERRα target gene activation (Ariazi, Kraus et al. 2007). These observations suggest that ERRα phosphorylation provides a mechanism of enhanced transactivation function in breast cancer cells. Recently, using a mouse model of ErbB2-initiated mammary tumorigenesis found that ablation of ERRα significantly delays ErbB2-induced tumor development, lowers the levels of ErbB2 and co-amplifies transcripts within the 17q12-21 chromosomal region (the ErbB2 amplicon) (Deblois, Chahrour et al. 2010). The minimal 17q12 amplicon houses not only the ErbB2 gene; it also includes those involved in signal transduction, transcription, cell migration and invasion, inhibition of apotosis, genomic instability and tamoxifen resistance. ERRα binds to those genes and directs the recruitment of co-activators PGC-1β and RNA polymerase II to their promoters (Deblois, Chahrour et al. 2010). Furthermore, ERRα antagonists repress the effect of ERα on the ErbB2 promoter which leads to the development of tamoxifen resistance in breast cancer cells.

2.5 ERRα and AIB1

Comparing the co-activators along with the expression of various nuclear receptors in 48 primary breast tumor samples, a positive correlation between ERRα and AIB1 (amplified in breast cancer-1) (Anzick, Kononen et al. 1997) was found. AIB1 is an oncogenic co-activator of ERα that is frequently amplified and over expressed in human breast carcinomas (Anzick, Kononen et al. 1997; Liao, Kuang et al. 2002). In addition, these two proteins were abundant in the tumor samples and a direct interaction of the receptor and co-activator was demonstrated by fluorescence-resonance energy transfer, mammalian two-hybrid, and coimmunoprecipitation assay with endogenous proteins. On the other hand, the levels of PGC-1α (a well characterized ERRα co-activator) in primary breast carcinoma was low and no detectable association with ERRα was found (Heck, Rom et al. 2009). The enhanced association of ERRα with AIB1 underscores the functional significance of ERRα/AIB1 rather than the ERRα/PGC-1α interaction for breast tumor development and progression.

2.6 ERRγ and PGC-1β

Although direct evidence between cellular metabolism and breast cancer development is lacking, switching from aerobic oxidative phosphorylation to glycolytic metabolism is a typical feature of cancer cells (Warburg 1956). Recent reports demonstrated that the expression of miR-378, an ErbB2-regulated microRNA, correlates with the progression of human breast cancer by inducing the metabolic shift from an oxidative to a glycolytic pathway (Eichner, Perry et al. 2010). The miR-378 is embedded within PGC-1β and when expressed, inhibits the expression of ERRγ and GABPA (PGC-1β partners), a function that is opposite to the PGC-1 family of co-activators. In view of the close relationship of ERRs and PGC-1 coactivator family in the context of energy metabolism (Giguere 2008; Villena and Kralli 2008), the finding that miR-378 targets ERRγ but not ERRα demonstrated again that the isoforms of ERR possess differential functions as well as overlapping activities either in regulating energy or in breast cancer biology.

3. The potential agonist and antagonist of ERRs

As mentioned earlier, the ERR-coactivator or corepressor interaction determines the receptor's functional activity. Any factor that interrupts this interaction has the ability to modulate ERR function (Huss, Kopp et al. 2002; Kamei, Ohizumi et al. 2003; Schreiber, Knutti et al. 2003;

Debevec, Christian et al. 2007), therefore could be a potential therapeutic target site. Small-molecule agonists for ERRβ and ERRγ have been identified and characterized. However, identifying an agonist for ERRα has proved to be difficult (Yu and Forman 2005; Hyatt, Lockamy et al. 2007). Nonetheless, novel synthetic antagonists of ERRs, especially for ERRα, are emerging (Yang and Chen 1999; Coward, Lee et al. 2001; Tremblay, Bergeron et al. 2001; Tremblay, Kunath et al. 2001; Busch, Stevens et al. 2004; Willy, Murray et al. 2004; Chisamore, Cunningham et al. 2009). By disrupting the constitutive ERR/co-activator interaction or by inducing proteosome-dependent protein degradation of the receptor, these small molecules inhibit the function of ERRs and thus tumor growth and progression (Ariazi and Jordan 2006; Stein, Chang et al. 2008; Chisamore, Wilkinson et al. 2009; Heck, Rom et al. 2009; Wu, Wang et al. 2009). Recently, a series of diaryl ether-based ligands for ERRα were developed and demonstrated in animal models to be antidiabetic agents (Patch, Searle et al. 2011). Taken together, these studies provide a basis for the further development of therapeutics to treat breast cancers based on suppressing ERRα expression and activity. Recently, environmental estrogenic compounds were found to modulate ERRα (Suetsugi, Su et al. 2003) and ERRγ (Matsushima, Kakuta et al. 2007; Takashima-Sasaki, Mori et al. 2007; Wang, Fang et al. 2009; Hirvonen, Rajalin et al. 2011) activities in either a positive or negative manner. The impact of environmental factors on breast cancer via ERRs is currently unclear.

4. ERRs in other cancers

Since the over expression of ERRα in breast cancer was discovered (Ariazi, Clark et al. 2002; Suzuki, Miki et al. 2004), additional studies have found an association between the abnormal expression of ERRs and a variety of tumors and cancers such as prostate (Cheung, Yu et al. 2005; Yu, Wang et al. 2007; Yu, Wong et al. 2008), ovarian (Sun, Sehouli et al. 2005), colon-rectal (Cavallini, Notarnicola et al. 2005) and endometrium (Gao, Sun et al. 2006). In neoplastic prostatic tissues, ERRβ and ERRγ show levels that are either reduced or undetectable as compared to normal prostatic epithelial cells (Cheung, Yu et al. 2005). This suggests a down-regulation of these two receptors in prostate cancer. In a series of experiments, the forced induction of ERRβ or ERRγ in androgen sensitive (LNCaP) and androgen-insensitive (DU145) prostate cancer cells demonstrated that over expression of these two receptors suppresses cell proliferation and tumorigenicity of the cancer cells. The inhibition of prostate cancer cell proliferation was due to cell cycle arrest as demonstrated by the induction of cyclin-dependent kinase inhibitor p21 by ERRβ and p21/p27 by ERRγ. Moreover, ERRβ and ERRγ-mediated growth inhibition could be potentiated by their specific agonist DY131 and reduced by siRNA (Yu, Wang et al. 2007; Yu, Wong et al. 2008). The expression of ERRβ and ERRγ in prostate cancer is in contrast to ERRα in breast cancer cells, colorectal tumor, and malignant colon cells (Cavallini, Notarnicola et al. 2005). ERRα expression in endometrial adenocarcinoma is positively correlated with myometrial invasion while a negative correlation was observed between the expression of ERRγ mRNA and nodal metastasis (Gao, Sun et al. 2006). Therefore, the expression levels of the subtype ERRs in cancer cells provides a potential prognostic strategy for the therapeutic treatment of the cancer.

5. Conclusion

The studies cited in this review demonstrate that ERRs are differentially expressed in normal and cancer cells. While many factors influence their expression, ERRs in turn, regulate many sets of genes involved in a wide variety of signaling pathways. As of today, the majority of studies are on ERRα and its relationship with breast cancer development and progression. How ERRα is involved in breast cancer biology is summarized in Figure 2.

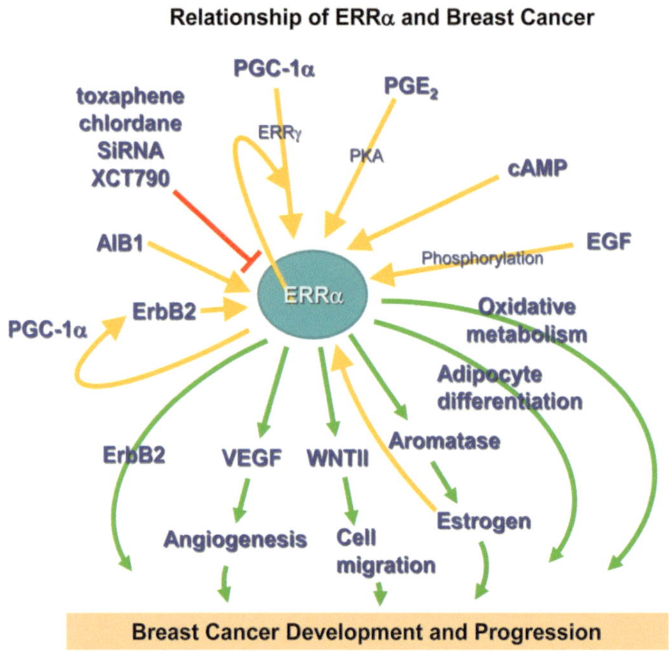

Fig. 2. Potential pathways that regulate ERRα expression and influences breast cancer development and progression. Yellow arrow, upregulates ERRα expression; red arrow, downregulates ERRα activity; green arrow, potential mechanisms of ERRα action on breast cancer.

The roles of ERRγ in breast cancer have yet to be established. While ERRγ targets the same metabolic gene network as ERRα, it may perform distinct physiological functions such as participation in the metabolic shift pathway in breast cancer cells. ERRγ was recently demonstrated as a target for endocrine disruptors, the estrogen-mimic of the environmental chemicals which may be involved in breast cancer development or progression. Compared to ERRα and ERRγ, the number of functional studies on ERRβ has been relatively slim. Nonetheless, the report on the repressive function of ERRβ in prostate cancer cells will certainly garner additional attention to this orphan receptor. Collectively, the role of these ERRs in this disease state is emerging and they could prove to be a viable therapeutic target in the treatment of breast cancer.

6. References

Anzick, S. L., J. Kononen, et al. (1997). "AIB1, a steroid receptor coactivator amplified in breast and ovarian cancer." *Science* 277(5328): 965-968.

Ariazi, E. A., G. M. Clark, et al. (2002). "Estrogen-related receptor alpha and estrogen-related receptor gamma associate with unfavorable and favorable biomarkers, respectively, in human breast cancer." *Cancer Res* 62(22): 6510-6518.

Ariazi, E. A. and V. C. Jordan (2006). "Estrogen-related receptors as emerging targets in cancer and metabolic disorders." *Curr Top Med Chem* 6(3): 203-215.

Ariazi, E. A., R. J. Kraus, et al. (2007). "Estrogen-related receptor alpha1 transcriptional activities are regulated in part via the ErbB2/HER2 signaling pathway." *Mol Cancer Res* 5(1): 71-85.

Barry, J. B. and V. Giguere (2005). "Epidermal growth factor-induced signaling in breast cancer cells results in selective target gene activation by orphan nuclear receptor estrogen-related receptor alpha." *Cancer Res* 65(14): 6120-6129.

Benoit, G., A. Cooney, et al. (2006). "International Union of Pharmacology. LXVI. Orphan nuclear receptors." *Pharmacological reviews* 58(4): 798-836.

Bombail, V., F. Collins, et al. (2010). "Modulation of ER alpha transcriptional activity by the orphan nuclear receptor ERR beta and evidence for differential effects of long- and short-form splice variants." *Molecular and cellular endocrinology* 314(1): 53-61.

Bonnelye, E. and J. E. Aubin (2002). "Differential expression of estrogen receptor-related receptor alpha and estrogen receptors alpha and beta in osteoblasts in vivo and in vitro." *J Bone Miner Res* 17(8): 1392-1400.

Bonnelye, E., V. Kung, et al. (2002). "Estrogen receptor-related receptor alpha impinges on the estrogen axis in bone: potential function in osteoporosis." *Endocrinology* 143(9): 3658-3670.

Bookout, A. L., Y. Jeong, et al. (2006). "Anatomical profiling of nuclear receptor expression reveals a hierarchical transcriptional network." *Cell* 126(4): 789-799.

Busch, B. B., W. C. Stevens, Jr., et al. (2004). "Identification of a selective inverse agonist for the orphan nuclear receptor estrogen-related receptor alpha." *J Med Chem* 47(23): 5593-5596.

Carroll, J. S., C. A. Meyer, et al. (2006). "Genome-wide analysis of estrogen receptor binding sites." *Nat Genet* 38(11): 1289-1297.

Cartoni, R., B. Leger, et al. (2005). "Mitofusins 1/2 and ERR{alpha} expression are increased in human skeletal muscle after physical exercise." *J Physiol.*

Castet, A., A. Herledan, et al. (2006). "Receptor-interacting protein 140 differentially regulates estrogen receptor-related receptor transactivation depending on target genes." *Molecular Endocrinology* 20(5): 1035-1047.

Cavallini, A., M. Notarnicola, et al. (2005). "Oestrogen receptor-related receptor alpha (ERRalpha) and oestrogen receptors (ERalpha and ERbeta) exhibit different gene expression in human colorectal tumour progression." *Eur J Cancer* 41(10): 1487-1494.

Chen, D., S. Reierstad, et al. (2009). "Regulation of breast cancer-associated aromatase promoters." *Cancer Lett* 273(1): 15-27.

Chen, S., D. Zhou, et al. (1999). "Breast tumor aromatase: functional role and transcriptional regulation." *Endocr Relat Cancer* 6(2): 149-156.

Cheung, C. P., S. Yu, et al. (2005). "Expression and functional study of estrogen receptor-related receptors in human prostatic cells and tissues." *J Clin Endocrinol Metab* 90(3): 1830-1844.

Chisamore, M. J., M. E. Cunningham, et al. (2009). "Characterization of a novel small molecule subtype specific estrogen-related receptor alpha antagonist in MCF-7 breast cancer cells." *PLoS One* 4(5): e5624.

Chisamore, M. J., H. A. Wilkinson, et al. (2009). "Estrogen-related receptor-alpha antagonist inhibits both estrogen receptor-positive and estrogen receptor-negative breast tumor growth in mouse xenografts." *Mol Cancer Ther* 8(3): 672-681.

Collin, R. W., E. Kalay, et al. (2008). "Mutations of ESRRB encoding estrogen-related receptor beta cause autosomal-recessive nonsyndromic hearing impairment DFNB35." *American journal of human genetics* 82(1): 125-138.

Conzen, S. D. (2008). "Minireview: nuclear receptors and breast cancer." *Mol Endocrinol* 22(10): 2215-2228.

Coward, P., D. Lee, et al. (2001). "4-Hydroxytamoxifen binds to and deactivates the estrogen-related receptor gamma." *Proc Natl Acad Sci U S A* 98(15): 8880-8884.

Debevec, D., M. Christian, et al. (2007). "Receptor interacting protein 140 regulates expression of uncoupling protein 1 in adipocytes through specific peroxisome proliferator activated receptor isoforms and estrogen-related receptor alpha." *Mol Endocrinol* 21(7): 1581-1592.

Deblois, G., G. Chahrour, et al. (2010). "Transcriptional control of the ERBB2 amplicon by ERRalpha and PGC-1beta promotes mammary gland tumorigenesis." *Cancer Res* 70(24): 10277-10287.

Deblois, G., J. A. Hall, et al. (2009). "Genome-wide identification of direct target genes implicates estrogen-related receptor alpha as a determinant of breast cancer heterogeneity." *Cancer Res* 69(15): 6149-6157.

Dwyer, M. A., J. D. Joseph, et al. (2010). "WNT11 expression is induced by estrogen-related receptor alpha and beta-catenin and acts in an autocrine manner to increase cancer cell migration." *Cancer Res* 70(22): 9298-9308.

Eichner, L. J., M. C. Perry, et al. (2010). "miR-378(*) mediates metabolic shift in breast cancer cells via the PGC-1beta/ERRgamma transcriptional pathway." *Cell Metab* 12(4): 352-361.

Eudy, J. D., S. Yao, et al. (1998). "Isolation of a gene encoding a novel member of the nuclear receptor superfamily from the critical region of Usher syndrome type IIa at 1q41." *Genomics* 50(3): 382-384.

Fu, M., T. Sun, et al. (2005). "A Nuclear Receptor Atlas: 3T3-L1 adipogenesis." *Molecular Endocrinology* 19(10): 2437-2450.

Gao, M., P. Sun, et al. (2006). "Expression of estrogen receptor-related receptor isoforms and clinical significance in endometrial adenocarcinoma." *Int J Gynecol Cancer* 16(2): 827-833.

Giguere, V. (2002). "To ERR in the estrogen pathway." *Trends Endocrinol Metab* 13(5): 220-225.

Giguere, V. (2008). "Transcriptional control of energy homeostasis by the estrogen-related receptors." *Endocr Rev* 29(6): 677-696.

Giguere, V., N. Yang, et al. (1988). "Identification of a new class of steroid hormone receptors." *Nature* 331: 91-94.

Glass, C. K., D. W. Rose, et al. (1997). "Nuclear receptor coactivators." *Current opinion in cell biology* 9(2): 222-232.

Greene, G. L., P. Gilna, et al. (1986). "Sequence and expression of human estrogen receptor complementary DNA." *Science* 231(4742): 1150-1154.

Greschik, H., J. M. Wurtz, et al. (2002). "Structural and functional evidence for ligand-independent transcriptional activation by the estrogen-related receptor 3." *Mol Cell* 9(2): 303-313.

Hayashi, S., T. Niwa, et al. (2009). "Estrogen signaling pathway and its imaging in human breast cancer." *Cancer Sci* 100(10): 1773-1778.

Heard, D. J., P. L. Norby, et al. (2000). "Human ERR gamma, a third member of the estrogen receptor- related receptor (ERR) subfamily of orphan nuclear receptors: Tissue-specific isoforms are expressed during development and in the adult." *Molecular Endocrinology* 14(3): 382-392.

Heck, S., J. Rom, et al. (2009). "Estrogen-related receptor alpha expression and function is associated with the transcriptional coregulator AIB1 in breast carcinoma." *Cancer Res* 69(12): 5186-5193.

Hirvonen, J., A.-M. Rajalin, et al. (2011). "Transcriptional activity of estrogen-related receptor [gamma] (ERR[gamma]) is stimulated by the phytoestrogen equol." *The Journal of Steroid Biochemistry and Molecular Biology* 123(1-2): 46-57.

Holbeck, S., J. Chang, et al. (2010). "Expression profiling of nuclear receptors in the NCI60 cancer cell panel reveals receptor-drug and receptor-gene interactions." *Mol Endocrinol* 24(6): 1287-1296.

Hong, H., L. Yang, et al. (1999). "Hormone-independent transcriptional activation and coactivator binding by novel orphan nuclear receptor ERR3." *J Biol Chem* 274(32): 22618-22626.

Horard, B., A. Castet, et al. (2004). "Dimerization is required for transactivation by estrogen-receptor-related (ERR) orphan receptors: evidence from amphioxus ERR." *J Mol Endocrinol* 33(2): 493-509.

Hu, P., H. K. Kinyamu, et al. (2008). "Estrogen induces estrogen-related receptor alpha gene expression and chromatin structural changes in estrogen receptor (ER)-positive and ER-negative breast cancer cells." *J Biol Chem* 283(11): 6752-6763.

Huss, J. M., R. P. Kopp, et al. (2002). "Peroxisome proliferator-activated receptor coactivator-1alpha (PGC-1alpha) coactivates the cardiac-enriched nuclear receptors estrogen-related receptor-alpha and -gamma. Identification of novel leucine-rich interaction motif within PGC-1alpha." *J Biol Chem* 277(43): 40265-40274.

Huss, J. M., I. P. Torra, et al. (2004). "Estrogen-related receptor alpha directs peroxisome proliferator-activated receptor alpha signaling in the transcriptional control of energy metabolism in cardiac and skeletal muscle." *Mol Cell Biol* 24(20): 9079-9091.

Hyatt, S. M., E. L. Lockamy, et al. (2007). "On the intractability of estrogen-related receptor alpha as a target for activation by small molecules." *J Med Chem* 50(26): 6722-6724.

Ichida, M., S. Nemoto, et al. (2002). "Identification of a specific molecular repressor of the peroxisome proliferator-activated receptor gamma Coactivator-1 alpha (PGC-1alpha)." *J Biol Chem* 277(52): 50991-50995.

Ijichi, N., T. Shigekawa, et al. (2011). "Estrogen-related receptor gamma modulates cell proliferation and estrogen signaling in breast cancer." *J Steroid Biochem Mol Biol* 123(1-2): 1-7.

Johnston, S. D., X. Liu, et al. (1997). "Estrogen-related receptor alpha 1 functionally binds as a monomer to extended half-site sequences including ones contained within estrogen- response elements." *Mol Endocrinol* 11(3): 342-352.

Kallen, J., J. M. Schlaeppi, et al. (2004). "Evidence for Ligand-independent Transcriptional Activation of the Human Estrogen-related Receptor {alpha} (ERR{alpha}): CRYSTAL STRUCTURE OF ERR{alpha} LIGAND BINDING DOMAIN IN

COMPLEX WITH PEROXISOME PROLIFERATOR-ACTIVATED RECEPTOR COACTIVATOR-1{alpha}." *J Biol Chem* 279(47): 49330-49337.

Kamei, Y., H. Ohizumi, et al. (2003). "PPARgamma coactivator 1beta/ERR ligand 1 is an ERR protein ligand, whose expression induces a high-energy expenditure and antagonizes obesity." *Proc Natl Acad Sci U S A* 100(21): 12378-12383.

Kelly, D. P. and R. C. Scarpulla (2004). "Transcriptional regulatory circuits controlling mitochondrial biogenesis and function." *Genes & development* 18(4): 357-368.

Kelsey, J. L. and L. Bernstein (1996). "Epidemiology and prevention of breast cancer." *Annu Rev Public Health* 17: 47-67.

Kraus, R. J., E. A. Ariazi, et al. (2002). "Estrogen-related receptor alpha 1 actively antagonizes estrogen receptor-regulated transcription in MCF-7 mammary cells." *J Biol Chem* 277(27): 24826-24834.

Kuiper, G. G., E. Enmark, et al. (1996). "Cloning of a novel receptor expressed in rat prostate and ovary." *Proc Natl Acad Sci U S A* 93(12): 5925-5930.

Laganiere, J., G. B. Tremblay, et al. (2004). "A Polymorphic Autoregulatory Hormone Response Element in the Human Estrogen-related Receptor {alpha} (ERR{alpha}) Promoter Dictates Peroxisome Proliferator-activated Receptor {gamma} Coactivator-1{alpha} Control of ERR{alpha} Expression." *J Biol Chem* 279(18): 18504-18510.

Li, Y., L. Birnbaumer, et al. (2010). "Regulation of ERRalpha gene expression by estrogen receptor agonists and antagonists in SKBR3 breast cancer cells: differential molecular mechanisms mediated by g protein-coupled receptor GPR30/GPER-1." *Molecular Endocrinology* 24(5): 969-980.

Liao, L., S. Q. Kuang, et al. (2002). "Molecular structure and biological function of the cancer-amplified nuclear receptor coactivator SRC-3/AIB1." *J Steroid Biochem Mol Biol* 83(1-5): 3-14.

Lipton, A., R. J. Santen, et al. (1992). "Prognostic value of breast cancer aromatase." *Cancer* 70(7): 1951-1955.

Liu, D., H. Benlhabib, et al. (2009). "cAMP Enhances estrogen-related receptor {alpha} (ERR{alpha}) transcriptional activity at the SP-A promoter by increasing its interaction with protein kinase A and steroid receptor coactivator 2 (SRC-2)." *Mol Endocrinol* 23(6): 772-783.

Liu, D., Z. Zhang, et al. (2003). "Estrogen Stimulates Estrogen-Related Receptor {alpha} Gene Expression Through Conserved Hormone Response Elements." *Endocrinology* 144(11): 4894-4904.

Liu, D., Z. Zhang, et al. (2005). "Estrogen-related receptor-gamma and peroxisome proliferator-activated receptor-gamma coactivator-1alpha regulate estrogen-related receptor-alpha gene expression via a conserved multi-hormone response element." *J Mol Endocrinol* 34(2): 473-487.

Luo, J., R. Sladek, et al. (1997). "Placental abnormalities in mouse embryos lacking the orphan nuclear receptor ERR-beta." *Nature* 388(6644): 778-782.

Matsushima, A., Y. Kakuta, et al. (2007). "Structural evidence for endocrine disruptor bisphenol A binding to human nuclear receptor ERR gamma." *J Biochem* 142(4): 517-524.

McKenna, N. J., R. B. Lanz, et al. (1999). "Nuclear receptor coregulators: cellular and molecular biology." *Endocrine reviews* 20(3): 321-344.

Miao, L., J. Shi, et al. (2010). "Estrogen receptor-related receptor alpha mediates up-regulation of aromatase expression by prostaglandin E2 in prostate stromal cells." *Mol Endocrinol* 24(6): 1175-1186.

Miki, Y., T. Suzuki, et al. (2007). "Aromatase localization in human breast cancer tissues: possible interactions between intratumoral stromal and parenchymal cells." *Cancer Res* 67(8): 3945-3954.

Miller, W. R., T. J. Anderson, et al. (1990). "Relationship between tumour aromatase activity, tumour characteristics and response to therapy." *J Steroid Biochem Mol Biol* 37(6): 1055-1059.

Miller, W. R. and J. O'Neill (1987). "The importance of local synthesis of estrogen within the breast." *Steroids* 50(4-6): 537-548.

Mootha, V. K., C. Handschin, et al. (2004). "Err{alpha} and Gabpa/b specify PGC-1{alpha}-dependent oxidative phosphorylation gene expression that is altered in diabetic muscle." *Proc Natl Acad Sci U S A.*

Nettles, K. W. and G. L. Greene (2005). "Ligand control of coregulator recruitment to nuclear receptors." *Annual review of physiology* 67: 309-333.

Park, Y. Y., S. W. Ahn, et al. (2005). "An autoregulatory loop controlling orphan nuclear receptor DAX-1 gene expression by orphan nuclear receptor ERRgamma." *Nucleic acids research* 33(21): 6756-6768.

Patch, R. J., L. L. Searle, et al. (2011). "Identification of Diaryl Ether-Based Ligands for Estrogen-Related Receptor alpha as Potential Antidiabetic Agents." *J Med Chem.*

Puigserver, P. and B. M. Spiegelman (2003). "Peroxisome proliferator-activated receptor-gamma coactivator 1 alpha (PGC-1 alpha): transcriptional coactivator and metabolic regulator." *Endocr Rev* 24(1): 78-90.

Riggins, R. B., J. P. Lan, et al. (2008). "ERR{gamma} Mediates Tamoxifen Resistance in Novel Models of Invasive Lobular Breast Cancer." *Cancer Res* 68(21): 8908-8917.

Riggins, R. B., M. M. Mazzotta, et al. (2010). "Orphan nuclear receptors in breast cancer pathogenesis and therapeutic response." *Endocr Relat Cancer* 17(3): R213-231.

Russo, J., Y. F. Hu, et al. (2000). "Developmental, cellular, and molecular basis of human breast cancer." *J Natl Cancer Inst Monogr*(27): 17-37.

Sanyal, S., J. Y. Kim, et al. (2002). "Differential regulation of the orphan nuclear receptor small heterodimer partner (SHP) gene promoter by orphan nuclear receptor ERR isoforms." *The Journal of biological chemistry* 277(3): 1739-1748.

Sasano, H. and N. Harada (1998). "Intratumoral aromatase in human breast, endometrial, and ovarian malignancies." *Endocr Rev* 19(5): 593-607.

Schreiber, S. N., R. Emter, et al. (2004). "The estrogen-related receptor {alpha} (ERR{alpha}) functions in PPAR{gamma} coactivator 1{alpha} (PGC-1{alpha})-induced mitochondrial biogenesis." *Proc Natl Acad Sci U S A.*

Schreiber, S. N., D. Knutti, et al. (2003). "The transcriptional coactivator PGC-1 regulates the expression and activity of the orphan nuclear receptor ERRalpha." *J Biol Chem.*

Schulz, H. (1991). "Beta oxidation of fatty acids." *Biochimica et biophysica acta* 1081(2): 109-120.

Shi, H., H. Shigeta, et al. (1997). "Human estrogen receptor-like 1 (ESRL1) gene: genomic organization, chromosomal localization, and promoter characterization." *Genomics* 44(1): 52-60.

Shigeta, H., W. Zuo, et al. (1997). "The mouse estrogen receptor-related orphan receptor alpha 1: molecular cloning and estrogen responsiveness." *J Mol Endocrinol* 19(3): 299-309.

Silva, M. C., M. G. Rowlands, et al. (1989). "Intratumoral aromatase as a prognostic factor in human breast carcinoma." *Cancer Res* 49(10): 2588-2591.

Sladek, R., J. A. Bader, et al. (1997). "The orphan nuclear receptor estrogen-related receptor alpha is a transcriptional regulator of the human medium-chain acyl coenzyme A dehydrogenase gene." *Mol Cell Biol* 17(9): 5400-5409.

Sladek, R., B. Beatty, et al. (1997). "Chromosomal mapping of the human and murine orphan receptors ERR alpha (ESRRA) and ERR beta (ESRRB) and identification of a novel human ERR alpha-related pseudogene." *Genomics* 45(2): 320-326.

Sonoda, J., J. Laganiere, et al. (2007). "Nuclear receptor ERR alpha and coactivator PGC-1 beta are effectors of IFN-gamma-induced host defense." *Genes & development* 21(15): 1909-1920.

Stein, R. A., C. Y. Chang, et al. (2008). "Estrogen-Related Receptor {alpha} Is Critical for the Growth of Estrogen Receptor-Negative Breast Cancer." *Cancer Res* 68(21): 8805-8812.

Stein, R. A., S. Gaillard, et al. (2009). "Estrogen-related receptor alpha induces the expression of vascular endothelial growth factor in breast cancer cells." *J Steroid Biochem Mol Biol* 114(1-2): 106-112.

Suetsugi, M., L. Su, et al. (2003). "Flavone and isoflavone phytoestrogens are agonists of estrogen-related receptors." *Mol Cancer Res* 1(13): 981-991.

Sumi, D. and L. J. Ignarro (2003). "Estrogen-related receptor {alpha}1 up-regulates endothelial nitric oxide synthase expression." *Proc Natl Acad Sci U S A* 100(24): 14451-14456.

Sun, P., J. Sehouli, et al. (2005). "Expression of estrogen receptor-related receptors, a subfamily of orphan nuclear receptors, as new tumor biomarkers in ovarian cancer cells." *J Mol Med* 83(6): 457-467.

Suzuki, T., Y. Miki, et al. (2004). "Estrogen-related receptor alpha in human breast carcinoma as a potent prognostic factor." *Cancer Res* 64(13): 4670-4676.

Takashima-Sasaki, K., C. Mori, et al. (2007). "Exposure of juvenile female mice to isoflavone causes lowered expression of estrogen-related receptor gamma gene in vagina." *Reprod Toxicol* 23(4): 507-512.

Thorsen, T., M. Tangen, et al. (1982). "Concentration of endogenous oestradiol as related to oestradiol receptor sites in breast tumor cytosol." *Eur J Cancer Clin Oncol* 18(4): 333-337.

Trapp, T. and F. Holsboer (1996). "Nuclear orphan receptor as a repressor of glucocorticoid receptor transcriptional activity." *The Journal of biological chemistry* 271(17): 9879-9882.

Tremblay, G. B., D. Bergeron, et al. (2001). "4-Hydroxytamoxifen is an isoform-specific inhibitor of orphan estrogen-receptor-related (ERR) nuclear receptors beta and gamma." *Endocrinology* 142(10): 4572-4575.

Tremblay, G. B., T. Kunath, et al. (2001). "Diethylstilbestrol regulates trophoblast stem cell differentiation as a ligand of orphan nuclear receptor ERR beta." *Genes Dev* 15(7): 833-838.

van Landeghem, A. A., J. Poortman, et al. (1985). "Endogenous concentration and subcellular distribution of estrogens in normal and malignant human breast tissue." *Cancer Res* 45(6): 2900-2906.

Vanacker, J. M., E. Bonnelye, et al. (1998). "Activation of the thyroid hormone receptor alpha gene promoter by the orphan nuclear receptor ERR alpha." *Oncogene* 17(19): 2429-2435.

Vanacker, J. M., C. Delmarre, et al. (1998). "Activation of the osteopontin promoter by the orphan nuclear receptor estrogen receptor related alpha." *Cell Growth Differ* 9(12): 1007-1014.

Vanacker, J. M., K. Pettersson, et al. (1999). "Transcriptional targets shared by estrogen receptor- related receptors (ERRs) and estrogen receptor (ER) alpha, but not by ERbeta." *Embo J* 18(15): 4270-4279.

Vega, R. B. and D. P. Kelly (1997). "A role for estrogen-related receptor alpha in the control of mitochondrial fatty acid beta-oxidation during brown adipocyte differentiation." *J Biol Chem* 272(50): 31693-31699.

Villena, J. A. and A. Kralli (2008). "ERRalpha: a metabolic function for the oldest orphan." *Trends Endocrinol Metab* 19(8): 269-276.

Wang, J., F. Fang, et al. (2009). "Kaempferol is an estrogen-related receptor alpha and gamma inverse agonist." *FEBS Lett* 583(4): 643-647.

Wang, L., Y. Li, et al. (2008). "PGC-1 alpha induces dynamic protein interactions on the ERR alpha gene multi-hormone response element nucleosome in kidney cells." *Biochem J* 416: 407-419.

Warburg, O. (1956). "On respiratory impairment in cancer cells." *Science* 124(3215): 269-270.

Willy, P. J., I. R. Murray, et al. (2004). "Regulation of PPARgamma coactivator 1alpha (PGC-1alpha) signaling by an estrogen-related receptor alpha (ERRalpha) ligand." *Proc Natl Acad Sci U S A* 101(24): 8912-8917.

Wu, F., J. Wang, et al. (2009). "Estrogen-related receptor alpha (ERRalpha) inverse agonist XCT-790 induces cell death in chemotherapeutic resistant cancer cells." *Chem Biol Interact* 181(2): 236-242.

Xie, C. Q., Y. Jeong, et al. (2009). "Expression profiling of nuclear receptors in human and mouse embryonic stem cells." *Molecular Endocrinology* 23(5): 724-733.

Xie, W., H. Hong, et al. (1999). "Constitutive activation of transcription and binding of coactivator by estrogen-related receptors 1 and 2." *Mol Endocrinol* 13(12): 2151-2162.

Yang, C. and S. Chen (1999). "Two organochlorine pesticides, toxaphene and chlordane, are antagonists for estrogen-related receptor alpha-1 orphan receptor." *Cancer Res* 59(18): 4519-4524.

Yang, C., D. Zhou, et al. (1998). "Modulation of aromatase expression in the breast tissue by ERR alpha-1 orphan receptor." *Cancer Res* 58(24): 5695-5700.

Yang, N., H. Shigeta, et al. (1996). "Estrogen-related receptor, hERR1, modulates estrogen receptor-mediated response of human lactoferrin gene promoter." *J Biol Chem* 271(10): 5795-5804.

Yang, X., M. Downes, et al. (2006). "Nuclear receptor expression links the circadian clock to metabolism." *Cell* 126(4): 801-810.

Yarden, Y. and M. X. Sliwkowski (2001). "Untangling the ErbB signalling network." *Nat Rev Mol Cell Biol* 2(2): 127-137.

Yu, D. D. and B. M. Forman (2005). "Identification of an agonist ligand for estrogen-related receptors ERRbeta/gamma." *Bioorg Med Chem Lett* 15(5): 1311-1313.

Yu, S., X. Wang, et al. (2007). "ERRgamma suppresses cell proliferation and tumor growth of androgen-sensitive and androgen-insensitive prostate cancer cells and its implication as a therapeutic target for prostate cancer." *Cancer Res* 67(10): 4904-4914.

Yu, S., Y. C. Wong, et al. (2008). "Orphan nuclear receptor estrogen-related receptor-beta suppresses in vitro and in vivo growth of prostate cancer cells via p21(WAF1/CIP1) induction and as a potential therapeutic target in prostate cancer." *Oncogene* 27(23): 3313-3328.

Zhang, Z., K. Chen, et al. (2006). "Estrogen-related receptors-stimulated monoamine oxidase B promoter activity is down-regulated by estrogen receptors." *Mol Endocrinol* 20(7): 1547-1561.

Zhang, Z. and C. T. Teng (2000). "Estrogen receptor-related receptor alpha 1 interacts with coactivator and constitutively activates the estrogen response elements of the human lactoferrin gene." *J Biol Chem* 275(27): 20837-20846.

Zhang, Z. and C. T. Teng (2001). "Estrogen receptor alpha and estrogen receptor-related receptor alpha1 compete for binding and coactivator." *Mol Cell Endocrinol* 172(1-2): 223-233.

Zhang, Z. and C. T. Teng (2007). "Interplay between estrogen-related receptor alpha (ERRalpha) and gamma (ERRgamma) on the regulation of ERRalpha gene expression." *Mol Cell Endocrinol* 264(1-2): 128-141.

Zhou, W., Z. Liu, et al. (2006). "Identification and characterization of two novel splicing isoforms of human estrogen-related receptor beta." *The Journal of clinical endocrinology and metabolism* 91(2): 569-579.

Zhou, W., S. C. Lo, et al. (2007). "ERRbeta: a potent inhibitor of Nrf2 transcriptional activity." *Molecular and cellular endocrinology* 278(1-2): 52-62.

15

The Role of MicroRNAs in Estrogen Receptor α-Positive Human Breast Cancer

Hiroko Yamashita, Tatsuya Toyama, Nobuyasu Yoshimoto, Yumi Endo, Mai Iwasa and Yoshitaka Fujii
Oncology, Immunology and Surgery, Nagoya City University Graduate School of Medical Sciences, Japan

1. Introduction

MicroRNAs (miRNAs) are a class naturally occurring small non-coding RNAs that control gene expression by targeting mRNAs for translational repression or cleavage (Krol et al., 2010). Recent evidence has shown that miRNA mutations or mis-expression correlate with various human cancers, and that loss- or gain-of function of specific miRNAs contributes to breast epithelial cellular transformation and tumorigenesis (Esquela-Kerscher et al., 2006). miRNA expression profiling also revealed that miRNAs are differently expressed among molecular subtypes in breast cancer (Blenkiron et al., 2007; Iorio et al., 2005).

There are large-scale molecular differences between estrogen receptor (ER) α-positive and ERα-negative breast cancers (Perou et al., 2000; Sorlie et al., 2003). Endocrine therapy has become the most important treatment option for women with ERα-positive breast cancer, and approximately 70% of primary breast cancers express ERα. ERα is essential for estrogen-dependent growth, and its level of expression is a crucial determinant of response to endocrine therapy and prognosis in ERα-positive breast cancer (Dowsett et al., 2008; Harvey et al., 1999; Yamashita et al., 2006). Multiple mechanisms involved in altering ERα gene expression in breast cancer have been proposed, including ERα gene amplification (Holst et al., 2007) as well as transcriptional silencing by DNA methylation of CpG islands within the ERα promoter (Giacinti et al., 2006) and mutations within the open reading frame of ERα (Herynk et al., 2004). However, expression levels of ERα in breast cancer tissues differ widely among patients (Yamashita et al., 2011), and frequently change during disease progression and in response to systemic therapies (Yamashita et al., 2009). It was reported that the microRNA miR-206 decreases endogenous ERα mRNA and protein levels in human MCF-7 breast cancer cells via two specific target sites within the 3′-untranslated region (UTR) of the human ERα transcript (Adams et al., 2007). We found that the expression levels of miR-206 were gradually decreased as ERα protein expression increased in breast cancer tissues, suggesting that miR-206 is a key factor for the regulation of ERα expression in human breast cancer (Kondo et al., 2008). Moreover, recent studies have shown that ERα-regulating miRNAs, miR-18a, miR-18b, miR-22, miR-193b, miR-302c, and miR-221/222, as well as miR-206, directly targeted ERα in 3′UTR reporter assays, and suggested that several miRNAs regulate ERα expression.

2. Estrogen receptor (ER) α expression in human breast cancer

2.1 Expression of ERα in human breast cancer tissues

2.1.1 ERα expression in normal and malignant breast epithelial cells

ERα expression in normal and premalignant breast epithelial cells has been assessed by immunohistochemistry. It was reported that on average, normal premenopausal terminal duct lobular units contain about 30% ERα-positive cells (Allred et al., 2004). In contrast, nearly all cells express very high levels of ERα in the majority of premalignant breast lesions, including atypical ductal hyperplasia, atypical lobular hyperplasia and lobular carcinoma in situ. DCIS (Ductal carcinoma in situ) shows various levels of ERα expression ranging from high levels of lower-grade lesions to low levels of higher-grade lesions, including entirely ERα-negative. Furthermore, the wide range of ERα expression is observed in invasive ductal carcinoma. There is a substantial (~25%) subset of invasive breast cancers that does not contain any ERα-expressing cells. The majority (~75%) of invasive breast cancers, however, does contain ERα-expressing cells, but the proportion varies ranging from very low, to intermediate, to very high. We examined ERα expression in breast cancer tissues by immunohistochemistry using Allred score (Allred et al., 1998), and demonstrated that breast tumors show a wide range of ERα expression levels (Yamashita et al., 2011). Moreover, intensity of ERα expression is not equal among breast cancer cells in an individual tumor. Eastern cooperative oncology group compared the distribution of ERα protein expression by immunohistochemistry and ERα mRNA expression by quantitative reverse transcription (RT)-PCR in ECOG 2197 study (Badve et al., 2008). They reported that ERα mRNA expression in breast cancer tissues also showed continuous and the wide range.

2.1.2 Role of expression levels of ERα in human breast cancer

It is well established that expression levels of ERα govern response to endocrine therapy and prognosis in ERα-positive human breast cancer. Allred and colleagues first reported that expression levels of ERα assessed by immunohistochemistry affected prognosis (Harvey et al., 1999). ERα status using Allred score was a highly significant predictor of disease-free survival for patients who received adjuvant endocrine therapy. Recently, relationship between expression levels of ERα and prognosis was analyzed in adjuvant endocrine therapy trials for postmenopausal breast cancer, and demonstrated that disease-free survival or time to recurrence were significantly different according to expression levels of ERα (Dowsett et al., 2008; Viale et al., 2007). It was reported that the use of a cutoff of 1% staining cells for ERα indicated a better prognosis and at least some degree of endocrine responsiveness (Hammond et al., 2010). In the neoadjuvant endocrine therapy trial for postmenopausal women, correlation between expression levels of ERα assessed by Allred score and response to neoadjuvant endocrine therapy was analyzed (Ellis et al., 2001). It showed that letrozole response rates were superior to tamoxifen response rates in every ERα Allred score from 3 to 8, indicating that letrozole is more effective than tamoxifen regardless of the level of ERα expression. We also studied expression levels of ERα on pretreatment biopsies and post-treatment surgical specimens in postmenopausal patients with ERα-positive primary breast cancer who were treated with aromatase inhibitors for 6 months (Yamashita et al., 2009). We showed that ERα expression was decreased in post-treatment tumors compared to pretreatment specimens. On the other hand, we analyzed expression levels of ERα in primary breast cancer specimens from 75 metastatic breast cancer patients who received endocrine therapy on relapse, and analyzed the correlation between expression levels of ERα and response to endocrine therapy and post-relapse survival (Yamashita et al., 2006). Our results indicated that patients with higher ERα expression responded significantly to endocrine therapy, and that patients with higher ERα expression had better survival after relapse. Moreover, we recently reported that patients whose breast tumors contained high ERα expression effectively responded to aromatase inhibitors and displayed longer time to progression during first-line endocrine therapy with aromatase inhibitors and time to endocrine therapy failure (Endo et al., 2011).

2.2 Regulation of expression levels of ERα

Multiple mechanisms involved in the regulation of ERα expression in breast cancer have been identified, including mutations of ERα gene (Herynk et al., 2004) and transcriptional silencing by DNA methylation within the ERα promoter (Gaudet et al., 2009; Giacinti et al., 2006; Iwase et al., 1999). It was recently reported ERα gene amplification in breast cancer (Holst et al., 2007; Tomita et al., 2009). Holst and colleagues demonstrated that ERα gene amplification was frequent and more than 20% of breast cancers harbored genomic amplification by FISH analysis. They reported that ESR1 amplification was tightly linked to ERα protein expression, and that ESR1 amplification was also found in benign and precancerous breast diseases, such as atypical ductal hyperplasia, ductal carcinoma in situ and lobular carcinoma in situ. However, breast cancer patients show a wide range of ERα expression levels (Yamashita et al., 2011), and the levels of expression in individual patients change during disease progression and in response to systemic therapies (Yamashita et al., 2009). Therefore, other mechanisms may also regulate ERα expression in breast cancer.

2.2.1 miRNA biogenesis and function

MicroRNAs (miRNAs) comprise a large family of ~21-nucleotide-long RNAs that have emerged as key post-transcriptional regulators of gene expression (Krol et al., 2010). In mammals, miRNAs are predicted to control the activity of ~50% of all protein-coding genes. Functional studies indicate that miRNAs participate in the regulation of almost every cellular process investigated so far and that changes in their expression are associated with many human pathologies. Primary miRNA transcripts are cleaved into 70- to 80-nucleotide precursor miRNA (pre-miRNA) hairpins by RNase III Drosha in the cell nucleus and transported to the cytoplasm, where pre-miRNAs are processed by RNA Dicer into 19- to 25-nucleotide miRNA duplexes. One strand of each duplex is degraded, and the other strands become mature miRNAs, which, incorporated into the RNA-induced silencing complex, recognize sites in the 3′-UTR of the target mRNAs and cause translational repression or mRNA cleavage. miRNAs are a new player among gene regulation mechanisms, and their functions have not been fully explored but are known to include the regulation of cellular differentiation, proliferation and apoptosis. Recent evidence has shown that miRNA mutations or mis-expression are associated with various human cancers (Esquela-Kerscher et al., 2006).

2.2.2 Regulation of expression levels of ERα by miRNAs

Adams and colleagues first identified two potential miRNA miR-206 target sites within the 3'-UTR of ERα mRNA via in Silico analysis (Adams et al., 2007). The validation assay revealed that both miR-206 target sites specifically interacted with miR-206, which in turn repressed the corresponding ERα mRNA and protein expression. They also demonstrated that expression levels of endogenous miR-206 were significantly higher in ERα-negative MDA-MB-231 cells than in ERα-positive MCF-7 cells. Moreover, they showed that miR-206 repressed ERα mRNA and protein expression in MCF-7 and T47D cells. We showed that miR-206 expression assayed by quantitative RT-PCR analysis was inversely correlated with ERα but not ERβ mRNA expression in human breast cancer tissues (Kondo et al., 2008). Moreover, miR-206 expression levels were gradually decreased as ERα protein expression increased in human breast cancer. Transfection experiments revealed that introduction of miR-206 in estrogen dependent MCF-7 cells inhibited cell growth. Transfection of miR-206 into MCF-7 cells suppressed ERα expression and inhibited cell growth in a dose-dependent manner. Furthermore, introduction of miR-206 produced a dose-dependent decrease of mRNA expression of ERα-target genes, such as progesterone receptor, cyclin D1 and pS2. Adams and colleagues recently reported that miR-206 coordinately targeted mRNAs encoding the coactivator proteins SRC-1 and SRC-3, and the transcription factor GATA-3, all of which contribute to estrogenic signaling and a luminal A phenotype (Adams et al., 2009). Furthermore, they identified that miR-206 contributed to the epidermal growth factor (EGF) induced repression of ERα signaling in MCF-7 cells.

2.2.3 MiRNAs that directly target ERα in human breast cancer

Zhao and colleagues demonstrated that miR-221 and miR-222 were highly expressed in ERα-negative breast cancer cells, and that miRNA in situ hybridization analyses also showed overexpression of miR-221 and miR-222 in ERα-negative breast tumors (Zhao et al., 2008). Recently, two groups reported several miRNAs that down-regulated ERα in breast cancer cells. They identified the target sites of miRNAs, such as miR-18a and b, miR-302, miR-193b, miR-22, and miR221/222 as well as miR-206, in the ERα 3'-UTR, and showed that these miRNAs inhibited estrogen signaling by directly targeting ERα mRNA (Leivonen et al., 2009; Pandey et al., 2009) (Fig.1).

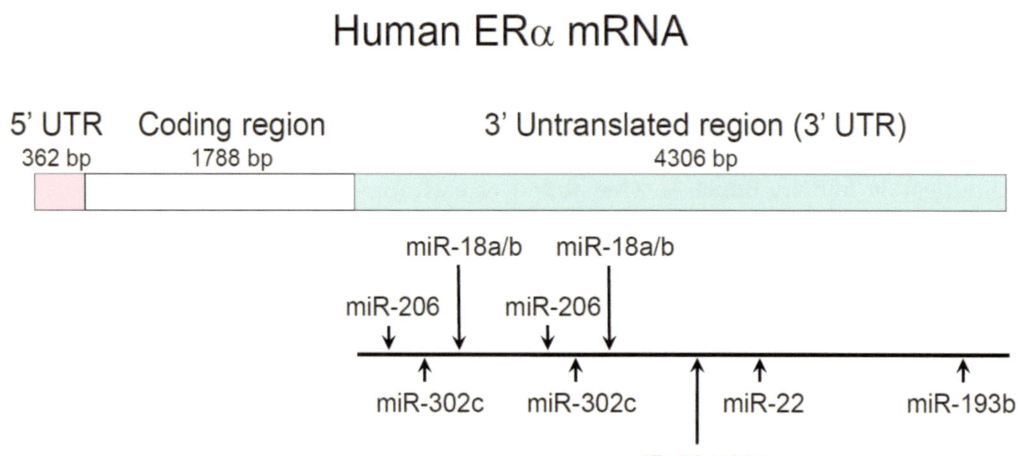

Fig. 1. Schematic representation of the human ERα mRNA and the predicted miRNA target sites.

We recently analyzed expression levels of miRNAs that directly target ERα, including miR-18a, miR-18b, miR-22, miR-193b, miR-221/222 and miR-302c in human breast cancer samples by quantitative RT-PCR analysis (Yoshimoto et al., 2011). Our results showed that miR-18a expression was much higher in ERα-negative than ERα-positive tumors, with the expression levels of miR-18a not differing in ERα-positive breast cancer as a function of ERα protein level. Surprisingly, expression levels of miR-193b and miR-221 were significantly lower in ERα-negative than ERα-positive tumors, and the levels of these miRNAs gradually increased as ERα protein expression increased. There was no statistically significant association between miR-22 and ERα expression, and miR-302c expression was minimal in human breast cancer samples. Prognostic analysis showed that low miR-18b expression was significantly associated with improved survival in HER2-negative breast cancer. Our results suggest that miRNAs that directly target ERα have distinct roles in not only regulating ERα but also regulating other target genes in human breast cancer, and that some miRNAs might be associated with characteristics of ERα-positive breast cancer.

2.3 Role of miRNAs in breast cancer

miRNAs can function as tumor suppressors and oncogenes (Esquela-Kerscher et al., 2006). The reduction or deletion of a miRNA that functions as a tumor suppressor leads to tumor formation. On the other hand, the amplification or overexpression of a miRNA that function as an oncogene results in tumor formation. Lu and colleagues first analyzed miRNA expression profiling in normal and tumor samples, and revealed global changes in miRNA expression (Lu et al., 2005). It was found that miRNA expression seems globally higher in normal tissues compared with tumors. Moreover, miRNAs are differentially expressed in various cancers. miRNA expression profiling also revealed that miRNAs are differently expressed among molecular subtypes in breast cancer (Blenkiron et al., 2007; Iorio et al., 2005). Iorio and colleagues first reported the miRNA gene expression profile in human breast cancer (Iorio et al., 2005). Compared with normal breast tissue, miRNAs are aberrantly expressed in human breast cancer. They also reported differentially expressed miRNAs associated with ERα expression, including miR-206. Blenkiron and colleagues analyzed miRNA expression in human breast cancer, and found that many miRNAs were differently expressed between breast cancer subtypes, such as luminal A, luminal B, HER2-positive, basal-like and normal-like (Blenkiron et al., 2007). They also found significant association between miRNA expression profiling and clinicopathological factors such as ERα status and tumor grade. Furthermore, recent studies have demonstrated that loss- or gain-of function of specific miRNAs contributes to breast epithelial cellular transformation and tumorigenesis. The interconnections between miRNAs and tumor suppressor genes and oncogenes in breast cancer were summarized by Zoon and colleagues (Zoon et al., 2009).

3. Conclusion

It is well recognized that individual miRNA sequences can suppress the production of hundreds of proteins (Krol et al., 2010). Reduction of protein levels in this way is often modest, however, and many such RNAs probably collectively fine-tune gene expression. Accumulating evidence supports the hypothesis that the ability of miRNAs to simultaneously regulate many target genes makes them attractive candidates for regulating normal and cancer cells. miRNAs are potential therapeutic targets for more tailored treatment strategies for breast cancer.

4. References

Adams BD, Cowee DM & White BA (2009). The role of miR-206 in the epidermal growth factor (EGF) induced repression of estrogen receptor-alpha (ERalpha) signaling and a luminal phenotype in MCF-7 breast cancer cells. *Mol Endocrinol,* Vol.23, No.8, pp. 1215-1230, ISSN 1944-9917

Adams BD, Furneaux H & White BA (2007). The micro-ribonucleic acid (miRNA) miR-206 targets the human estrogen receptor-alpha (ERalpha) and represses ERalpha messenger RNA and protein expression in breast cancer cell lines. *Mol Endocrinol,* Vol.21, No.5, pp. 1132-1147, ISSN 0888-8809

Allred DC, Brown P & Medina D (2004). The origins of estrogen receptor alpha-positive and estrogen receptor alpha-negative human breast cancer. *Breast Cancer Res,* Vol. 6, No. 6, pp. 240-245, ISSN 1465-542X

Allred DC, Harvey JM, Berardo M & Clark GM (1998). Prognostic and predictive factors in breast cancer by immunohistochemical analysis. *Mod Pathol,* Vol.11, No. 2, pp. 155-168, ISSN 0893-3952

Badve SS, Baehner FL, Gray RP, Childs BH, Maddala T, Liu ML, Rowley SC, Shak S, Perez EA, Shulman LJ, Martino S, Davidson NE, Sledge GW, Goldstein LJ & Sparano JA (2008). Estrogen- and progesterone-receptor status in ECOG 2197: comparison of immunohistochemistry by local and central laboratories and quantitative reverse transcription polymerase chain reaction by central laboratory. *J Clin Oncol,* Vol.26, No. 15, pp. 2473-2481, ISSN 1527-7755

Blenkiron C, Goldstein LD, Thorne NP, Spiteri I, Chin SF, Dunning MJ, Barbosa-Morais NL, Teschendorff AE, Green AR, Ellis IO, Tavare S, Caldas C & Miska EA (2007). MicroRNA expression profiling of human breast cancer identifies new markers of tumor subtype. *Genome Biol,* Vol.8, No. 10, pp. R214

Dowsett M, Allred C, Knox J, Quinn E, Salter J, Wale C, Cuzick J, Houghton J, Williams N, Mallon E, Bishop H, Ellis I, Larsimont D, Sasano H, Carder P, Cussac AL, Knox F, Speirs V, Forbes J & Buzdar A (2008). Relationship between quantitative estrogen and progesterone receptor expression and human epidermal growth factor receptor 2 (HER-2) status with recurrence in the Arimidex, Tamoxifen, Alone or in Combination trial. *J Clin Oncol,* Vol. 26, No. 7, pp. 1059-1065

Ellis MJ, Coop A, Singh B, Mauriac L, Llombert-Cussac A, Janicke F, Miller WR, Evans DB, Dugan M, Brady C, Quebe-Fehling E & Borgs M (2001). Letrozole is more effective neoadjuvant endocrine therapy than tamoxifen for ErbB-1- and/or ErbB-2-positive, estrogen receptor-positive primary breast cancer: evidence from a phase III randomized trial. *J Clin Oncol,* Vol. 19, No. 18, pp. 3808-3816

Endo Y, Toyama T, Takahashi S, Sugiura H, Yoshimoto N, Iwasa M, Kobayashi S, Fujii Y & Yamashita H (2011). High estrogen receptor expression and low Ki67 expression are associated with improved time to progression during first-line endocrine therapy with aromatase inhibitors in breast cancer. *Int J Clin Oncol*, ISSN 2547-7772, DOI 10.1007/s10147-011-0215-5

Esquela-Kerscher A & Slack FJ (2006). Oncomirs - microRNAs with a role in cancer. *Nat Rev Cancer,* Vol. 6, No. 4, pp. 259-269

Gaudet MM, Campan M, Figueroa JD, Yang XR, Lissowska J, Peplonska B, Brinton LA, Rimm DL, Laird PW, Garcia-Closas M & Sherman ME (2009). DNA hypermethylation of ESR1 and PGR in breast cancer: pathologic and epidemiologic associations. *Cancer Epidemiol Biomarkers Prev,* Vol. 18, No. 22, pp. 3036-3043, ISSN 1538-7755

Giacinti L, Claudio PP, Lopez M & Giordano A (2006). Epigenetic information and estrogen receptor alpha expression in breast cancer. *Oncologist,* Vol. 11, No. 1, pp. 1-8

Hammond ME, Hayes DF, Dowsett M, Allred DC, Hagerty KL, Badve S, Fitzgibbons PL, Francis G, Goldstein NS, Hayes M, Hicks DG, Lester S, Love R, Mangu PB, McShane L, Miller K, Osborne CK, Paik S, Perlmutter J, Rhodes A, Sasano H, Schwartz JN, Sweep FC, Taube S, Torlakovic EE, Valenstein P, Viale G, Visscher D, Wheeler T, Williams RB, Wittliff JL & Wolff AC (2010). American society of clinical oncology/college of american pathologists guideline recommendations for immunohistochemical testing of estrogen and progesterone receptors in breast cancer. *J Clin Oncol,* Vol. 28, No. 16, pp. 2784-2795

Harvey JM, Clark GM, Osborne CK & Allred DC (1999). Estrogen receptor status by immunohistochemistry is superior to the ligand-binding assay for predicting response to adjuvant endocrine therapy in breast cancer. *J Clin Oncol,* Vol. 17, No. 5, pp. 1474-1481, ISSN 0732-183X

Herynk MH & Fuqua SA (2004). Estrogen receptor mutations in human disease. *Endocr Rev,* Vol. 25, No. 6, pp. 869-898

Holst F, Stahl PR, Ruiz C, Hellwinkel O, Jehan Z, Wendland M, Lebeau A, Terracciano L, Al-Kuraya K, Janicke F, Sauter G & Simon R (2007). Estrogen receptor alpha (ESR1) gene amplification is frequent in breast cancer. *Nat Genet,* Vol. 39, No. 5, pp. 655-660

Iorio MV, Ferracin M, Liu CG, Veronese A, Spizzo R, Sabbioni S, Magri E, Pedriali M, Fabbri M, Campiglio M, Menard S, Palazzo JP, Rosenberg A, Musiani P, Volinia S, Nenci I, Calin GA, Querzoli P, Negrini M & Croce CM (2005). MicroRNA gene expression deregulation in human breast cancer. *Cancer Res,* Vol. 65, No. 16, pp. 7065-7070, ISSN 0008-5472

Iwase H, Omoto Y, Iwata H, Toyama T, Hara Y, Ando Y, Ito Y, Fujii Y & Kobayashi S (1999). DNA methylation analysis at distal and proximal promoter regions of the oestrogen receptor gene in breast cancers. *Br J Cancer,* Vol. 80, No. 12, pp. 1982-1986, ISSN 0007-0920

Kondo N, Toyama T, Sugiura H, Fujii Y & Yamashita H (2008). miR-206 Expression is down-regulated in estrogen receptor alpha-positive human breast cancer. *Cancer Res,* Vol. 68, No. 13, pp. 5004-5008, ISSN 1538-7445

Krol J, Loedige I & Filipowicz W (2010). The widespread regulation of microRNA biogenesis, function and decay. *Nat Rev Genet,* Vol. 11, No. 9, pp. 597-610, ISSN 1471-0064

Leivonen SK, Makela R, Ostling P, Kohonen P, Haapa-Paananen S, Kleivi K, Enerly E, Aakula A, Hellstrom K, Sahlberg N, Kristensen VN, Borresen-Dale AL, Saviranta P, Perala M & Kallioniemi O (2009). Protein lysate microarray analysis to identify microRNAs regulating estrogen receptor signaling in breast cancer cell lines. *Oncogene,* Vol. 28, No. 44, pp. 3926-3936, ISSN 1476-5594

Lu J, Getz G, Miska EA, Alvarez-Saavedra E, Lamb J, Peck D, Sweet-Cordero A, Ebert BL, Mak RH, Ferrando AA, Downing JR, Jacks T, Horvitz HR & Golub TR (2005). MicroRNA expression profiles classify human cancers. *Nature,* Vol. 435, No. 7043, pp. 834-838, ISSN 1476-4687

Pandey DP & Picard D (2009). miR-22 inhibits estrogen signaling by directly targeting the estrogen receptor alpha mRNA. *Mol Cell Biol,* Vol.29, No. 13, pp. 3783-3790, ISSN 1098-5549

Perou CM, Sorlie T, Eisen MB, van de Rijn M, Jeffrey SS, Rees CA, Pollack JR, Ross DT, Johnsen H, Akslen LA, Fluge O, Pergamenschikov A, Williams C, Zhu SX, Lonning PE, Borresen-Dale AL, Brown PO & Botstein D (2000). Molecular portraits of human breast tumours. *Nature,* Vol. 406, No. 6797, pp. 747-752

Sorlie T, Tibshirani R, Parker J, Hastie T, Marron JS, Nobel A, Deng S, Johnsen H, Pesich R, Geisler S, Demeter J, Perou CM, Lonning PE, Brown PO, Borresen-Dale AL & Botstein D (2003). Repeated observation of breast tumor subtypes in independent gene expression data sets. *Proc Natl Acad Sci U S A,* Vol. 100, No. 14, pp. 8418-8423

Tomita S, Zhang Z, Nakano M, Ibusuki M, Kawazoe T, Yamamoto Y & Iwase H (2009). Estrogen receptor alpha gene ESR1 amplification may predict endocrine therapy responsiveness in breast cancer patients. *Cancer Sci,* Vol. 100, No. 6, pp. 1012-1017, ISSN 1349-7006

Viale G, Regan MM, Maiorano E, Mastropasqua MG, Dell'Orto P, Rasmussen BB, Raffoul J, Neven P, Orosz Z, Braye S, Ohlschlegel C, Thurlimann B, Gelber RD, Castiglione-Gertsch M, Price KN, Goldhirsch A, Gusterson BA & Coates AS (2007). Prognostic and predictive value of centrally reviewed expression of estrogen and progesterone receptors in a randomized trial comparing letrozole and tamoxifen adjuvant therapy for postmenopausal early breast cancer: BIG 1-98. *J Clin Oncol,* Vol. 25, No. 25, pp. 3846-3852, ISSN 1527-7755

Yamashita H, Iwase H, Toyama T, Takahashi S, Sugiura H, Yoshimoto N, Endo Y, Fujii Y & Kobayashi S (2011). Estrogen receptor-positive breast cancer in Japanese women: trends in incidence, characteristics, and prognosis. *Ann Oncol*, Vol. 22, No. 6, pp. 1318-1325, ISSN 1569-8041

Yamashita H, Takahashi S, Ito Y, Yamashita T, Ando Y, Toyama T, Sugiura H, Yoshimoto N, Kobayashi S, Fujii Y & Iwase H (2009). Predictors of response to exemestane as primary endocrine therapy in estrogen receptor-positive breast cancer. *Cancer Sci,* Vol. 100, No. 11, pp. 2028-2033, ISSN 1349-7006

Yamashita H, Ando Y, Nishio M, Zhang Z, Hamaguchi M, Mita K, Kobayashi S, Fujii Y & Iwase H (2006). Immunohistochemical evaluation of hormone receptor status for predicting response to endocrine therapy in metastatic breast cancer. *Breast Cancer,* Vol. 13, No. 1, pp. 74-83, ISSN 1340-6868

Yoshimoto N, Toyama T, Takahashi S, Sugiura H, Endo Y, Iwasa M, Fujii Y & Yamashita H (2011). Distinct expressions of microRNAs that directly target estrogen receptor α in human breast cancer. *Breast Cancer Res Treat,* online, DOI 10.1007/s10549-011-1672-2

Zhao JJ, Lin J, Yang H, Kong W, He L, Ma X, Coppola D & Cheng JQ (2008). MicroRNA-221/222 negatively regulates estrogen receptor alpha and is associated with tamoxifen resistance in breast cancer. *J Biol Chem,* Vol. 283, No. 45, pp. 31079-31086, ISSN 0021-9258

Zoon CK, Starker EQ, Wilson AM, Emmert-Buck MR, Libutti SK & Tangrea MA (2009). Current molecular diagnostics of breast cancer and the potential incorporation of microRNA. *Expert Rev Mol Diagn,* Vol. 9, No. 5, pp. 455-467, ISSN 1744-8352

Part 3

Cell Growth Regulation, Carcinogenesis

16

Roles of SWI/SNF Complex Genes in Breast Cancer

Esra Gunduz[1], Mehmet Gunduz[2], Bunyamin Isik[3] and Omer Faruk Hatipoglu[4]
[1]Departments of Medical Genetics, School of Medicine, Fatih University, Ankara,
[2]Departments of Medical Genetics and Otolaryngology, School of Medicine, Fatih University, Ankara
[3]Department of Family Medicine, School of Medicine, Fatih University, Ankara
[4]Department of Molecular Biology and Biochemistry, Graduate School of Medicine, Dentistry and Pharmaceutical Sciences, Okayama
[1,2,3]Turkey
[4]Japan

1. Introduction

Cancer is a multifactorial genetic disease which is characterized by uncontrolled proliferation of the cells. Cells undergo mutational changes in a multistep process. Cancer developes from a tumor clone though the firstly mutated cell doesn't present all the features of a cancer cell. Accumulation of the mutations lead cells to display the properties of the cancer. The proliferating cells which have the capacity to survive and invade result in hyperplasia followed by dysplasia and invasion and metastasis at the end [1].

Breast cancer is the most common cancer type and one of the leading cause of cancer mortality in women. Various factors including estrogens and its signaling, EGFR signaling pathway, other oncogenes and tumor suppressor genes including chromatin remodeling factors contribute to development of breast cancer.

At molecular level two major group of genes are responsible for cancer development. These genes, proto- oncogenes and tumor suppressor genes (TSG) control cell growth together in cells at a balance. They are normally required for cell survival and have a direct role in carcinogenesis and cancer progression. When the balance is broken between oncogenes and TSGs due to activation of proto-oncogene or inactivation tumor suppressor genes, cancer develops (**Figure 1, 2**).

In cellular functions proto-oncogenes serve as growth factors, growth factor receptors, transcription factors and signal transduction elements. The mutated proto-oncogenes are named as oncogenes. An oncogene, when mutated or altered, contributes to conversion of a normal cell into a cancer cell. The activation of a proto-oncogene may occur during replication; by a translocation; by gene amplification or by the alterations in mRNA expression. TSGs are also normal cellular genes taking part in regulation of the cell cycle,

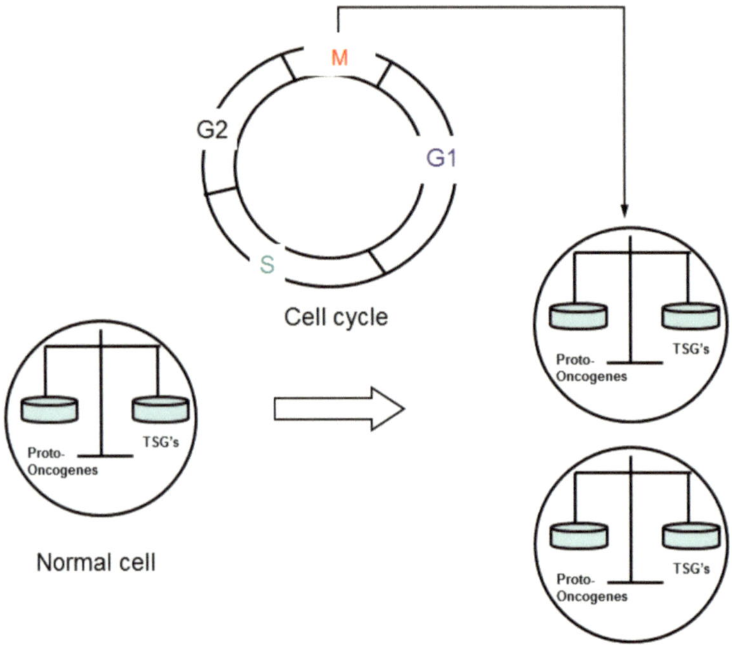

Fig. 1. In human cells proto-oncogenes and tumor suppressor genes are at a balance. There exists a controlled cell division and proliferation.

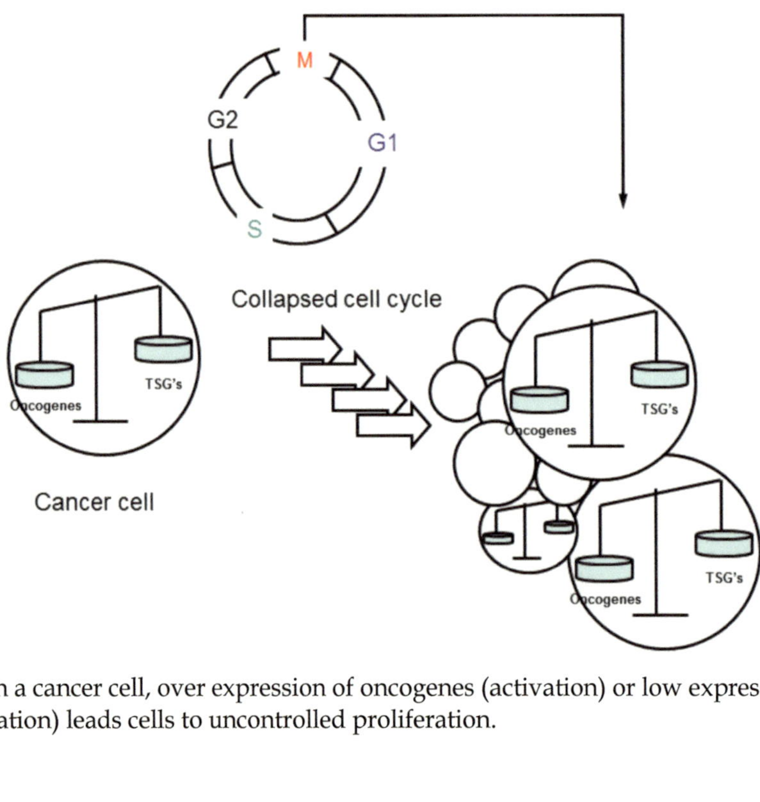

Fig. 2. In a cancer cell, over expression of oncogenes (activation) or low expression of TSGs (inactivation) leads cells to uncontrolled proliferation.

apoptosis, differentiation, surveillance of genomic integrity and repair of DNA errors, chromatin remodeling, signal transduction, and cell adhesion. The activation of the oncogenes and the inactivation of tumor suppressor genes lead cells to proliferate in an uncontrolled manner. Usually one mutation is sufficient for the activation mechanism of oncogenes whereas two hits are necessary for the inactivation of tumor suppressor genes [2,3]. However, a new class of tumor suppressor gene, in which one of the alleles is lost while the rest allele is kept, has recently been defined. Such a tumor suppressor gene is called as haploinsufficient and supposed to be in a cancer-prone state [4-6]. These patients develop cancer when they are exposed to the various carcinogens such as smoking, x-ray and chemicals.

In eukaryotic cells, genetic information encoded by DNA is packaged into chromatin and kept in the nucleus. Thus chromatin is composed of DNA and proteins. The primary proteins of chromatin are histones. A nucleosome, basic unit of chromatin, consists of 146 base-pairs of duplex DNA wrapped around a histone octamer composed of two of each of the conventional histone proteins: H2A, H2B, H3 and H4. Another histon, H1, provides compaction of neighboring nucleosomes by linking them. These compact situation of chromatin reversibly changes in an open and closed situation by various molecules such as histon acetyl transferases (HAT), histon deacetyl transferases (HDAC) and chromatin remodeling molecules, which then influence on transcriptional regulation of gene expression through accesibility of transcription factors by these molecules.

Transcription is an important step to control gene expression from the very early step of life to the end. To maintain transcription every human cell has to deal with the step of an access to DNA either through histone acetylases or chromating remodelling complexes. Many activator proteins of transcription use both of these mechanisms. Histone Acetyl Transferases (HATs) add acetyl groups to the tails of the histones that protrude out of nucleosomes which lead to the binding of the transcription factors. Chromatin remodeling complexes use ATP to open or close the chromatin (**Figure 3**).

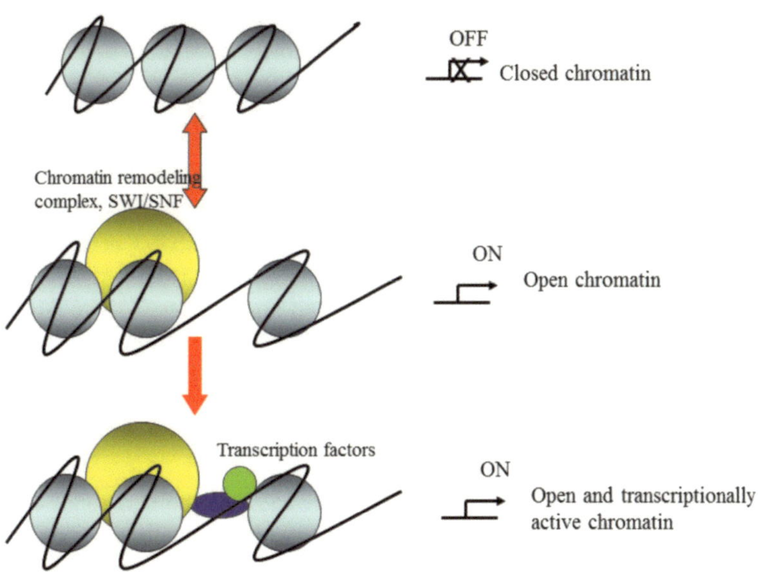

Fig. 3. The binding of chromatin remodeling complex changes conformationally closed chromatin to open chromatin that enables the transcription factors to bind and start transcription.

By cooperation of members of these two classes of complexes, the structure of chromatin is dynamically regulated and thus they play important roles in the control of gene expression. ATP-dependent chromatin remodelers are divided into families according to the subunit composition and biochemical activity such as SWI/SNF, ISWI, INO80, SWR1 and NURD/Mi2/CHD complexes. Of these in particular, some of the members SWI/SNF complexes are emerging tumor suppressors, as genetic and epigenetic inactivation events in several SWI/SNF subunits have been detected in various human cancers [7-10].

2. Function of SWI/SNF family members

Transcription factor action and then the targeted gene expression are mainly regulated by SWI/SNF family of chromatin remodeling complexes. SWI/SNF complexes are large 2-MDa (1.14 MDa in yeast) multi-subunit conglomerates that are involved in either enhancement or suppression of the downstream genes [7-12]. SWI/SNF complex genes were identified through two screens in yeast Saccharomyces cerevisiae. The first identified gene that is required for the expression of SUC2 for sucrose metabolism (sucrose non-fermenting (SNF) mutants), and the second screen showed another gene required for the activation of HO for mating-type switching (switch (SWI) mutants [7, 13-15].

SWI/SNF complex is composed of three groups of subunits; 1) enzymatic (ATPase), 2) core subunits, and 3) accessory subunits [8,11]. Though the exact mechanisms for modification of chromatin structure by SWI/SNF complexes remain incompletely understood, current knowledge suggests that ATPase-dependent disruption of histone-DNA association and resultant nucleosome "sliding" is the main mechanism [8,12]. The mammalian genome encodes 29 different SWI/SNF-like ATPases [12]. Accordingly, each SWI/SNF complex consists of only one of two ATPases, BRM (Brahma) or BRG1 (Brahma-Related Gene 1), which show 74% homology.

SWI/SNF complexes are classified into two major classes as BAF (BRG1 or BRM-Associated Factor; also known as SWI/SNF-A) or PBAF (Polybromo-Associated BAF; also known as SWI/SNF-B) complexes (**Figure 4**). BAF complexes contain either BRG1 (also known as SMARCA4, SNF2b, BAF190) or BRM (also known as SMARCA2, SNF2a) and PBAF complexes include only BRG1 as ATPase subunit. Each ATPase is accompanied with 10 to 12 proteins as core and accessory subunits. The core subunits include BAF155 (also known as SWI3, SRG3, SMARC1), BAF170 (also known as SMARCC2), and SNF5 (also known as SMARCB1, BAF47, INI1). Accessory subunits consist of BAF45 (a,b,c,d; encoded gene names PHF10, DPF1, DPF2, DPF3), BAF53 (a,b; encoded gene names ACTL6A, ACTL6B), BAF57 (encoded gene name SMARCE1), BAF60 (a,b,c; encoded gene name SMARCD1, SMARCD2, SMARCD3), BAF180 (encoded gene name PBRM1), BAF200 (encoded gene name ARID2), BRD7 and BAF250 (a,b; a: also known as ARID1A, SMARCF1, OSA1; b: also known as ARID1B, OSA2) [7,8]. ARID1A (BAF250a) and ARID1B (BAF250b) subunits are mutually exclusive and exist only in BAF complexes. BAF180, BAF200 and BRD7 are exclusively present in PBAF complexes [7,8] [**Figure 4**].

SWI/SNF complexes were found to be based on their roles in the transcription activation. However, studies show that mammalian SWI/SNF complexes have function to both repression and activation of the targeted genes. For development of mammalian T lymphocyte, BRG1 and BAF57 are necessary both for silencing CD4 and activating CD8 expression [7,16,17]. Specific combinations of individual SWI/SNF components were reported to generate sub-complexes with specialized functions that are involved in

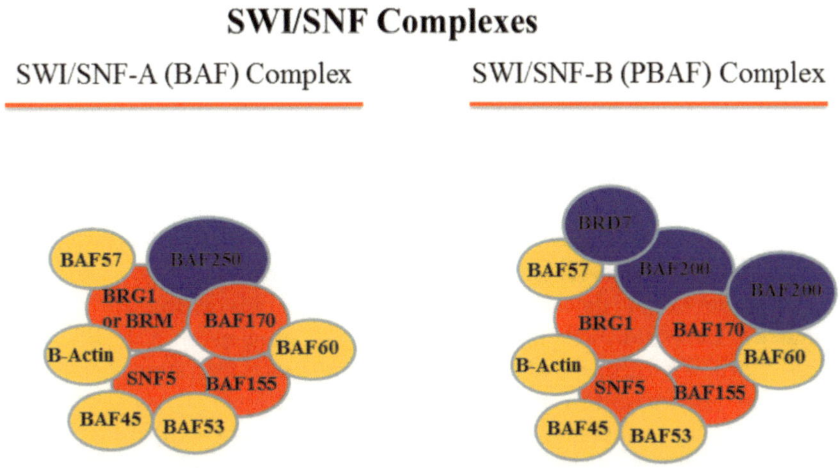

Fig. 4. SWI/SNF complexes are classified into two major classes as BAF (SWI/SNF-A) or PBAF (SWI/SNF-B) complexes. BAF complexes contain either BRG1 or BRM and PBAF complexes include only BRG1 as ATPase subunit. The core subunits include BAF155, BAF170, and SNF5. Accessory subunits consist of BAF45, BAF53, BAF57, BAF60, BAF180, BAF200, BRD7 and BAF250. BAF250a and BAF250b subunits are mutually exclusive and exist only in BAF complexes. BAF180, BAF200 and BRD7 are exclusively present in PBAF complexes.

sequential stages of muscle-gene activation--i.e., initial displacement of the nucleosome followed by the loading of the complete myogenic transcriptosome that promotes gene transcription [18]. Immunoprecipitation analysis of osteocalcin promoter showed that BRM- and BRG1-containing complexes have different roles on it. BRG1 complexes were associated with the promoter induction, while BRM-specific complexes were present only on the repressed promoter and were required for association of the co-repressor HDAC1 [19]. In embryonic stem (ES) cells, BRG1 was reported to act as a repressor to inhibit programmes that are associated with differentiation. On the other hand, it also facilitates the expression of core pluripotency programmes [20,21]. Loss of *Snf5* in murine fibroblasts results in more genes being activated such as E2F targeted genes than repressed [22]. Another example of repression of gene expression is recruitment histone deacetylases (HDACs), which remove activating acetyl marks from histone tails, by SWI/SNF complexes. By this mechanism, SNF5 suppresses cyclin expression in an HDAC1-dependent manner [23]. In conclusion, mammalian SWI/SNF complexes are composed of dynamic units with essential roles in regulating both the activation and the repression of gene expression programmes.

3. Roles of SWI/SNF proteins in cancer

Findings of abnormalities at genetic, epigenetic as well as protein levels of SWI/SNF complexes in various cancers provide a link between chromatin remodelling and tumour suppression. Tumor suppressor role of SWI/SNF complexes was first demonstrated with loss of BRG1 and BRM expression in many cancer cell lines and arrest of growth or slower growth after introduction of BRG1 or hBRM [24]. Brg mutant mice die at early embryonic days due to growth arrest of the inner cell mass and trophoblast [25,26]. Mice with Brg 1 heterozygosity develop mammary adenocarcinomas, suggesting an occurrence of cancer prone state due to haploinsufficiency of Brg1. On the other hand, the mouse with inactivation of BRM by homologous recombination (BRM-/- mice) is born alive and develops normally. Adult mutant mice were approximately 15% heavier than control littermates. This phenomenon was suggested to be caused by increased cell proliferation, because a higher mitotic index was detected in mutant livers and it was further supported by the observation that mutant embryonic fibroblasts were significantly deficient in their ability to arrest in the G0/G1 phase of the cell cycle in response to cell confluency or DNA damage. These studies suggested that BRM plays a role in the regulation of cell proliferation in adult mice and have some defects in control of cellular proliferation [27].

Chromosome transfer studies mapped tumor suppressor gene(s) at 19p13 chromosome locus [28,29]. Studies with microsatellite analysis and functional as well as cancer tissue examination for abnormalities of candidate tumor suppressor gene indicated that chromosome 19p13 locus includes at least two putative tumor suppressor genes namely STK11/LKB1 and BRG1 [30]. STK11 maps about 8.5 Mb distally from BRG1. Loss of heterozygosity of 19p13 was reported in various cancers including thyroid cancer, sex cord stromal tumors, breast cancer, oral carcinoma, prostate cancer, pancreas carcinoma, brain tumors, colorectal carcinoma, gynecological tumors, lung cancers and ovarian carcinoma [31-46]. Some of the studies included genetic analysis of STK11/LKB1 and showed mutation in a subset of tumors especially related with Peutz-Jeugher Syndrome such as breast, colorectal, lung, pancreatic, biliary and ovarian cancer [41-49]. On the other hand, quite a lot of studies reported mutations and/or loss or various alterations of BRG1 in human cancer lines and primary tumors [50-61]. Thus genes at this chromosomal locus may involve in various type cancer exclusively or in cooperation in some cancer types. It should be also noticed that some studies showed only LOH without alteration of either one of these genes. In this situation, each of them can still be involved in carcinogenesis due to haploinsufficiency. At least haploinsufficiency of BRG1 is recognized [25-27,62], while further studies are necessary whether such a role exists for STK11/LKB1 or not. Similar to BRG1, abnormalities of BRM in various cancers have been reported [58-61,63-69].

Though the early studies of cell lines and animal models strongly suggested subunits of SWI/SNF proteins as tumor suppressor, the first definitive evidence that members of these complexes function as tumor suppressive was shown by Versteege and colleagues. They demonstrated occurrence of LOH of BAF47 (SNF5) in almost all cases of pediatric rhabdoid sarcoma, in which the other allele was mutated or silenced by methylation [70]. Inactivation of SNF5 subunit of SWI/SNF is via biallelic mutations, including deletion, nonsense, mis-sense and frameshift mutations was also shown by other studies, supporting SNF5 as a strong tumor suppressor gene at least in this kind of tumors [71-73].

SNF5 alterations have also been shown in other types of tumors though it is much rare as compared to malignant rhabdoid tumors. In a recent study, the effects of Ini1 haploinsufficiency (loss of one allele) on cell growth and immortalization in mouse embryonic fibroblasts were examined. Their results revealed that heterozygosity for Ini1 up-regulated cell growth and immortalization and that exogenous Ini1 down-regulated the growth of primary cells in a Rb-dependent manner. Furthermore, loss of Ini1 was redundant with loss of Rb function in the formation of pituitary tumors in Rb heterozygous mice and gave rise to the formation of large, atypical Rb(+/-) tumor cells lacking adrenocorticotropic hormone expression, confirming in vivo the relationship between Rb and Ini1 in tumor suppression [74]. Mutations and alterations of SNF5 were also reported in familial schwannomatosis and other cancer types [75-84]. Germ line mutations of SNF5 were detected in brain tumors and rhabdoid tumors, suggesting its link with familial cancers [85-88]. In some other tumors, no alteration of SNF was detected [89,90].

Complete loss of Snf5 in genetically engineered mouse leads to early embryonic death. However, heterozygote mice with haploinsufficient Snf5 (snf5+/-) develop tumors similar to malignant rhabdoid tumors in about one third of the animals [91-93]. On the other hand, conditional biallelic inactivation of Snf5 (Snf5-/- mice) resulted in tumors including lymphomas and rhabdoid tumors in 100% of mice [94]. Onset of these tumors occurred in a median period of 11 weeks for a single gene inactivation. When compared to this period with most commonly mutated genes in human cancer i.e. p53 and RB1, p53 loss gave rise to lymphomas and sarcomas at 20 weeks and RB1 heterozygosity together with p53 deficiency resulted in similar tumors and other cancers at 16 weeks [95]. Thus shorter onset time for tumor occurrence in Snf5 inactivation as compared to other well-known tumor suppressors indicates strong tumor suppressor character of this gene. Tumor formation in the absence of SNF5 has been supposed to be due to loss of function of the SWI/SNF complex. However, this view has been challenged by several findings of a recent research. Using both human cell lines and mouse models, Wang et al. [96] showed that cancer formation in the absence of SNF5 does not result from SWI/SNF inactivation but rather that oncogenesis is dependent on continued presence of BRG1 activation than tumor suppressor loss. Thus Snf5 loss would lead to effects more frequently associated with oncogene activation than tumor suppressor loss.

Other than BRG1 and SNF5, alterations of other member of SWI/SNF complexes have been reported in various cancer types. For example mutations of BAF180 (PBRM1) were identified in 41% of renal cell carcinomas, making this gene as the second most frequently mutated gene in these cancers after VHL50 [97]. The ARID1A subunit of SWI/SNF complexes was also recently shown to have mutation or loss of protein in primary human cancers including ovarian clear cell carcinomas, low and high grade endometrioid carcinomas [98-101].ARID1A was also rarely mutated in medulloblastoma, breast and lung cancer [102,103].

4. Alterations and roles of SWI/SNF proteins in breast cancer

Breast cancer is among the most common tumors affecting women. It is characterized by a number of genetic aberrations. Some 5-10% of cases are thought to be inherited. Estrogen plays an important role in normal physiology and malignancy of breast tissue. Biological functions of estrogen are mediated by estrogen receptor (ER). ER controls transcription of ER targeted genes by binding to estrogen responsive elements in their promoters. ATP-dependent chromatin remodeling complexes also influence this signaling pathway by changing the chromatin open/close state. In this respect, heterozygous state of a SWI/SNF subunit, Brg1 in mice leads to mammary carcinomas, indicating roles of SWI/SNF proteins in breast cancer [25]. On the other hand, BRCA1 and BRCA2 genes are already known to have roles both in familial and sporadic breast cancers [104-106]. Breast tumors of patients with germ-line mutations in the BRCA1 and BRCA2 genes have more genetic defects than sporadic breast tumors.

Bochar et al. [107] isolated a predominant form of a multiprotein BRCA1-containing complex from human cells displaying chromatin-remodeling activity using a combination of affinity- and conventional chromatographic techniques. Mass spectrometric sequencing of components of this complex proved that BRCA1 is associated with a SWI/SNF-related complex. They also demonstrated that BRCA1 directly interacts with the BRG1 subunit of the SWI/SNF complex. Furthermore, p53-mediated stimulation of transcription by BRCA1 was completely abrogated by either a dominant-negative mutant of BRG1 or the cancer-causing deletion in exon 11 of BRCA1, revealing that BRCA1 has a direct function in transcriptional control through modulation of chromatin structure [107].

To investigate abnormalities SWI/SNF complex subunits in breast cancer, Decristofaro et al. [108] determined the protein status of the core subunits of BAF170, BAF155, BAF57, BAF53a, and BAF47 in 21 breast cancer cell lines. The authors also determined the protein status of the BRM, BRG1 as well as two other proteins found in human SWI/SNF complexes, BAF180 and BAF250. A breast cancer cell line negative for the BAF57 protein was identified [108].

Deficiency of p270 protein (ARID1A) was shown in a subset of breast cancer. BAF180, a subunit of the PBAP type SWI/SNF chromatin remodeling complex maps to 3p21, in a region where frequent allele loss has been detected in various cancers. A study which used screening for tumor suppressor genes in breast cancer revealed multiple truncating mutations of PB1, which encodes the BAF180 subunit and the mutation was associated with loss of heterozygosity of the wild-type allele [109]. Functional studies showed binding of endogenous wild-type BAF180 to the p21 promoter, which was required for proper p21 expression and G1 arrest after transforming growth factor-beta and gamma-radiation treatment, making BAF180 as a physiologic mediator of p21 expression [109].

In a study, Wang et al. [110] examined the role of BAF57 in breast cancer using the cell line, BT549, which is an invasive human breast carcinoma cell line that lacks expression of BAF57 [111]. They prepared a BT549 stable cell line with expression of the full-length BAF57 protein. The results showed that BT549 clones expressing BAF57 revealed remarkable phenotypic changes, slow growth kinetics, and restoration of contact inhibition. Moreover, microarray analysis showed that BAF57-mediated cell death was associated with up-regulation of proapoptotic genes including the tumor suppressor familial cylindromatosis (CYLD). CYLD was found to be a direct target of BAF57 by chromatin immunoprecipitation analysis. Increased expression of CYLD in BT549 cells induced apoptosis, while its suppression by small interfering RNA inhibited cell death in BAF57 expressing BT549 cells, suggesting the crucial role of BAF57 in cell growth regulation and provided a novel link between hSWI/SNF chromatin remodeling factors and apoptosis [112]. P270 subunit of SWI/SNF complexes was found to be essential for normal cell cycle arrest, providing a direct biological basis to support the implication from tumor tissue screens that deficiency of p270 plays a causative role in carcinogenesis [113]. In a separate study, BAF57 was found to be an ER subtype-selective modulator that specifically regulates ERalpha-mediated transcription, linking ER with SWI/SNF proteins [114].

Harte et al. [115] identified BRD7 as a novel binding partner of BRCA1 with a yeast two-hybrid screen using a BRCA1 bait composed of amino acids 1 to 1142. To determine the functional consequences of the BRCA1-BRD7 interaction, they examined the role of BRD7 in BRCA1-dependent transcription with microarray-based expression profiling. A variety of target genes such as ERalpha was found to be coordinately regulated by BRCA1 and BRD7 complex [115]. In a recent study, two novel mutations were found in one out of 95 breast cancer samples by sequencing BAF57 gene [116].

5. Conclusion and future aspects

Important function of subunits of SWI/SNF complexes arises from their roles in chromatin remodeling and trancription regulation. Mutation and other alterations of these proteins lead to cancer development. Researches on roles of SWI/SNF subunits in development and cancer are increasingly performed yet much work is necessary for clarifying the exact functions of these genes to provide therapy for various human cancers. Promising results are noticed at the moment for usability of some of these genes as a therapeutic and diagnostic target. Thus progress on the knowledge of functions of subunits of SWI/SNF complexes as well as the relationship with other breast cancer-related molecules such as BRCA1-2 and p53 will clarify their roles in human cancer including breast cancer, which will result in their uses in cancer diagnostics as well as therapy in near future.

6. References

[1] Renan MJ. How many mutations are required for tumorigenesis? Implications from human cancer data. Mol Carcinog 7: 139-146, 1993

[2] Hinds PW and Weinberg RA. Tumor suppressor genes. Curr Opin Genet Dev 4: 135-141, 1994

[3] Knudson AG Jr. Mutation and cancer: statistical study of retinoblastoma. Proc Natl Acad Sci USA 68: 820-823, 1971

[4] Mduff FK, Hook CE, Tooze RM, Huntly BJ, Pandolfi PP, Turner SD. Determining the contribution of NPM1 heterozygosity to NPM-ALK-induced lymphomagenesis. Lab Invest. 2011 Jun 27. doi: 10.1038/labinvest.2011.96. [Epub ahead of print]

[5] Zhou XZ, Huang P, Shi R, Lee TH, Lu G, Zhang Z, Bronson R, Lu KP. The telomerase inhibitor PinX1 is a major haploinsufficient tumor suppressor essential for chromosome stability in mice. J Clin Invest 121(4):1266-82, 2011

[6] Bouwman P, Drost R, Klijn C, Pieterse M, van der Gulden H, Song JY, Szuhai K, Jonkers J. Loss of p53 partially rescues embryonic development of Palb2 knockout mice but does not foster haploinsufficiency of Palb2 in tumour suppression. J Pathol 224:10-21, 2011

[7] Wilson BG, Roberts CW. SWI/SNF nucleosome remodellers and cancer. Nat Rev Cancer 11:481-92, 2011

[8] Weissman B, Knudsen KE. Hijacking the chromatin remodeling machinery: impact of SWI/SNF perturbations in cancer. Cancer Res 69:8223-30, 2009

[9] Hargreaves DC, Crabtree GR. ATP-dependent chromatin remodeling: genetics, genomics and mechanisms. Cell Res 21:396-420, 2011

[10] Reisman D, Glaros S, Thompson EA. The SWI/SNF complex and cancer. Oncogene 28:1653-68, 2009

[11] Wu JI, Lessard J, Crabtree GR. Understanding the words of chromatin regulation. Cell 136:200-6, 2009

[12] Lessard J, Wu JI, Ranish JA, Wan M, Winslow MM, Staahl BT, Wu H, Aebersold R, Graef IA, Crabtree GR. An essential switch in subunit composition of a chromatin remodeling complex during neural development. Neuron 55:201-15, 2007

[13] Neigeborn L, Carlson M. Genes affecting the regulation of SUC2 gene expression by glucose repression in Saccharomyces cerevisiae. Genetics 108:845–858, 1984

[14] Stern M, Jensen R, Herskowitz I. Five SWI genes are required for expression of the HO gene in yeast. J Mol Biol 178:853–868, 1984

[15] Breeden L, Nasmyth K. Cell cycle control of the yeast HO gene: cis- and trans-acting regulators. Cell 48:389–397, 1987

[16] Chi TH, Wan M, Zhao K, Taniuchi I, Chen L, Littman DR, Crabtree GR. Reciprocal regulation of CD4/CD8 expression by SWI/SNF-like BAF complexes. Nature 418:195-9, 2002

[17] Wan M, Zhang J, Lai D, Jani A, Prestone-Hurlburt P, Zhao L, Ramachandran A, Schnitzler GR, Chi T. Molecular basis of CD4 repression by the Swi/Snf-like BAF chromatin remodeling complex. Eur J Immunol 39:580-8, 2009

[18] Albini S, Puri PL. SWI/SNF complexes, chromatin remodeling and skeletal myogenesis: it's time to exchange!. Exp Cell Res 316:3073-80, 2010

[19] Flowers S, Nagl NG Jr, Beck GR Jr, Moran E. Antagonistic roles for BRM and BRG1 SWI/SNF complexes in differentiation. J Biol Chem 284:10067-75, 2009

[20] Ho L, Ronan JL, Wu J, Staahl BT, Chen L, Kuo A, Lessard J, Nesvizhskii AI, Ranish J, Crabtree GR. An embryonic stem cell chromatin remodeling complex, esBAF, is essential for embryonic stem cell self-renewal and pluripotency. Proc Natl Acad Sci U S A 106:5181-6, 2009

[21] Ho L, Jothi R, Ronan JL, Cui K, Zhao K, Crabtree GR. An embryonic stem cell chromatin remodeling complex, esBAF, is an essential component of the core pluripotency transcriptional network. Proc Natl Acad Sci U S A 106:5187-91, 2009

[22] Isakoff MS, Sansam CG, Tamayo P, Subramanian A, Evans JA, Fillmore CM, Wang X, Biegel JA, Pomeroy SL, Mesirov JP, Roberts CW. Inactivation of the Snf5 tumor suppressor stimulates cell cycle progression and cooperates with p53 loss in oncogenic transformation. Proc Natl Acad Sci U S A 102:17745-50, 2005

[23] Zhang ZK, Davies KP, Allen J, Zhu L, Pestell RG, Zagzag D, Kalpana GV. Cell cycle arrest and repression of cyclin D1 transcription by INI1/hSNF5. Mol Cell Biol 22:5975-88, 2002

[24] Dunaief JL, Strober BE, Guha S, Khavari PA, Alin K, Luban J, Begemann M, Crabtree GR, Goff SP. The retinoblastoma protein and BRG1 form a complex and cooperate to induce cell cycle arrest. Cell 79:119-30, 1994

[25] Bultman, S. J. Herschkowitz JI, Godfrey V, Gebuhr TC, Yaniv M, Perou CM, Magnuson T. Characterization of mammary tumors from Brg1 heterozygous mice. Oncogene 27:460–468, 2008

[26] Bultman, S. Gebuhr T, Yee D, La Mantia C, Nicholson J, Gilliam A, Randazzo F, Metzger D, Chambon P, Crabtree G, Magnuson T. A Brg1 null mutation in the mouse reveals functional differences among mammalian SWI/ SNF complexes. Mol Cell 6:1287–1295, 2000

[27] Reyes JC, Barra J, Muchardt C, Camus A, Babinet C, Yaniv M. Altered control of cellular proliferation in the absence of mammalian brahma (SNF2alpha). EMBO J 17:6979-91, 1998

[28] Astbury C, Jackson-Cook CK, Culp SH, Paisley TE, Ware JL. Suppression of tumorigenicity in the human prostate cancer cell line M12 via microcell-mediated restoration of chromosome 19. Genes Chromosomes Cancer 31:143 - 55, 2011

[29] Gao AC, Lou W, Ichikawa T, Denmeade SR, Barrett JC, Isaacs JT. Suppression of the tumorigenicity of prostatic cancer cells by gene(s) located on human chromosome 19p13.1 - 13.2. Prostate 38:46 - 54, 1999

[30] Rodriguez-Nieto S, Sanchez-Cespedes M. BRG1 and LKB1: tales of two tumor suppressor genes on chromosome 19p and lung cancer. Carcinogenesis 30:547-54, 2009

[31] Prazeres HJ, Rodrigues F, Soares P, Naidenov P, Figueiredo P, Campos B, Lacerda M, Martins TC. Loss of heterozygosity at 19p13.2 and 2q21 in tumours from familial clusters of non-medullary thyroid carcinoma. Fam Cancer 7:141-9, 2008
[32] Kato N, Romero M, Catasus L, Prat J. The STK11/LKB1 Peutz-Jegher gene is not involved in the pathogenesis of sporadic sex cord-stromal tumors, although loss of heterozygosity at 19p13.3 indicates other gene alteration in these tumors. Hum Pathol 35:1101-4, 2004
[33] Yang TL, Su YR, Huang CS, Yu JC, Lo YL, Wu PE, Shen CY. High-resolution 19p13.2-13.3 allelotyping of breast carcinomas demonstrates frequent loss of heterozygosity. Genes Chromosomes Cancer 41:250-6, 2004
[34] Dumur CI, Dechsukhum C, Ware JL, Cofield SS, Best AM, Wilkinson DS, Garrett CT, Ferreira-Gonzalez A. Genome-wide detection of LOH in prostate cancer using human SNP microarray technology. Genomics 81:260-9, 2003
[35] Sobottka SB, Haase M, Fitze G, Hahn M, Schackert HK, Schackert G. Frequent loss of heterozygosity at the 19p13.3 locus without LKB1/STK11 mutations in human carcinoma metastases to the brain. J Neurooncol 49:187-95, 2000
[36] Oesterreich S, Allredl DC, Mohsin SK, Zhang Q, Wong H, Lee AV, Osborne CK, O'Connell P. High rates of loss of heterozygosity on chromosome 19p13 in human breast cancer. Br J Cancer 84:493-8, 2001
[37] Connolly DC, Katabuchi H, Cliby WA, Cho KR. Somatic mutations in the STK11/LKB1 gene are uncommon in rare gynecological tumor types associated with Peutz-Jegher's syndrome. Am J Pathol 156:339-45, 2000
[38] Gunduz E, Gunduz M, Ouchida M, Nagatsuka H, Beder L, Tsujigiwa H, Fukushima K, Nishizaki K, Shimizu K, Nagai N. Genetic and epigenetic alterations of BRG1 promote oral cancer development. Int J Oncol 26:201-10, 2005
[39] Sentani K, Oue N, Kondo H, Kuraoka K, Motoshita J, Ito R, Yokozaki H, Yasui W. Increased expression but not genetic alteration of BRG1, a component of the SWI/SNF complex, is associated with the advanced stage of human gastric carcinomas. Pathobiology 69:315-20, 2001
[40] Valdman A, Nordenskjöld A, Fang X, Naito A, Al-Shukri S, Larsson C, Ekman P, Li C. Mutation analysis of the BRG1 gene in prostate cancer clinical samples. Int J Oncol 22:1003-7, 2003
[41] Sato N, Rosty C, Jansen M, Fukushima N, Ueki T, Yeo CJ, Cameron JL, Iacobuzio-Donahue CA, Hruban RH, Goggins M. STK11/LKB1 Peutz-Jeghers gene inactivation in intraductal papillary-mucinous neoplasms of the pancreas. Am J Pathol 159:2017-22, 2001
[42] Trojan J, Brieger A, Raedle J, Esteller M, Zeuzem S. 5'-CpG island methylation of the LKB1/STK11 promoter and allelic loss at chromosome 19p13.3 in sporadic colorectal cancer. Gut 47:272-6, 2000
[43] Nishioka Y, Kobayashi K, Sagae S, Sugimura M, Ishioka S, Nagata M, Terasawa K, Tokino T, Kudo R. Mutational analysis of STK11 gene in ovarian carcinomas. Jpn J Cancer Res 90:629-32, 1999
[44] Wang ZJ, Churchman M, Campbell IG, Xu WH, Yan ZY, McCluggage WG, Foulkes WD, Tomlinson IP. Allele loss and mutation screen at the Peutz-Jeghers (LKB1) locus (19p13.3) in sporadic ovarian tumours. Br J Cancer 80:70-2, 1999

[45] Gill RK, Yang SH, Meerzaman D, et al. Frequent homozygous deletion of the LKB1/STK11 gene in non-small cell lung cancer. Oncogene. 2011 May 2. [Epub ahead of print]

[46] Papp J, Kovacs ME, Solyom S, Kasler M, Børresen-Dale AL, Olah E. High prevalence of germline STK11 mutations in Hungarian Peutz-Jeghers Syndrome patients. BMC Med Genet 11:169, 2010

[47] Su GH, Hruban RH, Bansal RK, Bova GS, Tang DJ, Shekher MC, Westerman AM, Entius MM, Goggins M, Yeo CJ, Kern SE. Germline and somatic mutations of the STK11/LKB1 Peutz-Jeghers gene in pancreatic and biliary cancers. Am J Pathol 154:1835-40, 1999

[48] Nakanishi C, Yamaguchi T, Iijima T, Saji S, Toi M, Mori T, Miyaki M. Germline mutation of the LKB1/STK11 gene with loss of the normal allele in an aggressive breast cancer of Peutz-Jeghers syndrome. Oncology 67:476-9, 2004

[49] McCarthy A, Lord CJ, Savage K, Grigoriadis A, Smith DP, Weigelt B, Reis-Filho JS, Ashworth A. Conditional deletion of the Lkb1 gene in the mouse mammary gland induces tumour formation. J Pathol 219:306-16, 2009

[50] Wong AK, Shanahan F, Chen Y, et al. BRG1, a component of the SWI-SNF complex, is mutated in multiple human tumor cell lines. Cancer Res 60:6171 - 7, 2000

[51] Rodriguez-Nieto S, Cañada A, Pros E, Pinto AI, Torres-Lanzas J, Lopez-Rios F, Sanchez-Verde L, Pisano DG, Sanchez-Cespedes M. Massive parallel DNA pyrosequencing analysis of the tumor suppressor BRG1/SMARCA4 in lung primary tumors. Hum Mutat 32:E1999-2017, 2011

[52] Schneppenheim R, Frühwald MC, Gesk S, Hasselblatt M, Jeibmann A, Kordes U, Kreuz M, Leuschner I, Martin Subero JI, Obser T, Oyen F, Vater I, Siebert R. Germline nonsense mutation and somatic inactivation of SMARCA4/BRG1 in a family with rhabdoid tumor predisposition syndrome. Am J Hum Genet 86:279-84, 2010

[53] Bartlett C, Orvis TJ, Rosson GS, Weissman BE. BRG1 mutations found in human cancer cell lines inactivate Rb-mediated cell-cycle arrest. J Cell Physiol 226:1989-97, 2011

[54] Medina PP, Romero OA, Kohno T, Montuenga LM, Pio R, Yokota J, Sanchez-Cespedes M. Frequent BRG1/SMARCA4-inactivating mutations in human lung cancer cell lines. Hum Mutat 29:617-22, 2008

[55] Gunduz E, Gunduz M, Nagatsuka H, Beder L, Demircan K, Tamamura R, Hatipoglu OF, Mahmut N, Katase N, Naomoto Y, Nagai N. Epigenetic alterations of BRG1 leads to cancer development through its nuclear-cytoplasmic shuttling abnormalities. Med Hypotheses 67:1313-6, 2006

[56] Medina PP, Carretero J, Fraga MF, Esteller M, Sidransky D, Sanchez-Cespedes M. Genetic and epigenetic screening for gene alterations of the chromatin-remodeling factor, SMARCA4/BRG1, in lung tumors. Genes Chromosomes Cancer 41:170-7, 2004. Erratum in: Genes Chromosomes Cancer. 2005 Feb;42(2):211.

[57] Decristofaro MF, Betz BL, Rorie CJ, Reisman DN, Wang W, Weissman BE. Characterization of SWI/SNF protein expression in human breast cancer cell lines and other malignancies. J Cell Physiol 186:136 - 45, 2001

[58] Fukuoka J, Fujii T, Shih JH, Dracheva T, Meerzaman D, Player A, Hong K, Settnek S, Gupta A, Buetow K, Hewitt S, Travis WD, Jen J. Chromatin remodeling factors and BRM/BRG1 expression as prognostic indicators in non-small cell lung cancer. Clin Cancer Res 10:4314 - 24, 2004

[59] Reisman DN, Sciarrotta J, Wang W, Funkhouser WK, Weissman BE. Loss of BRG1/BRM in human lung cancer cell lines and primary lung cancers: correlation with poor prognosis. Cancer Res 63:560 - 6, 2003
[60] Reisman DN, Strobeck MW, Betz BL, Sciariotta J, Funkhouser W Jr, Murchardt C, Yaniv M, Sherman LS, Knudsen ES, Weissman BE. Concomitant down-regulation of BRM and BRG1 in human tumor cell lines: differential effects on RB-mediated growth arrest vs CD44 expression. Oncogene 21:1196 - 207, 2002
[61] Bock VL, Lyons JG, Huang XX, Jones AM, McDonald LA, Scolyer RA, Moloney FJ, Barnetson RS, Halliday GM. BRM and BRG1 subunits of the SWI/SNF chromatin remodelling complex are downregulated upon progression of benign skin lesions into invasive tumours. Br J Dermatol 164:1221-7, 2011
[62] Glaros S, Cirrincione GM, Palanca A, Metzger D, Reisman D. Targeted knockout of BRG1 potentiates lung cancer development. Cancer Res 68:3689-96, 2008
[63] Liu G, Gramling S, Munoz D, Cheng D, Azad AK, Mirshams M, Chen Z, Xu W, Roberts H, Shepherd FA, Tsao MS, Reisman D. Two novel BRM insertion promoter sequence variants are associated with loss of BRM expression and lung cancer risk. Oncogene. 2011 Apr 11. [Epub ahead of print]
[64] Glaros S, Cirrincione GM, Muchardt C, Kleer CG, Michael CW, Reisman D. The reversible epigenetic silencing of BRM: implications for clinical targeted therapy. Oncogene 26:7058 - 66, 2007
[65] Gunduz E, Gunduz M, Ali MA, Beder L, Tamamura R, Katase N, Tominaga S, Yamanaka N, Shimizu K, Nagatsuka H. Loss of heterozygosity at the 9p21-24 region and identification of BRM as a candidate tumor suppressor gene in head and neck squamous cell carcinoma. Cancer Invest 27:661-8, 2009
[66] Shen H, Powers N, Saini N, et al. The SWI/SNF ATPase Brm is a gatekeeper of proliferative control in prostate cancer. Cancer Res 68:10154-62, 2008
[67] Moloney FJ, Lyons JG, Bock VL, Huang XX, Bugeja MJ, Halliday GM. Hotspot mutation of Brahma in non-melanoma skin cancer. J Invest Dermatol 129:1012-5, 2009
[68] Yamamichi N, Inada K, Ichinose M, et al. Frequent loss of Brm expression in gastric cancer correlates with histologic features and differentiation state. Cancer Res 67:10727-35, 2007
[69] Strobeck MW, Reisman DN, Gunawardena RW, Betz BL, Angus SP, Knudsen KE, Kowalik TF, Weissman BE, Knudsen ES. Compensation of BRG-1 function by Brm: insight into the role of the core SWI-SNF subunits in retinoblastoma tumor suppressor signaling. J Biol Chem 277:4782-9, 2002
[70] Versteege I, Sévenet N, Lange J, Rousseau-Merck MF, Ambros P, Handgretinger R, Aurias A, Delattre O. Truncating mutations of hSNF5/INI1 in aggressive paediatric cancer. Nature 394:203-6, 1998
[71] Eaton KW, Tooke LS, Wainwright LM, Judkins AR, Biegel JA. Spectrum of SMARCB1/INI1 mutations in familial and sporadic rhabdoid tumors. Pediatr Blood Cancer. 56:7-15, 2011
[72] Jackson, E. M. Sievert AJ, Gai X, Hakonarson H, Judkins AR, Tooke L, Perin JC, Xie H, Shaikh TH, Biegel JA Genomic analysis using high-density single nucleotide polymorphism-based oligonucleotide arrays and multiplex ligation-dependent probe amplification provides a comprehensive analysis of INI1/SMARCB1 in malignant rhabdoid tumors. Clin Cancer Res 15:1923–1930, 2009

[73] Biegel, J. A. Zhou JY, Rorke LB, Stenstrom C, Wainwright LM, Fogelgren B. Germ-line and acquired mutations of INI1 in atypical teratoid and rhabdoid tumors. Cancer Res 59:74–79, 1999

[74] Guidi CJ, Mudhasani R, Hoover K, Koff A, Leav I, Imbalzano AN, Jones SN. Functional interaction of the retinoblastoma and Ini1/Snf5 tumor suppressors in cell growth and pituitary tumorigenesis. Cancer Res 66:8076-82, 2006

[75] Sevenet N, Lellouch-Tubiana A, Schofield D, Hoang-Xuan K, Gessler M, Birnbaum D, Jeanpierre C, Jouvet A, Delattre O. Constitutional mutations of the hSNF5/INI1 gene predispose to a variety of cancers. Am J Hum Genet 65:1342–1348, 1999

[76] Trobaugh-Lotrario AD, Tomlinson GE, Finegold MJ, Gore L, Feusner JH. Small cell undifferentiated variant of hepatoblastoma: adverse clinical and molecular features similar to rhabdoid tumors. Pediatr Blood Cancer 52:328–334, 2009

[77] Kohashi K, Izumi T, Oda Y, Yamamoto H, Tamiya S, Taguchi T, Iwamoto Y, Hasegawa T, Tsuneyoshi M. Infrequent SMARCB1/INI1 gene alteration in epithelioid sarcoma: a useful tool in distinguishing epithelioid sarcoma from malignant rhabdoid tumor. Hum Pathol 40:349-55, 2009

[78] Kohashi, K. Oda Y, Yamamoto H, Tamiya S, Oshiro Y, Izumi T, Taguchi T, Tsuneyoshi M. SMARCB1/INI1 protein expression in round cell soft tissue sarcomas associated with chromosomal translocations involving EWS: a special reference to SMARCB1/INI1 negative variant extraskeletal myxoid chondrosarcoma. Am J Surg Pathol 32:1168–1174, 2008

[79] Kreiger PA, Judkins AR, Russo PA, Biegel JA, Lestini BJ, Assanasen C, Pawel BR. Loss of INI1 expression defines a unique subset of pediatric undifferentiated soft tissue sarcomas. Mod Pathol 22:142–150, 2009

[80] Modena P, Lualdi E, Facchinetti F, Galli L, Teixeira MR, Pilotti S, Sozzi G. SMARCB1/INI1 tumor suppressor gene is frequently inactivated in epithelioid sarcomas. Cancer Res. 65:4012–4019, 2005

[81] Schmitz U, Mueller W, Weber M, Sévenet N, Delattre O, von Deimling A. INI1 mutations in meningiomas at a potential hotspot in exon 9. Br J Cancer 84:199-201, 2001

[82] Lin H, Wong RP, Martinka M, Li G. Loss of SNF5 expression correlates with poor patient survival in melanoma. Clin Cancer Res 15:6404-11, 2009

[83] Mobley BC, McKenney JK, Bangs CD, Callahan K, Yeom KW, Schneppenheim R, Hayden MG, Cherry AM, Gokden M, Edwards MS, Fisher PG, Vogel H. Loss of SMARCB1/INI1 expression in poorly differentiated chordomas. Acta Neuropathol 120:745–753, 2010

[84] Gessi M, Giangaspero F, Pietsch T. Atypical teratoid/rhabdoid tumors and choroid plexus tumors: when genetics "surprise" pathology. Brain Pathol 13:409-1, 2003

[85] Hulsebos TJ, Plomp AS, Wolterman RA, Robanus-Maandag EC, Baas F, Wesseling P. Germline mutation of INI1/ SMARCB1 in familial schwannomatosis. Am J Hum Genet 80:805–810, 2007

[86] Christiaans I, Kenter SB, Brink HC, van Os TA, Baas F, van den Munckhof P, Kidd AM, Hulsebos TJ. Germline SMARCB1 mutation and somatic NF2 mutations in familial multiple meningiomas. J Med Genet 48:93-7, 2011

[87] Bourdeaut F, Lequin D, Brugières L, et al. Frequent hSNF5/INI1 germline mutations in patients with rhabdoid tumor. Clin Cancer Res 17:31-8, 2011

[88] Rousseau G, Noguchi T, Bourdon V, Sobol H, Olschwang S. SMARCB1/INI1 germline mutations contribute to 10% of sporadic schwannomatosis. BMC Neurol 11:9, 2011
[89] Yamamoto H, Kohashi K, Tsuneyoshi M, Oda Y. Heterozygosity Loss at 22q and Lack of INI1 Gene Mutation in Gastrointestinal Stromal Tumor. Pathobiology 78:132-9, 2011
[90] Mori N, Inoue K, Okada M, Motoji T. Absence of Mutations on the SNF5 Gene in Hematological Neoplasms with Chromosome 22 Abnormalities. Acta Haematol 126:69-75, 2011
[91] Roberts CW, Galusha SA, McMenamin ME, Fletcher CD, Orkin SH. Haploinsufficiency of Snf5 (integrase interactor 1) predisposes to malignant rhabdoid tumors in mice. Proc Natl Acad Sci USA 97:13796–13800, 2000
[92] Klochendler-Yeivin, A. Fiette L, Barra J, Muchardt C, Babinet C, Yaniv M. The murine SNF5/INI1 chromatin remodeling factor is essential for embryonic development and tumor suppression. EMBO Rep 1:500–506, 2000
[93] Guidi, C. J. Sands AT, Zambrowicz BP, Turner TK, Demers DA, Webster W, Smith TW, Imbalzano AN, Jones SN. Disruption of Ini1 leads to peri-implantation lethality and tumorigenesis in mice. Mol Cell Biol 21:3598–3603, 2001
[94] Roberts CW, Leroux MM, Fleming MD, Orkin SH. Highly penetrant, rapid tumorigenesis through conditional inversion of the tumor suppressor gene Snf5. Cancer Cell 2:415–425, 2002
[95] Williams BO, Remington L, Albert DM, Mukai S, Bronson RT, Jacks T. Cooperative tumorigenic effects of germline mutations in Rb and p53. Nat Genet 7:480-4, 1994
[96] Wang X, Sansam CG, Thom CS, Metzger D, Evans JA, Nguyen PT, Roberts CW. Oncogenesis caused by loss of the SNF5 tumor suppressor is dependent on activity of BRG1, the ATPase of the SWI/SNF chromatin remodeling complex. Cancer Res 69:8094-101, 2009
[97] Varela I, Tarpey P, Raine K, et al. Exome sequencing identifies frequent mutation of the SWI/SNF complex gene PBRM1 in renal carcinoma. Nature 469:539-42, 2011
[98] Wiegand KC, Lee AF, Al-Agha OM, Chow C, Kalloger SE, Scott DW, Steidl C, Wiseman SM, Gascoyne RD, Gilks B, Huntsman DG. Loss of BAF250a (ARID1A) is frequent in high-grade endometrial carcinomas. J Pathol 224:328-33, 2011
[99] Guan B, Mao TL, Panuganti PK, Kuhn E, Kurman RJ, Maeda D, Chen E, Jeng YM, Wang TL, Shih IeM. Mutation and loss of expression of ARID1A in uterine low-grade endometrioid carcinoma. Am J Surg Pathol 35:625-32, 2011
[100] Wiegand KC, Shah SP, Al-Agha OM et al. ARID1A mutations in endometriosis-associated ovarian carcinomas. N Engl J Med 363:1532–1543, 2010
[101] Jones, S. Wang TL, Shih IeM, et al. Frequent mutations of chromatin remodeling gene ARID1A in ovarian clear carcinoma. Science 330:228–231, 2010
[102] Parsons, D. W. Li M, Zhang X, et al. The Genetic Landscape of the Childhood Cancer Medulloblastoma. Science 331:435–439, 2011
[103] Huang J, Zhao YL, Li Y, Fletcher JA, Xiao S. Genomic and functional evidence for an ARID1A tumor suppressor role. Genes Chromosom Cancer 46:745–750, 2007
[104] Wang F, Fang Q, Ge Z, Yu N, Xu S, Fan X. Common BRCA1 and BRCA2 mutations in breast cancer families: a meta-analysis from systematic review. Mol Biol Rep. 2011 Jun 4. [Epub ahead of print]

[105] Nanda R. Targeting" triple-negative breast cancer: the lessons learned from BRCA1-associated breast cancers. Semin Oncol 38:254-62, 2011
[106] Milne RL, Antoniou AC. Genetic modifiers of cancer risk for BRCA1 and BRCA2 mutation carriers. Ann Oncol Suppl 1:i11-7, 2011
[107] Bochar DA, Wang L, Beniya H, Kinev A, Xue Y, Lane WS, Wang W, Kashanchi F, Shiekhattar R. BRCA1 is associated with a human SWI/SNF-related complex: linking chromatin remodeling to breast cancer. Cell 102:257-65, 2000
[108] Decristofaro MF, Betz BL, Rorie CJ, Reisman DN, Wang W, Weissman BE. Characterization of SWI/SNF protein expression in human breast cancer cell lines and other malignancies. J Cell Physiol 186:136-45, 2001
[109] Wang X, Nagl NG Jr, Flowers S, Zweitzig D, Dallas PB, Moran E. Expression of p270 (ARID1A), a component of human SWI/SNF complexes, in human tumors. Int J Cancer 112:636, 2004
[110] Xia W, Nagase S, Montia AG, Kalachikov SM, Keniry M, Su T, Memeo L, Hibshoosh H, Parsons R. BAF180 is a critical regulator of p21 induction and a tumor suppressor mutated in breast cancer. Cancer Res 68:1667-74, 2008
[111] Kiskinis E, García-Pedrero JM, Villaronga MA, Parker MG, Belandia B. Identification of BAF57 mutations in human breast cancer cell lines. Breast Cancer Res Treat 98:191-8, 2006
[112] Wang L, Baiocchi RA, Pal S, Mosialos G, Caligiuri M, Sif S. The BRG1- and hBRM-associated factor BAF57 induces apoptosis by stimulating expression of the cylindromatosis tumor suppressor gene. Mol Cell Biol 25:7953-65, 2005
[113] Nagl NG Jr, Patsialou A, Haines DS, Dallas PB, Beck GR Jr, Moran E. The p270 (ARID1A/SMARCF1) subunit of mammalian SWI/SNF-related complexes is essential for normal cell cycle arrest. Cancer Res 65:9236-44, 2005
[114] García-Pedrero JM, Kiskinis E, Parker MG, Belandia B. The SWI/SNF chromatin remodeling subunit BAF57 is a critical regulator of estrogen receptor function in breast cancer cells. J Biol Chem 281:22656-64, 2006
[115] Harte MT, O'Brien GJ, Ryan NM, Gorski JJ, Savage KI, Crawford NT, Mullan PB, Harkin DP. BRD7, a subunit of SWI/SNF complexes, binds directly to BRCA1 and regulates BRCA1-dependent transcription. Cancer Res 70:2538-47, 2010
[116] Villaronga MA, López-Mateo I, Markert L, Espinosa E, Fresno Vara JA, Belandia B. Identification and characterization of novel potentially oncogenic mutations in the human BAF57 gene in a breast cancer patient.Breast Cancer Res Treat. 2011 Apr 5. [Epub ahead of print]

17

p53, p63 and p73 Network in Breast Cancers

Chee-Onn Leong
International Medical University,
Malaysia

1. Introduction

Inactivation of the tumor suppressor p53 is the single most common genetic defect in all human cancers. The p53 tumor suppressor is critically important in regulation of cell cycle progression, senescence, differentiation, DNA repair and apoptosis. The discovery of two closely related homologues, p63 and p73, in 1997 generated instant excitement and quick expectations about their tumor suppressor functions. However, despite a remarkable structural and partial functional similarity among p53, initial p63 and p73 mouse knockout studies revealed an unexpected functional diversity among them. p63 and p73 knockouts exhibit severe developmental abnormalities but no increased cancer susceptibility. While p53 is frequently mutated during tumorigenesis (in over 50% of human tumors), p63 and p73 are rarely mutated. Instead, the p63 locus is amplified in squamous cell carcinomas (Bjorkqvist et al., 1998; Massion et al., 2003) and p73 is overexpressed in many tumor types including breast cancers (Moll and Slade, 2004; Zaika and El-Rifai, 2006; Zaika et al., 1999). Although p63 and p73 can activate apoptosis *in vitro,* it is clear that they are not classic Knudson-like tumor suppressors like p53.

Throughout the years, impressive number of evidences has been uncovered, suggesting that the p53-family play an important role in breast cancers. The emerging picture is that of an interconnected pathway, in which all p53-family proteins are involved in the response to oncogenic stress and physiological inputs. The p53/p63/p73 family members are capable of interacting in many ways that involve direct or indirect protein interactions, regulation of same target gene promoter and regulation of each other's promoters. As such, fluctuations in the levels of selected p53 family members (or their isoforms) might change the relative availability of shared protein partners, as multiple p53-family proteins compete for interaction. Also, differential expression of selected interactors - linked with genetic variation - may distinguish the response of the p53 pathway to the same potentially oncogenic stimuli in diverse individuals.

Despite the recent advances in understanding the unique roles of p53 family protein in breast cancers, there are many outstanding questions. What are the unique functions of the TA and ΔN isoforms of p63 and p73? How is individual p53 family member mediates gene expression regulated by the interaction with mutant p53 and other family member and their splicing variants in the cell? What are the patterns of p53 family isoform expression during normal development and tumorigenesis? What are the upstream signaling pathways that regulate individual p53 family member? What are the p53, p63 and p73 target genes? Do p53, p63 and p73 regulate distinct and/or overlapping sets of genes? Understanding the complexity of these interactions allow us to delineate the function of p53 family in human tumorigenesis and enable the development of new cancer therapeutics.

2. The origins and gene architecture of the p53 family proteins

The tumor suppressor gene, p53, was discovered in 1979 (Lane and Crawford, 1979; Linzer and Levine, 1979). Until recently, *p53* was thought to be a unique gene with no genetic paralogues. In 1997, however, Caput and coworkers serendiptiously identified a human homolog of p53 which they called p73 (Irwin and Kaelin, 2001; Kaelin, 1999; Kaghad et al., 1997). Shortly thereafter, several groups identified a third member of the family variably called Ket, p40, p51, p73L and p63 (Irwin and Kaelin, 2001; Kaelin, 1999; Osada et al., 1998; Schmale and Bamberger, 1997; Senoo et al., 1998; Trink et al., 1998; Yang et al., 1998). While p53 was discovered first, evolutionary conservation of DNA sequence suggests that p63 arose first during evolution, then p73 and finally p53 (Johnson et al., 2005).

Like many transcription factors, p53 are modular proteins with a conserved N-terminal transcriptional activation domain (TA), central DNA-binding domain (DBD) and a C-terminal oligomerization domain (OD) (Fig. 1) (Arrowsmith, 1999). The DBD has the highest degree of homology, where p63 and p73 share 65% amino-acid identity with p53, and even higher identity with each other. All three genes express many spliced isoforms – a feature that was thought to be unique for p63 and p73 but has recently found to be true for p53.

The existence of an internal promoter within the p53 family was first discovered in *p63* (Yang et al., 1998). The human and mouse *p63* genes express at least three alternatively spliced C-terminal isoforms (α, β, γ), and can be transcribed from an alternative promoter located in the intron 3 (Fig. 1). The transactivating isoforms (TAp63) are generated using the promoter upstream of exon 1 while the alternative promoter in intron 3 leads to the expression of N-terminal truncated isoforms (ΔNp63) lacking the transactivation domain. Altogether, the *p63* gene expresses at least six mRNA variants which encode for six different p63 protein isoforms (TAp63α, TAp63β, TAp63γ, ΔNp63α, ΔNp63β, and ΔNp63γ) (Murray-Zmijewski et al., 2006).

The p73 gene expresses at least seven alternatively spliced C-terminal isoforms (α, β, γ, δ, ε, ζ and η) and at least four alternatively spliced N-terminal isoforms (Melino et al., 2003; Moll and Slade, 2004; Stiewe et al., 2002b). Like p63, the p73 gene can be transcribed from an alternative promoter located in the intron 3 (Fig. 1). The transactivating isoforms are generated by the activity of the promoter upstream of exon 1 while the alternative promoter in intron 3 leads to the expression of the N-terminal truncated isoforms (ΔNp73) lacking the transactivation domain. Altogether, the p73 gene expresses at least 35 mRNA variants, which can encode theoretically 29 different p73 protein isoforms (Fig. 1). So far, 14 different p73 protein isoforms have been described. In contrast to p63, p73 isoforms can be initiated from different ATG and contain different part of the N-terminal domain, suggesting that they can have distinct protein interactions and specific activities (Murray-Zmijewski et al., 2006).

3. Developmental phenotypes of p53, p63 and p73 knockout mice

Since p53 is a powerful tumor suppressor gene, its loss in mice predisposes the animals to cancers of various organs (involving tissues such as blood, muscle and bone) with no visible developmental defects. Similarly, human patients with Li Fraumeni syndrome, the disease

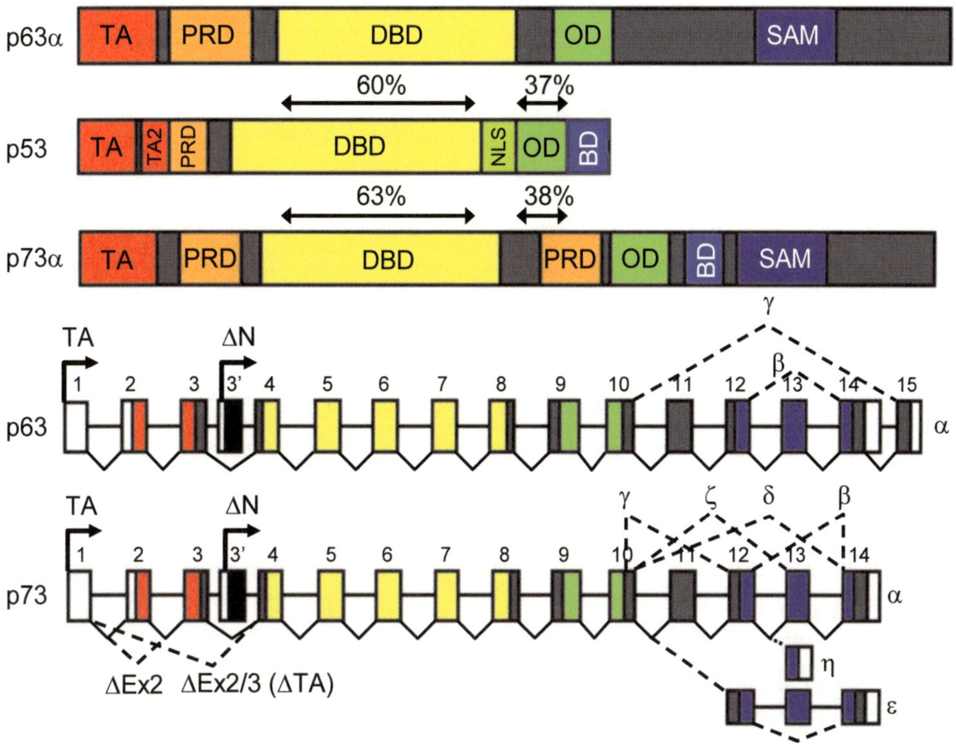

Fig. 1. **Gene architecture of the p53 family.** The p53 family includes the three genes p53, p63, and p73. Each of them has a modular structure consisting of the transactivation domain (TA), the DNA binding domain (DBD), and the oligomerization domain (OD). In addition to the 3 common domains, p63 and p73 also harbor a C-terminal sterile alpha-motif (SAM) domain in the α isoform. All p53 family genes are expressed as two major types: the full-length proteins containing the TA domain and ΔN proteins missing the TA domain. The P1 promoter in the 5′-untranslated region produces TA proteins that are transcriptionally active, whereas the P2 promoter produces ΔN proteins with dominant-negative functions toward themselves and toward wild-type p53. In addition, both p63 and p73 also undergo extensive C-terminal alternative splicing generating a myriad of isoforms with different transcriptional activity and specificity.

caused by germ line mutation of human p53, also predisposes to various cancer especially breast cancers (Johnson et al., 2005). While p53 seems to play little role in embryonic development, the p63 and p73 deficient mice have severe developmental abnormalities (Westfall and Pietenpol, 2004).

3.1 p63 in development: Role in epithelial differentiation and proliferation

p63-deficient mice are born alive but the limbs are absent or truncated owing to a malfunction of the apical ectodermal ridge (Mills et al., 1999; Yang et al., 1999). They fail to develop a stratified epidermis and most epithelial tissues (for example, hair follicles, teeth, prostate, lacrimal and salivary glands, and mammary glands), and eventually die from dehydration within hours of birth (Stiewe, 2007). Reminiscent of the knockout phenotype in mice, heterozygous germ line point mutations of p63 in humans also cause striking autosomal dominant developmental disorders including ectrodactyly-ectodermal dysplasia (EEC) (Celli et al., 1999), ankyloblepharon-ectodermal dysplasia clefting (Hay-Wells Syndrome) (Fomenkov et al., 2003), acro-dermato-ungual-lacrimal-tooth (ADULT) syndrome (Duijf et al., 2002), limb-mammary syndrome (LMF) (van Bokhoven et al., 2001), Rapp-Hodgkin syndrome (Chan et al., 2005), and split hand-split foot malformation syndrome (Brunner et al., 2002; Johnson et al., 2005; van Bokhoven et al., 2001).

Although the p63-deficient mice and human cases showed prominent phenotypes, the actual function of p63 in developmental processes remain controversial. The two groups that generated the p63-deficient mice reported identical phenotypes, the conclusions drawn from examination of the murine tissues differed (Westfall and Pietenpol, 2004). In one case clumps of differentiated cells were detected in the epidermis (Yang et al., 1999), whereas in the other, uncommitted ectodermal cells covered the body surface (Mills et al., 1999). This lead to two divergent points of view emerged from these analyses: one group attributed the p63-null phenotype to an absence of lineage commitment and an early block in epithelial differentiation (Mills et al., 1999); the other postulated that the phenotype was secondary to a defect in epithelial stem-cell renewal (Yang et al., 1999). It thus remained uncertain whether the primary function of p63 was in control of differentiation or self-renewal, or both (Blanpain and Fuchs, 2007).

Subsequent studies on p63 attempted to clarify this issue, but were further complicated with the discovery that the two principal isoforms of p63, ΔNp63 and TAp63, each of which have distinct roles in epithelial development. When transgenic mice expressing either TAp63 and/or ΔNp63 were bred on the p63-null background, mice expressing ΔNp63, but not TAp63, partially rescued basal epidermal gene expression, whereas only mice coexpressing both isoforms presented a significant improvement in expression of terminal differentiation marker. This data is consistent with the notion that ΔNp63 governs basal-epidermal gene expression, whereas TAp63 (possibly together with ΔNp63) promote terminal differentiation. Taken together, these studies supported a role for p63 in differentiation and not self-renewal. However, a later study by Senoo et al. (2007) demonstrated that p63 is not required for lineage commitment and differentiation of epithelial cells, as these cells present the typical markers for epithelial development and, in the case of the thymic epithelia, are fully competent to support the maturation of developing T cells in the thymus (Senoo et al., 2007). The study provides compelling evidence that p63 functions specifically to maintain the extraordinary proliferative capacity of the epithelial stem cells of the thymus and epidermis, suggesting a general function of the p63 transcription factor in maintaining the stem cells of a broad array of stratified epithelia. Thus, the question whether p63 functions in control of differentiation, self-renewal, or both remain debatable.

3.2 p73 in development: Role in neuronal and pheromonal pathways

The p73 knock-out mice have profound developmental defects including hippocampal dysgenesis, hydrocephalus, chronic infections and inflammation (Abraham and Meyer, 2003). They also exhibit abnormal reproductive and social behavior due to defects in pheromone detection, attributed to a dysfunctional nasal organ that normally expresses high levels of p73 (Johnson et al., 2005). The tissue specificity of the p73 deficient phenotype (concentrated to the brain and related structures) may be associated with variable patterns of isoforms expressed in brain vs. other tissues (Hu et al., 2000; Johnson et al., 2005).

ΔNp73 is the predominant isoform in the developing mouse brain and might act as a transcriptional repressor (Pozniak et al., 2000; Yang et al., 1998). *In situ* hybridization reveals strong ΔNp73 expression in E12.5 fetal mouse brain in the preplate layer, bed nucleus of stria terminalis, choroid plexus, vomeronasal area, and preoptic area (Yang et al., 2000). Moreover, ΔNp73 is the only form of p73 found in mouse brain and the sympathetic superior cervical ganglia in P10 neonatal mice (Pozniak et al., 2000). Functional studies and knockout mice showed ΔNp73 is required to counteract p53-mediated neuronal death during the normal development of the mouse neuronal system (Pozniak et al., 2000). Withdrawal of nerve growth factor, an obligate survival factor for mouse sympathetic neurons, leads to p53 induction and p53-dependent cell death. In pull-down assays, mixed protein complexes of p53/ΔNp73 were demonstrated, suggesting one biochemical basis for transdominance in addition to possible promoter competition. Together, these data demonstrated that ΔNp73 is downstream of nerve growth factor in the nerve growth factor survival pathway and explains why p73-deficient mice, missing all forms of p73 including protective ΔNp73, undergo accelerated neuronal death in postnatal superior cervical ganglia (Moll and Slade, 2004; Pozniak et al., 2000).

To date, there are no human developmental syndromes associated with germ line p73 mutations (Johnson et al., 2005). Unlike p53-decifiency, p73 knock-out mice show no increased susceptibility to spontaneous tumorigenesis (Stiewe and Putzer, 2002; Yang et al., 2000).

4. Role of p53 family in breast malignancy: Tumor suppressor or oncogene?

p53 is a powerful tumor suppressor, as proven by a wealth of in vivo models and dramatically confirmed by frequent mutation in human cancers. However, the role of p63 and p73 in tumor suppression is less obvious, because they are rarely deleted or mutated in cancer and the respective homozygous knockout mice die tumor-free from developmental defects in the initial studies.

4.1 p63 and cancer

p63, mainly its ΔN isoform, is highly expressed in embryonic epidermis and act as a molecular switch for initiation of an epithelial stratification program (Koster et al., 2004). In postnatal epidermis, ΔNp63 expression is restricted to the nuclei of basal cells of normal epithelia (skin, esophagus, tonsil, prostate, urothelium, ectocervix, and vagina) and to certain populations of basal cells in glandular structures of prostate, breast, and bronchi (Di Como et al., 2002; Yang et al., 1998). Specifically, p63 is expressed in myoepithelial cells of the breast that play an important role in differentiation and carcinogenesis of the breast (Davis et al., 2002; Garraway et al., 2003; Moll and Slade, 2004; Reis-Filho et al., 2003a; Ribeiro-Silva et al., 2003). p63 expression was not detected in mesenchymal, neural, endothelial, smooth muscle or adipose cells consistent with restricted p63 expression in squamous and basal epithelial tissues (Reis-Filho et al., 2003b; Westfall and Pietenpol, 2004).

The initial findings showed that ΔNp63α can act antagonistically toward p53 (Yang et al., 1998). Subsequent studies found dysregulated expression of p63, sometimes in conjunction with amplification of its genomic region at 3q27-28 in a many human epithelial cancers (Crook et al., 2000; Hibi et al., 2000; Massion et al., 2003; Park et al., 2000; Yamaguchi et al., 2000). Amplification of the p63 gene frequently leads to overexpression of the ΔNp63α variant (Hibi et al., 2000). Regardless, ΔNp63α have been reported to be frequently overexpressed in bladder, breast, cervix, head and neck, lung, prostate and nasopharyngeal carcinoma (Crook et al., 2000; Moll and Slade, 2004; Westfall and Pietenpol, 2004). Overexpression of the ΔNp63 variant in Rat 1a cells have also been shown to increase growth of these cells in soft agar and as xenograft tumors (Hibi et al., 2000). Thus, the maintenance of the ΔNp63 isoforms in squamous cancers may contribute to keeping the cells in a stem cell-like phenotype, thereby promoting tumor growth. Of note, analysis of p63 sequence isolated from various human tumors and numerous human cancer cell lines showed that p63 rarely, if ever, mutated (Hagiwara et al., 1999; Osada et al., 1998). Collectively these data suggest that p63 does not function as a tumor suppressor but rather as an oncogene (Westfall and Pietenpol, 2004).

Nevertheless, studies on the TA isoform of p63 suggest an opposite view. Transient transfection of TAp63 has been shown to induce cell cycle arrest and apoptosis (Osada et al., 1998; Westfall and Pietenpol, 2004; Yang et al., 1998). The TAp63 isoforms are able to bind to DNA through p53 response element (p53RE) and activate transcription of a subset of p53 target genes (Murray-Zmijewski et al., 2006). Interestingly, TAp63γ had the greatest transactivation activity and TAp63α had the minimal activity (Westfall and Pietenpol, 2004). The ΔNp63 isoforms can also bind DNA through p53RE and can exert dominant-negative effects over p53, p73 and p63 activities by either competing for DNA binding sites or by direct protein interaction (Benard et al., 2003). Moreover, ΔNp63 isoforms were also shown to directly activate specific gene targets not induced by TA isoforms (Dohn et al., 2001; Wu et al., 2003). Thus, p63 has the ability to regulate a number of genes with diverse roles and possesses opposing regulatory effect by expressing different amount of TAp63 and ΔNp63 isoforms. Thus, an abnormal alteration in expression of these isoforms is likely to play an important role in tumorigenesis.

4.2 p73 and cancer

Like p63, p73 is rarely, if ever mutated in cancers. Unlike p63 which is frequently amplified in epithelial cancers, p73 frequently undergoes loss of heterozygosity in breast and colon cancer, neuroblastoma, oligodendroglioma, and melanoma. This fact, in conjunction with the functional similarity to p53, originally led to the proposal that p73 is a tumor suppressor gene (Kaghad et al., 1997). Genetic data on most cancer types, however, exclude p73 as a classic Knudson-type tumor suppressor, which by definition is targeted to undergo loss of expression or function during tumorigenesis. To date, loss of function mutations in p73 are vanishingly rare (0.6%). Moreover, imprinting of the p73 locus, initially thought to be an epigenetic explanation to satisfy the two-hit hypothesis, is rather uncommon and, if present, varies from tissue to tissue and person to person and does not correlate with p73 expression levels (Kovalev et al., 1998; Moll and Slade, 2004; Nomoto et al., 1998; Tsao et al., 1999; Zaika et al., 1999).

In fact, TAp73 overexpression has been found in different tumor types including tumors of breast (Leong et al., 2007; Zaika et al., 1999), neuroblastoma (Kovalev et al., 1998), lung (Mai et al., 1998; Tokuchi et al., 1999), esophagus (Cai et al., 2000), stomach (Kang et al., 2000), colon (Sunahara et al., 1998), bladder (Chi et al., 1999; Yokomizo et al., 1999), ovarian cancer (Chen et al., 2000; Ng et al., 2000; Zwahlen et al., 2000), liver cancer (Tannapfel et al., 1999b), cholangiocellular carcinoma (Tannapfel et al., 1999a), colon carcinoma (Sun, 2002), and head and neck squamous carcinoma (Choi et al., 2002; Rocco et al., 2006; Weber et al., 2002). Of note, primary tumors and tumor cell lines with p73 overexpression tend to simultaneously overexpress a complex profile of shorter C-terminal splice variants (p73γ, p73δ, p73δ, and p73ϕ), whereas the normal tissue of origin is limited to the expression of p73α and p73β (Zaika et al., 1999). Importantly, patients with high global p73 protein expression had a worse survival than patients with undetectable levels (Moll and Slade, 2004; Sun, 2002; Tannapfel et al., 1999b).

Little is known about which genes are regulated specifically by p73 under physiological conditions. When overexpressed p73 also binds to p53 DNA target sites, transactivates p53-responsive genes and is capable of inducing cell cycle arrest and apoptosis in mammalian cells in a p53-like manner (Jost et al., 1997; Kaghad et al., 1997; Stiewe and Putzer, 2002). For example, p73 can activate the promoters of several p53-responsive genes, including *p21, BAX, PUMA, MDM2, GADD45, 14-3-3σ, cyclin G, IGFBP3,* and *p53R2* (Irwin and Kaelin, 2001; Jost et al., 1997; Kaghad et al., 1997; Lee and La Thangue, 1999; Nakano et al., 2000; Ueda et al., 1999; Vikhanskaya et al., 2001; Yang et al., 1998; Yu et al., 1999; Zhu et al., 1998). Nonetheless, there is evidence that p73 can activate many other genes which are not p53 target genes. For example, aquaporin 3 (AQP3), a glycerol and water transporter, has been shown to be a specific p73-responsive gene. It is speculated, that in p73-deficient mice lack of AQP3 induction accounts for the defects in production or reabsorption of cerebrospinal fluid, resulting in hydrocephalus (Stiewe and Putzer, 2002; Zheng and Chen, 2001).

Numerous reports also indicating a quantitative difference in the transcriptional activity of the various p73 splice variants. For example, the TAp73β is a more potent transcriptional activator than TAp73α (De Laurenzi et al., 1998; Lee and La Thangue, 1999; Yu et al., 1999; Zhu et al., 1998). Likewise TAp73β is more potent than TAp73α as an inducer of apoptosis, suggesting that TAp73α contains an 'inhibitory' region not included in the β-isoform. Consistently, a C-terminal deletion mutant of TAp73α lacking the putative inhibitory region showed a significantly higher level of transcriptional activity than wild-type TAp73α (Ozaki et al., 1999; Ueda et al., 2001). Moreover, the transcriptional activity of TAp73β was reduced *in trans* by co-expression with either TAp73α or p73ε, which bears an identical C-terminal structure as TAp73α (Ueda et al., 2001). This suppression effect is most likely mediated by inter-variant associations as it depends on the presence of the oligomerization domain. These observations indicate that p73-mediated gene expression is regulated by the interaction of all p73 isoforms present in the cell. The current data therefore indicate the existence of transciptional specificity among the p53-family members with pronounced differences between p53 and p73 on the one hand and between the various p73 isoforms on the other hand (Stiewe and Putzer, 2002).

5. Regulation of p53 family functions

The p53 family proteins are entangled in a regulatory network with positive or negative modulators. Many regulatory pathways may be shared by multiple p53-family proteins, with similar or different effects (Fig. 2).

5.1 Upstream regulation of p53 family members

One of the clear differences that discriminate p53 family members is the fact that they response to viral oncoproteins differently. Adenovirus E1B55, human papilloma virus E6 protein, and SV40 T antigen bind to and inactivate p53 during viral transformation (Fig. 2)

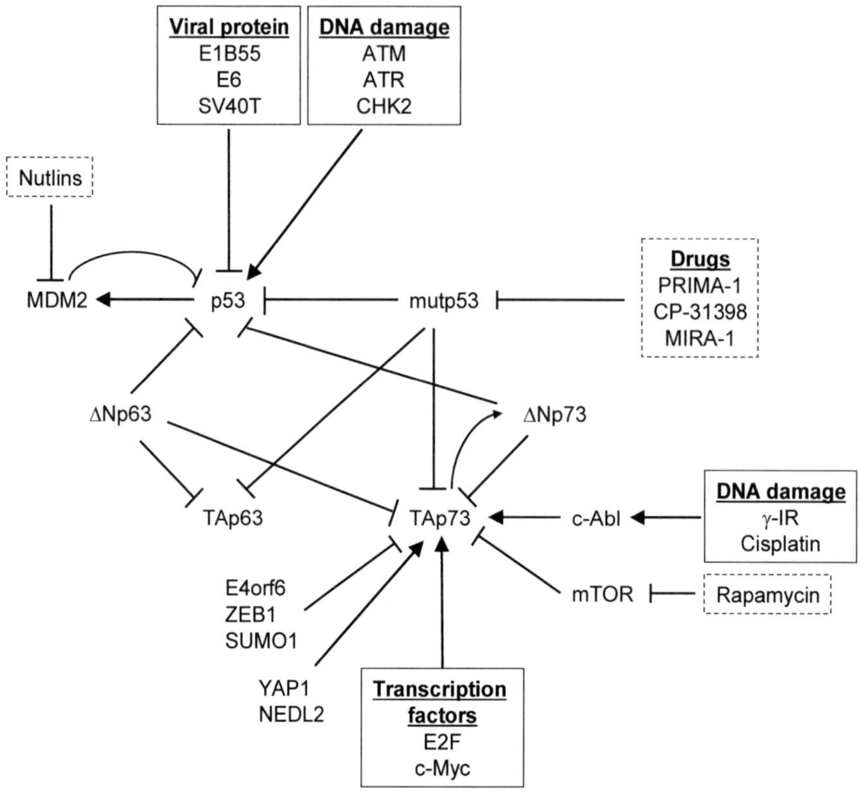

Fig. 2. The p53 family network and its regulation.

(Lechner et al., 1992; Linzer and Levine, 1979; Sarnow et al., 1982; Yew and Berk, 1992). These three proteins, however, do not bind to p73 (Dobbelstein and Roth, 1998; Marin et al., 1998; Roth et al., 1998; Steegenga et al., 1999). In fact, p73β can induce growth inhibition and apoptosis in cancer cells that produce E6 (Prabhu et al., 1998). Likewise, E6 and SV40 T antigen do not interact with p63 (Roth and Dobbelstein, 1999). The adenoviral protein E4orf6 also binds to and antagonizes p53, but there have been conflicting reports as to whether it interacts with p73. Roth *et al.* (1998) reported that E4orf6 does not affect p73 stability or the ability of p73 to activate transcription (Roth et al., 1998). Two other groups reported that E4orf6 binds to the C-terminus of p73 and blocks transcriptional activation and colony suppression by p73 (Higashino et al., 1998; Steegenga et al., 1999). Thus, certain viral oncoproteins preferentially inactivate p53 while sparing p63 and p73, despite the high degree of similarity between these three proteins (Fig. 2).

Several reports have shown that the cellular oncogenes E2F1 and c-Myc can induce and activate the endogenous TAp73α and TAp73β proteins for target gene transactivation, apoptosis, and growth suppression in p53-deficient human tumor cells (Irwin et al., 2000; Lissy et al., 2000; Stiewe and Putzer, 2000; Zaika et al., 2001). E2F1 is a specific and direct transcriptional activator of TAp73 but not p63 (Fig. 2) (Irwin et al., 2000; Stiewe and Putzer, 2000). Because oncogene deregulation of E2F1 and c-Myc are one of the most common genetic alterations in human tumors, these findings might provide a physiologic mechanism for TAp73 overexpression in tumors.

In a recent study, we showed that TAp73 is selective upregulated in BRCA1-associated ovarian tumors. Interestingly, we found that BRCA1-deficient ovarian carcinoma cells exhibit hypermethylation within a p73 regulatory region, which includes the binding site for the transcriptional repressor ZEB1. This hypermethylation leads to the abrogation of ZEB1 binding and hence increased expression of TAp73. Similarly, ZEB1 binding site methylation and TAp73 expression correlated with BRCA1 status in primary ovarian carcinomas and with clinical response to cisplatin (Fig. 2) (Ibrahim et al., 2010). Together, these data establish another important link between p73 and human cancer.

5.2 Regulation of p53 family protein stability

p53 is a short-lived protein, and its stability is very tightly regulated by ubiquitination under physiological condition (Haupt et al., 1997; Honda et al., 1997; Kubbutat et al., 1997). Polyubiquitination of p53 is carried out by the ubiquitin ligase MDM2. The polyubiquitination and degradation of p53 is influenced by a variety of factors including regulated changes in the subcellular localization of p53 and MDM2. Moreover, *MDM2* itself is a p53-inducible gene, and thus activation of p53 establishes a negative feedback loop wherein MDM2 limits p53 accumulation (Fig. 2) (Barak et al., 1993; Irwin and Kaelin, 2001).

In addition to its role in p53 degradation, MDM2 also binds to a sequence in the transactivation domain of p53 (amino acid residues 17–27) and thereby inhibits p53-dependent transactivation (Momand et al., 1992). The MDM2 binding site in p53 is well conserved in both p63 and p73. Several groups have shown that MDM2 bind to p73 and prevent it from binding to the transcriptional coactivators p300 and CBP (Balint et al., 1999; Ongkeko et al., 1999; Zeng et al., 1999; Zeng et al., 2000). This leads to impaired p73-dependent transcriptional activation and diminished apoptosis. Of note, like p53, p73 can activate the *MDM2* promoter (Wang et al., 2001b; Zeng et al., 1999; Zhu et al., 1998). Although MDM2 does not target p73 for polyubiquitination, p73 stability is indirectly dependent upon the activity of the proteasome. Specifically, many proteosome inhibitors have been shown to increase p73 levels (Balint et al., 1999; Irwin and Kaelin, 2001; Ongkeko et al., 1999). Thus, it is possible that p73 is polyubiquitinated in cells by a yet unknown E3 ligase.

Unlike p73 and p53, p63 does not bind to either MDM2 (Wang et al., 2001a). Although there are no data implicating ubiquitination pathways in p63 degradation, Ratovitski *et al.* (2001) showed that p63 abundance could be regulated by caspase-dependent proteolysis due to the presence of a caspase recognition site, YVED, in the amino acid sequence (Irwin and Kaelin, 2001; Ratovitski et al., 2001).

Besides MDM2, the degradation and protein stability of p53 family proteins might be regulated by small ubiquitin-related modifier-1 (SUMO-1) (Minty et al., 2000; Moll and Slade, 2004). Conjugation to SUMO-1 has been shown to affect p53 transcriptional activity but does not appear to influence p53 stability (Fig. 2) (Gostissa et al., 1999; Irwin and Kaelin, 2001; Rodriguez et al., 2001). Nevertheless, modification of p73α by SUMO-1 has been reported to alter p73 subcellular localization and increased the rate of p73 degradation. On the other hand, the novel Hect domain containing NEDD4-like E3 ubiquitin ligase, NEDL2, binds to p73 via its PY motif in the C-terminal region (Miyazaki et al., 2003). p53, which lacks the PY motif, does not bind to NEDL2. Overexpression of NEDL2 results in the ubiquitination of p73. However, rather than mediating degradation, ubiquitination by NEDL2 enhances the stability of p73 and its ability to transactivate p53/p73-responsive promoters (Fig. 2). The differential binding of NEDL2 to p53 family members is thus another factor that might contribute to their functional divergence. Likewise, the NAD(P)H:quinone oxidoreductase-1 (NQO1) stabilizes p73α (as well as p53) but not p73β by binding to the SAM domain of p73α and protect p73α from 20S proteasomal degradation.. This NQO1-mediated stabilization of p73α and p53 might explan why NQO1 knockout mice and human with inactive NQO1 polymorphisms are susceptible to cancer (Asher et al., 2002; Moll and Slade, 2004).

5.3 Regulation of p53 family protein transcriptional activity

The ankyrin-rich, Src holomogy 3 domain, proline-rich proteins, ASPP1 and ASPP2, stimulate the apoptotic function of p53, p63, and p73 (Bergamaschi et al., 2004; Samuels-Lev et al., 2001). By binding to the DBD of p53, p63, and p73, ASPP1 and ASPP2 stimulate the transactivation function of all three proteins on the promoters of *BAX*, *PIG3*, and *PUMA* but not *MDM2* or *p21*$^{WAF-1/CIP1}$. Hence, ASPP1 and ASPP2 are the first two identified common activators of all p53 family members.

The transcriptional coactivator Yes-associated protein (YAP) has also been shown to potentiate TAp73-mediated transactivation of BAX after DNA damage. Conversely, Akt phosphorylates YAP, which induces interaction with 14-3-3, relocation of YAP to the cytoplasm, and attenuation of p73-mediated apoptosis (Basu et al., 2003; Moll and Slade, 2004).

5.4 DNA damage response and postranslational modification

p53 stabilization and activation by genotoxic stress is associated with multiple post-translational modifications at the N- and C-termini of p53. Under genotoxic stress, activation of stress kinases such ATM, ATR, and Chk2 lead to phosphorylation of p53 at multiple residues at Ser15, Ser20, Ser33, Ser37, Ser46, Thr18, Thr81, Ser315 and Ser392 to stabilize the protein by interfering with MDM2 binding (Fig. 2). In addition, acetylation at Lys320, Lys373, and Lys382, and sumoylation at Lys386 have also been reported to activate the transcriptional activity of p53 (Appella, 2001).

p73 is also activated for apoptosis in response to various genotoxix agents including cisplatin, taxol, and γ-irradiation. The activation of p73 is highly dependent on the non-receptor tyrosine kinase c-abl (Agami et al., 1999; Gong et al., 1999; Moll and Slade, 2004; Yuan et al., 1999). In response to γ-irradiation and cisplatin, TAp73 undergoes phosphorylation at Tyr99 by c-abl (Fig. 2). This, in turn, lead to the stabilization of the protein and dissociation of TAp73 from the TAp73/ΔNp63 inhibitory complex followed by apoptosis (Agami et al., 1999; Leong et al., 2007; Tsai and Yuan, 2003; Yuan et al., 1999).

The activation and phosphorylation of p73 is mainly through the direct interaction between the PXXP motifs of p73 and the Src homology 3 domain of c-abl (Moll and Slade, 2004). Because c-abl is itself phosphorylated and activated by the ATM, ATM may also be involved in the pathway leading to c-abl-dependent p73 activation (Shaul, 2000). These findings suggest that p73 might participate in a mismatch-repair signaling pathway. Recent microarray gene expression profiles further support a role for p73 in response to and repair of DNA damage (Vikhanskaya et al., 2001). In addition to cisplatin, Taxol also increases p73 accumulation, but UV irradiation, actinomycin D, and methylmethane sulfonate do not (Irwin and Kaelin, 2001; Levrero et al., 1999). As p63 does not have the PXXP motifs, it is unlikely that c-abl will phosphorylate p63 (Moll and Slade, 2004).

In addition to c-abl, p73 proteins may also be regulated by cyclin-CDK complexes and play a role in the regulation of cell cycle. p73 physically interacts with various cyclins and certain cyclin-CDK complexes including cyclin A-CDK1/2, cyclin B-CDK1/ 2, and cyclin E-CDK2, which can phosphorylate various p73 isoforms in vitro at Thr86. This cell cycle–dependent phosphorylation inhibits p73 to induce endogenous p21 expression (Gaiddon et al., 2003). p73 is a physiologic target of the cyclin B-CDK1 mitotic kinase complex in vivo, which results in a decreased ability of p73 to bind DNA and activate transcription in mitotic cells. Thus, both p73α and p73β isoforms have been shown to be hyperphosphorylated in normal mitotic cells (Fulco et al., 2003).

DNA damage also induces acetylation of p73 at Lys321, Lys327, and Lys331 by the acetyltransferase p300/cAMP-responsive element binding protein. Non-acetylated p73 is defective in inducing proapoptotic genes such as p53AIP1 but retains the ability to activate other target genes such as p21. This indicates that DNA damage-dependent p73 acetylation, like in p53, potentiates the apoptotic function of p73 by selectively increasing its ability to induce the transcription of proapoptotic target genes (Costanzo et al., 2002; Moll and Slade, 2004).

Finally, the mammalian target of rapamycin (mTOR) was recently identified as a negative regulator of p73 (Fig. 2). Notably, pharmacologic inhibition of mTOR in primary human mammary epithelial cells resulted in differential regulation of p53 family members (Rosenbluth et al., 2008). Cells exhibited selective up-regulation of TAp73, whereas ΔNp63 and p53 levels were both decreased. Interestingly, inhibition of mTOR by rapamycin synergizes cisplatin sensitivity in breast cancer cells through upregulation of TAp73 (Wong et al., 2010). Since mTOR is a master regulator of energy homeostasis and cell growth, and is often active in tumors (Guertin and Sabatini, 2007), this suggests that mTOR may inhibit TAp73 in tumors. In general, cancer cells may use upstream kinases or cofactors to inhibit p53 family members in different cellular contexts, ultimately maintaining proliferation and survival (Rosenbluth and Pietenpol, 2008).

6. The p53 pathway as a network

The significance interplay between p53 family and their isoforms in tumor is demonstrated by the fact that p53 cannot induce apoptosis in response to DNA damage, without the presence of p63 and p73 (Flores et al., 2002). Various mechanisms by which p53/p63/p73 proteins and their isoforms determine the cell fate through formation of transdominant heterocomplex, promoter competition and autoregulatory feedback loop have been proposed. These mechanisms are likely to play an important role in the transition between normal cell cycling and the onset of tumor formation.

6.1 Homotypic and heterotypic interactions among p53 family members

Physical interaction between oncogenic and antioncogenic p53 family members have been demonstrated to interfere with the tumor suppressor functions of wild-type p53 and TAp73 (Nakagawa et al., 2002; Stiewe et al., 2003; Stiewe et al., 2002a; Zaika et al., 2002). Mixed protein complexes were found between endogenous ΔNp73α or ΔNp73β on the one hand and either wild-type p53, TAp73α, or TAp73β on the other hand in primary human tumors, cultured human tumor cells, and mouse neurons (Moll and Slade, 2004). In human head and neck suqamous cell carcinoma and triple-negative breast cancer, endogenous ΔNp63 was shown to physically interact with TAp73 and suppresses TAp73 tumor suppressor activities (Fig. 2) (Leong et al., 2007; Rocco et al., 2006).

In addition, physical interactions between certain human p53 mutants and TAp73 or TAp63 proteins have been reported in coimmunoprecipitation assays, and these interactions correlate with functional transdominance. In contrast, complexes between wild-type p53 and p73 are not observed in mammalian cells (Di Como et al., 1999; Marin et al., 2000; Pozniak et al., 2000; Vikhanskaya et al., 2000). Unexpectedly, protein contact occurs between the DBD of mutant p53 and the DBD and oligomerization domain of p73 rather than between the respective oligomerization domains (Davison et al., 1999; Gaiddon et al., 2001; Strano et al., 2000; Vikhanskaya et al., 2000). In cotransfection experiments, mixed heterocomplexes were shown between p53 mutants p53Ala143, p53Leu173, p53His175, p53Cys220, p53Trp248, or p53Gly281 and TAp73α, TAp73γ, TAp73δ and TAp63 (Di Como et al., 1999; Gaiddon et al., 2001; Marin et al., 2000; Strano et al., 2000). Physiologic complexes were found in five tumor cell lines between endogenous mutant p53 and p73 (Marin et al., 2000; Strano et al., 2000). Functionally, formation of such stable complexes leads to a loss of p73- and p63-mediated transactivation and proapoptotic abilities. Moreover, E2F1-induced p73 transactivation, apoptosis, and colony suppression was inhibited by coexpressed p53His175 (Stiewe and Putzer, 2000). Interestingly, the Arg/Pro polymorphism at codon 72 of mutant p53 is a biological determinant for binding and inactivation of p73, with 72R mutants of p53 being inhibitory, whereas 72P mutants are not (Fig. 2) (Bergamaschi et al., 2003; Marin et al., 2000; Moll and Slade, 2004).

This functional inhibition of TAp73 or TAp63 by some p53 mutants mirrors the ability of many transdominant missense p53 mutants to abrogate wild-type p53 function (Kern et al., 1992; Unger et al., 1992). It suggests that in tumors that express both TAp73 and mutant p53 (typically at very high levels due to deficient MDM2-mediated degradation), the function of TAp73 and TAp63 might be inactivated. If this occurs in primary human tumors, it might have far-reaching consequences because (a) it argues for a transdominant inhibition of the tumor suppressor function of TAp73 isoforms during tumor development, (b) it could be the underlying mechanism for the gain-of-function activity of certain p53 mutants, and (c) it might further increase chemoresistance in cancer therapy of established tumors.

p53 is exceptional among tumor suppressors in that it selects for the overexpression of missense mutants rather than for loss of expression as most other suppressor genes do. This gain-of function increased tumorigenicity compared with p53-null parental cells, increased resistance to cancer agents, and increased genomic instability due to abrogation of the mitotic spindle checkpoint (Dittmer et al., 1993; Halevy et al., 1990; Shaulsky et al., 1991). Conceivably, p63 might also participates in this network. A recent study shown that mutant p53His273 is required for survival of breast cancer cells as knock-down of endogenous mutant p53His273 in breast cancer cells induces massive apoptosis. Surprisingly, the survival effects of p53His273 is independent of TAp73 or TAp63 function as depletion of both isoforms did not rescue the cells from apoptosis following p53His273 knock-down (Lim et al., 2009). Therefore, it is important to note that not all p53 mutants have transdominant effects against TAp73 or TAp63. Some p53 mutants are clearly recessive toward TAp73 (e.g., p53His283, p53Tyr277 and p53His273) and do not interfere with its action (Gaiddon et al., 2001; Lim et al., 2009; Moll and Slade, 2004).

6.2 Promoter competition

Promoter competition by ΔNp73 and ΔNp63 at TAp73/p53 response elements has been reported previously (Kartasheva et al., 2002; Rocco et al., 2006; Stiewe et al., 2002a). It is conceivable that ΔNp73 or ΔNp63 homo-oligomers might have a stronger affinity to certain target gene promoters than wild-type p53 or TAp73. In those cases, p53 or TAp73 inhibition could occur due to competition at the level of target gene access. In the wild-type p53-containing ovarian carcinoma cell line A2780, coexpression of increasing amounts of either TAp73α, TAp73β, TAp73γ, or TAp73ε inhibits specific DNA binding and transcriptional activity of p53 in the absence of hetero-oligomer formation (Moll and Slade, 2004; Ueda et al., 1999; Vikhanskaya et al., 2000). These results suggest that promoter competition could be another mechanism for transdominance between p53 family proteins.

6.3 Autoregulatory feedback loop among p53, TAp73, and ΔNp73

p53 and TAp73 regulate ΔNp73 but not ΔNp63 levels by binding to the p73 P2 promoter and inducing its transcription (Fig. 2). A p73-specific responsive element was mapped within the P2 region (Nakagawa et al., 2002). This generates a negative feedback loop analogous negatively regulates the activity of p53 and p73 (Grob et al., 2001; Kartasheva et al., 2002; Nakagawa et al., 2002; Vossio et al., 2002). As mentioned earlier, ΔNp73 blocks p53 and TAp73 activity through heterocomplex formation (Nakagawa et al., 2002; Stiewe et al., 2002a; Zaika et al., 2002) or through promoter competition (Kartasheva et al., 2002; Stiewe et al., 2002a) and thus contributes to the termination of the p53/p73 response in cells. In contrast to ΔNp73, ΔNp63 expression is transcriptionally repressed by p53 (Moll and Slade, 2004; Waltermann et al., 2003).

7. Targeting the p53 family for treatment of breast cancers

As described above, activation of wild-type TAp73 (or TAp63) lead to cell death in cancer cells. This hypothesis is intriguing given the fact that p73 and p63 are rarely mutated in cancer. Instead, overexpression of TAp73 has been reported in many tumor types including breast cancers and head and neck squamous carcinoma (Leong et al., 2007; Rocco et al., 2006). As such, selective activaton of TAp73 (or TAp63) might induce tumor specific cell death. In principle, activation of the p53 family tumor suppressive pathways might be achieved in several ways (Kaelin, 1999).

First, induction and activation of TAp73 have been reported in response to wide variety of chemotherapeutic agents including Adriamycin, cisplatin, taxol, and etoposide in different tumor cell lines (Bergamaschi et al., 2003; Irwin et al., 2003; Moll and Slade, 2004). In particular, cisplatin treatment has been shown to induce c-abl dependent phosphorylation of TAp73 and lead to its dissociation from the TAp73/ΔNp63 inhibitory complex in head and neck squamous cell carcinoma and breast cancer cells (Fig. 2) (Leong et al., 2007; Rocco et al., 2006). Similarly, a recent clinical study also shown that cells that co-overexpressed TAp73 and ΔNp63 is more likely to response to cisplatin compare to tumors that have no TAp73 expression. These results suggest that certain chemotherapeutic agents can activate TAp73 even in the presence of high level of ΔN isoforms.

Second, a more detailed understanding of the upstream signals that impinge upon p73 and p63 might allow for the design of drugs that would activate the transcription of these genes or stabilize their protein products. For example, the mammalian target of rapamycin (mTOR) was recently identified as a negative regulator of p73 (Rosenbluth et al., 2008). Inhibition of mTOR in primary human mammary epithelial cells selectively up-regulate TAp73 (Rosenbluth et al., 2008; Rosenbluth and Pietenpol, 2008). Combination of cisplatin and mTOR inhibitor, rapamycin, has also been shown to synergizes cisplatin sensitivity in basal-like breast cancer cells through up-regulation of TAp73 recently (Fig. 2) (Wong et al.,

2010). Of note, a phase II neo-adjuvant clinical trial of cisplatin and mTOR inhibitor, everolimus, in patients with triple-negative breast cancer has recently opened for recruitment (ClinicalTrials.gov Identifier: NCT00930930) and will be able to directly address whether targeting these pathways will increase the sensitivity of tumors towards cisplatin chemotherapy.

Finally, it might be possible to design or discover drugs that block the interaction of mutant p53 with p73 or intreraction of MDM2 with p73 which has been shown to inhibit p73 transcription activity (Kaelin, 1999). In theory, molecules already in development that block the interaction of MDM2 with p53 or molecules that restore mutant p53 function might also function in this setting. For example, PRIMA-1, CP-31398 and MIRA-1 are molecules that have been shown to restore wild-type conformation and transcriptional transactivation to mutant p53 (Fig. 2) (Wiman, 2006). Similarly, MDM2 inhibitor such as Nutlins, might interfere MDM2-p73 binding and hence restore the tumor suppressor function of p73 (Ambrosini et al., 2007; Shangary and Wang, 2008). Whether these molecules will selectively activate TAp73 remain to be investigated.

8. Concluding remarks

In conclusion, studies of the newly identified p53 family members, p63 and p73, have revealed several structural and functional similarities. The p53 transactivation, DNA binding, and oligomerization domains are highly conserved among all family members. Like p53, p63 and p73 can form oligomers, bind DNA, and transactivate the promoters of a subset of p53 target genes and induce apoptosis. In addition, certain cellular and viral proteins known to bind and regulate p53 activity likewise can bind to p63 and p73.

Despite the fact that p63 and p73 mimic many p53 activities, more recent studies highlight significant differences between the family members. In contrast to *p53*, *p63* and *p73* give rise to multiple functionally distinct protein isoforms due to alternative promoter utilization and alternative mRNA splicing. The ΔN isoforms, which lack the N-terminal transactivation domain, can function as "dominant-negative" proteins, blocking certain activities of the corresponding full-length proteins.

Differences in the upstream signaling pathways involved in activation of each of the family members are also becoming apparent. Only a subset of the DNA-damaging agents that induce p53 also induce p73. Many cellular and viral oncoproteins also discriminate between p53 and the newer family members. Finally, it is becoming apparent that *p63* and *p73* are not classical Knudson-type tumor suppressor genes. In particular, these genes are not frequently mutated in tumors, and germ-line mutations in these genes do not cause tumors in mice. Instead, mice with deletions in *p63* and *p73* have significant developmental abnormalities.

Despite the significant advances in understanding the unique roles of p53, p63 and p73, there are still several outstanding questions. Understanding the complexity of p53 family members interactions may allow us to to delineate the function of the p53 family network in human tumorigenesis and facilitate the development of anticancer therapeutics that seek to induce the activation of "p53-responsive" genes in cells lacking wild-type p53.

9. References

Abraham, H., and Meyer, G. (2003). Reelin-expressing neurons in the postnatal and adult human hippocampal formation. Hippocampus *13*, 715-727.

Agami, R., Blandino, G., Oren, M., and Shaul, Y. (1999). Interaction of c-Abl and p73alpha and their collaboration to induce apoptosis. Nature *399*, 809-813.

Ambrosini, G., Sambol, E. B., Carvajal, D., Vassilev, L. T., Singer, S., and Schwartz, G. K. (2007). Mouse double minute antagonist Nutlin-3a enhances chemotherapy-induced apoptosis in cancer cells with mutant p53 by activating E2F1. Oncogene *26*, 3473-3481.

Appella, E. (2001). Modulation of p53 function in cellular regulation. Eur J Biochem *268*, 2763.

Arrowsmith, C. H. (1999). Structure and function in the p53 family. Cell Death Differ *6*, 1169-1173.

Asher, G., Lotem, J., Sachs, L., Kahana, C., and Shaul, Y. (2002). Mdm-2 and ubiquitin-independent p53 proteasomal degradation regulated by NQO1. Proc Natl Acad Sci U S A *99*, 13125-13130.

Balint, E., Bates, S., and Vousden, K. H. (1999). Mdm2 binds p73 alpha without targeting degradation. Oncogene *18*, 3923-3929.

Barak, Y., Juven, T., Haffner, R., and Oren, M. (1993). mdm2 expression is induced by wild type p53 activity. EMBO J *12*, 461-468.

Basu, S., Totty, N. F., Irwin, M. S., Sudol, M., and Downward, J. (2003). Akt phosphorylates the Yes-associated protein, YAP, to induce interaction with 14-3-3 and attenuation of p73-mediated apoptosis. Mol Cell *11*, 11-23.

Benard, J., Douc-Rasy, S., and Ahomadegbe, J. C. (2003). TP53 family members and human cancers. Hum Mutat *21*, 182-191.

Bergamaschi, D., Gasco, M., Hiller, L., Sullivan, A., Syed, N., Trigiante, G., Yulug, I., Merlano, M., Numico, G., Comino, A., *et al.* (2003). p53 polymorphism influences response in cancer chemotherapy via modulation of p73-dependent apoptosis. Cancer Cell *3*, 387-402.

Bergamaschi, D., Samuels, Y., Jin, B., Duraisingham, S., Crook, T., and Lu, X. (2004). ASPP1 and ASPP2: common activators of p53 family members. Mol Cell Biol *24*, 1341-1350.

Bjorkqvist, A. M., Husgafvel-Pursiainen, K., Anttila, S., Karjalainen, A., Tammilehto, L., Mattson, K., Vainio, H., and Knuutila, S. (1998). DNA gains in 3q occur frequently in squamous cell carcinoma of the lung, but not in adenocarcinoma. Genes Chromosomes Cancer *22*, 79-82.

Blanpain, C., and Fuchs, E. (2007). p63: revving up epithelial stem-cell potential. Nat Cell Biol *9*, 731-733.

Brunner, H. G., Hamel, B. C., and Bokhoven Hv, H. (2002). P63 gene mutations and human developmental syndromes. Am J Med Genet *112*, 284-290.

Cai, Y. C., Yang, G. Y., Nie, Y., Wang, L. D., Zhao, X., Song, Y. L., Seril, D. N., Liao, J., Xing, E. P., and Yang, C. S. (2000). Molecular alterations of p73 in human esophageal squamous cell carcinomas: loss of heterozygosity occurs frequently; loss of imprinting and elevation of p73 expression may be related to defective p53. Carcinogenesis *21*, 683-689.

Celli, J., Duijf, P., Hamel, B. C., Bamshad, M., Kramer, B., Smits, A. P., Newbury-Ecob, R., Hennekam, R. C., Van Buggenhout, G., van Haeringen, A., *et al.* (1999). Heterozygous germline mutations in the p53 homolog p63 are the cause of EEC syndrome. Cell *99*, 143-153.

Chan, I., McGrath, J. A., and Kivirikko, S. (2005). Rapp-Hodgkin syndrome and the tail of p63. Clin Exp Dermatol *30*, 183-186.

Chen, C. L., Ip, S. M., Cheng, D., Wong, L. C., and Ngan, H. Y. (2000). P73 gene expression in ovarian cancer tissues and cell lines. Clin Cancer Res *6*, 3910-3915.

Chi, S. G., Chang, S. G., Lee, S. J., Lee, C. H., Kim, J. I., and Park, J. H. (1999). Elevated and biallelic expression of p73 is associated withprogression of human bladder cancer. Cancer Res *59*, 2791-2793.

Choi, H. R., Batsakis, J. G., Zhan, F., Sturgis, E., Luna, M. A., and El-Naggar, A. K. (2002). Differential expression of p53 gene family members p63 and p73 in head and neck squamous tumorigenesis. Hum Pathol *33*, 158-164.

Costanzo, A., Merlo, P., Pediconi, N., Fulco, M., Sartorelli, V., Cole, P. A., Fontemaggi, G., Fanciulli, M., Schiltz, L., Blandino, G., *et al.* (2002). DNA damage-dependent acetylation of p73 dictates the selective activation of apoptotic target genes. Mol Cell *9*, 175-186.

Crook, T., Nicholls, J. M., Brooks, L., O'Nions, J., and Allday, M. J. (2000). High level expression of deltaN-p63: a mechanism for the inactivation of p53 in undifferentiated nasopharyngeal carcinoma (NPC)? Oncogene *19*, 3439-3444.

Davis, L. D., Zhang, W., Merseburger, A., Young, D., Xu, L., Rhim, J. S., Moul, J. W., Srivastava, S., and Sesterhenn, I. A. (2002). p63 expression profile in normal and malignant prostate epithelial cells. Anticancer Res *22*, 3819-3825.

Davison, T. S., Vagner, C., Kaghad, M., Ayed, A., Caput, D., and Arrowsmith, C. H. (1999). p73 and p63 are homotetramers capable of weak heterotypic interactions with each other but not with p53. J Biol Chem *274*, 18709-18714.

De Laurenzi, V., Costanzo, A., Barcaroli, D., Terrinoni, A., Falco, M., Annicchiarico-Petruzzelli, M., Levrero, M., and Melino, G. (1998). Two new p73 splice variants, gamma and delta, with different transcriptional activity. J Exp Med *188*, 1763-1768.

Di Como, C. J., Gaiddon, C., and Prives, C. (1999). p73 function is inhibited by tumor-derived p53 mutants in mammalian cells. Mol Cell Biol *19*, 1438-1449.

Di Como, C. J., Urist, M. J., Babayan, I., Drobnjak, M., Hedvat, C. V., Teruya-Feldstein, J., Pohar, K., Hoos, A., and Cordon-Cardo, C. (2002). p63 expression profiles in human normal and tumor tissues. Clin Cancer Res *8*, 494-501.

Dittmer, D., Pati, S., Zambetti, G., Chu, S., Teresky, A. K., Moore, M., Finlay, C., and Levine, A. J. (1993). Gain of function mutations in p53. Nat Genet *4*, 42-46.

Dobbelstein, M., and Roth, J. (1998). The large T antigen of simian virus 40 binds and inactivates p53 but not p73. J Gen Virol *79 (Pt 12)*, 3079-3083.

Dohn, M., Zhang, S., and Chen, X. (2001). p63alpha and DeltaNp63alpha can induce cell cycle arrest and apoptosis and differentially regulate p53 target genes. Oncogene *20*, 3193-3205.

Duijf, P. H., Vanmolkot, K. R., Propping, P., Friedl, W., Krieger, E., McKeon, F., Dotsch, V., Brunner, H. G., and van Bokhoven, H. (2002). Gain-of-function mutation in ADULT syndrome reveals the presence of a second transactivation domain in p63. Hum Mol Genet *11*, 799-804.

Flores, E. R., Tsai, K. Y., Crowley, D., Sengupta, S., Yang, A., McKeon, F., and Jacks, T. (2002). p63 and p73 are required for p53-dependent apoptosis in response to DNA damage. Nature *416*, 560-564.

Fomenkov, A., Huang, Y. P., Topaloglu, O., Brechman, A., Osada, M., Fomenkova, T., Yuriditsky, E., Trink, B., Sidransky, D., and Ratovitski, E. (2003). P63 alpha mutations lead to aberrant splicing of keratinocyte growth factor receptor in the Hay-Wells syndrome. J Biol Chem *278*, 23906-23914.

Fulco, M., Costanzo, A., Merlo, P., Mangiacasale, R., Strano, S., Blandino, G., Balsano, C., Lavia, P., and Levrero, M. (2003). p73 is regulated by phosphorylation at the G2/M transition. J Biol Chem *278*, 49196-49202.

Gaiddon, C., Lokshin, M., Ahn, J., Zhang, T., and Prives, C. (2001). A subset of tumor-derived mutant forms of p53 down-regulate p63 and p73 through a direct interaction with the p53 core domain. Mol Cell Biol *21*, 1874-1887.

Gaiddon, C., Lokshin, M., Gross, I., Levasseur, D., Taya, Y., Loeffler, J. P., and Prives, C. (2003). Cyclin-dependent kinases phosphorylate p73 at threonine 86 in a cell cycle-dependent manner and negatively regulate p73. J Biol Chem *278*, 27421-27431.

Garraway, L. A., Lin, D., Signoretti, S., Waltregny, D., Dilks, J., Bhattacharya, N., and Loda, M. (2003). Intermediate basal cells of the prostate: in vitro and in vivo characterization. Prostate *55*, 206-218.

Gong, J. G., Costanzo, A., Yang, H. Q., Melino, G., Kaelin, W. G., Jr., Levrero, M., and Wang, J. Y. (1999). The tyrosine kinase c-Abl regulates p73 in apoptotic response to cisplatin-induced DNA damage. Nature *399*, 806-809.

Gostissa, M., Hengstermann, A., Fogal, V., Sandy, P., Schwarz, S. E., Scheffner, M., and Del Sal, G. (1999). Activation of p53 by conjugation to the ubiquitin-like protein SUMO-1. EMBO J *18*, 6462-6471.

Grob, T. J., Novak, U., Maisse, C., Barcaroli, D., Luthi, A. U., Pirnia, F., Hugli, B., Graber, H. U., De Laurenzi, V., Fey, M. F., *et al.* (2001). Human delta Np73 regulates a dominant negative feedback loop for TAp73 and p53. Cell Death Differ *8*, 1213-1223.

Guertin, D. A., and Sabatini, D. M. (2007). Defining the role of mTOR in cancer. Cancer Cell *12*, 9-22.

Hagiwara, K., McMenamin, M. G., Miura, K., and Harris, C. C. (1999). Mutational analysis of the p63/p73L/p51/p40/CUSP/KET gene in human cancer cell lines using intronic primers. Cancer Res *59*, 4165-4169.

Halevy, O., Michalovitz, D., and Oren, M. (1990). Different tumor-derived p53 mutants exhibit distinct biological activities. Science *250*, 113-116.

Haupt, Y., Maya, R., Kazaz, A., and Oren, M. (1997). Mdm2 promotes the rapid degradation of p53. Nature *387*, 296-299.

Hibi, K., Trink, B., Patturajan, M., Westra, W. H., Caballero, O. L., Hill, D. E., Ratovitski, E. A., Jen, J., and Sidransky, D. (2000). AIS is an oncogene amplified in squamous cell carcinoma. Proc Natl Acad Sci U S A *97*, 5462-5467.

Higashino, F., Pipas, J. M., and Shenk, T. (1998). Adenovirus E4orf6 oncoprotein modulates the function of the p53-related protein, p73. Proc Natl Acad Sci U S A *95*, 15683-15687.

Honda, R., Tanaka, H., and Yasuda, H. (1997). Oncoprotein MDM2 is a ubiquitin ligase E3 for tumor suppressor p53. FEBS Lett *420*, 25-27.

Hu, J. F., Ulaner, G. A., Oruganti, H., Ivaturi, R. D., Balagura, K. A., Pham, J., Vu, T. H., and Hoffman, A. R. (2000). Allelic expression of the putative tumor suppressor gene p73 in human fetal tissues and tumor specimens. Biochim Biophys Acta *1491*, 49-56.

Ibrahim, N., He, L., Leong, C. O., Xing, D., Karlan, B. Y., Swisher, E. M., Rueda, B. R., Orsulic, S., and Ellisen, L. W. (2010). BRCA1-associated epigenetic regulation of p73 mediates an effector pathway for chemosensitivity in ovarian carcinoma. Cancer Res *70*, 7155-7165.

Irwin, M., Marin, M. C., Phillips, A. C., Seelan, R. S., Smith, D. I., Liu, W., Flores, E. R., Tsai, K. Y., Jacks, T., Vousden, K. H., and Kaelin, W. G., Jr. (2000). Role for the p53 homologue p73 in E2F-1-induced apoptosis. Nature *407*, 645-648.

Irwin, M. S., and Kaelin, W. G. (2001). p53 family update: p73 and p63 develop their own identities. Cell Growth Differ *12*, 337-349.

Irwin, M. S., Kondo, K., Marin, M. C., Cheng, L. S., Hahn, W. C., and Kaelin, W. G., Jr. (2003). Chemosensitivity linked to p73 function. Cancer Cell *3*, 403-410.

Johnson, J., Lagowski, J., Sundberg, A., and Kulesz-Martin, M. (2005). P53 family activities in development and cancer: relationship to melanocyte and keratinocyte carcinogenesis. J Invest Dermatol *125*, 857-864.

Jost, C. A., Marin, M. C., and Kaelin, W. G., Jr. (1997). p73 is a simian [correction of human] p53-related protein that can induce apoptosis. Nature *389*, 191-194.

Kaelin, W. G., Jr. (1999). The p53 gene family. Oncogene *18*, 7701-7705.

Kaghad, M., Bonnet, H., Yang, A., Creancier, L., Biscan, J. C., Valent, A., Minty, A., Chalon, P., Lelias, J. M., Dumont, X., *et al.* (1997). Monoallelically expressed gene related to p53 at 1p36, a region frequently deleted in neuroblastoma and other human cancers. Cell *90*, 809-819.

Kang, M. J., Park, B. J., Byun, D. S., Park, J. I., Kim, H. J., Park, J. H., and Chi, S. G. (2000). Loss of imprinting and elevated expression of wild-type p73 in human gastric adenocarcinoma. Clin Cancer Res *6*, 1767-1771.

Kartasheva, N. N., Contente, A., Lenz-Stoppler, C., Roth, J., and Dobbelstein, M. (2002). p53 induces the expression of its antagonist p73 Delta N, establishing an autoregulatory feedback loop. Oncogene *21*, 4715-4727.

Kern, S. E., Pietenpol, J. A., Thiagalingam, S., Seymour, A., Kinzler, K. W., and Vogelstein, B. (1992). Oncogenic forms of p53 inhibit p53-regulated gene expression. Science *256*, 827-830.

Koster, M. I., Kim, S., Mills, A. A., DeMayo, F. J., and Roop, D. R. (2004). p63 is the molecular switch for initiation of an epithelial stratification program. Genes Dev *18*, 126-131.

Kovalev, S., Marchenko, N., Swendeman, S., LaQuaglia, M., and Moll, U. M. (1998). Expression level, allelic origin, and mutation analysis of the p73 gene in neuroblastoma tumors and cell lines. Cell Growth Differ *9*, 897-903.

Kubbutat, M. H., Jones, S. N., and Vousden, K. H. (1997). Regulation of p53 stability by Mdm2. Nature *387*, 299-303.

Lane, D. P., and Crawford, L. V. (1979). T antigen is bound to a host protein in SV40-transformed cells. Nature *278*, 261-263.

Lechner, M. S., Mack, D. H., Finicle, A. B., Crook, T., Vousden, K. H., and Laimins, L. A. (1992). Human papillomavirus E6 proteins bind p53 in vivo and abrogate p53-mediated repression of transcription. EMBO J *11*, 3045-3052.

Lee, C. W., and La Thangue, N. B. (1999). Promoter specificity and stability control of the p53-related protein p73. Oncogene *18*, 4171-4181.

Leong, C. O., Vidnovic, N., DeYoung, M. P., Sgroi, D., and Ellisen, L. W. (2007). The p63/p73 network mediates chemosensitivity to cisplatin in a biologically defined subset of primary breast cancers. J Clin Invest *117*, 1370-1380.

Levrero, M., De Laurenzi, V., Costanzo, A., Gong, J., Melino, G., and Wang, J. Y. (1999). Structure, function and regulation of p63 and p73. Cell Death Differ *6*, 1146-1153.

Lim, L. Y., Vidnovic, N., Ellisen, L. W., and Leong, C. O. (2009). Mutant p53 mediates survival of breast cancer cells. Br J Cancer *101*, 1606-1612.

Linzer, D. I., and Levine, A. J. (1979). Characterization of a 54K dalton cellular SV40 tumor antigen present in SV40-transformed cells and uninfected embryonal carcinoma cells. Cell *17*, 43-52.

Lissy, N. A., Davis, P. K., Irwin, M., Kaelin, W. G., and Dowdy, S. F. (2000). A common E2F-1 and p73 pathway mediates cell death induced by TCR activation. Nature *407*, 642-645.

Mai, M., Yokomizo, A., Qian, C., Yang, P., Tindall, D. J., Smith, D. I., and Liu, W. (1998). Activation of p73 silent allele in lung cancer. Cancer Res *58*, 2347-2349.

Marin, M. C., Jost, C. A., Brooks, L. A., Irwin, M. S., O'Nions, J., Tidy, J. A., James, N., McGregor, J. M., Harwood, C. A., Yulug, I. G., *et al.* (2000). A common polymorphism acts as an intragenic modifier of mutant p53 behaviour. Nat Genet *25*, 47-54.

Marin, M. C., Jost, C. A., Irwin, M. S., DeCaprio, J. A., Caput, D., and Kaelin, W. G., Jr. (1998). Viral oncoproteins discriminate between p53 and the p53 homolog p73. Mol Cell Biol *18*, 6316-6324.

Massion, P. P., Taflan, P. M., Jamshedur Rahman, S. M., Yildiz, P., Shyr, Y., Edgerton, M. E., Westfall, M. D., Roberts, J. R., Pietenpol, J. A., Carbone, D. P., and Gonzalez, A. L. (2003). Significance of p63 amplification and overexpression in lung cancer development and prognosis. Cancer Res *63*, 7113-7121.

Melino, G., Lu, X., Gasco, M., Crook, T., and Knight, R. A. (2003). Functional regulation of p73 and p63: development and cancer. Trends Biochem Sci *28*, 663-670.

Mills, A. A., Zheng, B., Wang, X. J., Vogel, H., Roop, D. R., and Bradley, A. (1999). p63 is a p53 homologue required for limb and epidermal morphogenesis. Nature *398*, 708-713.

Minty, A., Dumont, X., Kaghad, M., and Caput, D. (2000). Covalent modification of p73alpha by SUMO-1. Two-hybrid screening with p73 identifies novel SUMO-1-interacting proteins and a SUMO-1 interaction motif. J Biol Chem *275*, 36316-36323.

Miyazaki, K., Ozaki, T., Kato, C., Hanamoto, T., Fujita, T., Irino, S., Watanabe, K., Nakagawa, T., and Nakagawara, A. (2003). A novel HECT-type E3 ubiquitin ligase, NEDL2, stabilizes p73 and enhances its transcriptional activity. Biochem Biophys Res Commun *308*, 106-113.

Moll, U. M., and Slade, N. (2004). p63 and p73: roles in development and tumor formation. Mol Cancer Res *2*, 371-386.

Momand, J., Zambetti, G. P., Olson, D. C., George, D., and Levine, A. J. (1992). The mdm-2 oncogene product forms a complex with the p53 protein and inhibits p53-mediated transactivation. Cell *69*, 1237-1245.

Murray-Zmijewski, F., Lane, D. P., and Bourdon, J. C. (2006). p53/p63/p73 isoforms: an orchestra of isoforms to harmonise cell differentiation and response to stress. Cell Death Differ *13*, 962-972.

Nakagawa, T., Takahashi, M., Ozaki, T., Watanabe Ki, K., Todo, S., Mizuguchi, H., Hayakawa, T., and Nakagawara, A. (2002). Autoinhibitory regulation of p73 by Delta Np73 to modulate cell survival and death through a p73-specific target element within the Delta Np73 promoter. Mol Cell Biol *22*, 2575-2585.

Nakano, K., Balint, E., Ashcroft, M., and Vousden, K. H. (2000). A ribonucleotide reductase gene is a transcriptional target of p53 and p73. Oncogene *19*, 4283-4289.

Ng, S. W., Yiu, G. K., Liu, Y., Huang, L. W., Palnati, M., Jun, S. H., Berkowitz, R. S., and Mok, S. C. (2000). Analysis of p73 in human borderline and invasive ovarian tumor. Oncogene *19*, 1885-1890.

Nomoto, S., Haruki, N., Kondo, M., Konishi, H., and Takahashi, T. (1998). Search for mutations and examination of allelic expression imbalance of the p73 gene at 1p36.33 in human lung cancers. Cancer Res *58*, 1380-1383.

Ongkeko, W. M., Wang, X. Q., Siu, W. Y., Lau, A. W., Yamashita, K., Harris, A. L., Cox, L. S., and Poon, R. Y. (1999). MDM2 and MDMX bind and stabilize the p53-related protein p73. Curr Biol *9*, 829-832.

Osada, M., Ohba, M., Kawahara, C., Ishioka, C., Kanamaru, R., Katoh, I., Ikawa, Y., Nimura, Y., Nakagawara, A., Obinata, M., and Ikawa, S. (1998). Cloning and functional analysis of human p51, which structurally and functionally resembles p53. Nat Med *4*, 839-843.

Ozaki, T., Naka, M., Takada, N., Tada, M., Sakiyama, S., and Nakagawara, A. (1999). Deletion of the COOH-terminal region of p73alpha enhances both its transactivation function and DNA-binding activity but inhibits induction of apoptosis in mammalian cells. Cancer Res *59*, 5902-5907.

Park, B. J., Lee, S. J., Kim, J. I., Lee, C. H., Chang, S. G., Park, J. H., and Chi, S. G. (2000). Frequent alteration of p63 expression in human primary bladder carcinomas. Cancer Res *60*, 3370-3374.

Pozniak, C. D., Radinovic, S., Yang, A., McKeon, F., Kaplan, D. R., and Miller, F. D. (2000). An anti-apoptotic role for the p53 family member, p73, during developmental neuron death. Science *289*, 304-306.

Prabhu, N. S., Somasundaram, K., Satyamoorthy, K., Herlyn, M., and El-Deiry, W. S. (1998). p73beta, unlike p53, suppresses growth and induces apoptosis of human papillomavirus E6-expressing cancer cells. Int J Oncol *13*, 5-9.

Ratovitski, E. A., Patturajan, M., Hibi, K., Trink, B., Yamaguchi, K., and Sidransky, D. (2001). p53 associates with and targets Delta Np63 into a protein degradation pathway. Proc Natl Acad Sci U S A *98*, 1817-1822.

Reis-Filho, J. S., Milanezi, F., Amendoeira, I., Albergaria, A., and Schmitt, F. C. (2003a). Distribution of p63, a novel myoepithelial marker, in fine-needle aspiration biopsies of the breast: an analysis of 82 samples. Cancer *99*, 172-179.

Reis-Filho, J. S., Simpson, P. T., Martins, A., Preto, A., Gartner, F., and Schmitt, F. C. (2003b). Distribution of p63, cytokeratins 5/6 and cytokeratin 14 in 51 normal and 400 neoplastic human tissue samples using TARP-4 multi-tumor tissue microarray. Virchows Arch *443*, 122-132.

Ribeiro-Silva, A., Zambelli Ramalho, L. N., Britto Garcia, S., and Zucoloto, S. (2003). The relationship between p63 and p53 expression in normal and neoplastic breast tissue. Arch Pathol Lab Med *127*, 336-340.

Rocco, J. W., Leong, C. O., Kuperwasser, N., DeYoung, M. P., and Ellisen, L. W. (2006). p63 mediates survival in squamous cell carcinoma by suppression of p73-dependent apoptosis. Cancer Cell *9*, 45-56.

Rodriguez, M. S., Dargemont, C., and Hay, R. T. (2001). SUMO-1 conjugation in vivo requires both a consensus modification motif and nuclear targeting. J Biol Chem *276*, 12654-12659.

Rosenbluth, J. M., Mays, D. J., Pino, M. F., Tang, L. J., and Pietenpol, J. A. (2008). A gene signature-based approach identifies mTOR as a regulator of p73. Mol Cell Biol *28*, 5951-5964.

Rosenbluth, J. M., and Pietenpol, J. A. (2008). The jury is in: p73 is a tumor suppressor after all. Genes Dev *22*, 2591-2595.

Roth, J., and Dobbelstein, M. (1999). Failure of viral oncoproteins to target the p53-homologue p51A. J Gen Virol *80 (Pt 12)*, 3251-3255.

Roth, J., Konig, C., Wienzek, S., Weigel, S., Ristea, S., and Dobbelstein, M. (1998). Inactivation of p53 but not p73 by adenovirus type 5 E1B 55-kilodalton and E4 34-kilodalton oncoproteins. J Virol *72*, 8510-8516.

Samuels-Lev, Y., O'Connor, D. J., Bergamaschi, D., Trigiante, G., Hsieh, J. K., Zhong, S., Campargue, I., Naumovski, L., Crook, T., and Lu, X. (2001). ASPP proteins specifically stimulate the apoptotic function of p53. Mol Cell *8*, 781-794.

Sarnow, P., Ho, Y. S., Williams, J., and Levine, A. J. (1982). Adenovirus E1b-58kd tumor antigen and SV40 large tumor antigen are physically associated with the same 54 kd cellular protein in transformed cells. Cell *28*, 387-394.

Schmale, H., and Bamberger, C. (1997). A novel protein with strong homology to the tumor suppressor p53. Oncogene *15*, 1363-1367.

Senoo, M., Pinto, F., Crum, C. P., and McKeon, F. (2007). p63 Is essential for the proliferative potential of stem cells in stratified epithelia. Cell *129*, 523-536.

Senoo, M., Seki, N., Ohira, M., Sugano, S., Watanabe, M., Inuzuka, S., Okamoto, T., Tachibana, M., Tanaka, T., Shinkai, Y., and Kato, H. (1998). A second p53-related protein, p73L, with high homology to p73. Biochem Biophys Res Commun *248*, 603-607.

Shangary, S., and Wang, S. (2008). Targeting the MDM2-p53 interaction for cancer therapy. Clin Cancer Res *14*, 5318-5324.

Shaul, Y. (2000). c-Abl: activation and nuclear targets. Cell Death Differ *7*, 10-16.

Shaulsky, G., Goldfinger, N., and Rotter, V. (1991). Alterations in tumor development in vivo mediated by expression of wild type or mutant p53 proteins. Cancer Res *51*, 5232-5237.

Steegenga, W. T., Shvarts, A., Riteco, N., Bos, J. L., and Jochemsen, A. G. (1999). Distinct regulation of p53 and p73 activity by adenovirus E1A, E1B, and E4orf6 proteins. Mol Cell Biol *19*, 3885-3894.

Stiewe, T. (2007). The p53 family in differentiation and tumorigenesis. Nat Rev Cancer *7*, 165-168.

Stiewe, T., and Putzer, B. M. (2000). Role of the p53-homologue p73 in E2F1-induced apoptosis. Nat Genet *26*, 464-469.

Stiewe, T., and Putzer, B. M. (2002). Role of p73 in malignancy: tumor suppressor or oncogene? Cell Death Differ *9*, 237-245.

Stiewe, T., Stanelle, J., Theseling, C. C., Pollmeier, B., Beitzinger, M., and Putzer, B. M. (2003). Inactivation of retinoblastoma (RB) tumor suppressor by oncogenic isoforms of the p53 family member p73. J Biol Chem *278*, 14230-14236.

Stiewe, T., Theseling, C. C., and Putzer, B. M. (2002a). Transactivation-deficient Delta TA-p73 inhibits p53 by direct competition for DNA binding: implications for tumorigenesis. J Biol Chem *277*, 14177-14185.

Stiewe, T., Zimmermann, S., Frilling, A., Esche, H., and Putzer, B. M. (2002b). Transactivation-deficient DeltaTA-p73 acts as an oncogene. Cancer Res *62*, 3598-3602.

Strano, S., Munarriz, E., Rossi, M., Cristofanelli, B., Shaul, Y., Castagnoli, L., Levine, A. J., Sacchi, A., Cesareni, G., Oren, M., and Blandino, G. (2000). Physical and functional interaction between p53 mutants and different isoforms of p73. J Biol Chem *275*, 29503-29512.

Sun, X. F. (2002). p73 overexpression is a prognostic factor in patients with colorectal adenocarcinoma. Clin Cancer Res *8*, 165-170.

Sunahara, M., Ichimiya, S., Nimura, Y., Takada, N., Sakiyama, S., Sato, Y., Todo, S., Adachi, W., Amano, J., and Nakagawara, A. (1998). Mutational analysis of the p73 gene localized at chromosome 1p36.3 in colorectal carcinomas. Int J Oncol *13*, 319-323.

Tannapfel, A., Engeland, K., Weinans, L., Katalinic, A., Hauss, J., Mossner, J., and Wittekind, C. (1999a). Expression of p73, a novel protein related to the p53 tumour suppressor p53, and apoptosis in cholangiocellular carcinoma of the liver. Br J Cancer *80*, 1069-1074.

Tannapfel, A., Wasner, M., Krause, K., Geissler, F., Katalinic, A., Hauss, J., Mossner, J., Engeland, K., and Wittekind, C. (1999b). Expression of p73 and its relation to histopathology and prognosis in hepatocellular carcinoma. J Natl Cancer Inst *91*, 1154-1158.

Tokuchi, Y., Hashimoto, T., Kobayashi, Y., Hayashi, M., Nishida, K., Hayashi, S., Imai, K., Nakachi, K., Ishikawa, Y., Nakagawa, K., *et al.* (1999). The expression of p73 is increased in lung cancer, independent of p53 gene alteration. Br J Cancer *80*, 1623-1629.

Trink, B., Okami, K., Wu, L., Sriuranpong, V., Jen, J., and Sidransky, D. (1998). A new human p53 homologue. Nat Med *4*, 747-748.

Tsai, K. K., and Yuan, Z. M. (2003). c-Abl stabilizes p73 by a phosphorylation-augmented interaction. Cancer Res *63*, 3418-3424.

Tsao, H., Zhang, X., Majewski, P., and Haluska, F. G. (1999). Mutational and expression analysis of the p73 gene in melanoma cell lines. Cancer Res *59*, 172-174.

Ueda, Y., Hijikata, M., Takagi, S., Chiba, T., and Shimotohno, K. (1999). New p73 variants with altered C-terminal structures have varied transcriptional activities. Oncogene *18*, 4993-4998.

Ueda, Y., Hijikata, M., Takagi, S., Chiba, T., and Shimotohno, K. (2001). Transcriptional activities of p73 splicing variants are regulated by inter-variant association. Biochem J *356*, 859-866.

Unger, T., Nau, M. M., Segal, S., and Minna, J. D. (1992). p53: a transdominant regulator of transcription whose function is ablated by mutations occurring in human cancer. EMBO J *11*, 1383-1390.

van Bokhoven, H., Hamel, B. C., Bamshad, M., Sangiorgi, E., Gurrieri, F., Duijf, P. H., Vanmolkot, K. R., van Beusekom, E., van Beersum, S. E., Celli, J., *et al.* (2001). p63 Gene mutations in eec syndrome, limb-mammary syndrome, and isolated split hand-split foot malformation suggest a genotype-phenotype correlation. Am J Hum Genet *69*, 481-492.

Vikhanskaya, F., D'Incalci, M., and Broggini, M. (2000). p73 competes with p53 and attenuates its response in a human ovarian cancer cell line. Nucleic Acids Res *28*, 513-519.

Vikhanskaya, F., Marchini, S., Marabese, M., Galliera, E., and Broggini, M. (2001). P73a overexpression is associated with resistance to treatment with DNA-damaging agents in a human ovarian cancer cell line. Cancer Res *61*, 935-938.

Vossio, S., Palescandolo, E., Pediconi, N., Moretti, F., Balsano, C., Levrero, M., and Costanzo, A. (2002). DN-p73 is activated after DNA damage in a p53-dependent manner to regulate p53-induced cell cycle arrest. Oncogene *21*, 3796-3803.

Waltermann, A., Kartasheva, N. N., and Dobbelstein, M. (2003). Differential regulation of p63 and p73 expression. Oncogene *22*, 5686-5693.

Wang, X., Arooz, T., Siu, W. Y., Chiu, C. H., Lau, A., Yamashita, K., and Poon, R. Y. (2001a). MDM2 and MDMX can interact differently with ARF and members of the p53 family. FEBS Lett *490*, 202-208.

Wang, X. Q., Ongkeko, W. M., Lau, A. W., Leung, K. M., and Poon, R. Y. (2001b). A possible role of p73 on the modulation of p53 level through MDM2. Cancer Res *61*, 1598-1603.

Weber, A., Bellmann, U., Bootz, F., Wittekind, C., and Tannapfel, A. (2002). Expression of p53 and its homologues in primary and recurrent squamous cell carcinomas of the head and neck. Int J Cancer *99*, 22-28.

Westfall, M. D., and Pietenpol, J. A. (2004). p63: Molecular complexity in development and cancer. Carcinogenesis *25*, 857-864.

Wiman, K. G. (2006). Strategies for therapeutic targeting of the p53 pathway in cancer. Cell Death Differ *13*, 921-926.

Wong, S. W., Tiong, K. H., Kong, W. Y., Yue, Y. C., Chua, C. H., Lim, J. Y., Lee, C. Y., Quah, S. I., Fow, C., Chung, C., *et al.* (2010). Rapamycin synergizes cisplatin sensitivity in basal-like breast cancer cells through up-regulation of p73. Breast Cancer Res Treat.

Wu, G., Nomoto, S., Hoque, M. O., Dracheva, T., Osada, M., Lee, C. C., Dong, S. M., Guo, Z., Benoit, N., Cohen, Y., *et al.* (2003). DeltaNp63alpha and TAp63alpha regulate transcription of genes with distinct biological functions in cancer and development. Cancer Res *63*, 2351-2357.

Yamaguchi, K., Wu, L., Caballero, O. L., Hibi, K., Trink, B., Resto, V., Cairns, P., Okami, K., Koch, W. M., Sidransky, D., and Jen, J. (2000). Frequent gain of the p40/p51/p63 gene locus in primary head and neck squamous cell carcinoma. Int J Cancer *86*, 684-689.

Yang, A., Kaghad, M., Wang, Y., Gillett, E., Fleming, M. D., Dotsch, V., Andrews, N. C., Caput, D., and McKeon, F. (1998). p63, a p53 homolog at 3q27-29, encodes multiple products with transactivating, death-inducing, and dominant-negative activities. Mol Cell *2*, 305-316.

Yang, A., Schweitzer, R., Sun, D., Kaghad, M., Walker, N., Bronson, R. T., Tabin, C., Sharpe, A., Caput, D., Crum, C., and McKeon, F. (1999). p63 is essential for regenerative proliferation in limb, craniofacial and epithelial development. Nature *398*, 714-718.

Yang, A., Walker, N., Bronson, R., Kaghad, M., Oosterwegel, M., Bonnin, J., Vagner, C., Bonnet, H., Dikkes, P., Sharpe, A., *et al.* (2000). p73-deficient mice have neurological, pheromonal and inflammatory defects but lack spontaneous tumours. Nature *404*, 99-103.

Yew, P. R., and Berk, A. J. (1992). Inhibition of p53 transactivation required for transformation by adenovirus early 1B protein. Nature *357*, 82-85.

Yokomizo, A., Mai, M., Tindall, D. J., Cheng, L., Bostwick, D. G., Naito, S., Smith, D. I., and Liu, W. (1999). Overexpression of the wild type p73 gene in human bladder cancer. Oncogene *18*, 1629-1633.

Yu, J., Zhang, L., Hwang, P. M., Rago, C., Kinzler, K. W., and Vogelstein, B. (1999). Identification and classification of p53-regulated genes. Proc Natl Acad Sci U S A *96*, 14517-14522.

Yuan, Z. M., Shioya, H., Ishiko, T., Sun, X., Gu, J., Huang, Y. Y., Lu, H., Kharbanda, S., Weichselbaum, R., and Kufe, D. (1999). p73 is regulated by tyrosine kinase c-Abl in the apoptotic response to DNA damage. Nature *399*, 814-817.

Zaika, A., Irwin, M., Sansome, C., and Moll, U. M. (2001). Oncogenes induce and activate endogenous p73 protein. J Biol Chem *276*, 11310-11316.

Zaika, A. I., and El-Rifai, W. (2006). The role of p53 protein family in gastrointestinal malignancies. Cell Death Differ *13*, 935-940.

Zaika, A. I., Kovalev, S., Marchenko, N. D., and Moll, U. M. (1999). Overexpression of the wild type p73 gene in breast cancer tissues and cell lines. Cancer Res *59*, 3257-3263.

Zaika, A. I., Slade, N., Erster, S. H., Sansome, C., Joseph, T. W., Pearl, M., Chalas, E., and Moll, U. M. (2002). DeltaNp73, a dominant-negative inhibitor of wild-type p53 and TAp73, is up-regulated in human tumors. J Exp Med *196*, 765-780.

Zeng, X., Chen, L., Jost, C. A., Maya, R., Keller, D., Wang, X., Kaelin, W. G., Jr., Oren, M., Chen, J., and Lu, H. (1999). MDM2 suppresses p73 function without promoting p73 degradation. Mol Cell Biol *19*, 3257-3266.

Zeng, X., Li, X., Miller, A., Yuan, Z., Yuan, W., Kwok, R. P., Goodman, R., and Lu, H. (2000). The N-terminal domain of p73 interacts with the CH1 domain of p300/CREB binding protein and mediates transcriptional activation and apoptosis. Mol Cell Biol *20*, 1299-1310.

Zheng, X., and Chen, X. (2001). Aquaporin 3, a glycerol and water transporter, is regulated by p73 of the p53 family. FEBS Lett *489*, 4-7.

Zhu, J., Jiang, J., Zhou, W., and Chen, X. (1998). The potential tumor suppressor p73 differentially regulates cellular p53 target genes. Cancer Res *58*, 5061-5065.

Zwahlen, D., Tschan, M. P., Grob, T. J., Peters, U. R., Fink, D., Haenggi, W., Altermatt, H. J., Cajot, J. F., Tobler, A., Fey, M. F., and Aebi, S. (2000). Differential expression of p73 splice variants and protein in benign and malignant ovarian tumours. Int J Cancer *88*, 66-70.

18

Role of ING Family Tumor Suppressors in Breast Cancer

Mehmet Gunduz[1], Esra Gunduz[2], Mikdat Bozer[3] and Ramazan Yigitoglu[4]
[1]Departments of Medical Genetics and Otolaryngology,
[2]Department of Medical Genetics,
[3]Department of General Surgery-Surgical Oncology Section,
[4]Department of Medical Biochemistry,
School of Medicine, Fatih University, Ankara,
Turkey

1. Introduction

Today cancer is one of the leading diseases, which treat human life and enormous efforts are being done for its eradication. Currently many cancer types including breast cancer are treated by extensive surgery as well as chemo-radiotherapy. These treatment modalities usually present extensive damage to the patient both anatomically, physiologically and psychologically. In addition, chemo-radiotherapy shows extreme side effects of the other system in the body and their efficiencies are quite limited especially in disseminated metastatic cases. Recent developments and progress in human genome technology provided us to develop novel therapeutic methods. This progress also provided novel biomarkers, which early diagnose the cancer and predict the sensitivity of the current chemo-radiation therapies.

Tight control by various regulatory mechanisms is applied on cell proliferation and growth in normal cells. However, certain genetic and epigenetic alterations permit the normal cells to avoid these mechanisms allowing indefinite cellular activities. Cancer is basically a genetic disease. The collection of genetic and epigenetic alterations of multiple genes and chromosomes lead to the development of cancer. In this regard, two major groups of tumor-associated genes, oncogenes and tumor suppressor genes (TSGs), have been implicated in the carcinogenic process **(Figure 1).**

TSGs have been defined as genetic elements whose loss or mutational inactivation allows cell to display one or more phenotypes of neoplastic growth [1]. TSG protein products are known to be involved in negative regulation of the cell cycle and proliferation and induction of apoptosis by different mechanisms. Thus inactivation of TSGs is one of the crucial steps during carcinogenetic process. In this process according to Knudson two-hit hypothesis for inactivation of TSGs [2], the deletion of targeted chromosomal regions (location of TSGs) eliminates one allele, while inactivating events (mutation, deletion, or epigenetic events such as promoter hypermethylation) affect the other allele of a concerning TSG [2]. The detection of frequent loss of heterozygosity (LOH) in a chromosomal locus is considered to be critical evidence for the localization of a TSG.

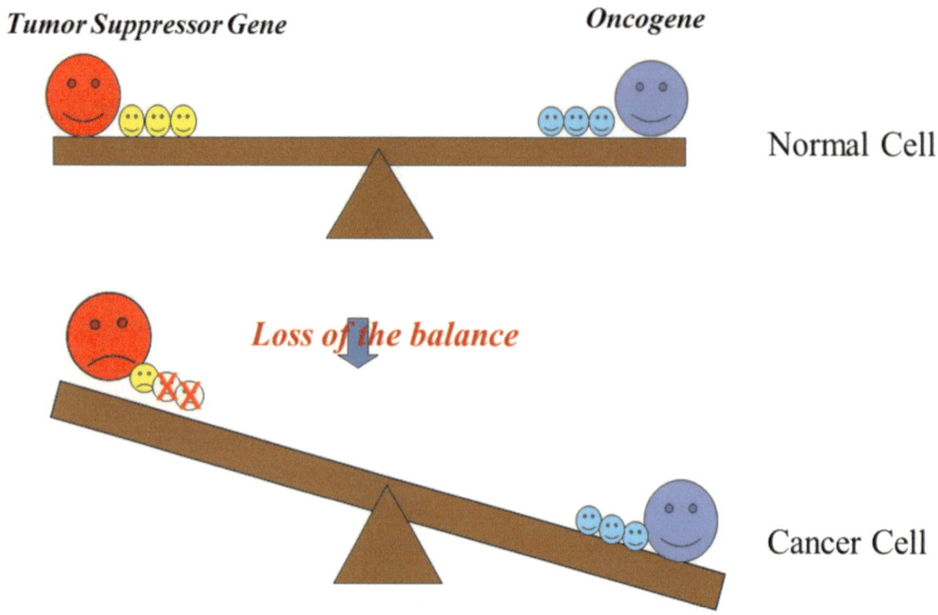

Fig. 1. Role of Oncogene and Tumor Suppressor Gene in Cancer.
Two group of genes (oncogene and tumor suppressor gene) influence on physiological cell proliferation and growth. In cancer development, balance between these two groups of genes is broken. Either oncogene activation or tumor suppressor gene inactivation promotes cancer development.

In fact many TSGs including well-known p53, RB1, p16, p21, and FHIT etc have been recently identified by using LOH analysis and then positional cloning. Inactivation of these classical TSGs usually occurs through deletion of one of its allele and mutation in the rest allele (Class I TSG, Knudson hypothesis). However, a novel class of TSGs with haploid insufficiency, in which one allele is lost and the remaining allele is haplo-insufficient, has been described recently, and the patients with these hemizygous TSGs in their genome are accepted as carriers for deficient allele of a TSG and they show a tumor-prone phenotype especially when challenged with carcinogens such as smoking, alcohol, x-ray, chemicals etc (Class II TSG) [3-7] **(Figure 2)**.

The novel TSG family, inhibitor of growth (ING), belongs to the group of genes that encodes proteins containing structural motifs involved in chromatin remodeling and transcription regulation. The ING family is classified as type II tumor suppressor since its inactivation has been implicated in neoplastic growth of various tumors [8-10]. Five human ING genes (ING1-5) have been identified and among them, ING1 is the founding member and the most widely studied. ING1 was first isolated using subtractive hybridization between short segments of cDNAs from normal and a number of breast cancer cell lines [11]. These randomly fragmented cDNAs interfered with the activity of tumor suppressors by either blocking protein production through anti-sense sequences or abrogating function in a dominant-negative fashion through truncated sense fragments [11]. Acute expression of transfected constructs encoding this gene inhibited cell growth while chronic expression of

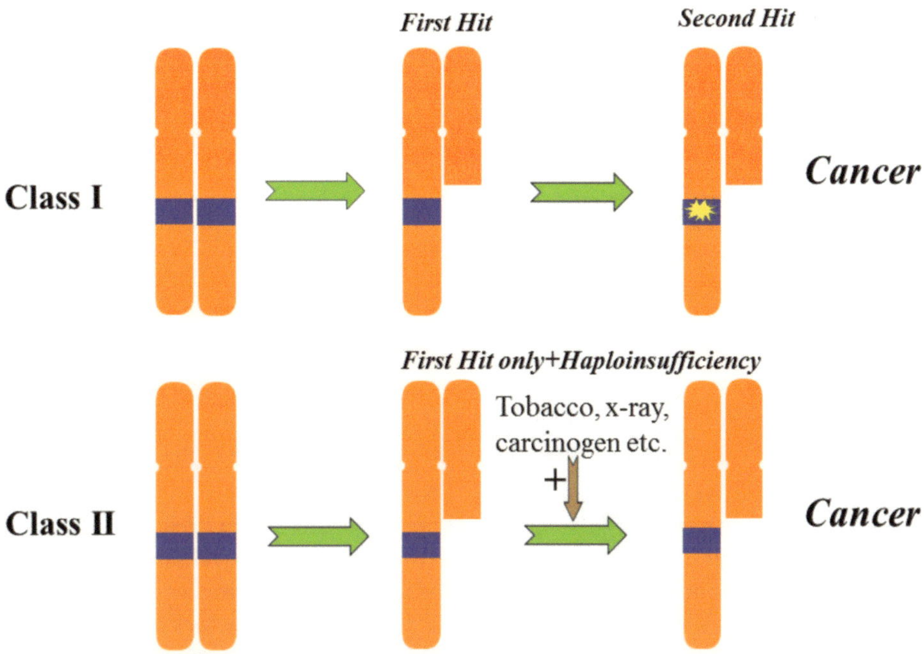

Fig. 2. Cancer Development through Inactivation of Tumor Suppressor Genes.
Knudson two-hit hypothesis for inactivation of TSGs, the deletion of targeted chromosomal regions (location of TSGs) eliminates one allele, while inactivating events (mutation, deletion, or epigenetic events such as promoter hypermethylation) affect the other allele of a concerning TSG (Class I). TSG with haploid insufficiency, in which one allele is lost and the remaining hemizygous allele is not enough to provide full suppression on cellular proliferation. These patients are carrier for deficient allele of a TSG and they show a tumor-prone phenotype especially when challenged with carcinogens such as smoking, alcohol, x-ray, chemicals etc (Class II).

antisense ING1 constructs promoted transformation of mouse breast epithelial cells and increased the frequency of focus formation with NIH3T3 cells and protected cells from apoptosis [11, 12]. Using radiation hybrid analysis, ING1 gene was mapped on human chromosome 13q33-34 [13]. The other four members have been disclosed through sequence homologies with ING1, followed by functional in-vitro and then in-vivo cancer patient tissue analysis [9, 10, 14-16]. However, recent researches demonstrated opposite findings for some of ING family members such as ING2 as a possible oncogene in specific conditions. In fact, ING2 expression was found to be increased in colorectal cancer and knock-down of ING2 suppressed cell growth and induced cell cycle arrest or apoptosis [17].

2. Structure and function of ING family genes

All members of ING family have distinct N-termini, which dictate the specific role of the ING members and, in certain instances, their antagonistic regulatory function [9,10,14-16]. Also all ING family members exhibit a highly conserved C-terminal plant homeodomain (PHD) that is commonly found in various chromatin remodeling proteins [9,10,14-22]

(Figure 3). The PHD motif consists of about 60 amino acids and shows a C4HC3 ring structure that typically binds two Zn2+ ions [16]. Approximately 150 distinct PHD domain-bearing proteins have been predicted to occur in humans [16]. PHD domains have been implicated in chromatin remodeling due to presence of their proteins as known components of larger chromatin remodeling complexes, and may function by strengthening a separate chromatin-binding activity of either the same protein or an associated protein [16]. Mutations within the PHD fingers of numerous proteins have been reported to be linked to tumorigenesis, immuno-deficiency syndromes, autoimmune syndromes, and several other genetic disorders [15, 23-26]. These mutations mainly occur at zinc-coordinating residues, suggesting that zinc ligation and hence integrity of the PHD finger fold are critical for the function of PHD finger-containing proteins [15].

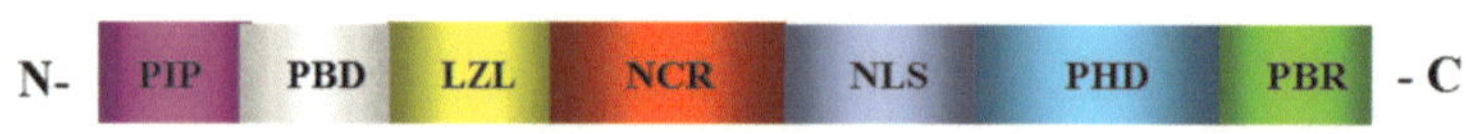

Fig. 3. Structure and Interacting Domains of ING Family Proteins.
All ING family proteins have a highly conserved plant homeodomain (PHD) finger motif, Novel Conserved Region (NCR) and Nuclear Localization Sequence (NLS). NLS directs ING to the nucleus through binding of the karyopherin/importins. NCR serves as an interacting site for lamin A as well as HAT/HDACs. The PHD finger binds to histone H3 and has a role in chromatin regulation. PCNA-interacting motif (PIP) and Partial Bromodomain (PBD) are specific to ING1. The PIP motif binds to PCNA and promotes ING1-mediated apoptosis. PBD domain binds SAP30 of mSin3A-HDAC1 and has a role in transcription regulation. All ING proteins except ING1 include LZL domain, which has roles in apoptosis and nucleotide excision repair of DNA. Both ING1 and ING2 include a short polybasic region called as PBR, to which PtdIns3P and PtdIns4P bind.

All ING proteins contain nuclear conserved region (NCR) domain, which was identified by sequence analyses and is the second most highly conserved domain in the ING family proteins [15]. This N-terminal region of ING1 has been reported to interact directly with lamin A, suggesting that the association with nuclear lamina is a common feature of this family [27].
All ING proteins contain a nuclear localization signal (NLS) at the carboxy terminal, and some of ING proteins have multiple NLS. Deletion of the NLS of ING1 resulted in cytoplasmic accumulation of the protein [28,29]. Translocation of ING proteins into the nucleus has been thought to be critical for their function because these molecules are nuclear proteins, and also it is clearly considered to be so by the observation of loss of nuclear ING1 staining in a number of cancers [16, 30]. Deletion of the entire NLS of ING4 resulted in a protein that could no longer bind p53 in co-transfection experiments [31]. Moreover, two copies of a putative nucleolar translocation signal (NTS) were found within the NLS of ING1, and translocation of ING1 into the nucleolus following exposure to UV light was suggested to be required for ING1-associated apoptosis [16,28].
All ING proteins, except ING1, contain leucine zipper-like (LZL) domain at the N-terminus. LZL domain forms a hydrophobic patch consisting of four to five conserved leucine or isoleucine residues spanning every seven amino acids. Similar leucine distribution has also been reported for ING3 to ING5 [15,32,33]. There is few information about the function of LZL and it been has reported that the LZL domain of ING2 is required for the induction of apoptosis and NER [34]. ING2 deletion mutants lacking the LZL domain do not show

increased apoptosis following UV exposure, suggesting that this domain is necessary for ING2-mediated apoptosis [34]. RNAi-mediated knockdown of ING2 has also been reported to abrogate the nucleotide excision repair (NER) capacity of melanoma cells [35].

Within ING family members, only ING1 includes PCNA binding domain called as PIP box in a DNA damage-inducible manner at N-terminus. This domain indicates the role of ING1 in DNA repair since PCNA has roles for DNA replication and repair. The interaction of this domain is specifically induced upon UV damage and has been thought to change PCNA activity away from DNA replication towards DNA repair [36]. Another unique domain present only in ING1b is called as PBD (partial bromodomain because of its sequence homology to bromodomains), which binds SAP30 of mSin3A-HDAC1, suggesting its role in transcriptional regulation of some genes [37].

Both ING1 and ING2 include a short polybasic region called as PBR at C-terminus. Though exact functions of this domain remain unknown, it has been reported that PtdIns3P and PtdIns4P can bind to the PBR [10,38], while PtdIns5P binds to the PHD motif of ING2 [10,39].

3. Genomic location, structure and expression of ING family genes

Most ING family genes are ubiquitously expressed in human tissues. We characterized genomic structure of human ING1 gene, and demonstrated that the human ING1 gene contains three exons (1a, 1b and 2) and two introns [8]. The gene has been mapped to chromosome 13 (13q33-34), and it has been found to encode 4 different mRNA variants. ING1 is ubiquitously expressed in various tissues [8]. The second member of the ING family, ING2 gene, has been mapped on chromosome 4 (4q35.1) and has been known to have 2 variants; ING2a and ING2b [40]. ING2 has 3 exons including ex1a, ex1b and 2 [41]. Our group identified the ING3 gene on chromosome 7 (7q31). The ING3 also encodes 2 different variants [9,10,41,42]. ING3 has 12 exons at its genomic location. The ING4 gene has been mapped on chromosome 12 (12q13.3) and encodes 8 variants with 8 exons [9,10,43,44]. The ING5 gene has been mapped on chromosome 2 (2q37.3) and encodes at least 5 different splicing variants with 8 exons [9,10,45].

4. Biological functions of ING family genes

ING proteins are involved in regulation of various cellular processes and signaling pathways such as angiogenesis, growth regulation, senescence, apoptosis, chemosensitivity, cell cycle, cell migration and DNA repair through p53-dependent and -independent pathways. ING proteins form complexes with HAT/HDAC [9,10,46]. After discovery of ING family genes prototype ING1, most of the functional studies have been conducted using ING1 variants, but fewer recently increasing studies, involving other ING family members, have also identified similar roles for these ING proteins. In addition, inhibition of ING proteins has been shown to increase cell spreading as well as migration, and relieve contact inhibition.

p33ING1b physically associates with the p53 tumor suppressor protein and seems to be a critical cofactor in p53-mediated regulation of cell growth and apoptosis [9,10,46,47]. However in a separate study, p37Ing1, mouse variant of human p33ING1b, blocked cell proliferation regardless of p53 and did not affect p53-mediated cell growth arrest following DNA damage [48]. p37Ing1 in mice regulated Bax levels in a negative way and worked as a prosurvival molecule following DNA damage independent of p53 status, complicating the function of ING1 in mouse and human and in various other circumstances. Moreover, recent experiments have also suggested that there are p53-independent functions for the ING proteins, including regulation of the NF-kB and hypoxia inducible factor (HIF) pathways [49-52].

ING2 shows a high rate of homology with ING1 about 70% [9,10,30,34,53]. Similar to other members of the ING family, ING2 is reported to have function in cooperation with p53, which is important for modulation of p53-mediated chromatin remodeling [54]. p33ING2 induces G1 phase cell cycle arrest or apoptosis in a p53-dependent manner following DNA damage [53]. ING2 has important roles in senescence, cellular response to DNA damage and DNA repair [34, 54]. Recently ING2 was also shown to interact with members of the transforming growth factor (TGF)-β signaling pathways enhancing transcription of target genes and cell cycle arrest [55]. However, overexpression of ING2 in colorectal cancer, burkitt lymphoma and cervical cancer and decreased expression in others such as head and neck carcinoma suggested that ING2 might have different function in various cancers [9,10,19,41,56,57]. Moreover, ING2 has 2 splicing variants and knockout experiments suggested oncogenic function of this gene [40,41]. In a recent study, a new function of ING2 was identified for the control of DNA replication and the maintenance of genome stability [58].

We identified ING3 for the first time by a homology search in human genome and showed ING3 as a candidate tumor suppressor in head and neck cancer [42]. Overexpression of p47ING3 protein resulted in a decreased population of cells in S phase, a diminished colony-forming efficiency, and induced apoptosis in RKO cells with wild type p53, but not in RKO-E6 cells with inactivated p53, suggesting necessity of p53 protein for at least some of its functions [59]. Histone acetyl transferase (HAT) complexes are important regulators of gene expression and among these, the NuA4 complex, first characterized in yeast, stands out as it controls multiple key nuclear functions in eukaryotic cells such as regulation of transcription, cell-cycle progression as well as the process of DNA repair [60]. p47ING3 activates p53-transactivated promoters, including promoters of p21/waf1 [61] and ING3 has been a stable component of Tip60/NuA4 HAT complex that cooperates with p53 and blocked cell cycle by activating the p21/waf1 gene [9,10,62,63]. Tip60 is an important transcriptional cofactor for p53-, NF-kB- and Myc-dependent transcription activation, suggesting that ING3 might have functions for many processes such as apoptosis and metastasis suppression at the transcription level through its association with the Tip60/NuA4 complex [63]. ING3 expression significantly promoted apoptosis by activating the Fas/caspase-8 pathway, suggesting that ING3 may also be involved in the death-receptor pathways [9,10,15,64]. Recently ING3 has been reported to be degraded by the ubiquitin-proteasome pathway through the SCF (Skp2) complex and interruption of ING3 degradation enhanced the tumor-suppressive function of ING3 [65].

p29ING4 was identified by Shiseki et al [66]. Overexpression of ING4 protein resulted in a diminished colony-forming efficiency, a decreased cell population in S phase, and the induction of apoptosis in a p53-dependent manner. p29ING4 also activated the p21/waf1 promoter, and induce p21/WAF1 expression [66].

ING4 has been proposed to regulate cell cycling and apoptosis. ING4 has been reported to inhibit angiogenesis by various studies besides its role for cellular processes common for all ING family members [67-69]. It has been demonstrated that ING4 physically interacts with p65 (RelA), a subunit of nuclear factor NF-kB, and that ING4 regulates angiogenesis through transcriptional repression of NF-kB-responsive genes in brain tumors [70]. ING4 functional studies suggest that this gene in addition to the common functions of the ING proteins could play a completely different role in tumorigenesis. Actually, ING4 is likely to be involved in inhibition of the cell's spreading and migration as well as tumor angiogenesis. Indeed, its loss results in loss of contact inhibition, activation of NF-kB transcriptional activity and enhanced cell migration. Thus ING4 deficiency may be a crucial step in malignant progression, especially for glioblastoma [9,10,15,16,66,71-75].

ING4 also associates with HBO1 (HAT binding to ORC1)/HAT complex [63,76]. It was shown that interaction between ING4 and H3K4me3 augments HBO1 acetylation activity on H3 tails and drives H3 acetylation at ING4 target promoters, which facilitates apoptosis in response to genotoxic stress and inhibits anchorage-independent cell growth, and these functions depend on ING4 interaction with H3K4me3 [77]. ING4 was recently reported to interact with tumor suppressor p53 through interaction with NLS domain and negatively regulate the cell growth with significant G2/M arrest of cell cycle in HepG2 cells through up-regulation of p53-inducible gene p21 [31,78].

Similar to ING4, ING5 was also identified by Shiseki et al [66]. Overexpression of ING5 protein also resulted in a diminished colony-forming efficiency, a decreased cell population in S phase, and the induction of apoptosis in a p53-dependent manner. p28ING5 protein activated the p21/waf1 promoter, and induced p21/WAF1 expression [66]. Relatively little information is available in the literature for ING5. Doyon et al. recently identified MOZ (monocytic leukemia zinc finger protein)/MORF (MOZ related factor) and HBO1 to be catalytic native subunits of ING5 complexes, which are necessary for their activity [63]. The MOZ, and the related factor MORF also form tetrameric complexes with Esa1-associated factor 6 ortholog (EAF6), and the bromodomain- and PHD finger protein (BRPF)-1, -2, or -3. BRPF proteins are rich in domains found in chromatin-associated factors, like PHD fingers and bromodomain. Ullah and his group found that BRPF proteins bridge the association of MOZ and MORF with ING5 and a homolog of yeast Esa-1 associated factor 6 (EAF6) [9,10,79]. ING5 as an adapter molecule links the MOZ/MORF and HBO1/HAT complexes. PHD fingers of ING proteins recognize histone H3 methylated at lysine 4 at the chromatin, suggesting the functional role of ING5 in the chromatin remodeling process [79, 80].

5. Disorders of ING family genes in human tumors

Rearrangement of ING1 gene locus was demonstrated in one neuroblastoma cell line and reduced expression in primary cancers and cell lines in early clinical studies at the time of ING1 cloning [8-11]. Following ING1 cDNA cloning, we identified the genomic structure of the human ING1 gene and showed its tumor suppressor character for the first time by finding its chromosomal deletion at the 13q34 locus and tumor-specific mutations in a number of head and neck squamous cell carcinoma (HNSCC) samples [8].

Few studies have analyzed the mRNA expression status of ING family genes in various human cancers. Toyama et al. found decrease of ING1 mRNA expression in about half of breast cancer samples and all of the breast cancer cell lines they examined [47]. Another study also revealed reduced expression of breast cancer samples [81]. Down-regulation of ING1 mRNA has also been demonstrated in various other cancer types, including lymphoid malignancies, gastric tumors, brain tumors, lung cancer, ovarian cancer and esophagogastric carcinomas, though no comprehensive clinical correlation was performed [9,10,15,16,82-90]. Uncommon missense mutations and reduced protein expression of ING1 have also been detected in esophageal carcinomas [91], and colon cancer cell lines [83] while no mutation was detected in leukemia [84,92], oral cancers [93] and lymphoid malignancies [82].

For loss of ING gene and their protein functions, loss of heterozygosity (LOH), promoter CpG hypermetylation and nucleo-cytoplasmic protein mislocalization have been proposed [9,10,15,16]. Using methylation-specific PCR, the p33ING1b promoter was methylated and silenced in almost a quarter of all cases in primary ovarian tumors [89]. No differences or increased expression of ING1 were observed in recent studies of myeloid leukemia or melanoma [92,94].

Recently reduced expression of ING2 mRNA as well as protein was observed in hepatocellular carcinoma (HCC) [95]. Decreased ING2 expression (but not ING2 mutation) has been observed in lung cancer [96]. Decrease of nuclear ING2 protein was observed in melanoma [57]. On the other hand increased expression of ING2 mRNA was shown in colon cancer [97]. We recently demonstrated that frequent deletion of ING2 locus at 4q35.1 associated with advanced tumor stage in HNSCC [98]. Moreover, ING2 may play a role in melanoma initiation, since reduction of nuclear ING2 has been reported in radial as well as vertical growth phases, and metastatic melanoma as compared to dysplastic nevi [57]. On the other hand, reduced ING2 expression was associated with tumor progression and shortened survival time in HCC [95]. These epidemiological studies suggest that ING2 loss or reduction may be important for tumor initiation and/or progression [9,10,15,16].

We showed frequent allelic loss of ING3 in HNSCC [42]. But ING3 mutation was very rare in our study (a sole missense mutation of ING3 at codon 20). In another recent study using a large study population, we revealed that down-regulation of ING3 was more evident in late-stage tumors as compared with early stage patients, and patients with low ING3 mRNA expression demonstrated worse survival rates as compared to the patients with normal-high ING3 expression [99]. As shown for ING2, decreased nuclear ING3 protein expression was associated with a poor survival rate. The survival rate was 93% for the patients with strong nuclear ING3 staining, whereas it declined to 44% for the patients with negative-to-moderate nuclear staining [100]. In a recent study, we also demonstrated frequent deletion of chromosomal locus of each of ING family member including ING3 in ameloblastomas [101].

ING4 mRNA was decreased in glioblastoma and associated with tumor progression [70]. Decreased ING4 has been associated with increased expression of IL-8 and osteopontin (OPN) in myeloma [9,102]. In both reports, decreased ING4 expression was associated with higher tumor grade and increased tumor angiogenesis. In myeloma, it was also associated with increased expression of interleukin-8 and osteopontin [9,102]. Expression of ING4 was decreased in malignant melanoma as compared to dysplastic nevi, and was found to be an independent poor prognostic factor for the patients [73]. ING4 was found to suppress the loss of contact inhibition and growth. Moreover some mutation and deletion were detected in cell lines derived from human cancers such as breast and lung [103].

We reported reduced expression level of ING4 and frequent LOH of the ING4 locus in HNSCC [43]. No mutation of the ING4 gene was found in head and neck cancers. Significant reduced expression of ING4 was detected in gliomas as compared with normal human brain tissue, and the extent of reduction correlated with the progression from lower to higher grades of tumours [70]. Klironomos et al. investigated immunohistochemically the expression pattern of ING-4, NF-kappaB and the NF-kappaB downstream targets MMP-2, MMP-9 and u-PA in human astrocytomas from 101 patients. They found that ING-4 expression was significantly reduced in astrocytomas, and it was associated with tumor grade progression. Expression of a NF-kappaB subunit p65 was significantly higher in grade

IV than in grade III and grade I/II tumors, and a statistical significant negative correlation between expression of ING-4 and expression of nuclear p65 was noticed [104].

Recently Nagahama et al. reported up-regulation of ING4 in a human gastric carcinoma cell line (MKN-1) by promoting mitochondria-mediated apoptosis via the activation of p53 [105]. Both mRNA and protein of ING4 expression were down regulated in hepatocellular carcinoma tissues. ING4 expression level correlated with prognosis and metastatic potential of hepatocellular carcinoma [106]. In another recent study, ING4 mRNA and protein expression were examined in gastric adenocarcinoma tissues and human gastric adenocarcinoma cell lines by RT-PCR, real-time RT-PCR, tissue microarray immunohistochemistry, and western blot analysis [107]. Their data showed that ING4 mRNA and protein were dramatically reduced in stomach adenocarcinoma cell lines and tissues, and significantly less in female than in male patients. Decrease of ING4 mRNA expression was found to correlate with the stage of the tumour [107]. Wang et al. examined ING4 protein expression in 246 lung cancer samples and overall reduced ING4 expression and higher ING4 expression in cytoplasm than in nucleus of tumour cells were detected, suggesting its involvement in the initiation and progression of lung cancers [108].

In a recent study, nuclear expression of ING4 was found to gradually decrease from non-cancerous epithelium and dysplasia to HNSCC and was negatively correlated with a poorly-differentiated status, T staging, and TNM staging in HNSCC. On the other hand, cytoplasmic expression of ING4 was significantly enhanced in HNSCC and was significantly associated with lymph node metastasis and 14-3-3η expression. Moreover, nuclear expression of ING4 was positively correlated with p21 and p300 expression and with the apoptotic index. Their results suggested that the decreases in nuclear ING4 and cytoplasmic translocation of ING4 protein play important roles in tumorigenesis, progression and tumor differentiation in HNSCC [109].

Examination of ING4 protein expression levels in colorectal cancer samples from 97 patients showed that ING4 protein was down regulated in adenoma relative to normal mucosa and further reduced in colorectal cancer tissues. Decrease of ING4 protein expression was also related to the more advanced Dukes' stages and ING4 expression levels in patients with lymphatic metastasis were lower than those without metastasis, suggesting that ING4 play a role in colorectal carcinoma progression [110].

Our group reported the first study linking ING5 chromosome locus to a human cancer. We demonstrated a high ratio of LOH in oral cancer using 16 microsatellite markers on the long arm of chromosome 2q21-37.3 [111]. ING5 appeared to be a strong candidate tumor suppressor in this study though several other candidate TSGs including ILKAP, HDAC4, PPP1R7, DTYMK, STK25, BOK are also localized at the area, where frequent deletion has been detected [9,10,111]. Moreover, our recent study revealed decreased expression of ING5 mRNA and mutations in oral cancer samples as compared to their corresponding normal controls, suggesting its tumor suppressive role in cancer [45]. Examination of 172 cases of HNSCC for ING5 protein by immunohistochemistry using tissue microarray, and in 3 oral SCC cell lines by immunohistochemistry and Western blot showed that a decrease in nuclear ING5 localization and cytoplasmic translocation were detected, supporting the previous studies and strong involvement of ING5 in tumorigenesis and tumor differentiation in HNSCC [112].

Xing et al. analyzed ING5 expression in gastric carcinoma tissues and cell lines (MKN28, MKN45, AGS, GT-3 TKB, and KATO-III) by Western blot and reverse transcriptase-polymerase chain reaction. An increased expression of ING5 messenger RNA was found in gastric carcinoma in comparison with paired mucosa and lower expression of nuclear ING5 protein and cytoplasmic translocation was detected in gastric dysplasia and carcinoma than that in nonneoplastic mucosa [113]. Nuclear ING5 expression was negatively correlated with tumor size, depth of invasion, lymph node metastasis, and clinicopathologic staging, whereas cytoplasmic ING5 was positively associated with depth of invasion, venous invasion, lymph node metastasis, and clinicopathologic staging [113].

6. Abnormalities of ING family genes in breast cancer

Abnormalities of ING family members are linked to etiopathogenesis of various cancers including breast cancer. In fact, ING1, the founding member, was first isolated using a method that combined PCR-mediated subtractive hybridization of cDNAs from normal and breast cancerous cells [11]. Later same group examined ING1 mutation and mRNA expression in breast cancer cell lines and in a large number of primary breast cancers [47]. Within 377 breast cancer patients analyzed for mutation of ING1, one germ-line missense and three germ-line silent alterations were detected. Then mRNA analysis was randomly examined in 48 breast cancer samples. Their results showed that ING1 mRNA expression was decreased (2-10-fold) in 44% (21 out of 48 cases) of breast cancer tissues compared to adjacent normal tissues, while 33% (16/48) of the tumors demonstrated levels similar to control sample and 23% (11/48) showed increases in ING1 mRNA. All of the 10 breast cancer lines displayed decreased ING1 mRNA expression. Using in situ hybridization, decrease of mRNA in breast cancer cells was also confirmed as compared to adjacent normal cells. Using a monoclonal antibody against ING1, similar levels of the protein was also demonstrated in randomly selected 10 breast cancer samples [47]. When the relationship between ING1 mRNA expression levels and clinicopathological factors of breast cancer samples was examined, probability of metastasis to regional lymph nodes was significantly increased in ING1-decreased samples. Only one of 11 tumors (%9) with increased ING1 mRNA expression metastasized to lymph nodes, whereas 11 of 19 cases (58%) with decreased expression of ING1 showed metastasis to lymph nodes [47].

Tokunaga et al. examined the expression of ING1 mRNA in breast cancer cell lines and clinical breast cancer tissues, using quantitative RT-PCR and real-time TaqMan™ technology [81]. Decreased expression of ING1 mRNA was found in 71% of the breast cancer samples as compared to adjacent normal tissues. The authors has also examined p53 mutation status by immunohistochemistry and decreased ING1 expression was detected in 9 of 15 tumors that were negative for p53 immunostaining (i.e, wild type). Decrease of ING1 mRNA was speculated to be responsible for malfunction of p53 in these cases [9,10,81].

In an immunohistochemical study performed by Nouman et al, 69 (80%) out of 86 breast cancer cases showed reduced expression of p33ING1b protein. On the other hand, strong nuclear expression of ING1 protein was detected in normal breast lobules and adjacent stroma. Correlation of each of estrogen and progesterone receptor status demonstrated a positive response with nuclear expression of p33ING1b protein. Nuclear loss of ING1 protein was associated with a concomitant enhancement of cytoplasmic p33ING1b expression in a proportion of the cases, suggesting as a cause for loss of normal function of the ING1 protein [114]. Similar reduced nuclear expression of p33ING1b protein was also shown in acute lymphoblastic leukemia [115], melanoma [116].

Toyama et al. reported that p33ING1b increased ERα transcriptional activity stimulated by estrogen through AF2 domain [10, 117]. In another research, p40, a protein highly homologous to breast carcinoma metastasis suppressor 1 (BRMS1), was found to be unit of the mammalian Sin3A co-repressor complex including RBP1 and p33ING1b and overexpression of p40 in human cells inhibited cell growth by recruiting the HDAC1 deacetylase complex. When tethered to the promoter by Gal-DNA binding domain, p40 can repress transcription of the luciferase reporter gene [118].

Kim et al. tried to identify genes that can suppress oncogenic properties such as loss of contact inhibition elicited by overexpression of MYCN. Their screen data revealed ING4 as a suppressor of loss of contact inhibition. Then they hypothesized that a deficiency of ING4 may play a role in tumorigenesis. For this aim, they examined ING4 transcripts in human cancer cell lines. They found a common deletion in various cancer cell lines including a breast cancer cell, T47D. Deletion of the four highly charged amino acid residues (KGKK) would result in mislocalization of the ING4 protein, thereby impairing its function [103]. Later this deletion was reported to be a source of alternative splicing variants of ING4 and was linked to abnormalities of subcellular localization of ING4 [71]. Besides Kim et al. also performed southern blot analysis for ING4 locus deletion in 55 breast cancer cell lines using 2 BAC probe within ING4 locus at 12p13.31. These probes, BAC RP11-272L6 and BAC RP11-59H1, were shown to be deleted in 24% and 11% of the cells including T47D breast cancer cell line, respectively [103].

In a recent study, ING4 was found to suppress an initial hyperplastic response to the oncogene MYC in a mouse model of breast cancer. In addition, they showed that a C-terminal truncation mutant of ING4 found in a human neuroblastoma cell line induced mammary hyperplasia and exacerbated MYC-initiated mammary tumorigenesis, suggesting that ING4 can function as a tumor suppressor gene in breast tissue [119].

In another recent report, therapeutic effect of adenovirus-mediated ING4 (Ad-ING4) gene therapy was investigated in human breast cancers in vitro and in vivo in an athymic nude mouse model, using two human breast carcinoma cell lines MDA-MB-231 (mutant p53) and MCF-7 (wild-type p53). The results displayed that Ad-ING4 treatment could induce in vitro significant growth suppression in both mutant p53 MDA-MB-231 and wild-type p53 MCF-7 breast carcinoma cells despite p53 status. Moreover the study further revealed that Ad-ING4 gene transfer resulted in G2/M phase arrest and apoptosis, upregulation of p21, p27, and Bax, downregulation of Bcl-2, IL-8, and Ang-1, promoted cytochrome c release from mitochondria into cytosol, and activated caspase-9, caspase-3, and PARP in mutant p53 MDA-MB-231 breast carcinoma cells. Furthermore, intratumoral injections of Ad-ING4 in nude mice bearing mutant p53 MDA-MB-231 breast tumors clearly inhibited the human breast xenografted tumor growth and decreased CD34 expression of tumor vessels and microvessel density. All these results suggest that Ad-ING4 is a potential candidate for breast cancer gene therapy [120].

ING4 was detected to be deleted in 170 (16.5%) of 1033 breast cancer samples using two color FISH with a probe of BAC RP11-433J6 including ING4 locus. Comparison of clinicopathological variables with ING4 deletion status in these breast cancer samples showed significant difference for Her2 expression status. Thirty- nine (23.8%) of 164 of tumors with ING4 deletion were HER2 positive, as compared with 115 (14.1%) of 814 of tumors without deletion. In another way, 25.3% (39/ 154) of HER2-positive tumors harbored ING4 deletion as compared to 15.1% (125/824) of HER2-negative tumors, indicating that ING4 deletion is more common in HER2- positive tumors [121]. In breast cancer, there is no report yet regarding with other members of ING family, ING2, 3 and 5. A summary of alterations of ING family genes in breast cancer is shown in table 1.

ING Gene	Alteration	Reference
ING1	Mutation, ↓ mRNA expression, ↓ protein expression	47
ING1	↓ mRNA expression	81
ING1	↓ Nuclear protein, ↑ Cytoplasmic protein	114
ING1	Induction of ERα activity	117
ING4	Deletion at chromosomal locus	103
ING4	Suppression of MYC-induced carcinogenesis	119
ING4	Ad-ING4-treated suppression of cancer cells and tumor growth	120
ING4	Deletion at chromosomal locus	121

Table 1. Alterations of ING Family Genes in Breast Cancer.

7. Future prospects

Nearly 15 years of research after discovery of the first member of ING family gene, ING1, there are more accumulating data which show importance of these gene family in multiple cellular functions such as transcription, chromatin regulation, cell cycling, angiogenesis, cell transformation, apoptosis, growth regulation, senescence, DNA repair and tumorigenesis etc. Recent knowledge on this family displays that the family members have common and separate functions in human cancer. Though at the beginning, all members were considered to be tumor suppressor, recent evidences show a complex situation with oncogenic functions for at least some of the members and in some specific conditions. Thus both diagnostic and therapeutic approach should be revisited according to their functional roles in various conditions and tumor types. Though much work is necessary for clarifying the exact functions of these genes to provide therapy for various human cancers, promising results are noticed at the moment for usability of these genes as a therapeutic and diagnostic target. Thus progress on the knowledge of functions of ING family genes as well as the relationship with p53 and other unknown molecules will clarify their roles in cancer, which will result in their uses in cancer diagnostics as well as therapy soon.

8. References

[1] Hinds PW and Weinberg RA. Tumor suppressor genes. Curr Opin Genet Dev 4: 135-141, 1994

[2] Knudson AG Jr. Mutation and cancer: statistical study of retinoblastoma. Proc Natl Acad Sci USA 68: 820-823, 1971

[3] Tang B, Bottinger EP, Jakowlew SB, Bagnall KM, Mariano J, Anver MR, Letterio JJ and Wakefield LM. Transforming growth factor-b1 is a new form of tumor suppressor with true haploid insufficiency. Nat Med 4: 802-807, 1998

[4] Bai F, Pei XH, Godfrey VL and Xiong Y. Haploinsufficiency of p18 (INK4c) sensitizes mice to carcinogen-induced tumorigenesis. Mol Cell Biol 23: 1269-1277, 2003
[5] Mduff FK, Hook CE, Tooze RM, Huntly BJ, Pandolfi PP, Turner SD. Determining the contribution of NPM1 heterozygosity to NPM-ALK-induced lymphomagenesis. Lab Invest. 2011 Jun 27. doi: 10.1038/labinvest.2011.96. [Epub ahead of print]
[6] Huang H, Wei X, Su X, Qiao F, Xu Z, Gu D, Fan H, Chen J. Clinical significance of expression of Hint1 and potential epigenetic mechanism in gastric cancer. Int J Oncol 38:1557-64, 2011
[7] Zhou XZ, Huang P, Shi R, Lee TH, Lu G, Zhang Z, Bronson R, Lu KP. The telomerase inhibitor PinX1 is a major haploinsufficient tumor suppressor essential for chromosome stability in mice. J Clin Invest 121(4):1266-82, 2011
[8] Gunduz M, Ouchida M, Fukushima K, Hanafusa H, Etani T, Nishioka S, Nishizaki K and Shimizu K. Genomic structure of the human ING1 gene and tumor-specific mutations detected in head and neck squamous cell carcinomas. Cancer Res 60: 3143-3146, 2000
[9] Gunduz M, Gunduz E, Rivera RS, Nagatsuka H. The inhibitor of growth (ING) gene family: potential role in cancer therapy. Curr Cancer Drug Targets 8:275-84, 2008
[10] Gunduz M, Demircan K, Gunduz E, Katase N, Tamamura R, Nagatsuka H. Potential usage of ING family members in cancer diagnostics and molecular therapy. Curr Drug Targets. 10(5):465-76, 2009
[11] Garkavtsev I, Kazarov A, Gudkov A and Riabowol K. Suppression of the novel growth inhibitor p33ING1 promotes neoplastic transformation. Nat Genet 14: 415-420, 1996
[12] Helbing CC, Veilette C, Riabowol K, Johnston RN and Garkavtsev I. A novel candidate tumor suppressor gene, ING1, is involved in the regulation of apoptosis. Cancer Res 57: 1255-1258, 1997
[13] Zeremski M, Horrigan SK, Grigorian IA, Westbrook CA and Gudkov AV. Localization of the candidate tumor suppressor gene ING1 to human chromosome 13q34. Somatic Cell Mol Genet 23: 233-236, 1997
[14] Feng X, Hara Y and Riabowol K. Different HATS of the ING1 gene family. Trends Cell Biol 12: 532-538, 2002
[15] Aguissa-Touré AH, Wong RP, Li G. Cell Mol Life Sci. The ING family tumor suppressors: from structure to function. 68:45-54, 2011
[16] Coles AH, Jones SN. The ING gene family in the regulation of cell growth and tumorigenesis. J Cell Physiol 218:45-57, 2009
[17] Unoki M, Kumamoto K, Harris CC. ING proteins as potential anticancer drug targets. Curr Drug Targets 10:442-54, 2009
[18] Aasland R, Gibson TJ, Stewart AF. The PHD finger: implications for chromatin-mediated transcriptional regulation. Trends Biochem Sci 20:56-59, 1995
[19] Shimada Y, Saito A, Suzuki M, Takahashi E, Horie M. Cloning of a novel gene (ING1L) homologous to ING1, a candidate tumor suppressor. Cytogenet Cell Genet 83:232-235, 1998
[20] Ha S, Park S, Yun CH, Choi Y. Characterization of nuclear localization signal in mouse ING1 homolog protein. Biochem Biophys Res Commun 293:163-166, 2002
[21] Scott M, Boisvert FM, Vieyra D, Johnston RN, Bazett-Jones DP, Riabowol K. UV induces nucleolar translocation of ING1 through two distinct nucleolar targeting sequences. Nucleic Acids Re 29:2052-2058, 2001

[22] Zeremski M, Hill JE, Kwek SS, Grigorian IA, Gurova KV, Garkavtsev IV, Diatchenko L, Koonin EV, Gudkov AV. Structure and regulation of the mouse ing1 gene. Three alternative transcripts encode two phd finger proteins that have opposite effects on p53 function. J Biol Chem 274:32172-32181, 1999

[23] Pascual J, Martinez-Yamout M, Dyson HJ, Wright PE. Structure of the PHD zinc finger from human Williams-Beuren syndrome transcription factor. J Mol Biol 304:723-9, 2000

[24] Gibbons RJ, Bachoo S, Picketts DJ, Aftimos S, Asenbauer B, Bergoffen J, Berry SA, Dahl N, Fryer A, Keppler K, Kurosawa K, Levin ML, Masuno M, Neri G, Pierpont ME, Slaney SF, Higgs DR. Mutations in transcriptional regulator ATRX establish the functional significance of a PHD-like domain. Nat Genet 17:146-8, 1997

[25] Saugier-Veber P, Drouot N, Wolf LM, Kuhn JM, Frébourg T, Lefebvre H. Identification of a novel mutation in the autoimmune regulator (AIRE-1) gene in a French family with autoimmune polyendocrinopathy-candidiasis-ectodermal dystrophy. Eur J Endocrinol 144:347-51, 2001

[26] Elkin SK, Ivanov D, Ewalt M, Ferguson CG, Hyberts SG, Sun ZY, Prestwich GD, Yuan J, Wagner G, Oettinger MA, Gozani OP. A PHD finger motif in the C terminus of RAG2 modulates recombination activity. J Biol Chem 280:28701-10, 2005

[27] Han X, Feng X, Rattner JB, Smith H, Bose P, Suzuki K, Soliman MA, Scott MS, Burke BE, Riabowol K. Tethering by lamin A stabilizes and targets the ING1 tumour suppressor. Nat Cell Biol 10:1333–1340, 2008

[28] Scott M, Boisvert FM, Vieyra D, Johnston RN, Bazett-Jones DP, Riabowol K. UV induces nucleolar translocation of ING1 through two distinct nucleolar targeting sequences. Nucleic Acids Res 29:2052–2058, 2001

[29] Ha S, Park S, Yun CH, Choi Y. Characterization of nuclear localization signal in mouse ING1 homolog protein. Biochem Biophys Res Commun 293:163–166, 2002

[30] Gong W, Suzuki K, Russell M, Riabowol K. Function of the ING family of PHD proteins in cancer. Int J Biochem Cell Biol 37:1054–1065, 2005

[31] Zhang X, Wang KS, Wang ZQ, Xu LS, Wang QW, Chen F, Wei DZ, Han ZG. Nuclear localization signal of ING4 plays a key role in its binding to p53. Biochem Biophys Res Commun 331:1032–1038, 2005

[32] Soliman MA, Riabowol K. After a decade of study-ING, a PHD for a versatile family of proteins. Trends Biochem Sci 32:509–519, 2007

[33] He GH, Helbing CC, Wagner MJ, Sensen CW, Riabowol K. Phylogenetic analysis of the ING family of PHD finger proteins. Mol Biol Evol 22:104–116, 2005

[34] Wang Y, Wang J, Li G. Leucine zipper-like domain is required for tumor suppressor ING2-mediated nucleotide excision repair and apoptosis. FEBS Lett 580:3787–3793, 2006

[35] Wang J, Chin MY, Li G. The novel tumor suppressor p33ING2 enhances nucleotide excision repair via inducement of histone H4 acetylation and chromatin relaxation. Cancer Res 66:1906–1911, 2006

[36] Scott M, Bonnefin P, Vieyra D, Boisvert FM, Young D, Bazett- Jones DP, Riabowol K. UV-induced binding of ING1 to PCNA regulates the induction of apoptosis. J Cell Sci 114:3455–3462, 2001

[37] Kuzmichev A, Zhang Y, Erdjument-Bromage H, Tempst P, Reinberg D. Role of the Sin3-histone deacetylase com- plex in growth regulation by the candidate tumor suppressor p33(ING1). Mol Cell Biol 22:835–848, 2002
[38] Kaadige MR, Ayer DE. The polybasic region that follows the plant homeodomain zinc finger 1 of Pf1 is necessary and sufficient for specific phosphoinositide binding. J Biol Chem 281:28831–28836, 2006
[39] Huang W, Zhang H, Davrazou F, Kutateladze TG, Shi X, Gozani O, Prestwich GD. Stabilized phosphatidylinositol- 5-phosphate analogues as ligands for the nuclear protein ING2: chemistry, biology, and molecular modeling. J Am Chem Soc 129:6498–6506, 2007
[40] Unoki M, Kumamoto K, Robles AI, Shen JC, Zheng ZM, Harris CC. A novel ING2 isoform, ING2b, synergizes with ING2a to prevent cell cycle arrest and apoptosis. FEBS Lett 582:3868-74, 2008
[41] Unoki M, Kumamoto K, Takenoshita S, Harris CC. Reviewing the current classification of inhibitor of growth family proteins. Cancer Sci 100:1173-9, 2009
[42] Gunduz M, Ouchida M, Fukushima K, Ito S, Jitsumori Y, Nakashima T, Nagai N, Nishizaki K, Shimizu K. Allelic loss and reduced expression of the ING3, a candidate tumor suppressor gene at 7q31, in human head and neck cancers. Oncogene 21:4462-70, 2002
[43] Gunduz M, Nagatsuka H, Demircan K, Gunduz E, Cengiz B, Ouchida M, Tsujigiwa H, Yamachika E, Fukushima K, Beder L, Hirohata S, Ninomiya Y, Nishizaki K, Shimizu K, Nagai N. Frequent deletion and down-regulation of ING4, a candidate tumor suppressor gene at 12p13, in head and neck squamous cell carcinomas. Gene 15;356:109-117, 2005
[44] Ythier D, Larrieu D, Brambilla C, Brambilla E, Pedeux R. The new tumor suppressor genes ING: genomic structure and status in cancer. Int J Cancer 123:1483-90, 2008
[45] Cengiz B, Gunduz E, Gunduz M, Beder LB, Tamamura R, Bagci C, Yamanaka N, Shimizu K, Nagatsuka H. Tumor-specific mutation and downregulation of ING5 detected in oral squamous cell carcinoma. Int J Cancer 127:2088-94, 2010
[46] Campos EI, Chin MY, Kuo WH, Li G. Biological functions of the ING family tumor suppressors. Cell Mol Life Sci 61(19-20):2597-613, 2004
[47] Toyama T, Iwase H, Watson P, Muzik H, Saettler E, Magliocco A, DiFrancesco L, Forsyth P, Garkavtsev I, Kobayashi S, Riabowol K. Suppression of ING1 expression in sporadic breast cancer. Oncogene 18:5187-93, 1999
[48] Coles AH, Liang H, Zhu Z, Marfella CG, Kang J, Imbalzano AN, Jones SN. Deletion of p37Ing1 in mice reveals a p53-independent role for Ing1 in the suppression of cell proliferation, apoptosis, and tumorigenesis. Cancer Res 67:2054-61, 2007
[49] Ozer A, Bruick RK. Regulation of HIF by prolyl hydroxylases: recruitment of the candidate tumor suppressor protein ING4. Cell Cycle 4:1153-6, 2005
[50] Ozer A, Wu LC, Bruick RK. The candidate tumor suppressor ING4 represses activation of the hypoxia inducible factor (HIF). Proc Natl Acad Sci U S A 102:7481-6, 2005
[51] Coles AH, Gannon H, Cerny A, Kurt-Jones E, Jones SN. Inhibitor of growth-4 promotes IkappaB promoter activation to suppress NF-kappaB signaling and innate immunity. Proc Natl Acad Sci U S A 107:11423-8, 2010

[52] Nozell S, Laver T, Moseley D, Nowoslawski L, De Vos M, Atkinson GP, Harrison K, Nabors LB, Benveniste EN. The ING4 tumor suppressor attenuates NF-kappaB activity at the promoters of target genes. Mol Cell Biol 28:6632-45, 2008
[53] Nagashima M, Shiseki M, Miura K, Hagiwara K, Linke SP, Pedeux R, Wang XW, Yokota J, Riabowol K, Harris CC. DNA damage-inducible gene p33ING2 negatively regulates cell proliferation through acetylation of p53. Proc Natl Acad Sci U S A 98:9671-6, 2001
[54] Pedeux R, Sengupta S, Shen JC, Demidov ON, Saito S, Onogi H, Kumamoto K, Wincovitch S, Garfield SH, McMenamin M, Nagashima M, Grossman SR, Appella E, Harris CC. ING2 regulates the onset of replicative senescence by induction of p300-dependent p53 acetylation. Mol Cell Biol 25:6639-48, 2005
[55] Sarker KP, Kataoka H, Chan A, Netherton SJ, Pot I, Huynh MA, Feng X, Bonni A, Riabowol K, Bonni S. ING2 as a novel mediator of transforming growth factor-beta-dependent responses in epithelial cells. J Biol Chem 283:13269-79, 2008
[56] Borkosky SS, Gunduz M, Nagatsuka H, Beder LB, Gunduz E, Ali MA, Rodriguez AP, Cilek MZ, Tominaga S, Yamanaka N, Shimizu K, Nagai N. Frequent deletion of ING2 locus at 4q35.1 associates with advanced tumor stage in head and neck squamous cell carcinoma. J Cancer Res Clin Oncol 135:703-13, 2009
[57] Lu F, Dai DL, Martinka M, Ho V, Li G. Nuclear ING2 expression is reduced in human cutaneous melanomas. Br J Cancer 95:80-6, 2006
[58] Larrieu D, Ythier D, Binet R, Brambilla C, Brambilla E, Sengupta S, Pedeux R. ING2 controls the progression of DNA replication forks to maintain genome stability. EMBO Rep 10:1168-74, 2009
[59] Nagashima M, Shiseki M, Pedeux RM, Okamura S, Kitahama-Shiseki M, Miura K, Yokota J, Harris CC. A novel PHD-finger motif protein, p47ING3, modulates p53-mediated transcription, cell cycle control, and apoptosis. Oncogene 22:343-50, 2003
[60] Doyon Y, Côté J.The highly conserved and multifunctional NuA4 HAT complex. Curr Opin Genet Dev 14:147-5, 2004
[61] Kataoka H, Bonnefin P, Vieyra D, Feng X, Hara Y, Miura Y, Joh T, Nakabayashi H, Vaziri H, Harris CC, Riabowol K. ING1 represses transcription by direct DNA binding and through effects on p53. Cancer Res 63:5785-92, 2003
[62] Doyon Y, Selleck W, Lane WS, Tan S, Côté J. Structural and functional conservation of the NuA4 histone acetyltransferase complex from yeast to humans. Mol Cell Biol 24:1884-9, 2004
[63] Doyon Y, Cayrou C, Ullah M, Landry AJ, Côté V, Selleck W, Lane WS, Tan S, Yang XJ, Côté J. ING tumor suppressor proteins are critical regulators of chromatin acetylation required for genome expression and perpetuation. Mol Cell 21:51-64, 2006
[64] Wang Y, Li G. J. ING3 promotes UV-induced apoptosis via Fas/caspase-8 pathway in melanoma cells. Biol Chem 281:11887-93, 2006
[65] Chen G, Wang Y, Garate M, Zhou J, Li G. The tumor suppressor ING3 is degraded by SCF (Skp2)-mediated ubiquitin-proteasome system. Oncogene 29:1498-508, 2010
[66] Shiseki M, Nagashima M, Pedeux RM, Kitahama-Shiseki M, Miura K, Okamura S, Onogi H, Higashimoto Y, Appella E, Yokota J, Harris CC. p29ING4 and p28ING5 bind to p53 and p300, and enhance p53 activity. Cancer Res 63:2373-8, 2003
[67] Li J, Li G. Cell cycle regulator ING4 is a suppressor of melanoma angiogenesis that is regulated by the metastasis suppressor BRMS1. Cancer Res 70:10445-53, 2010

[68] Xie YF, Sheng W, Xiang J, Zhang H, Ye Z, Yang J. Adenovirus-mediated ING4 expression suppresses pancreatic carcinoma cell growth via induction of cell-cycle alteration, apoptosis, and inhibition of tumor angiogenesis. Cancer Biother Radiopharm 24:261-9, 2009

[69] Zhu Y, Lv H, Xie Y, Sheng W, Xiang J, Yang J. Enhanced tumor suppression by an ING4/IL-24 bicistronic adenovirus-mediated gene cotransfer in human non-small cell lung cancer cells. Cancer Gene Ther. 2011 Jun 10. doi: 10.1038/cgt.2011.31. [Epub ahead of print]

[70] Garkavtsev I, Kozin SV, Chernova O, Xu L, Winkler F, Brown E, Barnett GH, Jain RK. The candidate tumour suppressor protein ING4 regulates brain tumour growth and angiogenesis. Nature 428:328-32, 2004

[71] Unoki M, Shen JC, Zheng ZM, Harris CC. Novel splice variants of ING4 and their possible roles in the regulation of cell growth and motility. J Biol Chem 281:34677-86, 2006

[72] Shen JC, Unoki M, Ythier D, Duperray A, Varticovski L, Kumamoto K, Pedeux R, Harris CC. Inhibitor of growth 4 suppresses cell spreading and cell migration by interacting with a novel binding partner, liprin alpha1. Cancer Res 67:2552-8, 2007

[73] Li J, Martinka M, Li G. Role of ING4 in human melanoma cell migration, invasion and patient survival. Carcinogenesis 29:1373-9, 2008

[74] Cai L, Li X, Zheng S, Wang Y, Wang Y, Li H, Yang J, Sun J. Inhibitor of growth 4 is involved in melanomagenesis and induces growth suppression and apoptosis in melanoma cell line M14. Melanoma Res 19:1-7, 2009

[75] Li X, Cai L, Chen H, Zhang Q, Zhang S, Wang Y, Dong Y, Cheng H, Qi J. Inhibitor of growth 4 induces growth suppression and apoptosis in glioma U87MG. Pathobiology 76:181-92, 2009

[76] Saksouk N, Avvakumov N, Champagne KS, Hung T, Doyon Y, Cayrou C, Paquet E, Ullah M, Landry AJ, Côté V, Yang XJ, Gozani O, Kutateladze TG, Côté J. HBO1 HAT complexes target chromatin throughout gene coding regions via multiple PHD finger interactions with histone H3 tail. Mol Cell 33:257-65, 2009

[77] Hung T, Binda O, Champagne KS, Kuo AJ, Johnson K, Chang HY, Simon MD, Kutateladze TG, Gozani O. ING4 mediates crosstalk between histone H3 K4 trimethylation and H3 acetylation to attenuate cellular transformation. Mol Cell 33:248-56, 2009

[78] Zhang X, Xu LS, Wang ZQ, Wang KS, Li N, Cheng ZH, Huang SZ, Wei DZ, Han ZG. ING4 induces G2/M cell cycle arrest and enhances the chemosensitivity to DNA-damage agents in HepG2 cells. FEBS Lett 570:7-12, 2004

[79] Ullah M, Pelletier N, Xiao L, Zhao SP, Wang K, Degerny C, Tahmasebi S, Cayrou C, Doyon Y, Goh SL, Champagne N, Côté J, Yang XJ. Molecular architecture of quartet MOZ/MORF histone acetyltransferase complexes. Mol Cell Biol 28:6828-43, 2008 Erratum in: Mol Cell Biol. 2009 Feb;29:942

[80] Champagne KS, Saksouk N, Peña PV, Johnson K, Ullah M, Yang XJ, Côté J, Kutateladze TG. The crystal structure of the ING5 PHD finger in complex with an H3K4me3 histone peptide. Proteins 72:1371-6, 2008

[81] Tokunaga E, Maehara Y, Oki E, Kitamura K, Kakeji Y, Ohno S, Sugimachi K. Diminished expression of ING1 mRNA and the correlation with p53 expression in breast cancers. Cancer Lett 152:15-22, 2000

[82] Ohmori M, Nagai M, Tasaka T, Koeffler HP, Toyama T, Riabowol K, Takahara J. Decreased expression of p33ING1 mRNA in lymphoid malignancies. Am J Hematol 62:118-9, 1999 Erratum in: Am J Hematol 2000 May;64(1):82.
[83] Oki E, Maehara Y, Tokunaga E, Kakeji Y, Sugimachi K. Reduced expression of p33 (ING1) and the relationship with p53 expression in human gastric cancer. Cancer Lett 147:157-62, 1999
[84] Ito K, Kinjo K, Nakazato T, Ikeda Y, Kizaki M. Expression and sequence analyses of p33(ING1) gene in myeloid leukemia. Am J Hematol 69:141-3, 2002
[85] Hara Y, Zheng Z, Evans SC, Malatjalian D, Riddell DC, Guernsey DL, Wang LD, Riabowol K, Casson AG. ING1 and p53 tumor suppressor gene alterations in adenocarcinomas of the esophagogastric junction. Cancer Lett 192:109-16, 2003
[86] Tallen G, Riabowol K, Wolff JE. Expression of p33ING1 mRNA and chemosensitivity in brain tumor cells. Anticancer Res 23(2B):1631-5, 2003
[87] Tallen G, Kaiser I, Krabbe S, Lass U, Hartmann C, Henze G, Riabowol K, von Deimling A. No ING1 mutations in human brain tumours but reduced expression in high malignancy grades of astrocytoma. Int J Cancer 109:476-9, 2004
[88] Takahashi M, Ozaki T, Todo S, Nakagawara A. Decreased expression of the candidate tumor suppressor gene ING1 is associated with poor prognosis in advanced neuroblastomas. Oncol Rep 12:811-6, 2004
[89] Shen DH, Chan KY, Khoo US, Ngan HY, Xue WC, Chiu PM, Ip P, Cheung AN. Epigenetic and genetic alterations of p33ING1b in ovarian cancer. Carcinogenesis 26:855-63, 2005
[90] Kameyama K, Huang CL, Liu D, Masuya D, Nakashima T, Sumitomo S, Takami Y, Kinoshita M, Yokomise H. Reduced ING1b gene expression plays an important role in carcinogenesis of non-small cell lung cancer patients. Clin Cancer Res 9:4926-34, 2003
[91] Chen L, Matsubara N, Yoshino T, Nagasaka T, Hoshizima N, Shirakawa Y, Naomoto Y, Isozaki H, Riabowol K, Tanaka N. Genetic alterations of candidate tumor suppressor ING1 in human esophageal squamous cell cancer. Cancer Res 61:4345-9, 2001
[92] Bromidge T, Lynas C. Relative levels of alternative transcripts of the ING1 gene and lack of mutations of p33/ING1 in haematological malignancies. Leuk Res 26:631-5, 2002
[93] Krishnamurthy J, Kannan K, Feng J, Mohanprasad BK, Tsuchida N, Shanmugam G. Mutational analysis of the candidate tumor suppressor gene ING1 in Indian oral squamous cell carcinoma. Oral Oncol 37:222-4, 2001
[94] Stark M, Puig-Butille JA, Walker G, Badenas C, Malvehy J, Hayward N, Puig S. Mutation of the tumour suppressor p33ING1b is rare in melanoma. Br J Dermatol 155:94-9, 2006
[95] Zhang HK, Pan K, Wang H, Weng DS, Song HF, Zhou J, Huang W, Li JJ, Chen MS, Xia JC. Decreased expression of ING2 gene and its clinicopathological significance in hepatocellular carcinoma. Cancer Lett 261:183-92, 2008
[96] Okano T, Gemma A, Hosoya Y, Hosomi Y, Nara M, Kokubo Y, Yoshimura A, Shibuya M, Nagashima M, Harris CC, Kudoh S. Alterations in novel candidate tumor suppressor genes, ING1 and ING2 in human lung cancer. Oncol Rep 15:545-9, 2006

[97] Kumamoto K, Fujita K, Kurotani R, Saito M, Unoki M, Hagiwara N, Shiga H, Bowman ED, Yanaihara N, Okamura S, Nagashima M, Miyamoto K, Takenoshita S, Yokota J, Harris CC. ING2 is upregulated in colon cancer and increases invasion by enhanced MMP13 expression. Int J Cancer 125:1306-15, 2009

[98] Borkosky SS, Gunduz M, Nagatsuka H, Beder LB, Gunduz E, Ali MA, Rodriguez AP, Cilek MZ, Tominaga S, Yamanaka N, Shimizu K, Nagai N. Frequent deletion of ING2 locus at 4q35.1 associates with advanced tumor stage in head and neck squamous cell carcinoma. J Cancer Res Clin Oncol 135:703-13, 2009

[99] Gunduz M, Beder LB, Gunduz E, Nagatsuka H, Fukushima K, Pehlivan D, Cetin E, Yamanaka N, Nishizaki K, Shimizu K, Nagai N. Downregulation of ING3 mRNA expression predicts poor prognosis in head and neck cancer. Cancer Sci 99:531-8, 2008

[100] Wang Y, Dai DL, Martinka M, Li G. Prognostic significance of nuclear ING3 expression in human cutaneous melanoma. Clin Cancer Res 13:4111-6, 2007

[101] Borkosky SS, Gunduz M, Beder L, Tsujigiwa H, Tamamura R, Gunduz E, Katase N, Rodriguez AP, Sasaki A, Nagai N, Nagatsuka H. Allelic loss of the ING gene family loci is a frequent event in ameloblastoma. Oncol Res 18:509-18, 2010

[102] Colla S, Tagliaferri S, Morandi F, Lunghi P, Donofrio G, Martorana D, Mancini C, Lazzaretti M, Mazzera L, Ravanetti L, Bonomini S, Ferrari L, Miranda C, Ladetto M, Neri TM, Neri A, Greco A, Mangoni M, Bonati A, Rizzoli V, Giuliani N. The new tumor-suppressor gene inhibitor of growth family member 4 (ING4) regulates the production of proangiogenic molecules by myeloma cells and suppresses hypoxia-inducible factor-1 alpha (HIF-1alpha) activity: involvement in myeloma-induced angiogenesis. Blood 110:4464-75, 2007. Epub 2007 Sep 11. Erratum in Blood. 2008 Sep 1;112:2170.

[103] Kim S, Chin K, Gray JW, Bishop JM. A screen for genes that suppress loss of contact inhibition: identification of ING4 as a candidate tumor suppressor gene in human cancer. Proc Natl Acad Sci U S A 101:16251-6, 2004

[104] Klironomos G, Bravou V, Papachristou DJ, Gatzounis G, Varakis J, Parassi E, Repanti M, Papadaki H. Loss of inhibitor of growth (ING-4) is implicated in the pathogenesis and progression of human astrocytomas. Brain Pathol 20:490-7, 2010

[105] Nagahama Y, Ishimaru M, Osaki M, Inoue T, Maeda A, Nakada C, Moriyama M, Sato K, Oshimura M, Ito H. Apoptotic pathway induced by transduction of RUNX3 in the human gastric carcinoma cell line MKN-1. Cancer Sci 99:23-30, 2008

[106] Fang F, Luo LB, Tao YM, Wu F, Yang LY. Decreased expression of inhibitor of growth 4 correlated with poor prognosis of hepatocellular carcinoma. Cancer Epidemiol Biomarkers Prev 18:409-16, 2009

[107] Li M, Jin Y, Sun WJ, Yu Y, Bai J, Tong DD, Qi JP, Du JR, Geng JS, Huang Q, Huang XY, Huang Y, Han FF, Meng XN, Rosales JL, Lee KY, Fu SB. Reduced expression and novel splice variants of ING4 in human gastric adenocarcinoma. J Pathol 219:87-95, 2009

[108] Wang QS, Li M, Zhang LY, Jin Y, Tong DD, Yu Y, Bai J, Huang Q, Liu FL, Liu A, Lee KY, Fu SB. Down-regulation of ING4 is associated with initiation and progression of lung cancer. Histopathology 57:271-81, 2010

[109] Li XH, Kikuchi K, Zheng Y, Noguchi A, Takahashi H, Nishida T, Masuda S, Yang XH, Takano Y. Downregulation and translocation of nuclear ING4 is correlated with

tumorigenesis and progression of head and neck squamous cell carcinoma. Oral Oncol 47:217-23, 2011

[110] You Q, Wang XS, Fu SB, Jin XM. Downregulated Expression of Inhibitor of Growth 4 (ING4) in Advanced Colorectal Cancers: A Non-Randomized Experimental Study. Pathol Oncol Res. 2011 May 31. [Epub ahead of print]

[111] Cengiz B, Gunduz M, Nagatsuka H, Beder L, Gunduz E, Tamamura R, Mahmut N, Fukushima K, Ali MA, Naomoto Y, Shimizu K, Nagai N. Fine deletion mapping of chromosome 2q21-37 shows three preferentially deleted regions in oral cancer. Oral Oncol 43:241-7, 2007

[112] Li X, Nishida T, Noguchi A, Zheng Y, Takahashi H, Yang X, Masuda S, Takano Y. Decreased nuclear expression and increased cytoplasmic expression of ING5 may be linked to tumorigenesis and progression in human head and neck squamous cell carcinoma. J Cancer Res Clin Oncol 136:1573-83, 2010

[113] Xing YN, Yang X, Xu XY, Zheng Y, Xu HM, Takano Y, Zheng HC. The altered expression of ING5 protein is involved in gastric carcinogenesis and subsequent progression. Hum Pathol 42:25-35, 2011

[114] Zheng HC, Xia P, Xu XY, Takahashi H, Takano Y. The nuclear to cytoplasmic shift of ING5 protein during colorectal carcinogenesis with their distinct links to pathologic behaviors of carcinomas. Hum Pathol 42:424-33, 2011

[115] Nouman GS, Anderson JJ, Crosier S, Shrimankar J, Lunec J, Angus B. Downregulation of nuclear expression of the p33(ING1b) inhibitor of growth protein in invasive carcinoma of the breast. J Clin Pathol 56:507-11, 2003

[116] Nouman GS, Anderson JJ, Wood KM, Lunec J, Hall AG, Reid MM, Angus B. Loss of nuclear expression of the p33(ING1b) inhibitor of growth protein in childhood acute lymphoblastic leukaemia. J Clin Pathol 55:596-601, 2002

[117] Nouman GS, Anderson JJ, Mathers ME, Leonard N, Crosier S, Lunec J, Angus B. Nuclear to cytoplasmic compartment shift of the p33ING1b tumour suppressor protein is associated with malignancy in melanocytic lesions. Histopathology 40:360-6, 2002

[118] Toyama T, Iwase H, Yamashita H, Hara Y, Sugiura H, Zhang Z, Fukai I, Miura Y, Riabowol K, Fujii Y. p33(ING1b) stimulates the transcriptional activity of the estrogen receptor alpha via its activation function (AF) 2 domain. J Steroid Biochem Mol Biol 87:57-63, 2003

[119] Nikolaev AY, Papanikolaou NA, Li M, Qin J, Gu W. Identification of a novel BRMS1-homologue protein p40 as a component of the mSin3A/p33(ING1b)/HDAC1 deacetylase complex. Biochem Biophys Res Commun 323:1216-22, 2004

[120] Kim S, Welm AL, Bishop JM. A dominant mutant allele of the ING4 tumor suppressor found in human cancer cells exacerbates MYC-initiated mouse mammary tumorigenesis. Cancer Res 70:5155-62, 2010

[121] Li Z, Xie Y, Sheng W, Miao J, Xiang J, Yang J. Tumor-suppressive effect of adenovirus-mediated inhibitor of growth 4 gene transfer in breast carcinoma cells in vitro and in vivo. Cancer Biother Radiopharm 25:427-37, 2010

[122] Tapia C, Zlobec I, Schneider S, Kilic E, Güth U, Bubendorf L, Kim S. Deletion of the inhibitor of growth 4 (ING4) tumor suppressor gene is prevalent in human epidermal growth factor 2 (HER2)-positive breast cancer. Hum Pathol 42:983-90, 2011

19

Lipid Rafts as Master Regulators of Breast Cancer Cell Function

Irina S. Babina[1], Simona Donatello[1], Ivan R. Nabi[2] and Ann M. Hopkins[1]
[1]*Royal College of Surgeons in Ireland, Beaumont Hospital, Dublin*
[2]*University of British Columbia, Vancouver*
[1]*Ireland*
[2]*Canada*

1. Introduction

Cancer is a leading cause of death in developed countries, and is on the rise in developing countries due in part to a lack of prophylactic screening and non-universal access to medical care (Jemal et al., 2011). Breast cancer is initiated when breast epithelial cells escape growth arrest and form a proliferating tumour mass. Numerous cellular mechanisms are dysregulated in breast tumour cells, including modified cell fate, altered protein signalling and trafficking, and enhanced cell migratory potential. Although these events are complex and subject to regulation by multiple elements, recent evidence has suggested that specialised cell membrane domains termed lipid rafts are actively involved in each of these processes (Cary & Cooper, 2000; Nabi & Le, 2003; Simons & Toomre, 2000). This chapter will therefore focus on the contribution of lipid rafts to breast cancer initiation and progression under these headings.

Lipid rafts are sub-domains of the cell membrane enriched in cholesterol and glycosphingolipids (Le Moyec et al., 1992; Nohara et al., 1998). These microdomains cluster together proteins involved in the regulation of crucial cellular processes; many of which are altered in cancer cells (Pike, 2003; de Laurentiis et al., 2007). Furthermore, lipid rafts are readily modified by diet and nutrition (Schley et al., 2007; Yaqoob, 2009), and studies have shown that fatty acid supplementation sensitises human mammary tumour cells to the cytotoxic effects of anti-cancer agents *in vitro* and *in vivo* (Germain et al., 1998; Menendez et al., 2005; Colas et al., 2006). This chapter will focus on the potential regulatory functions of lipid rafts as a novel approach towards understanding mechanisms of cancer initiation, progression and cell migration, a key event preceding metastatic progression. Finally it will discuss the potential of lipid rafts as novel therapeutic targets in breast cancer.

2. What are lipid rafts?

The discovery of glycosphingolipid clustering in the Golgi apparatus and at the apical surface of polarised epithelial cells led to the hypothesis of non-random membrane compartmentalisation (Simons & Ikonen, 1997; van Meer et al., 2008). These "compartments" were termed lipid rafts.

The structure and function of lipid raft domains depend on their lipid and protein compositions. An example of this is the sub-population of lipid rafts first identified in endothelial cells as flask-shaped membrane invaginations termed caveolae, or "little caves" (Yamada, 1955), which subsequent characterisation revealed to be enriched in proteins from the caveolin family (Rothberg, K G et al., 1992). Caveolins localise in the cytoplasmic leaflet of the cell membrane, and, together with high concentrations of cholesterol, are responsible for the characteristic curvature of caveolar membranes. Lipid rafts and caveolae have different structural protein markers and different proteins associated with them (Table 1), but their lipid composition and the mechanisms of protein targeting to them are very similar.

	Lipids	Protein Markers	Receptor Proteins	Signalling Proteins	References
Non-caveolar lipid rafts	Cholesterol Glycosphingolipid Sphingomyelin Ganglioside GM1 Ganglioside GM3	Flotillin-1, -2	Fas EGFR HER2 IGF-1R CD44 ER	Ras Src Erk2 Shc	(Nohara et al., 1998; de Laurentiis et al., 2007; Patra, 2008)
Caveolae	Cholesterol Glycosphingolipid Sphingomyelin Ganglioside GM1	Caveolin-1, -2 and -3	Fas EGFR HER2 IGF-1R CD44 ER uPAR MMP-1, -2, -9	Ras Src eNOS PI3 kinase Phospho-lipase C	

Table 1. Lipid and protein contents of caveolae and non-caveolar lipid rafts.

2.1 Lipid composition of membrane rafts

The functional properties of raft sub-populations differ according to subtle variations in the types of lipid and quantities of cholesterol they contain. This has permitted differential detergent extraction of various types of lipid rafts. The cholesterol concentration in detergent-resistant membranes (rafts) is 3-5 times higher than that in total membranes (Brown & Rose, 1992; Pike & Casey, 2002), sphingomyelin represents 10-15% of total lipid content, while glycosphingolipids such as cerebrosides and gangliosides account for a further 10-20% (Brown & Rose, 1992; Prinetti et al., 2000). In contrast, glycerophospholipids (including membrane phospholipids) comprise less than 30% of raft lipids despite accounting for approximately 60% of total membrane lipids (Brown & Rose, 1992; Pike & Casey, 2002). Raft-enriched lipids localise preferentially on the outer leaflet of the cell membrane, unlike glycerophospholipids (Pike, 2003). These observations suggest that lipid rafts are bilayer structures and that a variable composition of the cell membrane leaflets may play a role in recruitment of various proteins into lipid rafts. Accordingly, proteins can be targeted to rafts in many dynamically-regulated ways, including attachment of glycosylphosphatidylinositol (GPI) anchors or via lipid modifications such as prenylation and palmitoylation.

2.2 Protein targeting to lipid rafts

Perhaps the best-characterised system of protein association with lipid rafts is via modification with GPI anchors. The GPI anchor is a conserved oligosaccharide core covalently linked to a lipid moiety embedded in the outer leaflet of the cell membrane through acyl or alkyl chains (Levental et al., 2010). These anchors are added to soluble polypeptides in the lumen of the endoplasmic reticulum (ER), promoting membrane raft affiliation (Brown & Rose, 1992). Partitioning of GPI-anchored proteins into lipid rafts may allow sorting to the apical surface of polarised epithelial cells (Fiedler et al., 1993).

Another way in which proteins are targeted to lipid rafts is through addition of prenyl groups. Two types of prenyl groups, C_{15} farnesyl and C_{20} geranylgeranyl, are added on to C-terminal cysteine-rich domains of cytoplasmic proteins by prenyl transferases (Casey & Seabra, 1996). Although prenylated proteins are reportedly enriched in lipid rafts (Prior & Hancock, 2001; Parmryd et al., 2003), it is thought that the prenyl groups interact with raft-affiliated proteins rather than being directly incorporated into rafts (Magee & Seabra, 2003).

Another lipid post-translational modification, palmitoylation, is dynamically regulated by enzymes (Kang et al., 2008; Wan et al., 2007), and controls raft targeting of certain proteins in physiological and pathophysiological settings. Palmitoylation involves the addition of palmitic acid moieties to integral and peripheral membrane proteins through esterification (Bhatnagar & Gordon, 1997). Membrane-associated palmitoyl acyltransferases (PATs) are the most studied palmitoylation enzymes (Planey & Zacharias, 2009), while the palmitoyl thioesterase family removes palmitate groups (Camp & Hofmann, 1995). Close proximity of protein cysteine residues to the membrane is thought to facilitate palmitoylation by PATs, whereas membrane-distal residues are more likely to be prenylated or N-myristoylated (Bijlmakers & Marsh, 2003). PAT activity has been linked to lipid rafts (Dunphy et al., 2001), with palmitoylated proteins found either at the cell membrane or on intracellular membranes (Lobo et al., 2002; Roth et al., 2002). Palmitoylated proteins are naturally more lipophilic, thus their affinity for lipid rafts is increased. Many proteins are targeted to lipid rafts through palmitoylation, including flotillins, Src family kinases, endothelial nitric oxide synthase and various transmembrane receptors (Ghosh et al., 1998; Gong et al., 2003).

2.2.1 Flotillin-1 and -2 mark non-caveolar lipid rafts

Non-caveolar lipid rafts are associated with expression of the reggie family of proteins, flotillin-1 and flotillin-2 (Figure 1a). Palmitoylation of flotillin-1 is essential for localisation to lipid rafts (Morrow et al., 2002), while two hydrophobic stretches also contribute to its raft affiliation (Liu et al., 2005). On the other hand, flotillin-2 is raft-targeted via both myristoylation and palmitoylation. Flotillins were originally thought to be localised in caveolae (Bickel et al., 1997), however later studies excluded this (Neumann-Giesen et al., 2004; Stuermer et al., 2004). Much remains to be determined about the functionality of flotillins in lipid rafts, in particular, the significance of their highly conserved N-terminal domain (Babuke & Tikkanen, 2007; Tavernarakis et al., 1999).

2.2.2 Caveolins – selective markers for caveolar lipid rafts

Along with glycosphingolipids (Tran et al., 1987) and increased cholesterol (Rothberg, K. G. et al., 1990), caveolae are enriched in the family of 21-24 kDa integral membrane proteins known as caveolins. There are three known caveolins: caveolin-1 (Rothberg, J. M. & Artavanis-Tsakonas, 1992), caveolin-2 (Okamoto et al., 1998) and caveolin-3 (Tang et al., 1996).

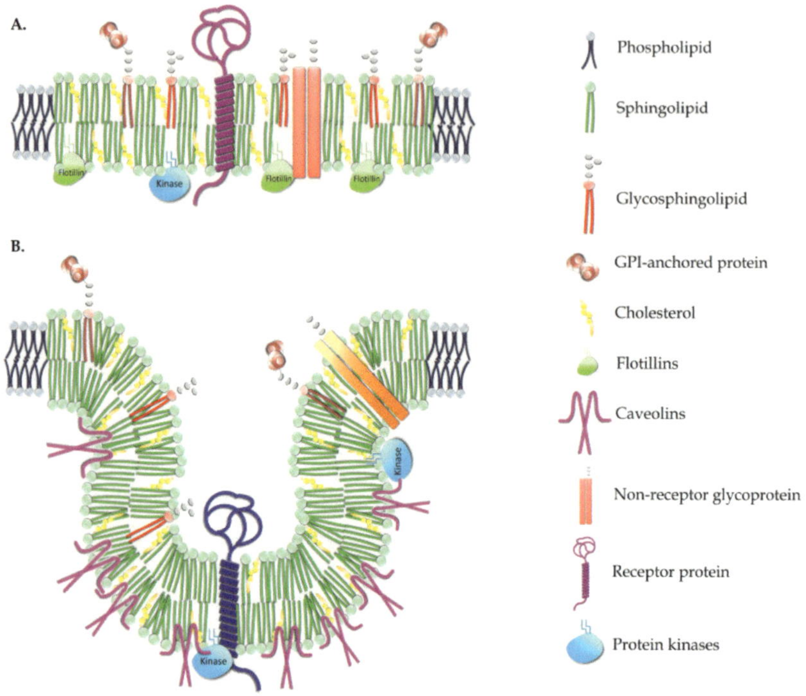

Fig. 1. Lipid and protein components of (A.) non-caveolar lipid rafts and (B.) caveolae.

Caveolins form "omega" structures in the membrane via cytoplasmic localization of both their N- and C-termini (Figure 1b). Aside from palmitoylation, the ability of caveolins to bind sphingolipids (Fra et al., 1995) and cholesterol (Murata et al., 1995) can also explain their high affinity for caveolar lipid rafts. Caveolins -1 and -2 are abundantly expressed in most cell types, including adipocytes, fibroblasts, endothelial and epithelial cells (Fan et al., 1983; Galbiati et al., 2001). Caveolin-3 expression however is restricted to muscle (Rubin et al., 2007). The N-terminal region of caveolin-1 contains a scaffolding domain which aids interactions with various signalling molecules, illustrating the potential importance of caveolin-1 for the signalling functions of caveolar lipid rafts (Everson & Smart, 2006).

2.3 Physiological functions of lipid rafts

Lipid rafts and caveolae are often viewed as organisation centres or signalling platforms, and Table 1 outlines examples of raft-associated proteins which will be discussed in the text. In this chapter, we will concentrate on dynamic raft regulation of a variety of physiological processes, including membrane trafficking, cell polarisation and signal transduction.

2.3.1 Membrane trafficking and cell polarity

Membrane trafficking allows exchange of cellular components between cell sites and cellular organelles. In polarised epithelial cells the trafficking machinery is highly polarised, targeting plasma membrane proteins to separate apical and basolateral domains (Mellman & Nelson, 2008). Following lipid and protein synthesis in the ER, vesicular transfer mediates transport to subsequent or final destinations (Rodriguez-Boulan et al., 2005). The formation and distribution of vesicles requires organised stabilisation of the membrane to allow deformation and fusion with the target compartment. The most studied mechanism involves coating of the vesicle with clathrin oligomers (Gorelick & Shugrue, 2001), which is thought to be vital in basolateral protein sorting (Deborde et al., 2008; Folsch et al., 2009). Apical trafficking is less understood, but lipid rafts have been proposed to play a decisive role (Schuck & Simons, 2004). Conformational changes in the membrane are proposed to occur via oligomerisation and fusion of many small lipid raft domains (Lipowsky, 1993). Attachment of GPI anchors may also contribute to the polarisation of membrane trafficking (Paladino et al., 2008).

2.3.2 Cell signalling

Lipid raft-mediated trafficking of lipids and proteins facilitates dynamic regulation of cellular signalling cascades. Several frameworks have been suggested to link rafts to signal transduction. The simplest interpretation views lipid rafts as platforms where signalling molecules are co-localised, aiding their structural interactions and influencing downstream signalling (Lingwood et al., 2009). The nature of a signal may be modified by the type of lipid raft the target molecule is localised in and also the primary location of the raft, which in turn enhances the specificity of the signal. Rafts can also control cellular signalling by altering the function of their affiliated proteins. Accumulating evidence suggests that raft-associated proteins behave differently whether localized inside or outside of rafts. Modified signal transduction following lipid raft/caveolar disruption has been reported in the case of several signalling cascades involving Erk (Furuchi & Anderson, 1998), EGFR (Ringerike et al., 2002; Schley et al., 2007), insulin receptor (Parpal et al., 2001), and PDGF receptor (McGuire et al., 1993).

Finally, some lipid rafts are actively involved in endocytosis (reviewed in Lajoie & Nabi, 2010), which promotes internalisation of receptors and signalling molecules. This process may be facilitated by clustering of caveolin or receptor proteins (Paladino et al., 2004). Internalisation of ligands or receptors modifies downstream signal transduction, and is associated with the termination of extracellular ligand-driven signalling events via transient receptor desensitisation.

The ability of lipid rafts to traffic proteins, control cell polarity and alter cell signalling underlies their emerging roles as crucial regulators of cellular processes including cell fate, growth, adhesion and migration. Since all are dysregulated in cancer, it is reasonable to suggest that lipid rafts may modify tumorigenic processes. This will next be addressed.

3. Lipid raft regulation of key processes in breast cancer cells

Alterations in cell fate, growth, adhesion and migration play central roles in the initiation and progression of breast cancer. We next outline how lipid rafts may regulate such processes during the initial stages of cancer development, during tumour growth and during the possible progression to a migratory and metastatic phenotype.

3.1 Apoptosis and regulation of cell fate

Defects in apoptosis allow tumour cells to escape growth-inhibitory signals and to progress through the cell cycle. Two major apoptotic pathways have been described, extrinsic (mediated by activation of death receptors) and intrinsic (mediated by mitochondria). Both may require lipid rafts for successful signal transduction (Li et al., 1998).

Death receptors are located at the cell membrane, and once activated, trigger apoptotic signal transduction. Perhaps the best-characterised death receptor is Fas (CD95 or APO-1), which has been implicated in the apoptotic events that drive physiological remodelling of the mammary gland after breast feeding (Song et al., 2000). Down-regulation of Fas has also been associated with poor prognosis in breast cancer patients (Reimer et al., 2000), and inhibition of Fas activity has been linked to drug resistance (Landowski et al., 1997). Activation of Fas results in receptor aggregation, and recruitment of procaspase-8 to form the death-inducing signalling complex DISC (Peter & Krammer, 2003) (Figure 3a). Recent studies have shown that Fas is translocated into lipid rafts, where apoptotic receptor aggregation takes place (Gajate et al., 2004; Gajate & Mollinedo, 2005). This is the mode of action of a pro-apoptotic drug, edelfosine; with cholesterol depletion being shown to abolish apoptosis (Gajate & Mollinedo, 2001; Gajate & Mollinedo, 2007; Gajate et al., 2009).

Whether rafts could be used as targets to re-trigger Fas-dependent apoptosis in tumour cells is an intriguing concept. A recent study demonstrated that nitric oxide (NO) can reverse apoptotic resistance via increasing Fas S-nitrosylation (Leon et al., 2011). In breast cancer cells that overexpressed wild-type Fas, NO incubation resulted in enhanced recruitment of the receptor into lipid rafts, which in turn sensitized cancer cells to the death-inducing Fas ligand. In fact, DISC formation is impaired in cells expressing nitrosylation (Leon et al., 2011) and palmitoylation (Chakrabandhu et al., 2007) mutants of Fas.

Acquired resistance of breast cancer cells to Fas-induced apoptosis may alternatively result from activation of survival pathways, such as the PI3 kinase pathway. Its engagement leads to activation of the serine-threonine kinase Akt, which negatively regulates apoptosis by inactivating pro-apoptotic proteins such as Bad and caspase-9 (Datta et al., 1999). Lipid raft localisation of Akt has been implicated in facilitating its activation (Hill et al., 2002; Elhyany et al., 2004). Raft disruption has been reported to reduce the sensitivity of normal-like MCF-10a cells to apoptosis, suggesting that tumour cells rely on cholesterol for growth and malignant signalling (Li et al., 2006). Interestingly the cholesterol analogue ginsenoside Rh2 has been shown to reduce lipid raft abundance and increase internalisation, decreasing Akt-dependent survival signalling (Park et al., 2010). It has also been demonstrated that cholesterol depletion induces anoikis-like apoptosis via down-regulation of focal adhesion kinase and hypoxia inducible factor-1 (Lee et al., 2009; Park et al., 2009).

Another apoptotic death receptor is TNF-related apoptosis-inducing ligand (TRAIL) receptor 1 and 2, referred to as DR4 and DR5 respectively (Yang et al., 2010). Studies have demonstrated that translocation of these receptors into lipid rafts after TRAIL engagement is involved in apoptotic signal transduction (Merino et al., 2006; Dumitru et al., 2007; Song et al., 2007). In metastatic MDA-MB-231 cells, for instance, DR4 palmitoylation (Rossin et al., 2009) is crucial not only for its localisation into lipid rafts but also for receptor aggregation, both of which are essential for TRAIL-induced cell death (Merino et al., 2006). Therefore while much remains to be understood about the role of rafts in regulating apoptosis in breast cancer cells, it may offer a novel therapeutic target (see Section 4).

3.2 Growth and metabolism

In conjunction with altered apoptosis, abnormal signalling by growth factor receptors can facilitate breast tumour proliferation and growth. Lipid rafts modulate the signalling functions of several growth factor receptors, including the ErbB (HER) family of receptors.

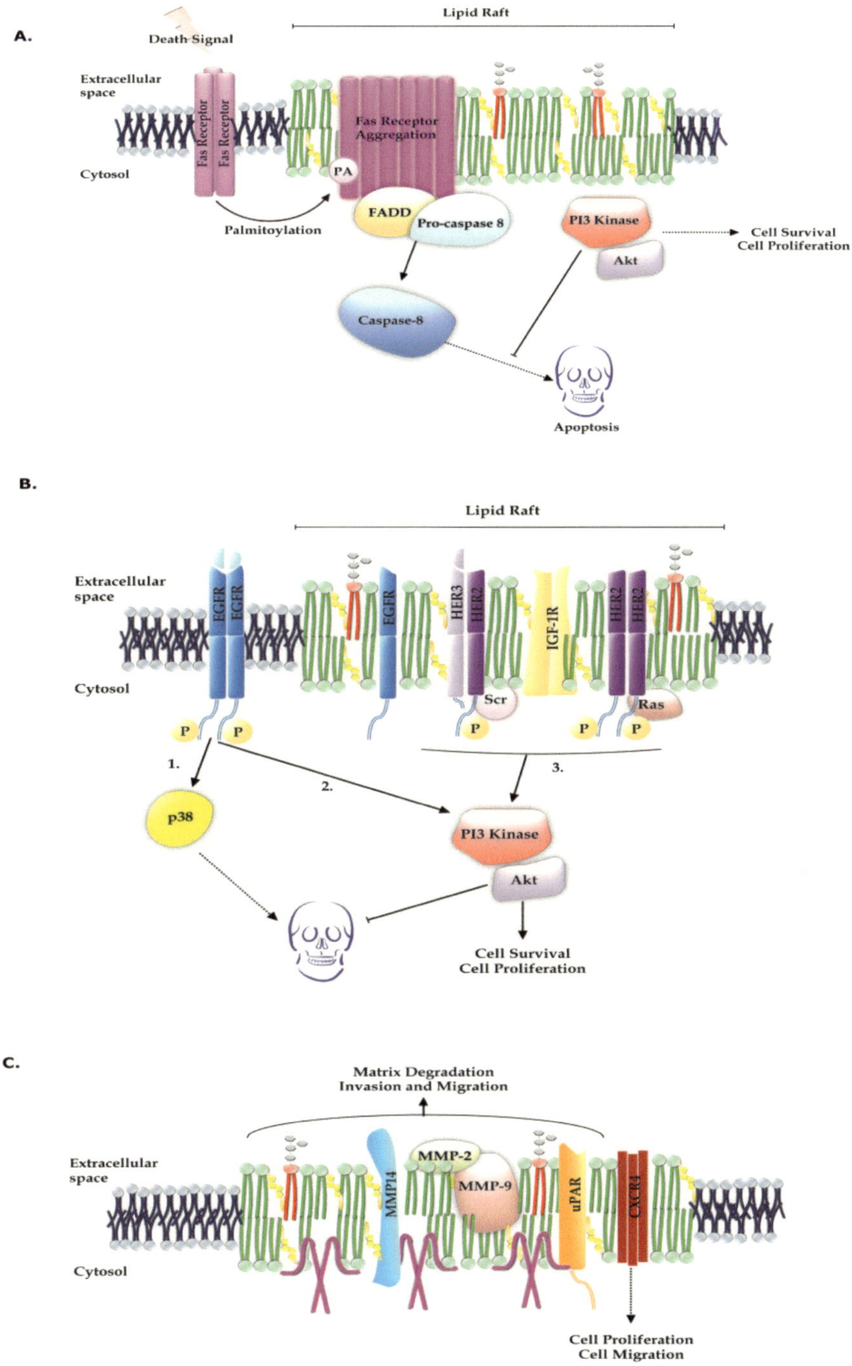

Fig. 2. Lipid raft regulation of breast cancer cell processes. (A.) Apoptotic signals are transduced via lipid rafts. (B.) EGFR signalling may induce apoptosis (1.) or proliferation (2.) outside of lipid rafts. Predominant oncogenic signalling is transduced through rafts (3.). (C.) Rafts cluster many degradation enzymes and proteins crucial for cell migration.

ErbB receptors are often mutated, amplified and/or overexpressed in breast cancer (Troyer & Lee, 2001). In particular, epidermal growth factor receptor, EGFR, and HER2 homo- and heterodimerisations have been described to promote oncogenic proliferation (Barros et al., 2010). Both of these receptors are associated with lipid rafts, and raft modifications can alter their signal transduction (Chen & Resh, 2002; Freeman et al., 2007).

EGFR functionality in particular is largely dependent upon its affiliation with rafts. Upon ligand binding, EGFR translocates out of caveolin-positive raft domains to stimulate downstream signalling (Mineo et al., 1999) and caveolin-1 raft domains negatively regulate EGFR activation (Lajoie et al., 2007). Accordingly, raft disruption via cholesterol depletion reportedly results in EGFR activation (Pike & Casey, 2002; Westover et al., 2003). Although EGFR phosphorylation is associated with oncogenic proliferation, sustained activation of EGFR outside of lipid rafts in fact correlates with increased p38 activation, which is pro-apoptotic. Potential modulations of EGFR activation status by dietary lipids will be discussed in Section 4.

Some studies have examined the activation of downstream targets of EGFR signalling, such as the small GTPase Ras (Rogers et al., 2010), after exposure to fatty acids. Ras associates with lipid rafts via palmitoylation (Calder & Yaqoob, 2007), and is involved in cell survival, growth and proliferation (Downward, 2006). Furthermore, enhanced anti-proliferative effects were seen upon co-treatment with an EGFR inhibitor and DHA (Rogers et al., 2010).

Another member of the ErbB family, HER2, is the favoured dimerisation partner of other ErbB proteins for receptor activation (Tzahar et al., 1996; Park, B. W. et al., 2000). Oncogenic HER2 dimerisation in breast cancer cells takes place in lipid rafts (Nagy et al., 2002), and forced exclusion of HER2 from rafts (via crosslinking of the raft-associated ganglioside GM1) has been shown to decrease HER2 dimerisation and tyrosine phosphorylation (Nagy et al., 2002). Another possible avenue of HER2 signalling regulation by lipid rafts relates to protein trafficking. HER2 is rapidly recycled back to the cell membrane if endocytosed (Worthylake et al., 1999), which maintains its overexpression at the cell membrane of breast cancer cells. Modulation of lipid metabolism may control HER2 overexpression by increasing its endocytosis and preventing redistribution back to the cell membrane (Paris et al., 2010). For instance, phospholipase C (PLC) has been shown to co-localise with HER2 in lipid raft domains of HER2-overexpressing breast cancer cell lines, and PLC antagonism enhances HER2 internalisation and delays its recycling to the cell membrane, reducing breast cancer cell proliferation (Paris et al., 2010). This implies that lipid rafts play a key role in transduction of this oncogenic signal.

Another protein known to localise in lipid rafts with HER2, in addition to EGFR, is the estrogen receptor (ER) (Marquez et al., 2006). Estrogen signalling is linked to lipid rafts, where ER co-localises with ErbB receptors to modulate growth events (Marquez et al., 2006). Both these receptors may be activated by membrane-bound ER (Razandi et al., 2003), resulting in MAP kinase-dependent ER phosphorylation (Pietras, 2003). As these receptors are reportedly lipid raft-affiliated, interference of this union with lipid rafts may prove to be useful in targeting endocrine resistance in breast cancer.

Insulin-like growth factor-1 receptor (IGF-1R) is another receptor tyrosine kinase whose activation leads to proliferation and differentiation via MAP kinase and PI3 kinase/Akt pathways (Adams et al., 2000). IGF-1R activity has been linked to lipid raft affiliation, particularly caveolae. Stable expression of caveolin-1 in MCF7 breast cancer cells, while decreasing cell attachment (Fiucci et al., 2002), results in enhanced matrix-independent cell survival via upregulation of IGF-1R and subsequent activation of p53 and p21 (Ravid et al., 2005). Caveolin-1 further drives IGF-1R-induced recruitment of β_1-integrin into lipid rafts (Salani et al., 2009), which could in turn regulate the influence of β_1-integrin on cell fate (Li et al., 2005). In fact segregation of IGF-1R in and out of rafts has been shown to dynamically regulate overall signalling potency of the protein (Remacle-Bonnet et al., 2005), which is emerging as a promising pharmaceutical target in breast cancer (Weroha & Haluska, 2008).

Sigma receptors are a novel family of receptors whose physiological and pathophysiological roles are only beginning to emerge. They inhibit proliferation, induce apoptosis and can decrease cell adhesion in mammary carcinoma cell lines (reviewed in Aydar et al., 2004). Sigma receptors were proposed to have the ability to remodel lipid rafts by modulating raft cholesterol levels via cholesterol-binding motifs (Gebreselassie & Bowen, 2004; Takebayashi et al., 2004). Accordingly, raft cholesterol levels are reduced following sigma-1 gene knockdown (Palmer et al., 2007). Sigma-1 receptors also form a complex with β_1-integrin in MDA-MB-231 cells, and their translocation outside rafts decreases breast cancer cell growth and adhesion (Palmer et al., 2007). Because cancer cells have elevated levels of lipid rafts and cholesterol (Li et al., 2006), and because many growth signalling molecules depend on rafts to exert their functions, dietary fat modifications could affect signal transduction in breast cancer cells (as will be further addressed in Section 4).

3.3 Cell migration and metastasis

Cancer progression does not depend solely on increased growth and reduced apoptosis, but also on the ability of tumours to seek out new niches to support their continued survival. Accordingly, cells often activate pathways that reduce adhesion and promote cell migration, increasing the likelihood of the metastatic spread of breast cancer.

Kinases play a significant role in regulating cell adhesion and migration. The Src family of kinases (SFK) integrates signal transduction from many receptor tyrosine kinases, including EGFR, IGF-1R and HER2 (Belsches-Jablonski et al., 2001; Parsons & Parsons, 2004) to multiple downstream targets including PI3-kinase, Ras and focal adhesion kinase (Parsons & Parsons, 2004). SFK activation has been linked to lipid rafts in breast cancer cells (Hitosugi et al., 2007), fuelling speculation that selective targeting of raft-affiliated SFK may offer a more potent therapy than conventional SFK inhibitors such as dasatinib. Src has also been shown to phosphorylate the raft marker flotillin-2 in an EGF-dependent manner, resulting in Src translocation into endosomes and the enhancement of cell spreading (Neumann-Giesen et al., 2007). Conversely, the finding that flotillin-2 knockdown reduces cell spreading further highlights the potential regulatory influence of lipid rafts on cell adhesion and actin dynamics (Neumann-Giesen et al., 2007).

Lipid rafts and caveolin-1 have also been shown to be crucial for the formation of invadopodia, membrane protrusions that penetrate the surrounding matrix through a combination of matrix remodelling and physical force (Buccione et al., 2009). Invadopodia cluster together proteins involved in actin cytoskeleton organisation, signalling, cell-ECM adhesion and membrane remodelling (Gimona et al., 2008). Lipid rafts have been reported to be concentrated at the leading edge of invadopodia in a panel of breast cancer cell lines, and disruption of lipid rafts may suppress invadopodia formation (Yamaguchi et al., 2009). Invasive potential has also been linked with the raft-affiliated proteins caveolin-1 and membrane type 1 matrix metalloproteinase (MMP14) in both breast (Annabi et al., 2001) and prostate (Wang et al., 2009) cancer cells. In fact caveolin-1 and MMP14 have been shown to co-associate (Labrecque et al., 2004) and to be co-trafficked in invasive breast cancer cell lines (Yamaguchi et al., 2009). Accordingly, a reduction in matrix degradation activity of MMP14 has been reported in MDA-MB-231 cells following disruption of lipid rafts by cholesterol depletion or after knockdown of caveolin-1 in MMP14-overexpressiong MDA-MB-231 cells (Yamaguchi et al., 2009). Together these results highlight that lipid rafts and caveolin-1 are important for invadopodia function in breast cancer cells.

MMP14 is not the only lipid raft-affiliated proteinase implicated in breast cancer progression. Aberrant expression of MMP2 and MMP9, which localize in rafts during cancer cell migration (Patra, 2008), have been associated with high-grade breast cancer (Mira et al., 2004). Downregulation of MMP2 and MMP9 has been shown to decrease tumour cell invasion (Patra, 2008). Similarly, the serine protease urokinase-type plasminogen activator (uPA) and its receptor (uPAR), which have been linked to breast cancer progression and metastasis (Patra, 2008; Sahores et al., 2008), localise to lipid rafts during cancer cell migration (Sahores et al., 2008). A recent study investigating the importance of lipid rafts in regulating uPAR and MMP9 functionality in breast cancer has demonstrated that cholesterol depletion reduces co-localisation of uPAR and MMP9 with lipid rafts and significantly decreases their total protein and mRNA levels (Raghu et al., 2010). Lipid raft disruption in breast cancer cells resulted in reduced amounts of active Src, FAK, Akt and ERK and increased uPAR co-localisation with lysosomal markers, which was reversed after cholesterol repletion (Raghu et al., 2010). This is in agreement with previous observations of differences in MMP9-driven cell migration according to its sub-cellular localisation inside or outside rafts (Mira et al., 2004).

Although controversial, another approach to understanding breast cancer metastasis comes from the observation that disseminated tumour cells have progenitor-like properties, termed "cancer stem cells" (Acconcia et al., 2004). Low expression of CD24, a ligand for P-selectin on cancer and myeloid cells (Aigner et al., 1997), has been proposed as a marker for cancer stem cells, and breast cancer patients with aggressive triple-negative disease reportedly have higher percentages of cancer stem-like cells (May et al., 2011; Reuben et al., 2011). CD24 appears to govern the localization and function of the chemokine receptor CXCR4, which regulates proliferation in primary and metastatic breast cancer (Smith et al., 2004). CXCR4 must localise in lipid rafts for effective signalling (Manes et al., 2001; Wysoczynski et al., 2005), and CD24 reportedly reduces cellular responsiveness to CXCR4 signalling in a metastatic breast cancer cell line by excluding the latter from lipid rafts (Schabath et al., 2006). Thus low CD24 levels in putative cancer stem cells would have a positive effect on CXCR4-driven proliferative signalling, via enhanced raft affiliation of CXCR4. Accordingly, high expression of CD24 has been shown to reduce tumour growth and spread in mice (Schabath et al., 2006). Therefore CXCR4 metastatic potential may be modulated by altering its affiliation with rafts independently of its expression levels.

Another proposed marker for breast cancer stem cells is CD44 (Blick et al., 2010; May et al., 2011), a multi-functional lipid raft-affiliated transmembrane glycoprotein expressed in a variety of tissues (Murai et al., 2011). CD44 is the major receptor for the extracellular matrix component hyaluronan (HA) (Herrera-Gayol & Jothy, 1999); but it can also act as a co-receptor for growth factors (Bourguignon et al., 1997; Orian-Rousseau et al., 2002) and organise the cellular actin cytoskeleton through cytoplasmic linker proteins (Ponta et al., 2003). CD44 abnormalities have been associated with aggressive histological features of breast cancer (Joensuu et al., 1993; Diaz et al., 2005), and the association of CD44 with MMP9 in breast tumour cells promotes tumour cell migration and invasion (Bourguignon et al., 1998). It is possible that this matrix-degrading association takes place in lipid rafts, where both CD44 and MMP9 localize. Interactions between CD44 and HA also stimulate a variety of events leading to tumour progression, including Rho kinase activation, Ras signalling and others (reviewed in Bourguignon, 2008). Although the exact mechanisms of these events have yet to be clarified, one proposed method involves CD44 interaction with ankyrin within lipid rafts (Singleton & Bourguignon, 2004). Another matrix glucosaminoglycan, osteopontin, can also activate CD44 to promote cell survival and increased endothelial adhesion by recruiting Src and integrins into lipid rafts (Lee et al., 2008).

The influence of CD44 on cancer progression also extends to other growth factor signalling pathways, since it has previously been demonstrated that the growth factor receptor c-Met cannot be activated by its ligand alone, but also requires CD44 co-expression (van der Voort et al., 1999). c-Met, which has been shown to localise in lipid rafts and whose signalling is sensitive to cholesterol depletion (Coleman et al., 2009), is frequently dysregulated in metastatic breast cancer (Gastaldi et al., 2010; Elnagar et al., 2011). It can thus be hypothesised that lipid rafts are required for successful transduction of growth factor-mediated oncogenic signals through formation of functional CD44 complexes.

Taken altogether, several key molecules frequently implicated in breast cancer initiation, growth and migration are regulated by lipid rafts via sequestration, endocytosis or termination of protein interactions. Considering the ongoing need to develop drugs which selectively attack cancer cells while leaving normal cells unaltered, the imbalance in lipid raft composition between tumour and normal cells may suggest rafts as attractive and novel pharmacological targets in the battle against breast cancer.

4. Lipid rafts as novel therapeutic targets in breast cancer

This section will focus on current cancer treatments targeting lipid rafts, the potential importance of lipid raft modulation to overcome mechanisms of drug resistance, and new mechanisms associated with lipid raft physiology that could be targeted by novel drugs. Finally it will discuss the importance of the diet in influencing lipid raft physiology as a potential mechanism to prevent or reduce cancer dissemination.

4.1 Current drug treatments targeting lipid rafts

There is growing interest in the possibility of targeting lipid rafts for cancer treatments due to their role in the regulation of many steps of tumour transformation and progression, such as the apoptotic pathways initiated by FasL and TRAIL. Current treatments targeting lipid rafts are mainly focused on activating these apoptotic pathways in cancer cells. However many classes of drugs routinely used in breast cancer chemotherapy have been shown to exert some of their effects by modulating lipid rafts.

One key example is cisplatin, whose mechanism of action is still incompletely understood, but which has been described to exert some of its actions through modulation of ceramide lipid rafts. In a human colon cancer cell line, cisplatin induced clustering of the Fas receptor in membrane lipid rafts by activating the acid sphingomyelinase (ASMase), which produces ceramide and is responsible for induction of apoptosis. Nystatin, a compound which disrupts lipid rafts, completely reversed this effect (Lacour et al., 2004). It has also been reported that a combination of cisplatin and an anti-Fas antibody in cells expressing sphingomyelinase induced marked apoptosis of cancer cells (Huang et al., 2010).

Moreover, histone deacetylase inhibitors (HDACi), powerful tumour suppressors for many different solid and hematologic cancers, have also been shown to modulate lipid raft physiology. These compounds act on tumour cells by inducing accumulation of acetylated proteins that can cause growth arrest, apoptosis and ROS-induced cell death (Marks & Xu, 2009). Since normal cells are resistant to these treatments, HDACi have been widely tested in clinical trials alone or in combination with other drugs (Marks & Xu, 2009). Van Oosten and colleagues observed a drastic increase in the expression and localization of TRAIL in lipid rafts after treatment of prostate cancer cells with a HDACi depsipeptide, inducing elevated cell apoptosis (Vanoosten et al., 2005). Similarly, in preclinical mouse breast cancer models the HDACi vorinostat, in combination with administration of monoclonal antibodies against the mouse TRAIL receptor (DR5), induced robust cell apoptosis (Frew et al., 2008).

Likewise, some derivatives of doxorubicin, an anthracycline widely used in breast cancer adjuvant chemotherapy, exercise their actions by activating lipid raft-associated pathways. Aroui and colleagues illustrated that treatment of MDA-MB-231 cells with Dox-CPP, obtained by conjugating doxorubicin to a cell-penetrating peptide, sensitised cells to TRAIL-induced apoptotic pathways by increasing TRAIL clustering and its inclusion in ceramide lipid rafts (Aroui et al., 2009). Lipid raft-mediated activation of TRAIL is also important because it reduces resistance mechanisms associated with doxorubicin resistance.

4.2 Overcoming drug resistance by targeting lipid rafts

One major drawback of current cancer treatment regimens is the development of drug resistance. Two main mechanisms have been described to be involved in this multifactorial process: 1) alterations in tumour cell physiology that cause either insensitivity to drug-induced apoptosis or induction of drug-detoxifying mechanisms; 2) expression of energy-dependent transporters that detect and eject anti-cancer drugs from cells (Wang et al., 2010).

Recent evidence points to the correlation of both mechanisms with lipid raft physiology. Mechanisms of breast cancer resistance to the anti-HER2 therapeutic antibody Herceptin/ Trastuzumab may involve compensatory signalling through dimerisation of HER2 with other ErbB family members, cross-talk between HER2 and the IGF-1R pathway, coverage of the antibody binding site by MUC4 overexpression, and constitutive activation of the PI3 kinase/Akt pathways (Nahta & Esteva, 2006). Interestingly, all these events take place in lipid raft compartments and are involved in the activation of alternative oncogenic pathways to overcome the inhibitory effects of cancer treatments. Therefore, treatments altering lipid raft physiology could provide hope in preventing or reducing mechanisms of resistance to specific anti-cancer drugs.

HER2 over-expression in breast cancer cells has also been reported to stimulate fatty acid synthase (FASyn) gene expression (Menendez et al., 2004). FASyn is a major lipogenic enzyme catalyzing the synthesis of long-chain saturated fatty acids, which localize to lipid rafts in epithelial cells. Accordingly, FASyn inhibitors work by altering lipid raft physiology through deregulation of fatty acid synthesis; and have been reported to re-sensitise cells to Trastuzumab, causing growth inhibition and apoptotic cell death. Since these inhibitors also affect EGFR1 localization to lipid rafts, they may also disrupt the cross-talk between HER2 and EGFR which is involved in Trastuzumab resistance (reviewed in Menendez, 2005).

Correspondingly, since ER can localize to lipid rafts through post-translational lipid modifications termed acylations, lipid rafts have been suggested as the possible location of interactions between ER and growth factor receptors which occur during resistance to endocrine therapy (Acconcia et al., 2004; Weinberg et al., 2005; Arpino et al., 2008). Mutations of ER acylation sites impair the ability of ER to activate transcription and cell proliferation in response to estradiol stimulation (Pietras et al., 2005). It is appealing to speculate that combinations of hormonal therapies and treatments altering ER localization to lipid rafts could prevent cross-talk between ER and EGFR pathways; and may be a future therapeutic strategy to reduce drug resistance arising in hormonal therapy. Furthermore, it has been shown that poor responsiveness of breast cancer cells to treatment with the EGFR inhibitor gefitinib may be due to increased localization of EGFR in lipid raft domains. Treatment of breast cells with lipid raft-disrupting agents (such as lovastatin) induced cellular sensitivity to gefitinib, and abrogated proliferative pathways initiated by Akt phosphorylation (Irwin et al., 2010).

However, along with single drug resistance in breast cancer therapy, the phenomenon of multidrug resistance has also been described (Ogretmen & Hannun, 2001). This occurs when resistance to one drug is accompanied by resistance to drugs whose structures and mechanisms of action may be completely different. Several studies have observed alterations of lipid raft components in multidrug-resistant cells, such as increased caveolin-1 expression, larger numbers of caveolae (Lavie et al., 1998) and elevated membrane cholesterol content (Gayet et al., 2005). Lavie and colleagues suggested that an increased number of caveolae may be more of a cause than an effect of multidrug resistance. In fact, caveolae, being capable of effluxing cholesterol, may be used by cancer cells to efflux lipophilic drugs. Since caveolar efficiency to efflux cholesterol or any cytotoxic drug is very low, they hypothesized that a higher number of caveolae is therefore necessary to compensate for drug cytotoxic effects and efflux them efficiently (Lavie et al., 1998).

Cellular lipid changes are also often accompanied by increased expression of ABC transporters which can localize to lipid rafts (Klappe et al., 2009). One member of this family, BCRP/ABCG2, which was discovered and cloned in breast cancer cells (Doyle et al., 1998), has been recently described to localize to lipid rafts. Interestingly, disruption of lipid rafts using methyl-β-cyclodextrin has been shown to cause a 40% decrease in BCRP activity (Storch et al., 2007); further highlighting the potential value of pharmacological raft targeting as a mechanism of reducing multi-drug resistance.

Overall these examples demonstrate the importance of lipid rafts in clustering oncogenic signalling molecules that are involved in breast cancer resistance to current conventional treatments. It is also evident that treatments aimed at preventing or disrupting the localisation of oncogenic signalling mediators (such as HER2, ER, IGF-1R or ABC transporters) in lipid rafts may prove therapeutically useful in combination with current treatments in order to prevent the development of resistance.

4.3 Novel lipid raft- mediated approaches in breast cancer treatment

Recently, glycomic studies have highlighted an emerging and critical importance of glycans in influencing lipid raft physiology. Therefore potential future cancer treatments may also indirectly target lipid rafts by targeting glycans. For example, in breast cancer cells, gangliosides (such as the ganglioside GM1 or the O-glycosylated protein MUC4) regulate the formation of EGFR growth factor-responsive heterodimer complexes in lipid rafts (Komatsu et al., 2001). Lipid rafts play a fundamental role in providing a microenvironment favouring functional interactions between glycans and HER2 / HER3, which drive tumour progression (Komatsu et al., 2001; Nagy et al., 2002). Antibodies targeting MUC4 or treatments targeting gangliosides (i.e. ceramide glycosylation inhibitors or ganglioside-targeted vaccines such as NeuGcGM3 and Theratope) may therefore be possible treatments to interfere with ErbB-driven proliferation of breast cancer cells via modulation of lipid raft physiology (Carr et al., 2003; Ibrahim & Murray, 2003; Julien et al., 2009; Mulens et al., 2010). Raft-dependent endocytosis of paclitaxel-conjugated autocrine motility factor is elevated in metastatic breast cancer cells and has been shown to induce tumour regression and promote survival of tumour-bearing mice (Kojic et al., 2008; Kojic et al., 2007). In addition, some new generation treatments have considered the use of nanoparticles to target lipid raft-affiliated proteins involved in tumour progression and invasion. Conjugated nanoparticles present the advantage of selectively targeting cancer cells without affecting the physiology of normal cells. For example, a study in glioma cells using magnetic nanoparticles conjugated to chlorotoxin (which targets MMP2, a protein highly expressed in glioma tumour cells) demonstrated the induction of lipid-raft mediated endocytosis of MMP2 together with Cl^- and K^+ channels (Veiseh et al., 2009), the latter proteins being involved in regulating cell volume during cell invasion. Using this system, a 98% reduction in invasion was observed in nanoparticle-treated cells compared to controls. In the same manner, MMP2 has also been shown to play a role in breast cancer progression and invasion and has been described as a marker for poor prognosis in ER- negative patients (Ma et al., 2009). Therefore, it is conceivable that an approach similar to the one used by Veiseh et al. might be useful as a companion drug strategy for breast cancer chemotherapy.

4.4 Lipid rafts and diet in cancer progression

Cancer cells generally possess higher levels of saturated fatty acids and cholesterol than normal cells (Li et al., 2006). Emerging evidence thus suggests the potential of diet to influence raft composition and the role of rafts in cancer pathophysiology (section 3.2).

Several studies have shown that polyunsaturated fatty acids (PUFAs) may have anti-carcinogenic properties (Sauer et al., 2007). The mechanism by which PUFAs work is still incompletely understood, but two mechanisms have been proposed. The first suggests that PUFAs affect the palmitoylation status of lipid raft proteins (Webb et al., 2000); while the second model suggests that PUFAs, having a low affinity for cholesterol due to their bulky structure, reduce raft cholesterol levels and cause displacement of raft proteins (Stulnig et al., 2001). In fact, it has been described that *in vivo* PUFA supplementation affects lipid raft composition by depleting up to 50% of cholesterol and by altering lipid raft/caveolar protein composition. In comparison to chemical disruption of lipid rafts (e.g. with methyl-β-cyclodextrin and nystatin), PUFA treatment is very selective and depletes only membrane cholesterol without affecting other cellular sources of cholesterol (Ma et al., 2004).

It has also been shown that PUFAs such as EPA and DHA inhibit protein palmitoylation of selected T cell lipid raft proteins (such as Fyn) similarly to the chemical compound 2-bromopalmitate (Webb et al., 2000). Interestingly, in MDA-MB-231 breast cancer cells, PUFAs have been shown to decrease cell proliferation and induce apoptotic cell death probably by decreasing Akt/NFκB signal transduction (Schley et al., 2005). Furthermore, PUFA treatment has been shown to increase EPA and DHA concentrations in lipid rafts, with a corresponding decrease of sphingomyelin, cholesterol and diacylglycerol (Schley et al., 2007). In particular, PUFAs reduce sphingomyelin levels by inducing its hydrolysis to ceramide, which (as discussed) activates pro-apoptotic pathways (Schley et al., 2005).

Section 3 discussed how lipid raft disruption negatively modulates EGFR localization and signalling, and, similarly, PUFAs have been shown to exert pro-apoptotic properties by reducing EGFR localization within lipid rafts, thus inducing a sustained activation of EGFR and p38 phosphorylation in breast cancer cells (Schley et al., 2007). In the same way, (-)-epigallocatechin-3-gallate (EGCG), the active compound contained in green tea, can alter lipid raft domain composition. EGCG has been described to prevent EGF interactions with its receptor, to prevent EGFR dimerisation and to inhibit its localisation within rafts. This would promote pro-apoptotic signalling via p38. Altogether, EGFR translocation alters its activation status and may have anti-cancer effects (Patra et al., 2008). EGCG also exerts further anti-cancer activity by suppressing proliferation and enhancing apoptosis by interfering with lipid raft remodelling (Patra et al., 2008). Indeed, EGCG has been described to block the laminin-1 receptor, a raft-affiliated protein (Tachibana et al., 2004) whose activation is connected with a kinase/phosphatase cascade involved in tumour progression (Patra et al., 2008). Interestingly, EGCG also seems to play a role in modulating multidrug resistance. In fact it has been described that EGCG causes a dose-dependent increase in apoptosis in Trastuzumab- (Eddy et al., 2007), Tamoxifen- and multidrug-resistant breast cancer cells (Farabegoli et al., 2010).

Taken together, we have summarized putative anti-tumour mechanisms involving interference with lipid rafts, and highlighted the importance of rafts as targets for cancer therapy. Development of drugs directed to specific raft components could facilitate widespread use of these treatments; while dietary modification alone could influence tumorigenic behaviour through modulation of lipid raft composition. Overall we suggest that lipid rafts play a key role both in the prevention and treatment of breast cancer, and are confident that further studies in this area will prove highly fruitful in the future.

5. References

Acconcia, F, Ascenzi, P, Fabozzi, G, Visca, P & Marino, M (2004). S-palmitoylation modulates human estrogen receptor-alpha functions. *Biochem Biophys Res Commun*, Vol. 316, No. 3, (2004), pp 878-83

Adams, TE, Epa, VC, Garrett, TP & Ward, CW (2000). Structure and function of the type 1 insulin-like growth factor receptor. *Cell Mol Life Sci*, Vol. 57, No. 7, (2000), pp 1050-93

Aigner, S, Sthoeger, ZM, Fogel, M, Weber, E, Zarn, J et al. (1997). CD24, a mucin-type glycoprotein, is a ligand for P-selectin on human tumor cells. *Blood*, Vol. 89, No. 9, (1997), pp 3385-95

Annabi, B, Lachambre, M, Bousquet-Gagnon, N, Page, M, Gingras, D et al. (2001). Localization of membrane-type 1 matrix metalloproteinase in caveolae membrane domains. *Biochem J*, Vol. 353, No. Pt 3, (2001), pp 547-53

Aroui, S, Brahim, S, Hamelin, J, De Waard, M, Breard, J et al. (2009). Conjugation of doxorubicin to cell penetrating peptides sensitizes human breast MDA-MB 231 cancer cells to endogenous TRAIL-induced apoptosis. *Apoptosis*, Vol. 14, No. 11, (2009), pp 1352-65

Arpino, G, Wiechmann, L, Osborne, CK & Schiff, R (2008). Crosstalk between the estrogen receptor and the HER tyrosine kinase receptor family: molecular mechanism and clinical implications for endocrine therapy resistance. *Endocr Rev*, Vol. 29, No. 2, (2008), pp 217-33

Aydar, E, Palmer, CP & Djamgoz, MB (2004). Sigma receptors and cancer: possible involvement of ion channels. *Cancer Res*, Vol. 64, No. 15, (2004), pp 5029-35

Babuke, T & Tikkanen, R (2007). Dissecting the molecular function of reggie/flotillin proteins. *Eur J Cell Biol*, Vol. 86, No. 9, (2007), pp 525-32

Barros, FF, Powe, DG, Ellis, IO & Green, AR (2010). Understanding the HER family in breast cancer: interaction with ligands, dimerization and treatments. *Histopathology*, Vol. 56, No. 5, (2010), pp 560-72

Belsches-Jablonski, AP, Biscardi, JS, Peavy, DR, Tice, DA, Romney, DA et al. (2001). Src family kinases and HER2 interactions in human breast cancer cell growth and survival. *Oncogene*, Vol. 20, No. 12, (2001), pp 1465-75

Bhatnagar, RS & Gordon, JI (1997). Understanding covalent modifications of proteins by lipids: where cell biology and biophysics mingle. *Trends Cell Biol*, Vol. 7, No. 1, (1997), pp 14-20

Bickel, PE, Scherer, PE, Schnitzer, JE, Oh, P, Lisanti, MP et al. (1997). Flotillin and epidermal surface antigen define a new family of caveolae-associated integral membrane proteins. *J Biol Chem*, Vol. 272, No. 21, (1997), pp 13793-802

Bijlmakers, MJ & Marsh, M (2003). The on-off story of protein palmitoylation. *Trends Cell Biol*, Vol. 13, No. 1, (2003), pp 32-42

Blick, T, Hugo, H, Widodo, E, Waltham, M, Pinto, C et al. (2010). Epithelial mesenchymal transition traits in human breast cancer cell lines parallel the CD44(hi/)CD24 (lo/-) stem cell phenotype in human breast cancer. *J Mammary Gland Biol Neoplasia*, Vol. 15, No. 2, (2010), pp 235-52

Bourguignon, LY (2008). Hyaluronan-mediated CD44 activation of RhoGTPase signaling and cytoskeleton function promotes tumor progression. *Semin Cancer Biol*, Vol. 18, No. 4, (2008), pp 251-9

Bourguignon, LY, Zhu, D & Zhu, H (1998). CD44 isoform-cytoskeleton interaction in oncogenic signaling and tumor progression. *Front Biosci*, Vol. 3, No. (1998), pp d637-49

Bourguignon, LY, Zhu, H, Chu, A, Iida, N, Zhang, L et al. (1997). Interaction between the adhesion receptor, CD44, and the oncogene product, p185HER2, promotes human ovarian tumor cell activation. *J Biol Chem*, Vol. 272, No. 44, (1997), pp 27913-8

Brown, DA & Rose, JK (1992). Sorting of GPI-anchored proteins to glycolipid-enriched membrane subdomains during transport to the apical cell surface. *Cell*, Vol. 68, No. 3, (1992), pp 533-44

Buccione, R, Caldieri, G & Ayala, I (2009). Invadopodia: specialized tumor cell structures for the focal degradation of the extracellular matrix. *Cancer Metastasis Rev*, Vol. 28, No. 1-2, (2009), pp 137-49

Calder, PC & Yaqoob, P (2007). Lipid rafts--composition, characterization, and controversies. *J Nutr*, Vol. 137, No. 3, (2007), pp 545-7

Camp, LA & Hofmann, SL (1995). Assay and isolation of palmitoyl-protein thioesterase from bovine brain using palmitoylated H-Ras as substrate. *Methods Enzymol*, Vol. 250, No. (1995), pp 336-47

Carr, A, Rodriguez, E, Arango Mdel, C, Camacho, R, Osorio, M et al. (2003). Immunotherapy of advanced breast cancer with a heterophilic ganglioside (NeuGcGM3) cancer vaccine. *J Clin Oncol*, Vol. 21, No. 6, (2003), pp 1015-21

Cary, LA & Cooper, JA (2000). Molecular switches in lipid rafts. *Nature*, Vol. 404, No. 6781, (2000), pp 945, 947

Casey, PJ & Seabra, MC (1996). Protein prenyltransferases. *J Biol Chem*, Vol. 271, No. 10, (1996), pp 5289-92

Chakrabandhu, K, Herincs, Z, Huault, S, Dost, B, Peng, L et al. (2007). Palmitoylation is required for efficient Fas cell death signaling. *EMBO J*, Vol. 26, No. 1, (2007), pp 209-20

Chen, X & Resh, MD (2002). Cholesterol depletion from the plasma membrane triggers ligand-independent activation of the epidermal growth factor receptor. *J Biol Chem*, Vol. 277, No. 51, (2002), pp 49631-7

Colas, S, Maheo, K, Denis, F, Goupille, C, Hoinard, C et al. (2006). Sensitization by dietary docosahexaenoic acid of rat mammary carcinoma to anthracycline: a role for tumor vascularization. *Clin Cancer Res*, Vol. 12, No. 19, (2006), pp 5879-86

Coleman, DT, Bigelow, R & Cardelli, JA (2009). Inhibition of fatty acid synthase by luteolin post-transcriptionally down-regulates c-Met expression independent of proteosomal/lysosomal degradation. *Mol Cancer Ther*, Vol. 8, No. 1, (2009), pp 214-24

Datta, SR, Brunet, A & Greenberg, ME (1999). Cellular survival: a play in three Akts. *Genes Dev*, Vol. 13, No. 22, (1999), pp 2905-27

de Laurentiis, A, Donovan, L & Arcaro, A (2007). Lipid rafts and caveolae in signaling by growth factor receptors. *Open Biochem J*, Vol. 1, No. (2007), pp 12-32

Deborde, S, Perret, E, Gravotta, D, Deora, A, Salvarezza, S et al. (2008). Clathrin is a key regulator of basolateral polarity. *Nature*, Vol. 452, No. 7188, (2008), pp 719-23

Diaz, LK, Zhou, X, Wright, ET, Cristofanilli, M, Smith, T et al. (2005). CD44 expression is associated with increased survival in node-negative invasive breast carcinoma. *Clin Cancer Res*, Vol. 11, No. 9, (2005), pp 3309-14

Downward, J (2006). Signal transduction. Prelude to an anniversary for the RAS oncogene. *Science*, Vol. 314, No. 5798, (2006), pp 433-4

Doyle, LA, Yang, W, Abruzzo, LV, Krogmann, T, Gao, Y et al. (1998). A multidrug resistance transporter from human MCF-7 breast cancer cells. *Proc Natl Acad Sci U S A*, Vol. 95, No. 26, (1998), pp 15665-70

Dumitru, CA, Carpinteiro, A, Trarbach, T, Hengge, UR & Gulbins, E (2007). Doxorubicin enhances TRAIL-induced cell death via ceramide-enriched membrane platforms. *Apoptosis*, Vol. 12, No. 8, (2007), pp 1533-41

Dunphy, JT, Greentree, WK & Linder, ME (2001). Enrichment of G-protein palmitoyltransferase activity in low density membranes: in vitro reconstitution of Galphai to these domains requires palmitoyltransferase activity. *J Biol Chem*, Vol. 276, No. 46, (2001), pp 43300-4

Eddy, SF, Kane, SE & Sonenshein, GE (2007). Trastuzumab-resistant HER2-driven breast cancer cells are sensitive to epigallocatechin-3 gallate. *Cancer Res*, Vol. 67, No. 19, (2007), pp 9018-23

Elhyany, S, Assa-Kunik, E, Tsory, S, Muller, T, Fedida, S et al. (2004). The integrity of cholesterol-enriched microdomains is essential for the constitutive high activity of protein kinase B in tumour cells. *Biochem Soc Trans*, Vol. 32, No. Pt 5, (2004), pp 837-9

Elnagar, AY, Sylvester, PW & El Sayed, KA (2011). (-)-Oleocanthal as a c-Met Inhibitor for the Control of Metastatic Breast and Prostate Cancers. *Planta Med*, Vol. No. (2011), 1439-0221

Everson, WV & Smart, EJ. (2006). *Caveolin and its Role in Intracellular Chaperone Complexes* (edition), Wiley-VCH Verlag GmbH & Co. KGaA, 9783527608072,

Fan, JY, Carpentier, JL, van Obberghen, E, Grunfeld, C, Gorden, P et al. (1983). Morphological changes of the 3T3-L1 fibroblast plasma membrane upon differentiation to the adipocyte form. *J Cell Sci*, Vol. 61, No. (1983), pp 219-30

Farabegoli, F, Papi, A, Bartolini, G, Ostan, R & Orlandi, M (2010). (-)-Epigallocatechin-3-gallate downregulates Pg-P and BCRP in a tamoxifen resistant MCF-7 cell line. *Phytomedicine*, Vol. 17, No. 5, (2010), pp 356-62

Fiedler, K, Kobayashi, T, Kurzchalia, TV & Simons, K (1993). Glycosphingolipid-enriched, detergent-insoluble complexes in protein sorting in epithelial cells. *Biochemistry*, Vol. 32, No. 25, (1993), pp 6365-73

Fiucci, G, Ravid, D, Reich, R & Liscovitch, M (2002). Caveolin-1 inhibits anchorage-independent growth, anoikis and invasiveness in MCF-7 human breast cancer cells. *Oncogene*, Vol. 21, No. 15, (2002), pp 2365-75

Folsch, H, Mattila, PE & Weisz, OA (2009). Taking the scenic route: biosynthetic traffic to the plasma membrane in polarized epithelial cells. *Traffic*, Vol. 10, No. 8, (2009), pp 972-81

Fra, AM, Williamson, E, Simons, K & Parton, RG (1995). De novo formation of caveolae in lymphocytes by expression of VIP21-caveolin. *Proc Natl Acad Sci U S A*, Vol. 92, No. 19, (1995), pp 8655-9

Freeman, MR, Cinar, B, Kim, J, Mukhopadhyay, NK, Di Vizio, D et al. (2007). Transit of hormonal and EGF receptor-dependent signals through cholesterol-rich membranes. *Steroids*, Vol. 72, No. 2, (2007), pp 210-7

Frew, AJ, Lindemann, RK, Martin, BP, Clarke, CJ, Sharkey, J et al. (2008). Combination therapy of established cancer using a histone deacetylase inhibitor and a TRAIL receptor agonist. *Proc Natl Acad Sci U S A*, Vol. 105, No. 32, (2008), pp 11317-22

Furuchi, T & Anderson, RG (1998). Cholesterol depletion of caveolae causes hyperactivation of extracellular signal-related kinase (ERK). *J Biol Chem*, Vol. 273, No. 33, (1998), pp 21099-104

Gajate, C, Del Canto-Janez, E, Acuna, AU, Amat-Guerri, F, Geijo, E et al. (2004). Intracellular triggering of Fas aggregation and recruitment of apoptotic molecules into Fas-enriched rafts in selective tumor cell apoptosis. *J Exp Med*, Vol. 200, No. 3, (2004), pp 353-65

Gajate, C, Gonzalez-Camacho, F & Mollinedo, F (2009). Lipid raft connection between extrinsic and intrinsic apoptotic pathways. *Biochem Biophys Res Commun*, Vol. 380, No. 4, (2009), pp 780-4

Gajate, C & Mollinedo, F (2001). The antitumor ether lipid ET-18-OCH(3) induces apoptosis through translocation and capping of Fas/CD95 into membrane rafts in human leukemic cells. *Blood*, Vol. 98, No. 13, (2001), pp 3860-3

Gajate, C & Mollinedo, F (2005). Cytoskeleton-mediated death receptor and ligand concentration in lipid rafts forms apoptosis-promoting clusters in cancer chemotherapy. *J Biol Chem*, Vol. 280, No. 12, (2005), pp 11641-7

Gajate, C & Mollinedo, F (2007). Edelfosine and perifosine induce selective apoptosis in multiple myeloma by recruitment of death receptors and downstream signaling molecules into lipid rafts. *Blood*, Vol. 109, No. 2, (2007), pp 711-9

Galbiati, F, Engelman, JA, Volonte, D, Zhang, XL, Minetti, C et al. (2001). Caveolin-3 null mice show a loss of caveolae, changes in the microdomain distribution of the dystrophin-glycoprotein complex, and t-tubule abnormalities. *J Biol Chem*, Vol. 276, No. 24, (2001), pp 21425-33

Gastaldi, S, Comoglio, PM & Trusolino, L (2010). The Met oncogene and basal-like breast cancer: another culprit to watch out for? *Breast Cancer Res*, Vol. 12, No. 4, (2010), pp 208

Gayet, L, Dayan, G, Barakat, S, Labialle, S, Michaud, M et al. (2005). Control of P-glycoprotein activity by membrane cholesterol amounts and their relation to multidrug resistance in human CEM leukemia cells. *Biochemistry*, Vol. 44, No. 11, (2005), pp 4499-509

Gebreselassie, D & Bowen, WD (2004). Sigma-2 receptors are specifically localized to lipid rafts in rat liver membranes. *Eur J Pharmacol*, Vol. 493, No. 1-3, (2004), pp 19-28

Germain, E, Chajes, V, Cognault, S, Lhuillery, C & Bougnoux, P (1998). Enhancement of doxorubicin cytotoxicity by polyunsaturated fatty acids in the human breast tumor cell line MDA-MB-231: relationship to lipid peroxidation. *Int J Cancer*, Vol. 75, No. 4, (1998), pp 578-83

Ghosh, RN, Mallet, WG, Soe, TT, McGraw, TE & Maxfield, FR (1998). An endocytosed TGN38 chimeric protein is delivered to the TGN after trafficking through the endocytic recycling compartment in CHO cells. *J Cell Biol*, Vol. 142, No. 4, (1998), pp 923-36

Gimona, M, Buccione, R, Courtneidge, SA & Linder, S (2008). Assembly and biological role of podosomes and invadopodia. *Curr Opin Cell Biol*, Vol. 20, No. 2, (2008), pp 235-41

Gong, M, Wilson, M, Kelly, T, Su, W, Dressman, J et al. (2003). HDL-associated estradiol stimulates endothelial NO synthase and vasodilation in an SR-BI-dependent manner. *J Clin Invest*, Vol. 111, No. 10, (2003), pp 1579-87

Gorelick, FS & Shugrue, C (2001). Exiting the endoplasmic reticulum. *Mol Cell Endocrinol*, Vol. 177, No. 1-2, (2001), pp 13-8

Herrera-Gayol, A & Jothy, S (1999). Adhesion proteins in the biology of breast cancer: contribution of CD44. *Exp Mol Pathol*, Vol. 66, No. 2, (1999), pp 149-56

Hill, MM, Feng, J & Hemmings, BA (2002). Identification of a plasma membrane Raft-associated PKB Ser473 kinase activity that is distinct from ILK and PDK1. *Curr Biol*, Vol. 12, No. 14, (2002), pp 1251-5

Hitosugi, T, Sato, M, Sasaki, K & Umezawa, Y (2007). Lipid raft specific knockdown of SRC family kinase activity inhibits cell adhesion and cell cycle progression of breast cancer cells. *Cancer Res*, Vol. 67, No. 17, (2007), pp 8139-48

Huang, CR, Jin, ZX, Dong, L, Tong, XP, Yue, S et al. (2010). Cisplatin augments FAS-mediated apoptosis through lipid rafts. *Anticancer Res*, Vol. 30, No. 6, (2010), pp 2065-71

Ibrahim, NK & Murray, JL (2003). Clinical development of the STn-KLH vaccine (Theratope). *Clin Breast Cancer*, Vol. 3 Suppl 4, No. (2003), pp S139-43

Irwin, ME, Mueller, KL, Bohin, N, Ge, Y & Boerner, JL (2010). Lipid raft localization of EGFR alters the response of cancer cells to the EGFR tyrosine kinase inhibitor gefitinib. *J Cell Physiol*, Vol. No. (2010), 1097-4652

Jemal, A, Bray, F, Center, MM, Ferlay, J, Ward, E et al. (2011). Global cancer statistics. *CA Cancer J Clin*, Vol. 61, No. 2, (2011), pp 69-90

Joensuu, H, Klemi, PJ, Toikkanen, S & Jalkanen, S (1993). Glycoprotein CD44 expression and its association with survival in breast cancer. *Am J Pathol*, Vol. 143, No. 3, (1993), pp 867-74

Julien, S, Picco, G, Sewell, R, Vercoutter-Edouart, AS, Tarp, M et al. (2009). Sialyl-Tn vaccine induces antibody-mediated tumour protection in a relevant murine model. *Br J Cancer*, Vol. 100, No. 11, (2009), pp 1746-54

Kang, R, Wan, J, Arstikaitis, P, Takahashi, H, Huang, K et al. (2008). Neural palmitoyl-proteomics reveals dynamic synaptic palmitoylation. *Nature*, Vol. 456, No. 7224, (2008), pp 904-9

Klappe, K, Hummel, I, Hoekstra, D & Kok, JW (2009). Lipid dependence of ABC transporter localization and function. *Chem Phys Lipids*, Vol. 161, No. 2, (2009), pp 57-64

Komatsu, M, Jepson, S, Arango, ME, Carothers Carraway, CA & Carraway, KL (2001). Muc4/sialomucin complex, an intramembrane modulator of ErbB2/HER2/Neu, potentiates primary tumor growth and suppresses apoptosis in a xenotransplanted tumor. *Oncogene*, Vol. 20, No. 4, (2001), pp 461-70

Labrecque, L, Nyalendo, C, Langlois, S, Durocher, Y, Roghi, C et al. (2004). Src-mediated tyrosine phosphorylation of caveolin-1 induces its association with membrane type 1 matrix metalloproteinase. *J Biol Chem*, Vol. 279, No. 50, (2004), pp 52132-40

Lacour, S, Hammann, A, Grazide, S, Lagadic-Gossmann, D, Athias, A et al. (2004). Cisplatin-induced CD95 redistribution into membrane lipid rafts of HT29 human colon cancer cells. *Cancer Res*, Vol. 64, No. 10, (2004), pp 3593-8

Lajoie, P & Nabi, IR (2010). Lipid rafts, caveolae, and their endocytosis. *Int Rev Cell Mol Biol*, Vol. 282, No. (2010), pp 135-63

Lajoie, P, Partridge, EA, Guay, G, S., N, Goetz, JG et al. (2007). Plasma membrane domain organization regulates EGFR signaling in tumor cells. *J Cell Biol*, Vol. 179, No. 2, (2007), pp 341-56

Landowski, TH, Gleason-Guzman, MC & Dalton, WS (1997). Selection for drug resistance results in resistance to Fas-mediated apoptosis. *Blood*, Vol. 89, No. 6, (1997), pp 1854-61

Lavie, Y, Fiucci, G & Liscovitch, M (1998). Up-regulation of caveolae and caveolar constituents in multidrug-resistant cancer cells. *J Biol Chem*, Vol. 273, No. 49, (1998), pp 32380-3

Le Moyec, L, Tatoud, R, Eugene, M, Gauville, C, Primot, I et al. (1992). Cell and membrane lipid analysis by proton magnetic resonance spectroscopy in five breast cancer cell lines. *Br J Cancer*, Vol. 66, No. 4, (1992), pp 623-8

Lee, JL, Wang, MJ, Sudhir, PR & Chen, JY (2008). CD44 engagement promotes matrix-derived survival through the CD44-SRC-integrin axis in lipid rafts. *Mol Cell Biol*, Vol. 28, No. 18, (2008), pp 5710-23

Lee, SH, Koo, KH, Park, JW, Kim, HJ, Ye, SK et al. (2009). HIF-1 is induced via EGFR activation and mediates resistance to anoikis-like cell death under lipid rafts/caveolae-disrupting stress. *Carcinogenesis*, Vol. 30, No. 12, (2009), pp 1997-2004

Leon, L, Subramaniam, S, Cauvard, O, Plenchette-Colas, S, Paul, C et al. (2011). S-Nitrosylation of the Death Receptor Fas Promotes Fas Ligand-Mediated Apoptosis in Cancer Cells. *Gastroenterology*, Vol. No. (2011), 1528-0012

Levental, I, Grzybek, M & Simons, K (2010). Greasing their way: lipid modifications determine protein association with membrane rafts. *Biochemistry*, Vol. 49, No. 30, (2010), pp 6305-16

Li, H, Zhu, H, Xu, CJ & Yuan, J (1998). Cleavage of BID by caspase 8 mediates the mitochondrial damage in the Fas pathway of apoptosis. *Cell*, Vol. 94, No. 4, (1998), pp 491-501

Li, N, Zhang, Y, Naylor, MJ, Schatzmann, F, Maurer, F et al. (2005). Beta1 integrins regulate mammary gland proliferation and maintain the integrity of mammary alveoli. *EMBO J*, Vol. 24, No. 11, (2005), pp 1942-53

Li, YC, Park, MJ, Ye, SK, Kim, CW & Kim, YN (2006). Elevated levels of cholesterol-rich lipid rafts in cancer cells are correlated with apoptosis sensitivity induced by cholesterol-depleting agents. *Am J Pathol*, Vol. 168, No. 4, (2006), pp 1107-18

Lingwood, D, Kaiser, HJ, Levental, I & Simons, K (2009). Lipid rafts as functional heterogeneity in cell membranes. *Biochem Soc Trans*, Vol. 37, No. Pt 5, (2009), pp 955-60

Lipowsky, R (1993). Domain-induced budding of fluid membranes. *Biophys J*, Vol. 64, No. 4, (1993), pp 1133-8

Liu, J, Deyoung, SM, Zhang, M, Dold, LH & Saltiel, AR (2005). The stomatin/prohibitin/flotillin/HflK/C domain of flotillin-1 contains distinct sequences that direct plasma membrane localization and protein interactions in 3T3-L1 adipocytes. *J Biol Chem*, Vol. 280, No. 16, (2005), pp 16125-34

Lobo, S, Greentree, WK, Linder, ME & Deschenes, RJ (2002). Identification of a Ras palmitoyltransferase in Saccharomyces cerevisiae. *J Biol Chem*, Vol. 277, No. 43, (2002), pp 41268-73

Ma, DW, Seo, J, Switzer, KC, Fan, YY, McMurray, DN et al. (2004). n-3 PUFA and membrane microdomains: a new frontier in bioactive lipid research. *J Nutr Biochem*, Vol. 15, No. 11, (2004), pp 700-6

Ma, XJ, Dahiya, S, Richardson, E, Erlander, M & Sgroi, DC (2009). Gene expression profiling of the tumor microenvironment during breast cancer progression. *Breast Cancer Res*, Vol. 11, No. 1, (2009), pp R7, 1465-542X

Magee, AI & Seabra, MC (2003). Are prenyl groups on proteins sticky fingers or greasy handles? *Biochem J*, Vol. 376, No. Pt 2, (2003), pp e3-4

Manes, S, Lacalle, RA, Gomez-Mouton, C, del Real, G, Mira, E et al. (2001). Membrane raft microdomains in chemokine receptor function. *Semin Immunol*, Vol. 13, No. 2, (2001), pp 147-57

Marks, PA & Xu, WS (2009). Histone deacetylase inhibitors: Potential in cancer therapy. *J Cell Biochem*, Vol. 107, No. 4, (2009), pp 600-8

Marquez, DC, Chen, HW, Curran, EM, Welshons, WV & Pietras, RJ (2006). Estrogen receptors in membrane lipid rafts and signal transduction in breast cancer. *Mol Cell Endocrinol*, Vol. 246, No. 1-2, (2006), pp 91-100

May, CD, Sphyris, N, Evans, KW, Werden, SJ, Guo, W et al. (2011). Epithelial-mesenchymal transition and cancer stem cells: a dangerously dynamic duo in breast cancer progression. *Breast Cancer Res*, Vol. 13, No. 1, (2011), pp 202

McGuire, TF, Corey, SJ & Sebti, SM (1993). Lovastatin inhibits platelet-derived growth factor (PDGF) stimulation of phosphatidylinositol 3-kinase activity as well as association of p85 subunit to tyrosine-phosphorylated PDGF receptor. *J Biol Chem*, Vol. 268, No. 30, (1993), pp 22227-30

Mellman, I & Nelson, WJ (2008). Coordinated protein sorting, targeting and distribution in polarized cells. *Nat Rev Mol Cell Biol*, Vol. 9, No. 11, (2008), pp 833-45

Menendez, JA, Lupu, R & Colomer, R (2005). Exogenous supplementation with omega-3 polyunsaturated fatty acid docosahexaenoic acid (DHA; 22:6n-3) synergistically enhances taxane cytotoxicity and downregulates Her-2/neu (c-erbB-2) oncogene expression in human breast cancer cells. *Eur J Cancer Prev*, Vol. 14, No. 3, (2005), pp 263-70

Menendez, JA, Vellon, L, Mehmi, I, Oza, BP, Ropero, S et al. (2004). Inhibition of fatty acid synthase (FAS) suppresses HER2/neu (erbB-2) oncogene overexpression in cancer cells. *Proc Natl Acad Sci U S A*, Vol. 101, No. 29, (2004), pp 10715-20

Merino, D, Lalaoui, N, Morizot, A, Schneider, P, Solary, E et al. (2006). Differential inhibition of TRAIL-mediated DR5-DISC formation by decoy receptors 1 and 2. *Mol Cell Biol*, Vol. 26, No. 19, (2006), pp 7046-55

Mineo, C, Gill, GN & Anderson, RG (1999). Regulated migration of epidermal growth factor receptor from caveolae. *J Biol Chem*, Vol. 274, No. 43, (1999), pp 30636-43

Mira, E, Lacalle, RA, Buesa, JM, de Buitrago, GG, Jimenez-Baranda, S et al. (2004). Secreted MMP9 promotes angiogenesis more efficiently than constitutive active MMP9 bound to the tumor cell surface. *J Cell Sci*, Vol. 117, No. Pt 9, (2004), pp 1847-57

Morrow, IC, Rea, S, Martin, S, Prior, IA, Prohaska, R et al. (2002). Flotillin-1/reggie-2 traffics to surface raft domains via a novel golgi-independent pathway. Identification of a novel membrane targeting domain and a role for palmitoylation. *J Biol Chem*, Vol. 277, No. 50, (2002), pp 48834-41

Mulens, V, de la Torre, A, Marinello, P, Rodriguez, R, Cardoso, J et al. (2010). Immunogenicity and safety of a NeuGcGM3 based cancer vaccine: Results from a controlled study in metastatic breast cancer patients. *Hum Vaccin*, Vol. 6, No. 9, (2010), 1554-8619

Murai, T, Maruyama, Y, Mio, K, Nishiyama, H, Suga, M et al. (2011). Low cholesterol triggers membrane microdomain-dependent CD44 shedding and suppresses tumor cell migration. *J Biol Chem*, Vol. 286, No. 3, (2011), pp 1999-2007

Murata, M, Peranen, J, Schreiner, R, Wieland, F, Kurzchalia, TV et al. (1995). VIP21/caveolin is a cholesterol-binding protein. *Proc Natl Acad Sci U S A*, Vol. 92, No. 22, (1995), pp 10339-43

Nabi, IR & Le, PU (2003). Caveolae/raft-dependent endocytosis. *J Cell Biol*, Vol. 161, No. 4, (2003), pp 673-7

Nagy, P, Vereb, G, Sebestyen, Z, Horvath, G, Lockett, SJ et al. (2002). Lipid rafts and the local density of ErbB proteins influence the biological role of homo- and heteroassociations of ErbB2. *J Cell Sci*, Vol. 115, No. Pt 22, (2002), pp 4251-62

Nahta, R & Esteva, FJ (2006). HER2 therapy: molecular mechanisms of trastuzumab resistance. *Breast Cancer Res*, Vol. 8, No. 6, (2006), pp 215, 1465-542X

Neumann-Giesen, C, Falkenbach, B, Beicht, P, Claasen, S, Luers, G et al. (2004). Membrane and raft association of reggie-1/flotillin-2: role of myristoylation, palmitoylation and oligomerization and induction of filopodia by overexpression. *Biochem J*, Vol. 378, No. Pt 2, (2004), pp 509-18

Neumann-Giesen, C, Fernow, I, Amaddii, M & Tikkanen, R (2007). Role of EGF-induced tyrosine phosphorylation of reggie-1/flotillin-2 in cell spreading and signaling to the actin cytoskeleton. *J Cell Sci*, Vol. 120, No. Pt 3, (2007), pp 395-406

Nohara, K, Wang, F & Spiegel, S (1998). Glycosphingolipid composition of MDA-MB-231 and MCF-7 human breast cancer cell lines. *Breast Cancer Res Treat*, Vol. 48, No. 2, (1998), pp 149-57

Ogretmen, B & Hannun, YA (2001). Updates on functions of ceramide in chemotherapy-induced cell death and in multidrug resistance. *Drug Resist Updat*, Vol. 4, No. 6, (2001), pp 368-77

Okamoto, T, Schlegel, A, Scherer, PE & Lisanti, MP (1998). Caveolins, a family of scaffolding proteins for organizing "preassembled signaling complexes" at the plasma membrane. *J Biol Chem*, Vol. 273, No. 10, (1998), pp 5419-22

Orian-Rousseau, V, Chen, L, Sleeman, JP, Herrlich, P & Ponta, H (2002). CD44 is required for two consecutive steps in HGF/c-Met signaling. *Genes Dev*, Vol. 16, No. 23, (2002), pp 3074-86

Paladino, S, Lebreton, S, Tivodar, S, Campana, V, Tempre, R et al. (2008). Different GPI-attachment signals affect the oligomerisation of GPI-anchored proteins and their apical sorting. *J Cell Sci*, Vol. 121, No. Pt 24, (2008), pp 4001-7

Paladino, S, Sarnataro, D, Pillich, R, Tivodar, S, Nitsch, L et al. (2004). Protein oligomerization modulates raft partitioning and apical sorting of GPI-anchored proteins. *J Cell Biol*, Vol. 167, No. 4, (2004), pp 699-709

Palmer, CP, Mahen, R, Schnell, E, Djamgoz, MB & Aydar, E (2007). Sigma-1 receptors bind cholesterol and remodel lipid rafts in breast cancer cell lines. *Cancer Res*, Vol. 67, No. 23, (2007), pp 11166-75

Paris, L, Cecchetti, S, Spadaro, F, Abalsamo, L, Lugini, L et al. (2010). Inhibition of phosphatidylcholine-specific phospholipase C downregulates HER2 overexpression on plasma membrane of breast cancer cells. *Breast Cancer Res*, Vol. 12, No. 3, (2010), pp R27, 1465-542X

Park, BW, Zhang, HT, Wu, C, Berezov, A, Zhang, X et al. (2000). Rationally designed anti-HER2/neu peptide mimetic disables P185HER2/neu tyrosine kinases in vitro and in vivo. *Nat Biotechnol*, Vol. 18, No. 2, (2000), pp 194-8

Park, EK, Lee, EJ, Lee, SH, Koo, KH, Sung, JY et al. (2010). Induction of apoptosis by the ginsenoside Rh2 by internalization of lipid rafts and caveolae and inactivation of Akt. *Br J Pharmacol*, Vol. 160, No. 5, (2010), pp 1212-23

Park, EK, Park, MJ, Lee, SH, Li, YC, Kim, J et al. (2009). Cholesterol depletion induces anoikis-like apoptosis via FAK down-regulation and caveolae internalization. *J Pathol*, Vol. 218, No. 3, (2009), pp 337-49

Parmryd, I, Adler, J, Patel, R & Magee, AI (2003). Imaging metabolism of phosphatidylinositol 4,5-bisphosphate in T-cell GM1-enriched domains containing Ras proteins. *Exp Cell Res*, Vol. 285, No. 1, (2003), pp 27-38

Parpal, S, Karlsson, M, Thorn, H & Stralfors, P (2001). Cholesterol depletion disrupts caveolae and insulin receptor signaling for metabolic control via insulin receptor substrate-1, but not for mitogen-activated protein kinase control. *J Biol Chem*, Vol. 276, No. 13, (2001), pp 9670-8

Parsons, SJ & Parsons, JT (2004). Src family kinases, key regulators of signal transduction. *Oncogene*, Vol. 23, No. 48, (2004), pp 7906-9

Patra, SK (2008). Dissecting lipid raft facilitated cell signaling pathways in cancer. *Biochim Biophys Acta*, Vol. 1785, No. 2, (2008), pp 182-206

Patra, SK, Rizzi, F, Silva, A, Rugina, DO & Bettuzzi, S (2008). Molecular targets of (-)-epigallocatechin-3-gallate (EGCG): specificity and interaction with membrane lipid rafts. *J Physiol Pharmacol*, Vol. 59 Suppl 9, No. (2008), pp 217-35

Peter, ME & Krammer, PH (2003). The CD95(APO-1/Fas) DISC and beyond. *Cell Death Differ*, Vol. 10, No. 1, (2003), pp 26-35

Pietras, RJ (2003). Interactions between estrogen and growth factor receptors in human breast cancers and the tumor-associated vasculature. *Breast J*, Vol. 9, No. 5, (2003), pp 361-73

Pietras, RJ, Marquez, DC, Chen, HW, Tsai, E, Weinberg, O et al. (2005). Estrogen and growth factor receptor interactions in human breast and non-small cell lung cancer cells. *Steroids*, Vol. 70, No. 5-7, (2005), pp 372-81

Pike, LJ (2003). Lipid rafts: bringing order to chaos. *J Lipid Res*, Vol. 44, No. 4, (2003), pp 655-67

Pike, LJ & Casey, L (2002). Cholesterol levels modulate EGF receptor-mediated signaling by altering receptor function and trafficking. *Biochemistry*, Vol. 41, No. 32, (2002), pp 10315-22

Planey, SL & Zacharias, DA (2009). Palmitoyl acyltransferases, their substrates, and novel assays to connect them (Review). *Mol Membr Biol*, Vol. 26, No. 1, (2009), pp 14-31

Ponta, H, Sherman, L & Herrlich, PA (2003). CD44: from adhesion molecules to signalling regulators. *Nat Rev Mol Cell Biol*, Vol. 4, No. 1, (2003), pp 33-45

Prinetti, A, Chigorno, V, Tettamanti, G & Sonnino, S (2000). Sphingolipid-enriched membrane domains from rat cerebellar granule cells differentiated in culture. A compositional study. *J Biol Chem*, Vol. 275, No. 16, (2000), pp 11658-65

Prior, IA & Hancock, JF (2001). Compartmentalization of Ras proteins. *J Cell Sci*, Vol. 114, No. Pt 9, (2001), pp 1603-8

Raghu, H, Sodadasu, PK, Malla, RR, Gondi, CS, Estes, N et al. (2010). Localization of uPAR and MMP-9 in lipid rafts is critical for migration, invasion and angiogenesis in human breast cancer cells. *BMC Cancer*, Vol. 10, No. (2010), pp 647, 1471-2407

Ravid, D, Maor, S, Werner, H & Liscovitch, M (2005). Caveolin-1 inhibits cell detachment-induced p53 activation and anoikis by upregulation of insulin-like growth factor-I receptors and signaling. *Oncogene*, Vol. 24, No. 8, (2005), pp 1338-47

Razandi, M, Pedram, A, Park, ST & Levin, ER (2003). Proximal events in signaling by plasma membrane estrogen receptors. *J Biol Chem*, Vol. 278, No. 4, (2003), pp 2701-12

Reimer, T, Herrnring, C, Koczan, D, Richter, D, Gerber, B et al. (2000). FasL:Fas ratio--a prognostic factor in breast carcinomas. *Cancer Res*, Vol. 60, No. 4, (2000), pp 822-8

Remacle-Bonnet, M, Garrouste, F, Baillat, G, Andre, F, Marvaldi, J et al. (2005). Membrane rafts segregate pro- from anti-apoptotic insulin-like growth factor-I receptor signaling in colon carcinoma cells stimulated by members of the tumor necrosis factor superfamily. *Am J Pathol*, Vol. 167, No. 3, (2005), pp 761-73

Reuben, JM, Lee, BN, Gao, H, Cohen, EN, Mego, M et al. (2011). Primary breast cancer patients with high risk clinicopathologic features have high percentages of bone marrow epithelial cells with ALDH activity and CD44(+)CD24(lo) cancer stem cell phenotype. *Eur J Cancer*, Vol. No. (2011), 1879-0852

Ringerike, T, Blystad, FD, Levy, FO, Madshus, IH & Stang, E (2002). Cholesterol is important in control of EGF receptor kinase activity but EGF receptors are not concentrated in caveolae. *J Cell Sci*, Vol. 115, No. Pt 6, (2002), pp 1331-40

Rodriguez-Boulan, E, Kreitzer, G & Musch, A (2005). Organization of vesicular trafficking in epithelia. *Nat Rev Mol Cell Biol*, Vol. 6, No. 3, (2005), pp 233-47

Rogers, KR, Kikawa, KD, Mouradian, M, Hernandez, K, McKinnon, KM et al. (2010). Docosahexaenoic acid alters epidermal growth factor receptor-related signaling by disrupting its lipid raft association. *Carcinogenesis*, Vol. 31, No. 9, (2010), pp 1523-30

Rossin, A, Derouet, M, Abdel-Sater, F & Hueber, AO (2009). Palmitoylation of the TRAIL receptor DR4 confers an efficient TRAIL-induced cell death signalling. *Biochem J*, Vol. 419, No. 1, (2009), pp 185-92

Roth, AF, Feng, Y, Chen, L & Davis, NG (2002). The yeast DHHC cysteine-rich domain protein Akr1p is a palmitoyl transferase. *J Cell Biol*, Vol. 159, No. 1, (2002), pp 23-8

Rothberg, JM & Artavanis-Tsakonas, S (1992). Modularity of the slit protein. Characterization of a conserved carboxy-terminal sequence in secreted proteins and a motif implicated in extracellular protein interactions. *J Mol Biol*, Vol. 227, No. 2, (1992), pp 367-70

Rothberg, KG, Heuser, JE, Donzell, WC, Ying, Y-S, Glenney, JR et al. (1992). Caveolin, a protein component of caveolae membrane coats. *Cell*, Vol. 68, No. (1992), pp 673-682

Rothberg, KG, Ying, YS, Kolhouse, JF, Kamen, BA & Anderson, RG (1990). The glycophospholipid-linked folate receptor internalizes folate without entering the clathrin-coated pit endocytic pathway. *J Cell Biol*, Vol. 110, No. 3, (1990), pp 637-49

Rubin, J, Schwartz, Z, Boyan, BD, Fan, X, Case, N et al. (2007). Caveolin-1 knockout mice have increased bone size and stiffness. *J Bone Miner Res*, Vol. 22, No. 9, (2007), pp 1408-18

Sahores, M, Prinetti, A, Chiabrando, G, Blasi, F & Sonnino, S (2008). uPA binding increases UPAR localization to lipid rafts and modifies the receptor microdomain composition. *Biochim Biophys Acta*, Vol. 1778, No. 1, (2008), pp 250-9

Salani, B, Briatore, L, Contini, P, Passalacqua, M, Melloni, E et al. (2009). IGF-I induced rapid recruitment of integrin beta1 to lipid rafts is Caveolin-1 dependent. *Biochem Biophys Res Commun*, Vol. 380, No. 3, (2009), pp 489-92

Sauer, LA, Blask, DE & Dauchy, RT (2007). Dietary factors and growth and metabolism in experimental tumors. *J Nutr Biochem*, Vol. 18, No. 10, (2007), pp 637-49

Schabath, H, Runz, S, Joumaa, S & Altevogt, P (2006). CD24 affects CXCR4 function in pre-B lymphocytes and breast carcinoma cells. *J Cell Sci*, Vol. 119, No. Pt 2, (2006), pp 314-25

Schley, PD, Brindley, DN & Field, CJ (2007). (n-3) PUFA alter raft lipid composition and decrease epidermal growth factor receptor levels in lipid rafts of human breast cancer cells. *J Nutr*, Vol. 137, No. 3, (2007), pp 548-53

Schley, PD, Jijon, HB, Robinson, LE & Field, CJ (2005). Mechanisms of omega-3 fatty acid-induced growth inhibition in MDA-MB-231 human breast cancer cells. *Breast Cancer Res Treat*, Vol. 92, No. 2, (2005), pp 187-95

Schuck, S & Simons, K (2004). Polarized sorting in epithelial cells: raft clustering and the biogenesis of the apical membrane. *J Cell Sci*, Vol. 117, No. Pt 25, (2004), pp 5955-64

Simons, K & Ikonen, E (1997). Functional rafts in cell membranes. *Nature*, Vol. 387, No. 6633, (1997), pp 569-72

Simons, K & Toomre, D (2000). Lipid rafts and signal transduction. *Nat Rev Mol Cell Biol*, Vol. 1, No. 1, (2000), pp 31-9

Singleton, PA & Bourguignon, LY (2004). CD44 interaction with ankyrin and IP3 receptor in lipid rafts promotes hyaluronan-mediated Ca^{2+} signaling leading to nitric oxide production and endothelial cell adhesion and proliferation. *Exp Cell Res*, Vol. 295, No. 1, (2004), pp 102-18

Smith, MC, Luker, KE, Garbow, JR, Prior, JL, Jackson, E et al. (2004). CXCR4 regulates growth of both primary and metastatic breast cancer. *Cancer Res*, Vol. 64, No. 23, (2004), pp 8604-12

Song, J, Sapi, E, Brown, W, Nilsen, J, Tartaro, K et al. (2000). Roles of Fas and Fas ligand during mammary gland remodeling. *J Clin Invest*, Vol. 106, No. 10, (2000), pp 1209-20

Song, JH, Tse, MC, Bellail, A, Phuphanich, S, Khuri, F et al. (2007). Lipid rafts and nonrafts mediate tumor necrosis factor related apoptosis-inducing ligand induced apoptotic and nonapoptotic signals in non small cell lung carcinoma cells. *Cancer Res*, Vol. 67, No. 14, (2007), pp 6946-55

Storch, CH, Ehehalt, R, Haefeli, WE & Weiss, J (2007). Localization of the human breast cancer resistance protein (BCRP/ABCG2) in lipid rafts/caveolae and modulation of its activity by cholesterol in vitro. *J Pharmacol Exp Ther*, Vol. 323, No. 1, (2007), pp 257-64

Stuermer, CA, Langhorst, MF, Wiechers, MF, Legler, DF, Von Hanwehr, SH et al. (2004). PrPc capping in T cells promotes its association with the lipid raft proteins reggie-1 and reggie-2 and leads to signal transduction. *FASEB J*, Vol. 18, No. 14, (2004), pp 1731-3

Stulnig, TM, Huber, J, Leitinger, N, Imre, EM, Angelisova, P et al. (2001). Polyunsaturated eicosapentaenoic acid displaces proteins from membrane rafts by altering raft lipid composition. *J Biol Chem*, Vol. 276, No. 40, (2001), pp 37335-40

Tachibana, H, Koga, K, Fujimura, Y & Yamada, K (2004). A receptor for green tea polyphenol EGCG. *Nat Struct Mol Biol*, Vol. 11, No. 4, (2004), pp 380-1

Takebayashi, M, Hayashi, T & Su, TP (2004). Sigma-1 receptors potentiate epidermal growth factor signaling towards neuritogenesis in PC12 cells: potential relation to lipid raft reconstitution. *Synapse*, Vol. 53, No. 2, (2004), pp 90-103

Tang, Z, Scherer, PE, Okamoto, T, Song, K, Chu, C et al. (1996). Molecular cloning of caveolin-3, a novel member of the caveolin gene family expressed predominantly in muscle. *J Biol Chem*, Vol. 271, No. 4, (1996), pp 2255-61

Tavernarakis, N, Driscoll, M & Kyrpides, NC (1999). The SPFH domain: implicated in regulating targeted protein turnover in stomatins and other membrane-associated proteins. *Trends Biochem Sci*, Vol. 24, No. 11, (1999), pp 425-7

Tran, D, Carpentier, JL, Sawano, F, Gorden, P & Orci, L (1987). Ligands internalized through coated or noncoated invaginations follow a common intracellular pathway. *Proc Natl Acad Sci U S A*, Vol. 84, No. 22, (1987), pp 7957-61

Troyer, KL & Lee, DC (2001). Regulation of mouse mammary gland development and tumorigenesis by the ERBB signaling network. *J Mammary Gland Biol Neoplasia*, Vol. 6, No. 1, (2001), pp 7-21

Tzahar, E, Waterman, H, Chen, X, Levkowitz, G, Karunagaran, D et al. (1996). A hierarchical network of interreceptor interactions determines signal transduction by Neu differentiation factor/neuregulin and epidermal growth factor. *Mol Cell Biol*, Vol. 16, No. 10, (1996), pp 5276-87

van der Voort, R, Taher, TE, Wielenga, VJ, Spaargaren, M, Prevo, R et al. (1999). Heparan sulfate-modified CD44 promotes hepatocyte growth factor/scatter factor-induced signal transduction through the receptor tyrosine kinase c-Met. *J Biol Chem*, Vol. 274, No. 10, (1999), pp 6499-506

van Meer, G, Voelker, DR & Feigenson, GW (2008). Membrane lipids: where they are and how they behave. *Nat Rev Mol Cell Biol*, Vol. 9, No. 2, (2008), pp 112-24

Vanoosten, RL, Moore, JM, Ludwig, AT & Griffith, TS (2005). Depsipeptide (FR901228) enhances the cytotoxic activity of TRAIL by redistributing TRAIL receptor to membrane lipid rafts. *Mol Ther*, Vol. 11, No. 4, (2005), pp 542-52

Veiseh, O, Gunn, JW, Kievit, FM, Sun, C, Fang, C et al. (2009). Inhibition of tumor-cell invasion with chlorotoxin-bound superparamagnetic nanoparticles. *Small*, Vol. 5, No. 2, (2009), pp 256-64

Wan, J, Roth, AF, Bailey, AO & Davis, NG (2007). Palmitoylated proteins: purification and identification. *Nat Protoc*, Vol. 2, No. 7, (2007), pp 1573-84

Wang, B, Rosano, JM, Cheheltani, R, Achary, MP & Kiani, MF (2010). Towards a targeted multi-drug delivery approach to improve therapeutic efficacy in breast cancer. *Expert Opin Drug Deliv*, Vol. 7, No. 10, (2010), pp 1159-73

Wang, X, Wilson, MJ, Slaton, JW, Sinha, AA, Ewing, SL et al. (2009). Increased aggressiveness of human prostate PC-3 tumor cells expressing cell surface localized membrane type-1 matrix metalloproteinase (MT1-MMP). *J Androl*, Vol. 30, No. 3, (2009), pp 259-74

Webb, Y, Hermida-Matsumoto, L & Resh, MD (2000). Inhibition of protein palmitoylation, raft localization, and T cell signaling by 2-bromopalmitate and polyunsaturated fatty acids. *J Biol Chem*, Vol. 275, No. 1, (2000), pp 261-70

Weinberg, OK, Marquez-Garban, DC & Pietras, RJ (2005). New approaches to reverse resistance to hormonal therapy in human breast cancer. *Drug Resist Updat*, Vol. 8, No. 4, (2005), pp 219-33

Weroha, SJ & Haluska, P (2008). IGF-1 receptor inhibitors in clinical trials--early lessons. *J Mammary Gland Biol Neoplasia*, Vol. 13, No. 4, (2008), pp 471-83

Westover, EJ, Covey, DF, Brockman, HL, Brown, RE & Pike, LJ (2003). Cholesterol depletion results in site-specific increases in epidermal growth factor receptor phosphorylation due to membrane level effects. Studies with cholesterol enantiomers. *J Biol Chem*, Vol. 278, No. 51, (2003), pp 51125-33

Worthylake, R, Opresko, LK & Wiley, HS (1999). ErbB-2 amplification inhibits down-regulation and induces constitutive activation of both ErbB-2 and epidermal growth factor receptors. *J Biol Chem*, Vol. 274, No. 13, (1999), pp 8865-74

Wysoczynski, M, Reca, R, Ratajczak, J, Kucia, M, Shirvaikar, N et al. (2005). Incorporation of CXCR4 into membrane lipid rafts primes homing-related responses of hematopoietic stem/progenitor cells to an SDF-1 gradient. *Blood*, Vol. 105, No. 1, (2005), pp 40-8

Yamada, E (1955). The fine structure of the renal glomerulus of the mouse. *J Biophys Biochem Cytol*, Vol. 1, No. 6, (1955), pp 551-66

Yamaguchi, H, Takeo, Y, Yoshida, S, Kouchi, Z, Nakamura, Y et al. (2009). Lipid rafts and caveolin-1 are required for invadopodia formation and extracellular matrix degradation by human breast cancer cells. *Cancer Res*, Vol. 69, No. 22, (2009), pp 8594-602

Yang, A, Wilson, NS & Ashkenazi, A (2010). Proapoptotic DR4 and DR5 signaling in cancer cells: toward clinical translation. *Curr Opin Cell Biol*, Vol. 22, No. 6, (2010), pp 837-44

Yaqoob, P (2009). The nutritional significance of lipid rafts. *Annu Rev Nutr*, Vol. 29, No. (2009), pp 257-82

20

Differences in Membrane Composition and Organization of Crucial Molecules Define the Invasive Properties of MCF-7 Breast Cancer Cells

Van slambrouck Séverine and Steelant Wim
New Mexico Institute of Mining and Technology,
St. Thomas University,
USA

1. Introduction

Breast cancer is the leading cause of cancer deaths among women in the United States and Europe [Jemal et al., 2011]. Most of these women die from their metastases, also known as the spread of primary breast cancer cells, to distant organs such as lung, brain and bone [Mehrotra et al., 2004]. Metastatic development comprises a complex series of linked, sequential steps. These steps include disconnection of intercellular adhesions and separation of single cells within a primary tumour, interaction with the surrounding extracellular matrix, local migration and invasion, followed by intravasation, transit through blood vessels and extravasation at distant organs, where they establish secondary tumours or metastases. In other words, the most lethal aspects of breast cancer are the processes of tumour cell migration and invasion, both prerequisites for the formation of metastases [Yilmaz & Christofori, 2010]. At present, however, the mechanisms responsible for the acquisition of invasive and metastatic potential of tumour cells are poorly understood. Thus, a better understanding of the biology and molecular interactions that regulate and coordinate the steps of tumour cell migration and invasion, is required to effectively treat metastatic breast cancer and control the devastating nature of breast cancer. It is widely accepted that cancer cells, capable of initiating metastases acquire specific features and exert activities that are not shared with the primary tumour cells [Liotta & Kohn, 2001]. Over the past years, a number of particular complex invasion-associated cellular activities have been recognized and characterized, including variations in expression levels of cell-cell and cell-matrix adhesion molecules and proteases that degrade the surrounding extracellular matrix, along with changes in expression or activity levels of a variety of cellular proteins in multiple branched signalling pathways [Mareel & Leroy, 2003]. Additionally, previous studies have highlighted the importance of aberrant glycosylation as a crucial event in the induction of invasion and metastasis [Hakomori, 2002], including altered glycosylation of cell-surface glycoproteins [Kim & Varki, 1997] and GSLs (glycosphingolipids) [Hakomori, 1998]. GSLs are common components of cell membranes. In malignant cells, they have been identified as tumour-associated antigens as defined by specific monoclonal antibodies [Hakomori, 1996]. Essentially all GSLs, in tumour and normal cells, can cluster and assemble with specific membrane proteins and signal transducers. Of importance is that clustering of particular GSLs may affect cellular activities associated with tumour cell migration and invasion, since they are recognized to mediate cell-cell and cell-matrix adhesion and initiate signal transduction, induced by stimulation of GSLs [Hakomori et al., 1998]. Roles for GSLs in invasion were demonstrated recently for GM3 (monosialoganglioside 3) in mouse melanoma B16 cells [Iwabuchi et al., 1998; Iwabuchi et al., 1998] and in human bladder KK47 cells [Mitsuzuka et al., 2005], for GM1 in mouse Lewis lung cancer cells [Zhang et al., 2006], for DSGG (diasyl-GalNAcLc4) in renal cell carcinoma [Satoh et al., 2000; Ito et al., 2001] and for GD3 (disialoganglioside 3) in melanoma cells [Hamamura et al., 2005]. The glycosphingolipid, MSGb5 (monosialyl-Gb5), also known as SSEA-4 (stage-specific embryonic antigen-4) [Kannagi et al., 1983], is found maximally expressed in human renal cell carcinomas and correlates with metastases [Saito et al., 1991; Saito et al., 1997]. The molecular mechanisms regulating synthesis of MSGb5 have been studied previously [Saito et al., 2003]; however, no clear functional role of MSGb5 in the invasive and metastatic behaviour of tumour cells has been demonstrated. In this chapter, we present data on a functional role of the glycosphingolipid MSGb5 in the human mammary carcinoma variant cell line MCF-7/AZ, showing increased invasiveness and motility in response to stimulation of MSGb5 by its monoclonal antibody RM1 or through induced clustering of MSGb5 by ET-18-OMe. ET-18-OMe is a synthetic ether lipid analogue shown to induce loss of cell-cell adhesion and to stimulate invasion of MCF-7/AZ breast cancer cells [Steelant et al., 2001] and was used as a molecular probe in the presented study.

2. TLC patterns of GSLs from cell extracts of MCF-7AZ and MCF-7/6 cells

The major GSLs identified in the two human breast cancer cell lines, MCF-7/AZ and MCF-7/6, were characterized as: globo-series Gb3, Gb4, MsGb5 and ganglio-series structure GM2, by TLC developed in a solvent system of chloroform/methanol/aqueous $CaCl_2$ and visualized with orcinol staining (Figure 1) [Saito et al., 1971]. Lacto-series structures were presumably below the detection limit.

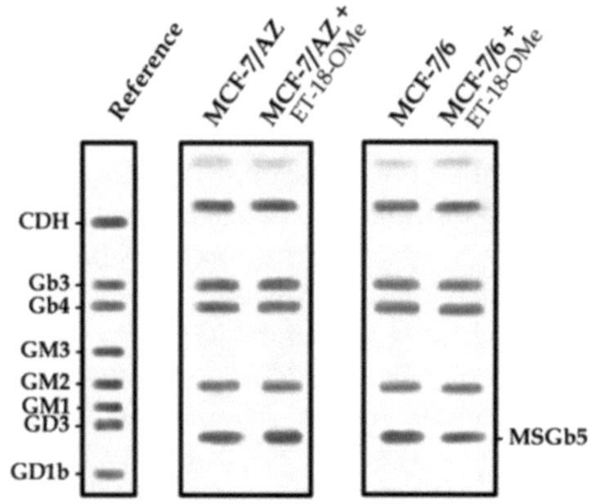

Fig. 1. TLC pattern of GSLs from whole cell extracts of MCF-7/AZ and MCF-7/6 cells with or without ET-18-OMe. GSLs were extracted from cells of the same protein weight, spotted onto TLC plates, developed in a solvent system of chloroform/methanol/0.2% aqueous $CaCl_2$, visualized by spraying with 0.5% orcinol in 2M sulfuric acid. CDH (lactosylceramide), Gb3, Gb4, MSGb5, GM3, GM1, GD3 and GD1b were used as reference markers.

All identified GSLs were present in the insoluble low-density fractions, as prepared after elimination of sucrose by dialysis and detected by TLC immunostaining with specific monoclonal antibodies (mouse IgM 1A4 to Gb3, mouse IgM 9G7 to Gb4, mouse IgM SSEA-3 to Gb5, mouse IgM RM1 to MSGb5, mouse IgM MBr1 to globo-H ($\alpha 1 \rightarrow 2$ fucosyl-Gb5), mouse IgM MK1-8 to GM2, mouse IgG_3 DH2 to GM3 and mouse IgM 5F3 to disialyl-Gb5) [Kannagi & Hakomori, 2001; Ito et al., 2001] (Figure 2). The cell variants in this study lack the abundant presence of GM3 and GM1 as was reported by Nohara et al. (1998) in MCF-7 cells, but show a comparable expression pattern for Gb3 and other globo-series structures similar to Gb5 and globo-H. Furthermore, we found that treatment with the ether lipid ET-18-OMe did not alter the expression levels of GSLs present in these cell lines.

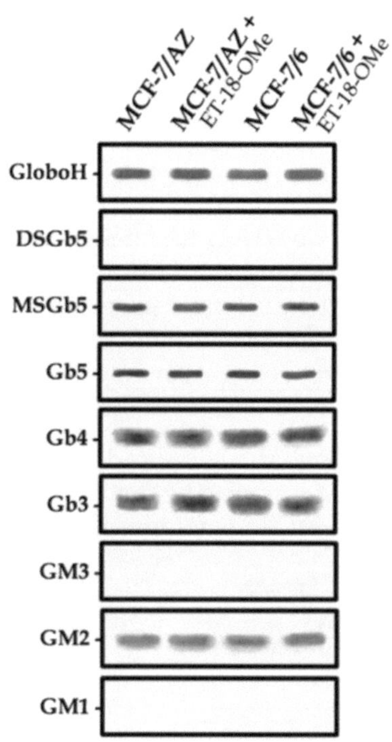

Fig. 2. TLC pattern of GSLs in low-density fractions of MCF-7/AZ and MCF-7/6 cells with or without ET-18-OMe. GSL fractions were prepared after elimination of sucrose by dialysis using C_{18} columns. Immunostaining of various GLS structures present in the low-density fractions were detected by using nine antibodies directed against the respective structures.

3. RM1 and ET-18-OMe stimulate motility and invasion through clustering of MsGb5 in MCF-7/AZ cells

The two human breast cancer cell variants, MCF-7/AZ and MCF-7/6, are non-invasive into a collagen type I gel-layer as determined by a method using specific assembly [Bracke et al., 1999] and the motility of the two variants as revealed by wound migration assay is basically the same. When MCF-7/AZ cells were treated with monoclonal anti-MSGb5 antibody RM1 or with ET-18-OMe, their invasiveness into collagen I layer was greatly enhanced, while no such effect could be observed on MCF-7/6 cells. Control IgM antibodies from normal mouse serum and antibodies to other GSLs (anti-globo-H MBr-1, anti-Gb3 1A4, anti-Gb5 SSEA-3, anti-GM2 MK1-8) [Steelant et al., 2002], did not increase invasiveness of either cell variant (Figure 3).

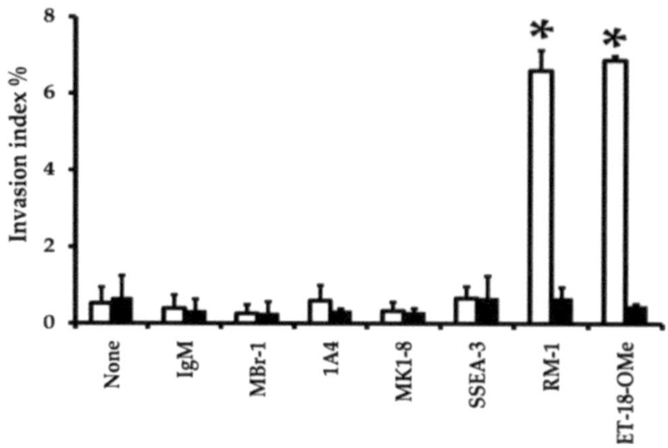

Fig. 3. Invasiveness of MCF-7/AZ cells and MCF-7/6 cells. Effect of mouse IgM or antibodies against Globo-H (MBr-1), Gb3 (1A4), Gb5 (SSEA-3), GM2 (MK1-8), MSGb5 (RM1) and ET-18-OMe on invasion into collagen type I of MCF-7/AZ cells (open columns) and MCF-7/6 cells (black columns). The invasion index expresses the percentage of cells invading into collagen type I over the total number of cells after 24 h. Results are means + S.D., * indicate statistical difference from control conditions, untreated MCF-7/AZ and MCF-7/6 cells, $p < 0.05$.

The motility of MCF-7/AZ cells was also enhanced upon treatment with anti-MSGb5 monoclonal antibody RM1, and again similar treatment did not influence the migratory capacity of the other variant cell line, MCF-7/6 (Figure 4).

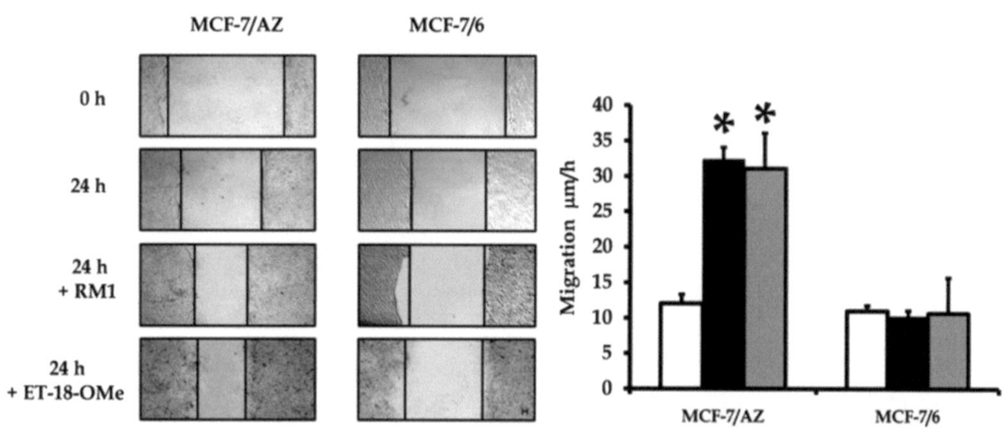

Fig. 4. Migration of MCF-7/AZ and MCF-7/6 cells. Effect of MSGb5 antibody RM1 and ET-18-OMe on MCF-7/AZ and MCF-7/6 cells in wound migration assay. Confluent cells were wounded, measured and allowed to grow in the presence of RM1 and ET-18-OMe. Scale bar = 250 µm. After 24 h, the distances over which the cells migrated were measured and results are expressed as migratory velocity (µm/h). *, indicate statistical difference from untreated MCF-7/AZ and MCF-7/6 cells ($p<0.05$).

Although both cell lines displayed no differences in their GSL composition upon treatment with ET-18-OMe, the possibility arose that changes in organization and clustering of GSLs could be responsible for the observed biological activity and this presumably through assembly with and activation of associated signal transducers. Such an activation model was reported for disialylgalactosylgloboside, DSGG, in the renal cell carcinoma cell line TOS-1 [Satoh et al., 2000] and for GM3 in B16 melanoma cells [Iwabuchi et al., 1998; Iwabuchi et al., 1998]. Alterations in the organization pattern of MSGb5 were observed by immunofluoresescence and confocal microscopy (Figure 5). MSGb5 was detected in both variant cell lines MCF-7/AZ and MCF-7/6, which was consistent with the TLC data. Fluorescence examination of MCF-7/AZ cells treated with ET-18-OMe revealed clustering of MSGb5 at the membrane within minutes. Clustering of MSGb5 in MCF-7/6 cells was not observed (data not shown), nor clustering of other GSLs, for example Gb3 and Gb5 in MCF-7/AZ cells after ET-18-OMe treatment.

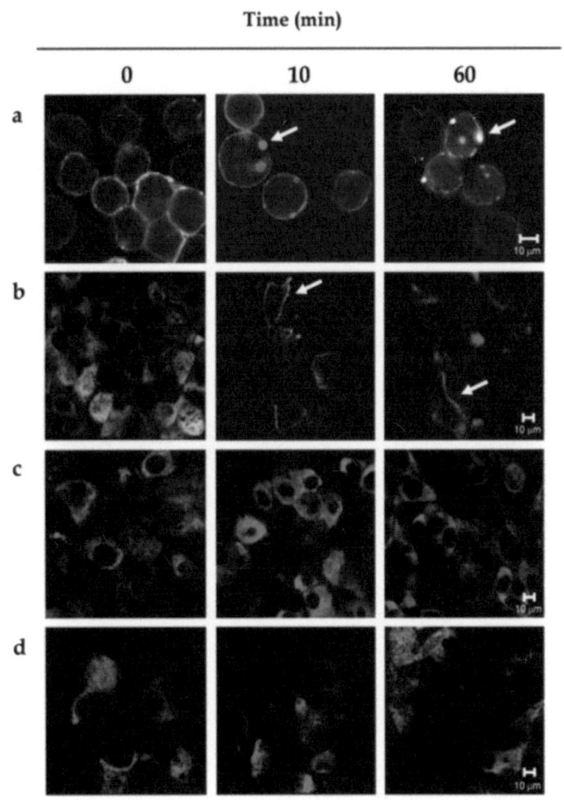

Fig. 5. Clustering of MSGb5 in MCF-7/AZ cells. The organizational pattern of MSGb5 by fluorescence(a) and confocal microscopy(b). Cells in suspension (a) or grown on glass coverslips (b-d), and analysed using antibodies against MSGb5, Gb3 and Gb5 and detected with FITC-labeled anti-mouse antibody. (a) and (b) show the homogenous organization of MSGb5, in untreated MCF-7/AZ cells; arrows indicate clustering of MSGb5 on the membrane of MCF-7/AZ cells after 10 and 60 min ET-18-OMe treatment. Organizational pattern of Gb3 (c) and Gb5 (d) by confocal microscopy, by using antibodies 1A4 against Gb3 and SSEA-3 against Gb5, followed by FITC-labeled mouse antibodies. Scale bar = 10 μm.

4. Src, the FAK-src signalling complex and the activation of the downstream pathway mediating invasion and motility in MCF-7/AZ cells

Several studies provide evidence that the non-receptor tyrosine kinase, src, is implicated in cancer progression of several cancer types. Changes in its expression and tyrosine phosphorylation correlate with the acquisition of an invasive cell phenotype [Guarino, 2010]. The motility and invasion promoting effects of RM1 and ET-18-OMe on MCF-7/AZ cells in our studies suggested that RM1 and ET-18-OMe initiate signalling pathways in MCF-7/AZ cells but not in MCF-7/6 cells. The possible involvement of src kinase in the signalling pathway leading to enhanced migration and invasion could be demonstrated by pretreating MCF-7/AZ cells with PP1, a pharmacological inhibitor of src kinase activity in the collagen I and wound migration assays (Figure 6).

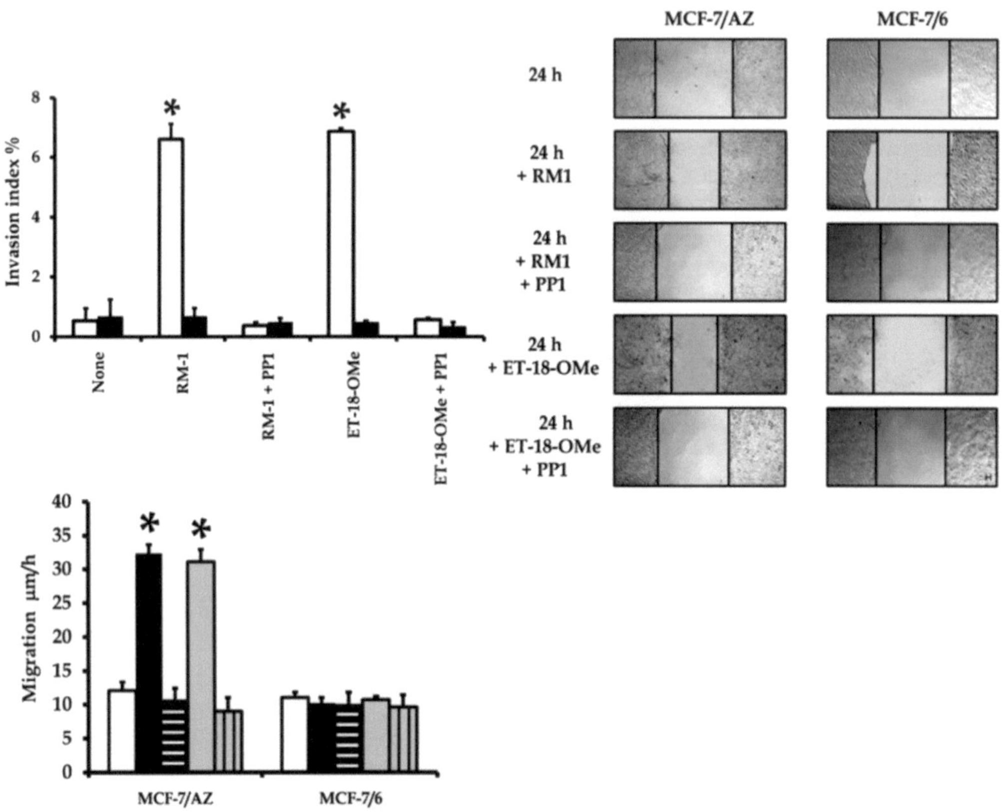

Fig. 6. Invasion and migration of MCF-7/AZ and MCF-7/6 cells. Effect of pharmacological inhibitor PP1 on RM1 or ET-18-OMe-mediated enhanced invasiveness (left panel) and migration of MCF-7/AZ cells (Right panel). Left: Invasion into collagen type I of MCF-7/AZ (open columns) and MCF-7/6 cells (black columns). The invasion index expresses the percentage of cells invading into collagen type I over the total number of cells. Right: Wound migration assay of MCF-7/AZ and MCF-7/6 cells. Scale bar = 250 µm. After 24 h, the distances over which the cells migrated were measured and results are expressed as migratory velocity (µm/h). *, indicate statistical difference from untreated MCF-7/AZ and MCF-7/6 cells ($p<0.05$).

Accordingly, western blotting results revealed that src kinase activity in MCF-7/AZ cells was greatly increased within minutes of RM1 or ET-18-OMe treatment, and abolished by pretreatment with PP1, while there was no such activation of src by both treatments in MCF-7/6 cells. In addition, expression levels of src were left unaltered (Figure 7).

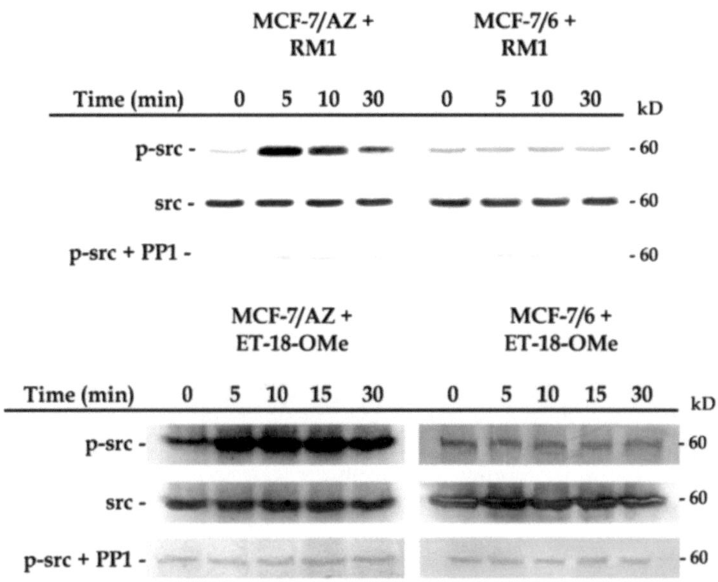

Fig. 7. Expression levels of phosphorylated src (Tyr416) upon RM1, RM1 + PP1, ET-18-OMe and ET-18-OMe + PP1 treatment in MCF-7/AZ and MCF-7/6 cells. Cells of 70% confluency were treated for indicated times, and lysed. Cell lysates, containing 30 μg of proteins, were analysed by SDS-PAGE (7.5% gels) and immunoblotted with antibody against src (Tyr416). The membrane was stripped at 50°C for 30 min in stripping buffer (100 mM 2-mercapto-ethanol, 2% (w/v) SDS, 62.5 mM Tris-HCl (pH 6.8)) and reblotted with anti-src antibody, for src total expression levels and equal loading.

These results clearly demonstrated a prominent role for src in motility and invasion induced by RM1 and ET-18-OMe. A possible mechanism by which src further promotes invasive behavior is through formation of a transient complex with focal adhesion kinase (FAK) [Hauck et al., 2002; Hsia et al., 2003]. FAK is another non-receptor tyrosine kinase recognized in cancer progression since it is found upregulated in malignant human tumour samples [Chatzizacharias et al., 2008]. Correspondingly, in our western blotting studies, RM1 and ET-18-OMe treatment increased the activity of FAK at tyrosine residue 397 (FAK Tyr397), the major autophosphorylation site [Parsons, 2003], in MCF-7/AZ cells and this also within minutes of treatment, while chemical levels of FAK remained unchanged (Figure 8). Similar treatment of MCF-7/6 cells did not change the activation of FAK Tyr397.

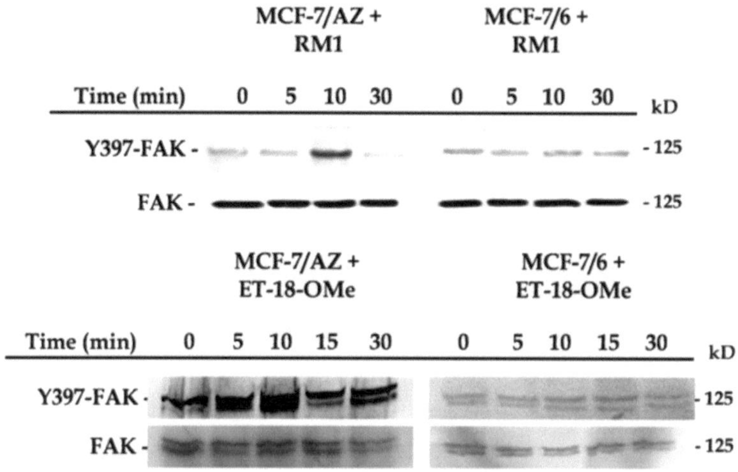

Fig. 8. Expression levels of phosphorylated FAK (Tyr397) upon RM1 and ET-18- OMe treatment in MCF-7/AZ and MCF-7/6 cells. Cells of 70% confluency were treated for indicated times, and lysed. Cell lysates, containing 30 μg of proteins, were analysed by SDS-PAGE (7.5% gels) and immunoblotted with antibody against FAK (Tyr397). The membrane was stripped and reblotted with anti-FAK, for FAK total expression levels and equal loading.

FAK plays an important role in relaying signals to intracellular targets, such as src, generated by cellular adhesion molecules and other cell surface molecules when they interact with the surrounding extracellular matrix [Parsons, 2003; Mitra et al., 2005]. The activation of FAK results in increased phosphorylation at Tyr397, the major autophosphorylation site, and subsequently in the recruitment and binding of src through its SH2 domain and further stabilization of the src-FAK interaction by src's SH3 domain [Thomas et al., 1998]. The formation of this transient bipartite kinase complex disrupts an inhibitory intramolecular interaction, resulting in increased activity of src [Schaller et al., 1994; Xing et al., 1994]. The specific organization plays a crucial role in src-dependent and mediated phosphorylation of other tyrosine residues on FAK within the kinase domain activation loop (Tyr576 and Tyr577) and at the C-terminal domain residues, Tyr861 and Tyr925 [Calalb et al., 1995; Calalb et al., 1996; Schlaepfer et al., 1996]. Interesting is that the activated FAK (Tyr397)-src signalling complex allows the activation of multiple different downstream pathways depending on which specific tyrosine residue on FAK is activated [Brunton et al., 2005]. As shown in scheme 1, the activated FAK-src complex can result in the activation of the mitogen-activated protein kinase (MAPK)-cascade through FAK Tyr925 [Schlaepfer et al. 1998], p130Cas via FAK Tyr861 [Lim et al., 2004] or paxillin by FAK Tyr576 [Calalb et al., 1995]. These three signalling pathways downstream of the FAK-src signalling complex, all lead to increased release of matrix metalloproteinase-2 (MMP-2) and MMP-9, the major proteinases responsible for the degradation of collagen type I [Kurata et al., 2000; Liu et al., 2000; Hsia et al., 2003; Brabek et al., 2004; Brabek et al., 2005; Bjorklund & Koivunen, 2005].

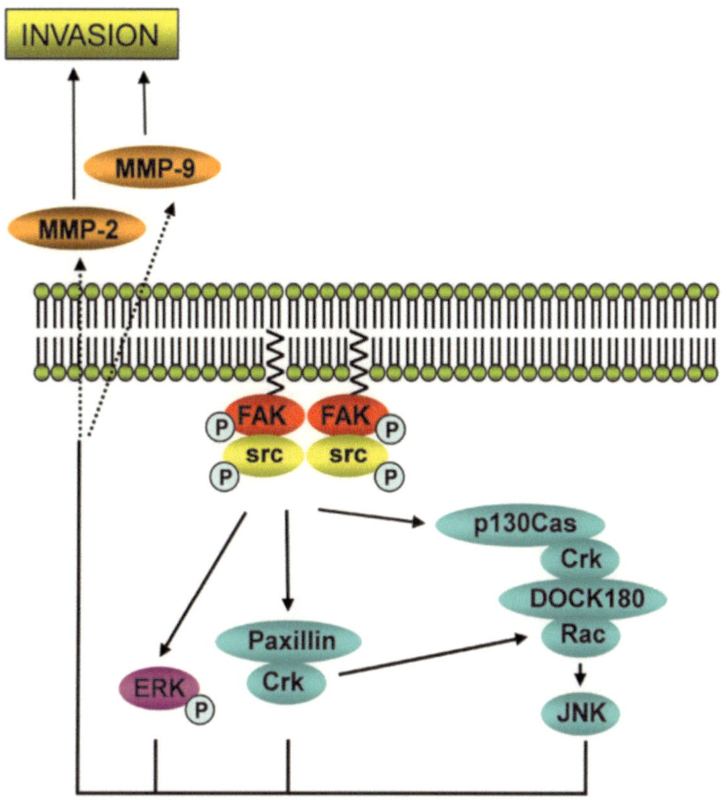

Scheme 1. Possible pathways downstream of the transient FAK-src complex leading to increased expression of MMPs, facilitating invasion into collagen type I layer.

Our results support that ET-18-OMe treatment results in the formation of a temporary FAK-src complex through FAK (Tyr397) activation and the subsequent src-dependent phosphorylation of FAK on Tyr925, since pretreatment of MCF-7/AZ cells with PP1, blocked the activation of src (Figure 7) and FAK Tyr925, while the activation of FAK at Tyr397 was only partially reduced (Figure 9). These results also point out that ET-18-OMe-mediated activation and autophosphorylation of FAK at Tyr397 is upstream and required for the activation of src and that src activity is responsible for the activation of the additional tyrosine residue 925 of FAK but not of FAK Tyr576 and 861 (Figure 9). Furthermore, we provide evidence linking FAK Tyr925 phosphorylation to the activation of the MAPK-pathway, since treatment of MCF-7/AZ cells with ET-18-OMe resulted in the downstream activation of extracellular signal-regulated kinase 1 and 2 (ERK1/2) and PP1 blocked the enhanced activation. In addition, we demonstrated that p130Cas and paxillin, which are known substrates of src associated with phosphorylation of FAK on Tyr861 and 576 respectively [Lim et al., 2004; Calalb et al., 1995], are not involved in the ET-18-OMe-induced effect and confirmed the lack of phosphorylation at FAK Tyr861 and 576 (Figure 10).

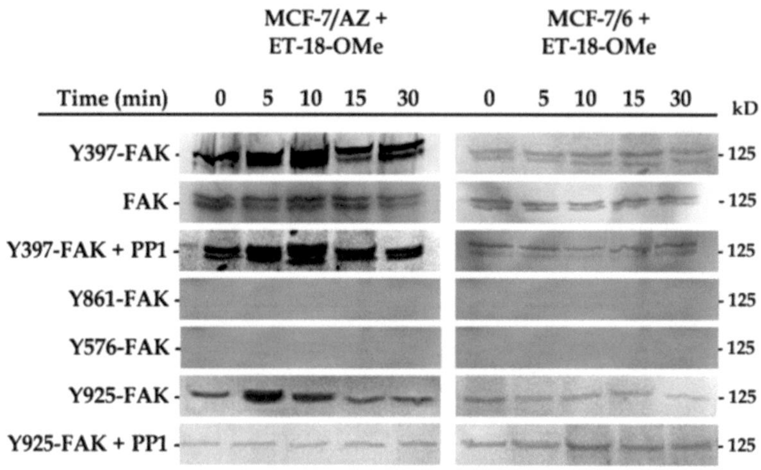

Fig. 9. Expression levels of FAK (Tyr397, Tyr925) upon ET-18-OMe and ET-18-OMe + PP1 treatment in MCF-7/AZ and MCF-7/6 cells. Cells of 70% confluency were treated for indicated times, and lysed. Cell lysates, containing 30 μg of proteins, were analysed by SDS-PAGE (7.5% gels) and immunoblotted with antibodies against FAK (Tyr397, Tyr576, Tyr861 and Tyr925). The membranes were stripped and reblotted with anti-FAK, for FAK total expression levels and equal loading.

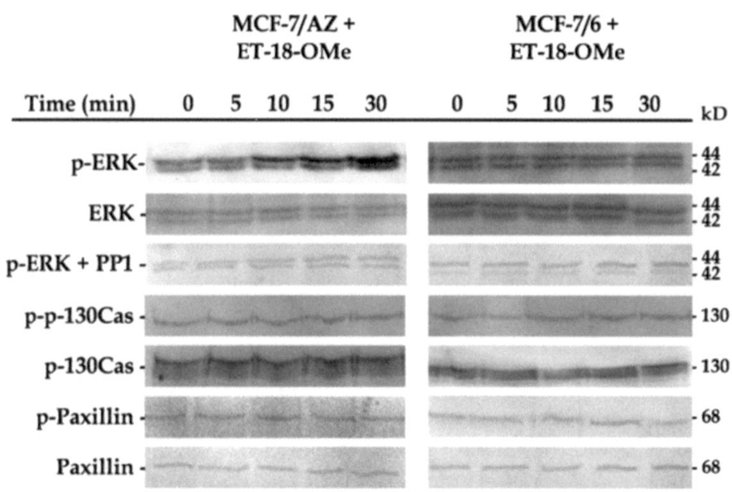

Fig. 10. Expression levels of ERK (Thr202/Tyr204) upon ET-18-OMe and ET-18-OMe + PP1 treatment in MCF-7/AZ and MCF-7/6 cells. Cells of 70% confluency were treated for indicated times, and lysed. Cell lysates, containing 30 μg of proteins, were analysed by SDS-PAGE (7.5% gels) and immunoblotted with antibodies against ERK (Thr202/Tyr204), p130Cas (Tyr410) and paxillin (Ser178). The membranes were stripped and reblotted with anti-ERK, anti-p130Cas and paxillin for total ERK, p130Cas and paxillin expression levels and equal loading.

5. MSGb5 activates the FAK-src signalling complex

Tumour cell invasion includes alterations of expression levels of integrin receptors. Integrin receptors are important upstream regulators of intracellular and downstream signalling events associated with cancer cell invasion. This family of heterodimeric α/β subunit receptors, expressed on every cell type, is capable of interacting with specific ligands in the surrounding extracellular matrix. Binding to these components results in clustering of integrin receptors in the plasmamembrane and recruitment and association of signalling proteins with integrin cytoplasmic domains to initiate downstream signalling events [Schwartz, 2001]. Since src and FAK are recognized as two critical mediators of integrin signalling, we addressed the question whether particular integrins were implicated in ET-18-OMe-induced activation of FAK and src and invasiveness of MCF-7/AZ cells. The integrin receptors α1β1 and α2β1 are the major receptors binding to collagen type I in the extracellular matrix [Gullberg et al., 1992]. Given that RM1 and ET-18-OMe induce invasiveness of MCF-7/AZ cells in collagen type I layer, we examined the expression levels of integrin subunits α1, β1 and α2 upon treatment with ET-18-OMe by Western blotting. Expression of the α1 and β1 subunits were found decreased over time in MCF-7/AZ cells, and no changes of either integrin subunit was observed in the variant cell line (Figure 11), whereas the integrin α2 subunit was not detectable in both cell lines (data not shown).

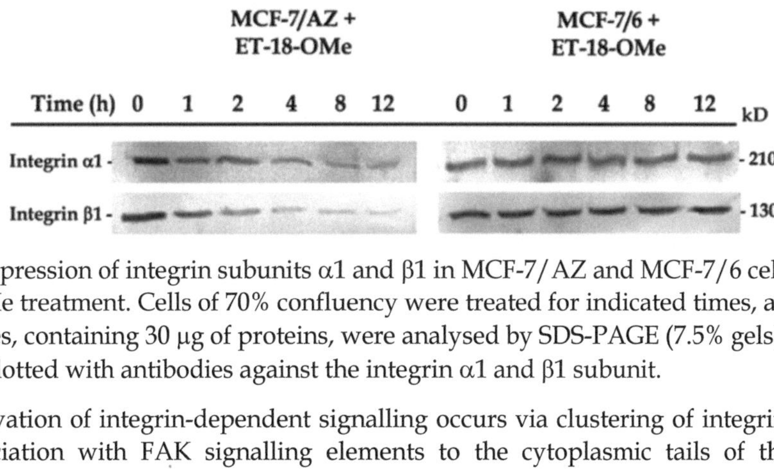

Fig. 11. Expression of integrin subunits α1 and β1 in MCF-7/AZ and MCF-7/6 cells upon ET-18-OMe treatment. Cells of 70% confluency were treated for indicated times, and lysed. Cell lysates, containing 30 μg of proteins, were analysed by SDS-PAGE (7.5% gels) and immunoblotted with antibodies against the integrin α1 and β1 subunit.

Since activation of integrin-dependent signalling occurs via clustering of integrin receptors and association with FAK signalling elements to the cytoplasmic tails of the receptor [Miyamoto et al., 1995], organizational patterns of the α1 and β1 subunits and co-clustering with signalling molecules FAK and src, upon ET-18-OMe treatment were examined by fluorescence microscopy and co-immunoprecipitation experiments. The microscopy data revealed that ET-18-OMe did not change the organization of the respective integrin subunits and the fact that signalling molecules FAK and src could not be detected in the immunoprecipitates of either integrin subunits confirmed that integrin receptors α1β1 and α2β1 were not of crucial importance in the activation of downstream signalling events in MCF-7/AZ cells mediated by ET-18-OMe or RM1 (data not shown). This was in sharp contrast with data reported by other investigators [Schaller et al., 1995]. However, the recognition that glycosphingolipids may influence cellular phenotype by clustering and assembly with signal transducing molecules, let us to explore the possible involvement of the glycosphingolipid MSGb5 in initiating the signalling events in MCF-7/AZ cells upon

RM1 or ET-18-OMe treatment. This idea was supported by two of our observations namely that RM1 and ET-18-OMe treatment resulted in clustering of MSGb5 in MCF-7/AZ cells and that similar treatment profoundly affected the cellular activities associated with the migratory and invasive capacity of MCF-7/AZ cells. A close connection between MSGb5 and signalling molecules was shown by co-immunoprecipitation experiments, in which aliquots of cell lysates were immunoprecipitated by incubation with anti-MSGb5 antibody and captured with protein G-Sepharose beads. The signalling molecules, FAK and src as well as their activated forms, src (Tyr416) and FAK (Tyr397), were detected in MSGb5 immunoprecipitates prepared from MCF-7/AZ cells treated with ET-18-OMe for indicated time points, and the obtained results were in line with the earlier performed kinase experiments. In MCF-7/6 cells, FAK and src were found associated with MSGb5, and as expected no kinase activity was observed upon ET-18-OMe treatment (Figure 12). The involvement of other glycosphingolipids could be excluded since no clustering and no association between FAK and src with Gb3, Gb5 or GM2 (data not shown) could be found in MCF-7/AZ cells. Equal levels of MSGb5 were detected in the immunoprecipitates of both cell lines.

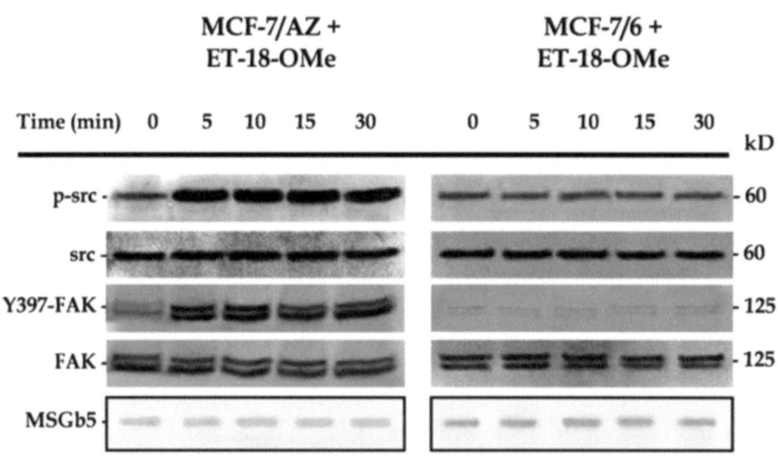

Fig. 12. MSGb5 associates with src (Tyr416) and FAK (Tyr397) in MCF-7/AZ cells after ET-18-OMe treatment. MSGb5 was immunoprecipitated from whole cell lysates with mouse IgG_3 anti-MSGb5 antibody. Aliquots of immunoprecipitates were electrophoresed, transferred and immunoblotted, with anti-src (Tyr416), anti-src, anti-FAK (Tyr397) and anti-FAK. MSGb5 content in the different immunoprecipitates was determined by TLC.

6. Concept of "Glycosynapse"

Glycosphingolipids are highly expressed during defined stages of development and after oncogenic transformation and are referred to as stage-specific embryonic antigen and tumour-associated antigens respectively [Hakomori, 1998]. Most studies, however, use the presence of GSLs as markers of low-density membrane fractions and are neither focused on their structural variety nor their possible functional roles. In this chapter, we present data supporting a functional role for MSGb5 in migration and invasion of MCF-7/AZ cells upon stimulation with RM1 or treatment with ET-18-OMe, resulting in MSGb5 clustering and activation of associated signalling molecules. These observations can be placed in the concept of the 'glycosynapse' [Hakomori, 2002]. This term defines glycosylation-dependent adhesion and signalling, mediated via glycosylepitopes of GSLs in microenvironments where tumour cells interface with other tumour cells, host cells or the surrounding matrix, in analogy to the 'immune synapse' which on its turn controls functional adhesion and signalling between immunocytes [Ilangumaran et al., 2000]. In addition to glycosylation-dependent adhesion of GSLs between interfacing glycosynapses, conversion of phenotypes is highly controlled by the presence, interactions and organization of other crucial molecules in the glycosynapse, such as growth factor receptors, integrin receptors, tetraspanins, mucins and gangliosides [Hakomori & Handa, 2002]. Furthermore, this new concept has been extended to phenotypic conversion induced through the deletion or addition of a single component, resulting in a disorganized glycosynapse framework and initiating altered signalling events [Mitsuzuka et al., 2005]. We can relate our observations to the latter revised glycosynapse concept and more specifically to the formation of a disorganized glycosynapse framework. We conclude that phenotypic conversion from non-invasive to invasive MCF-7/AZ breast cancer cells is induced by: (i) an aberrant MSGb5 pattern; (ii) loss of integrin receptor subunits $\alpha 1$ and $\beta 1$; and (iii) high tetraspanin CD9 expression levels [Steelant et al., 2002], all of which are responsible for the formation of disorganized glycosynapse framework interfaces, thereby inducing activation of FAK, src and downstream ERK, with consequent enhanced secretion and activity of MMP-2 and MMP-9, and thus leading to invasion.

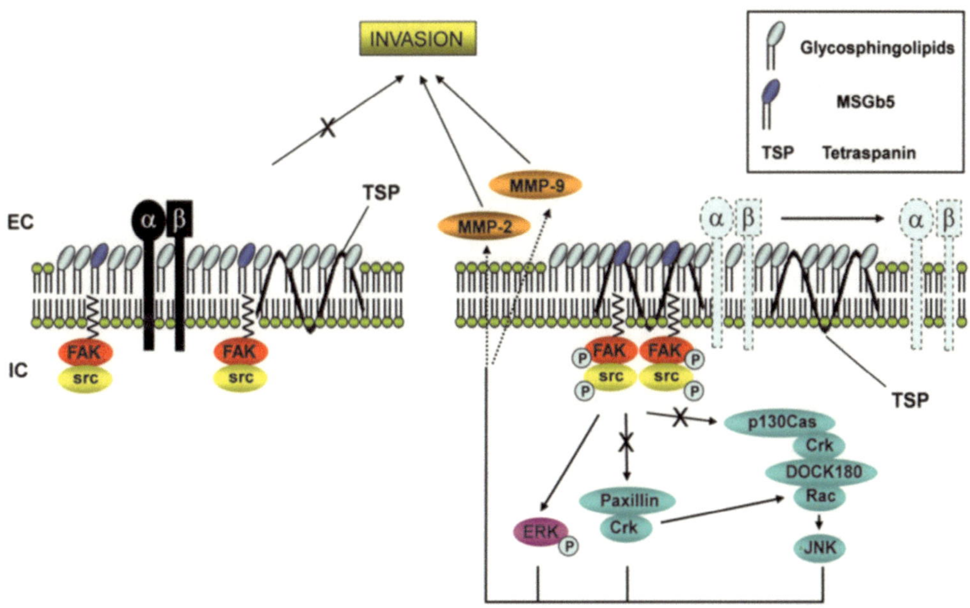

Scheme 2. Cancer cell invasion revised. In non-invasive MCF-7/AZ cells integrin subunits α1 and β1 form a stable complex with tetraspanin CD9 and GLSs, associated with non-active signalling molecules, FAK and src. In invasive MCF-7/AZ cells clustering of MSGb5 and loss of integrin subunits α1 and β1 disorganize the glycosynapse framework, resulting in activation of downstream signalling to invasion. EC, extracellular; IC, intracellular; TSP, tetraspanin.

7. Conclusion

In conclusion, our studies are an extension of previous work on the glycosynapse [Hakomori, 2002], re-formulating the classic concept of integrin-dependent invasion of tumour cells and providing evidence that phenotypic conversion can be explained by differences in composition and organization of crucial molecules in the glycosynapse. At present, only a few studies have appeared that focus, in particular, on GM3 [Mitsuzuka et al., 2005, Toledo et al., 2005]. The present study reveals a novel insight into the composition and organization of the glycosynapses in MCF-7/AZ breast cancer cells, which explain phenotypic changes. Further studies along this line are necessary to understand the complex interplay of distinct molecules in invasion, as well as other basic cellular mechanisms, and their implications on disease processes, which will be expected to lead to novel therapeutic approaches.

8. Acknowledgements

These studies were supported by the Belgian Federation Against Cancer, the US National Institutes of Health [RR-16480] under the BRIN/INBRE program of the National Center for Research Resources and the New Mexico Tech startup funds and the New Mexico Department of Veteran Services.

9. References

Bjorklund, M. & Koivunen, E. (2005) Gelatinase-mediated migration and invasion of cancer cells. *Biochimica et Biophysica Acta*, 1755, 1, 37-69.

Brabek, J.; Constancio, S.S.; Shin, N.Y.; Pozzi, A.; Weaver, A.M. & Hanks, S.K. (2004). CAS promotes invasiveness of Src-transformed cells. *Oncogene*, 23, 44, 7406–7415.

Brabek, J.; Constancio, S.S.; Siesser, P.F.; Shin, N.Y.; Pozzi, A. & Hanks, S.K. (2005). Crk-associated substrate tyrosine phosphorylation sites are critical for invasion and metastasis of SRC-transformed cells. *Molecular Cancer Research*, 3, 6, 307–315.

Bracke, M.E.; Boterberg, T.; Bruyneel, E.A. & Mareel, M.M. (2001). Collagen invasion assay. In: *Metastasis Research Protocols*, Brooks, S. & Schumacher, U. (eds.) , Humana Press, Totowa, pp. 81–89,

Brunton, V.G.; Avizienyte, E.; Fincham, V.J.; Serrels, B.; Metcalf, C.A. 3rd; Sawyer, T.K. & Frame, M.C. (2005). Identification of Src-specific phosphorylation site on focal adhesion kinase: dissection of the role of Src SH2 and catalytic functions and their consequences for tumor cell behaviour. *Cancer Research*, 65, 4, 1335–1342.

Calalb, M.B.; Polte, T.R. & Hanks, S.K. (1995). Tyrosine phosphorylation of focal adhesion kinase at sites in the catalytic domain regulates kinase activity: a role for Src family kinases. *Molecular and Cellular Biology*, 15, 2, 954-963.

Calalb, M.B.; Zhang, X.; Polte, T.R. & Hanks, S.K. (1996). Focal adhesion kinase tyrosine-861 is a major site of phosphorylation by Src. *Biochemical and Biophysical Research Communications*, 228, 3, 662-668.

Chatzizacharias, N.A.; Kouraklis , G.P. & Theocharis, S.E. (2008). Clinical significance of FAK expression in human neoplasia. *Histology and Histopathology*, 23, 5, 629-650.

Guarino, M. (2010). Src signaling in cancer cell invasion. *Journal of Cellular Physiology*, 223, 1, 14-26.

Gullberg, D., Gehlsen, K.R., Turner, D.C., Ahlén, K., Zijenah, L.S., Barnes, M.J. & Rubin, K. (1992). Analysis of alpha 1 beta 1, alpha2 beta 1 and alpha3 beta 1 integrins in cell-collagen interactions: identification of conformation dependent aplhal beta 1 binding sites in collagen type I. *EMBO Journal*, 11, 11, 3863-3873.

Hakomori, S. (1996). Tumor malignancy defined by aberrant glycosylation and sphingo(glycol)lipid metabolism. *Cancer Research*, 56, 23, 5309-5318.

Hakomori, S. (1998). Cancer-associated glycosphingolipid antigens: their structure, organization, and function. *Acta Anatomica*, 161, 1-4, 79–90.

Hakomori, S.; Yamamura, S. & Handa, A.K. (1998). Signal transduction through glyco(sphingo)lipids: introduction and recent studies on glyco(sphingo)lipid-enriched microdomains. *Annals of the New York Academy of Sciences*, 845, 1–10.

Hakomori, S. (2002). Glycosylation defining cancer malignancy: new wine in an old bottle. *Proceedings of the National Academy of Sciences of the United States of America*, 99, 6, 10231–10233.

Hakomori, S. & Handa, K. (2002). Glycosphingolipid-dependent cross-talk between glycosynapses interfacing tumor cells with their host cells: essential basis to define tumor malignancy. *FEBS Letters*, 531, 1, 88–92.

Hakomori, S. (2002) The glycosynapse. *Proceedings of the National Academy of Sciences of the United States of America*, 99, 1, 225–232.

Hamamura, K.; Furakawa, K.; Hayashi, T.; Hattori, T.; Nakano, J.; Nakashima, H.; Okuda, T.; Mizutani, H.; Hattori, H.; Ueda, M.; Urano, T.; Lloyd, K.O. & Furakawa, K. (2005). Ganglioside GD3 promotes cell growth and invasion through p130Cas and paxillin in malignant melanoma cells. *Proceedings of the National Academy of Sciences of the United States of America*, 102, 31, 11041–11046.

Hauck, C.R.; Hsia, D.A.; Puente, X.S.; Cheresh, D.A. & Schlaepfer, D.D. (2002). FRNK blocks v-Src-stimulated invasion and experimental metastases without effects on cell motility or growth. *EMBO Journal*, 21, 23, 6289–6302.

Hsia, D.A.; Mitra, S.K.; Hauck, C.R.; Streblow, D.N.; Nelson, J. A.; Ilic, D.; Huang, S.; Li, E.; Nemerow, G.R.; Leng, J.; Spencer, K.S.; Cheresh, D.A. & Schlaepfer, D.D. (2003). Differential regulation of cell motility and invasion by FAK. *The Journal of Cell Biology*, 160, 5, 753–767.

Ilangumaran, S.; He, H.T. & Hoessli, D.C. (2000). Microdomains in lymphocyte signalling: beyond GPI-anchored proteins. *Immunology Today*, 21, 1, 2-7.

Ito, A.; Saito, S.; Masuko, T.; Oh-eda, M.; Matsuura, T.; Satoh, M.; Nejad, F.M.; Enomoto, T.; Orikasa, S. & Hakomori, S. I. (2001). Monoclonal antibody (5F3) defining renal cell carcinoma-associated antigen disialosyl globopentaosylceramide (V3NeuAcIV6NeuAcGb5), and distribution pattern of the antigen in tumor and normal tissues. *Glycoconjugate Journal*, 18, 6, 475–485.

Ito, A.; Levery, S.B.; Saito, S.; Satoh, M. & Hakomori, S. (2001). A novel ganglioside isolated from renal cell carcinoma. *Journal of Biological Chemistry*, 276, 20, 16695–16703.

Iwabuchi, K.; Yamamura, S.; Prinetti, A.; Handa, K. & Hakomori, S. (1998). GM3-enriched microdomain involved in cell adhesion and signal transduction through carbohydrate-carbohydrate interaction in mouse melanoma B16 cells. *Journal of Biological Chemistry*, 273, 15, 9130–9138.

Iwabuchi, K.; Handa, K. & Hakomori, S. (1998). Separation of "glycosphingolipid signaling domain" from caveolin-containing membrane fraction in mouse melanoma B16 cells and its role in cell adhesion coupled with signaling. *Journal of Biological Chemistry*, 273, 50, 33766–33773.

Jemal, A.; Bray, F., Center, M.M.; Ferlay, J.; Ward, E. & Forman, D. (2011). Global cancer statistics. *CA: a Cancer Journal for Clinicians*, 61, 2, 69-90.

Kannagi, R.; Cohran, N.A.; Ishigami, F.; Hakomori, S.; Andrews, P.W.; Knowles, B.B. & Solter, D. (1983). Stage-specific embryonic antigens (SSEA-3 and -4) are epitopes of a unique globo-series ganglioside isolated from human teratocarcinoma cells. *EMBO Journal*, 2, 12, 2355–2361.

Kannagi, R. & Hakomori, S. (2001). A guide to monoclonal antibodies directed to glycotopes. *Advances in Experimental Medicine and Biology*, 491, 587–630.

Kim, Y.J. & Varki, A. (1997). Perspectives on the significance of altered glycosylation of glycoproteins in cancer. *Glycoconjugate Journal*, 14, 5, 569–576.

Kurata, H.; Thant, A.A.; Matsuo, S.; Senga, T.; Okazaki, K.; Hotta, N. & Hamaguchi, M. (2000). Constitutive activation of MAP kinase kinase (MEK1) is critical and sufficient for the activation of MMP-2. *Experimental Cell Research*, 254, 1, 180–188.

Liotta, L. & Kohn, E. (2001). The microenvironment of the tumor-host interface. *Nature*, 411, 6835, 375-379.

Lim, Y.; Han, I.; Jeon, J.; Park, H.; Bahk, Y.Y. & Oh E.S. (2004). Phosphorylation of focal adhesion kinase at tyrosine 861 is crucial for Ras transformation of fibroblasts. *Journal of Biological Chemistry*, 279, 28, 29060-29065.

Liu, E.; Thant, A.A.; Kikkawa, F.; Kurata, H.; Tanaka, S.; Nawa, A.; Mizutani, S.; Matsuda, S.; Hanafusa, H. & Hamaguchi, M. (2000). The Ras-mitogen-activated protein kinase pathway is critical for the activation of matrix metalloproteinase secretion and the invasiveness in v-crk-transformed 3Y1. *Cancer Research*, 60, 9, 2361–2364.

Mareel, M. & Leroy, A. (2003). Clinical, cellular, and molecular aspects of cancer invasion. *Physiological Reviews*, 83, 2, 337–376.

Mehrotra J.; Vali, M.; McVeigh, M.; Kominsky, S.L.; Fackler, M.J.; Lahti-Domenici, J.; Polyak, K.; Sacchi, N.; Garrett-Mayer, E.; Argani, P. & Sukumar, S. (2004). Very high frequency of hypermethylated genes in breast cancer metastasis to the bone, brain and lung. *Clinical Cancer Research*, 10, 9, 3104-3109.

Mitra, S.K., Hanson, D.A. & Schlaepfer, D.D. (2005). Focal adhesion kinase: in command and control of cell motility. *Nature Reviews. Molecular Cell Biology*, 6, 1, 56-62.

Mitsuzuka, K.; Handa, K.; Satoh, M.; Arai, Y. & Hakomori, S. (2005). A specific microdomain ("glycosynapse 3") controls phenotypic conversion and reversion of bladder cancer cells through GM3-mediated interaction of $a3\beta1$ integrin with CD9. *Journal of Biological Chemistry*, 280, 42, 35545–35553.

Miyamoto, S.; Teramoto, H.; Coso, O.A.; Gutkind, J.S.; Burbelo, P.D.; Akiyama, S.K. & Yamada, K.M. (1995). Integrin function: molecular hierarchies of cytoskeletal and signaling molecules. *Journal of Cell Biology*, 131, 3, 791-805, 1995.

Nohara, K.; Wang, F. & Spiegel, S. (1998). Glycosphingolipid composition of MDA-MB-231 and MCF-7 human breast cancer cell lines. *Breast Cancer Research and Treatment*, 48, 2, 149–157.

Parsons, J. T. (2003). Focal adhesion kinase: the first ten years. *Journal of Cell Science*, 116, 8, 1409-1416.

Saito, S.; Orikasa, S.; Ohyama, C.; Satoh, M. & Fukushi, Y. (1991). Changes in glycolipids in human renal-cell carcinoma and their clinical significance. *International Journal of Cancer*, 49, 3, 329–334.

Saito, S.; Orikasa, S.; Satoh, M.; Ohyama, C.; Ito, A. & Takahashi, T. (1997). Expression of globo-series gangliosides in human renal cell carcinoma. *Japanese Journal of Cancer Research*, 88, 7, 652–659.

Saito, S.; Aiko, H.; Ito, A.; Ueno, S.,;Wada, T.; Mitsuzuka, K.; Satoh, M.; Arai, Y. & Miyagi, T. (2003). Human *a*2,3-sialyltransferase (ST3Gal II) is a stage-specific embryonic antigen-4 synthase. *Journal of Biological Chemistry*, 278, 29, 26474–26479.

Saito, T. & Hakomori, S. (1971). Quantitative isolation of total glycosphingolipids from animal cells. *Journal of Lipid Research*, 12, 2, 257–259.

Satoh, M.; Nejad, F.M.; Ohtani, H.; Ito, A.; Ohyama, C.; Saito, S.; Orikasa, S. & Hakomori, S. (2000). Association of renal cell carcinoma antigen, disialylgalactosylgloboside, with c-Src and RhoA in clustered domains at the surface membrane. *International Journal of Oncology*, 16, 3, 529–536.

Schaller, M.D.; Hildebrand, J.D.; Shannon, J.D.; Fox, J.W.; Vines, R.R. & Parsons, J.T. (1994) Autophosphorylation of the focal adhesion kinase, pp125FAK, directs SH2 dependent binding of pp60src. *Molecular and Cellular Biology*, 14, 3, 1680-1688.

Schaller, M.D.; Otey, C.A.; Hildebrand, J.D. & Parsons, J.T. (1995). Focal adhesion kinase and paxillin bind to peptides mimicking beta integrin cytoplasmic domains. *Journal of Cellular Biology*, 130, 5, 1181–1187.

Schlaepfer, D.D. & Hunter T (1996). Evidence for in vivo phosphorylation of the Grb2 SH2-domain binding site on focal adhesion kinase by Src-family protein-tyrosine kinases. *Molecular and Cellular Biology*, 16, 10, 5623-5633.

Schlaepfer, D.D.; Jones, K.C. & Hunter, T. (1998). Multiple Grb2-mediated integrin-stimulated signaling pathways to ERK2/mitogen-activated protein kinase: summation of both c-Src- and focal adhesion kinase-initiated tyrosine phosphorylation events. *Molecular and Cellular Biology*, 18, 5, 2571–2585.

Schwartz, M.A. (2001). Integrin signaling revisited. *Trends in Cell Biology*, 11, 12, 466-470.

Steelant, W.F.; Goeman, J.L.; Philippe, J.; Oomen, L.C.; Hilkens, J.; Krzewinski-Recchi, M.-A.; Huet, G.; Van der Eycken, J.; Delannoy, P.; Bruyneel, E.A. & Mareel, M.M. (2001). Alkyl-lysophospholipid 1-O-octadecyl-2-O-methyl-glycerophosphocholine induces invasion through episialin-mediated neutralization of E-cadherin in human mammary MCF-7 cells in vitro. *International Journal of Cancer*, 92, 4, 527–536.

Steelant, W.F.; Kawakami, Y.; Ito, A.; Handa, A.K.; Bruyneel, E.A.; Mareel, M. & Hakomori, S. (2002). Monosialyl-Gb5 organized with cSrc and FAK in GEM of human breast carcinoma MCF-7 cells defines their invasive properties. *FEBS Letters*, 531, 1, 93–98.

Thomas, J. W.; Ellis, B.; Boerner, R.J.; Knight, W.B.; White, G.C. 2nd & Schaller, M.D. (1998) SH2- and SH3-mediated interactions between focal adhesion kinase and Src. *Journal of Biological Chemistry*, 273, 1, 577-583.

Toledo, M.S.; Suzuki, E.; Handa, K. & Hakomori, S. (2005). Effect of ganglioside and tetraspanins in microdomains on interaction of integrins with fibroblast growth factor receptor. *Journal of Biological Chemistry*, 280, 16, 16227–16234.

Xing, Z.; Chen, H.C.; Nowlen, J.K.; Taylor, S.J., Shalloway, D. & Guan, J. L. (1994). Direct interaction of v-Src with the focal adhesion kinase mediated by the Src SH2 domain. *Molecular Biology of the Cell*, 5, 4, 413-421.

Yilmaz, M. & Christofori, G. (2010). Mechanisms of motility in metastasizing cells. *Molecular Cancer Research*, 8, 5, 629-642.

Zhang, Q.; Furukawa, K.; Chen, H.H.; Sakakibara, T.; Urano, T. & Furukawa, K. (2006). Metastatic potential of mouse Lewis lung cancer cells is regulated via ganglioside GM1 by modulating matrix metalloprotease-9 localization in lipid rafts. *Journal of Biological Chemistry*, 281, 26, 18145–18155.

21

Adipose Tissue and Desmoplastic Response in Breast Cancer

Jorge Martinez and Mariana Cifuentes
Laboratorio de Biología Celular y Molecular, INTA, Universidad de Chile, Santiago, Chile

1. Introduction

Breast tumors belong to a group of neoplastic lesions which, under the influence of tumoral cell products, originate a fibrous structure responsible for the dense and hard consistency of the tumoral mass. This trait also constitutes a factor that increases the relative risk of tumor recurrence (Hasabe et al., 1998). Myofibroblasts have been identified as major players in this phenomenon, acting either as producers of extracellular matrix (ECM) proteins and/or as functioning as elastic components of the tumor structure (Hinz B., 2007). Taken together, these pro-fibrotic processes are known as "tumoral desmoplastic reactions" (Shao et al., 2000).

The origin of the fibroblastic component in tumors is controversial. On one hand, it has been proposed that fibroblasts derive essentially from epithelia under an epithelial-to-mesenchymal transition (EMT) or, on the other, that the abundance of fibroblasts-like cells come from a dedifferentiation process by which mature adipose cells revert to fibroblastic -not lipid laden- cells (Taylor et al., 2010, Guerrero et al, 2010). In any case, the fibrotic outcome seems to be the result of a fluid cross-talk of signals among the predominant adipose stroma and epithelia. Epithelial control of mammary adipose cells is also observed under physiological conditions. During pregnancy and lactation, reproductive hormones induce the expansion and terminal differentiation of the mammary epithelium into secretory, milk-producing, lobular alveoli in a process that also includes the dedifferentiation of adipocytes into tiny preadipocytes (Wiseman and Werb, 2002). To further analyze the current hypothesis on the origin and possible fate or breast adipose tissue in the context of a tumoral breast, some aspects of breast adipose tissue need to be discussed in more detail.

2. Breast adipose tissue, obesity and cancer

Obesity, characterized by an excess of adipose tissue, has been linked in numerous epidemiological studies to an elevated risk of postmenopausal breast cancer (Petrelli et al., 2002, Calle et al., 2004, Pischon et al., 2008 and references therein). In general, the greater risk for several other cancers (such as colon, endometrium, kidney and esophagus) has been mechanistically linked to obesity via the metabolic and endocrine effects of the excess of adipose tissue, such as the alterations that it induces in the production of peptide and steroid hormones, as well as inflammatory factors. In addition to this role of total body adipose tissue, the case of breast cancer is of particular interest, because an important part of breast tissue is composed of the adipose stroma, whose active and direct influence on cancer cells is becoming an important focus of attention.

It is well known that the microenvironment of breast cancer cells greatly influences the growth and progression of the tumor, due to several elements such as cell-cell contact, soluble secreted factors, and the insoluble extracellular matrix (Celis et al., 2005 and references therein). Cells present in the stromal fraction such as fibroblasts, endothelial and various inflammatory cells can influence the phenotypic behavior of malignant cells. At the same time, tumor cells -or factors produced by them- can influence the surrounding stroma to generate a compatible microoenvironment that favors tumor survival and progression.

Among the many different cell types present in mammary tissue, the most abundant that surround breast cancer cells are those that make up adipose tissue, mainly mature adipocytes and their precursor cells, preadipocytes. An important number of primary breast tumors are originated by the transformation of ductal or intraductal epithelial cells. In many cases, these lesions develop in close contact with adipocytes, and in this microenvironment a reciprocal functional interaction takes place (Celis et al., 2005). In spite of this, adipose tissue has not received the attention it deserves in the context of breast cancer research. A possible reason for this may be that up until recent decades, the adipocyte was viewed as a rather inert, fat-storing cell with no other relevant physiological roles or capabilities. More recently, though, it has become evident that adipose tissue is a highly active endocrine organ, capable of secreting a vast number of hormones and other factors ("adipokines") including growth factors, several proinflammatory substances, hormone-like molecules, and extracellular matrix proteins (Deng and Scherer 2010, Karastergiou and Mohamed-Ali 2010). Moreover, adipose tissue may be infiltrated with other cell types, such as proinflammatory environment-inducing macrophages, thus elevating the number of local factors that may influence tumor progression. In this scenario, breast adipose tissue can constitute an important possible player influencing breast cancer development and progress. Some of the possible mechanisms involved are described below.

2.1 Adipose secretory products

The versatile endocrine organ nature of adipose tissue creates a complex local environment in the mammary tissue, influenced not only by circulating levels of different factors and hormones, but also to a great extent by the local production of mammary fat. Given the observation that tumor cells are in close contact spreading through fat tissue in high risk breast cancer, Celis et al. searched for secretory factors produced by adipocytes that may help elucidate the phenomena derived from this close association (Celis et al., 2005). Using a proteomics approach, the authors identified over 350 proteins within mammary adipose tissue from cancer patients undergoing mastectomy. These proteins included signaling molecules, hormones, cytokines and growth factors, which could be linked to various biological processes such as signal transduction, cell communication, cell metabolism and growth, immune response and apoptosis, among others. Their observations suggest that breast tumor cells and adipocytes provide each other with growth support by secreting factors that are mutually beneficial. This proteomics-based study provides interesting information regarding the gene products expressed by adipose tissue that helps define the tumor microenvironment.

In support of the role of adipokines influencing breast tumor growth, work by Iyengar and colleagues (Iyengar et al., 2003) provide further evidence to define molecular interactions between adipocytes and malignant breast ductal epithelial cells. In experiments using adipose conditioned media, they observed that adipose secretory products have relevant effects of breast cancer cell survival and proliferation. They showed that many genes promoting such events were upregulated, whereas genes that suppress growth and induce apoptosis are downregulated. Additionally, they observed that adipokines can induce the expression of oncogenes and other tumor-supporting factors such as AP1, cFOS and cJUN in MCF-7 cells. The effect on endothelial cells showed that they are able to promote angiogenesis in breast tumors. Adipose secretory products were also shown to have an impact on the invasive/metastasic potential, as they were able to increase motility of breast cancer cells.

2.2 Estrogen and aromatase

Estrogen, especially 17β-estradiol, plays an important role in the development of hormone dependent breast cancer. In postmenopausal women, the biosynthesis of estrogens occurs mainly through aromatase-mediated metabolism of androgen precursors. Adipose tissue is a relevant site of this conversion, and its occurrence is directly proportional to the degree of adiposity. The concentration of 17β-estradiol in breast cancer tissues from postmenopausal women has been observed to be 10-fold greater than those in plasma, and increased presence of aromatase and/or estrogen biosynthesis has been associated with the development of postmenopausal breast cancer (Sasano et al., 1998). Moreover, it has been proposed that most of the relationship between obesity and breast cancer can be explained by the adiposity-related increase in endogenous estrogen levels (Calle et al., 2004).

Besides the direct influence that adipose-secreted factors have on the different aspects of tumor development and progression (Maccio et al., 2009 and references therein), there is a series of interactions between adipokines and estrogens. Such cross-talk becomes of great relevance in hormone-dependent breast cancer, and may influence the outcome of pharmacological treatment. Leptin, for example, can modulate the influence of estrogen on tumor cells at different levels; it can induce estrogen receptor expression, induce aromatase activity and interfere with the effect of anti-estrogen drugs (Catalano et al., 2004, Garofalo et al., 2004).

Interestingly, the tumor itself also influences local aromatase expression and thus estrogen production by the surrounding adipose tissue. In breast cancer, there is a switch in promoter utilization for the transcription of the aromatase gene, from the weaker adipose-specific I.4 promoter to the more potent ovary-specific PII, leading to elevated aromatase expression and subsequent estrogen production. One possible factor leading to this induction in PII aromatase expression is prostaglandin E2 produced by malignant breast epithelium and macrophages within the tumor (Simpson et al., 2002).

The above-mentioned factors may act independently or in concert to elevate the risk for the development or progression of breast tumors. Recently, Subbaramaiah and collaborators evaluated the connections between obesity, inflammation and aromatase through interactions between the different cell types present in adipose tissue; adipocytes, macrophages and epithelial cells. In mammary fat from mice models of obesity, they observed necrotic adipocytes surrounded by macrophages, forming the so-called "crown like structures" (CLS) that are well known in human obesity and its detrimental consequences. The presence of CLS was associated with elevated levels of proinflammatory mediators as well as aromatase expression and activity in the mammary gland. Moreover, the proinflammatory mediators induced aromatase and estrogen-dependent gene expression in adipocytes. These authors thus have established important paracrine interactions between adipocytes and macrophages that may explain elevated local levels of aromatase.

2.3 Extracellular matrix

The extracellular matrix (ECM) is assembled by stromal cells within the mammary tissue. An altered ECM composition leads to tissue stiffness, which is characteristic of some solid tumors that develop desmoplastic reaction. Breast tumors are stiffer than the surrounding tissue. It has been proposed that this is the result of the recruitment and differentiation of tumoral myofibroblasts, cells that together with some elastic properties, provide the tumor environment with the capacity to generate a dense extracellular collagenous matrix scaffold (Egebland et al, 2005). In breast tumors, collagen is upregulated and densely crosslinked, and fibronectin -a molecule critical for collagen turnover- is also upregulated and associated with tumor malignancy (Chandler et al., 2011).

Adipocytes generate a basement membrane that promotes mammary tumor progression through collagen VI, and adipose-derived stem cells deposit an ECM rich in fibronectin. Collagen VI, which is abundantly expressed by adipocytes, seems to be an important factor contributing to the supportive role of adipose tissue in breast tumor survival. Iyengar and colleagues (Iyengar et al., 2005) showed in MCF-7 cells that adipocyte-derived collagen VI induces pro-mitogenic signals through the NG2/chondroitin sulfate proteoglycan receptor expressed on the surface of malignant ductal epithelial cells, to stabilize β-catenin and upregulate cyclin D1. The effects of collagen VI on breast cancer were also confirmed with *in vivo* experiments. Adipocytes thus play a vital role in defining the ECM environment for normal and tumor-derived ductal epithelial cells, and contribute significantly to tumor growth at early stages through secretion and processing of collagen VI. Immunohistochemistry studies of human mammary carcinoma tissue showed strong collagen VI staining around the tumors and the adipocytes whereas normal human mammary tissue showed low staining. This demonstration of collagen VI protein upregulation in human breast tumors, further suggests its relevance to human breast cancer.

Another mammary extracellular matrix component whose expression and assembly is modified by tumoral factors is fibronectin. The regulation of fibronectin matrix assembly and stiffness as a result of paracrine communication between breast cancer and adipose progenitor cells was recently assessed by Chandler and colleagues (Chandler et al., 2011). These authors evaluated the fibronectin assembled by 3T3-L1 preadipocytes that were treated with secretory products from MDA-MB231 breast cancer cells. Cultures exposed to the cancer cell-conditioned media produced a denser and more fibrilar fibronectin matrix, with increased fibronectin mRNA and protein levels. The results suggest that adipose-derived stem cells in the breast cancer microenvironment have enhanced fibronectin transcription and matrix assembly. In other experiments, they showed that adipose stromal cells enhanced fibronectin deposition and remodeling in the mammary tumor microenvironment, and that the factors derived from the tumor can alter the phenotype of the adipose cells, thus contributing to the changes. These data are yet another example of how paracrine signals from breast adipose tissue regulates mammary tumors, in this case by enhancing its rigidity.

3. TGF-β as a prototype of an epithelial factor that induces stromal reaction

It has been proposed that Transforming growth factor-beta (TGF-β), mainly produced by tumoral epithelial cells, plays a central role in the maintenance of a tumor-promoting stroma, acting as a key player in the stromal-epithelial dialogue (Derynck et al., 2001). In the advanced stages of the carcinogenic process, TGF-β acts either as a promoter of EMT or as an active stimulus in the fibroblastic activation to myofibroblasts (Stover et al., 2007). Because TGF-β is produced abundantly in malignant breast cancer cells as part of an autocrine repertoire, it is expected that this factor, in a paracrine manner, would exert a marked influence in the circumvent stroma and for that reason, would play a role in the mammary adipose structure (Guerrero et al, 2010). In the epithelial context, TGF-β is a multifunctional cytokine that displays a paradoxical behavior in carcinogenesis. During the premalignant phase, it inhibits epithelial cell proliferation and induces apoptosis. At more advanced steps of the process, this growth factor stimulates cancer progression in a manner strongly dependent of the tissue context, as it has been demonstrated in the bone metastasis model (Onishi et al 2010).

Our laboratory has provided evidence that at least part of the enhancement in tumor fibroblast abundance derives from a reversion process, in which mammary adipocytes lose their lipid load and become a typical elongated fibroblastic cell (Guerrero et al, 2010). We have proposed that this phenomenon is stimulated by soluble factors arising from epithelial tumoral cells among which TGF-β1 plays a relevant role. Human mammary adipose cells cultured in semi solid conditions in the presence of media conditioned by human tumoral mammary cell lines that secrete a different amount of TGF-β, showed an adipose reversion that is manifested in a high proportion of mammary fatty cells losing their lipid content and acquiring a fibroblast-like shape (Fig 1). The lipid loss also occurs when adipose cells are cultured in the presence of TGF-β1 and TNF-α that in these fatty cells are also able to inhibit the expression of the transcription factors C/EBPα and PPARγ, which are involved in the maintenance of the adipose phenotype. These data led us to propose that, in the tumoral microenvironment, TGF-β1 and TNF-α activate signaling routes that bring about the predominance of the fibroblastic over the adipocyte phenotype, which is concordant with the fibrotic response present in desmoplastic tumors. Moreover, the role of TGF-β1 on regulation of fibroblast/adipocyte ratio in mammary stroma was previously analyzed in studies that demonstrated that TGF-β1 strongly decreased adipogenesis, diminishing the cell-surface availability of TGF-β1 receptors (Choy, 2000).

In breast cancer models, it has been demonstrated that inflammatory mechanisms influence tumorigenesis and metastatic progression. This, despite that the etiology of breast cancer does not involve a pre-existing inflammation event (Grivennikov et al, 2010). Moreover, infiltration of inflammatory cells that include T cells, neutrophils and macrophages, among others, is a very common feature in breast cancer lesions. (Yang, 2010).

Current data allow us to suggest that in the tumoral environment, TGF-β1 not only regulates the abundance and activity of the fibroblastic compartment but also the relative amount and activity of the majority of infiltrated cells, such as immune cells, acting as an immunosuppressive cytokine. In this case, TGF-β1 suppresses the activity of cytotoxic T lymphocytes, through transcriptional repression of genes encoding key proteins engaged in the elimination of tumoral cells, counteracting in this manner the immunological surveillance against the tumor (Yang et al. 2010).

A) B)

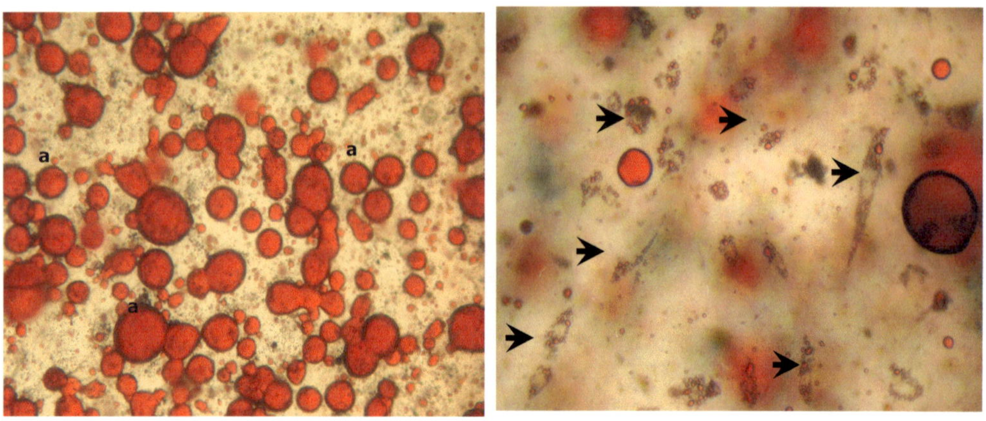

Fig. 1. Adipocyte reversion in three-dimensional collagen gel culture.
Human mature mammary adipocytes (10^5) were cultured in 1.5 ml semisolid collagen gel for 10 days in the absence (A) or presence (B) of 50% medium conditioned by human mammary MDA-MB-231 cells. Cells were stained with oil red O that identified lipid content in mature spherical adipocytes (a) and elongated cells with a fibroblast phenotype (b).

Macrophages frequently infiltrate tumors. In fact, a percentage of the tumoral mass is made up of the so-called tumor-associated macrophages (TAM) and their presence in the tumor environment correlate with poor prognosis (Flavell, 2010). However, depending on the type and specificities of tumoral microenvironments, TAMS may also have antitumor activity (Flavell, 2010). Besides active fibroblasts, these TAMs are among the main stromal components on desmoplastic breast tumors. Moreover, it has been proposed that tumor-associated fibroblasts are avid attractors for circulating monocytes (Silzle et al, 2003). It is plausible to suggest that macrophages play a relevant role in the mammary tumor-dependent fibrotic process. In adipose tissue, it has been demonstrated that soluble factors derived from macrophages promote a profibrotic phenotype which is the consequence of a significant overexpression of extracellular matrix (ECM) genes in inflammatory preadipocytes (Keophiphath et al, 2009).

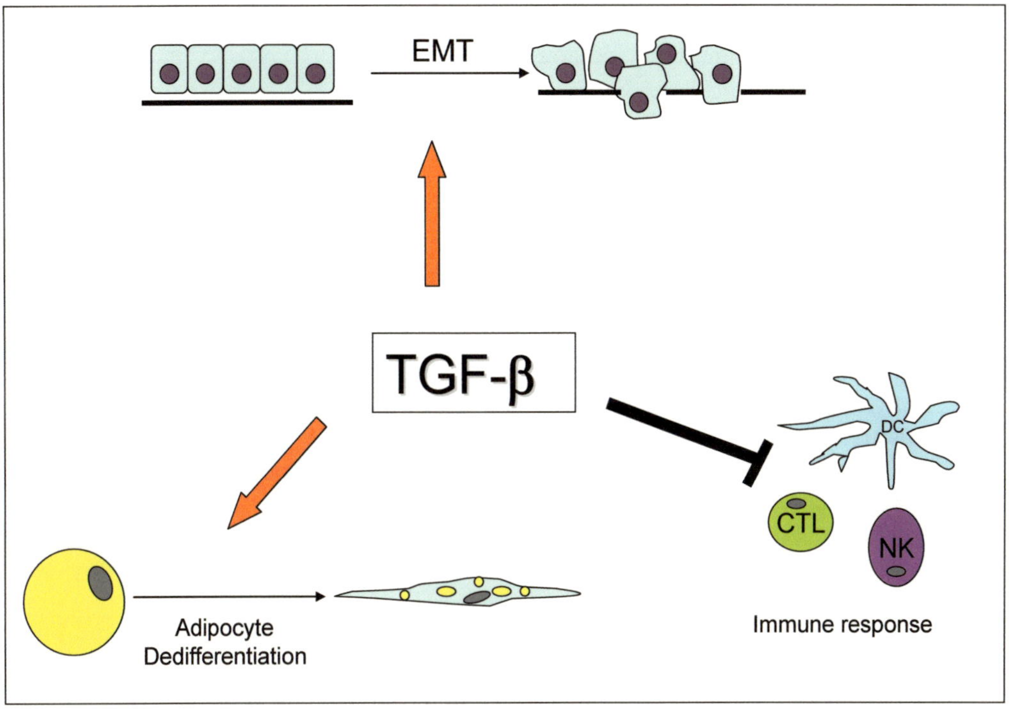

Fig. 2. TGF-β affects multiple components on tumoral environment.
TGF-β induces the reversion of adipose cells to a fibroblast-like phenotype, the epithelial-to-mesenchymal transition and the cytotoxic activity of immune cells. EMT: epithelial to mesenchymal transition; DC: dendritic cell; CTL: citotoxic T lymphocyte; NK: natural killer cell.

4. Concluding remarks

The desmoplastic reaction is one of the most common features of human breast cancer. Considering that mammary adipose cells are an important source of fibroblastic cells, which characterize desmoplastic tumors, it is relevant to take into account that some of the well-known physiological clues that regulate adipose tissue metabolism in other depots, can be also valid in the breast. Results from our laboratory propose that, in breast cancer, the fibrotic microenvironment that allows the expansion and progression of tumoral epithelia, has an original substratum in the adipose mammary tissue. We believe that different soluble factors derived from epithelia, among which TGF- β1 is one of the most important, collaborate in different ways to constitute a fibrotic tumoral microenvironment. TGF-β1 is one of the more abundant factors released by tumoral cells, and a determinant factor in the epithelial-to-mesenchymal transition, the reversion of adipose to a fibroblastic phenotype and the inhibition of local tumoral immunosurveillance. In light of that, it is clear that TGF-β1, a well known antiadipogenic factor, constitutes a key player in the regulation and function of tumor microenvironment. This justifies the attention that has led to different clinical trials based in the inhibition of its signaling.

5. References

[1] Calle EE, Kaaks R. Overweight, obesity and cancer: epidemiological evidence and proposed mechanisms. Nat Rev Cancer. 2004; 4(8):579-91.

[2] Catalano S, Mauro L, Marsico S, Giordano C, Rizza P, Rago V, Montanaro D, Maggiolini M, Panno ML, Andó S. Leptin induces, via ERK1/ERK2 signal, functional activation of estrogen receptor alpha in MCF-7 cells. J Biol Chem. 2004; 279(19):19908-15.

[3] Celis JE, Moreira JM, Cabezón T, Gromov P, Friis E, Rank F, Gromova I. Identification of extracellular and intracellular signaling components of the mammary adipose tissue and its interstitial fluid in high risk breast cancer patients: toward dissecting the molecular circuitry of epithelial-adipocyte stromal cell interactions. Mol Cell Proteomics. 2005; 4(4):492-522.

[4] Chandler EM, Saunders MP, Yoon CJ, Gourdon D, Fischbach C. Adipose progenitor cells increase fibronectin matrix strain and unfolding in breast tumors. Phys Biol. 2011; 8(1):015008.

[5] Choy L. Skillington J. and Derynck R. Roles of Autocrine TGFβ Receptor and Smad Signaling in Adipocyte Differentiation J. Cell Biol. 2000; 149: 667–681

[6] Deng Y, Scherer PE. Adipokines as novel biomarkers and regulators of the metabolic syndrome. Ann N Y Acad Sci. 2010; 1212:E1-E19.

[7] Derynck R., Akhurst R.J. and Ballmain A. TGF-β1 signaling in tumor suppression and cancer progression. Nature Genetics 2001; 29: 117-129

[8] Egeblad M., Littlepage L.E, and Werb Z. The Fibroblastic Coconspirator in Cancer Progression Cold Spring Harbor Lab. Press 2005; vol LXX: 383-387

[9] Flavell RA, Sanjabi S, Wrzesinski SH, Licona-Limón P. The polarization of immune cells in the tumour environment by TGFbeta. Nat Rev Immunol. 2010; 10:554-67.

[10] Garofalo C, Sisci D, Surmacz E. Leptin interferes with the effects of the antiestrogen ICI 182,780 in MCF-7 breast cancer cells. Clin Cancer Res. 2004; 10: 6466–6475

[11] Grivennikov, S. I., Greten, F. R. & Karin, M. Immunity, inflammation, and cancer. Cell 2010; 140: 883–899

[12] Guerrero J., Tobar N., Caceres M., Espinoza L., Escobar P., Dotor J., Smith P.C. and Martınez J. Soluble factors derived from tumor mammary cell lines induce a stromal mammary adipose reversion in human and mice adipose cells. Possible role of TGF-β1 and TNF-α. Breast Cancer Res Treat 2010; 119:497–508

[13] Hasebe T, Tsuda H, Hirohashi S, Shimosato Y, Tsubono Y, Yamamoto H, Mukai K. Fibrotic focus in infiltrating ductal carcinoma of the breast: a significant histopathological prognostic parameter for predicting the long-term survival of the patients. Breast Cancer Res Treat 1998; 49:195–208

[14] Hinz B., Phan S.H. Thannickal V.J., Galli A., Bonachaton-Piallat M-L., Gabbiani G. The Myofibroblast. One function, multiple origins. Am. J. Pathol 2007; 170: 1807-1816
[15] Iyengar P, Combs TP, Shah SJ, Gouon-Evans V, Pollard JW, Albanese C, Flanagan L, Tenniswood MP, Guha C, Lisanti MP, Pestell RG, Scherer PE. Adipocyte-secreted factors synergistically promote mammary tumorigenesis through induction of anti-apoptotic transcriptional programs and proto-oncogene stabilization. Oncogene. 2003;22(41):6408-23.
[16] Iyengar P, Espina V, Williams TW, Lin Y, Berry D, Jelicks LA, Lee H, Temple K, Graves R, Pollard J, Chopra N, Russell RG, Sasisekharan R, Trock BJ, Lippman M, Calvert VS, Petricoin EF 3rd, Liotta L, Dadachova E, Pestell RG, Lisanti MP, Bonaldo P, Scherer PE. Adipocyte-derived collagen VI affects early mammary tumor progression in vivo, demonstrating a critical interaction in the tumor/stroma microenvironment. J Clin Invest. 2005;115(5):1163-76.
[17] Karastergiou K, Mohamed-Ali V. The autocrine and paracrine roles of adipokines. Mol Cell Endocrinol. 2010;318(1-2):69-78
[18] Keophiphath M, Achard V, Henegar C, Rouault C, Clément K, Lacasa D. Macrophage-secreted factors promote a profibrotic phenotype in human preadipocytes. Mol Endocrinol. 2009; 23:11-24.
[19] Macciò A, Madeddu C, Mantovani G. Adipose tissue as target organ in the treatment of hormone-dependent breast cancer: new therapeutic perspectives. Obes Rev. 2009;10(6):660-70.
[20] Onishi T, Hayashi N, Theriault RL, Hortobagyi GN, Ueno NT. Future directions of bone-targeted therapy for metastatic breast cancer. Nat Rev Clin Oncol. 2010; 7:641-51 (2010)
[21] Petrelli JM, Calle EE, Rodriguez C, Thun MJ. Body mass index, height, and postmenopausal breast cancer mortality in a prospective cohort of US women. Cancer Causes Control. 2002;13(4):325-32.
[22] Pischon T, Nöthlings U, Boeing H. Obesity and cancer. Proc Nutr Soc. 2008; 67(2):128-45.
[23] Sasano H, Harada N. Intratumoral aromatase in human breast, endometrial, and ovarian malignancies. Endocr Rev. 1998;19(5):593-607.
[24] Shao ZM, Nguyen M, Barsky SH. Human breast carcinoma desmoplasia is PDGF initiated. Oncogene 2000; 19:4337–4345
[25] Silzle T, Kreutz M, Dobler MA, Brockhoff G, Knuechel R, Kunz-Schughart LA. Tumor-associated fibroblasts recruit blood monocytes into tumor tissue. Eur J Immunol. 2003;33(5):1311-20
[26] Simpson ER, Clyne C, Rubin G, Boon WC, Robertson K, Britt K, Speed C, Jones M. Aromatase--a brief overview. Annu Rev Physiol. 2002;64:93-127.
[27] Stover D.G., Bierie B. and Moses H.L. A delicate balance: TGF-β1 and tumor microenvironment. J. Cell Biochem 2007; 101: 851-861
[28] Taylor M.A, Parvani J. G and & William P. Schiemann W.P The Pathophysiology of Epithelial-Mesenchymal Transition Induced by Transforming Growth Factor-β in Normal and Malignant Mammary Epithelial Cells. J Mammary Gland Biol Neoplasia 2010; 15:169–190
[29] Wiseman BS, Werb Z. Stromal effects on mammary gland development and breast cancer. Science 2002; 296:1046–1049

[30] Yang L., Yanli Pang Y. and Moses H.L. TGF-b and immune cells: an important regulatory axis in the tumor microenvironment and progression Trends in Immunology 2010; 31: 220-227

22

Cross-Talk of Breast Cancer Cells with the Immune System

Sandra Demaria, Karsten A. Pilones and Sylvia Adams
New York University School of Medicine and NYU Langone Medical Center, New York, NY, United States

1. Introduction

Understanding the pathogenesis of breast and other cancers requires an improved understanding of the local microenvironment in which cancer develops and progresses (Hanahan and Weinberg, 2011). Many cell types have been defined as key components of the tumor stroma that contributes to tumor growth and metastasis, and modulates the response to treatment. In this chapter we will focus on cells of the immune system, critical players with dual function comprising cells that can foster a pro-tumorigenic inflammatory environment as well as reject tumors (Demaria et al., 2010). Importantly, the therapeutic manipulation of the host immune system has a tremendous potential to enhance the response of breast cancer patients to treatment. Therefore, it is imperative to understand the cross-talk between breast cancer cells and cells of the innate and adaptive immune system.

Several cell communication systems are involved in this cross-talk, including pro-inflammatory and immunosuppressive cytokines, chemokines and endogenous danger signals, known as damage-associated molecular pattern (DAMP) molecules that bind to Toll-like Receptors (TLR). Some of these factors represent interesting targets for immunotherapy strategies based on their known ability to stimulate the immune system, but in the context of the tumor microenvironment these immune stimulatory agents may also produce unwanted pro-tumorigenic effects by binding to receptors ectopically expressed on the cancer cells. Others are involved in recruiting to the tumor immune cells with regulatory and immune suppressive functions that protect the tumor from immune rejection. Clearly, the cross-talk between epithelial cells and the immune system is distorted in cancer to promote tumor growth and progression.

We will review pre-clinical and clinical data in support of the concept that the cross-talk between neoplastic and immune cells is a key determinant of tumor behavior and treatment outcomes. The mediators of this cross-talk that have been identified in breast cancer will be discussed. Ultimately, improved understanding of the potential double-edge sword quality of therapies targeting mediators of this cross-talk is essential for a cautious use of immune response modifiers to harness the positive (anti-tumor immune reactivity) without promoting the negative (tumor growth, immune suppression) effects.

2. Immune cells infiltrating breast cancer

The presence of an inflammatory infiltrate in benign breast is not uncommon and may be seen in association with a variety of fibrocystic changes or conditions such as mammary duct ectasia. However, for the most part immune cells are not a significant component of the normal breast stroma. In contrast, a marked increase in adaptive and innate immune cells often accompanies the process of carcinogenesis, with prominent inflammatory infiltrates seen around ducts involved by in situ carcinoma, as well as within invasive breast cancers (figure 1) (DeNardo and Coussens, 2007). The innate immune system plays a major role in maintenance of tissue homeostasis and reacts to tissue disruption, including physiological tissue disruption that occurs in the breast during branching morphogenesis at puberty and pregnancy, and in post-weaning involution. Macrophages, for example, have been shown to be important regulators of these processes (Gyorki and Lindeman, 2008). These physiological processes are self-limiting and the inflammation associated with them resolves once tissue homeostasis is restored. In contrast, carcinogenesis is a chronic process, often characterized by disorderly proliferation and death of the neoplastic cells, such as seen in ductal carcinoma in situ (DCIS). Deregulated cell death can foster a status of chronic inflammation, possibly due to the release of DAMPs from the dying cells (Mantovani et al., 2008; Zeh and Lotze, 2005). Death of epithelial cells that have undergone or are undergoing transformation also releases tumor-associated antigens and can result in activation of tumor-specific T and B cell responses. These immune responses can prevent tumor outgrowth, but eventually genetically unstable cancer cells give rise to variants that have become resistant to the recognition and/or killing by immune effector cells, a process defined as immunoediting (Schreiber et al., 2011). Escape from immune control does not necessarily require the loss of the antigen(s) recognized by T cells, but it is a complex process involving the production of immunosuppressive cytokines and the recruitment of regulatory innate and adaptive immune cells that protect the tumor from rejection. Key players in development and maintenance of the pro-tumorigenic environment are myeloid cells and subsets of CD4 T cells functionally differentiated towards T-helper type 2 (Th2) and regulatory (Treg) phenotypes that actively maintain a state of tolerance to the tumor (Disis, 2010). The contribution of Th2 CD4 cells has been recently demonstrated in an experimental study showing that interleukin (IL)-4 produced by Th2 CD4 T cells regulates the function of macrophages and promotes their pro-tumorigenic M2 phenotype in a mouse breast cancer model (Allavena et al., 2008; DeNardo et al., 2009). Interestingly, IL-4 has also been shown to be produced by primary epithelial breast cancer cells and to serve as an autocrine survival factor (Todaro et al., 2008). Another Th2 cytokine, IL-13, was shown to be involved in growth of human breast cancer cells (Aspord et al., 2007). Finally, a correlation between the number of Treg infiltrating human breast cancer and worse prognosis was reported in a study of 62 patients with DCIS and 237 patients with invasive breast cancer (Bates et al., 2006).

Conversely, evidence of effective anti-tumor immunity limiting tumor growth has been reported in several studies. Presence of a gene signature rich in Th1 and CD8 T cell markers was associated with a better outcome regardless of the type of epithelial malignancy in a study analyzing the stroma of primary breast cancers (Finak et al., 2008). Other studies, however, found that the prognostic value of immune signatures is different depending on the molecular subtype of breast cancer, and is a dominant factor in hormone receptors- and human epidermal growth factor receptor (Her)-2-negative (triple negative) cancers (Calabrò et al., 2009; Desmedt et al., 2008; Kreike et al., 2007; Mahmoud et al., 2011).

Overall, accumulating data support the concept that the balance between pro-tumorigenic and anti-tumor immune reactions is a key determinant of breast cancer progression. As detailed below, the neoplastic epithelial cells both secrete and respond to cytokines, chemokines and other bioactive molecules that regulate the recruitment and function of immune cells.

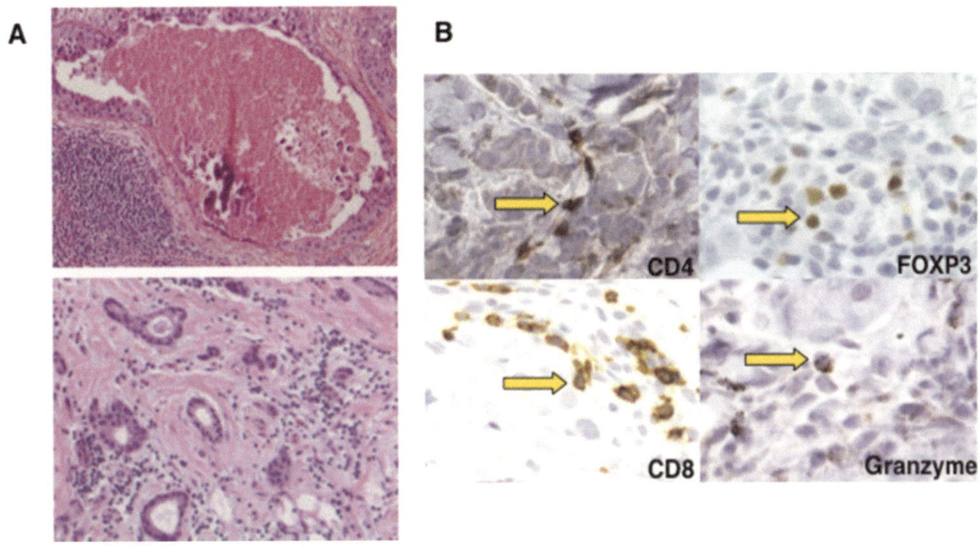

Fig. 1. Example of immune infiltrate in breast cancer. (A) Lymphocytic infiltrate as seen in H&E-stained sections. Ductal carcinoma in situ (DCIS) with comedo necrosis (upper panel), well differentiated invasive ductal carcinoma (lower panel). (B) Immunohistochemical staining of intratumoral T cells for markers of helper T cells (CD4), regulatory T cells (FoxP3), and effector T cells (CD8 and granzyme).

3. Chemokines and cytokines produced by breast cancer cells

A large network of chemokines and their receptors regulate trafficking and recruitment of innate and adaptive immune cells to different tissues in response to inflammation (Kunkel and Butcher, 2002). Signaling *via* chemokine receptors regulates processes such as cell migration, invasion, interaction with the endothelium and extracellular matrix, as well as survival. Interestingly, many epithelial cells acquire the expression of chemokine receptors and/or secrete chemokines when they undergo neoplastic transformation (Balkwill, 2004). The production of chemokines by cancer cells has been shown to influence the degree and phenotype of the inflammatory infiltrate. For example, the chemokine CCL2 (also known as monocyte chemotactic protein-1, MCP-1) is frequently secreted by breast cancer cells and is primarily responsible for recruitment of monocytes to tumors (Ueno et al., 2000; Valković et al., 1998). Within the tumor microenvironment monocytes differentiate into tumor-associated macrophages (TAM), which play a role in cancer progression and metastasis by producing immunosuppressive cytokines and pro-angiogenic factors (Pollard, 2004; Ueno et al., 2000). In human breast cancer levels of CCL2 correlate with a poor prognosis (Saji et al., 2001; Ueno et al., 2000) and recent evidence indicates that CCL2 plays a key role in pulmonary metastases of breast cancer by recruiting $Gr1^+$ inflammatory monocytes (Qian et al., 2011). Another chemokine produced by breast cancer cells and implicated in recruitment of monocytes is CCL5 (also known as Rantes) (Luboshits et al., 1999). Co-expression of CCL5 with CCL2 was reported to be associated with more advanced breast cancer stage (Soria et al., 2008).

Levels of two pro-inflammatory and pro-angiogenic chemokines, CXCL8 (also known as IL-8) and CXCL1 (also known as Growth-related oncogene, GRO) were found to be significantly elevated in sera of metastatic breast cancer patients with Her-2-positive compared with Her-2-negative cancers (Vazquez-Martin et al., 2007). *In vitro*, over-expression of Her-2 in human breast cancer cells MCF7 led to a marked increase in release of CXCL8 and CXCL1 that was abrogated by treatment with the tyrosine kinase inhibitor geftinib (Iressa), suggesting that these chemokines may play a role in the aggressive behavior of Her-2-positive breast cancers (Vazquez-Martin et al., 2007). CXCL1 and CXCL8 recruit neutrophils to tumors, and there is evidence that in the tumor microenvironment these cells acquire a pro-tumor phenotype in response to transforming growth factor (TGF)β (Fridlender et al., 2009).

Secretion of the chemokines CCL20 (also known as macrophage inflammatory protein, MIP-3α) and CCL19 (MIP-3β) by human breast cancer cells has been implicated in the recruitment of immature dendritic cells (DC) to breast cancer but the prognostic value remains uncertain (Bell et al., 1999; Treilleux et al., 2004). Interestingly, infiltration of breast cancer by Treg cells, which are recruited by CCL22 produced by approximately 60% of breast cancers (Gobert et al., 2009), was found to be associated with increased risk of relapse (Bates et al., 2006).

Conversely, some chemokines produced by breast cancer cells enhance recruitment of anti-tumor T cells. One such example is CXCL16, a chemokine that is up-regulated during inflammation in peripheral tissues and promotes recruitment of activated CD8 and Th1 T cells (Sato et al., 2005; Yamauchi et al., 2004). This may explain why the levels of expression of CXCL16 in colorectal carcinoma correlate with increased infiltration of tumors by T cells and better prognosis (Hojo et al., 2007). We were the first to report the expression of CXCL16 by human and mouse breast cancer cells, and to show that CXCL16 is markedly induced *in vitro* and *in vivo* by treatment with radiotherapy (Matsumura et al., 2008). We also showed in a mouse model of metastatic breast cancer that induction of CXCL16 by radiotherapy enhanced tumor infiltration by CD8 T cells elicited by immunotherapy promoting immune-mediated tumor rejection (Matsumura et al., 2008). Data in the preclinical model suggest that CXCL16 may play a role in response to treatment with radiotherapy and immunotherapy. Although the prognostic value of the expression of CXCL16 in breast cancer remains to be determined, it is possible that in the absence of treatment-induced anti-tumor CD8 T cells the lymphocytes recruited to CXCL16$^+$ tumors may instead promote pro-tumorigenic inflammation, as suggested in prostate cancer (Darash-Yahana et al., 2009). Whether the pro- or anti-tumor effects of CXCL16 prevail may be determined by expression of the cognate receptor, CXCR6, by the cancer cells, as discussed in the next section. Overall, chemokines expressed by breast cancer cells play critical roles in shaping the tumor immune infiltrate and likely influence tumor progression and response to treatment.

Among cytokines produced by breast cancer cells, the role of TGFβ in tumor development and progression has been extensively studied. Acting as a tumor suppressor early on, TGFβ later becomes a key factor in promoting tumor progression, metastases, and resistance to treatment (Barcellos-Hoff and Akhurst, 2009). Relevant to the focus of this chapter, in addition to direct effects on the neoplastic cells, TGFβ acts on innate and adaptive immune cells suppressing their function (Gorelik and Flavell, 2001; Wrzesinski et al., 2007). DCs

(Kobie et al., 2003) and effector CD8 T cells (Gorelik and Flavell, 2001; Thomas and J., 2005; Wrzesinski et al., 2007) are key targets of TGFβ suppressive effects in cancer leading to defects in activation and function of anti-tumor effector cells. Interestingly, an unexpected tumor-promoting effect of TGFβ was shown to be mediated by induction of production of the pro-inflammatory cytokine IL-17 by CD8 T cells (Nam et al., 2008). IL-17 acted as a survival factor for tumor cells, including mouse breast cancer cell lines that ectopically expressed the IL-17 receptor (Nam et al., 2008). These intriguing observations emphasize the complexity of interactions between tumor cells and immune system. Breast cancer cells also produce IL-4 and use it as an autocrine survival factor (Todaro et al., 2008).

The expression and production of IL-10 and IL-12 p40, but not of IL-12 p70, by human breast tumor cells was recently reported (Heckel et al., 2011). IL-10 has immunosuppressive anti-inflammatory effects, and IL-12p40 can bind to IL-12 receptor on immune cells and work as an antagonist of IL-12p70, a cytokine that promotes Th1 T cell differentiation. Although the contribution of IL-10 and IL-12p40 produced by breast cancer cells to generation of an immune suppressive tumor microenvironment remains to be further studied, data support the concept that tumors that become clinically apparent have undergone multiple changes to escape immune rejection (Schreiber et al., 2011).

4. Chemokine receptors expressed by breast cancer cells

Cancer cells express several chemokine receptors, and exploit the chemokine system to home to bone marrow and different organs that are sites of metastases. An example is CXCR4, the chemokine receptor most commonly found on cancer cells and the role of which has been more extensively characterized (Balkwill, 2004). *In vitro,* binding of CXCR4 to its ligand, the chemokine CXCL12 (also known as stromal derived factor -1, SDF-1) activates migration and invasion of cancer cells. *In vivo,* expression of CXCR4 is associated with metastatic capacity in melanoma, breast, and other cancers (Balkwill, 2004; Muller et al., 2001). Another chemokine receptor that is required for homing of lymphocytes and DCs to lymph nodes, CCR7, has been shown to be expressed by breast cancer cells and guide their metastases to lymph nodes (Muller et al., 2001).

CXCR3, a chemokine receptor expressed by activated Th1 and effector CD8 T and natural killer (NK) cells, binds to three chemokines, CXCL9, CXCL10 and CXCL11. Overexpression of CXCL10 (also known as interferon (IFN)-γ inducible protein 10, IP-10), or CXCL9 (also known as monokine induced by IFN-γ, Mig) by genetic engineering of tumor cells in experimental mouse tumor models enhanced recruitment of T and NK cells and promoted immune-mediated tumor rejection (Luster and Leder, 1993; Walser et al., 2007). However, CXCR3 is also expressed by human and mouse breast cancer cell lines (Goldberg-Bittman et al., 2004; Walser et al., 2006), and more recently it was found in all human primary breast cancers tested (N=75). Importantly, high CXCR3 expression, found in 24% of the tumors, was associated with poor overall survival (Ma et al., 2009). In experimental mouse models, blocking CXCR3 with a small molecule inhibitor prior to i.v. injection of the tumor cells, or by gene silencing in the tumor cells inhibited metastases (Ma et al., 2009; Walser et al., 2006). Intriguingly, inhibition of lung metastases by CXCR3 gene silencing required NK cells and was compromised in IFN-γ-deficient mice (Ma et al., 2009). These data highlight the complexity of the interactions between tumor and host, and caution that the systemic use of CXCR3 inhibitors could elicit mixed effects by reducing metastases while potentially interfering also with recruitment of immune cells that are required for metastasis control.

Similarly to CXCR3, CXCR6 is expressed on immune cells with anti-tumor effector function, namely activated CD8 and Th1 CD4 T cells, NK cells, and NKT cells (Kim et al., 2002; Kim et al., 2001; Nakayama et al., 2003; Unutmaz et al., 2000). CXCL16, the only ligand for CXCR6, was first shown to be expressed by immune cells with antigen-presenting function, and to be up-regulated during inflammation in different organs (Sato et al., 2005; Yamauchi et al., 2004). As mentioned above, expression of CXCL16 was recently described in several tumors, including breast cancer. Autocrine effects of CXCL16 binding to CXCR6 expressed on the same cancer cells were described in prostate cancer, where signaling via CXCR6 induced the activation of AKT/mammalian target of rapamycin (mTOR) pathway and promoted tumor cell invasion, growth and angiogenesis (Wang et al., 2008). In contrast, in renal cell carcinoma, CXCL16 expression was associated with better prognosis in patients. Endogenous CXCL16 appeared to inhibit growth and migration by interacting with CXCR6 expressed by the same tumor cells (Gutwein et al., 2009). Whether the pro- or anti-tumor effects of the CXCL16/CXCR6 pathway depend on the levels of CXCR6 expression on the tumor cells or its interaction with different forms of CXCL16 remains to be clarified. CXCL16 is one of only two chemokines that is released by cleavage of the chemokine domain from a transmembrane molecule by the activity of the disintegrin-like metalloproteinase ADAM10 (Abel et al., 2004). Soluble CXCL16 has chemotactic activity, while the transmembrane form can mediate adhesion to CXCR6^{+} cells, as well as function as a scavenger receptor for oxidized low density lipoproteins, phosphatidylserine, and dextran sulfate (Shimaoka et al., 2003). Therefore, it is possible that interaction of CXCR6 expressed on tumor cells with the soluble chemokine domain or the transmembrane form of CXCL16 has different consequences. Expression of CXCR6 was initially reported in mouse breast cancer cell lines (Wang et al., 2006). A recent report in human breast cancer cells shows that CXCR6 can mediate chemotaxis in response to soluble CXCL16. Interestingly, expression of CXCR6 was regulated by hypoxia via hypoxia inducible factor (HIF)-1α, suggesting a role of CXCR6 expressed in breast cancer cells in cell migration in response to hypoxia (Lin et al., 2009). Although intriguing, these findings need confirmation in functional experiments assessing the role of CXCR6 in breast cancer metastasis. Overall, more data is required to clarify the expression and function of CXCR6 in breast cancer.

Another chemokine receptor, CCR5, has been implicated in breast cancer metastases promoted by mesenchymal stem cells. Intriguingly, the increased metastatic ability was dependent on the production of CCL5 by mesenchymal stem cells, which was induced de novo by the breast cancer cells, highlighting the importance of the tumor microenvironment in the cross-talk between neoplastic and stromal cells (Karnoub et al., 2007).

5. TLR and their ligands

Immune surveillance by cells of the innate immune system is mediated in large part by pattern recognition receptors (PRRs) that allow sensing of the invading pathogens and initiation of the inflammatory cascade (Kopp and Medzhitov, 2003). PRRs represent a family of evolutionarily conserved, germline-encoded proteins that recognize structural motifs found in bacteria and viruses known as pathogen-associated molecular patterns (PAMPs) (Barton and Medzhitov, 2002). TLRs constitute the most well-studied and characterized family of PRRs. To date, 11 TLRs and their cognate ligands have been identified in humans. TLRs are predominantly expressed in DCs, macrophages and NK cells. TLR activation by their respective PAMPs induces the release of pro-inflammatory cytokines, chemokines as well as adhesion molecules that collectively enhance phagocytosis, microbial killing as well as recruitment of adaptive immunity (Iwasaki and Medzhitov, 2004).

In addition to sensing microbial pathogens, TLRs are also activated by endogenous ligands and trigger a sterile form of inflammation. First described by Matzinger as DAMP, these endogenous danger signals are often released or expressed in the context of tissue injury by both normal and neoplastic cells (Bianchi, 2007; Gallucci et al., 1999). Several recently identified DAMPs include heat- shock proteins (Ohashi et al., 2000; Roelofs et al., 2006; Vabulas et al., 2002), uric acid crystals (Liu-Bryan et al., 2005) and extracellular matrix proteins (Okamura et al., 2001) (Figure 2).

DAMP-TLR interactions have been implicated in the pathogenesis of immune dysfunction in autoimmune diseases and atherosclerosis, as well as in the chronic inflammation often associated with cancer (Marshak-Rothstein, 2006).

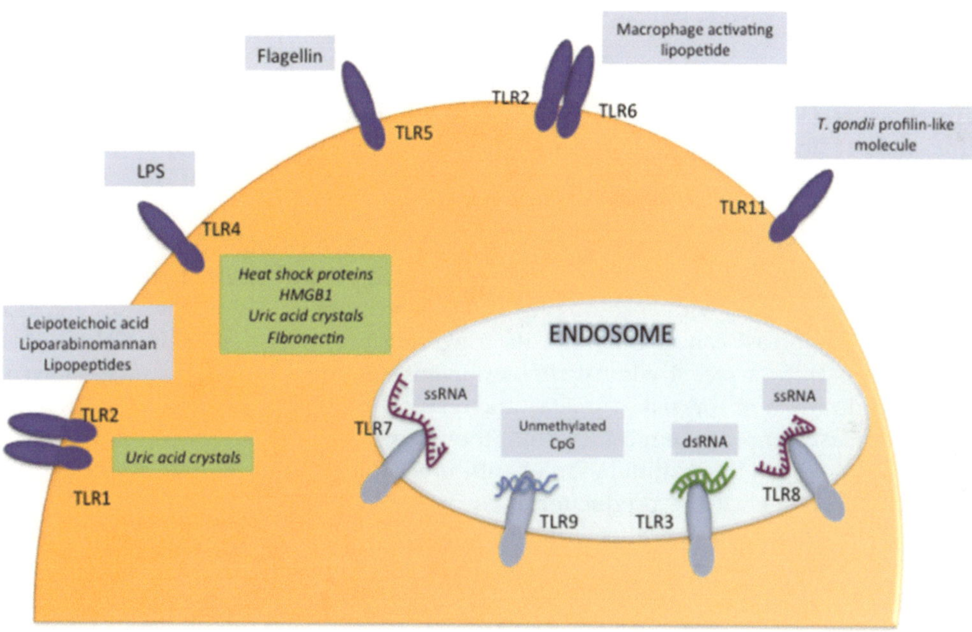

Fig. 2. Overview of toll-like receptors (TLRs) and their ligands. Activation of TLRs can be induced by exogenous microbial-derived ligands (PAMPs) as well as endogenous ligands (DAMPs) which are released from tissues in response to injury and inflammation.

Importantly, DAMP-TLR interactions have also been shown to play a decisive role in shaping anti-tumor immune responses (Apetoh et al., 2007a). Tumor cell death induced by some chemotherapy drugs and ionizing radiation resulted in release of copious amounts of the DAMP high-mobility-group box 1 (HMGB1) that binds to TLR4 expressed by DC and promotes the cross-presentation of tumor-derived antigens to T cells (Apetoh et al., 2007b). The ability of TLR engagement to activate innate immune cells to promote a defense response by inducing adaptive anti-tumor responses has spurred efforts to exploit TLR agonists as novel adjuvants for cancer therapy (Adams, 2009). Both purified natural and synthetic TLR ligands have been used in a variety of vaccination regimens designed to overcome tolerance and sustain tumor-specific T-cell responses. Evidence from pre-clinical and clinical studies has shown the benefit of TLR stimulation when combined with conventional cancer treatment modalities such as radiotherapy and/or chemotherapy (Manegold et al., 2008; Mason et al., 2006). The discovery that many epithelial cells, including carcinoma cells, do express at least some TLRs, however, has raised the question about the effect of TLR stimulation on the tumor cells (Yu and Chen, 2008), and the effects of their therapeutic use (Huang et al., 2008). For instance, data from both mouse and human cancer cells show that while activation of some TLRs can increase susceptibility of tumor cells to apoptosis (Salaun et al., 2006), the ligation of other TLRs promotes tumorigenesis on several levels. Indeed, in a variety of tumor models, TLR stimulation has been shown to enhance proliferation, diminish tumor susceptibility to apoptosis, stimulate migratory capacity and invasiveness as well as promote angiogenesis (Harmey et al., 2002; Jego et al., 2006; Pidgeon et al., 1999). In the following section, we summarize data about the function of the main TLRs known to be expressed by breast cancer cells.

5.1 TLR3

Several TLRs (TLR 3,7,8 and 9) that recognize nucleic acid ligands are expressed intracellularly in the endosomal compartment, thus allowing for rapid detection of foreign nucleic acid material (Liu et al., 2008). TLR3 is an important detector of viral infection since it binds viral double-stranded RNA (dsRNA) and initiates a strong IFN type I response. Synthetic dsRNA agonists for TLR3, such as polyadenylic-polyuridylic acid [poly(A:U)], have been developed and tested in clinical trials in several cancers, including breast cancer, with encouraging results (Lacour et al., 1980). Interestingly, TLR3 is expressed by breast cancer cells and its triggering promotes apoptosis (Salaun et al., 2006) (Figure 3). In a recent clinical trial, adjuvant treatment with poly(A:U) showed a significant decrease in the risk of metastatic relapse in TLR3 positive but not in TLR3-negative breast cancers, suggesting that the direct anti-tumor effect may be more important than the indirect stimulation of anti-tumor immunity (Salaun et al., 2011). TLR3 triggering can also elicit the production by some tumor cells of chemokines that recruit immune cells with opposing effects (Conforti et al., 2010). Therefore, the use of TLR3 agonists should be combined with strategies to enhance anti-tumor Th1 responses and/or decrease immunosuppressive cells responsive to CCL5.

5.2 TLR4

The prototypical and best-characterized agonist for TLR4 activation is lipopolysaccharide (LPS), a structural component of Gram-negative bacteria. TLR4 can also be stimulated by viral components derived, for example, from respiratory syncytial virus (Kurt-Jones et al., 2000) or the murine retrovirus MMTV (Rassa et al., 2002). Additionally, endogenous DAMPs such as heat-shock proteins and HMGB-1 are ligands for TLR4 (Apetoh et al., 2007b; Ohashi et al., 2000). A synthetic derivative, i.e., monophospohryl lipid A (MPL), is used as a vaccine adjuvant for hepatitis B (Fendrix) and human papilloma virus (Cervarix) (reviewed in (Adams, 2009)). In the 1990's, MPL was included as a component of DETOX adjuvant in tumor vaccines for skin, lung and breast malignancies, with promising results in Phase II/III clinical trials (Eton et al., 1998; He et al., 2007; MacLean et al., 1993). On the other hand, recent evidence has implicated TLR4 expression in tumor cells as having a profound impact on tumor cell survival by evading host anti-tumor responses (He et al., 2007) or promoting

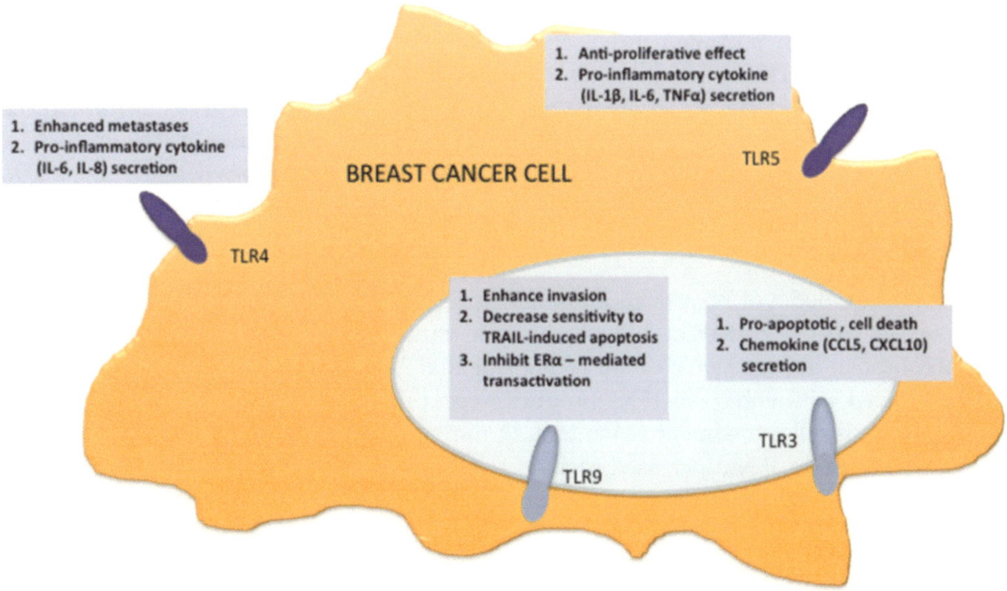

Fig. 3. Documented effects of TLR ligation on breast cancer cells. TLR activation in breast cancer cells is complex since it can either promote tumor cell death or enhance its growth and invasive potential. Like most other epithelial malignancies, breast cancer cells express several TLRs although the endogenous ligands for many of these TLRs remain unknown.

chemoresistance (Kelly et al., 2006). Expression of TLR4 by a large majority (~90%) of primary breast cancers was detected by immunohistochemistry in a study of 133 cases, but there was no significant association between TLR4-positivity and outcome (Petricevic et al., 2011). On the other hand, another study reported an interesting correlation between metastatic propensity and expression of TLR4 among stromal cells (i.e mononuclear inflammatory cells), which are found in abundance in primary breast tumors (Gonzalez-Reyes et al., 2010). These findings reiterate the complexity of the role that stromal cells play in tumor progression and suggest that TLR4 expression may be a critical mediator in these events. Furthermore, TLR4 was the predominant TLR detected in the immortalized human breast cancer cell line MDA-MB-231 (Yang et al., 2010). Knockdown of TLR4 significantly inhibited growth and secretion of IL-6 and IL-8 by these breast cancer cells, suggesting that TLR4 could be a therapeutic target. Overall, while stimulation of TLR4 in the cancer cells themselves may have deleterious effects, stimulation of TLR4 in innate immune cells could have opposite effects, depending on the tumor microenvironment, the type of myeloid cells involved (e.g., macrophages versus DC) and the availability of other signals that have to be integrated by DC to promote, rather than suppress, anti-tumor immune responses (Zitvogel et al., 2010).

5.3 TLR5

TLR5 is a cell surface receptor that recognizes bacterial flagellin and is unique among TLRs in that it is highly expressed in DCs within the lamina propria of the gut epithelium. It has also been detected in carcinomas of the gastro-intestinal tract, where it has been hypothesized that it may interact with bacterial pathogens linked to cancer development such as Helicobacter pylori (Schmausser et al., 2005). Interestingly, a functional TLR5 is also expressed by human prostate cancer cells and its stimulation triggers the production of chemokines that recruit immune cells, although it is unclear whether recruited cells contribute to pro-tumorigenic inflammation or tumor rejection (Galli et al., 2010). On the other hand, the pro-inflammatory effects of TLR5 activation, particularly IL-6 and CCL2 release, were implicated in tumor progression of ovarian malignancies (Zhou et al., 2009). Indeed, early studies comparing TLR5 expression in normal and ovarian cancer have suggested that TLR5 could be a promising biomarker for malignant changes (Kim et al., 2008).

In a preclinical model of breast cancer, administration of flagellin to mice with established tumors inhibited the growth of an immunogenic variant expressing human Her-2 but not the parental non-immunogenic tumor (Sfondrini et al., 2006). TLR5 stimulation by flagellin was associated with enhanced IFNγ production and diminished infiltration of Treg cells. Interestingly, flagellin treatment at the time of tumor implantation had the opposite effect, leading to decreased IFNγ, increased frequency of Treg cells and accelerated tumor growth, indicating that opposing effects may be elicited depending on the tumor/host environment at time of administration (Sfondrini et al., 2006). However, since TLR5 expression in tumor cells themselves was not definitively established, no conclusions could be drawn whether the pro- or anti-tumorigenic effects of flagellin treatment resulted from direct effects on carcinoma cells.

A recent study in human primary breast cancer specimens from 75 patients demonstrated that TLR5 is expressed in normal ductal epithelium and in 80% of breast cancers examined (Cai et al., 2011). TLR5 was also expressed in 6 human breast cancer cell lines, and flagellin treatment inhibited tumor cell proliferation *in vitro* and *in vivo*, in a xenograft model. In MCF7 cells, flagellin stimulation induced tumor necrosis factor (TNF)-α, IL-1β, IL-6, and IL-8 mRNA, suggesting that flagellin activates TLR5-dependent signaling pathway in breast cancer cells. The production of several chemokines was also increased by flagellin, including MIP-3α, MCP-1, macrophage-derived chemokine (MDC), IL-6, Gro-α, and osteoprotegerin. *In vivo*, flagellin-treated MCF7 and MDA-MB-468 tumors growing in nude (T cell deficient) mice showed increased infiltration by neutrophils (Cai et al., 2011). It will be important to establish, however, if these anti-tumor effects can be achieved in immunocompetent mice.

5.4 TLR9

TLR9 is located intracellularly in the endoplasmic reticulum and binding induces translocation to the endosomal/lysosomal compartment. In humans, TLR9 is abundantly expressed in plasmacytoid DC (pDCs) and B cells. Until recently, TLR9 has been thought to recognize hypomethylated CpG deoxynucleotides (CpG-ODN) motifs characteristic of bacterial DNA but molecular studies have definitively shown that TLR9 binds instead to the 2′-deoxyribose sugar backbone (Haas et al., 2008). TLR9 activation in pDC enhances their maturation into more efficient antigen presenting cells and producers of powerful pro-inflammatory cytokines such as type I IFN (Gilliet et al., 2008). Furthermore, the activation of TLR9 in B cells promotes their proliferation and polyclonal immunoglobulin synthesis, thus generating a robust humoral response as well (Chiron et al., 2008). The broad spectrum of immunoactivating effects of TLR9 stimulation on both innate and adaptive responses have spurred efforts to use synthetic TLR9 ligands as an immunotherapeutic for both solid tumors and hematological malignancies (Krieg, 2008). Initially, TLR9 expression was thought to be restricted to immune cells, but recent studies have conclusively showed that a variety of tumor cell types also express functional TLR9 molecules. Indeed, expression of TLR9 has been confirmed in both frozen breast tumor specimens (Berger et al., 2010)as well as breast cancer cell lines (Berger et al., 2010; Merrell et al., 2006; Qiu et al., 2009). A study of 124 frozen breast tissue specimen from women diagnosed with breast cancer found a positive correlation (Spearman rank p=0.04) between TLR9 mRNA expression and increasing tumor grade, suggesting that TLR9 expression may be a molecular marker for poorly differentiated breast cancers (Berger et al., 2010).

The direct effects of TLR9 stimulation on tumor cells, however, remains decidedly complex. In 2006, Selander and colleagues showed that CpG-ODN stimulation of the TLR9-positive MDA-MB-231 but not TLR9-negative MCF-7 human breast cancer cells induced their migration across a matrigel matrix (Merrell et al., 2006), suggesting that TLR9 signaling plays a role in cancer progression and metastasis. TLR9 overexpression in BT-20 breast cancer cells has similarly been found to enhance invasiveness *in vitro* (Berger et al., 2010). In both studies, CpG-ODN stimulation did not affect cellular proliferation, thus negating the possibility that the enhanced migration could be attributed to increased cell division. TLR9 expression may also be a mechanism that tumors employ to evade host immune responses such as tumor necrosis factor-related apoptosis inducing ligand (TRAIL)-induced apoptosis. The TRAIL/TRAIL receptor interaction is an important mechanism by which anti-tumor effectors such as CD8 T cells, NK cells and NKT cells mediate tumor-directed cell kill. In an *in vitro* study using TLR9-expressing breast cancer cell lines HCC1569 and Cal51, CpG-ODN stimulation resulted in a significant decrease in the sensitivity of tumor cells to lexatumumab, an anti-DR5 agonist antibody that stimulates the TRAIL pathway (Chiron et al., 2009; Ohta et al., 2006) . Using a synthetic TLR9 ligand in which the phosphate backbone was modified to increase resistance to nucleases and enhance circulating half-life, Chiron and co-workers showed that the phosphorothioate-modified TLR9 agonist could bind directly to the DR5 receptor on tumor cells and inhibit TRAIL-dependent killing by NK cells. These findings have important implications for the use of TLR9-directed therapies using synthetic CpG-ODNs which may potentially attenuate tumor immunosurveillance. Conversely, a recent study suggest that CpG-ODN stimulation may hold therapeutic promise in estrogen-responsive breast cancer cells (Qiu et al., 2009). TLR9 activation in T47D and MCF-7 breast cancer cells inhibited estrogen-receptor alpha (ERα)-mediated transactivation through the NF-κB pathway. Although these findings need to be confirmed in primary breast tumor tissues, it is intriguing to investigate whether CpG-ODN stimulation can synergize with hormonal therapy for ER^+ breast cancers.

6. The cross-talk between regulatory T cells and breast cancer cells (RANKL)

Receptor activator of NF-kB (RANK) is a type I membrane protein, which shares high homology with CD40. RANK ligand (RANKL, also called TRANCE (TNF-related activation-induced cytokine) or osteoclast differentiation factor (ODF) is a type II membrane protein with belongs to the TNF superfamily originally identified as a dendritic cell survival factor. RANKL is predominately expressed in activated T cells, as well as the thymus, lymph node and bone marrow. RANK/RANKL are essential regulators of bone remodeling, body temperature, lymph node and thymus formation as well as mammary gland development during pregnancy (Leibbrandt and Penninger, 2008). Furthermore, the RANK/RANKL axis has been linked to progestin-driven breast carcinomas and bone metastases (Schramek et al., 2010).

In addition to the expression of RANK on hematopoietic osteoclast precursors and DC, the receptor is also expressed by some tumor cell types, including melanoma, osteosarcomas, breast and prostate cancers (Jones et al., 2006; Mori et al., 2007a; Mori et al., 2007b). RANK expression has been reported in 6-57% of invasive human breast cancers, depending upon the parameters used to define positivity and antibodies utilized for staining (Gonzalez-Suarez et al., 2010; Santini et al., 2011). Stimulation of RANK+ human breast cancer cells with recombinant RANKL induces actin polymerization and migration without affecting cell proliferation (Jones et al., 2006). Preclinical models of Her-2+ mammary carcinoma (MMTV-neu transgenic mouse) have shown that metastatic spread is dependent on RANK signaling and that pharmacological inhibition of RANKL reduces tumor growth and lung metastases (Gonzalez-Suarez et al., 2010; Tan et al., 2011).

While only a subgroup of breast cancers expresses RANKL and there is no evidence for co-localization of RANK and its ligand in the carcinoma epithelium (Gonzalez-Suarez et al., 2010; Van Poznak et al., 2006), RANKL is expressed by infiltrating immune cells. In one study, RANKL was detected in tumor-infiltrating mononuclear cells (not further characterized) and occasionally in fibroblast-like stromal cells (Gonzalez-Suarez et al., 2010). Another report showed that the majority of RANKL-producing cells infiltrating breast cancers were T cells expressing FOXP3, a transcription factor produced by Treg cells (Tan et al., 2011). Importantly, RANK signaling mediated the metastatic behavior of RANK-expressing mouse breast cancer cells, and RANKL was produced by Treg cells (Tan et al., 2011). Therefore, in addition to suppressing anti-tumor immune responses, Treg cells might promote the metastatic behaviors of some tumors by producing RANKL, explaining why Treg cells have been shown to have prognostic significance in breast cancers. In 237 patients with operable breast cancers, Treg cell numbers in the primary tumor correlated with relapse-free survival independently of nodal involvement, tumor size and grade (Bates et al., 2006). Therefore, it will be of great interest to determine if tumor infiltration by Treg cells and/or Th17 cells, another T cell subset that has been shown to express high levels of RANKL (Sato et al., 2006), predicts for increased metastases of RANK+ breast cancers, and whether RANKL inhibition will be effective at inhibiting metastasis and risk of recurrence and death from breast cancer.

7. Therapeutic implications

The role of interactions between tumor cells and host immune system is increasingly appreciated as critical for tumor development and progression, as well as therapeutic response. As discussed above, the type and density of immune cells infiltrating breast cancers is associated with prognosis, with high density of macrophages forecasting a worse outcome (Bingle et al., 2002) while high numbers of $CD8^+$ T cells predict a better outcome (Mahmoud et al., 2011). Importantly, the presence of a brisk lymphocytic infiltrate in pre-treatment biopsies of more than one thousand primary breast cancers was significantly associated with pathological complete response (pCR) to neoadjuvant anthracycline/taxane treatment (Denkert et al., 2010). A significant association was found between markers of T cells (CD3) and effector T-cell recruitment (CXCL9) and pCR (Denkert et al., 2010). These data in patients support the concept that the anti-cancer immune response is essential for therapeutic success (Zitvogel et al., 2008), and suggest that immune infiltrates can provide predictive information. Indeed, if cytocidal treatments work, in part, by causing an immunogenic tumor cell death and generating an *in situ* vaccine, the presence of a less immunosuppressive microenvironment will favor development of anti-tumor immunity post-treatment (Apetoh et al., 2007c; Formenti and Demaria, 2009; Ghiringhelli et al., 2009; Obeid et al., 2007). Conversely, immune cells and their receptors become attractive targets for improving response to chemo- and radio-therapy. For example, we have shown in a mouse model of metastatic breast cancer that targeting the co-inhibitory receptor CTLA-4 on T cells synergizes with local radiotherapy in inducing the immune-mediated regression of the irradiated tumor and metastases outside of the radiation field (Demaria et al., 2005). In a different mouse model of breast cancer targeting colony stimulating factor (CSF)-1 receptor with an antagonist blocked macrophage recruitment to paclitaxel-treated tumors leading to improved therapeutic response, longer survival and reduced metastases (DeNardo et al., 2011).

Strategies to deplete Treg cells in breast cancer patients (Dannull et al., 2005; Rech and Vonderheide, 2009) may also be beneficial by reducing local immunosuppression as well as removing a main source of RANKL production. Increased accumulation of Treg cells is also seen in sentinel lymph nodes of breast cancer patients and it correlates with the size of the primary tumor (Gupta et al., 2011). Since anti-tumor T cells are activated in sentinel lymph nodes (Kim et al., 2006) the increased Treg cell presence might limit the efficacy of pre-operative chemotherapy for locally advanced breast cancer by inhibiting the activation of tumor-specific T cells (Boissonnas et al., 2010).

Multiple additional strategies for manipulating the immune environment of breast cancer are being studied, including TLR agonists (Lu et al., 2010), immunomodulatory drugs and vaccines (Emens et al., 2009). A critical question that will need to be addressed is how we predict response to treatment with agents that target the immune system, whether directly such as antibodies against co-stimulatory or co-inhibitory T cell receptors, or indirectly such as chemotherapy drugs that induce an immunogenic cell death. In fact, polymorphisms of TLR4 and P2X7, receptors that play a key role in development of anti-tumor immunity following chemotherapy-induced immunogenic tumor cell death, are present in the population and have been shown to impact response to treatment with anthracyclines and radiotherapy (Apetoh et al., 2007c; Ghiringhelli et al., 2009). Therefore, as recently proposed by Zitvogel and colleagues (Zitvogel et al., 2011), immune-relevant biomarkers will need to be considered together with tumor cell biomarkers in tailoring treatment for patients towards a personalized therapeutic approach.

8. Conclusions

This chapter summarizes the recent advances in our understanding of the interplay between breast cancer and the immune system. Cancer cells secrete and respond to cytokines, chemokines, and DAMPs influencing the nature and quantity of the immune infiltrate. In turn, the type of immune cells present within breast cancer can have a major impact on tumor progression, prognosis and response to treatment. Immune cells can foster a pro-tumorigenic inflammatory environment as well as inhibit tumors (Figure 4). To achieve therapeutic success, any treatment strategy will need to include an approach to shift the balance of pro-tumorigenic and anti-tumor immunity in favor of the latter. The good news is that enlisting the power of the immune system to synergize with cytocidal tumor therapy holds the promise to revolutionize treatment and the hope to achieve long-term tumor control and perhaps cure (Schreiber et al., 2011).

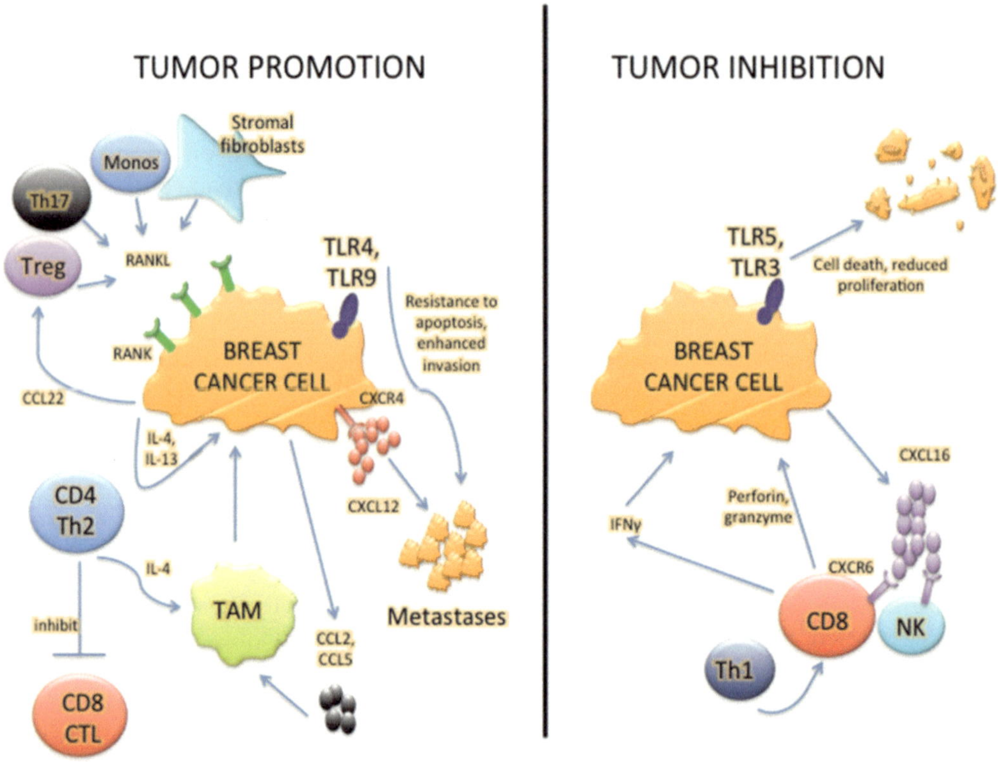

Fig. 4. Immune cells infiltrating breast cancer play a dual role, promoting (left) or inhibiting (right) tumor growth and metastases. Breast cancer cells produce chemokines, such as CCL5 and MCP-1, that recruit monocytic cells which, in the presence of IL-4 secreted by Th2 T cells differentiate into pro-tumorigenic macrophages (TAMs). Breast cancer cells also express chemokine receptors, such as CXCR4, that promote their migration in response to CXCL12, guiding metastases to distant organs. In contrast, other chemokines produced by breast cancer cells, such as CXCL16, promote the recruitment of CXCR6+ anti-tumor CD8 T cells. Activation of TLRs on the surface of breast cancer cells has differential effects that can either promote or inhibit tumor growth. The recruitment of Treg cells by breast tumor cells via secretion of CCL22 contributes to create an immunosuppressive milieu. In addition, RANKL production by Treg and Th17 cells, and possibly other stromal cells, promotes metastases of RANK+ breast cancer cells.

9. Acknowledgments

Sandra Demaria is supported, in part, by NIH R01 CA113851 and a grant from the Chemotherapy Foundation. Karsten A. Pilones is supported by DOD BCRP Post-doctoral fellowship W81XWH-10-1-0007. Sylvia Adams is supported, in part, by NCI K23 CA125205.

10. References

Abel, S., Hundhausen, C., Mentlein, R., Schulte, A., Berkhout, T.A., Broadway, N., Hartmann, D., Sedlacek, R., Dietrich, S., Muetze, B., Schuster, B., Kallen, K.J., Saftig, P., Rose-John, S., &Ludwig, A.(2004) The transmembrane CXC-chemokine ligand 16 is induced by IFN-gamma and TNF-alpha and shed by the activity of the disintegrin-like metalloproteinase ADAM10. *J Immunol*. Vol. 172:pp6362-6372.

Adams, S.(2009) Toll-like receptor agonists in cancer therapy. *Immunotherapy*. Vol. 1:pp949-964.

Allavena, P., Sica, A., Garlanda, C., &Mantovani, A.(2008) The Yin-Yang of tumor-associated macrophages in neoplastic progression and immune surveillance. *Immunol Rev*. Vol. 222:pp155-161.

Apetoh, L., Ghiringhelli, F., Tesniere, A., Criollo, A., Ortiz, C., Lidereau, R., Mariette, C., Chaput, N., Mira, J.-P., Delaloge, S., Andre, F., Tursz, T., Kroemer, G., &Zitvogel, L.(2007a) The interaction between HMGB1 and TLR4 dictates the outcome of anticancer chemotherapy and radiotherapy. *Immunological Reviews*. Vol. 220:pp47-59.

Apetoh, L., Ghiringhelli, F., Tesniere, A., Obeid, M., Ortiz, C., Criollo, A., Mignot, G., Maiuri, M.C., Ullrich, E., Saulnier, P., Yang, H., Amigorena, S., Ryffel, B., Barrat, F.J., Saftig, P., Levi, F., Lidereau, R., Nogues, C., Mira, J.-P., Chompret, A., Joulin, V., Clavel-Chapelon, F., Bourhis, J., Andre, F., Delaloge, S., Tursz, T., Kroemer, G., &Zitvogel, L.(2007b) Toll-like receptor 4-dependent contribution of the immune system to anticancer chemotherapy and radiotherapy. *Nat Med*. Vol. 13:pp1050-1059.

Apetoh, L., Ghiringhelli, F., Tesniere, A., Obeid, M., Ortiz, C., Criollo, A., Mignot, G., Maiuri, M.C., Ullrich, E., Saulnier, P., Yang, H., Amigorena, S., Ryffel, B., Barrat, F.J., Saftig, P., Levi, F., Lidereau, R., Nogues, C., Mira, J.P., Chompret, A., Joulin, V., Clavel-Chapelon, F., Bourhis, J., André, F., Delaloge, S., Tursz, T., Kroemer, G., &Zitvogel, L.(2007c) Toll-like receptor 4-dependent contribution of the immune system to anticancer chemotherapy and radiotherapy. *Nat Med*. Vol. 13:pp1050-1059.

Aspord, C., Pedroza-Gonzalez, A., Gallegos, M., Tindle, S., Burton, E.C., Su, D., Marches, F., Banchereau, J., &Palucka, A.K.(2007) Breast cancer instructs dendritic cells to prime interleukin 13-secreting CD4+ T cells that facilitate tumor development. *J Exp Med*. Vol. 204:pp1037-1047.

Balkwill, F.(2004) Cancer and the chemokine network. *Nat Rev Cancer*. Vol. 4:pp540-550.

Barcellos-Hoff, M.H., &Akhurst, R.J.(2009) Transforming growth factor-beta in breast cancer: too much, too late. *Breast Cancer Res*. Vol. 11:pp202.

Barton, G.M., &Medzhitov, R.(2002) Toll-like receptors and their ligands. *Current Topics in Microbiology & Immunology*. Vol. 270:pp81-92.

Bates, G.J., Fox, S.B., Han, C., Leek, R.D., Garcia, J.F., Harris, A.L., &Banham, A.H.(2006) Quantification of regulatory T cells enables the identification of high-risk breast cancer patients and those at risk of late relapse. *J Clin Oncol*. Vol. 24:pp5373-5380.

Bell, D., Chomarat, P., Broyles, D., Netto, G., Harb, G.M., Lebecque, S., Valladeau, J., Davoust, J., Palucka, K.A., &Banchereau, J.(1999) In breast carcinoma tissue, immature dendritic cells reside within the tumor, whereas mature dendritic cells are located in peritumoral areas. *J Exp Med*. Vol. 190:pp1417-1426.

Berger, R., Fiegl, H., Goebel, G., Obexer, P., Ausserlechner, M., Doppler, W., Hauser-Kronberger, C., Reitsamer, R., Egle, D., Reimer, D., Muller-Holzner, E., Jones, A., &Widschwendter, M.(2010) Toll-like receptor 9 expression in breast and ovarian cancer is associated with poorly differentiated tumors. *Cancer Science*. Vol. 101:pp1059-1066.

Bianchi, M.E.(2007) DAMPs, PAMPs and alarmins: all we need to know about danger. *J Leukoc Biol*. Vol. 81:pp1-5.

Bingle, L., Brown, N.J., &Lewis, C.E.(2002) The role of tumour-associated macrophages in tumour progression: implications for new anticancer therapies. *J Pathol*. Vol. 196:pp254-265.

Boissonnas, A., Scholer-Dahirel, A., Simon-Blancal, V., Pace, L., Valet, F., Kissenpfennig, A., Sparwasser, T., Malissen, B., Fetler, L., &Amigorena, S.(2010) Foxp3+ T cells induce perforin-dependent dendritic cell death in tumor-draining lymph nodes. *Immunity*. Vol. 32:pp266-278.

Cai, Z., Sanchez, A., Shi, Z., Zhang, T., Liu, M., &Zhang, D.(2011) Activation of Toll-like Receptor 5 on Breast Cancer Cells by Flagellin Suppresses Cell Proliferation and Tumor Growth. *Cancer Research*. Vol. 71:pp2466-2475.

Calabrò, A., Beissbarth, T., Kuner, R., Stojanov, M., Benner, A., Asslaber, M., Ploner, F., Zatloukal, K., Samonigg, H., Poustka, A., &Sültmann, H.(2009) Effects of infiltrating lymphocytes and estrogen receptor on gene expression and prognosis in breast cancer. *Breast Cancer Res Treat*. Vol. 116:pp69-77.

Chiron, D., Bekeredjian-Ding, I., Pellat-Deceunynck, C., Bataille, R., &Jego, G.(2008) Toll-like receptors: lessons to learn from normal and malignant human B cells. *Blood*. Vol. 112:pp2205-2213.

Chiron, D., Pellat-Deceunynck, C., Maillasson, M., Bataille, R., &Jego, G.(2009) Phosphorothioate-modified TLR9 ligands protect cancer cells against TRAIL-induced apoptosis. *J Immunol*. Vol. 183:pp4371-4377.

Conforti, R., Ma, Y., Morel, Y., Paturel, C., Terme, M., Viaud, S., Ryffel, B., Ferrantini, M., Uppaluri, R., Schreiber, R., Combadiere, C., Chaput, N., Andre, F., Kroemer, G., &Zitvogel, L.(2010) Opposing effects of toll-like receptor (TLR3) signaling in tumors can be therapeutically uncoupled to optimize the anticancer efficacy of TLR3 ligands. *Cancer Research*. Vol. 70:pp490-500.

Dannull, J., Su, Z., Rizzieri, D., Yang, B.K., Coleman, D., Yancey, D., Zhang, A., Dahm, P., Chao, N., Gilboa, E., &Vieweg, J.(2005) Enhancement of vaccine-mediated antitumor immunity in cancer patients after depletion of regulatory T cells. *J Clin Invest*. Vol. 115:pp3623-3633.

Darash-Yahana, M., Gillespie, J.W., Hewitt, S.M., Chen, Y.Y., Maeda, S., Stein, I., Singh, S.P., Bedolla, R.B., Peled, A., Troyer, D.A., Pikarsky, E., Karin, M., &Farber, J.M.(2009) The chemokine CXCL16 and its receptor, CXCR6, as markers and promoters of inflammation-associated cancers. *PLoS One*. Vol. 4:ppe6695.

Demaria, S., Kawashima, N., Yang, A.M., Devitt, M.-L., Babb, J.S., Allison, J.P., &Formenti, S.C.(2005) Immune-mediated inhibition of metastases following treatment with local radiation and CTLA-4 blockade in a mouse model of breast cancer. *Clin Cancer Res*. Vol. 11:pp728-734.

Demaria, S., Pikarsky, E., Karin, M., Coussens, L.M., Chen, Y.C., El-Omar, E.M., Trinchieri, G., Dubinett, S.M., Mao, J.T., Szabo, E., Krieg, A., Weiner, G.J., Fox, B.A., Coukos, G., Wang, E., Abraham, R.T., Carbone, M., &Lotze, M.T.(2010) Cancer and inflammation: promise for biologic therapy. *J Immunother*. Vol. 33:pp335-351.

DeNardo, D.G., Barreto, J.B., Andreu, P., Vasquez, L., Tawfik, D., Kolhatkar, N., &Coussens, L.M.(2009) CD4(+) T cells regulate pulmonary metastasis of mammary carcinomas by enhancing protumor properties of macrophages. *Cancer Cell*. Vol. 16:pp91-102.

DeNardo, D.G., &Coussens, L.M.(2007) Inflammation and breast cancer. Balancing immune response: crosstalk between adaptive and innate immune cells during breast cancer progression. *Breast Cancer Res*. Vol. 9:pp212.

DeNardo, D.G., Donal J. Brennan, D.J., Rexhepaj, E., Ruffell, B., Shiao, S.L., Madden, S.F., Gallagher, W.M., Wadhwani, N., Scott D. Keil, S.D., Junaid, S.A., Rugo, H.S., Hwang, E.S., Jirström, K., West, B.L., &Coussens, L.M.(2011) Leukocyte Complexity Predicts Breast Cancer Survival and Functionally Regulates Response to Chemotherapy. *Cancer Discov*. Vol. doi:10.1158/2159-8274.CD-10-0028.

Denkert, C., Loibl, S., Noske, A., Roller, M., Muller, B.M., Komor, M., Budczies, J., Darb-Esfahani, S., Kronenwett, R., Hanusch, C., von Torne, C., Weichert, W., Engels, K., Solbach, C., Schrader, I., Dietel, M., &von Minckwitz, G.(2010) Tumor-associated lymphocytes as an independent predictor of response to neoadjuvant chemotherapy in breast cancer.[Erratum appears in J Clin Oncol. 2010 Feb 1;28(4):708]. *Journal of Clinical Oncology*. Vol. 28:pp105-113.

Desmedt, C., Haibe-Kains, B., Wirapati, P., Buyse, M., Larsimont, D., Bontempi, G., Delorenzi, M., Piccart, M., &Sotiriou, C.(2008) Biological processes associated with breast cancer clinical outcome depend on the molecular subtypes. *Clin Cancer Res*. Vol. 14:pp5158-5165.

Disis, M.L.(2010) Immune regulation of cancer. *J Clin Oncol*. Vol. 28:pp4531-4538.

Emens, L.A., Asquith, J.M., Leatherman, J.M., Kobrin, B.J., Petrik, S., Laiko, M., Levi, J., Daphtary, M.M., Biedrzycki, B., Wolff, A.C., Stearns, V., Disis, M.L., Ye, X., Piantadosi, S., Fetting, J.H., Davidson, N.E., &Jaffee, E.M.(2009) Timed sequential treatment with cyclophosphamide, doxorubicin, and an allogeneic granulocyte-macrophage colony-stimulating factor-secreting breast tumor vaccine: a chemotherapy dose-ranging factorial study of safety and immune activation. *Journal of Clinical Oncology*. Vol. 27:pp5911-5918.

Eton, O., Kharkevitch, D.D., Gianan, M.A., Ross, M.I., Itoh, K., Pride, M.W., Donawho, C., Buzaid, A.C., Mansfield, P.F., Lee, J.E., Legha, S.S., Plager, C., Papadopoulos, N.E., Bedikian, A.Y., Benjamin, R.S., &Balch, C.M.(1998) Active immunotherapy with ultraviolet B-irradiated autologous whole melanoma cells plus DETOX in patients with metastatic melanoma. *Clinical Cancer Research*. Vol. 4:pp619-627.

Finak, G., Bertos, N., Pepin, F., Sadekova, S., Souleimanova, M., Zhao, H., Chen, H., Omeroglu, G., Meterissian, S., Omeroglu, A., Hallett, M., &Park, M.(2008) Stromal gene expression predicts clinical outcome in breast cancer. *Nat Med*. Vol. 14:pp518-527.

Formenti, S.C., &Demaria, S.(2009) Systemic effects of local radiotherapy. *Lancet Oncol*. Vol. 10:pp718-726.

Fridlender, Z.G., Sun, J., Kim, S., Kapoor, V., Cheng, G., Ling, L., Worthen, G.S., &Albelda, S.M.(2009) Polarization of tumor-associated neutrophil phenotype by TGF-beta: "N1" versus "N2" TAN. *Cancer Cell*. Vol. 16:pp183-194.

Galli, R., Starace, D., Busa, R., Angelini, D.F., Paone, A., De Cesaris, P., Filippini, A., Sette, C., Battistini, L., Ziparo, E., &Riccioli, A.(2010) TLR stimulation of prostate tumor cells induces chemokine-mediated recruitment of specific immune cell types. *Journal of Immunology*. Vol. 184:pp6658-6669.

Gallucci, S., Lolkema, M., &Matzinger, P.(1999) Natural adjuvants: endogenous activators of dendritic cells. *Nat Med*. Vol. 5:pp1249-1255.

Ghiringhelli, F., Apetoh, L., Tesniere, A., Aymeric, L., Ma, Y., Ortiz, C., Vermaelen, K., Panaretakis, T., Mignot, G., Ullrich, E., Perfettini, J.L., Schlemmer, F., Tasdemir, E., Uhl, M., Génin, P., Civas, A., Ryffel, B., Kanellopoulos, J., Tschopp, J., André, F., Lidereau, R., McLaughlin, N.M., Haynes, N.M., Smyth, M.J., Kroemer, G., &Zitvogel, L.(2009) Activation of the NLRP3 inflammasome in dendritic cells induces IL-1beta-dependent adaptive immunity against tumors. *Nat Med*. Vol. 15:pp1170-1178.

Gilliet, M., Cao, W., &Liu, Y.-J.(2008) Plasmacytoid dendritic cells: sensing nucleic acids in viral infection and autoimmune diseases. *Nature Reviews Immunology*. Vol. 8:pp594-606.

Gobert, M., Treilleux, I., Bendriss-Vermare, N., Bachelot, T., Goddard-Leon, S., Arfi, V., Biota, C., Doffin, A.C., Durand, I., Olive, D., Perez, S., Pasqual, N., Faure, C., Ray-Coquard, I., Puisieux, A., Caux, C., Blay, J.Y., &Ménétrier-Caux, C.(2009) Regulatory T cells recruited through CCL22/CCR4 are selectively activated in lymphoid infiltrates surrounding primary breast tumors and lead to an adverse clinical outcome. *Cancer Res*. Vol. 69:pp2000-2009.

Goldberg-Bittman, L., Neumark, E., Sagi-Assif, O., Azenshtein, E., Meshel, T., Witz, I.P., &Ben-Baruch, A.(2004) The expression of the chemokine receptor CXCR3 and its ligand, CXCL10, in human breast adenocarcinoma cell lines. *Immunol Lett*. Vol. 92:pp171-178.

Gonzalez-Reyes, S., Marin, L., Gonzalez, L., Gonzalez, L.O., del Casar, J.M., Lamelas, M.L., Gonzalez-Quintana, J.M., &Vizoso, F.J.(2010) Study of TLR3, TLR4 and TLR9 in breast carcinomas and their association with metastasis. *BMC Cancer*. Vol. 10:pp665.

Gonzalez-Suarez, E., Jacob, A.P., Jones, J., Miller, R., Roudier-Meyer, M.P., Erwert, R., Pinkas, J., Branstetter, D., &Dougall, W.C.(2010) RANK ligand mediates progestin-induced mammary epithelial proliferation and carcinogenesis. *Nature*. Vol. 468:pp103-107.

Gorelik, L., &Flavell, R.A.(2001) Immune-mediated eradication of tumors through the blockade of transforming growth factor-beta signaling in T cells. *Nat Med*. Vol. 7:pp1118-1122.

Gupta, R., Babb, J.S., Singh, B., Chiriboga, L., Liebes, L., Adams, S., &Demaria, S.(2011) The Numbers of FoxP3+ Lymphocytes in Sentinel Lymph Nodes of Breast Cancer Patients Correlate With Primary Tumor Size but Not Nodal Status. *Cancer Invest*. Vol. 29:pp419-425.

Gutwein, P., Schramme, A., Sinke, N., Abdel-Bakky, M.S., Voss, B., Obermüller, N., Doberstein, K., Koziolek, M., Fritzsche, F., Johannsen, M., Jung, K., Schaider, H., Altevogt, P., Ludwig, A., Pfeilschifter, J., &Kristiansen, G.(2009) Tumoural CXCL16 expression is a novel prognostic marker of longer survival times in renal cell cancer patients. *Eur J Cancer*. Vol. 45:pp478-489.

Gyorki, D.E., &Lindeman, G.J.(2008) Macrophages, more than just scavengers: their role in breast development and cancer. *ANZ J Surg*. Vol. 78:pp432-436.

Haas, T., Metzger, J., Schmitz, F., Heit, A., Muller, T., Latz, E., &Wagner, H.(2008) The DNA sugar backbone 2' deoxyribose determines toll-like receptor 9 activation. *Immunity*. Vol. 28:pp315-323.

Hanahan, D., &Weinberg, R.A.(2011) Hallmarks of cancer: the next generation. *Cell*. Vol. 144:pp646-674.

Harmey, J.H., Bucana, C.D., Lu, W., Byrne, A.M., McDonnell, S., Lynch, C., Bouchier-Hayes, D., &Dong, Z.(2002) Lipopolysaccharide-induced metastatic growth is associated with increased angiogenesis, vascular permeability and tumor cell invasion. *International Journal of Cancer*. Vol. 101:pp415-422.

He, W., Liu, Q., Wang, L., Chen, W., Li, N., &Cao, X.(2007) TLR4 signaling promotes immune escape of human lung cancer cells by inducing immunosuppressive cytokines and apoptosis resistance. *Mol Immunol*. Vol. 44:pp2850-2859.

Heckel, M.C., Wolfson, A., Slachta, C.A., Schwarting, R., Salgame, P., Katsetos, C.D., &Platsoucas, C.D.(2011) Human breast tumor cells express IL-10 and IL-12p40 transcripts and proteins, but do not produce IL-12p70. *Cell Immunol*. Vol. 266:pp143-153.

Hojo, S., Koizumi, K., Tsuneyama, K., Arita, Y., Cui, Z., Shinohara, K., Minami, T., Hashimoto, I., Nakayama, T., Sakurai, H., Takano, Y., Yoshie, O., Tsukada, K., &Saiki, I.(2007) High-level expression of chemokine CXCL16 by tumor cells correlates with a good prognosis and increased tumor-infiltrating lymphocytes in colorectal cancer. *Cancer Res*. Vol. 67:pp4725-4731.

Huang, B., Zhao, J., Unkeless, J.C., Feng, Z.H., &Xiong, H.(2008) TLR signaling by tumor and immune cells: a double-edged sword. *Oncogene*. Vol. 27:pp218-224.

Iwasaki, A., &Medzhitov, R.(2004) Toll-like receptor control of the adaptive immune responses. *Nature Immunology*. Vol. 5:pp987-995.

Jego, G., Bataille, R., Geffroy-Luseau, A., Descamps, G., &Pellat-Deceunynck, C.(2006) Pathogen-associated molecular patterns are growth and survival factors for human myeloma cells through Toll-like receptors. *Leukemia*. Vol. 20:pp1130-1137.

Jones, D.H., Nakashima, T., Sanchez, O.H., Kozieradzki, I., Komarova, S.V., Sarosi, I., Morony, S., Rubin, E., Sarao, R., Hojilla, C.V., Komnenovic, V., Kong, Y.-Y., Schreiber, M., Dixon, S.J., Sims, S.M., Khokha, R., Wada, T., &Penninger, J.M.(2006) Regulation of cancer cell migration and bone metastasis by RANKL. *Nature*. Vol. 440:pp692-696.

Karnoub, A.E., Dash, A.B., Vo, A.P., Sullivan, A., Brooks, M.W., Bell, G.W., Richardson, A.L., Polyak, K., Tubo, R., &Weinberg, R.A.(2007) Mesenchymal stem cells within tumour stroma promote breast cancer metastasis. *Nature*. Vol. 449:pp557-563.

Kelly, M.G., Alvero, A.B., Chen, R., Silasi, D.-A., Abrahams, V.M., Chan, S., Visintin, I., Rutherford, T., &Mor, G.(2006) TLR-4 signaling promotes tumor growth and paclitaxel chemoresistance in ovarian cancer. *Cancer Research*. Vol. 66:pp3859-3868.

Kim, C.H., Johnston, B., &Butcher, E.C.(2002) Trafficking machinery of NKT cells: shared and differential chemokine receptor expression among V alpha 24(+)V beta 11(+) NKT cell subsets with distinct cytokine-producing capacity. *Blood*. Vol. 100:pp11-16.

Kim, C.H., Kunkel, E.J., Boisvert, J., Johnston, B., Campbell, J.J., Genovese, M.C., Greenberg, H.B., &Butcher, E.C.(2001) Bonzo/CXCR6 expression defines type 1-polarized T-cell subsets with extralymphoid tissue homing potential. *J Clin Invest*. Vol. 107:pp595-601.

Kim, R., Emi, M., Tanabe, K., &Arihiro, K.(2006) Immunobiology of the sentinel lymph node and its potential role for antitumour immunity. *Lancet Oncol*. Vol. 7:pp1006-1016.

Kim, W.Y., Lee, J.W., Choi, J.J., Choi, C.H., Kim, T.J., Kim, B.G., Song, S.Y., &Bae, D.S.(2008) Increased expression of Toll-like receptor 5 during progression of cervical neoplasia. *Int J Gynecol Cancer*. Vol. 18:pp300-305.

Kobie, J.J., Wu, R.S., Kurt, R.A., Lou, S., Adelman, M.K., Whitesell, L.J., Ramanathapuram, L.V., Arteaga, C.L., &Akporiave, E.T.(2003) Transforming growth factor beta inhibits the antigen-presenting functions and antitumor activity of dendritic cell vaccines. *Cancer Res*. Vol. 63:pp1860-1864.

Kopp, E., &Medzhitov, R.(2003) Recognition of microbial infection by Toll-like receptors. *Current Opinion in Immunology*. Vol. 15:pp396-401.

Kreike, B., van Kouwenhove, M., Horlings, H., Weigelt, B., Peterse, H., Bartelink, H., &van de Vijver, M.J.(2007) Gene expression profiling and histopathological characterization of triple-negative/basal-like breast carcinomas. *Breast Cancer Res*. Vol. 9:ppR65.

Krieg, A.M.(2008) Toll-like receptor 9 (TLR9) agonists in the treatment of cancer. *Oncogene*. Vol. 27:pp161-167.

Kunkel, E.J., &Butcher, E.C.(2002) Chemokines and the tissue-specific migration of lymphocytes. *Immunity*. Vol. 16:pp1-4.

Kurt-Jones, E.A., Popova, L., Kwinn, L., Haynes, L.M., Jones, L.P., Tripp, R.A., Walsh, E.E., Freeman, M.W., Golenbock, D.T., Anderson, L.J., &Finberg, R.W.(2000) Pattern recognition receptors TLR4 and CD14 mediate response to respiratory syncytial virus. *Nature Immunology*. Vol. 1:pp398-401.

Lacour, J., Lacour, F., Spira, A., Michelson, M., Petit, J.Y., Delage, G., Sarrazin, D., Contesso, G., &Viguier, J.(1980) Adjuvant treatment with polyadenylic-polyuridylic acid (Polya.Polyu) in operable breast cancer. *Lancet*. Vol. 2:pp161-164.

Leibbrandt, A., &Penninger, J.M.(2008) RANK/RANKL: regulators of immune responses and bone physiology. *Ann N Y Acad Sci*. Vol. 1143:pp123-150.

Lin, S., Sun, L., Hu, J., Wan, S., Zhao, R., Yuan, S., &Zhang, L.(2009) Chemokine C-X-C motif receptor 6 contributes to cell migration during hypoxia. *Cancer Lett*. Vol. 279:pp108-117.

Liu, L., Botos, I., Wang, Y., Leonard, J.N., Shiloach, J., Segal, D.M., &Davies, D.R.(2008) Structural basis of toll-like receptor 3 signaling with double-stranded RNA. *Science*. Vol. 320:pp379-381.

Liu-Bryan, R., Scott, P., Sydlaske, A., Rose, D.M., &Terkeltaub, R.(2005) Innate immunity conferred by Toll-like receptors 2 and 4 and myeloid differentiation factor 88 expression is pivotal to monosodium urate monohydrate crystal-induced inflammation. *Arthritis & Rheumatism*. Vol. 52:pp2936-2946.

Lu, H., Wagner, W.M., Gad, E., Yang, Y., Duan, H., Amon, L.M., Van Denend, N., Larson, E.R., Chang, A., Tufvesson, H., &Disis, M.L.(2010) Treatment failure of a TLR-7 agonist occurs due to self-regulation of acute inflammation and can be overcome by IL-10 blockade. *J Immunol*. Vol. 184:pp5360-5367.

Luboshits, G., Shina, S., Kaplan, O., Engelberg, S., Nass, D., Lifshitz-Mercer, B., Chaitchik, S., Keydar, I., &Ben-Baruch, A.(1999) Elevated expression of the CC chemokine regulated on activation, normal T cell expressed and secreted (RANTES) in advanced breast carcinoma. *Cancer Res*. Vol. 59:pp4681-4687.

Luster, A.D., &Leder, P.(1993) IP-10, a -C-X-C- chemokine, elicits a potent thymus-dependent antitumor response in vivo. *J Exp Med*. Vol. 178:pp1057-1065.

Ma, X., Norsworthy, K., Kundu, N., Rodgers, W.H., Gimotty, P.A., Goloubeva, O., Lipsky, M., Li, Y., Holt, D., &Fulton, A.(2009) CXCR3 expression is associated with poor survival in breast cancer and promotes metastasis in a murine model. *Mol Cancer Ther*. Vol. 8:pp490-498.

MacLean, G.D., Reddish, M., Koganty, R.R., Wong, T., Gandhi, S., Smolenski, M., Samuel, J., Nabholtz, J.M., &Longenecker, B.M.(1993) Immunization of breast cancer patients using a synthetic sialyl-Tn glycoconjugate plus Detox adjuvant. *Cancer Immunol Immunother*. Vol. 36:pp215-222.

Mahmoud, S.M., Paish, E.C., Powe, D.G., Macmillan, R.D., Grainge, M.J., Lee, A.H., Ellis, I.O., &Green, A.R.(2011) Tumor-Infiltrating CD8+ Lymphocytes Predict Clinical Outcome in Breast Cancer. *J Clin Oncol*. Vol. 29:pp1949-1955.

Manegold, C., Gravenor, D., Woytowitz, D., Mezger, J., Hirsh, V., Albert, G., Al-Adhami, M., Readett, D., Krieg, A.M., &Leichman, C.G.(2008) Randomized phase II trial of a toll-like receptor 9 agonist oligodeoxynucleotide, PF-3512676, in combination with first-line taxane plus platinum chemotherapy for advanced-stage non-small-cell lung cancer. *Journal of Clinical Oncology*. Vol. 26:pp3979-3986.

Mantovani, A., Allavena, P., Sica, A., &Balkwill, F.(2008) Cancer-related inflammation. *Nature*. Vol. 454:pp436-444.

Marshak-Rothstein, A.(2006) Toll-like receptors in systemic autoimmune disease. *Nature Reviews. Immunology*. Vol. 6:pp823-835.

Mason, K.A., Neal, R., Hunter, N., Ariga, H., Ang, K., &Milas, L.(2006) CpG oligodeoxynucleotides are potent enhancers of radio- and chemoresponses of murine tumors. *Radiotherapy & Oncology*. Vol. 80:pp192-198.

Matsumura, S., Wang, B., Kawashima, N., Braunstein, S., Badura, M., Cameron, T.O., Babb, J.S., Schneider, R.J., Formenti, S.C., Dustin, M.L., &Demaria, S.(2008) Radiation-induced CXCL16 release by breast cancer cells attracts effector T cells. *J Immunol*. Vol. 181:pp3099-3107.

Merrell, M.A., Ilvesaro, J.M., Lehtonen, N., Sorsa, T., Gehrs, B., Rosenthal, E., Chen, D., Shackley, B., Harris, K.W., &Selander, K.S.(2006) Toll-like receptor 9 agonists promote cellular invasion by increasing matrix metalloproteinase activity. *Molecular Cancer Research: MCR*. Vol. 4:pp437-447.

Mori, K., Le Goff, B., Berreur, M., Riet, A., Moreau, A., Blanchard, F., Chevalier, C., Guisle-Marsollier, I., Leger, J., Guicheux, J., Masson, M., Gouin, F., Redini, F., &Heymann, D.(2007a) Human osteosarcoma cells express functional receptor activator of nuclear factor-kappa B. *J Pathol.* Vol. 211:pp555-562.

Mori, K., Le Goff, B., Charrier, C., Battaglia, S., Heymann, D., &Redini, F.(2007b) DU145 human prostate cancer cells express functional receptor activator of NFkappaB: new insights in the prostate cancer bone metastasis process. *Bone.* Vol. 40:pp981-990.

Muller, A., Homey, B., Soto, H., Ge, N., Catron, D., Buchanan, M.E., McClanahan, T., Murphy, E., Yuan, W., Wagner, S.N., Barrera, J.L., Mohar, A., Verastegui, E., &Zlotnik, A.(2001) Involvement of chemokine receptors in breast cancer metastasis. *Nature.* Vol. 410:pp50-56.

Nakayama, T., Hieshima, K., Izawa, D., Tatsumi, Y., Kanamaru, A., &Yoshie, O.(2003) Cutting edge: profile of chemokine receptor expression on human plasma cells accounts for their efficient recruitment to target tissues. *J Immunol.* Vol. 170:pp1136-1140.

Nam, J.S., Terabe, M., Kang, M.J., Chae, H., Voong, N., Yang, Y.A., Laurence, A., Michalowska, A., Mamura, M., Lonning, S., Berzofsky, J.A., &Wakefield, L.M.(2008) Transforming growth factor beta subverts the immune system into directly promoting tumor growth through interleukin-17. *Cancer research.* Vol. 68:pp3915-3923.

Obeid, M., Tesniere, A., Ghiringhelli, F., Fimia, G.M., Apetoh, L., Perfettini, J.L., Castedo, M., Mignot, G., Panaretakis, T., Casares, N., Metivier, D., Larochette, N., van Endert, P., Ciccosanti, F., Piacentini, M., Zitvogel, L., &Kroemer, G.(2007) Calreticulin exposure dictates the immunogenicity of cancer cell death. *Nat Med.* Vol. 13:pp54-61.

Ohashi, K., Burkart, V., Flohe, S., &Kolb, H.(2000) Cutting edge: heat shock protein 60 is a putative endogenous ligand of the toll-like receptor-4 complex. *Journal of Immunology.* Vol. 164:pp558-561.

Ohta, A., Gorelik, E., Prasad, S.J., Ronchese, F., Lukashev, D., Wong, M.K., Huang, X., Caldwell, S., Liu, K., Smith, P., Chen, J.F., Jackson, E.K., Apasov, S., Abrams, S., &Sitkovsky, M.(2006) A2A adenosine receptor protects tumors from antitumor T cells. *Proc Natl Acad Sci U S A.* Vol. 103:pp13132-13137.

Okamura, Y., Watari, M., Jerud, E.S., Young, D.W., Ishizaka, S.T., Rose, J., Chow, J.C., &Strauss, J.F., 3rd.(2001) The extra domain A of fibronectin activates Toll-like receptor 4. *Journal of Biological Chemistry.* Vol. 276:pp10229-10233.

Petricevic, B., Vrbanec, D., Jakic-Razumovic, J., Brcic, I., Rabic, D., Badovinac, T., Ozimec, E., &Bali, V.(2011) Expression of Toll-like receptor 4 and beta 1 integrin in breast cancer. *Medical Oncology.* Vol.:pp1-9.

Pidgeon, G.P., Harmey, J.H., Kay, E., Da Costa, M., Redmond, H.P., &Bouchier-Hayes, D.J.(1999) The role of endotoxin/lipopolysaccharide in surgically induced tumour growth in a murine model of metastatic disease. *British Journal of Cancer.* Vol. 81:pp1311-1317.

Pollard, J.W.(2004) Tumour-educated macrophages promote tumour progression and metastasis. *Nat Rev Cancer.* Vol. 4:pp71-78.

Qian, B.Z., Li, J., Zhang, H., Kitamura, T., Zhang, J., Campion, L.R., Kaiser, E.A., Snyder, L.A., &Pollard, J.W.(2011) CCL2 recruits inflammatory monocytes to facilitate breast-tumour metastasis. *Nature*. Vol. Jun 8. doi: 10.1038/nature10138. [Epub ahead of print]

Qiu, J., Wang, X., Guo, X., Zhao, C., Wu, X., &Zhang, Y.(2009) Toll-like receptor 9 agonist inhibits ERalpha-mediated transactivation by activating NF-kappaB in breast cancer cell lines. *Oncology Reports*. Vol. 22:pp935-941.

Rassa, J.C., Meyers, J.L., Zhang, Y., Kudaravalli, R., &Ross, S.R.(2002) Murine retroviruses activate B cells via interaction with toll-like receptor 4. *Proceedings of the National Academy of Sciences of the United States of America*. Vol. 99:pp2281-2286.

Rech, A.J., &Vonderheide, R.H.(2009) Clinical use of anti-CD25 antibody daclizumab to enhance immune responses to tumor antigen vaccination by targeting regulatory T cells. *Ann N Y Acad Sci*. Vol. 1174:pp99-106.

Roelofs, M.F., Boelens, W.C., Joosten, L.A.B., Abdollahi-Roodsaz, S., Geurts, J., Wunderink, L.U., Schreurs, B.W., van den Berg, W.B., &Radstake, T.R.D.J.(2006) Identification of small heat shock protein B8 (HSP22) as a novel TLR4 ligand and potential involvement in the pathogenesis of rheumatoid arthritis. *Journal of Immunology*. Vol. 176:pp7021-7027.

Saji, H., Koike, M., Yamori, T., Saji, S., Seiki, M., Matsushima, K., &Toi, M.(2001) Significant correlation of monocyte chemoattractant protein-1 expression with neovascularization and progression of breast carcinoma. *Cancer*. Vol. 92:pp1085-1091.

Salaun, B., Coste, I., Rissoan, M.-C., Lebecque, S.J., &Renno, T.(2006) TLR3 can directly trigger apoptosis in human cancer cells. *Journal of Immunology*. Vol. 176:pp4894-4901.

Salaun, B., Zitvogel, L., Asselin-Paturel, C., Morel, Y., Chemin, K., Dubois, C., Massacrier, C., Conforti, R., Chenard, M.P., Sabourin, J.-C., Goubar, A., Lebecque, S., Pierres, M., Rimoldi, D., Romero, P., &Andre, F.(2011) TLR3 as a biomarker for the therapeutic efficacy of double-stranded RNA in breast cancer. *Cancer Research*. Vol. 71:pp1607-1614.

Santini, D., Perrone, G., Roato, I., Godio, L., Pantano, F., Grasso, D., Russo, A., Vincenzi, B., Fratto, M.E., Sabbatini, R., Della Pepa, C., Porta, C., Del Conte, A., Schiavon, G., Berruti, A., Tomasino, R.M., Papotti, M., Papapietro, N., Onetti Muda, A., Denaro, V., &Tonini, G.(2011) Expression pattern of receptor activator of NFkappaB (RANK) in a series of primary solid tumors and related bone metastases. *J Cell Physiol*. Vol. 226:pp780-784.

Sato, K., Suematsu, A., Okamoto, K., Yamaguchi, A., Morishita, Y., Kadono, Y., Tanaka, S., Kodama, T., Akira, S., Iwakura, Y., Cua, D.J., &Takayanagi, H.(2006) Th17 functions as an osteoclastogenic helper T cell subset that links T cell activation and bone destruction. *Journal of Experimental Medicine*. Vol. 203:pp2673-2682.

Sato, T., Thorlacius, H., Johnston, B., Staton, T.L., Xiang, W., Littman, D.R., &Butcher, E.C.(2005) Role for CXCR6 in recruitment of activated CD8+ lymphocytes to inflamed liver. *J Immunol*. Vol. 174:pp277-283.

Schmausser, B., Andrulis, M., Endrich, S., Muller-Hermelink, H.-K., &Eck, M.(2005) Toll-like receptors TLR4, TLR5 and TLR9 on gastric carcinoma cells: an implication for interaction with Helicobacter pylori. *Ijmm International Journal of Medical Microbiology*. Vol. 295:pp179-185.

Schramek, D., Leibbrandt, A., Sigl, V., Kenner, L., Pospisilik, J.A., Lee, H.J., Hanada, R., Joshi, P.A., Aliprantis, A., Glimcher, L., Pasparakis, M., Khokha, R., Ormandy, C.J., Widschwendter, M., Schett, G., &Penninger, J.M.(2010) Osteoclast differentiation factor RANKL controls development of progestin-driven mammary cancer. *Nature*. Vol. 468:pp98-102.

Schreiber, R.D., Old, L.J., &Smyth, M.J.(2011) Cancer immunoediting: integrating immunity's roles in cancer suppression and promotion. *Science*. Vol. 331:pp1565-1570.

Sfondrini, L., Rossini, A., Besusso, D., Merlo, A., Tagliabue, E., Menard, S., &Balsari, A.(2006) Antitumor activity of the TLR-5 ligand flagellin in mouse models of cancer. *Journal of Immunology*. Vol. 176:pp6624-6630.

Shimaoka, T., nakayama, T., Kume, N., Takahashi, S., Yamaguchi, J., Minami, M., Hayashida, K., Kita, T., Ohsumi, J., Yoshie, O., &Yonehara, S.(2003) Cutting edge: SR-PSOX/CXC chemokine ligand 16 mediates bacterial phagocytosis by APCs through its chemokine domain. *J Immunol*. Vol. 171:pp1647-1651.

Soria, G., Yaal-Hahoshen, N., Azenshtein, E., Shina, S., Leider-Trejo, L., Ryvo, L., Cohen-Hillel, E., Shtabsky, A., Ehrlich, M., Meshel, T., Keydar, I., &Ben-Baruch, A.(2008) Concomitant expression of the chemokines RANTES and MCP-1 in human breast cancer: a basis for tumor-promoting interactions. *Cytokine*. Vol. 44:pp191-200.

Tan, W., Zhang, W., Strasner, A., Grivennikov, S., Cheng, J.Q., Hoffman, R.M., &Karin, M.(2011) Tumour-infiltrating regulatory T cells stimulate mammary cancer metastasis through RANKL-RANK signalling. *Nature*. Vol. 470:pp548-553.

Thomas, D.A., &J., M.(2005) TGF-β directly targets cytotoxic T cell functions during tumor evasion of immune surveillance *Cancer Cell*. Vol. 8:pp369-380.

Todaro, M., Lombardo, Y., Francipane, M.G., Alea, M.P., Cammareri, P., Iovino, F., Di Stefano, A.B., Di Bernardo, C., Agrusa, A., Condorelli, G., Walczak, H., &Stassi, G.(2008) Apoptosis resistance in epithelial tumors is mediated by tumor-cell-derived interleukin-4. *Cell Death Differ*. Vol. 15:pp762-772.

Treilleux, I., Blay, J.Y., Bendriss-Vermare, N., Ray-Coquard, I., Bachelot, T., Guastalla, J.P., Bremond, A., Goddard, S., Pin, J.J., Barthelemy-Dubois, C., &Lebecque, S.(2004) Dendritic cell infiltration and prognosis of early stage breast cancer. *Clin Cancer Res*. Vol. 10:pp7466-7474.

Ueno, T., Toi, M., Saji, H., Muta, M., Bando, H., Kuroi, K., Koike, M., Inadera, H., &Matsushima, K.(2000) Significance of macrophage chemoattractant protein-1 in macrophage recruitment, angiogenesis, and survival in human breast cancer. *Clin Cancer Res*. Vol. 6:pp3282-3289.

Unutmaz, D., Xiang, W., Sunshine, M.J., Campbell, J., Butcher, E., &Littman, D.R.(2000) The primate lentiviral receptor Bonzo/STRL33 is coordinately regulated with CCR5 and its expression pattern is conserved between human and mouse. *J Immunol*. Vol. 165:pp3284-3292.

Vabulas, R.M., Braedel, S., Hilf, N., Singh-Jasuja, H., Herter, S., Ahmad-Nejad, P., Kirschning, C.J., Da Costa, C., Rammensee, H.-G., Wagner, H., &Schild, H.(2002) The endoplasmic reticulum-resident heat shock protein Gp96 activates dendritic cells via the Toll-like receptor 2/4 pathway. *Journal of Biological Chemistry*. Vol. 277:pp20847-20853

Valković, T., Lucin, K., Krstulja, M., Dobi-Babić, R., &Jonjić, N.(1998) Expression of monocyte chemotactic protein-1 in human invasive ductal breast cancer. *Pathol Res Pract*. Vol. 194:pp335-340.

Van Poznak, C., Cross, S.S., Saggese, M., Hudis, C., Panageas, K.S., Norton, L., Coleman, R.E., &Holen, I.(2006) Expression of osteoprotegerin (OPG), TNF related apoptosis inducing ligand (TRAIL), and receptor activator of nuclear factor kappaB ligand (RANKL) in human breast tumours. *J Clin Pathol*. Vol. 59:pp56-63.

Vazquez-Martin, A., Colomer, R., &Menendez, J.A.(2007) Protein array technology to detect HER2 (erbB-2)-induced 'cytokine signature' in breast cancer. *Eur J Cancer*. Vol. 43:pp1117-1124.

Walser, T.C., Ma, X., Kundu, N., Dorsey, R., Goloubeva, O., &Fulton, A.M.(2007) Immune-mediated modulation of breast cancer growth and metastasis by the chemokine Mig (CXCL9) in a murine model. *J Immunother*. Vol. 30:pp490-498.

Walser, T.C., Rifat, S., Ma, X., Kundu, N., Ward, C., Goloubeva, O., Johnson, M.G., Medina, J.C., Collins, T.L., &Fulton, A.(2006) Antagonism of CXCR3 inhibits lung metastasis in a murine model of metastatic breast cancer. *Cancer Res*. Vol. 66:pp7701-7707.

Wang, B., Badura, M., He, C., Cameron, T., Dustin, M., Formenti, S.C., Schneider, R.J., &Demaria, S.(2006) CXCR6 and CXCL16 are expressed by breast cancer cells and may play a dual role in tumor progression *Breast Cancer Res Treat*. Vol. 100:ppS299.

Wang, J., Lu, Y., Wang, J., Koch, A.E., Zhang, J., &Taichman, R.S.(2008) CXCR6 induces prostate cancer progression by the AKT/mammalian target of rapamycin signaling pathway. *Cancer Res*. Vol. 68:pp10367-10376.

Wrzesinski, S.H., Wan, Y.Y., &Flavell, R.A.(2007) Transforming growth factor-beta and the immune response: implications for anticancer therapy. *Clin Cancer Res*. Vol. 13:pp5262-5270.

Yamauchi, R., Tanaka, M., Kume, N., Minami, M., Kawamoto, T., Togi, K., Shimaoka, T., Takahashi, S., Yamaguchi, J., Nishina, T., Kitaichi, M., Komeda, M., Manabe, T., Yonehara, S., &Kita, T.(2004) Upregulation of SR-PSOX/CXCL16 and recruitment of CD8+ T cells in cardiac valves during inflammatory valvular heart disease. *Arterioscler Thromb Vasc Biol*. Vol. 24:pp282-287.

Yang, H., Zhou, H., Feng, P., Zhou, X., Wen, H., Xie, X., Shen, H., &Zhu, X.(2010) Reduced expression of Toll-like receptor 4 inhibits human breast cancer cells proliferation and inflammatory cytokines secretion. *Journal of Experimental & Clinical Cancer Research*. Vol. 29:pp92.

Yu, L., &Chen, S.(2008) Toll-like receptors expressed in tumor cells: targets for therapy. *Cancer Immunol Immunother*. Vol. 57:pp1271-1278.

Zeh, H.J.r., &Lotze, M.T.(2005) Addicted to death: invasive cancer and the immune response to unscheduled cell death. *J Immunother*. Vol. 28:pp1-9.

Zhou, M., McFarland-Mancini, M.M., Funk, H.M., Husseinzadeh, N., Mounajjed, T., &Drew, A.F.(2009) Toll-like receptor expression in normal ovary and ovarian tumors. *Cancer Immunol Immunother*. Vol. 58:pp1375-1385.

Zitvogel, L., Apetoh, L., Ghiringhelli, F., André, F., Tesniere, A., &Kroemer, G.(2008) The anticancer immune response: indispensable for therapeutic success? *J Clin Invest.* Vol. 118:pp1991-2001.

Zitvogel, L., Kepp, O., &Kroemer, G.(2010) Decoding cell death signals in inflammation and immunity. *Cell.* Vol. 140:pp798-804.

Zitvogel, L., Kepp, O., &Kroemer, G.(2011) Immune parameters affecting the efficacy of chemotherapeutic regimens. *Nat Rev Clin Oncol.* Vol. 8:pp151-160,I S S N

23

Engineering Transcription Factors in Breast Cancer Stem Cells

Pilar Blancafort, Karla Oyuky Juarez,
Sabine Stolzenburg and Adriana S. Beltran
*Department of Pharmacology, the University of North Carolina at Chapel Hill,
Chapel Hill, NC
United States of America*

1. Introduction

Breast cancers are classified in at least six different subtypes (normal-like, luminal A, luminal B, Her2, basal-like, claudin-low), which are characterized by distinct genome-wide transcriptional profiles and response to therapy [1]. Recently, it has been shown that these intrinsic types of breast cancers are associated with unique DNA-methylation patterns [2,3,4]. In 2009, a large-scale genomic analysis of breast cancer cohorts has identified a novel subtype of breast cancer enriched in putative cancer stem-cell (CSC) markers, named claudin-low [5]. In addition to cancer or stem cell signatures, claudin-low tumors are enriched in Epithelial-to-Mesenchymal transition (EMT) markers, such as high expression of the Transcription Factors (TFs) Twist and Snail, and loss of epithelial junction proteins, such as cadherins, claudins and ocludins. Together with basal-like breast cancers, claudin-low carcinomas are mostly triple negative, hence their lack of expression of the Estrogen Receptor (ER), Progesterone Receptor (PR) and Her2. Consequently, these carcinomas are refractory to regimens to treat breast cancers, such as anti-estrogens and conventional chemotherapy. Similarly to these breast cancers, a subtype of serious epithelial ovarian cancers also appear to be poorly differentiated, high grade, and associated with poor clinical outcome. These serous epithelial ovarian tumors, named type II, are often associated with p53 and BRCA mutations [6]. Thus, there is a need to develop novel and more effective strategies to target poorly differentiated carcinomas. This will begin with a better understanding of molecular pathways that are activated in these tumors, which maintain aberrant proliferation and potentially, tumor initiation.

Little is known regarding the molecular determinants of tumor initiation and progression in poorly differentiated cancers. it has been proposed that claudin-low and basal-like breast tumors are originated by oncogenic transformation of bipotent stem and progenitor cells, respectively. Consistent with this idea, we found that many Transcription Factors (TFs) normally expressed in both, adult and embryonic stem cells (hESCs), are also over-expressed in poorly differentiated breast and ovarian carcinomas. In the first part of this chapter we will overview oncogenic TFs and TF networks that could play a role in maintaining aberrant self-renewal, with special focus on the OCT4-SOX2-NANOG embryonic TF network. In addition to abnormal reactivation of oncogenic TFs, tumor suppressor genes undergo epigenetic silencing processes during tumor initiation, such as $p16^{INK4A}$ a critical factor involved in immortalization of normal epithelial cells. *Mammary serine protease inhibitor* (*maspin*) is a tumor suppressor epigenetically silenced during metastatic progression of several epithelial cancers, including breast carcinomas. In the second part of the chapter we will describe the design of Artificial Transcription Factors (ATFs) and their potential applications to redirect or reprogram the epigenetic and transcriptional state of aggressive carcinomas towards a more benign or less aggressive phenotype. ATFs are typically composed of arrays of specific six Zinc Finger (ZF) domains, and are designed to bind, unique eighteen base pairs (bps) in targeted promoters. These ZFs are linked to several effector domain functions, which mediate activation, repression or epigenetic regulation of the gene of interest [7]. We will review ATFs generated in our laboratory and others, able to reprogram the epigenetic status of endogenous promoters, oncogenes and tumor suppressors, to revert some of the phenotypic hallmarks of aggressive cancer cells.

1.1 Overview of molecular subtypes of breast cancers

Large-scale genomic analyses of breast cancer patients have revealed that breast cancer is, clinically and biologically, a heterogeneous disease. Moreover, gene expression microarray technology has stratified breast cancer patients in distinct subtypes: normal-like, luminal A, luminal B, Her2, basal-like, claudin-low [1,8,9]. Recently, a novel subtype of breast cancer has been discovered, named claudin-low [5]. Although this subtype affects 5-10 % of all breast cancers, is associated with poor response to conventional therapy and with tumor relapse. Together with the basal-like subtype, the majority of claudin-low carcinomas are triple negative, (Estrogen Receptor (ER), Progesterone Receptor (PR) and Her2 negative [8,10].

One of the molecular hallmarks of claudin-low tumors is the down-regulation of tight junction proteins, such as claudin 3, 4, 7 and E-cadherin (CDH1), and an over-representation of mesenchymal proteins characteristic of stromal cells, such as vimentin. Claudin-low carcinomas express TFs associated with epithelial-to-mesenchymal transition (EMT), including Snail1/2, Twist1/2 and ZEB1/2. Additional characteristics of claudin-low tumors are the enrichment in putative cancer stem-cell signatures, such as high CD44 and low CD24 levels, high degree of lymphocyte infiltration, and resistance to chemotherapy [8,10,11,12].

The cell of origin of breast tumors. Although genome-wide expression analyses have clearly defined subtypes of breast cancer patients, the cell of origin that is target of transformation is still subject of intense investigation and debate. To isolate and characterize the target cell giving rise the distinct subtypes of breast cancer is crucial in order to develop effective, targeted, and tailored therapies. It is generally accepted that human mammary epithelial cell preparations are composed of a hierarchic organization of cell types, where more undifferentiated, multipotent stem cells, can either remain quiescent, self-renew (generating progeny of undifferentiated cells identical to the mother cells) or differentiate towards specific, defined lineages (Figure 1). In addition to specific transcriptional profiles, the subtypes of cells within the breast hierarchy are characterized by distinct epigenetic landscapes, including DNA-methylation [13], and possibly, histone modifications. In addition, stromal cells surrounding the epithelial ductal structures of the mammary gland highly influence the degree of self-renewal or differentiation of stem and progenitor cells. Stromal-tumor cell interactions are of critical importance during tumor formation and progression [14]. For example, Mesenchymal stem cells (MSCs) originated in the bone-

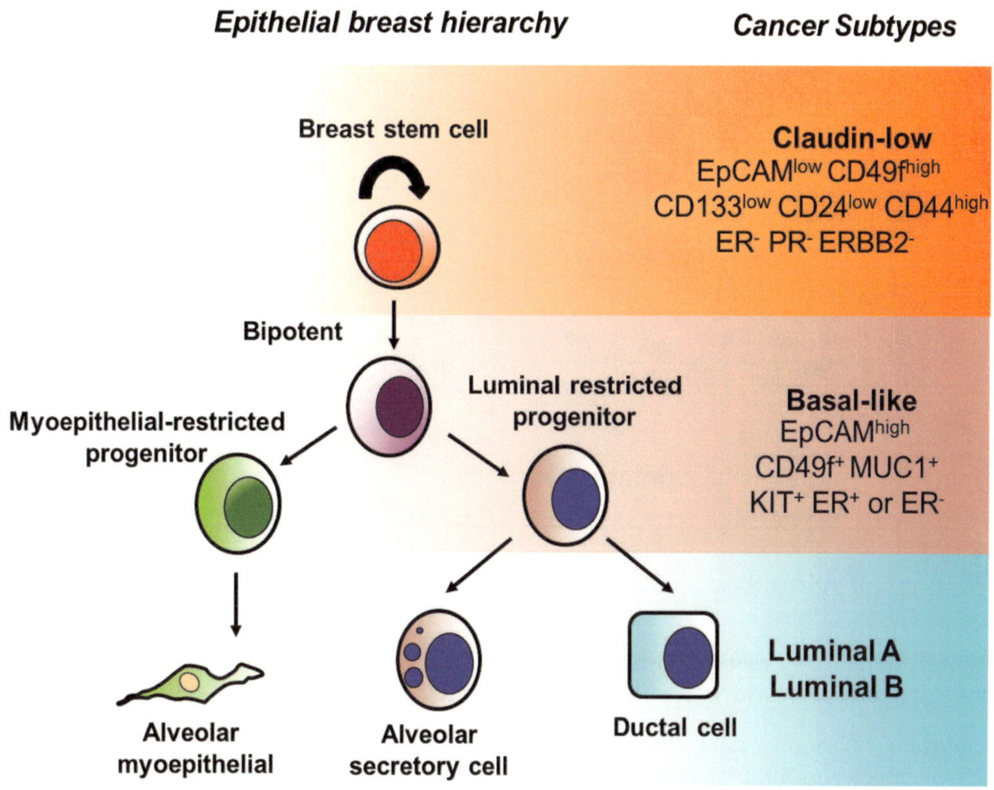

Fig. 1. Schematic representation of the human breast epithelial cell hierarchy and its association with the main breast cancer subtypes. Each subpopulation of breast cells is defined by the expression of selected cell surface markers. Gene expression profiles of these cell populations upon fractionation of the mammary gland and cell sorting, revealed similarities to specific subtypes of breast cancer. Modified from [25].

marrow can home to breast tumors and promote metastasis [15,16]. Fibroblasts or "tumor-associated fibroblasts" can similarly influence the growth and motility of breast epithelial cells [14,17].

Mammary stem cells (MSCs). The mammary epithelium is composed of two main lineages of epithelial cells: an inner layer of luminal cells and an outer sheath of myoepithelial cells (Figure 2). These cells compose the basic architecture of the human mammary gland, named terminal duct lobular units (TDLUs) [18,19]. MSCs are defined as cells having self-renewal ability and able to generate all the cell types of the mammary epithelium [20]. Progenitor cells are more restricted or committed cells having proliferative capabilities. Both stem and primitive progenitors are believed to reside within the ducts of the mammary gland, rather than in the terminal ductal lobular units. Bipotent epithelial cells are capable to fully differentiate in luminal and myoepithelial cells. These cells retain the ability to generate entire TDLUs both *in vitro* and also upon transplantation in nude mice [18,19,20,21]. These primitive cells occupy a suprabasal position *in vivo* and co-express the luminal keratin K19 and the basal-specific keratin K14. The most likely candidates for MSCs are basal positioned small electro-lucent (light) cells (SLCs), occurring at a frequency of 1-3% within the epithelium.

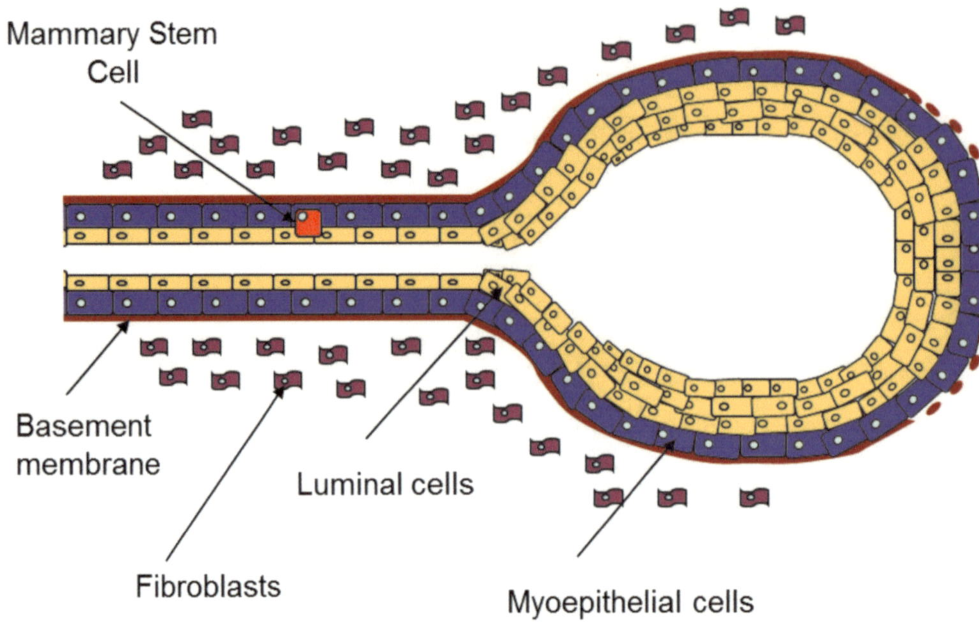

Fig. 2. Schematic representation of a terminal end duct in the mammary gland. Expansion (shown in red) occurs during puberty and pregnancy.

Dontu and colleagues have developed a culture system to isolate and propagate *in vitro* human breast multipotent stem/progenitor cells in a non-differentiated state. They have generated mammospheres (MMS), or non-adherent spherical cell clusters, clonally derived from single cells possessing self-renewal ability. Primary MMS contain eight-times more of bi-potent progenitors than freshly cultured human mammary cells [22,23]. The majority of bi-potent progenitors are able to generate colonies in 3D matrigel cultures containing all the main lineages of the mammary gland [24].

To date, combination of markers for the isolation of human stem/progenitor cells have been proposed based on the ability of the resulting populations to regenerate TDLUs by *in vivo* transplantation experiments. Based on prospective cell surface fractionation markers the current model of breast hierarchy is shown in Figure 1. In this model, the putative human MSC is a $CD49f^{hi}$ $EpCAM^{-/low}$ $CD24^{-}$ $CD133^{-/low}$ ER^{-} PR^{-} ERBB2- and the luminal progenitor is a $CD49f^{+}EpCAM^{+}$ cell [25,26].

In a seminal experiment by Lim *et al.*, gene expression microarray studies of specific (sorted) populations of human breast revealed that the "prospective stem cell population" closely resembles claudin-low tumors (Figure 1). This has intrigued investigators and indicated that the cell of origin target of transformation in claudin-low carcinomas is possibly an early, undifferentiated $EpCAM^{-}$ stem cell. Basal-like breast cancers, which are highly proliferative, mostly triple negative and associated with BRCA mutation carriers, are possibly target of transformation of a more downstream, luminal-restricted, EpCAM+ progenitor. Finally, it has been proposed that both, luminal A and luminal B breast carcinomas are originated from "more" differentiated luminal cells [25].

Stem/progenitor cells as potential targets of transformation. Stem and primitive progenitor cells exhibit the ubiquitous feature of either remaining quiescent or sustaining self-renewal in response to their microenvironment. These cells also undergo an asymmetric cell division and differentiate towards more committed cell lineages [18,21,27,28]. The identification of factors regulating self-renewal and differentiation in the mammary gland is of primary importance, as these factors could be potentially involved in oncogenesis. Unlike somatic cells, which undergo senescence, adult stem cells exist in the period of a life-time of an individual. These "long lived" cells have the potential to accumulate genetic and epigenetic aberrations contributing to oncogenesis [19]. The BRCA1 gene, a major tumor suppressor associated with basal breast cancer, has been shown to regulate human mammary stem/progenitor cell fate. Knock-down of BRCA in primary breast cells leads to an increase in cells displaying the stem/progenitor cell marker ALDH1 and a decrease in cells expressing luminal epithelial markers and estrogen receptor [29]. Similarly, the protein Musashi (Msi1) has been shown to modulate mammary progenitor cell expansion by activation of Wnt and Notch pathways, which are often dys-regulated in breast cancers [30].

Breast Cancer Stem Cells (breast CSCs). It has been demonstrated that only a small population of cancer cells (named "Tumor Initiating Cells, TICs, or Cancer Stem Cells, CSCs) retains the ability to form new tumors after transplantation in immunodeficient mice [31,32,33]. TICs display stem/progenitor cells properties, namely competence for self-renewal and capacity to re-establish tumor heterogeneicity [18]. Like normal stem/progenitor cells, CSCs can be propagated as spheroids cultures, named tumorspheres, when grown in low adherence conditions. Tumorspheres isolated from human cancer cell lines and patients are resistant to chemotherapy agents, such as paclitaxel and 5-fluorouracil [24,34]. Given their capability to promote tumor formation and the fact that these cells are refractory to chemotherapy, CSCs are primordial targets in breast cancer therapeutics. Very active research aims to the identification of prospective CSC markers for the isolation and study of these tumor-initiating cells. In a seminal study reported by Al-Hajj and colleagues, CSCs from breast cancer patients were identified by isolating the $Lin^{-}CD44^{+}CD24^{-/low}$ population (where Lin^{-} refers the lineage negative population) [35]. As little as 100 cells of the sorted population formed palpable tumors when injected in immunodeficient animals. Recently, the same $CD44^{+}CD24^{-/low}$ signature was identified in a panel of eight different human cancer cell lines. Importantly, the highest percentage of $CD44^{+}CD24^{-/low}$ positive cells was found in basal-like breast cancer lines, whereas that more differentiated breast cancer cell lines, such as luminal and luminal-mix lines, showed significantly less percentage of cells expressing this signature. [34]. Reciprocally, TICs have also been isolated from three breast cancer lesions using the tumorsphere method. The resulting breast carcinoma lines exhibited the $CD44^{+}CD24^{-/low}$ signature, over-expressed cytoprotective factors (including Survivin) and were able to self-renew and differentiate into both, luminal and basal lineages, indicating that these cells could arise from a bi-potent progenitor. Importantly, these cells expressed the OCT4 stem cell marker, and as few as 1000 cells generated tumors in nude mice [36]. In addition to the $CD44^{+}CD24^{-/low}$ signature, another potential marker for CSCs is the aldefluor (ALDH1). ALDH1 is a detoxifying enzyme responsible for the oxidation of intracellular aldehydes and thought to play a role in stem cell differentiation through metabolism of retinal to retinoic acid. Two recent publications have demonstrated that the ALDH1 positive population (which is typically 1% of the total tumor cell lines) displayed CSC characteristics and were able to promote tumor formation in immunodeficient mice [31,37].

In summary, the above results suggest that cancer cell lines contain a hierarchical organization of cell populations, and that rare CSCs exhibiting tumor-initiating capabilities can be isolated with at least two defined molecular signatures.

Basal-like (BL) and claudin-low (CL) breast cancers are enriched in putative Cancer Stem Cell (CSC) signatures. Recent studies suggest that basal-like and claudin-low breast cancers are enriched in gene signatures associated with Cancer Stem Cells (CSCs). First, Honeth et al. performed immunohistochemistry with the CD44 and CD24 antibodies in 240 human breast tumors, and demonstrated that the $CD44^{+}CD24^{-}$ phenotype was enriched in the basal-like subtype. From all $BRCA^{-}$ breast cancers analyzed, 94% contained the $CD44^{+}CD24^{-}$ signature. However, this phenotype was detected in 31% of the all breast tumors scored, hence not all the basal-like tumors, and very few Her2+ tumors, contained this signature. Thus, is likely than other molecular signatures remain to be discovered for these tumors [38]. Second, characterization of mammary TICs revealed expression of many proteins that are up-regulated in basal-like and claudin-low tumors: CK5, CK14, α6 integrin, and αB-crystallin in the case of basal-like tumors [1], and ALDH1 in the case of claudin-low tumors [5]. Third, immunohistochemistry analyses indicate that basal-like tumors express both luminal and basal CKs, suggesting that the cell type of origin of these tumors is bi-potent [39]. Finally, histo-pathological analysis of basal-like tumors reveals a poorly differentiated phenotype, nuclear atypia and mitotic index that are reminiscent to stem cells [40]. The recently identified claudin-low breast cancer subtype is characterized by a high enrichment of epithelial-mesenchymal transition (EMT) markers, such as high TWIST1, SNAI1, ZEB2 and Vimentin. More importantly, a hallmark of these tumors is the presence of $CD44+/CD24^{-/low}$ CSC signature and also poor response to chemotherapy or hormonotherapy [41]. Overall, these findings suggest that this novel mesenchymal subtype is potentially enriched with CSCs that might be resistant to standard therapy.

Targeting claudin-low and basal-like breast cancers. As expressed above, both claudin-low and basal-like breast cancers are triple negative and associated with poor prognosis. Basal breast cancers are currently treated with a combination of chemotherapeutic and anti-angiogenic regimens [12]. However, because claudin-low tumors are refractory to chemotherapy and biologic therapy, there is an urgency to develop novel strategies to target these patients.

The first targeting genetic approach consists in down-regulating potential oncogenes that are over-expressed in CSCs. This can be achieved by knock-down strategies, including siRNA, and repressive Artificial Transcription Factors, which will be discussed more in detail in the following sections. The second strategy is the forced up-regulation of tumor suppressors, which are often silenced in tumor cells. This can be achieved by over-expression of tumor suppressors, by epigenetic remodeling drugs, which target repressive chromatin, and Artificial Transcription Factors (Figure 3).

In the following sections we will overview first, embryonic TFs and their regulatory networks in stem and CSCs, and second, we will focus on the biology of selected tumor suppressor genes. Finally we will review recent investigations aiming to characterize ATFs targeting the tumor suppressor gene *mammary serine protease inhibitor* (*maspin*), which is down-regulated in claudin-low carcinomas.

2. Targeting self-renewal transcription factors, TFs

Because claudin-low tumors are possibly originated from primitive stem cells, dys-regulation of self-renewal and differentiation gene pathways might be at the basis of their oncogenic potential. In that regard, it is possible that claudin-low/basal breast cancers use an operational machinery of transcription factors (TFs), which regulates self-renewal in stem

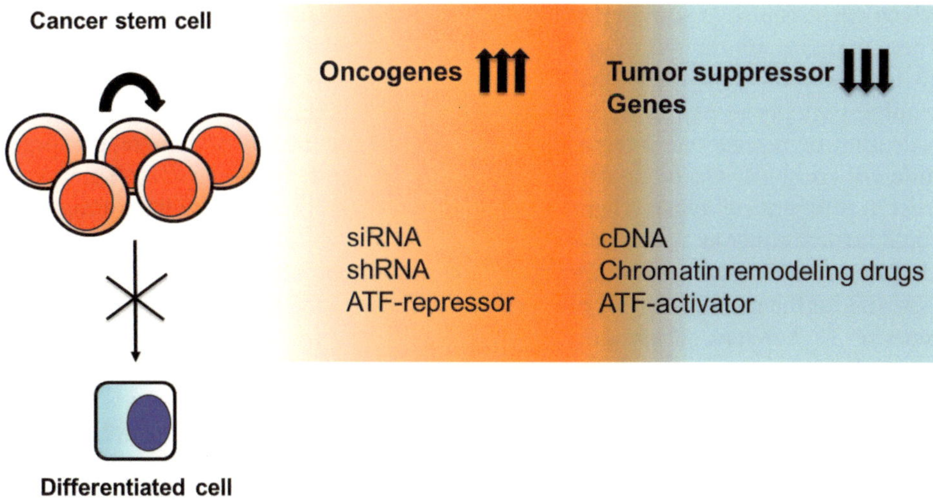

Fig. 3. Current approaches to target tumor initiating cells by down-regulation of potential oncogenes and up-regulation of tumor suppressors.

cells. The improper function of this circuitry could unbalance a delicate equilibrium between self-renewal and differentiation, thereby locking stem/early progenitor cells in an aberrant, excessive self-renewal stage. Aberrant self-renewal could prevent or limit stem cells from undertaking downstream differentiation gene programs. The initial pool of self-renewal cells could accumulate subsequent genetic and epigenetic aberrations, particularly in patients associated with mutations in the BRCA tumor suppressor gene (basal and claudin-low breast cancer). How is self-renewal dys-regulated in cancer stem cells? Can we learn some lessons from stem cell biology? Is there a network of TFs over-activated/operative in cancer stem cells?

The self-renewal TF network of human embryonic stem cells (hESCs). The self-renewal TF network has been characterized in hESCs by ChIP-chip and Chip-seq. This network involves the transcriptional activation as well as the physical association of multiple TFs. The "heart" or "core" of this network is composed of three master regulators TFs: OCT4, SOX2 and NANOG. Interactions between these TFs results on an autoregulatory feed-forward feedback loop [42]. The OCT4-SOX2-NANOG circuit functions as an epigenetic switch, which controls the maintenance of the self-renewal state. In hESCs DNA-methylation of the OCT4, SOX2 and NANOG promoters acts as an "irreversible switch" promoting differentiation gene programs [43]. Are OCT4, SOX2 and NANOG, and downstream self-renewal TFs activated in breast cancers? If so, a very attractive approach would consist in promoting persistent, imprinted, and inherited silencing on these upstream master regulators to force tumor cells to switch from a "proliferative" towards a "differentiation" stage. OCT4 positive cells have been reported in breast cancer cell lines derived from tumors [36,44]. The SOX2 gene is over-expressed in basal breast cancer specimens and cell lines, and thus, represents a potential cancer stem cell/progenitor marker [44]. In the following sections we will describe the OCT4 and SOX2 TF targets and their functional importance in hESCs and potentially in CSCs.

OCT4/POU5F1 (Octamer binding transcription factor 4). As a member of the POU transcription factor family (Pit, Oct, Unc), OCT4 contains a bipartite DNA-binding domain, which consists of two sub-domains, namely the POU-specific and the POU-homeodomain. These domains are connected by a flexible linker of variable length. The POU proteins have an intrinsic ability to bind DNA with sequence specificity. They interact with different binding partners as well as transcriptional co-activators or co-repressors, which mediate the activation or repression of their targets [45], [46]. This has a fundamental importance as different constellations of co-activator, co-repressors and chromatin remodeling complexes exist in different cell types. Thereby, depending on the chromatin microenvironment OCT4 could behave either as an activator or a repressor.

OCT4 was the first gene to be identified as a master regulator of pluripotency [47]. OCT4 is essential for the maintenance of pluripotency and this is mediated by up-regulation of a self-renewal TF network. These downstream TF targets of OCT4 coordinately activate self-renewal gene programs, while preventing the expression of genes that are activated during stem cell differentiation [48],[42,49].

The regulatory core network in embryonic cells comprises OCT4, SOX2, and NANOG transcription factors. The transcription factors OCT4, SOX2 and NANOG form the basic core of the self-renewal TF network. OCT4, SOX2 and NANOG are able to physically associate with different TFs as well as with large co-activators/co-repressor complexes, and co-occupy a set of 179 target promoters, namely the "NOS" gene set. This mediates the activation of self-renewal transcription factors, while it represses targets associated with differentiation gene programs [42] [50]. The results reported by Boyer *et al.* [42] suggested a model of ESCs transcriptional regulation. Some of the OCT4, SOX2, and NANOG targets include genes involved maintenance of self-renewal (e.g. *OCT4, SOX2, NANOG, STAT3* and *ZIC3*), members of the Wnt (*DKK1, FRAT1/2*) and TGFβ *(TDGF1, LEFTY2/EBAF)* signaling pathways, and histone-modifying and chromatin remodelers, such as *SMARCAD1, MYST3* and *SET*. Genes that encoded for homeodomain proteins, such as *DLX5, HOXB1, LHX5, TITF1, LBX1* and *HOP* implicated in developmental gene programs were repressed [42]. Importantly, genome-wide studies have shown that NOS targets are over-represented in poorly differentiated carcinomas, such as breast carcinomas and gliomas, which suggest that embryonic TFs could similarly play an important role in maintaining aberrant self-renewal in these tumors [51].

OCT4 in cancer stem cells (CSCs). In humans, CSCs have been associated with multiple malignancies, including breast [35], ovarian [52] and prostate cancer [53]. The role of OCT4 in CSCs has been a subject of intense investigation. Several studies suggest that OCT4 is critical for tumor cell survival and for the formation of tumor-initiation units *in vitro,* or tumor-spheroids. High expression of OCT4 has been reported *in vitro* in Lewis lung carcinoma 3LL and human breast cancer MCF7 cells. Silencing of Oct4 by siRNA resulted in cell apoptosis, suggesting that OCT4 is essential for cell survival [54]. Furthermore, human breast cancer cell lines have been isolated that exhibit the CSC signature $CD44^{+}CD24^{-}$ and these cells express high levels of OCT4 [36]. In the same line, another group has shown a 60% reduction in cell viability in epithelial ovarian cancer PA-1 cells transfected with siRNA specific for OCT4, and the reduction in cell viability was in part due to an increase of apoptosis [55].

SRY (Sex determining Region Y) Box 2 (SOX2). SOX2 is a member of the SRY-related High Mobility Group (HMG) box transcription factor. SOX2 is key regulator of cell fate and is necessary for the maintenance of self-renewal in embryonic stem cells. SOX2 has been proposed to be a marker of CSCs (together with other genes, e.g. OCT4, CD133, CD44) in several tumor types, including glioblastoma, prostate, lung, liver and breast carcinomas [51], [56], [57], [58], [59], [60]. Gene-expression microarrays revealed that SOX2 up-regulated

Cyclin D1, which contributes to cell cycle progression. Consistently, Cyclin D1 over-expression is observed in a variety of tumors [61]. However, the functional role of SOX2 in breast organogenesis remains still unexplored. SOX2 is over-expressed in breast cancer cells with increasing levels of expression in poorly differentiated cancer cells [62],[44]. Loss of function studies using SOX2-specific shRNA resulted in an inhibition of tumorigenic phenotype of MCF-7 breast cancer cells in xenograft studies in nude mice ([63]). These results give evidence that down-regulation of SOX2 in breast cancer cells can be used for clinical applications for the treatment of aggressive breast cancers.

3. Targeting tumor suppressors in breast cancers

In addition to activation of oncogenes, aggressive carcinomas inactivate multiple panels of tumor suppressor genes. The $p16^{INK4A}$, p53, and BRCA tumor suppressor genes are commonly inactivated in breast cancers. As expressed earlier, BRCA mutation carriers are associated with risk to develop basal-like breast cancers [26]. Loss of p53 and $p16^{INK4A}$ tumor suppressor genes, which are also a main blockade for reprogramming of somatic cells, occurs in the earliest steps of mammary carcinogenesis [64,65,66]. Together with up-regulation of telomerase reverse transcriptase (hTERT), loss of $p16^{INK4A}$ is involved in immortalization of normal epithelial cells [64]. Loss of $p16^{INK4A}$ gene function could thus be a critical initial stem for prospective cancers stem cells to bypass the senescence pathway. In addition to the above described tumor suppressor genes, DKK1 inactivation has been associated with claudin-low tumors [67,68]. DKK1 functions as an antagonist of the Wnt signaling pathway, which plays an essential role in maintaining self-renewal and in stem cells, and possibly, in cancer stem cells.

The loss of tumor suppressive functions associated with self-renewal of stem cells could result in further genetic and epigenetic instability leading to tumor initiation. In addition to mutations and/or re-arrangements of tumor suppressors, epigenetic silencing mechanisms, for example DNA- and histone-methylation, and histone deacetylation, are very often observed in tumors. Some tumor suppressor genes named Class II tumor suppressors, such as the gene *maspin,* are ideal epigenetic targets because are solely down-regulated by epigenetic mechanisms in aggressive cancer cells.

The maspin tumor suppressor. *Mammary serine protease inhibitor* (*maspin* or *SERPIN B5*) is a multifaced protein able to induce apoptosis and suppress cell motility and metastasis [69,70,71,72,73,74]. The mechanisms by which *maspin* exert their functions are still under investigation but recent evidence suggest that the tumor suppressive and possibly the anti-metastatic responses are associated with the nuclear localization of this protein [75]. It has been demonstrated that *maspin* physically associates with chromatin and functions as a histone-deacetylase (HDAC) inhibitor [75,76]. The function of *maspin* as metastasis suppressor has been associated with the regulation of the urokinase-type plasminogen activator (uPA) and receptor (uPAR) protein system [77,78]. In addition to enhanced tumor cell apoptosis and inhibition of tumor cell motility, ectopic expression of *maspin* results in decreased angiogenesis, which as been attributed to regulation of endothelial cell migration and adhesion [79], as well as induction of endothelial apoptosis [80].

Maspin expression is regulated at many levels, including TFs (p53, p63, AP1/2) [81], microRNAs (mirRNA-21; [82]) and lastly, by promoter epigenetic regulation [83]. Epigenetic inhibitors, affecting both DNA- and histone methylation (for example 5-Aza-2′dC) and histone deacetylation (for example, SAHA) are commonly used to re-activate silenced tumor suppressors, including *maspin*. These inhibitors are presently in clinical trials particularly for non-solid malignancies. However, the problem of using these inhibitors in a clinical setting is their high toxicity due to their lack of targeted specificity. Thus, novel strategies are required to target more specifically tumor suppressor genes.

Our laboratory has developed Artificial Transcription Factors (ATFs), able to specifically bind the regulatory regions of both, oncogenes and tumor suppressors, to repress or activate gene expression. A hallmark or unique property of ATFs is their ability to revert the epigenetic state of the targeted genes, thereby reprogramming the phenotype of the tumor cell. This is particularly important for silencing oncogenes; the induction of epigenetic silencing by ATF has the unique capacity to promote inherited and stable changes in the tumor cell, which entails epigenetic, transcriptional and phenotypic memory. In the following sections we will describe the anatomical constituents of ATFs, the recent advances in the technology, and their potential to modulate gene expression in the breast cancer field.

4. Artificial transcription factors for targeting cancer-associated genes

Designer zinc finger transcription factors or Artificial Transcription factors (ATFs) are engineered proteins composed of a DNA-binding-domain (DBD) and an effector domain (ED). The DBD is designated to recognize specific DNA sequences, while the ED enables to edit or modify DNA. EDs comprise transcriptional activators or repressors, as well as enzymatic domains, such as methyltransferases, recombinases, and site-specific nucleases. Thus, unique features of ATFs comprise their capability to bind specific regions of the genome, as well as to edit, modify and sculpt the chromatin landscape of the cell. These technologies facilitate the directed and specific modification of the genome for gene therapy purposes.

Design of the DNA binding domain (DBD). The DBD is designed to bind specific DNA sequences, typically in the promoter region of the gene of interest. Most of the DBDs used to engineer ATFs are based on zinc finger (ZF) scaffolds, because of their modular nature and the simplicity of their DNA–protein interactions. Cys2-His2 ZF domains are compact, 30 amino acids units composed of a recognition α-helix and two antiparallel β-strands stabilized by a zinc ion [84,85]. Each ZF α-helix recognizes 3 base-pairs (bps) of DNA in an antiparallel manner [84]. Importantly, each ZF recognize the DNA in a quasi-independent manner, which has facilitated the selection and rational design of multimodular ("polydactyl" ZF proteins). Novel DNA-binding specificities are generated by mutagenesis of the recognition α-helix, without altering the rest of the scaffold. This has facilitated the construction of arrays of ZFs to recognize large DNA sequences using simple and relatively quick molecular biology approaches. Nevertheless, proteins of improved DNA-binding specificity can be further optimized by randomization and subsequent selection of the ZF backbone, using both *in vitro* and *in vivo* approaches (for an overview of these, see references [7,86,87]). Our laboratory has focused on six-ZF arrays recognizing 18-bp sequences because of the high affinity of these proteins (with K_ds in the picomolar range). In addition, 6ZF proteins are capable of binding and regulating single genes in complex genomes and thus, possess higher selectivity than three ZF proteins [88].

Effector domains linked to the DNA binding domain (DBD). The effector domain (ED) mediates the ATF function by either modulating transcription or by modifying or editing the chromatin. The VP16 [89], VP64 [90] and p65 [91] are common transcriptional activators that interact with the Mediator protein recruiting the polymerase-II transcriptional complex and associated enzymes to facilitate transcription. Additional activator domains used to

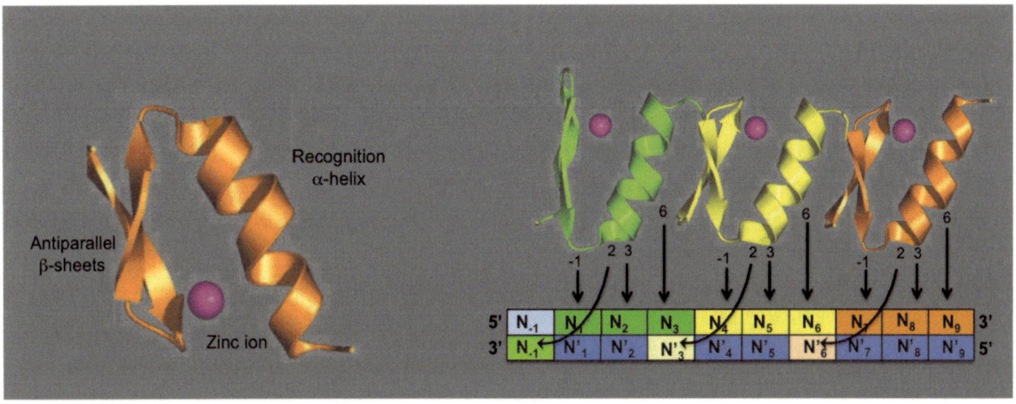

Fig. 4. Structure of Cys2Hys2 ZF proteins and their DNA-recognition mode. (a) Crystal structure of a ZF protein illustrating the recognition α-helix, the two antiparallel β-strands, and the zinc ion. (b) ZF-DNA interactions of a prototype 3ZF protein binding a 9-bp target.

construct ATFs comprise the S3H domain [92] and the $(FDTDL)_{11}$ domain derived from the C-terminal transcriptional activator domain of β-catenin [93].

Commonly used repressor domains include the Krüppel-associated box domain of KOX1 (KRAB) [94] and the SID domain (derived from the amino acid residues 1- 36 of the Mad mSIN3 interaction domain [95]). These EDs repress transcription by interacting with transcriptional co-repressors and chromatin condensing enzymes, resulting in a decreased accessibility of the promoter, which impedes the access of transcription factors and the polymerase II complex. Additional repressor domains include the ERD domain (comprising the residues 473-530 of the est2 repressor factor) [96], the vErbA (the ligand-binding domain of the thyroid hormone receptor v-erbA) [97], and the SRDX domain, derived from the transcription factor SUPERMAN of *Arabidopsis thaliana* [93].

Recently, DBDs have been linked to methyltransferase domains to silence promoter activity [98]; this fusion induced an epigenetic modification conferring stably and inherited gene silencing. DNA-methyltransferases catalyze the incorporation of methyl groups in position 5 of a cytosine base in CpG dinucleotides. In the cell, DNA methylation marks are "read" by methyl-binding-proteins (MBPs) proteins, which recruit large repressive complexes resulting in chromatin compaction and gene silencing. ZFs have been also linked to the Histone methyltransferase G9a to promote H3K9 methylation in the VEGF-A promoter [98]. Our laboratory has recently found that the VP64 activator domain can directionally de-methylate the *maspin* promoter [99]. Overall, these results hold great promise to develop novel ATFs able to alter the epigenetic code at specific promoter contexts, thereby promoting stable and inherited phenotypic changes in target cells.

Construction of Artificial Transcription Factors. Two main strategies have been developed to engineer ZF proteins, namely the modular assembly and the combinatorial-selection. The modular strategy involves the assembly of a basic repertoire of ZF building blocks of pre-characterized DNA-binding specificities. The modular approach is commonly performed by the "helix grafting" method ([90,100,101,102,103]). The combinatorial method produces ZFs with high specificity and binding affinity after the interrogation of randomized libraries and selection techniques. Here again, several strategies are available for investigators to select for ZF DBDs, such us as Phage display [104,105,106,107,108], ribosome display [109], two hybrids [110,111], and more recently the OPEN [112] and CODA systems [113]. The selection of the specific ZF units is a first critical step, and researchers can take advantage of several web-based tools available for designing their suitable array of ZFs, such as Zinc Finger Tools, (http://www.scripps.edu/mb/barbas/zfdesign/zfdesignhome.php) [114]; Zinc Finger Targeter, ZiFiT (http://bindr.gdcb.iastate.edu:8080/ZiFDB/) [115]; and ZFNGenome (http://bindr.gdcb.iastate.edu/ZFNGenome) [116]. These web-based tools are user-friendly interfaces that identify potential ZF binding sites on the target gene and provide scores for each ZF protein.

Endogenous gene regulation by Artificial Transcription Factors. In 1997 at the Barbas' lab demonstrated that 6ZF ATFs coupled either with the VP16 or KRAB-A box EDs were able to regulate the expression of an ErbB2-driven reporter gene [117]. The same group later demonstrated that an ATF was able to target the endogenous ErbB2 promoter [90]. For the purpose of modulating gene expression in mammalian cells, ATFs are cloned either in transient expression vectors (pcDNA), or retroviral expression vectors. These constructs facilitate the expression of ATFs in primary and transformed mammalian cells. Some of the genes successfully regulated by ATFs are listed on **Table I**. Recently regulated genes include: *mammary serine protease inhibitor* (*maspin*) [103,118], dystrophin-related gene *utrophin* [119], *vascular endothelial growth factor A* (*VEGF-A*) [120,121], *gamma-globin* [122], *heme oxygenase-1 gene* (*HMOX1*) [123], *glial cell line-derived neurotrophic factor gene* (*GDNF*) [124], derived tyrosine kinase receptors *ErbB2* [90,125], and *ErbB3* [100,125]. Genes that were successfully down-regulated by ATFs comprise: *VEGF-A* [120,121], *ErbB2* [90,125], *ErbB3* [100], the human telomerase reverse transcriptase (*hTERT*) [126], the nuclear hormone receptor PPARγ gene (*PPARγ*) [127], and the repression of the checkpoint kinase 2 (*CHK2*) gene [88].

The most recent application of engineered ZF DBDs embrace the ability to specifically modify the genome using zinc finger nucleases (ZFNs). These ZFNs are composed of 2-4 ZF arrays linked to DNA-cleavage domain of Fok-I. Gene correction has been successfully demonstrated in human embryonic and hematopoietic cells [128].

Regulation of cancer associated genes by ATFs. ATFs are versatile tools, which offer a unique therapeutic strategy to modulate the expression of oncogenes and tumor suppressors. Currently, several ATFs have been constructed to regulate cancer genes. Falke *et al.* reported an ATF up-regulating the pro-apoptotic *Bax* gene. Upon transfection in Saos-2 cells this ATF promoted a 40% reduction in cell viability and apoptosis induction [130].

High levels of VEGF-A protein expression have been associated with tumor vascularization. In 2003 Snowden et al. [97] generated an ATF coupled with the repressor domain v-ErbA targeting the *VEGF-A* gene. Transfection of this ATF into tumorigenic HEK293 cells resulted in a 50% reduction of protein expression.

Several cancers are associated with the over-expression of the ErbB-family of receptors (e.g. breast, prostate, colon, pancreas and ovary). The ErbB2 receptor has an important role in tumor cell proliferation and metastasis, particularly in breast cancer cell models. ATFs designed to up- and down-regulate this gene in A431 cells, derived from an epidermoid squamous cell carcinoma line, caused an increase in cell migration when ErbB2 was over-expressed, while its down-regulation led to a significant reduction in cell migration [125]. Recently Lund CV. *et al.* described the generation of a single twelve-ZF construct designed to down-regulate the ErbB2 and ErbB3 genes. This ZF protein was properly expressed in the cells, co-regulated both targets, and was able decrease breast tumor cell proliferation *in vitro* [125].

Endogenous gene	Regulation	Target site length (bp)	Effector Domain	Reference
CCK2R	↑	9	VP16	Liu et al. 2004 [129]
Utrophin	↑	9	VP16	Corbi et al. 2000 [119]
Bax	↑	15	VP16	Falke et al. 2003 [130]
Human erythropoietin	↑	9	VP16	Zhang et al. 2000 [131]
EPO-1	↑	9	VP64	Zhang et al. 2000 [131]
γ-Globin	↑	18	VP64	Blau et al. 2005 [122]
Maspin	↑	18	VP64	Beltran et al. 2007 [103]
HMOX1	↑	18	p65	Guo et al. 2010 [123]
GDNF	↑	18	p65	Laganiere et al. 2010 [124]
PEDF	↑	18	p65	Yokoi et al. 2007 [132]
PTHR1	↑	9	VP16/p65	Liu et al 2005 [133]
VEGF-A	↑	9	VP16/p65	Liu et al. 2001, Mori et al. 2008 [121,134]
IGF2/H19	↑↓	9	VP16/p65/v-ErbA	Jouvenot et al. 2003 [132]
ErbB2/ErbB3	↑↓	9	VP16, VP64 KRAB, ERD, SID	Beerli et al, 1998, 2000 [90,100]
ErbB2/ErbB3	↑↓	18	VP64/KRAB	Lund et al. 2005 [125]
ErbB2	↑↓	18	VP64/KRAB	Beerli et al. 2000 [100]
OCT-4	↑↓	18	VP16/KRAB	Bartsevich et al. 2003 [135]
MDR1	↑↓	15	VP16/KRAB	Bartsevich et al. 2000 [136]
hTERT	↓	12	KRAB	Sohn et al. 2010 [126]
PPARγ	↓	18	KRAB	Ren et al. 2002 [127]
CHK2	↓	18	KRAB	Tan et al. 2003 [88]

Table 1. Genes regulated by Artificial Transcription Factors.

Targeting the maspin tumor suppressor gene. Recently, our laboratory has targeted the gene *maspin*, a tumor suppressor silenced by epigenetic mechanisms in aggressive cancer cells. We have constructed three six-ZF ATFs designed to bind 18-pbs sites in the *maspin* proximal promoter. These ATFs were fused to the VP64 transactivator domain and designed to awake the silenced gene. These ATFs offer a versatile strategy to study the phenotypic consequences of re-expressing the endogenous gene in different cancer cell models. ATFs -97 and -126 strongly reactivated *maspin* in highly metastatic breast and lung cancer cell lines [99,103,118]. The up-regulation of *maspin* decreased cell motility and induced tumor-cell apoptosis in approximately 60% of the transfected cells; the remaining cell population restored cell junction proteins, such as E-cadherin, and other normal-like features. When ATF-126 was expressed in MDA-MB-231 cells using inducible retroviral vectors, ATF induction resulted in 50% of tumor burden reduction and totally abolished metastatic colonization in nude mice. Furthermore, gene expression microarrays demonstrated that the ATF-responsive genes predicted normal-like cell behavior, better prognosis and therapeutic response of breast cancer patients. These data point to the future clinical application of ATFs targeting *maspin* in breast cancers.

Subsequent studies with *maspin*-specific ATFs in several cancer cell backgrounds revealed that the re-activation of the gene was partially compromised by the epigenetic status of its promoter. Maspin is aberrantly silenced in metastatic tumors by epigenetic mechanisms including DNA methylation, H3K9 methylation, and histone de-acetylation. Co-treatment of low-maspin expressing breast and lung cancer cell lines with ATF-126 with either methyltransferase or HDAC inhibitors resulted in a synergistic interaction in re-activating *maspin* expression, and cell death induction. Furthermore, the triple combination (ATF-126 + methyltransferase + HDAC inhibitor) was far more potent in re-activating *maspin* and in inducing cell death as compared to single or double treatments, even at low concentration of inhibitors. These observations demonstrated the importance of the promoter context, particularly promoter methylation, in the reactivation of *maspin* by ATFs.
Later experiments have demonstrated that both ATFs, ATF-126 and ATF-97, were able to re-activate *maspin* in non-small cell lung carcinoma (NSCLC) cancer cells carrying a hypermethylated *maspin* promoter. Sodium bisulfate methylation studies in ATF-97 and ATF-126 transfected cells demonstrated substantial DNA demethylation upstream the ATF-binding sites (~70% reduction relative to control cells). This unidirectional, site-specific, de-methylation effect was dependent on the positioning of VP64 along the promoter. The VP64 transactivator domain interacts with the mediator protein to recruit RNA polymerase complex and chromatin remodeling enzymes in the *maspin* promoter, which acts to relax the chromatin and to ignite transcription. Although the mechanism by which ATFs de-methylate the *maspin* promoter remains elusive, these results demonstrate that ATFs can be target DNA demethylation in specific promoters.
ATFs designed against the *maspin* promoter resulted in successful target gene regulation. The next step involves the delivery of the ATFs into tumors and metastasis in a pre-clinical setting. To this end, our laboratory and others are developing targeted nanoparticles and adenoviral delivery systems. Although these delivery systems are at this time under development, an ATF made to target the Vascular Endothelial Growth Factor (VEGF-A) gene is currently in clinical trials. Nevertheless, the forthcoming engineering of ATFs will benefit from EDs that actively shape the chromatin to either compact or relax its native architecture. In addition, combinations of ATFs to target both, oncogenes and tumor suppressors, are anticipated to achieve more potent therapeutic outcomes. The development of ATFs able to alter the chromatin landscape of multiple loci represents a powerful novel genetic tool to target malignant breast cancer.

5. Acknowledgements and funding

This work was supported from NCI/NIH grants 1R01CA125273, 3R01CA125273-03S1 and Department of Defense W81XWH-10-1-0265 (PB).

6. References

[1] Sorlie T, Perou CM, Tibshirani R, Aas T, Geisler S, et al. (2001) Gene expression patterns of breast carcinomas distinguish tumor subclasses with clinical implications. Proc Natl Acad Sci U S A 98: 10869-10874.

[2] Kamalakaran S, Varadan V, Giercksky Russnes HE, Levy D, Kendall J, et al. (2011) DNA methylation patterns in luminal breast cancers differ from non-luminal subtypes

and can identify relapse risk independent of other clinical variables. Mol Oncol 5: 77-92.
[3] Holm K, Hegardt C, Staaf J, Vallon-Christersson J, Jonsson G, et al. (2010) Molecular subtypes of breast cancer are associated with characteristic DNA methylation patterns. Breast Cancer Res 12: R36.
[4] Killian JK, Bilke S, Davis S, Walker RL, Jaeger E, et al. (2011) A methyl-deviator epigenotype of estrogen receptor-positive breast carcinoma is associated with malignant biology. Am J Pathol 179: 55-65.
[5] Hennessy BT, Gonzalez-Angulo AM, Stemke-Hale K, Gilcrease MZ, Krishnamurthy S, et al. (2009) Characterization of a naturally occurring breast cancer subset enriched in epithelial-to-mesenchymal transition and stem cell characteristics. Cancer Res 69: 4116-4124.
[6] Kurman RJ, Shih Ie M (2011) Molecular pathogenesis and extraovarian origin of epithelial ovarian cancer-Shifting the paradigm. Hum Pathol 42: 918-931.
[7] Blancafort P, Beltran AS (2008) Rational design, selection and specificity of artificial transcription factors (ATFs): the influence of chromatin in target gene regulation. Comb Chem High Throughput Screen 11: 146-158.
[8] Prat A, Parker JS, Karginova O, Fan C, Livasy C, et al. (2010) Phenotypic and molecular characterization of the claudin-low intrinsic subtype of breast cancer. Breast Cancer Res 12: R68.
[9] Perou CM, Sorlie T, Eisen MB, van de Rijn M, Jeffrey SS, et al. (2000) Molecular portraits of human breast tumours. Nature 406: 747-752.
[10] Creighton CJ, Li X, Landis M, Dixon JM, Neumeister VM, et al. (2009) Residual breast cancers after conventional therapy display mesenchymal as well as tumor-initiating features. Proc Natl Acad Sci U S A 106: 13820-13825.
[11] Herschkowitz JI, Zhao W, Zhang M, Usary J, Murrow G, et al. (2011) Breast Cancer Special Feature: Comparative oncogenomics identifies breast tumors enriched in functional tumor-initiating cells. Proc Natl Acad Sci U S A.
[12] Perou CM (2010) Molecular stratification of triple-negative breast cancers. Oncologist 15 Suppl 5: 39-48.
[13] Bloushtain-Qimron N, Yao J, Snyder EL, Shipitsin M, Campbell LL, et al. (2008) Cell type-specific DNA methylation patterns in the human breast. Proc Natl Acad Sci U S A 105: 14076-14081.
[14] McCave EJ, Cass CA, Burg KJ, Booth BW (2010) The normal microenvironment directs mammary gland development. J Mammary Gland Biol Neoplasia 15: 291-299.
[15] Goldstein RH, Reagan MR, Anderson K, Kaplan DL, Rosenblatt M (2010) Human bone marrow-derived MSCs can home to orthotopic breast cancer tumors and promote bone metastasis. Cancer Res 70: 10044-10050.
[16] Karnoub AE, Dash AB, Vo AP, Sullivan A, Brooks MW, et al. (2007) Mesenchymal stem cells within tumour stroma promote breast cancer metastasis. Nature 449: 557-563.
[17] Orimo A, Gupta PB, Sgroi DC, Arenzana-Seisdedos F, Delaunay T, et al. (2005) Stromal fibroblasts present in invasive human breast carcinomas promote tumor growth and angiogenesis through elevated SDF-1/CXCL12 secretion. Cell 121: 335-348.
[18] Stingl J (2009) Detection and analysis of mammary gland stem cells. J Pathol 217: 229-241.

[19] Dontu G, Al-Hajj M, Abdallah WM, Clarke MF, Wicha MS (2003) Stem cells in normal breast development and breast cancer. Cell Prolif 36 Suppl 1: 59-72.
[20] Shackleton M, Vaillant F, Simpson KJ, Stingl J, Smyth GK, et al. (2006) Generation of a functional mammary gland from a single stem cell. Nature 439: 84-88.
[21] Clarke RB, Anderson E, Howell A, Potten CS (2003) Regulation of human breast epithelial stem cells. Cell Prolif 36 Suppl 1: 45-58.
[22] Dontu G, Abdallah WM, Foley JM, Jackson KW, Clarke MF, et al. (2003) In vitro propagation and transcriptional profiling of human mammary stem/progenitor cells. Genes Dev 17: 1253-1270.
[23] Dey D, Saxena M, Paranjape AN, Krishnan V, Giraddi R, et al. (2009) Phenotypic and functional characterization of human mammary stem/progenitor cells in long term culture. PLoS ONE 4: e5329.
[24] Grimshaw MJ, Cooper L, Papazisis K, Coleman JA, Bohnenkamp HR, et al. (2008) Mammosphere culture of metastatic breast cancer cells enriches for tumorigenic breast cancer cells. Breast Cancer Res 10: R52.
[25] Lim E, Vaillant F, Wu D, Forrest NC, Pal B, et al. (2009) Aberrant luminal progenitors as the candidate target population for basal tumor development in BRCA1 mutation carriers. Nat Med 15: 907-913.
[26] Visvader JE (2009) Keeping abreast of the mammary epithelial hierarchy and breast tumorigenesis. Genes Dev 23: 2563-2577.
[27] Cariati M, Purushotham AD (2008) Stem cells and breast cancer. Histopathology 52: 99-107.
[28] Ponti D, Zaffaroni N, Capelli C, Daidone MG (2006) Breast cancer stem cells: an overview. Eur J Cancer 42: 1219-1224.
[29] Liu S, Ginestier C, Charafe-Jauffret E, Foco H, Kleer CG, et al. (2008) BRCA1 regulates human mammary stem/progenitor cell fate. Proc Natl Acad Sci U S A 105: 1680-1685.
[30] Wang XY, Yin Y, Yuan H, Sakamaki T, Okano H, et al. (2008) Musashi1 modulates mammary progenitor cell expansion through proliferin-mediated activation of the Wnt and Notch pathways. Mol Cell Biol 28: 3589-3599.
[31] Charafe-Jauffret E, Ginestier C, Iovino F, Wicinski J, Cervera N, et al. (2009) Breast cancer cell lines contain functional cancer stem cells with metastatic capacity and a distinct molecular signature. Cancer Res 69: 1302-1313.
[32] Wright MH, Calcagno AM, Salcido CD, Carlson MD, Ambudkar SV, et al. (2008) Brca1 breast tumors contain distinct CD44+/CD24- and CD133+ cells with cancer stem cell characteristics. Breast Cancer Res 10: R10.
[33] Wright MH, Robles AI, Herschkowitz JI, Hollingshead MG, Anver MR, et al. (2008) Molecular analysis reveals heterogeneity of mouse mammary tumors conditionally mutant for Brca1. Mol Cancer 7: 29.
[34] Fillmore CM, Kuperwasser C (2008) Human breast cancer cell lines contain stem-like cells that self-renew, give rise to phenotypically diverse progeny and survive chemotherapy. Breast Cancer Res 10: R25.
[35] Al-Hajj M, Wicha MS, Benito-Hernandez A, Morrison SJ, Clarke MF (2003) Prospective identification of tumorigenic breast cancer cells. Proc Natl Acad Sci U S A 100: 3983-3988.

[36] Ponti D, Costa A, Zaffaroni N, Pratesi G, Petrangolini G, et al. (2005) Isolation and in vitro propagation of tumorigenic breast cancer cells with stem/progenitor cell properties. Cancer Res 65: 5506-5511.
[37] Croker AK, Goodale D, Chu J, Postenka C, Hedley BD, et al. (2008) High aldehyde dehydrogenase and expression of cancer stem cell markers selects for breast cancer cells with enhanced malignant and metastatic ability. J Cell Mol Med.
[38] Honeth G, Bendahl PO, Ringner M, Saal LH, Gruvberger-Saal SK, et al. (2008) The CD44+/CD24- phenotype is enriched in basal-like breast tumors. Breast Cancer Res 10: R53.
[39] Bocker W, Moll R, Poremba C, Holland R, Van Diest P, et al. (2002) Common adult stem cells in the human breast give rise to glandular and myoepithelial cell lineages: a new cell biological concept. Lab Invest 82: 737-746.
[40] Rakha EA, Reis-Filho JS, Ellis IO (2008) Basal-like breast cancer: a critical review. J Clin Oncol 26: 2568-2581.
[41] Chang J, Creighton C, Landis M, Lewis M, Pavlick A, et al. (2008) Gene signature of cancer stem cells in an intrinsic subgroup of breast cancers with mesenchymal properties. Proc Am Soc Clin Oncol, abstract 11009.
[42] Boyer LA, Lee TI, Cole MF, Johnstone SE, Levine SS, et al. (2005) Core transcriptional regulatory circuitry in human embryonic stem cells. Cell 122: 947-956.
[43] Hochedlinger K, Plath K (2009) Epigenetic reprogramming and induced pluripotency. Development 136: 509-523.
[44] Lengerke C, Fehm T, Kurth R, Neubauer H, Scheble V, et al. (2011) Expression of the embryonic stem cell marker SOX2 in early-stage breast carcinoma. BMC Cancer 11: 42.
[45] Scholer HR, Ruppert S, Suzuki N, Chowdhury K, Gruss P (1990) New type of POU domain in germ line-specific protein Oct-4. Nature 344: 435-439.
[46] Herr W, Cleary MA (1995) The POU domain: versatility in transcriptional regulation by a flexible two-in-one DNA-binding domain. Genes Dev 9: 1679-1693.
[47] Nichols J, Zevnik B, Anastassiadis K, Niwa H, Klewe-Nebenius D, et al. (1998) Formation of pluripotent stem cells in the mammalian embryo depends on the POU transcription factor Oct4. Cell 95: 379-391.
[48] Pesce M, Scholer HR (2000) Oct-4: control of totipotency and germline determination. Mol Reprod Dev 55: 452-457.
[49] Rizzino A (2009) Sox2 and Oct-3/4: a versatile pair of master regulators that orchestrate the self-renewal and pluripotency of embryonic stem cells. Wiley Interdiscip Rev Syst Biol Med 1: 228-236.
[50] Walker E, Ohishi M, Davey RE, Zhang W, Cassar PA, et al. (2007) Prediction and testing of novel transcriptional networks regulating embryonic stem cell self-renewal and commitment. Cell Stem Cell 1: 71-86.
[51] Ben-Porath I, Thomson MW, Carey VJ, Ge R, Bell GW, et al. (2008) An embryonic stem cell-like gene expression signature in poorly differentiated aggressive human tumors. Nat Genet 40: 499-507.
[52] Alvero AB, Chen R, Fu HH, Montagna M, Schwartz PE, et al. (2009) Molecular phenotyping of human ovarian cancer stem cells unravels the mechanisms for repair and chemoresistance. Cell Cycle 8: 158-166.

[53] Collins AT, Berry PA, Hyde C, Stower MJ, Maitland NJ (2005) Prospective identification of tumorigenic prostate cancer stem cells. Cancer Res 65: 10946-10951.
[54] Leemhuis H, Nightingale KP, Hollfelder F (2008) Directed evolution of a histone acetyltransferase--enhancing thermostability, whilst maintaining catalytic activity and substrate specificity. FEBS J 275: 5635-5647.
[55] Peng S, Maihle NJ, Huang Y (2010) Pluripotency factors Lin28 and Oct4 identify a sub-population of stem cell-like cells in ovarian cancer. Oncogene 29: 2153-2159.
[56] Gangemi RM, Griffero F, Marubbi D, Perera M, Capra MC, et al. (2009) SOX2 silencing in glioblastoma tumor-initiating cells causes stop of proliferation and loss of tumorigenicity. Stem Cells 27: 40-48.
[57] Liu A, Cheng L, Du J, Peng Y, Allan RW, et al. (2010) Diagnostic utility of novel stem cell markers SALL4, OCT4, NANOG, SOX2, UTF1, and TCL1 in primary mediastinal germ cell tumors. Am J Surg Pathol 34: 697-706.
[58] Leung EL, Fiscus RR, Tung JW, Tin VP, Cheng LC, et al. (2010) Non-small cell lung cancer cells expressing CD44 are enriched for stem cell-like properties. PLoS One 5: e14062.
[59] Yang XR, Xu Y, Yu B, Zhou J, Qiu SJ, et al. (2010) High expression levels of putative hepatic stem/progenitor cell biomarkers related to tumour angiogenesis and poor prognosis of hepatocellular carcinoma. Gut 59: 953-962.
[60] Zhang HZ, Lin XG, Hua P, Wang M, Ao X, et al. (2010) The study of the tumor stem cell properties of CD133+CD44+ cells in the human lung adenocarcinoma cell line A549. Cell Mol Biol (Noisy-le-grand) 56 Suppl: OL1350-1358.
[61] Chen Y, Shi L, Zhang L, Li R, Liang J, et al. (2008) The molecular mechanism governing the oncogenic potential of SOX2 in breast cancer. J Biol Chem 283: 17969-17978.
[62] Rodriguez-Pinilla SM, Sarrio D, Moreno-Bueno G, Rodriguez-Gil Y, Martinez MA, et al. (2007) Sox2: a possible driver of the basal-like phenotype in sporadic breast cancer. Mod Pathol 20: 474-481.
[63] Cheng GZ, Zhang WZ, Sun M, Wang Q, Coppola D, et al. (2008) Twist is transcriptionally induced by activation of STAT3 and mediates STAT3 oncogenic function. J Biol Chem 283: 14665-14673.
[64] Novak P, Jensen TJ, Garbe JC, Stampfer MR, Futscher BW (2009) Stepwise DNA methylation changes are linked to escape from defined proliferation barriers and mammary epithelial cell immortalization. Cancer Res 69: 5251-5258.
[65] Kawamura T, Suzuki J, Wang YV, Menendez S, Morera LB, et al. (2009) Linking the p53 tumour suppressor pathway to somatic cell reprogramming. Nature 460: 1140-1144.
[66] Li H, Collado M, Villasante A, Strati K, Ortega S, et al. (2009) The Ink4/Arf locus is a barrier for iPS cell reprogramming. Nature 460: 1136-1139.
[67] DiMeo TA, Anderson K, Phadke P, Fan C, Perou CM, et al. (2009) A novel lung metastasis signature links Wnt signaling with cancer cell self-renewal and epithelial-mesenchymal transition in basal-like breast cancer. Cancer Res 69: 5364-5373.
[68] Mikheev AM, Mikheeva SA, Maxwell JP, Rivo JV, Rostomily R, et al. (2008) Dickkopf-1 mediated tumor suppression in human breast carcinoma cells. Breast Cancer Res Treat 112: 263-273.
[69] Hopkins PC, Whisstock J (1994) Function of maspin. Science 265: 1893-1894.
[70] Seftor RE, Seftor EA, Sheng S, Pemberton PA, Sager R, et al. (1998) maspin suppresses the invasive phenotype of human breast carcinoma. Cancer Res 58: 5681-5685.

[71] Zou Z, Anisowicz A, Hendrix MJ, Thor A, Neveu M, et al. (1994) Maspin, a serpin with tumor-suppressing activity in human mammary epithelial cells. Science 263: 526-529.
[72] Hall DC, Johnson-Pais TL, Grubbs B, Bernal R, Leach RJ, et al. (2008) Maspin reduces prostate cancer metastasis to bone. Urol Oncol 26: 652-658.
[73] Sheng S, Carey J, Seftor EA, Dias L, Hendrix MJ, et al. (1996) Maspin acts at the cell membrane to inhibit invasion and motility of mammary and prostatic cancer cells. Proc Natl Acad Sci USA 93: 11669-11674.
[74] Khalkhali-Ellis Z (2006) Maspin: the new frontier. Clin Cancer Res 12: 7279-7283.
[75] Goulet B, Kennette W, Ablack A, Postenka CO, Hague MN, et al. (2011) Nuclear localization of maspin is essential for its inhibition of tumor growth and metastasis. Lab Invest.
[76] Li X, Yin S, Meng Y, Sakr W, Sheng S (2006) Endogenous inhibition of histone deacetylase 1 by tumor-suppressive maspin. Cancer Res 66: 9323-9329.
[77] Schaefer JS, Zhang M (2005) Hypoxia effects: implications for maspin regulation of the uPA/uPAR complex. Cancer Biol Ther 4: 1033-1035.
[78] Amir S, Margaryan NV, Odero-Marah V, Khalkhali-Ellis Z, Hendrix MJ (2005) Maspin regulates hypoxia-mediated stimulation of uPA/uPAR complex in invasive breast cancer cells. Cancer Biol Ther 4: 400-406.
[79] Qin L, Zhang M (2010) Maspin regulates endothelial cell adhesion and migration through an integrin signaling pathway. J Biol Chem 285: 32360-32369.
[80] Schaefer JS, Zhang M (2006) Targeting maspin in endothelial cells to induce cell apoptosis. Expert Opin Ther Targets 10: 401-408.
[81] Bailey CM, Margaryan NV, Abbott DE, Schutte BC, Yang B, et al. (2009) Temporal and spatial expression patterns for the tumor suppressor Maspin and its binding partner interferon regulatory factor 6 during breast development. Dev Growth Differ 51: 473-481.
[82] Zhu S, Wu H, Wu F, Nie D, Sheng S, et al. (2008) MicroRNA-21 targets tumor suppressor genes in invasion and metastasis. Cell Res 18: 350-359.
[83] Futscher BW, Oshiro MM, Wozniak RJ, Holtan N, Hanigan CL, et al. (2002) Role for DNA methylation in the control of cell type specific maspin expression. Nat Genet 31: 175-179.
[84] Pavletich NP, Pabo CO (1991) Zinc finger-DNA recognition: crystal structure of a Zif268-DNA complex at 2.1 A. Science 252: 809-817.
[85] Elrod-Erickson M, Rould MA, Nekludova L, Pabo CO (1996) Zif268 protein-DNA complex refined at 1.6 A: a model system for understanding zinc finger-DNA interactions. Structure 4: 1171-1180.
[86] Beltran A, Liu Y, Parikh S, Temple B, Blancafort P (2006) Interrogating genomes with combinatorial artificial transcription factor libraries: asking zinc finger questions. Assay Drug Dev Technol 4: 317-331.
[87] Beltran AS, Blancafort P (2010) Remodeling genomes with artificial transcription factors (ATFs). Methods Mol Biol 649: 163-182.
[88] Tan S, Guschin D, Davalos A, Lee YL, Snowden AW, et al. (2003) Zinc-finger protein-targeted gene regulation: genomewide single-gene specificity. Proc Natl Acad Sci U S A 100: 11997-12002.
[89] Triezenberg SJ, Kingsbury RC, McKnight SL (1988) Functional dissection of VP16, the trans-activator of herpes simplex virus immediate early gene expression. Genes Dev 2: 718-729.

[90] Beerli RR, Segal DJ, Dreier B, Barbas CF, 3rd (1998) Toward controlling gene expression at will: specific regulation of the erbB-2/HER-2 promoter by using polydactyl zinc finger proteins constructed from modular building blocks. Proc Natl Acad Sci U S A 95: 14628-14633.

[91] Ruben SM, Dillon PJ, Schreck R, Henkel T, Chen CH, et al. (1991) Isolation of a rel-related human cDNA that potentially encodes the 65-kD subunit of NF-kappa B. Science 254: 11.

[92] Pollock R, Issner R, Zoller K, Natesan S, Rivera VM, et al. (2000) Delivery of a stringent dimerizer-regulated gene expression system in a single retroviral vector. Proc Natl Acad Sci U S A 97: 13221-13226.

[93] Tachikawa K, Schroder O, Frey G, Briggs SP, Sera T (2004) Regulation of the endogenous VEGF-A gene by exogenous designed regulatory proteins. Proc Natl Acad Sci U S A 101: 15225-15230.

[94] Margolin JF, Friedman JR, Meyer WK, Vissing H, Thiesen HJ, et al. (1994) Kruppel-associated boxes are potent transcriptional repression domains. Proc Natl Acad Sci U S A 91: 4509-4513.

[95] Ayer DE, Laherty CD, Lawrence QA, Armstrong AP, Eisenman RN (1996) Mad proteins contain a dominant transcription repression domain. Mol Cell Biol 16: 5772-5781.

[96] Sgouras DN, Athanasiou MA, Beal GJ, Jr., Fisher RJ, Blair DG, et al. (1995) ERF: an ETS domain protein with strong transcriptional repressor activity, can suppress ets-associated tumorigenesis and is regulated by phosphorylation during cell cycle and mitogenic stimulation. EMBO J 14: 4781-4793.

[97] Snowden AW, Zhang L, Urnov F, Dent C, Jouvenot Y, et al. (2003) Repression of vascular endothelial growth factor A in glioblastoma cells using engineered zinc finger transcription factors. Cancer Res 63: 8968-8976.

[98] Snowden AW, Gregory PD, Case CC, Pabo CO (2002) Gene-specific targeting of H3K9 methylation is sufficient for initiating repression in vivo. Curr Biol 12: 2159-2166.

[99] Beltran (2011) Reactivation of MASPIN in non-small cell lung carcinoma (NSCLC) cells by artificial transcription factors (ATFs). Epigenetics 6.

[100] Beerli RR, Dreier B, Barbas CF, 3rd (2000) Positive and negative regulation of endogenous genes by designed transcription factors. Proc Natl Acad Sci U S A 97: 1495-1500.

[101] Segal DJ, Beerli RR, Blancafort P, Dreier B, Effertz K, et al. (2003) Evaluation of a modular strategy for the construction of novel polydactyl zinc finger DNA-binding proteins. Biochemistry 42: 2137-2148.

[102] Blancafort P, Segal DJ, Barbas CF, 3rd (2004) Designing transcription factor architectures for drug discovery. Mol Pharmacol 66: 1361-1371.

[103] Beltran A, Parikh S, Liu Y, Cuevas BD, Johnson GL, et al. (2007) Re-activation of a dormant tumor suppressor gene maspin by designed transcription factors. Oncogene 26: 2791-2798.

[104] Rebar EJ, Pabo CO (1994) Zinc finger phage: affinity selection of fingers with new DNA-binding specificities. Science 263: 671-673.

[105] Jamieson AC, Kim SH, Wells JA (1994) In vitro selection of zinc fingers with altered DNA-binding specificity. Biochemistry 33: 5689-5695.

[106] Choo Y, Klug A (1994) Toward a code for the interactions of zinc fingers with DNA: selection of randomized fingers displayed on phage. Proc Natl Acad Sci U S A 91: 11163-11167.
[107] Isalan M, Klug A, Choo Y (2001) A rapid, generally applicable method to engineer zinc fingers illustrated by targeting the HIV-1 promoter. Nat Biotechnol 19: 656-660.
[108] Greisman HA, Pabo CO (1997) A general strategy for selecting high-affinity zinc finger proteins for diverse DNA target sites. Science 275: 657-661.
[109] Ihara H, Mie M, Funabashi H, Takahashi F, Sawasaki T, et al. (2006) In vitro selection of zinc finger DNA-binding proteins through ribosome display. Biochem Biophys Res Commun 345: 1149-1154.
[110] Joung JK, Ramm EI, Pabo CO (2000) A bacterial two-hybrid selection system for studying protein-DNA and protein-protein interactions. Proc Natl Acad Sci U S A 97: 7382-7387.
[111] Herrmann F, Garriga-Canut M, Baumstark R, Fajardo-Sanchez E, Cotterell J, et al. (2011) p53 Gene Repair with Zinc Finger Nucleases Optimised by Yeast 1-Hybrid and Validated by Solexa Sequencing. PLoS One 6: e20913.
[112] Maeder ML, Thibodeau-Beganny S, Osiak A, Wright DA, Anthony RM, et al. (2008) Rapid "open-source" engineering of customized zinc-finger nucleases for highly efficient gene modification. Mol Cell 31: 294-301.
[113] Sander JD, Dahlborg EJ, Goodwin MJ, Cade L, Zhang F, et al. (2011) Selection-free zinc-finger-nuclease engineering by context-dependent assembly (CoDA). Nat Methods 8: 67-69.
[114] Mandell JG, Barbas CF, 3rd (2006) Zinc Finger Tools: custom DNA-binding domains for transcription factors and nucleases. Nucleic Acids Res 34: W516-523.
[115] Sander JD, Zaback P, Joung JK, Voytas DF, Dobbs D (2007) Zinc Finger Targeter (ZiFiT): an engineered zinc finger/target site design tool. Nucleic Acids Res 35: W599-605.
[116] Reyon D, Kirkpatrick JR, Sander JD, Zhang F, Voytas DF, et al. (2011) ZFNGenome: a comprehensive resource for locating zinc finger nuclease target sites in model organisms. BMC Genomics 12: 83.
[117] Liu Q, Segal DJ, Ghiara JB, Barbas CF, 3rd (1997) Design of polydactyl zinc-finger proteins for unique addressing within complex genomes. Proc Natl Acad Sci U S A 94: 5525-5530.
[118] Beltran AS, Sun X, Lizardi PM, Blancafort P (2008) Reprogramming epigenetic silencing: artificial transcription factors synergize with chromatin remodeling drugs to reactivate the tumor suppressor mammary serine protease inhibitor. Mol Cancer Ther 7: 1080-1090.
[119] Corbi N, Libri V, Fanciulli M, Tinsley JM, Davies KE, et al. (2000) The artificial zinc finger coding gene 'Jazz' binds the utrophin promoter and activates transcription. Gene Ther 7: 1076-1083.
[120] Mori T, Sasaki J, Kanamori T, Aoyama Y, Sera T (2009) Hypoxia-specific upregulation of the endogenous human VEGF-A gene by hypoxia-driven expression of artificial transcription factor. Biochem Biophys Res Commun 390: 845-848.
[121] Mori T, Sasaki J, Aoyama Y, Sera T (2008) Modulation of endogenous VEGF-A expression under hypoxia by using artificial transcription factors. Nucleic Acids Symp Ser (Oxf): 187-188.

[122] Blau CA, Barbas CF, 3rd, Bomhoff AL, Neades R, Yan J, et al. (2005) {gamma}-Globin gene expression in chemical inducer of dimerization (CID)-dependent multipotential cells established from human {beta}-globin locus yeast artificial chromosome ({beta}-YAC) transgenic mice. J Biol Chem 280: 36642-36647.

[123] Guo H, Tian Y, Lu H, Wei Y, Ying D (2010) Upregulation of endogenous HMOX1 expression by a computer-designed artificial transcription factor. J Biomed Biotechnol 2010.

[124] Laganiere J, Kells AP, Lai JT, Guschin D, Paschon DE, et al. (2010) An engineered zinc finger protein activator of the endogenous glial cell line-derived neurotrophic factor gene provides functional neuroprotection in a rat model of Parkinson's disease. J Neurosci 30: 16469-16474.

[125] Lund CV, Popkov M, Magnenat L, Barbas CF, 3rd (2005) Zinc finger transcription factors designed for bispecific coregulation of ErbB2 and ErbB3 receptors: insights into ErbB receptor biology. Mol Cell Biol 25: 9082-9091.

[126] Sohn JH, Yeh BI, Choi JW, Yoon J, Namkung J, et al. (2010) Repression of human telomerase reverse transcriptase using artificial zinc finger transcription factors. Mol Cancer Res 8: 246-253.

[127] Ren D, Collingwood TN, Rebar EJ, Wolffe AP, Camp HS (2002) PPARgamma knockdown by engineered transcription factors: exogenous PPARgamma2 but not PPARgamma1 reactivates adipogenesis. Genes Dev 16: 27-32.

[128] Lombardo A, Genovese P, Beausejour CM, Colleoni S, Lee YL, et al. (2007) Gene editing in human stem cells using zinc finger nucleases and integrase-defective lentiviral vector delivery. Nat Biotechnol 25: 1298-1306.

[129] Liu PQ, Morton MF, Reik A, de la Rosa R, Mendel MC, et al. (2004) Cell lines for drug discovery: elevating target-protein levels using engineered transcription factors. J Biomol Screen 9: 44-51.

[130] Falke D, Fisher M, Ye D, Juliano RL (2003) Design of artificial transcription factors to selectively regulate the pro-apoptotic bax gene. Nucleic Acids Res 31: e10.

[131] Zhang L, Spratt SK, Liu Q, Johnstone B, Qi H, et al. (2000) Synthetic zinc finger transcription factor action at an endogenous chromosomal site. Activation of the human erythropoietin gene. J Biol Chem 275: 33850-33860.

[132] Yokoi K, Zhang HS, Kachi S, Balaggan KS, Yu Q, et al. (2007) Gene transfer of an engineered zinc finger protein enhances the anti-angiogenic defense system. Mol Ther 15: 1917-1923.

[133] Liu PQ, Tan S, Mendel MC, Murrills RJ, Bhat BM, et al. (2005) Isogenic human cell lines for drug discovery: regulation of target gene expression by engineered zinc-finger protein transcription factors. J Biomol Screen 10: 304-313.

[134] Liu PQ, Rebar EJ, Zhang L, Liu Q, Jamieson AC, et al. (2001) Regulation of an endogenous locus using a panel of designed zinc finger proteins targeted to accessible chromatin regions. Activation of vascular endothelial growth factor A. J Biol Chem 276: 11323-11334.

[135] Bartsevich VV, Miller JC, Case CC, Pabo CO (2003) Engineered zinc finger proteins for controlling stem cell fate. Stem Cells 21: 632-637.

[136] Bartsevich VV, Juliano RL (2000) Regulation of the MDR1 gene by transcriptional repressors selected using peptide combinatorial libraries. Mol Pharmacol 58: 1-10.

24

Breast Cancer Stem Cells – A Review

Julia S. Samaddar and Edmond Ritter
School of Medicine, Medical College of Georgia, Augusta,
Department of Surgery, School of Medicine, Medical College of Georgia, Augusta,
USA

1. Introduction

Breast cancer is a leading cause of morbidity and mortality among women. Much of the morbidity and mortality is associated with metastasis or local recurrence. There has been significant research on what can cause breast cancer progression and resistance to treatment. Carcinomas are made of transformed cells contained within stromal cells, fibroblasts, and immune cells. Difficulty in determining definite causal pathways of development of resistance and metastases is complicated by the heterogeneity of breast cancers. There are many different subtypes of breast cancer, each with certain unique phenotypes and genotypes. There has been shown 3 subsets of mammary cells: basal stem/progenitor cells, luminal progenitors, and non stem luminal cells. Although there is heterogeneity among the cell population of breast cancer tumors, there is generally a dominant cell type that allows classification of the tumor. There are at least four different breast cancer phenotypes. The first is the normal-like phenotype which resembles non cancerous breast cancer. The second is the luminal phenotype, generally ER positive and often divided into luminal A and luminal B categories. These breast cancers also express E-cadherein, KRT8, KRT18, and KRT19. The third category is HER-2 positive phenotype, which is generally ER negative. The fourth phenotype, designated as basal-like, generally overexpresses markers characteristic of normal mammary gland myoepithelium including EGF, p63, and basal cytokeratins KRT14, KRT17, and KRT5/6.

However, a poorly differentiated phenotype has been established as a hallmark for aggressive breast cancers, which has suggested a role of stem cells in breast cancers. Stem cells are defined as cells that have the ability to undergo unlimited cell cycle divisions to create new stem cells that retain their undifferentiated state and multipotent differentiating potential. There are two broad categories of stem cells, embryonic and adult, or somatic, stem cells. Embryonic stem cells are found in the inner cell mass of blastocysts and involved in the differentiation of the embryo. Somatic stem cells are found in various tissues after embryogenesis with the main function of normal tissue repair and renewal. Examples include mammary stem cells found in breast tissue and recently associated with breast carcinomas, as well as mesenchymal stem cells, found in various locations throughout the body, including the bone marrow, and involved in modulating immune response. Many believe that the somatic stem cells are not as pluripotent as embryonic stem cells and should therefore be considered more as progenitor cells rather than stem cells. Progenitor cells are similar to stem cells in their ability for self-renewal and ability to differentiate into multiple cell lineages but with a finite number of cell cycle division and more drive toward differentiation than embryonic stem cells. Somatic stem cells and progenitor cells are often used interchangeably, as will be the case in this chapter.

An increase in interest in stem cells began in 1997 when malignant stem cells were found in acute myeloid leukemia. Subsequent research revealed stem cells in various other solid tumors such as prostate, breast, lung, colon, and brain. The discovery of stem cells in breast cancer along with the heterogeneity of breast cancers and ability to develop resistance to treatment and relapse helped change the previous theory of each cell having equal tumorigenic potential to a preference for a theory suggesting that only certain cells within the tumor population allow progression of the tumor. Where these stem cells came from, however, is still up for debate. Breast cancers have a very heterogeneous set of phenotypes which leads to problems with generalizations of clonal origins of breast cancer stem cells (BCSC). As will be discussed in this chapter, there are several theories about breast cancer stem cell origins. Research about BCSC has captured the attention of scientists because of the undifferentiated character of aggressive breast cancer and the ability of stem cells for self-renewal, which may fuel breast cancer tumor progression and metastases. However, there are significant complicating variables that must be taken into consideration in BCSC research. BCSC are complicated with unknown origin, various pathways linked with a variety of physiologic processes as well as the uncertainty of isolating breast cancer stem cells due to lack of definite cell markers and BCSC definition. An additional roadblock in furthering research on BCSC is the possible need of these cells for a particular niche in which to grow. Not only must research concentrate on the characterization and pathways of BCSC but also take into account the normal physiologic processes and environmental conditions which influence the behaviors of cells and tissues . Additionally, it remains to be determined whether different subtypes of breast cancer harbor different types of BCSC.

In evaluating breast cancer, factors to be considered include subtype of breast cancer, prognosis, what causes relapse and why breast cancer tumors can develop resistance to therapy. Although stem cells have been suggested to be the culprit for possible relapse and resistance to therapy, which is often linked to a poor prognosis, the presence of stem cells alone is not indicative of poor prognosis. Indeed, mammary stem cells are found in normal breast tissue, shown by studies to be present in the basal epithelial compartment of mammary glands. Therefore, it is paramount to determine why stem cells become malignant or from where the malignant stem cells came. Despite that the exact nature and role of BCSC still remain elusive to researchers, much has been discovered about them since 1997, with every day giving more insight into their role in breast cancer. This chapter will give an overview of the major players in BCSC research in characterization, pathways, and treatments, all suggesting possible future directions in breast cancer research.

2. Characterizing breast cancer stem cells

One of the difficulties in research about BCSC remains the elusive definition of the cells. Although there is no concrete definition of cancer stem cells, generally, scientists include the following two characteristics in determining BCSC: the ability for self-renewal to generate another malignant cell and the ability to show lineage-specific differentiation. Even given these criteria, characterization of BCSC is further hindered by phenotypes linked to self-renewability such as ALDH1. These phenotypes will be further discussed later in the chapter. Other universally accepted characteristics of BSCS include undifferentiated phenotype and resistance to various breast cancer therapies. The resilience of these cells to less than optimal conditions has potentially been attributed to their low mitotic rates, when compared to the mitotic rates of their differentiated counterpart.

An important characteristic of stem cells is their inherent resistance to multiple drugs. This multiple drug resistance (MDR) profile is generally believed to be conferred to these cells mainly by ATP-binding cassette transporters. BCSC are thought to be associated with overexpression of these transporters and the most likely mechanism for failure of chemotherapy in these cells (Figure 1). The ATP-binding cassette transporters are able to efflux various, unrelated drugs out of cells on which they are present, thus conferring an MDR profile to these cancer cells. Multidrug resistance gene 1(MDR1) also is a major cause of breast cancer resistance to chemotherapy. Other multi drug resistance-linked genes include ABCB1, CCNE1, and MMP9. Although MDR is a significant obstacle to effective chemotherapy, MDR appears to be a normal protective function not only in malignant cancer cells, but also in their benign counterparts as studies have identified ATP-binding cassette transporters in normal tissue stem cells. Importantly, MDR activity is up regulated in response to chemotherapy. Of significant concern, these transporters have also been found in tumor cells that have not been exposed to chemotherapy, indicating a built in obstacle to antineoplastic treatment. Studies have shown that chemotherapy also

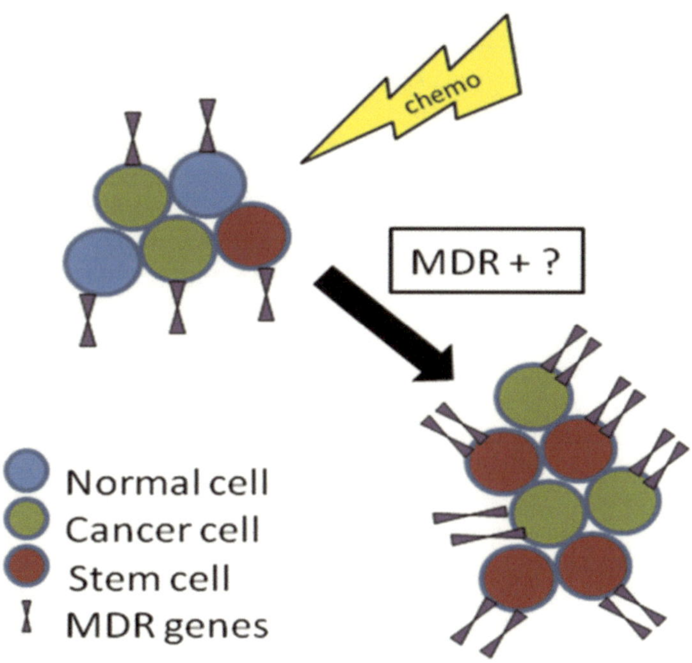

Fig. 1. MDR gene in breast cancer.
MDR is a natural defense mechanism in many, non-carcinogenic cells. However, MDR genes can be upregulated when exposed to chemotherapy, which can allow for tumor proliferation and an increasing stem cell phenotype. Nonetheless, expression of MDR genes is not the only factor in determining cancer progression or induced-stem cell phenotype after chemotherapy because sole upregulation of these genes do not result in stem cell phenotype, only treatment escape.

significantly increases tumor enrichment with stem cells, suggesting the idea that MDR genes may be involved in stem cell phenotype. However, singularly over expressing MDR genes showed that although MDR genes may allow escape from treatment, overexpression alone does not cause an increase in stem cell phenotype.

To help determine a concrete definition for BCSC, researchers have endeavored to find cells markers common, or more helpfully, exclusive, to BCSC. Cell markers that have garnered significant interest in research include CD44 and CD 24. CD44 is a transmembrane glycoprotein which is involved in cell adhesion and migration and has been shown to be upregulated in various cancers as well as their metastastes. Studies in which the blockage of CD44 led to inhibition of local growth and metastases suggest that CD44 is potentially a protective measure in breast cancer tumors. CD24 is a heavily glycosylated cell marker, which has been suggested to play a role in tumor migration due to its ability to bind P-selectin, a lectin expressed by endothelium and platelets. It has been suggested that the dynamic nature of the CD marker expression, however, prevents CD44 and CD24 from being definite markers for BCSC. Their expression can be influenced by epigenetic factors, genomic instability, and epithelial to mesenchymal transition, discussed later in this chapter. In addition, other studies have found that CD24 is not a consistent marker for breast cancer even though it has been and still continues to be used as a marker for BCSC. Therefore, the tide is potentially turning away from using these as the only markers for BCSC. However, they are still currently being used extensively by the scientific community to help identify BCSC. The usage is supported by studies which show that although the CD markers were not found to be consistently expressed in all breast cancer or with an increased stem cell-like phenotype, in mammospheres, the stem cell phenotype was present as was the ability to differentiate into luminal and basal phenotypes in human breast cancers.

Mammospheres are discrete clusters of cells that have the ability to survive and proliferate in non adherent, non differentiated culture conditions and are indicative of stem cell-like characteristics. Studies have shown that mammospheres may be more accurate in studying stem cells as more stem cell markers and characteristics were found in the spheroids rather than the adherent cultures. The spheroids were also found to be more malignant with greater altered chemo sensitivity than their adherent counterpart. Therefore, mammosphere formation may be used as a characteristic to help identify BCSC. These studies additionally showed that MAPK, Notch, Wnt genes, and aldehyde dehydrogenase (ALDH) are all over-expressed in breast cancer mammospheres. These markers and pathways have all been linked to BCSC by various studies and are accepted as potential BCSC markers.

Side populations are being investigated as a potential identification method for BCSC. Side populations were originally used to establish a population of hematopoietic cells enriched in hematopoietic stem cell. They are defined by their ability to efflux the dye Hoechst 33342 out of the cell determined to be due to ATP-binding cassette transporters. Importantly, this side population was also found in breast cancers and irradiated breast cancer tumors were discovered to contain side populations enriched in progenitor cells. However, the usage of this potential method of identification is hampered by the toxicity of the dye to non-side population cells.

ALDH1 is becoming more important for isolation of BCSC along with usage for identification of side populations of breast cancer cells with MDR proteins. ALDH1 is a member of a family of ALDH enzymes involved in the detoxification of a wide array of aldehydes. Functional enzymatic assays are utilized to detect the presence of ALDH enzymes due to the wide array of enzymes within the family. There are some contradictory

studies about the frequency of ALDH+ cells within a tumor with one study suggesting it is as low as 25% while another study reported finding ALDH+ cells in 23 out of the 33 breast cancer tumors tested. Although these studies may appear contradictory in the prevalence of ALDH+ cells in breast cancer tumors, studies have shown that ALDH- cells are far less tumorigenic than ALDH+ cells, especially the small subset that also displays stem cell markers CD44+/CD24-/low. In addition, the ALDH+ tumor exhibited preference for forming high-grade, HER2+, hormone receptor negative tumor, all indicative of poor overall prognosis. ALDH1 has also been rumored to be an independent prognostic factor in predicting metastases in inflammatory breast cancer with the associated BCSC having the ability to reconstruct the heterogeneity of the originating breast cancer at the distant site .
CD133, also known as Prominin-1, has been suggested to identify a subset of BCSC. A transmembrane glycoprotein, CD133 has been used in defining a wide array of somatic stem cells as well as being elevated in the peripheral blood of patients with metastatic disease. CD133 is considered a very important stem cell marker despite not much being know about it because of it greater restriction to cancer stem cells unlike CD44 and ALDH. Additionally, downregulation of CD133 has been shown to decrease cell growth, cell motility, ability to metastasize, and ability to form spheroids in stem cell-like conditions (Figure 2). CD133 may

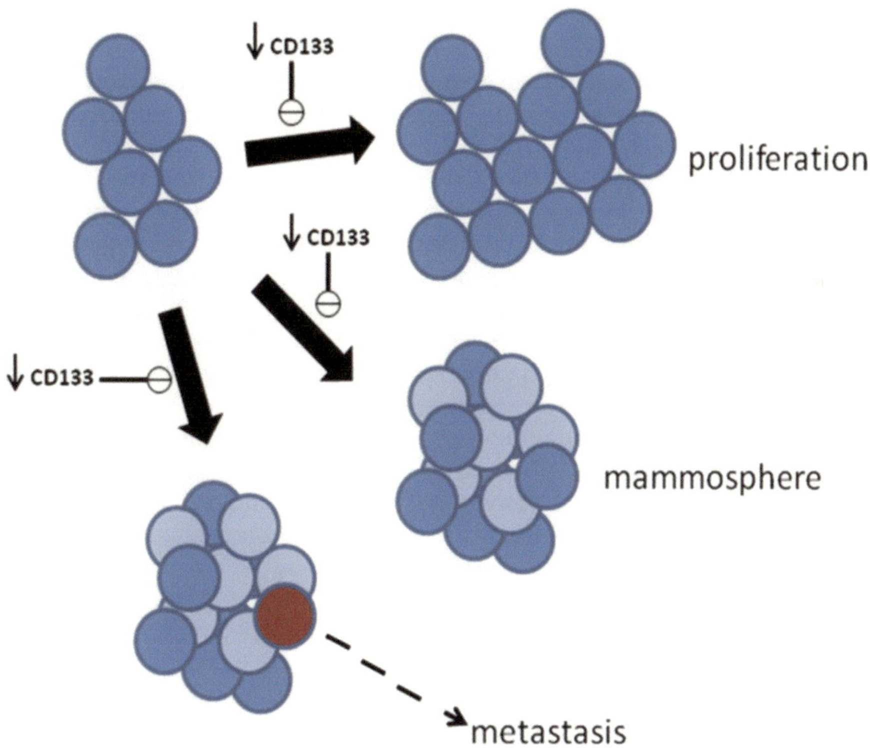

Fig. 2. Role of CD133 in breast cancer.
CD133 downregulation results in poor mammosphere formation, less metastasis, and less proliferation, suggesting a potential target for breast cancer treatment. Furthermore, CD133 is more specific to breast cancer stem cells than many other markers such as CD44, showing additional importance in the role of cancer progression and characterization.

also be a successful anti-neoplastic therapeutic target as shown in hepatocellular and gastric cancers in addition having a role as a cancer stem cell marker. CD133 is potentially a very important cancer stem cell marker in breast cancer specifically as shown by several labs. Cells from basal-like breast cancer and mammospheres from ductal carcinomas express high levels of CD133. Isolated CD133-specfic breast cancer cells from BRCA-1 lines have greater colony forming efficiency and increased proliferative potential, similar to stem cells. Finally, CD133 has been identified in a majority of inflammatory breast cancers, an aggressive form characterized by extensive lymphovascular invasion. A specific xenograft model of inflammatory breast cancer, MARY-X, has not only been shown to contain BCSC-enriched spheroids expressing CD133, but these spheroids have also been shown to contain BCSC profile of CD44+/CD24-/low and ALDH+.

3. Origin of breast cancer stem cells

The origins of BCSC to date still have not been fully elucidated. Indeed, prior to interest in stem cells, the theory of breast cancer progression was different as well. The traditional theory of breast cancer progression hypothesized that each breast cancer cell has the same tumorigenic potential and phenotypic heterogeneity, according to this stochastic model, was due to the accumulation of genetic insults in the progenitor cells. As more light was shed on the undifferentiated nature of aggressive breast cancer tumors and development of therapeutic resistance, a new hierarchical model was suggested. This newer theory believes that the progression of breast cancer is due to a subset of cells within the tumor with stem cell-like characteristics of self-renewal and multi-lineage differentiation potential, which also accounts for the heterogeneity of breast cancer (Figure 3). Further support of the hierarchical model is additionally shown by studies in which only a small portion of cells within a tumor is shown to lead to tumorigenesis. Moreover, the majority of breast cancer cells are very inefficient at tumorigenesis at a cellular level, therefore, only a subset within the tumor must be responsible for metastases by invading blood vessels and transversing the basement membrane. Within the hierarchical model, the subset of cells within breast cancer tumors leading to tumorigenesis has been suggested to be BCSC. This returns to the question about where these cells come from. There are a variety of theories on the subject. BCSC have been supposed to come from de-differentiation, progenitor cells or acquirement of genetic alterations by normal resident cells. Embryonic stem cells have been known to have undifferentiated phenotype and ability for multi lineage differentiation. BCSC are not quite the same although they have the same basic characteristics. In fact, the molecular mechanisms involved in the genesis of BCSC appear to point to a variety of pathways common to both stem cells and cancer biology, which will be discussed later. P53, a long known cell cycle regulator, has been identified as a key determinant in stem cell-like characteristics in breast cancer tumors. The mechanism by which p53 endows breast cancer tumors to develop tumor progression is by allowing reprogramming of tumor cells to become induced-pluripotent cells (Figure 4). These p53 mutations arise often late in tumor progression. There is a clear association between p53 inactivation and the presence of stem cell associated transcription factors in breast cancer. Furthermore, there is an increased incidence of decreased p53 function in malignant tumors, which implies that decreased p53 function leads to phenotypic plasticity and reprogramming of tumor cells. Additional support is seen in studies where induced p53 function led to an inhibition of induced-pluripotent cells from their differentiated counterpart. In addition, the involvement of epithelial to mesenchymal transition (EMT), discussed below, has been purported to be involved in the creation of BCSC.

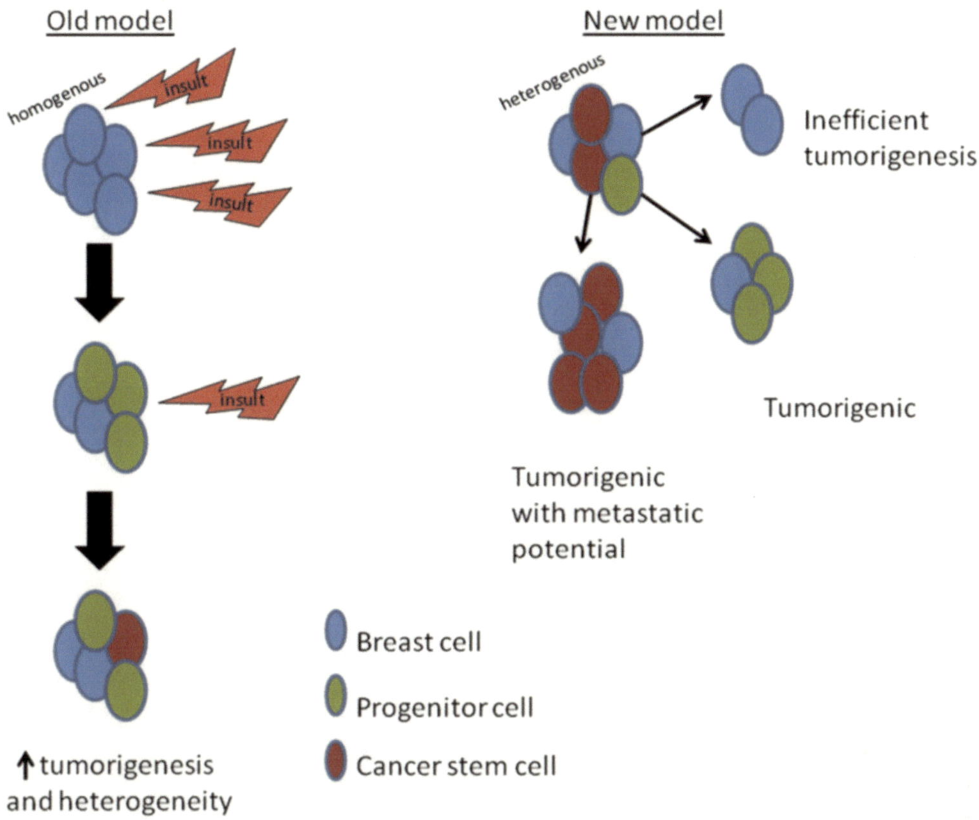

Fig. 3. Theories of breast cancer progression.
The old model of breast cancer progression assumed that all breast cells have equal potential to become tumorigenic with repetitive insults. The new model contends that the breast cells are heterogenous from the start with differing potentials for tumorigenesis, thus resulting in heterogenous breast cancers.

Epithelial to mesenchymal transition is defined as the loss of epithelial characteristics of a cell to adopt a more mesenchymal phenotype. EMT is a function of normal development, for example, involved in gastrulation of a chicken embryo. However, the mesenchymal phenotype typically allows more cell migration and invasion and is the reason EMT is being researched in relation to cancer progression and metastases. Although EMT has been researched for the past two decades, evidence showing EMT in vivo has been controversial. EMT has been identified in breast carcinomas and associated with poor prognosis at both the gene and subtype level. Features characterizing EMT include loss of cell to cell adhesion via E-cadherein in adherens junctions, occludins and claudins in tight junctions and desmoplakin in desmosomes. Aditionally, there is a down regulation of epithelial cytokeratins (KRT8, KRT18, KRT19), upregulation of mesenchymal proteins vimentin and ACTA2. Importantly, there is increased potential for migration and resistance due to an

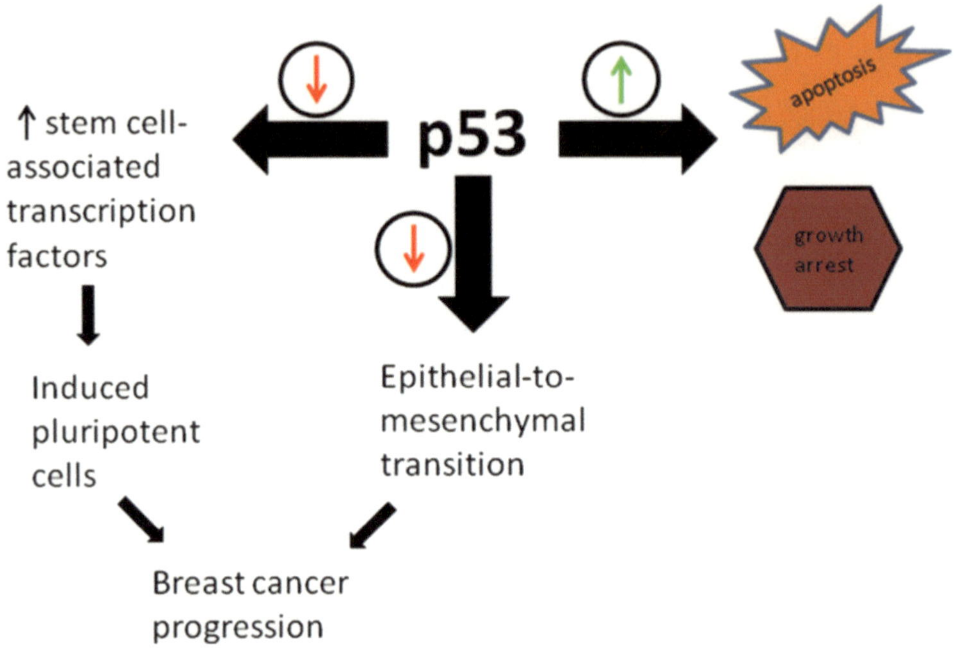

Fig. 4. p53 in breast cancer progression.
P53 is integral in regulating the normal cell cycle. Ordinarily, it eventually induces apoptosis and growth arrest through various caspases. With loss or mutation of p53, EMT and increased stem cell associated transcription factors result in breast cancer progression.

adoption of dynamic actin microfilament networks and increased resistance to apoptosis. EMT has also been shown to be induced by EGF, IGF-1, IGF-2, and TGFb, as well as though transcriptional control of E-cadherin by transcription factors such as SNA1, SNA2, ZEB1, ZEB2, TWIST, and GSC. Signal pathways such as Wnt, Hedgehog and Notch have also been implicated in EMT.
Cells that are the result of EMT and BCSC are not necessarily the same thing. EMT is considered distinct from BCSC generation but has some overlapping factors such as EMT cells demonstrate a CD44+/CD24-/low phenotype similar to BCSC. It has been suggested that EMT can help create BCSC as shown in studies where overexpression of Snail or TWIST lead to the creation of cells with CD44+/CD24-/low expression. EMT has been investigated in breast cancer and BCSC research because these cells have been associated with tumor metastases as well as aggressive breast cancer and a poor prognosis. Furthermore, EMT is implicated in the de-evolution of normal mammary cells to acquire stem cell-like properties. EMT is important in breast cancer research not only as a possible origin for BCSC but also for prognosis. EMT that may create BCSC promotes the development of refractory and resistant breast cancer because BCSC are often resistant to many cancer tx, which ultimately leads to breast cancer relapse. EMT can be induced by CD8+T cells with the resulting tumors having CD44+/CD24-/low phenotype, potent tumorigenicity, ability to re-estabilish an epithelial tumor and increased resistance to therapy further lending credence to the idea that EMT is involved in BCSC generation.
Not only do BCSC lend breast cancer the ability for tumor progression but breast cancer is also potentially affected by mesenchymal stem cells (MSC). MSC may have a role in being

protective for BCSC, thus affecting breast cancer progression. These cells have been shown to migrate to breast cancer tumor site and allow the breast cancer to become resistant to therapy. Importantly, MSC play an important role in helping BC cells evade the immune system, thus allowing tumor progression. MSC by itself has the ability to promote tumor progression by creating cancer associated fibroblasts (CAFs). These CAFs, characterized by SDF-1 are established in tumor stroma and leads to the creation of metastases, angiogenesis and other pro-tumorigenic factors; however, further details are beyond the scope of this chapter.

4. Pathways

Important pathways that have been implicated in BCSC include Hedgehog, Notch, Wnt, p53, and TGFB. TGFB, an immunosuppressive cytokine that is involved in wound healing, fibrosis, and cell cycle regulation has been shown to be critical in BCSC behavior. Importantly, loss of TGFB may enhance breast cancer motility (thus leading to metastases) via EMT, as discussed earlier. This increased motility may be due to the fact that TGFB is responsible for cell cycle inhibition and blocking de novo cancer formation. Loss of TGFB is associated with an increase the Sca1 marker, showing an increase in the luminal progenitor cells within the tumor. Additionally, TGFB results in a decrease in side population cells, characterized by the ability to efflux Horest dye, which is thought to be enriched with progenitor cells. Furthermore, TGFb was silenced in a cell population with the CD44+/CD24-/low phenotype, thus further supporting the fact that TGFb is a tumor suppressor.

Wnt pathway involves secreted growth factors involved in a wide range of cell processes and has been shown to be regulatory in nature of stem cell maintenance and carcinogenesis. There are two broad categories in this pathway: canonical and non-canonical pathways. The canonical pathway, including Wnt1, is b-catenin-dependent while the non-canonical pathway, including Wnt5a, is b-catenin-independent. The canonical pathway is associated with stem cell maintenance or expansion by suppressing differentiation and promoting self-renewal. Exogenous administration of Wnt to normal mammary stem cells results in an expansion of stem cells with an increase in self-renewal ability. Furthermore, Lp5, a receptor for Wnt signaling, is present in the same location as mammary stem cells in the basal-epithelial compartment of the mammary gland, as previously mentioned. A decreased in Lp5 results in the loss of stem cell activity in the mammary gland. The canonical pathway is b-catenin dependent, as previously mentioned, therefore, it follows that a gain of function mutation resulting in increased b-catenin activity results in increased mammary stem cell self renewal. Although the canonical Wnt pathway is involved in stem cell maintenance, it has also been implicated in tumorigenesis from stem cells and luminal progenitor cells as shown in studies where there is an increase in stem cells and Sca1, a marker for luminal progenitor cells, in tumors with overexpressed Wnt1. On the other hand, decreased Wnt5a in breast cancer tumors have been implicated in early relapse and poor prognosis. Wnt 1 of the canonical Wnt pathway is unregulated and Wnt5a is downregulated in breast cancer cells when compared to normal mammilary cells, indicating that the Wnt5a has tumor suppressive ability similar to TGFb (discussed above). The two opposing Wnt pathways appear to exert effects on each other to maintain normal cellular function. When the canonical pathway is suppressed by the non-canonical pathway, there is a decrease in stem cell phenotype.

Importantly, the Wnt pathway and TGFb are connected since TGFb tumor suppressive function appears to involve antagonism of the canonical Wnt pathway by Wnt5a. The two are interconnected further because TGFb regulates Wnt5a expression in mammary gland while Wnt1 of the canonical pathway mediates TGFb effects on branching during breast development. The data suggests that TGFb and Wnt5a can inhibit the canonical Wnt pathway, redirecting the mammilary tumor cells to adopt a more basal-like characteristic. The mechanism for this tumor suppression by TGFb has been reported to be due to the fact that TGFb acting through Wnt5a inhibits b-catenin, thus initiating tumor suppression by limiting stem/progenitor cell populations (Figure 5).

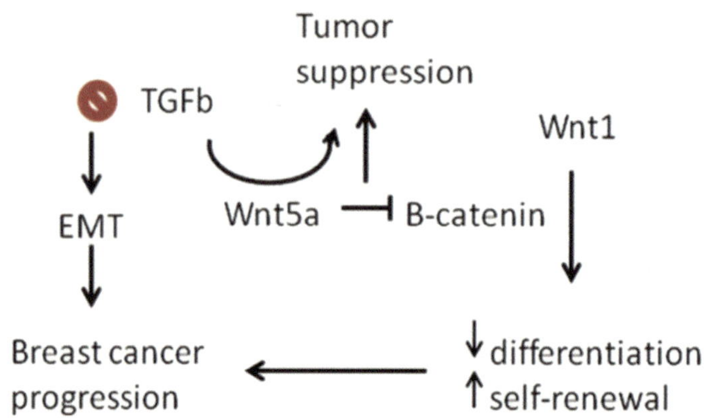

Fig. 5. TGFb and Wnt pathways interplay in breast cancer.
TGFb and Wnt5a both act as tumor suppressors. TGFb, when inhibited, induces epithelial-to-mesenchymal transition, leading to breast cancer progression. Wnt1 is normally inhibited by Wnt5a, leading to suppressed ability for self-reneal and de-differentiation. When b-catenin is not inhibited by Wnt5a, Wnt1 leads to increased self renewal and decreased differentiation, both of which lead to breast cancer progression. Therefore, Wnt1 and Wnt5a, along with TGFb, work against each other to help maintain normal cell physiology.

The hedgehog pathway has been implicated in sustaining cancer stem cells through self-renewal. The pathway was first discovered in Drosophila melanagaster and is a major regulator of cell proliferation, differentiation, and stem cell maintenance. The link to cancer was established while studying a rare familial disease, Gorlin syndrome, in 1996. Secreted Hedgehog ligands bind their transmembrane receptor Patch, which causes Smo release and dissociation of transcription factors Gil1, Gil2, and Gil 3 from Fu and SuFu. These transcription factors lead to transcription of cyclin D, cyclin E, Myc and EGF factors, enhancing carcinogenesis. In the absence of the Hedgehog ligands, the transmembrane receptor Patch associates with Smo, effectively blocking Smo function. Thus, Hedgehog inhibitors, such as cyclopamine, are being looked at as potential anti-neoplastic agents (Figure 6). Additionally, TFGb has been demonstrated to upregulate factors in the Hedgehog pathway. Further support of a role in cancer is shown by studies in which the hedgehog pathway has been implicated in progression from non-invasive phenotype to invasive phenotype in ductal carcinoma. An important fact of which to take note, however, is the fact that Hedgehog is also intimately involved in normal developmental processes as well, causing potential difficulties implementing Hedgehog inhibitors as anti-tumorigenic agents.

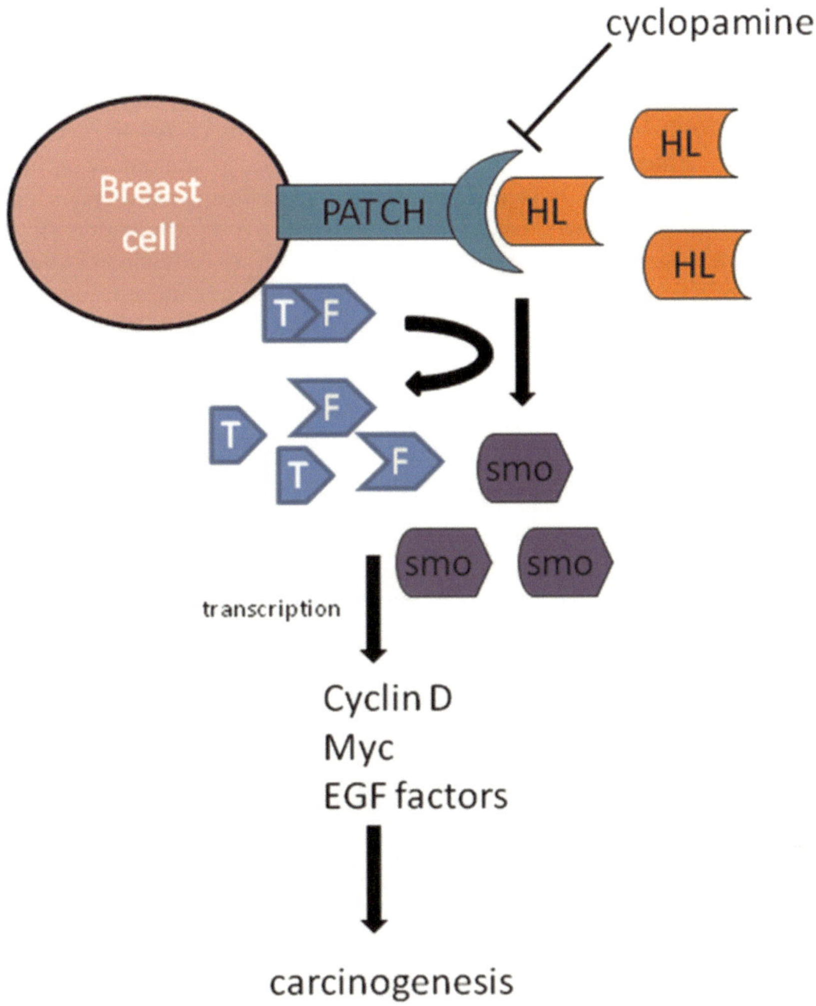

Fig. 6. Promotion of carcinogenesis through Hedgehog.
With Hedgehog ligand association with PATCH, smo is released, allowing smo to function causing dissociation of transcription factors. This causes an increase in transcriptional activity producing Cyclin D, Cyclin E, Myc and EFG factors, all of which lead to carcinongenesis. In the absence of Hedgehog ligand, PATCH associates with smo, effectively blocking smo function and ultimately inhibiting carcinogenesis, thus suggesting the utility of Hedgehog inhibitors such as cyclopamine in breast cancer treatment.

The Notch pathway has been implicated in normal cell proliferation control and apoptosis as well as the development of a variety of organs. This pathway has been demonstrated to be abnormally regulated in cancer stem cells, including BCSC, leading to uncontrolled BCSC self-renewal. The Notch receptors are bound by ligands called Delta-like and Jagged. The bound receptors are proteolytically cleaved by ADAM protease family and y-sectretase, allowing sequestration into the nucleus. Once in the nucleus, the transcription of genes inhibiting cell differentiation and increasing cell proliferation ensues. The released intracellular domain of Notch acts as a transcriptional co-activator to promote transcription of downstream targets of the recombination signal sequence binding protein Jk such as Myc and Cyclin D1 (Figure 7). Additionally, Notch transmembrane receptors for Notch proteins Notch 1-4 have been found in many stem cells. Studies have shown that treatment of ductal carcinomas with Notch inhibitors have led to the formation of fewer mammospheres, further supporting evidence of Notch playing a key role in mammary epithelial cell proliferation and differentiation. In fact, studies nearly a decade ago provided evidence for a role of Notch in breast cancer. These studies showed hyperproliferation of normally mammary cells in a dose-dependent manner by Notch pathway activation of constitutively active Notch receptors. Notch inhibitors are being considered in clinical trials also because Notch signaling has been implicated in breast cancer to resistance to radiation therapy.

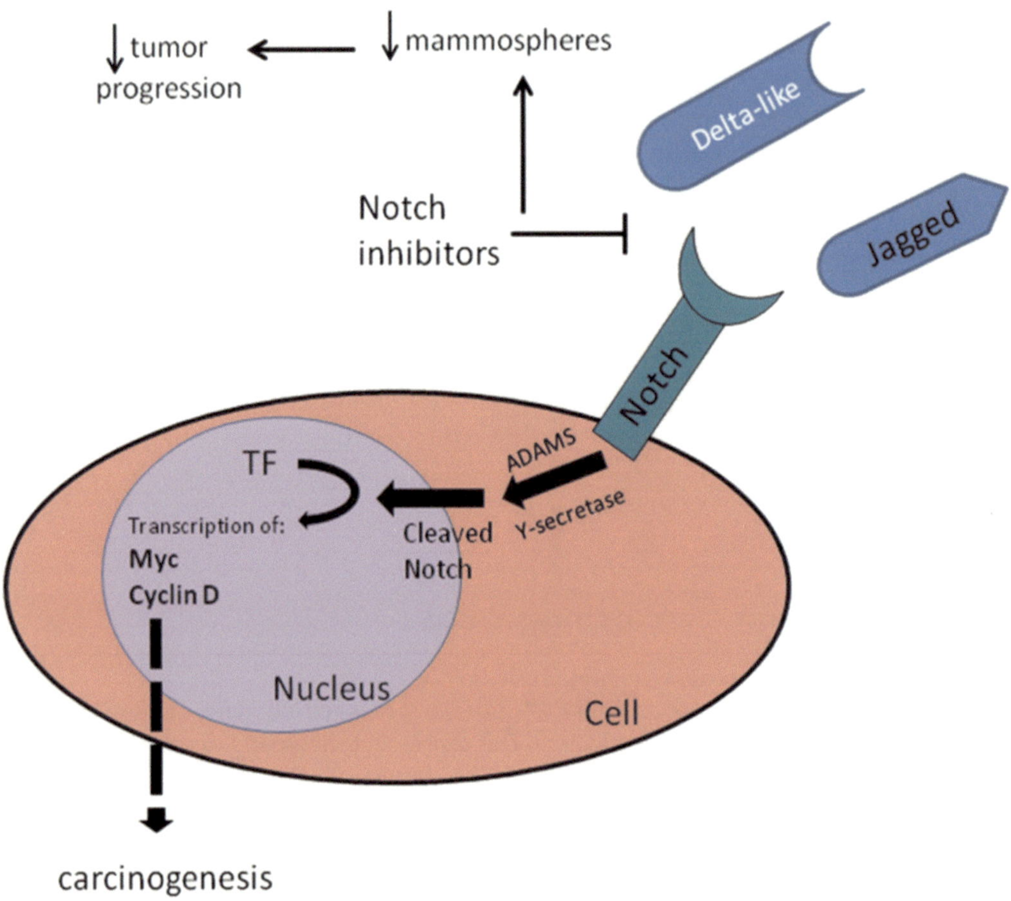

Fig. 7. Role of Notch in breast cancer.
The intracellular domain of Notch is cleaved by ADAMS and y -secretase after being bound by Delta-like and Jagged ligands. The cleaved portions are then sequestered in the nucleus where they act as transcription cofactors resulting in increased Myc and Cyclin D, promoting carcinogenesis. Also, Notch inhibitors have been demonstrated to decrease mammosphere formation, further suggesting the importance of Notch in breast cancer therapy.

5. Treatments

Since the discovery of stem cells in breast cancer, these cells have also been the focus of research as potential targets for anti-neoplastic treatment. If these cells allow cancer progression, resistance, and recurrence, it is logical that treatments concentrated on stem cell suppression would lead to more efficacious breast cancer treatment. Importantly, long-term efficacy is doubtful since renewal of stem cells is always a possibility. Nonetheless, there are have many proposed therapies targeted at BCSC and their pathways. To date, several potential treatments have been suggested against the MDR profile of BCSC including UHRF1, dofequidor fumarate, isotetrandrine. UHRF1 plays a role in treating breast cancer by inhibiting MDR1 promoter activity and expression. Studies have shown that overexpression of UHRF1 can induce deacetylation of histonesH3 and H4 on the MDR1 promoter. This deacetylation leads to a loss of binding to transcription factors MyoD, CBP, and p300, ultimately suppression MDR1. These cells have been shown to have increased sensitivity to chemotherapy agents that are transported by p-glycoprotein. Dofequidor fumarate, an orally active quinilone compound, has been shown to decrease MDR profile by inhibiting p-glygoprotein, MDR1 or both. Indeed, phase III clinical trials have shown a decrease in chemo-resistance in patients who have not previously received treatment. The compound is thought to work by inhibiting ABCG2/BCRP, which is higher in side populations than non side population cells, which results in an increased sensitivity to anti-neoplastic treatment. Another agent found to be efficacious against the MDR profile associated with BCSC is isotetrandrine, an isoquinoline alkaloid extracted from Caulis manhoniae. This agent has been discovered to result in MDR reversal through inhibition of p-glycoprotein-mediated MDR as has phenybutenoids derived from the rhizomes of Zingiber cassumunar, both acting as a potent chemo-sensitizing agent in the treatment against breast cancer. Additionally, IL-24 has recently gained attention as a potential anti-neoplastic treatment based on its anti-tumor effects via induction of apoptosis. Other anti-BCSC agents include salinomycin, an agent that targets cancer stem cells of epithelial origin. This agent has been shown to decrease the population of CD44+/CD24-/low within breast cancer. Although not specifically shown to inhibit breast cancer progression, cyclopamine has been demonstrated to inhibit progression of other cancers through the Hedgehog pathway, which is responsible for maintenance of CD44+/CD24-/low population in breast cancer.

Since de-differentiation is a major focus as a potential origin of BCSC and the de-differentiated phenotype is associated with aggressive breast cancers, it follows that agents that can induce differentiation could serve as possible agents antagonistic to stem cell creation and survival, leading to improved prognosis and treatment efficacy. Retinoids are the forerunners for differentiation therapy and has been shown to be successful as seen in acute myeloid leukemia M3 therapy where all-trans retinoic acid is currently being used. Of note, BRCA1 has been shown to be integral in differentiation in breast cancer. BRCA1 knockdown is present in breast cancers with increased mammosphere formation, increased ALDH1 cells and increased BCSC.

It is imperative also to consider the interaction of the immune system with breast cancer cells prior to initiating targeted treatment against BCSC. The helper T cell phenotype (Th1 phenotype), has been found to be more anti-neoplastic than the counterbalancing Th2 phenotype. Th1 phenotype have effects that may be bimodal, however, since the inflammatory nature of the Th1 response can cause DNA damage leading to malignant cell transformation, while also allowing anti-tumorigenic actions, perhaps to eliminate these malignant cells, as seen by micrometastases to sentinel lymph nodes creating an increased Th1 phenotype. The Th2 phenotype, which studies show to be more clearly linked to pro-tumorigenic processes, demonstrates a facilitative effect on cancer via release of Il-4, which prevents chemo-sensitivity and escape from immune detection.

Pathways associated with BCSC have also been targeted in breast cancer research. There is significant evidence of a role for Hedgehog and Wnt, on stem cells in breast cancer, however, there is difficulties associated with inhibiting these pathways because they are also involved in normal somatic stem cells required in development. Additionally, since Numb, an inhibitor of the Notch pathway, has been shown to have decreased activity in BCSC, targeted therapies against Notch have made it to clinical trials unfortunately however, with limited success. Much of the ineffectuality of the treatments has been attributed to potential cross talk with other pathways.

6. Conclusion

Breast cancer research has come a long way in uncovering the unique characteristics of stem cells found within breast cancers that make them an important aspect in breast cancers as both a reason for resistance and progression as well as a potential target for anti-neoplastic treatment. Although much has been discovered about BCSC since their introduction into breast cancer research back in 1997, there is still a lot to be figured out. There have been a lot of characteristic that have been found helping identify BCSC, however, there is still a lack of a concrete definition. Indeed, it may be not only unrealistic to determine a single definition of BCSC, but also counterproductive. Since there are such a variety of breast cancers and treatments vary accordingly, maybe it is only natural that the definition of these BCSC would also vary. Even after stem cells have been identified, it is difficult to specifically target these cells. Given that BCSC, whether or not they result directly from normal stem cells, have a lot of pathways common to both the abnormal and normal stem cells. This makes it difficult to inhibit these pathways without altering normal cellular processes necessary for normal cell survival as well. Determination of the development and origin of BCSC would be greatly helpful in establishing specific treatments focused on these malignant cells. Given the plethora of information already discovered about BCSC and the vast areas still being investigated, research has shown how critical BCSC are in the fight against breast cancer.

7. References

Alonso L, Fuchs E. Stem cells in the skin: waste not, Wnt not. Genes Dev. 2003;17(10):1189–200.

Badders NM, Goel S, Clark RJ, Klos KS, Kim S, Bafico A, et al. The Wnt receptor, Lrp5, is expressed by mouse mammary stem cells and is required to maintain the basal lineage. PLoS ONE. 2009;4(8):e6594.

Benhaj K, Akcali KC, Ozturk M. Redundant expression of canonical Wnt ligands in human breast cancer cell lines. Oncol Rep. 2006;15(3):701–7.

Bonnet D, Dick JE. Human acute myeloid leukemia is organized as a hierarchy that originates from a primitive hematopoietic cell. Nat Med. 1997;3(7):730–7.

Borggrefe T, Oswald F, The Notch signaling pathway: transcriptional regulation at Notch target genes, Cell Mol Life Sci 66 (2009), pp. 1631–1646.

Calcagno AM, Salcido CD, Gillet JP, Wu CP, Fostel JM, Mumau MD, Gottesman MM, Varticovski L, Ambudkar SV. Prolonged drug selection of breast cancer cells and enrichment of cancer stem cell characteristics. J Natl Cancer Inst. 2010 Nov 3;102(21):1637-52.

Callahan R, Raafat A, Notch signaling in mammary gland tumorigenesis, J. Mammary Gland Biol. Neoplasia 6 (2001), pp. 23–36.

Charafe-Jauffret E, Ginestier C, Iovino F, et al. Aldehyde dehydrogenase 1-positive cancer stem cells mediate metastasis and poor clinical outcome in inflammatory breast cancer. Clinical Cancer Research. 2010;16(1):45–55.

Charafe-Jauffret E, Ginestier C, Iovino F, et al. Breast cancer cell lines contain functional cancer stem sells with metastatic capacity and a distinct molecular signature. Cancer Research.2009;69(4):1302–1313.

Chen MS, Woodward WA, Behbod F, et al. Wnt/β-catenin mediates radiation resistance of Sca1+ progenitors in an immortalized mammary gland cell line. Journal of Cell Science. 2007;120(3):468–477.

Cho RW, Wang X, Diehn M, Shedden K, Chen GY, Sherlock G, et al. Isolation and molecular characterization of cancer stem cells in MMTV-Wnt-1 murine breast tumors. Stem Cells. 2008;26(2):364–71.

Chung SY, Han AR, Sung MK, Jung HJ, Nam JW, Seo EK, Lee HJ. Potent modulation of P-glycoprotein activity by naturally occurring phenylbutenoids from Zingiber cassumunar. Phytother Res. 2009 Apr;23(4):472-6.

Croker AK, Allan AL. Cancer stem cells: implications for the progression and treatment of metastatic disease. J Cell Mol Med. 2008;12(2):374–90.

Dabiri G, Tumbarello DA, Turner CE, Van de Water L. TGF-beta1 slows the growth of pathogenic myofibroblasts through a mechanism requiring the focal adhesion protein, Hic-5. *J Invest Dermatol.*2008;128(2):280–91

Donnenberg VS, Meyer EM, Donnenberg AD. Measurement of multiple drug resistance transporter activity in putative cancer stem/progenitor cells. Methods Mol Biol. 2009;568:261-79.

Farnie G, Clarke RB, Spence K, Pinnock N, Brennan K, Anderson NG, Bundred NJ, Novel cell culture technique for primary ductal carcinoma in situ: role of Notch and epidermal growth factor receptor signaling pathways, J. Natl. Cancer Inst. 99 (2007), pp. 616–627.

Ginestier C, Hur MH, Charafe-Jauffret E, et al. ALDH1 is a marker of normal and malignant human mammary stem cells and a predictor of poor clinical outcome. Cell Stem Cell.2007;1(5):555–567.

Goodell MA, Brose K, Paradis G, Conner AS, Mulligan RC. Isolation and functional properties of murine hematopoietic stem cells that are replicating in vivo. Journal of Experimental Medicine.1996;183(4):1797–1806.

Gupta PB, Onder TT, Jiang G, et al. Identification of selective inhibitors of cancer stem cells by high-throughput screening. Cell. 2009;138(4):645–59.

Hansen LA, Sigman CC, Andreola F, Ross SA, Kelloff GJ, De Luca LM. Retinoids in chemoprevention and differentiation therapy. Carcinogenesis. 2000;21(7):1271–9.

Hollier BG, Evans K, Mani SA. The epithelial-to-mesenchymal transition and cancer stem cells: a coalition against cancer therapies. J Mammary Gland Biol Neoplasia. 2009;14(1):29–43.

Ischenko I, Seeliger H, Schaffer M, Jauch KW, Bruns CJ. Cancer stem cells: how can we target them? Curr Med Chem. 2008;15(30):3171–84.

Jin W, Liu Y, Xu SG, Yin WJ, Li JJ, Yang JM, Shao ZM. UHRF1 inhibits MDR1 gene transcription and sensitizes breast cancer cells to anticancer drugs. Breast Cancer Res Treat. 2010 Nov;124(1):39-48.

Johnson RW, Nguyen MP, Padalecki SS, Grubbs BG, Merkel AR, Oyajobi BO, Matrisian LM, Mundy GR, Sterling JA. TGF-beta promotion of Gli2-induced expression of parathyroid hormone-related protein, an important osteolytic factor in bone metastasis, is independent of canonical Hedgehog signaling. Cancer Res. 2011 Feb 1;71(3):822-31.

Kang SK, Park JB, Cha SH. Multipotent, dedifferentiated cancer stem-like cells from brain gliomas.Stem Cells Dev. 2006;15(3):423–35.

Katayama R, Koike S, Sato S, Sugimoto Y, Tsuruo T, Fujita N. Dofequidar fumarate sensitizes cancer stem-like side population cells to chemotherapeutic drugs by inhibiting ABCG2/BCRP-mediated drug export. Cancer Sci. 2009 Nov;100(11):2060-8.

Kim HJ, Kim JB, Lee KM, et al. Isolation of CD24(high) and CD24(low/-) cells from MCF-7: CD24 expression is positively related with proliferation, adhesion and invasion in MCF-7. Cancer Letters.2007;258(1):98–108.

Korkaya H, Paulson A, Charafe-Jauffret E, Ginestier C, Brown M, Dutcher J, Clouthier SG, Wicha MS. Regulation of mammary stem/progenitor cells by PTEN/Akt/beta-catenin signaling. PLoS Biol.2009;7(6):e1000121.

Lewis M.T and Veltmaat J.M, Next stop, the twilight zone: hedgehog network regulation of mammary gland development, J Mammary Gland Biol Neoplasia 9 (2004), pp. 165–181.

Lim E, Vaillant F, Wu D, et al. Aberrant luminal progenitors as the candidate target population for basal tumor development in BRCA1 mutation carriers. Nat Med. 2009;15(8):907–13.

Linn SC, Van't Veer LJ. Clinical relevance of the triple-negative breast cancer concept: genetic basis and clinical utility of the concept. Eur J Cancer. 2009;45 (Suppl 1):11–26.

Liu BY, McDermott SP, Khwaja SS, Alexander CM. The transforming activity of Wnt effectors correlates with their ability to induce the accumulation of mammary progenitor cells. Proc Natl Acad Sci USA. 2004;101(12):4158–63.

Liu H, Gu D, Xie J. Clinical implications of hedgehog signaling pathway inhibitors. Chin J Cancer. 2011 Jan;30(1):13-26. PubMed PMID: 21192841.

Liu S, Ginestier C, Charafe-Jauffret E, et al. BRCA1 regulates human mammary stem/progenitor cell fate. *Proc Natl Acad Sci U S A.* 2008;105(5):1680–5.

Lorico A, Rappa G. Phenotypic heterogeneity of breast cancer stem cells. J Oncol. 2011;2011:135039.

Mani SA, Guo W, Liao MJ, et al. The epithelial-mesenchymal transition generates cells with properties of stem cells. *Cell.* 2008;133(4):704–15.

Matsuura K, Yamaguchi Y, Osaki A, et al. FOXP3 expression of micrometastasis-positive sentinel nodes in breast cancer patients. Oncol Rep. 2009;22(5):1181–7.

Mehra N, Penning M, Maas J, et al. Progenitor marker CD133 mRNA is elevated in peripheral blood of cancer patients with bone metastases. Clinical Cancer Research. 2006;12(16):4859–4866.

Melinkeri SR, Gupta RK, Dabadghao S. A Sweet-like syndrome manifesting as gingival hyperplasia and myositis without cutaneous involvement. Ann Hematol. 2002;81(7):397–8.

Mishra PJ, Merlino G. MicroRNA reexpression as differentiation therapy in cancer. *J Clin Invest.*2009;119(8):2119–23. [PMC free article] [PubMed]

Mishra PJ, Mishra PJ, Humeniuk R, et al. Carcinoma-associated fibroblast-like differentiation of human mesenchymal stem cells. *Cancer Res.* 2008;68(11):4331–9.

Mizrak D, Brittan M, Alison MR. CD 133: molecule of the moment. Journal of Pathology.2008;214(1):3–9.

Mizuno H, Spike BT, Wahl GM, Levine AJ. Inactivation of p53 in breast cancers correlates with stem cell transcriptional signatures. Proc Natl Acad Sci U S A. 2010 Dec 28;107(52):22745-50.

Modolell M, Choi BS, Ryan RO, et al. Local suppression of T cell responses by arginase-induced L-arginine depletion in nonhealing leishmaniasis. PLoS Negl Trop Dis. 2009;3(7):e480.

Moreno-Bueno G, Portillo F, Cano A: Transcriptional regulation of cell polarity in EMT and cancer. Oncogene 2008, 27:6958-6969.

Mumm JS, Kopan R, Notch signaling: from the outside in, Dev Biol 228 (2000), pp. 151–165.

Orian-Rousseau V. CD44, a therapeutic target for metastasising tumours. Eur J Cancer. 2010 May;46(7):1271-7.

Pasca di Magliano M. and Hebrok M., Hedgehog signalling in cancer formation and maintenance, Nat Rev Cancer 3 (2003), pp. 903–911.

Patel SA, Ndabahaliye A, Lim PK, Milton R, Rameshwar P. Challenges in the development of future treatments for breast cancer stem cells. Breast Cancer (London). 2010;2:1-11.

Patrawala L, Calhoun T, Schneider-Broussard R, Zhou J, Claypool K, Tang DG. Side population is enriched in tumorigenic, stem-like cancer cells, whereas ABCG2 and ABCG2 cancer cells are similarly tumorigenic. *Cancer Research.* 2005;65(14):6207–6219.

Pece S, Serresi M, Santolini E, et al. Loss of negative regulation by Numb over Notch is relevant to human breast carcinogenesis. J Cell Biol. 2004;167(2):215–21.

Rappa G, Fodstad O, Lorico A. The stem cell-associated antigen CD133 (Prominin-1) is a molecular therapeutic target for metastatic melanoma. Stem Cells. 2008;26(12):3008–3017.

Rhodes LV, Muir SE, Elliott S, et al. Adult human mesenchymal stem cells enhance breast tumorigenesis and promote hormone independence. *Breast Cancer Res Treat.* 2009.

Rizzo P, Osipo C, Foreman K, Golde T, Osborne B, Miele L. Rational targeting of Notch signaling in cancer. Oncogene. 2008;27(38):5124–31.

Roarty K, Baxley SE, Crowley MR, Frost AR, Serra R. Loss of TGF-beta or Wnt5a results in an increase in Wnt/beta-catenin activity and redirects mammary tumour phenotype. Breast Cancer Res. 2009;11(2):R19.

Sakariassen PO, Immervoll H, Chekenya M. Cancer stem cells as mediators of treatment resistance in brain tumors: status and controversies. *Neoplasia.* 2007;9(11):882–92.

Santisteban M, Reiman JM, Asiedu MK, et al. Immune-induced epithelial to mesenchymal transition in vivo generates breast cancer stem cells. *Cancer Res.* 2009;69(7):2887–95.

Schatton T, Frank NY, Frank MH. Identification and targeting of cancer stem cells. *Bioessays.*2009;31(10):1038–1049.

Scola L, Giacalone A, Marasà L, et al. Genetic determined downregulation of both type 1 and type 2 cytokine pathways might be protective against pancreatic cancer. Ann N Y Acad Sci.2009;1155:284–8.

Serra R, Easter SL, Jiang W, Baxley SE. Wnt5a as an Effector of TGFβ in Mammary Development and Cancer. J Mammary Gland Biol Neoplasia. 2011 Mar 18.

Shipitsin M, Campbell LL, Argani P, et al. Molecular definition of breast tumor heterogeneity.Cancer Cell. 2007;11(3):259–73.

Sjolund J, Manetopoulos C, Stockhausen MT, Axelson H, The Notch pathway in cancer: differentiation gone awry, Eur. J. Cancer 41 (2005), pp. 2620–2629.

Smith LM, Nesterova A, Ryan MC, et al. CD133/prominin-1 is a potential therapeutic target for antibody-drug conjugates in hepatocellular and gastric cancers. British Journal of Cancer.2008;99(1):100–109.

Sonnenberg M, van der Kuip H, Haubeis S, Fritz P, Schroth W, Friedel G, Simon W, Mürdter TE, Aulitzky WE. Highly variable response to cytotoxic chemotherapy in carcinoma-associated fibroblasts (CAFs) from lung and breast. BMC Cancer. 2008 Dec 11;8:364.

Souzaki M, Kubo M, Kai M, Kameda C, Tanaka H, Taguchi T, Tanaka M, Onishi H, Katano M. Hedgehog signaling pathway mediates the progression of non-invasive breast cancer to invasive breast cancer. Cancer Sci. 2011 Feb;102(2):37381.

Storci G, Sansone P, Trere D, et al. The basal-like breast carcinoma phenotype is regulated by SLUG gene expression. Journal of Pathology. 2008;214(1):25–37.

Tan AR, Alexe G, Reiss M. Transforming growth factor-beta signaling: emerging stem cell target in metastatic breast cancer? *Breast Cancer Res Treat.* 2009;115(3):453–95.

Tanaka H, Nakamura M, Kameda C, et al. The Hedgehog signaling pathway plays an essential role in maintaining the CD44+CD24−/low subpopulation and the side population of breast cancer cells. Anticancer Res. 2009;29(6):2147–57.

Tang B, Yoo N, Vu M, Mamura M, Nam JS, Ooshima A, et al. Transforming growth factor-beta can suppress tumorigenesis through effects on the putative cancer stem or early progenitor cell and committed progeny in a breast cancer xenograft model. Cancer Res. 2007;67(18):8643–52.

Thiery JP. Epithelial-mesenchymal transitions in tumour progression. Nat Rev Cancer 2002, 2:442-454.

Tomaskovic-Crook, E, Erik W Thompson, EW, Thiery, JP. Epithelial to mesenchymal transition and breast cancer. Breast Cancer Research 2009, 11:213.

Wang J, Wakeman TP, Lathia JD et al., Notch promotes radioresistance ofglioma stem cells, Stem Cells 28 (2009), pp. 17–28.

Wang TX, Yang XH. Reversal effect of isotetrandrine, an isoquinoline alkaloid extracted from Caulis Mahoniae, on P-glycoprotein-mediated doxorubicin-resistance in human breast cancer (MCF-7/DOX) cells. Yao Xue Xue Bao. 2008 May;43(5):461-6.

Wang Z, Li Y, Banerjee S., Sarkar F.H, Emerging role of Notch in stem cells and cancer, Cancer Lett 279 (2009), pp. 8–12.

Winquist RJ, Boucher DM, Wood M, Furey BF. Targeting cancer stem cells for more effective therapies: Taking out cancer's locomotive engine. Biochem Pharmacol. 2009;78(4):326–34.

Wright MH, Calcagno AM, Salcido CD, Carlson MD, Ambudkar SV, Varticovski L. Brca1 breast tumors contain distinct CD44+/CD24- and CD133+ cells with cancer stem cell characteristics. Breast Cancer Research. 2008;10(1, article R10)

Xiao YI, Ye Y, Yearsley K, Jones S, Barsky SH. The lymphovascular embolus of inflammatory breast cancer expresses a stem cell-like phenotype. American Journal of Pathology.2008;173(2):561–574.

Yang YJ, Chen DZ, Li LX, Sheng QS, Jin ZK, Zhao DF. Targeted IL-24 gene therapy inhibits cancer recurrence after liver tumor resection by inducing tumor cell apoptosis in nude mice. Hepatobiliary Pancreat Dis Int. 2009;8(2):174–8.

Zardawi SJ, O'Toole SA, Sutherland RL, Musgrove EA. Dysregulation of Hedgehog, Wnt and Notch signalling pathways in breast cancer. Histol Histopathol. 2009;24(3):385–98.

Zeng YA, Nusse R. Wnt proteins are self-renewal factors for mammary stem cells and promote their long-term expansion in culture. Cell Stem Cell. 2010;6(6):568–77.

25

Potential Roles of miR-106a in Breast Cancer

KuanHui E. Chen and Ameae M. Walker
University of California, Riverside, CA, USA

1. Introduction

The discovery of interfering RNAs uncovered a new level of regulation of gene expression. It is now believed that as much as 92% of gene expression may be regulated by interfering RNAs. Interfering RNAs may be micro RNAs (miRNAs) or small interfering RNAs (siRNAs). Our focus is on miRNAs. These are mostly coded in intronic or intergenic regions of DNA and are grouped into families on the basis that they likely evolved from a common ancestral gene. Among the miRNA families, the miR17-92 family has attracted attention because of its oncogenic activity. miRNAs in this family include the miR17-92 cluster and two paralogs, the miR-106a and miR-106b clusters. Expression of these miRNAs is markedly upregulated in several types of cancer, and they are considered oncomirs. The two paralogs derive from an ancient gene duplication event involving the miR17-92 cluster. They therefore share highly similar sequences with miR17-92 family members and each other. As a result, they also work on very similar targets, primarily inhibiting the translation of target mRNAs by binding to the 3′ untranslated region. The miR-106 paralogs are located on different chromosomes from the miR17-92 cluster: miR-106a is intriguingly located on the X chromosome, miR-106b on chromosome 7, and miR17-92 on chromosome 13. Regulation of expression of any of the paralogs can therefore occur without concomitant regulation of the other two. This review examines the thesis that miR-106a in particular may play an important role in the development and progression of breast cancer. Because relatively little attention has yet to be given to miR-106a, the potential role of miR-106a is often suggested on the basis of a known role of a related family member. Similarly, defined roles of miR-106a and family members in other neoplasms are used to suggest a role in breast cancer.

2. Small interfering RNAs

Interfering RNAs are small ribonucleic acids around 18-25 nucleotides in length. Depending on the author, between 60 and 92% of human genes are likely regulated by these small RNAs (Baek et al. 2008, Dai and Ahmed 2011). Interfering RNAs may be microRNAs (miRNAs) or small interfering RNAs (siRNAs). Both share a similar mechanism of action, but differ in their initial cellular processing. miRNAs are usually encoded by intergenic or intronic regions of DNA, but may be present in exonic regions of non-protein-coding genes or of protein coding genes subject to alternate splicing (Rodriguez et al. 2004 , (Kim et al., 2009). In the classical scheme for their production (Figure 1), miRNA regions of the genome are transcribed by RNA polymerase II as longer sequences including a region that forms a

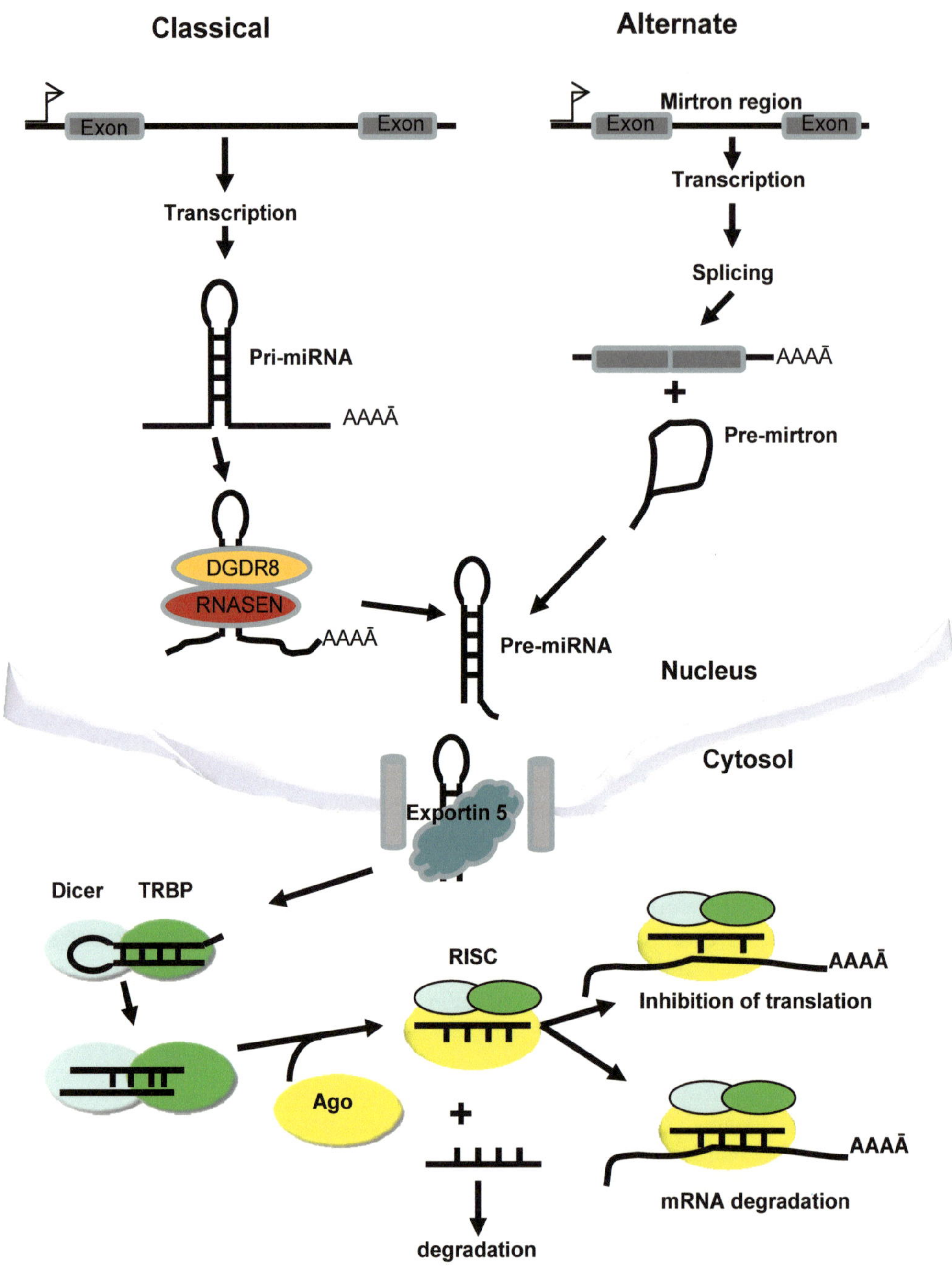

Fig. 1. Classical and alternate pathways of miRNA generation and the mechanisms of inhibition of target gene expression. Figure modified from one by Dai and Ahmed (2011).

hairpin or stem loop (pri-miRNA). This is then processed by binding to DGCR8 (DiGeorge Syndrome Critical Region protein 8) and cleavage by RNASEN (an RNAse III enzyme) to form a pre-miRNA of about 70 nucleotides in length. The pre-miRNA is exported from the nucleus by binding to exportin 5, which recognizes its double-stranded hairpin region. Once in the cytosol, the pre-miRNA is subject to further cleavage by the dicer complex. This removes the loop portion of the hairpin creating two complementary strands of miRNAs. These two strands, along with dicer and a binding protein then interact with Argonaute (Ago) to form RISC (RNA Induced Silencing Complex). One of the complementary strands is released and degraded. The other, now a single-stranded miRNA, is able to bind to its target sequence. At this point, the degree of complementarity between the miRNA and its target sequence determines whether it functions to inhibit translation or promote the degradation of mRNA. The less the complementarity, the more likely it will function to inhibit translation without effect on the level of mRNA. With greater complementarity, miRNAs function more like siRNAs and promote mRNA degradation (Lee et al. 1993, Bartel 2004, Carthew and Sontheimer 2009). To accomplish both of these endpoints, the miRNA binds to the 3′ untranslated region (UTR) of mRNAs (Yekta et al. 2004). Interaction with the 3′UTR relies on a 7 nucleotide "seed sequence" present in the miRNA (see table I).

An alternate pathway for miRNA synthesis exists in which splicing of a small intronic region (a microRNA intron region or mirtron region) out of pre-mRNA creates a lasso-like structure (a pre-mirtron) that subsequently loses its branch to form double-stranded pre-miRNA. This hairpin double-stranded pre-miRNA is then handled in the same manner as the RNASEN-processed variety.

SiRNAs, by contrast, originate via viral infection or are introduced into a cell experimentally. Either way, the cell gains long stretches of double-stranded RNA. These are recognized and bound by specific binding proteins which initiate cleavage by dicer into short 18-25 nucleotide lengths of double-stranded RNA that can interact with Ago. This interaction results in the release and degradation of one strand and the targeting of the specific complementary strand. Since SiRNAs have perfect complementarity, they result in mRNA degradation rather than inhibition of translation.

Having discussed the differences and similarities between these two forms of interfering RNA, focus is now on miRNAs. Although several miRNAs have been proposed to be of importance in breast cancer, the purpose of this review is to draw attention to the potential role of miR-106a.

3. The miR-106a cluster (paralog to miR-106b and miR-17-92 clusters)

To date, the best studied miRNAs implicated in carcinogenesis are in the miR-17-92 family. This family consists of six members : miR-17, miR-18a, miR-19a, miR-20a, miR-19b, and miR-92a. They are all transcribed from the same polycistronic cluster, the miR-17-92 cluster on chromosome 13. In addition in mammals, there are two paralogs, the miR-106b-25 cluster on chromosome 7, and the miR-106a-363 cluster on the X chromosome. These resulted from gene duplications of the miR-17-92 cluster during evolution. As mentioned earlier, miRNAs interact with the 3′UTR of target mRNAs through their seed sequence; hence miRNAs with the same seed sequence may share the same targets. Based on homology of the seed sequences, miRNAs in these paralogous clusters can be grouped into four different families, miR-17,miR-18, miR-19 and miR-92, as shown in table 1.

Seed Sequence	Members in miR-17-92 cluster	Members in miR-106a-363 cluster	Members in miR-106b-25 cluster
AAAGUG (miR-17 family)	miR-17, miR-20a	miR-20b, miR-106a	miR-106b, miR-93
AAGGUG (miR-18 family)	miR-18a	miR-18b	
GUGCAA (miR-19 family)	miR-19a, miR-19b-1	miR-19b-2	
AUUGCA (miR-92 family)	miR-92a-1	miR-92a-2, miR-363	miR-25

Table 1. miRNAs from miR-17-92, miR-106a-363 and miR-106b-25 clusters were grouped into 4 different families based on their seed sequences. Table adapted from Van Haaften et al. (2010).

According to this grouping, miR-106a, for example, may target the same mRNAs as miR-17,miR-20a, miR-20b, miR-106b and miR-93. Tanzer et al.(2004) analyzed the evolutionary history of these miRNAs, a history based on the seed sequence. Interestingly, while an ortholog of the miR-17-92 seed sequence family occurs in Drosophila and C. elegans, both the miR-17 and miR-19 seed sequence families seem to be vertebrate innovations. Moreover, miR-106a seems to exist only in mammals; it was found in mouse, rat, human, and chimp, but not in any non-mammalian vertebrates tested. This raises the possibility of a specific role for miR-106a in mammals where one defining feature is the presence of mammae.

4. Regulation of miRNAs

4.1 Regulation of miRNA by methylation

In addition to protein expression being regulated by miRNAs, formation of miRNAs can be regulated by hypermethylation. Thus, hypermethylation of CpG islands that encompass or are adjacent to miRNA regions can inhibit transcription, as can histone modification (Lehmann et al, 2008). In fact, the frequency of epigenetic regulation of miRNA regions on the genome is estimated to be about an order of magnitude greater than for protein-coding regions. The regions of miRs-124-1, 124-2, 124-3, 126, 141, 148a, 152, 199a-1, 199a-2, 200c, 34a, 663, and 9-1, previously associated with breast cancer, are epigenetically modified, showing an established role for regulation of miRNAs by methylation in breast cancer. The miR-106a region has also been reported to be epigenetically modified in colon cancer (Kunej et al, 2011). Although not yet specifically examined, it is possible therefore that miR-106a is also epigenetically modified in breast cancer, becoming either hypo- or hyper-methylated.

4.2 Regulation of miR-106a by myc and estrogen

In several cancers, upregulation of the oncogene, myc, is accompanied by the induction of many miRNAs, including several members from the miR-17-92, miR-106a-363, and miR-106b-25 clusters (O'Donnell et al. 2005). Evidence that myc directly regulated the expression of these miRNAs was produced by chromatin immunoprecipitation (ChIP). This showed that myc could interact with a fragment upstream of the miR-17-92 cluster. Though there were seven putative myc binding sites (CACGTG) upstream of the miR-106a-363 cluster, no interaction was found in the ChIP assay. However, the expression of miR-106a-363 was undetectable in their tested cell line, P493-6 B lymphoma cells. Castellano et al. (2009) expanded this study to breast cancer cells and included upstream regulation by estrogen. With estrogen stimulation, expression of myc, and both miR-17-92 and miR-106a-363 clusters was upregulated. There is an estrogen receptor response element 70 bp upstream of the c-myc binding site on the miR-17-92 promoter. However, no detectable interaction between the estrogen receptor and this DNA region was observed. Expression levels of miR106a were too low to make this determination. For miR-17-92, this suggests that estrogen induction of myc preceeds myc induction of the miR-17-92 cluster. Although an indirect induction, it is nevertheless an important link between estrogen, a known oncogene, and the miR-17-92 cluster. miR-106a expression can also be negatively regulated in some cancers. As reported in monocytopoiesis, the transcription factor, acute myeloid leukaemia-1 (AML-1), also known as Runt-related transcription factor 1 (Runx1) can bind to the promoter region of the miR-106a-363 cluster and repress the expression of miR-106a (Fontana et al. 2007).

5. The expression pattern of miR-106a correlates with breast tumor development and other tumor development

Table 2 illustrates the relative expression of miR-106a in tumors versus normal tissue and then in metastasized versus non-metastasized tumors. As can be appreciated, as breast cancer progresses, expression of miR-106a increases. This is also true for several other tumors in which the analysis was carried through to the metastatic stage. Wang et al. (2010), for example, examined breast tumors, matching serum and adjacent normal tissue from patients and showed that miR-106a was consistently and significantly overexpressed in both breast tumors and matching serum samples. The expression was gradually increased as the stage of breast cancer progressed. In addition, the expression was higher in progesterone receptor negative versus positive cancers, as well as in estrogen receptor negative versus ER

Tissue	Expression of miR-106a in tumor compared to non-tumor tissue	Expression of miR-106a in metastasized tumor to non-metastasized tumor
Gastric	Up-regulated	Increased
Colon	Up-regulated	decreased
Renal	Up-regulated	decreased
Pancreas/Liver	Up-regulated	ND
Lung	Up-regulated	Increased
Nervous system	Down-regulated	ND
Prostate	Up-regulated	Increased
Immune	Up-regulated	ND
Breast	Up-regulated	Increased

Table 2. Summary of expression pattern of miR-106a in different tissues and in metastasized tumors. ND, not determined.

positive cancers (Wang et al. 2010). An interesting experiment was performed by Fassan et al. (2009) during which they compared the miRNA expression profiles in male and female breast cancer patients. When compared to female breast tumors, the expression of miR-106a in male tumor samples was downregulated, indicating there might exist a different regulation mechanism between male and female breast cancer, perhaps resulting from a different X chromosome complement (see below).

Macrophages play a dual role in tumor development, acting first to present tumor antigens to T cells that kill transformed cells, and later contributing to tumor progression in a number of different ways (Lamagna et al, 2006). miR-106a inhibits monocyte and therefore macrophage development (Fontana et al 2007). This might be predicted to reduce initial clearing responses to transformed cells and therefore to increase the incidence of breast cancer.

6. Potential significance of X chromosome location of miR-106a

Group B retroviruses, like the mouse mammary tumor, share a common integration site on the X chromosome (Mueller et al. 1992). This is close to the promoter region for the miR-106a cluster. As a result,there is elevated expression of miR-106a.

Irregardless of virus involvement, there are multiple studies indicating reactivation of the silenced X chromosome in breast cancer, particularly basal-like breast cancers (Richardson et al. 2006). Such reactivation could elevate expression of the miR-106a cluster. Some features of the inactive X chromosome (Xi) have been identified. These include hypermethylation of DNA and hypoacetylation of Histones 3 and 4 (Lucchesi et al. 2005). Reactivation of Xi would therefore have to reverse these features. As we will discuss later, it is interesting to note that miR-106a may target SUV420H1, a DNA methyltransferase, and BRMS1-L, a component of the histone deacetylase complex (HDAC). Downregulation of these two proteins by targeting their mRNA by miR-106a would result in DNA hypomethylation and histone acetylation, thereby linking elevated miR106a to the possibility of X chromosome reactivation.

There is also another potential link between breast cancer and X reactivation, in this case related to BRCA1 functionality. Thus, BRCA1 has been reported to regulate Xist transcription from the X chromosome that should be inactive. When transcribed, BRCA1 then guides Xist to reinteract with and therefore re-silence the same chromosome (Ganesan et al., 2004; Ganesan et al., 2002; Silver et al., 2007). However, this is not a universal finding (Pageau et al., 2007; Xiao et al., 2007).

7. Potential targets of miR-106a

Although miR-106a has not been extensively investigated, there are several ways in which reports connect it to an influence on tumor progression. From results derived from a miRNA target search, for example, over 700 potential targets for miR-106a were identified (Sinha et al., 2008). These include cell cycle regulatory proteins, and proteins that regulate apoptosis, angiogenesis, autophagy, metastasis, and drug resistance.

7.1 Involvement in cell cycle regulation and apoptosis

Using a miRNA target search engine, Sinha et al.(2008) proposed that miR-106a had up to 40 targets involved in the regulation of cell proliferation, and up to 44 targets involved in the regulation of apoptosis (Table 3). Among these targets, the best studied example to date is the tumor suppressor protein, retinoblastoma 1(RB1). RB is a tumor suppressor whose inactivation is involved at some stage in many cancers. Phosphorylation of the Rb protein blocks progression of the cell cycle from G1 to S phase. Inactivation of RB therefore has a proliferative effect. Several studies have shown upregulation of miR-106a was accompanied by downregulation of Rb in a number of different cancers (Zhou et al. 2010, Xiao et al. 2009, Volinia et al. 2006). In addition, RB attenuation also appears to be important in the development of resistance to anti-estrogens, including Tamoxifen (Boscoe et al. 2007, (Lehn et al., 2011), Thangavel et al. 2011). Moreover, therapeutically activating RB has been shown to reestablish cell cycle control in endocrine therapy-resistant breast cancer (Thangavel et al. 2011).

Another important tumor suppressor is p21, also known as cyclin-dependent kinase inhibitor 1 (gene is CDKN1A on table 3). This also regulates cell cycle progression between the G1 and S phase and contains several putative miR-106a sites in its 3'-UTR. The importance of p21 specifically in breast cancer is currently unclear. However, it is widely accepted that loss of function of p21, caused by mutations, reduced expression, or abnormal cellular translocation, would promote breast cancer progression (Trimis et al. 2008, Winters et al. 2003, Balbín et al. 1996). Also, upregulation of miR-106a downregulates p21 expression, and transfection with an antimir of miR-106a restores expression (Ivanovska et al. 2008). Thus, p21 expression is clearly regulated by miR-106a even though direct demonstration of the use of the putative 3' UTR sites has yet to be reported.

There is a complicated and highly regulated interplay among the many pro- and anti-apoptotic proteins in a cell. Bim (gene called BCL2L11 in table) is a pro-apoptotic molecule, involved in regulating anoikis in the normal developing mammary gland to create a duct lumen (Whelan et al., 2010), as well as responses of breast cancer cells to chemotherapeutics such as paclitaxel (Kutuk and Letai, 2010). Early breast cancer is in many instances characterized by a duct lumen filled with cells that have not undergone normal anoikis. Caspase 6 is the direct activator of caspase 8 in the intrinsic pathway for initiation of apoptosis (Cowling and Downward, 2002). A reduction in expression of Bim, caspase 6 and caspase 8 brought about by elevations of miR-106a would therefore be expected to reduce anoikis/apoptosis leading to increased cell number. Increased proliferation and decreased apoptosis also predict poor prognosis in recurrent breast cancers (Vakkala et al. 1999).

Predicted targets of miR-106a associated with cell proliferation	Predicted targets of miR-106a associated with apoptosis
BCL11B, BCL6, BHLHB3, BMPR2, BTG1,BTG2, BTG3, **CDKN1A**, *COL4A3, CSF1,DERL2, E2F1, EBI3, EDD1, EDG1, EFNB1,EREG, FLT1, FZD3, GAB1, HDAC4, KLF11,LIF, MAP3K11, MAPRE1, PAFAH1B1, PCAF,PDGFRA, PPARD, PTEN, PTHLH, PURB,* **RB1**,*RBBP7, TAL1, TBX3, TGFB1, TOPORS,TSG101, TUSC2*	*ACIN1, ACVR1B, APBB2, APP,* **BCL2L11**,*BCL2L2, BCL6, BIRC4, BNIP2, BTG1,* **CASP6, CASP8**, *CDKN1A, CFLAR, COL4A3, DAPK2,DEDD, DNASE2, DNM2, E2F1, EGLN3,EP300, FASTK, FOXL2, HIF1A, INHBA,LALBA, MAP3K5, PAK7, PIK3R1, PLAGL2,PPARD, PPP2CA, PTEN, PURB, SQSTM1,STK17B, TAOK2, TAX1BP1, TIMP3,TMEM23, TNFRSF21, TOPORS, TP53INP1*

Table 3. Predicted targets of miR-106a involved in cell proliferation and apoptosis. Data from Sinha et al. (2008). Genes in bold type are those chosen as examples in the text.

The activation of oncogenes usually induces cellular apoptosis or senescence as a protective mechanism (Li et al. 2009a, Maes et al. 2008b). In an activated ras oncogene model, it was shown that overexpression of the miR-106a-363 cluster abolished ras-induced senescence. With further deletion analysis, only miR-106a and miR-20b were essential for this function (Hong et al. 2010). The upregulation of miR-106a in cancer therefore might play an important role in inhibition of oncogene-induced senescence, allowing cancer cells to escape this anti-tumor defensive pathway.

7.2 Involvement in metastasis /differentiation of tumors

As shown earlier in table 2, the expression of miR-106a increases with metastasis in breast cancer. This is also true of a number of other cancers and suggests a potential role for miR-106a in the metastatic process. Laminin 5 is a component of the basement membrane that mediates attachment of epithelial cells. Laminin 5 is a direct target of the tumor suppressor, smad4, and increased laminin 5 increases cell adhesion and reduces cancer cell migration (Zapatka et al. 2007). Moreover, epithelial cell interaction with the basement membrane promotes mammary differentiation (McCave et al. 2010). Overexpression of miR-106a down-regulates laminin 5 in the breast cancer cell line, MCF-7, and with an antimir to miR-106a expression is normalized (Wenrich et al. 2007). Thus, reduced laminin 5 is associated with reduced differentiation and reduced cell adhesion to the basement membrane. However, if laminin 5 is cleaved by matrix metalloproteases it becomes a tumor-promoting factor that stimulates cell motility (Carpenter et al. 2009). Thus, the end effect of miR-106a via laminin 5 will depend on the level of matrix metalloprotease activity.

BRMS1L (Breast Cancer Metastasis 1 Like) suppresses metastasis of human breast cancer. It is a component of the mSin3a family of histone deacetylase complexes (HDAC) and therefore suppresses transcription of genes (Meehan et al. 2004). As for the other examples, this protein has a potential binding site for miR-106a on its 3'-UTR. Edmonds et al. (2009) investigated the miRNA expression profile related to expression of the related protein, BRMS1, in breast cancer. Unfortunately, miR-106a was not within their tested array. Given the binding site, however, miR-106a may promote breast cancer metastasis through downregulation of BRMS1-L. Other than this function to suppress metastasis, the related protein, BRMS1, has also been reported to be involved in maintaining sensitivity of breast cancer to chemotherapy (Vaidya et al. 2009).

The protein product of the ARID4A (AT Rich Interactive Domain 4A) gene has been reported to interact with the tumor suppressor proteins, BRMS1 and RB, and therefore to participate in tumor suppression (Hurst et al. 2008). As a predicted target of miR-106a, downregulation of this protein would be expected to promote breast cancer progression.

7.3 Involvement in angiogenesis

The role of miR-106a in angiogenesis is hard to predict from the amount of information currently available. On the one hand, thrombospondin-1 (TSP-1) and connective tissue growth factor (CTGF/CCN2), both anti-angiogenic factors, are targeted by members of the same seed family and therefore would be predicted to be targeted by miR-106a. Downregulation of both contributes to endothelial cell migration and therefore tumor progression (Dews et al. 2006, Chien et al. 2011). On the other hand, vascular endothelial growth factor (VEGF), one of the most important pro-angiogenic factors (Delli Carpini et al., 2010) also has putative binding sites for miR-106a on the 3'UTR. Hua et al. (2006) made a reporter construct by connecting the 3'UTR of VEGF downstream of a luciferase reporter and then co-transfected this construct into cells with different miRNAs reported to act on this 3'UTR. Among the miRNAs examined (miR-106a, miR-106b, miR-17, miR-20a, miR-20b, miR-150, miR-29b), miR-106a showed the greatest inhibition of luciferase expression (Hua et al. 2006). Further analysis will therefore be required to identify all counterbalancing activities in regard to miR-106a, angiogenesis and breast cancer. All that can be said at present is that both miR-106a and VEGF are increased as a function of breast cancer progression and hence that other factors must influence the interaction between miR-106a and the 3'UTR of VEGF mRNA. PRDM6 (PR/SET Domain Protein 6) is another angiogenesis-related potential target protein. High expression of this protein inhibits endothelial cell proliferation and differentiation (Wu et al. 2008). Down regulation of this protein by miR-106a may initiate breast cancer metastasis through promotion of both endothelial cell differentiation and proliferation.

7.4 Other potential targets in breast cancer

7.4.1 SUV420H1, a DNA methyltransferase

DNA methylation governs the expression of genes and an abnormal epigenetic pattern may contribute to disease. DNA hypomethylation is associated with the worst stages of breast cancer (Soares et al. 1999), and the DNA methyltransferase, SUV420H1, is severely downregulated in human breast cancers (Tryndyak et al. 2006). As mentioned eariler, RB, which forms a complex with this methyltransferase, is also a target of miR-106a. Thus, an elevation of miR-106a would concurrently reduce expression of both RB and the methyltransferase, thereby enhancing hypomethylation.

7.4.2 Atg7 (autophagy-related protein 7)

Autophagy, or self eating, is a lysosomal process that occurs in all cells in order to recycle the components of worn out organelles, to reduce unecessary organelles or cytoplasmic constituents when physiological demands change, or upon cellular stress. Autophagy can serve as a tumor suppressor since defective autophagy provides an oncogenic stimulus, resulting in malignant transformation and spontaneous tumors (Dalby et al. 2010). At the same time, autophagy can function as a cell survival mechanism (Dalby et al. 2010). Atg7 (Autophagy-related protein 7) is a potential target of miR-106a. The effect of reduction in expression of Atg7, as assessed in a knockout mouse model, is increased cell survival (Xue et al. 2010), an effect that would be predicted to contribute to tumor progression.

7.5 Targets related to chemotherapy resistance

Xia et al. (2008) investigated the correlation between miRNA expression and the development of drug resistance in gastric cancers. The data showed that miR-106a was downregulated in the vincristine (VCR)-resistant gastric cancer cell line, SGC7901/VCR (Xia et al. 2008). However, in human breast cancer doxorubicin-resistant MCF-7 cells, there was an upregulation of miR-106a (Kovalchuk et al. 2008). There were no further experiments performed regarding the functional role of this altered expression of miR-106a in either cancer in these papers. Much drug resistance develops through increased expression of multidrug resistance transporter proteins such as MDR-1. In B cell lymphomas, Fu et al. (2009) examined the relationship between miRNAs and drug resistance. Based on the observation that patients with mantle cell lymphomas (MCL) express higher miR-17-92, he overexpressed miR-17-92 in MCL cells and exposed them to the chemotherapy drug, topotecan. The miR-17-92 overexpressing cells were more resistant to drug treatment. Interestingly, David et al. (2004) found an association between DNA hypomethylation in breast cancer and drug resistance that occurred through regulation of the multidrug resistance protein, MDR-1.

8. miR-106a in development

There are many correlates between early embryogenesis and tumor formation and progression. We therefore sought information concerning the role of miR-106a in development. Foshay et al. (2009) examined the expression of miR-17, miR-20a, miR-106a, and miR-93 (all members of the same seed sequence family) during mouse development. At an early stage of development (E 4.0), both miR-17 and miR-20a were expressed more in the trophectoderm. By contrast, miR-106a was expressed primarily in the inner cell mass, a region considered as the source of stem cells with the potential to differentiate into most cell types. The expression of miR-93 was seen in both the trophectoderm and primitive endoderm. As development progressed (E 6.5), the visceral endoderm had low expression of all four miRNAs, however, the expression of miR-106a and miR-20 was relatively higher. One might speculate therefore that miR-106a expression may be related to stem cell function and differentiation in endoderm-derived tissues. However, in regard to the latter none of the members of the miR-106a-363 cluster, including miR-106a, miR-18b, miR-20b and miR-363, was expressed in early embryonic lung (Lu et al. 2007). The role of miR-106a in development was best described by Ventura et al. who analyzed the consequences of miR-17-92, miR-106a-363 and miR-106b-25 cluster deletion, separately or in combination (Ventura et al. 2008). miR-17-92 deficient mice cannot survive due to severe lung failure. Furthermore, deletion of the miR-17-92 cluster caused defects in B-cell development. However, neither deletion of miR-106b-25 nor miR-106a-363 had any obvious effects. The combined deletion of miR-106b-25 and miR-106a-363 also showed no effect, but the double knockout of miR-106b-25 and miR-17-92 caused more serious problems than deletion of miR-17-92 alone. This analysis either implies a straightforward lack of importance of miR-106a-363 in development or perhaps a degree of subtlety of its effects not easily appreciated. If miR-106a is important to stem cell function, one might predict early tissue aging. Concordant with this suggestion is downregulated expression in human aging (Hackl et al. 2010).

9. Potential roles of miR-106a in other cancers

As shown in table 2, the expression of miR-106a was upregulated in gastric cancer. This was accompanied by low expression of RB1, mentioned previously as a direct target of miR-106a (Zhou et al. 2010, Xiao et al. 2009). Further analysis revealed a positive correlation between miR-106a expression and the stage of tumor-node-metastasis. Higher expression of miR-106a was associated with increasing gastric tumor size, and lymphatic and distant metastasis (Xiao et al. 2009), implying an important role of miR-106a in gastric tumor progression.

In colorectal cancer, miR-106a was overexpressed at both stages I and II, but was decreased at stages III and IV. In addition, high expression of miR-106a was inversely correlated with the cell proliferation-associated target, E2F1 (table 3) (Schetter et al. 2008, Guo et al. 2008). Late stage downregulation of miR-106a predicted shortened disease-free survival. (Díaz et al. 2008).

Slaby et al. (2010) studied miRNA expression in renal cell carcinoma (RCC) versus renal parenchyma from disease-free areas. They found a similar pattern as that described for colorectal cancer i.e. higher levels initially, followed by lower levels when metastasized.

In pancreatic and hepatocellular cancer, miR-106a was upregulated, but no further analysis has yet been performed (Volinia et al. 2006, Kutay et al. 2006).

Primary lung cancer can be classified into 2 types, non-small cell lung cancer (NSCLC) and small cell lung cancer (SCLC). SCLC is usually diagnosed when the cancer has already spread. The expression of miR-106a is higher in lung cancer compared to non-cancerous regions and higher still in SCLC than NSCLC (Navarro et al. 2009). In addition, it was also shown that patients with higher miR-106a expression had a significantly worse prognosis (Yanaihara et al. 2006).

In vitro analyses have shown that miRNAs in the miR-106a-363 cluster are overexpressed in both Hodgkins lymphoma cells and T cell leukemia (Gibcus et al. 2011, Landais et al. 2007). Targets in leukemia were also identified : myosin regulatory light chain–interacting protein, which regulates actin stress fibers and motility in non-muscle cells, and RB1-like protein, a known tumor suppressor (Landais et al. 2007). $p27^{kip1}$-deficient mice that are highly susceptible to viral infections and develop lymphomas were used to analyze effects in vivo. Among the miRNAs tested (188) that were overexpressed were members of the miR-106a-363 cluster. Their expression was even higher when there was a MMuLV integration at the Xpcl1 locus, the locus responsible for expression of the miR-106a-363 cluster on chromosome X (Kuppers et al. 2011).

In prostate cancer, expression of miR-106a was not merely increased but there was also in incremental increase that correlated with increasing cancer risk. Furthermore, there was a positive correlation between the expression of miR-106a and metastatic status (Moltzahn et al. 2011).

Schulte et al. (2008) examined the expression pattern of miRNAs at different stages of neuroblastoma. However, there was no correlation with the presence or absence of disease or stage of neuroblastoma. In contrast to neuroblastoma, when surgical samples of astrocytoma were compared to adjacent non-astrocytoma tissue, miR-106a was downregulated in astrocytomas when compared to normal tissue. In addition, patients with reduced miR-106a had a lower survival rate. These results imply a rather different and possibly protective role of miR-106a in the brain (Zhi et al. 2010).

10. Conclusion

In this review we have presented experimental, bioinformatic and correlative data and our speculations supporting a role for overexpression of miR-106a in breast cancer. We have discussed the potential role of miR-106a in cell proliferation, apoptosis, metastasis, angiogenesis, gene repression through DNA hypomethylation, and the development of resistance to therapies. From this perspective, we propose that knockdown of miR-106a may be therapeutically beneficial.

11. References

Baek D, Villen J, Shin C, Camargo FD, Gygi SP, Bartel DP. (2008). The impact of microRNAs on protein output. *Nature*, 455, pp. 64–71, ISSN 1476-4687

Balbín M, Hannon GJ, Pendás AM, Ferrando AA, Vizoso F, Fueyo A, López-Otín C. (1996). Functional analysis of a p21^{WAF1,CIP1,SDI1} mutant (Arg^{94}→Trp) identified in a human breast carcinoma. Evidence that the mutation impairs the ability of p21 to inhibit cyclin-dependent kinases. *J. Biol. Chem.*, 271, pp. 15782–15786, ISSN 0021-9258

Bartel DP. (2004). MicroRNAs: genomics, biogenesis, mechanism, and function. *Cell*, 116, pp. 281-297, ISSN 0092-8674

Bosco EE, Wang Y, Xu H, Zilfou JT, Knudsen KE, Aronow BJ, Lowe SW, Knudsen ES. (2007). The retinoblastoma tumor suppressor modifies the therapeutic response of breast cancer. *J Clin Invest*, 117, pp. 218-28, ISSN 0021-9738

Carpenter PM, Dao AV, Arain ZS, Chang MK, Nguyen HP, Arain S, Wang-Rodriguez J, Kwon SY, Wilczynski SP. Motility induction in breast carcinoma by mammary epithelial laminin 332 (laminin 5). Mol Cancer Res. 2009 Apr;7(4):462-75.

Carthew RW, and Sontheimer EJ. (2009). Origins and Mechanisms of miRNAs and siRNAs. *Cell*, 136, pp. 642-655, ISSN 1097-4172

Castellano L, Giamas G, Jacob J, Coombes RC, Lucchesi W, Thiruchelvam P, Barton G, Jiao LR, Wait R, Waxman J, Hannon GJ, Stebbing J. (2009). The estrogen receptor-alpha-induced microRNA signature regulates itself and its transcriptional response. *Proc Natl Acad Sci U S A.*, 106, 37, pp. 15732-7, ISSN 1091-6490

Chien W, O'Kelly J, Lu D, Leiter A, Sohn J, Yin D, Karlan B, Vadgama J, Lyons KM, Koeffler HP. (2011). Expression of connective tissue growth factor (CTGF/CCN2) in breast cancer cells is associated with increased migration and angiogenesis. *Int J Oncol.*, Epub, ISSN 1791-2423

Cowling, V., and Downward, J. (2002). Caspase-6 is the direct activator of caspase-8 in the cytochrome c-induced apoptosis pathway: absolute requirement for removal of caspase-6 prodomain. *Cell Death Differ*, 9, pp. 1046-1056, ISSN 1350-9047

Dai R and Ahmed SA. (2011). MicroRNA, a new paradigm for understanding immunoregulation, inflammation, and autoimmune diseases. *Transl Res.*, 157, 4 , pp. 163-79, ISSN 1878-1810

Dalby KN, Tekedereli I, Lopez-Berestein G, Ozpolat B. (2010). Targeting the prodeath and prosurvival functions of autophagy as novel therapeutic strategies in cancer. *Autophagy.* , 6, 3, pp. 322-9, ISSN 1554-8635

David GL, Yegnasubramanian S, Kumar A, Marchi VL, De Marzo AM, Lin X, Nelson WG. (2004). MDR1 promoter hypermethylation in MCF-7 human breast cancer cells: Changes in chromatin structure induced by treatment with 5-aza-cytidine. *Cancer Biol Ther*, 3, pp. 540-8. ISSN 1538-4047

Delli Carpini J, Karam AK, Montgomery L. (2010). Vascular endothelial growth factor and its relationship to the prognosis and treatment of breast, ovarian, and cervical cancer. *Angiogenesis.* ,13, 1, pp. 43-58, ISSN 1573-7209

Dews M, Homayouni A, Yu D, Murphy D, Sevignani C, Wentzel E, Furth EE, Lee WM, Enders GH, Mendell JT, Thomas-Tikhonenko A. (2006). Augmentation of tumor angiogenesis by a Myc-activated microRNA cluster. *Nat Genet.*, 38, 9, pp. 1060-5, ISSN 1061-4036

Díaz R, Silva J, García JM, Lorenzo Y, García V, Peña C, Rodríguez R, Muñoz C, García F, Bonilla F, Domínguez G. (2008). Deregulated expression of miR-106a predicts survival in human colon cancer patients. *Genes Chromosomes Cancer.*, 47, 9, pp. 794-802, ISSN 1098-2264

Edmonds MD, Hurst DR, Vaidya KS, Stafford LJ, Chen D, Welch DR. (2009). Breast cancer metastasis suppressor 1 coordinately regulates metastasis-associated microRNA expression. *Int J Cancer.*, 125, 8, pp. 1778-85, ISSN 1097-0215

Fassan M, Baffa R, Palazzo JP, Lloyd J, Crosariol M, Liu CG, Volinia S, Alder H, Rugge M, Croce CM, Rosenberg A. (2009). MicroRNA expression profiling of male breast cancer. *Breast Cancer Res.*,11, 4, pp. R58, ISSN 1465-542X

Fontana L, Pelosi E, Greco P, Racanicchi S, Testa U, Liuzzi F, Croce CM, Brunetti E, Grignani F, Peschle C. (2007). MicroRNAs 17-5p-20a-106a control monocytopoiesis through AML1 targeting and M-CSF receptor upregulation. *Nat Cell Biol.* , 9, 7, pp. 775-87, ISSN 1465-7392.

Foshay KM, Gallicano GI. (2009). miR-17 family miRNAs are expressed during early mammalian development and regulate stem cell differentiation. *Dev Biol.* , 326, 2, pp. 431-43, ISSN 1095-564X.

Fu K. Targeting the miR-17-92 miRNA cluster for treatment of mantle cell lymphoma. Mantle Cell Lymphoma Consortium (MCLC) Scientific Workshop. Atlanta, GA, March 30-31, 2009.

Ganesan, S., Silver, D. P., Drapkin, R., Greenberg, R., Feunteun, J., and Livingston, D. M. (2004). Association of BRCA1 with the inactive X chromosome and XIST RNA. *Philos Trans R Soc Lond B Biol Sci* ,359, pp. 123-128, ISSN 0092-8674

Ganesan, S., Silver, D. P., Greenberg, R. A., Avni, D., Drapkin, R., Miron, A., Mok, S. C., Randrianarison, V., Brodie, S., Salstrom, J., *et al.* (2002). BRCA1 supports XIST RNA concentration on the inactive X chromosome. *Cell* ,111, pp. 393-405,ISSN 0962-8436

Gibcus JH, Tan LP, Harms G, Schakel RN, de Jong D, Blokzijl T, Möller P, Poppema S, Kroesen BJ, van den Berg A. (2009). Hodgkin lymphoma cell lines are characterized by a specific miRNA expression profile. *Neoplasia.*;11, 2, pp. 167-76, ISSN 1476-5586.

Guo C, J. F. Sah, L. Beard, J. K. V. Willson, S. D. Markowitz, and K. Guda. (2008). "The noncoding RNA, miR-126, suppresses the growth of neoplastic cells by targeting phosphatidylinositol 3- kinase signaling and is frequently lost in colon cancers," *Genes Chromosomes and Cancer*, 47, 11, pp. 939–946, ISSN 1098-2264

Hackl M, Brunner S, Fortschegger K, Schreiner C, Micutkova L, Mück C, Laschober GT, Lepperdinger G, Sampson N, Berger P,Herndler-Brandstetter D, Wieser M, Kühnel H, Strasser A, Rinnerthaler M, Breitenbach M, Mildner M, Eckhart L, Tschachler E, Trost A, Bauer JW, Papak C, Trajanoski Z, Scheideler M, Grillari-Voglauer R, Grubeck-Loebenstein B, Jansen-Dürr P, Grillari J. (2010). miR-17, miR-19b, miR-20a, and miR-106a are down-regulated in human aging. *Aging Cell.*, 9, 2, pp. 291–296, ISSN 1474-9726

Hong L, Lai M, Chen M, Xie C, Liao R, Kang YJ, Xiao C, Hu WY, Han J, and Sun P. (2010). The miR-17-92 cluster of microRNAs confers tumorigenicity by inhibiting oncogene-induced senescence. *Cancer Res,* 70, pp. 8547-8557, ISSN 1538-7445

Hua Z, Lv Q, Ye W, Wong CK, Cai G, Gu D, Ji Y, Zhao C, Wang J, Yang BB, Zhang Y. (2006). MiRNA-directed regulation of VEGF and other angiogenic factors under hypoxia. *PLoS One.,* 1, pp. e116, ISSN 1932-6203

Hurst DR, Xie Y, Vaidya KS, Mehta A, Moore BP, Accavitti-Loper MA, Samant RS, Saxena R, Silveira AC, Welch DR. (2008). Alterations of BRMS1-ARID4A interaction modify gene expression but still suppress metastasis in human breast cancer cells. *J Biol Chem.*, 283,12, pp. 7438-44. ISSN 0021-9258

Ivanovska I, Ball AS, Diaz RL, Magnus JF, Kibukawa M, Schelter JM, Kobayashi SV, Lim L, Burchard J, Jackson AL, Linsley PS, Cleary MA. (2008). MicroRNAs in the miR-106b family regulate p21/CDKN1A and promote cell cycle progression. *Mol Cell Biol.;* 28, 7, pp. 2167-74, ISSN 1098-5549

Kim, V. N., Han, J., and Siomi, M. C. (2009). Biogenesis of small RNAs in animals. *Nat Rev Mol Cell Biol,* 10, pp. 126-139, ISSN 1471-0080

Kovalchuk O, Filkowski J, Meservy J, Ilnytskyy Y, Tryndyak VP, Chekhun VF, Pogribny IP. (2008). Involvement of microRNA-451 in resistance of the MCF-7 breast cancer cells to chemotherapeutic drug doxorubicin. *Mol Cancer Ther.,* 7, 7, pp. 2152-9, ISSN 1535-7163

Kunej T, Godnic I, Ferdin J, Horvat S, Dovc P, Calin GA. (2011). Epigenetic regulation of microRNAs in cancer: An integrated review of literature. *Mutat Res.*, pp. 110441-8, ISSN 0027-5107

Kuppers DA, Hwang HC, Jackson AL, Linsley PS, Clurman BE, Fero ML. (2011). Effect of Xpcl1 Activation and p27 Loss on Gene Expression in Murine Lymphoma. *PLOS One.*, 6, 3, pp. 14758, ISSN 1932-6203

Kutay H, Bai S, Datta J, Motiwala T, Pogribny I, Frankel W, Jacob ST, Ghoshal K. (2006). Downregulation of miR-122 in the rodent and human hepatocellular carcinomas. *J Cell Biochem.*,99, 3, pp. 671-8, ISSN 0730-2312

Kutuk, O., and Letai, A. (2010). Displacement of Bim by Bmf and Puma rather than increase in Bim level mediates paclitaxel-induced apoptosis in breast cancer cells. *Cell Death Differ* ,17, pp. 1624-1635, ISSN 1476-5403

Lamagna C, Aurrand-Lions M, Imhof BA. (2006). Dual role of macrophages in tumor growth and angiogenesis. *J Leukoc Biol ,80,* pp. 705-713, ISSN 0741-5400

Landais S, Landry S, Legault P, Rassart E. (2007). Oncogenic potential of the miR-106-363 cluster and its implication in human T-cell leukemia. *Cancer Res, 67,* pp. 5699-5707, ISSN 0008-5472

Lee RC, Feinbaum RL, Ambros V. (1993). The C. elegans heterochronic gene lin-4 encodes small RNAs with antisense complementarity to lin-14. *Cell.* , 75, 5, pp. 843-54, ISSN

Lehmann U, Hasemeier B, Christgen M, Müller M, Römermann D, Länger F, Kreipe H. (2008). Epigenetic inactivation of microRNA gene hsa-mir-9-1 in human breast cancer. *J Pathol.* , 214, 1, pp. 17-24, ISSN 0022-3417

Lehn, S., Fernö, M., Jirström, K., Rydén, L., and Landberg, G. (2011). A non-functional retinoblastoma tumor suppressor (RB) pathway in premenopausal breast cancer is associated with resistance to tamoxifen. *Cell Cycle* ,10,6, ISSN 1551-4005

Li G, Luna C, Qiu J, Epstein DL, Gonzalez P. (2009a). Alterations in microRNA expression in stress-induced cellular senescence. *Ageing Dev.;* 130, pp. 731–741, ISSN 1872-6216

Lu Y, Thomson JM, Wong HY, Hammond SM, Hogan BL. (2007). Transgenic over-expression of the microRNA miR-17-92 cluster promotes proliferation and inhibits differentiation of lung epithelial progenitor cells. *Dev Biol.;* 310, 2, pp. 442–453. ISSN 0012-1606

Lucchesi, J. C., Kelly, W. G., and Panning, B. (2005). Chromatin remodeling in dosage compensation. *Annu Rev Genet,* 39, pp. 615-651, ISSN 0066-4197

Maes OC, An J, Sarojini H, Wu H, Wang E. (2008). Changes in MicroRNA expression patterns in human fibroblasts after low-LET radiation. *J. Cell. Biochem.;*105, pp. 824–834, ISSN 1097-4644

McCave EJ, Cass CA, Burg KJ, Booth BW. (2010). The normal microenvironment directs mammary gland development. *J Mammary Gland Biol Neoplasia.* ,15, 3, pp. 291-9, ISSN 1573-7039

Meehan WJ, Samant RS, Hopper JE, Carrozza MJ, Shevde LA, Workman JL, Eckert KA, Verderame MF, Welch DR. (2004). Breast cancer metastasis suppressor 1 (BRMS1) forms complexes with retinoblastoma-binding protein 1 (RBP1) and the mSin3 histone deacetylase complex and represses transcription. *J Biol Chem.;*279, 2, pp. 1562-9, ISSN 0021-9258

Moltzahn F, Olshen AB, Baehner L, Peek A, Fong L, Stöppler H, Simko J, Hilton JF, Carroll P, Blelloch R. (2011). Microfluidic-based multiplex qRT-PCR identifies diagnostic and prognostic microRNA signatures in the sera of prostate cancer patients. *Cancer Res.;*71, 2, pp. 550-60, ISSN 1538-7445

Mueller RE, Baggio L, Kozak CA, Ball JK. (1992). A common integration locus in type B retrovirus-induced thymic lymphomas. *Virology,* 191, 2, pp. 628-37, ISSN 0042-6822

Navarro A, Marrades RM, Viñolas N, Quera A, Agustí C, Huerta A, Ramirez J, Torres A, Monzo M. (2009). MicroRNAs expressed during lung cancer development are expressed in human pseudoglandular lung embryogenesis. *Oncology.;* 76, 3, pp. 162-9, ISSN 1423-0232

O'Donnell KA, Wentzel EA, Zeller KI, Dang CV, Mendell JT. (2005). c-Myc-regulated microRNAs modulate E2F1 expression. *Nature,* 435, 7043, pp. 839-43, ISSN 1476-4687

Pageau, G. J., Hall, L. L., and Lawrence, J. B. (2007). BRCA1 does not paint the inactive X to localize XIST RNA but may contribute to broad changes in cancer that impact XIST and Xi heterochromatin. *J Cell Biochem* ,100, 835-850, ISSN 0730-2312

Richardson AL, Wang ZC, De Nicolo A, Lu X, Brown M, Miron A, Liao X, Iglehart JD, Livingston DM, Ganesan S. (2006). X chromosomal abnormalities in basal-like human breast cancer. *Cancer Cell.,* 9, 2, pp. 121-32, ISSN 1535-6108

Rodriguez, A., Griffiths-Jones, S., Ashurst, J. L., and Bradley, A. (2004). Identification of mammalian microRNA host genes and transcription units. *Genome Res,* 14, pp. 1902-1910, ISSN 1088-9051

Schetter AJ, Leung SY, Sohn JJ, Zanetti KA, Bowman ED, Yanaihara N, Yuen ST, Chan TL, Kwong DL, Au GK, Liu CG, Calin GA, Croce CM, Harris CC. (2008). MicroRNA expression profiles associated with prognosis and therapeutic outcome in colon adenocarcinoma. *JAMA.*, 299, 4, pp. 425-36, ISSN 1538-3598

Schulte JH, Horn S, Otto T, Samans B, Heukamp LC, Eilers UC, Krause M, Astrahantseff K, Klein-Hitpass L, Buettner R, Schramm A, Christiansen H, Eilers M, Eggert A, Berwanger B. (2008). MYCN regulates oncogenic MicroRNAs in neuroblastoma. *Int J Cancer,* 122, 3, pp. 699-704, ISSN 1097-0215

Silver, D. P., Dimitrov, S. D., Feunteun, J., Gelman, R., Drapkin, R., Lu, S. D., Shestakova, E., Velmurugan, S., Denunzio, N., Dragomir, S., *et al.* (2007). Further evidence for BRCA1 communication with the inactive X chromosome. *Cell* ,128, 991-1002, ISSN 0092-8674

Sinha, A. U., Kaimal, V., Chen, J., and Jegga, A. G. (2008). Dissecting microregulation of a master regulatory network. *BMC Genomics,* 9, pp. 88, ISSN 1471-2164

Slaby O, Jancovicova J, Lakomy R, Svoboda M, Poprach A, Fabian P, Kren L, Michalek J, Vyzula R. (2010). Expression of miRNA-106b in conventional renal cell carcinoma is a potential marker for prediction of early metastasis after nephrectomy. *J Exp Clin Cancer Res.*, 29, pp. 90 , ISSN 1756-9966

Soares J, Pinto AE, Cunha CV, Andre A, Barao I, Sousa JM, Cravo M. (1999). Global *DNA* hypomethylation in breast carcinoma (correlation with prognostic factors and tumor progression). *Cancer,* 85, pp. 112-8, ISSN 0008-543X

Tanzer A and Stadler PF. (2004). Molecular evolution of a microRNA cluster. *J Mol Biol.* ,339, 2, pp. 327-35, ISSN 0022-2836

Thangavel, C., Dean, J. L., Ertel, A., Knudsen, K. E., Aldaz, C. M., Witkiewicz, A. K., Clarke, R., and Knudsen, E. S. (2011). Therapeutically activating RB: reestablishing cell cycle control in endocrine therapy resistant breast cancer. *Endocr Relat Cancer.*, Epub, ISSN 1479-6821

Trimis G, Chatzistamou I, Politi K, Kiaris H, Papavassiliou AG. (2008). Expression of p21waf1/Cip1 in stromal fibroblasts of primary breast tumors. *Hum Mol Genet.,* 17, 22, pp. 3596-600, ISSN 1460-2083

Tryndyak V.P., Kovalchuk O., Pogribny I.P. (2006). Loss of DNA methylation and histone H4 lysine 20 trimethylation in human breast cancer cells is associated with aberrant expression of DNA methyltransferase 1, Suv4-20h2 histone methyltransferase and methyl-binding proteins. *Cancer Biol. Ther.* , 5, pp. 65-70, ISSN 1538-4047

Vaidya KS, Sanchez JJ, Kim EL, Welch DR. (2009). Expression of the Breast Cancer Metastasis Suppressor 1 (BRMS1) maintains in vitro chemosensitivity of breast cancer cells. *Cancer Lett.* , 281, 1, pp. 100-7, ISSN 1872-7980

Vakkala M., Lahteenmaki K., Raunio H., Paakko P., Soini Y. (1999). Apoptosis during breast carcinoma progression. Clin. *Cancer Res.,* 5, pp. 319-324, ISSN 0007-0920

Van Haaften G and Agami R. (2010). Tumorigenicity of the miR-17-92 cluster distilled. *Genes Dev.,* 24, 1, pp. 1–4, ISSN 1549-5477

Ventura A, Young AG, WinslowMM,Lintault L, Meissner A, Erkeland SJ, et al. (2008). Targeted deletion reveals essential and overlapping functions of the miR-17 through 92 family of miRNA clusters. *Cell,* 132, pp. 875–86, ISSN 1097-4172

Volinia S, Calin GA, Liu CG, Ambs S, Cimmino A, Petrocca F, Visone R, Iorio M, Roldo C, Ferracin M, Prueitt RL, Yanaihara N, Lanza G, Scarpa A, Vecchione A, Negrini M, Harris CC, Croce CM. (2006). A microRNA expression signature of human solid tumors defines cancer gene targets. *Proc Natl Acad Sci U S A.*; 103, 7, pp. 2257-61, ISSN 0027-8424

Wang F, Zheng Z, Guo J, Ding X. (2010). Correlation and quantitation of microRNA aberrant expression in tissues and sera from patients with breast tumor. *Gynecol Oncol.*; 119, 3, pp. 586-93, ISSN 1095-6859

Wenrich L, Liang X, Hajivandi MR, Love B, Adams C, Pope M. Correlation of miRNA and SILAC protein expression in a primary cancer cell line. AACR, Los Angeles, April, 2007.

Whelan, K. A., Caldwell, S. A., Shahriari, K. S., Jackson, S. R., Franchetti, L. D., Johannes, G. J., and Reginato, M. J. (2010). Hypoxia suppression of Bim and Bmf blocks anoikis and luminal clearing during mammary morphogenesis. *Mol Biol Cell* ,21,pp. 3829-3837, ISSN 1939-4586

Winters ZE, Leek RD, Bradburn MJ, Norbury CJ, Harris AL. (2003). Cytoplasmic p21WAF1/CIP1 expression is correlated with HER-2/ neu in breast cancer and is an independent predictor of prognosis. *Breast Cancer Res.*; 5, 6, pp. R242-9, ISSN 1465-542X

Wu Y, Ferguson JE 3rd, Wang H, Kelley R, Ren R, McDonough H, Meeker J, Charles PC, Wang H, Patterson C. (2008). PRDM6 is enriched in vascular precursors during development and inhibits endothelial cell proliferation, survival, and differentiation. *J Mol Cell Cardiol.*; 44, 1, pp. 47-58, ISSN 1095-8584

Xia L, Zhang D, Du R, Pan Y, Zhao L, Sun S, Hong L, Liu J, Fan D. (2008). miR-15b and miR-16 modulate multidrug resistance by targeting BCL2 in human gastric cancer cells. Int J Cancer., 123, 2, pp. 372-9, ISSN 1097-0215

Xiao B, Guo J, Miao Y, Jiang Z, Huan R, Zhang Y, Li D, Zhong J. (2009). Detection of miR-106a in gastric carcinoma and its clinical significance. *Clin Chim Acta, 400*, pp. 97-102, ISSN 1873-3492

Xiao, C., Sharp, J. A., Kawahara, M., Davalos, A. R., Difilippantonio, M. J., Hu, Y., Li, W., Cao, L., Buetow, K., Ried, T., *et al.* (2007). The XIST noncoding RNA functions independently of BRCA1 in X inactivation. *Cell* , 128, pp. 977-989, ISSN 0092-8674

Xue LY, Chiu SM, Oleinick NL. (2010). Atg7 deficiency increases resistance of MCF-7 human breast cancer cells to photodynamic therapy. *Autophagy.*, 6, 2, pp. 248-55, ISSN 1554-8635

Yanaihara N, Caplen N, Bowman E, Seike M, Kumamoto K, Yi M, Stephens RM, Okamoto A, Yokota J, Tanaka T, Calin GA, Liu CG, Croce CM, Harris CC. (2006). Unique microRNA molecular profiles in lung cancer diagnosis and prognosis. *Cancer Cell.*, 9, 3, pp.189-98, ISSN 1535-6108

Yekta S, Shih IH, Bartel DP. (2004). MicroRNA-directed cleavage of HOXB8 mRNA. *Science.*;304, pp. 594-596, ISSN 1095-9203

Zapatka M, Zboralski D, Radacz Y, Böckmann M, Arnold C, Schöneck A, Hoppe S, Tannapfel A, Schmiegel W, Simon-Assmann P, Schwarte-Waldhoff I. (2007).

Basement membrane component laminin-5 is a target of the tumor suppressor Smad4. *Oncogene.* ,26, 10,pp. 1417-27, ISSN 0950-9232

Zhi F, Chen X, Wang S, Xia X, Shi Y, Guan W, Shao N, Qu H, Yang C, Zhang Y, Wang Q, Wang R, Zen K, Zhang CY, Zhang J, Yang Y. (2010). The use of hsa-miR-21, hsa-miR-181b and hsa-miR-106a as prognostic indicators of astrocytoma. *Eur J Cancer.*, 46, 9, pp. 1640-9, ISSN 1879-0852

Zhou H, Guo JM, Lou YR, Zhang XJ, Zhong FD, Jiang Z, Cheng J, Xiao BX. (2010). Detection of circulating tumor cells in peripheral blood from patients with gastric cancer using microRNA as a marker. *J Mol Med,* 88, pp. 709-717, ISSN 1432-1440

26

Scleroderma and Breast Cancer

Adamantios Michalinos[1], Michalis Kontos[1] and Ian S. Fentiman[2]
[1]*First Department of Surgery of the University of Athens, Laiko General Hospital, Athens*
[2]*Research Oncology, 3rd Flooe Bermondsey Wing, Guy's Hospital, London*
[1]*Greece*
[2]*United Kingdom*

1. Introduction

The relationship between breast cancer and scleroderma is complex, involving aspects of epidemiological coexistence, pathophysiology and treatment. Increased risk of malignancy is known to occur in scleroderma patients particularly lung and breast cancer. Risk factors for breast cancer in scleroderma patients include older age and autoimmunity status (lack of ANA positivity). The sometimes close temporal relationship between breast cancer and scleroderma suggests the possible existence of a common pathophysiological mechanism. TGF- β and Caveolin-1 have been widely investigated, while researchers also examined estrogen receptors, common genetic background and other possible mechanisms.

Treatment for breast cancer with radiotherapy and taxanes can both induce scleroderma, morphea and sclerodermic skin lesions. The existence of scleroderma can affect breast cancer treatment and reversely. Breast conservation surgery is avoided in scleroderma patients and radiotherapy is also traditionally considered a relative contradiction due to more frequent and severe toxicity.

2. Epidemiology

There is an increased risk of malignancy in scleroderma patients with an incidence between 4 and 11% [1,2,3,4,5,6,7]. The exact characteristics of this relationship are difficult to assess due to the rarity of scleroderma and the consequent lack of statistical power to determine the importance of any comparison, the differences in methodology of the studies and the lack of knowledge of the detailed pathophysiology of scleroderma.

Several well-designed population studies have reported a correlation between scleroderma and different types of cancers. The results are summarized in Table 1. The majority of the studies reported a significantly elevated SIR of between 1-5 and 3.15 [1 2 3 4 8 5]. In contrast, Chatterjee *et al* [9] found no statistically significant increase in malignancy in patients with scleroderma compared with the normal population. The only malignancy with a significantly increased risk was liver cancer in black females. The commonest cancer type occurring in scleroderma is lung cancer, while data over other cancer types are not clear[1].

In terms of breast cancer risk, some studies such as those of Siau *et al* [2] and Abu - Shakra *et al* [4] found a statistically important correlation with SIRs 3,07 and 6,1 respectively, while others [3,8] reported a non statistically significant correlation or no correlation at all.[1, 5, 9]

Author	SIR	95% CI
Olesen	1.5	1.3-1.7
Siau	3.15	1.77-5.2
Hill	1.99	1.46-2.65
Abu-Shakra	2.1	
Derk	1.55	1.16-1.93
Rosenthal	2.4	1.5-3.6
Chatterjee	1.23	

Table 1. Scleroderma and Standardised Incidence Rate of malignancy.

The risk factors for malignancy in patients with scleroderma , in particular breast cancer are not determined. Siau *et al* [2] found age > 70 to be an important risk factor, while Abu - Shakra *et al* [4] found an increased risk for age > 65 for all cancer types. Derk *et al* reported that the diagnosis of scleroderma occurs in older patients with cancer in general [8] or breast cancer[10], while Lu *et al* [11] concluded that age of scleroderma diagnosis was irrelevant to age of breast cancer diagnosis. Kyndt [7] reported that scleroderma patients with breast cancer had their scleroderma diagnosis at a later age than patients with scleroderma only, but this difference was not statistically significant.

The role of the gender of the patients is not determined either. Most authors state that both male and female scleroderma patients are at higher risk of developing cancer in comparison to the general population, but there is no agreement as to whether the correlation is stronger for men [1,3,4,8] or women[5]. It is important to highlight that both breast cancer and scleroderma predominately affect women.

As for the scleroderma type, data are also equivocal. Some authors [9,11] believe that scleroderma type is not important while some others [4,7] find various differences that do not reach statistical importance. Siau *et al* [2] report that limited scleroderma is a risk factor for cancer development and Hill *et al* [3] states the same for diffuse scleroderma. Systemic sclerosis, morphea and breast cancer can coexist[12].

With regard to the autoimmune status of the patients, most authors [3,4,9,7] agree that ANA, Scl 70 and U1 - RNP antibody status do not constitute a risk factor for cancer development. Reports focusing on breast cancer however[10, 11] find the lack of ANA positivity to be a risk factor for breast cancer development. Family history is considered a risk factor for all cancer types in scleroderma patients [8] and also for breast cancer. On the other hand, scleroderma patients with breast cancer use Hormone Replacement Therapy less frequently than those without the disease but this finding may be biased[11, 10].

Breast cancer diagnosis can precede, follow or coincide with diagnosis of scleroderma. To evaluate this relationship, it has to be taken in consideration that authors use different definitions of "simultaneous", accepting a time lag from 1 to 6 months between the breast cancer and scleroderma diagnosis. Derk [10] studied two groups, one with breast cancer and scleroderma and another with scleroderma only (control group). The first group was the divided into two subgroups: those in whom breast cancer diagnosis followed the scleroderma diagnosis (48%) and those in which it preceded (52%). When these groups were compared for age at scleroderma diagnosis it emerged that patients with breast cancer diagnosis prior to scleroderma diagnosis were older than the ones with breast cancer after scleroderma. This difference was however not statistically significant. In contrast, for the group in which breast cancer was diagnosed prior to scleroderma with the control group, the difference reached statistical significance. This was not true for the group in which breast cancer diagnosis followed scleroderma diagnosis. The first subgroup of patients was ANA negative compared with patients with scleroderma only, and this attained statistical significance when the second subgroup were compared with the control subgroup. Not all researchers agree on the timing of diagnoses of the two conditions. In another study by Lu *et al* [11] cancer diagnosis predated scleroderma diagnosis in only 24% of the patients and followed in 76%.

Others[13,14] have underlined the close temporal relationship between scleroderma diagnosis and breast cancer diagnosis, and explored the possibility of a pathophysiological connection between them. Pineda et al [15] described a rare case of bilateral breast carcinoma and diffuse scleroderma. Possible aetiologies for this include scleroderma as a true paraneoplasmatic syndrome, a common background immunological abnormality, or a detection bias due to extensive investigation of unwell patients.[16]

3. Pathophysiology

While the epidemiological connection between cancer and scleroderma is well established, any pathophysiological relationship is not clear yet. Certain mechanisms such as lung fibrosis have been incriminated for lung cancer, the commonest coexisting cancer in scleroderma patients, but few data exist for other cancer types.

Epidemiological correlations do not necessarily mean aetiological correlation, since they can be attributed to higher prevalence of both diseases in older ages[17], female gender[18] or a diagnostic bias from close follow-up and extensive clinical investigation. Yet, there is some evidence that could support the existence of mechanisms that, in some extent, connect the two diseases. Hypotheses for these include a common genetic background, a common mechanism or finally scleroderma as a consequence of breast cancer radiotherapy and chemotherapy.

With regard to the common genetic background, scleroderma patients have been occasionally reported to have a breast cancer family history[11]. Genetic polymorphism has been incriminated and HLA-DR_2 haplotype is more frequent in scleroderma and breast cancer patients.[17] Explanations proposed include that this haplotype confers to a germline BRCA mutation or is at a genetic linkage to it.[11]

Mechanisms involving both conditions include TGF-β/Smad signaling pathway that is known to regulate many events in scleroderma, especially in the pathogenesis of fibrosis via upregulation of collagen expression [19]. On the other hand, increased collagen formation, expressed as greater mammographic density[20] is a recognized risk factor for breast cancer development. Interestingly TGF β is a known breast tumor suppressor[21] although certain reports refer both to proliferative and suppressive action[22]. TGF-β levels are increased in breast cancer patients and, in those having limited disease, they decrease after resection of the tumor[23]

Another piece of evidence that could potentially indicate common pathophysiology is the breast tumor associated antigen Ca 15-3 (MUC-1) which is increased in scleroderma patients, and correlates with more severe disease including renal and joint involvement, ANA positivity and elevated CRP[24]. Furthermore, scleroderma has sometimes evolved in women undergoing breast augmentation surgery and the proposed mechanism was fibroblastic actions of silica or a Graft versus Host disease[25]

Sex hormone changes are also involved in the pathophysiology of both diseases. Certain predisposing factors for breast cancer such as nulliparity [26] or protective factors like increasing number of births [27] alter the course of scleroderma disease. Existence of parity delays scleroderma onset and decreases disease mortality and morbidity but does not alter duration[26]. Not only estrogens but also genetic alterations in estrogen receptors (ER) are involved in the pathogenesis of scleroderma. Specifically ERa XbaI GG phenotype was significantly less frequent in systemic scleroderma patients than in healthy controls although no association with clinical manifestations was found[28]. Nevertheless, ERa up-regulation is an early event during mammary hyperplasia and adenocarcinoma development.[29]

The two conditions are also connected in studies focusing on certain mediators such as Caveolin I, a regulator that inhibits the baseline activity of several pro-proliferative and oncogenic proteins via the TGF-β/Smad signaling pathway[30]. Caveolin-1 is known to suppress collagen expression via interactions with TGF - β[31] and also has a variety of effects on breast cancer development such as up-regulation of ERa or molecular changes necessary in the development of metastasis as confirmed in mouse models. Caveolin-1 normally inhibits metastases via suppression of matrix metalloproteinase secretion that degrades the basement membrane of normal epithelia [32,33]. In humans loss of stromal caveolin-1 is a novel breast cancer biomarker that predicts early disease recurrence, metastasis, survival, and tamoxifen resistance.[34]

Post irradiation morphea was first described in 1905, the first large series in 1989[35]. Radiotherapy for breast cancer can induce scleroderma through various mechanisms. After radiotherapy morphea in the breast region is a relatively common manifestation, but systemic scleroderma has also been occasionally reported.[36] Its frequency is calculated at up to 1/500 [37,38]. The hypothesis of a systemic mechanism, triggered by radiotherapy is supported by the scleroderma appearance away from the radiated field. Possible mechanisms involve T cell activation [36] and clonal fibroblast population alteration. Selective local immune alteration, including TGF-β increase and endothelial alterations have also been proposed for radiation caused scleroderma[39, 37].

Research on predictive factors for breast cancer patients to develop scleroderma manifestations is inconclusive. Patient age, total dose of radiation, dose per fraction, severity of the acute reaction and tamoxifen use do not appear significant.[37] Several studies however indicate the severity of scleroderma is an important predictive factor[40]. Finally apart from radiotherapy, chemotherapy especially with docetaxel and paclitaxel has been reported to occasionally induce scleroderma[41,42,43,44].

4. Treatment

A possible relation between the two diseases could potentially lead to treatment alternations with dilemmas occurring mainly when scleroderma patients develop a breast cancer. No evidence exists in the literature that the core treatment - surgery - should be altered but questions over adjuvant chemotherapy and radiotherapy have been raised.

Finally, hormonal and biological therapies do not seem to interfere with the course of scleroderma.

Scleroderma is a relative contradiction for radiotherapy due to possible sensitivity of the tissue affected by the disease. Many doctors hesitate to treat breast cancer in scleroderma patients with breast conservation[45,46], although large studies failed to prove severe toxicity[48,49], such as grade III or IV toxicity (severe adverse events or life threatening or disabling adverse events respectively). It has been stated that clinicians consider radiotherapy to be contraindicated to scleroderma patients because mainly of publication bias, severe cases of toxicity being written up as case reports, while cases with mild toxicity or no toxicity are omitted [38].

A large study by Lin et al[50] found no differences in early toxicity, but differences were found in late toxicity. Proven prognostic factors for scleroderma patients developing toxicity effects are curative treatment, multi organ involvement of scleroderma for acute toxicity and negative antinuclear antibodies for late toxicity.[51]. However these results reach statistical importance for mild toxicity only (Grade 1 and 2 according to Common Terminology Criteria for Adverse Events version 3.0 grading scales).

Another implication of the coexistence of scleroderma and breast cancer is imaging surveillance after breast conservation. This may be difficult due to breast fibrosis and is sometimes achieved only by MRI.[47]

On the other hand, previously healthy patients who receive radiotherapy for breast cancer can develop sclerodermatic changes. The typical clinical picture includes sclerotic and pigmentary lesions in the breast, initially severe and painful but self - limited. [37] The initial calculation of its incidence at 0.2% is probably an overestimate. This situation is rare and is only reported in sparse case reports in the English literature[35,38,39].

In these cases the clinician can use the appropriate scleroderma therapy and topical steroids, calcineurin inhibitors or low doses of systemic immunosuppressants (steroids, methotrexate MTX cyclosporine) can be applied. Topical softening of the tissue can be achieved by means of heparin, hyaluronidase, UVA1 irradiation, PUVA irradiation, or the systemic administration of penicillamine with various success [54,52,55].

5. Conclusions

While the relationship between cancer and scleroderma is strongly suggested, its characteristics are not yet clarified and more research is required. Questions to be answered include underlying pathophysiological mechanisms and alterations in the treatment for scleroderma patients. Coexistence of scleroderma and breast cancer can be a challenging problem, involving general surgeons, rheumatologists, oncologists, radiologists and, last but not least, mental health professionals since the coexistence of two diseases can affect the patients' psychological status and their compliance with the treatment. A multidisciplinary approach with doctors, nurses and paramedics, high clinical vigilance and cooperation is required so to avoid undesirable consequences.

6. References

[1] Olesen AB, Svaerke C, Farkas DK, Sørensen HT. Systemic sclerosis and the risk of cancer: a nationwide population-based cohort study. *Br. J. Dermatol.* 2010;163(4):800-806.

[2] Siau K, Laversuch CJ, Creamer P, O'Rourke KP . Malignancy in scleroderma patients from south west England: a population-based cohort study. *Rheumatol. Int.* 2010.

[3] Hill CL, Nguyen A-M, Roder D, Roberts-Thomson P. Risk of cancer in patients with scleroderma: a population based cohort study. *Ann. Rheum. Dis.* 2003;62(8):728-731.

[4] Abu-Shakra M, Guillemin F, Lee P. Cancer in systemic sclerosis. *Arthritis Rheum.* 1993;36(4):460-464.

[5] Rosenthal AK, McLaughlin JK, Linet MS, Persson I. Scleroderma and malignancy: an epidemiological study. *Ann. Rheum. Dis.* 1993;52(7):531-533.

[6] Wooten M . Systemic sclerosis and malignancy: a review of the literature. *South. Med. J.* 2008;101(1):59-62.

[7] Kyndt X, Hebbar M, Queyrel V, κ.ά. [Systemic scleroderma and cancer. Search for predictive factors of cancer in 123 patients with scleroderma]. *Rev Med Interne.* 1997;18(7):528-532.

[8] Derk CT, Rasheed M, Artlett CM, Jimenez SA A cohort study of cancer incidence in systemic sclerosis. *J. Rheumatol.* 2006;33(6):1113-1116.

[9] Chatterjee S, Dombi GW, Severson RK, Mayes MD Risk of malignancy in scleroderma: a population-based cohort study. *Arthritis Rheum.* 2005;52(8):2415-2424.

[10] Derk CT Associations of breast cancer development in patients with systemic sclerosis: an exploratory study. *Clin. Rheumatol.* 2007;26(10):1615-1619.

[11] Lu TY-T, Hill CL, Pontifex EK, Roberts-Thomson PJ Breast cancer and systemic sclerosis: a clinical description of 21 patients in a population-based cohort study. *Rheumatol. Int.* 2008;28(9):895-899.

[12] Mittal G, Maddison P, Williams W Systemic sclerosis, morphoea and breast cancer. *Rheumatology (Oxford).* 2006;45(1):119-120.

[13] Launay D, Le Berre R, Hatron P-Y. Association between systemic sclerosis and breast cancer: eight new cases and review of the literature. *Clin. Rheumatol.* 2004;23(6):516-522.

[14] Forbes AM, Woodrow JC, Verbov JL, Graham RM Carcinoma of breast and scleroderma: four further cases and a literature review. *Br. J. Rheumatol.* 1989;28(1):65-69.

[15] Pineda V, Salvador R, Soriano J Bilateral breast cancer associated with diffuse scleroderma. *Breast.* 2003;12(3):217-219.

[16] Scope A, Sadetzki S, Sidi Y, κ.ά. Breast cancer and scleroderma. *Skinmed.* 2006;5(1):18-24.

[17] Wenzel J Scleroderma and malignancy. Mechanisms of interrelationship. *Eur J Dermatol.* 2002;12(3):296-300.

[18] Chifflot H, Fautrel B, Sordet C, Chatelus E, Sibilia J Incidence and prevalence of systemic sclerosis: a systematic literature review. *Semin. Arthritis Rheum.* 2008;37(4):223-235.

[19] Mori Y, Chen S-J, Varga J Expression and regulation of intracellular SMAD signaling in scleroderma skin fibroblasts. *Arthritis Rheum.* 2003;48(7):1964-1978.

[20] Martin LJ, Boyd NF Mammographic density. Potential mechanisms of breast cancer risk associated with mammographic density: hypotheses based on epidemiological evidence. *Breast Cancer Res.* 2008;10(1):201.

[21] Kretzschmar M Transforming growth factor-beta and breast cancer: Transforming growth factor-beta/SMAD signaling defects and cancer. *Breast Cancer Res.* 2000;2(2):107-115.

[22] Dumont N, Arteaga CL Transforming growth factor-beta and breast cancer: Tumor promoting effects of transforming growth factor-beta. *Breast Cancer Res.* 2000;2(2):125-132.

[23] Kong FM, Anscher MS, Murase T, κ.ά. Elevated plasma transforming growth factor-beta 1 levels in breast cancer patients decrease after surgical removal of the tumor. *Ann. Surg.* 1995;222(2):155-162.

[24] Szekanecz Z, Szekanecz E, Bakó G, Shoenfeld Y Malignancies in autoimmune rheumatic diseases - a mini-review. *Gerontology.* 2011;57(1):3-10.

[25] Kumagai Y, Abe C, Shiokawa Y Scleroderma after cosmetic surgery: four cases of human adjuvant disease. *Arthritis Rheum.* 1979;22(5):532-537.

[26] Artlett CM, Rasheed M, Russo-Stieglitz KE, Sawaya HHB, Jimenez SA Influence of prior pregnancies on disease course and cause of death in systemic sclerosis. *Ann. Rheum. Dis.* 2002;61(4):346-350.

[27] Lambe M, Björnådal L, Neregård P, Nyren O, Cooper GS Childbearing and the risk of scleroderma: a population-based study in Sweden. *Am. J. Epidemiol.* 2004;159(2):162-166.

[28] Hoshi M, Yasuoka H, Kuwana M Estrogen receptor gene polymorphisms in Japanese patients with systemic sclerosis. *Clin. Exp. Rheumatol.* 2008;26(5):914-917.

[29] Sotgia F, Rui H, Bonuccelli G. Caveolin-1, mammary stem cells, and estrogen-dependent breast cancers. *Cancer Res.* 2006;66(22):10647-10651.

[30] Qian N, Ueno T Is dysfunction of caveolin-1 a link between systemic sclerosis and breast cancer, opening a window on both etiologies? *Arch. Med. Res.* 2010;41(4):297-301.

[31] Tourkina E, Gooz P, Pannu J. Opposing effects of protein kinase Calpha and protein kinase Cepsilon on collagen expression by human lung fibroblasts are mediated via MEK/ERK and caveolin-1 signaling. *J. Biol. Chem.* 2005;280(14):13879-13887.

[32] Williams TM, Medina F, Badano I. Caveolin-1 gene disruption promotes mammary tumorigenesis and dramatically enhances lung metastasis in vivo. Role of Cav-1 in cell invasiveness and matrix metalloproteinase (MMP-2/9) secretion. *J. Biol. Chem.* 2004;279(49):51630-51646.

[33] Witkiewicz AK, Dasgupta A, Nguyen KH.. Stromal caveolin-1 levels predict early DCIS progression to invasive breast cancer. *Cancer Biol. Ther.* 2009;8(11):1071-1079.

[34] Witkiewicz AK, Dasgupta A, Sotgia F. An absence of stromal caveolin-1 expression predicts early tumor recurrence and poor clinical outcome in human breast cancers. *Am. J. Pathol.* 2009;174(6):2023-2034.

[35] Colver GB, Rodger A, Mortimer PS, κ.ά. Post-irradiation morphoea. *Br. J. Dermatol.* 1989;120(6):831-835.

[36] Ardern-Jones MR, Black MM Widespread morphoea following radiotherapy for carcinoma of the breast. *Clin. Exp. Dermatol.* 2003;28(2):160-162.

[37] Bleasel NR, Stapleton KM, Commens C, Ahern VA Radiation-induced localized scleroderma in breast cancer patients. *Australas. J. Dermatol.* 1999;40(2):99-102.

[38] Herrmann T, Günther C, Csere P Localized morphea--a rare but significant secondary complication following breast cancer radiotherapy. Case report and review of the

literature on radiation reaction among patients with scleroderma/morphea. *Strahlenther Onkol.* 2009;185(9):603-607.

[39] Davis DA, Cohen PR, McNeese MD, Duvic M Localized scleroderma in breast cancer patients treated with supervoltage external beam radiation: radiation port scleroderma. *J. Am. Acad. Dermatol.* 1996;35(6):923-927.

[40] Gold DG, Miller RC, Pinn ME, κ.ά. Chronic toxicity risk after radiotherapy for patients with systemic sclerosis (systemic scleroderma) or systemic lupus erythematosus: association with connective tissue disorder severity. *Radiother Oncol.* 2008;87(1):127-131.

[41] Hassett G, Harnett P, Manolios N Scleroderma in association with the use of docetaxel (taxotere) for breast cancer. *Clin. Exp. Rheumatol.* 2001;19(2):197-200.

[42] Farrant PBJ, Mortimer PS, Gore M Scleroderma and the taxanes. Is there really a link? *Clin. Exp. Dermatol.* 2004;29(4):360-362.

[43] Vignes S, Lebrun-Vignes B Sclerodermiform aspect of arm lymphoedema after treatment with docetaxel for breast cancer. *J Eur Acad Dermatol Venereol.* 2007;21(8):1131-1133.

[44] Itoh M, Yanaba K, Kobayashi T, Nakagawa H Taxane-induced scleroderma. *Br. J. Dermatol.* 2007;156(2):363-367.

[45] De Naeyer B, De Meerleer G, Braems S, Vakaet L, Huys J Collagen vascular diseases and radiation therapy: a critical review. *Int. J. Radiat. Oncol. Biol. Phys.* 1999;44(5):975-980.

[46] Chen AM, Obedian E, Haffty BG Breast-conserving therapy in the setting of collagen vascular disease. *Cancer J.* 2001;7(6):480-491.

[47] Phan C, Mindrum M, Silverman C, Paris K, Spanos W Matched-control retrospective study of the acute and late complications in patients with collagen vascular diseases treated with radiation therapy. *Cancer J.* 2003;9(6):461-466.

[48] Ross JG, Hussey DH, Mayr NA, Davis CS Acute and late reactions to radiation therapy in patients with collagen vascular diseases. *Cancer.* 1993;71(11):3744-3752.

[49] Lin A, Abu-Isa E, Griffith KA, Ben-Josef E Toxicity of radiotherapy in patients with collagen vascular disease. *Cancer.* 2008;113(3):648-653.

[50] Gold DG, Miller RC, Petersen IA, Osborn TG Radiotherapy for malignancy in patients with scleroderma: The Mayo Clinic experience. *Int. J. Radiat. Oncol. Biol. Phys.* 2007;67(2):559-567.

[51] Seale M, Koh W, Henderson M, Drummond R, Cawson J Imaging surveillance of the breast in a patient diagnosed with scleroderma after breast-conserving surgery and radiotherapy. *Breast J.* 2008;14(4):379-381.

[52] Schaffer JV, Carroll C, Dvoretsky I, Huether MJ, Girardi M Postirradiation morphea of the breast presentation of two cases and review of the literature. *Dermatology (Basel).* 2000;200(1):67-71.

[53] Walsh N, Rheaume D, Barnes P, Tremaine R, Reardon M Postirradiation morphea: an underrecognized complication of treatment for breast cancer. *Hum. Pathol.* 2008;39(11):1680-1688.

[54] Shetty G, Lewis F, Thrush S Morphea of the breast: case reports and review of literature. *Breast J.* 2007;13(3):302-304.

Part 4

Signaling Pathways (Others)

27

FZD7 in Triple Negative Breast Cancer Cells

Lixin Yang, Charles C.H. Kim and Yun Yen
Department of Molecular Pharmacology, Beckman Research Institute, City of Hope National Medical Center, Duarte, CA, USA

1. Introduction

Breast cancer is the most prevalent cancer in women. Although the survival rate of breast cancer has improved steadily in the past two decades, over 40,000 women die from breast cancer related complications each year. The heterogeneity of breast cancer makes the treatment of different subtypes difficult (Gonzalez-Angulo *et al.*, 2007; Perez *et al.*, 2010). Triple negative breast cancer (TNBC) is one of the subtypes. It is negative for both estrogen and progesterone hormone receptors and lack the overexpression of human epidermal growth factor receptor 2 (HER2). TNBC constitutes approximately 15% of all breast cancers. However, its death rate is disproportionately higher than any other subtype of breast cancer, especially among young Black, Asian and Hispanic patients (Anders and Carey, 2009; Kassam *et al.*, 2009; Rahman *et al.*, 2009). Although, HER2 antibody, Herceptin, estrogen receptor antagonist, and aromatase inhibitor have brought hope to breast cancer patients, the treatment of TNBC remains to be a great challenge (Amir *et al.*, 2010; Gluz *et al.*, 2009; Silver *et al.*, 2010). Thus it is imperative to investigate effective therapeutic targets for TNBC patients.

FZD7, a Wnt pathway receptor, is one of the most abundant Frizzled family proteins expressed in TNBC and its cell lines. Wnt canonical signaling regulates cell fate decision throughout embryonic development and is related to human disease (Clevers, 2006; MacDonald *et al.*, 2009; Reya and Clevers, 2005). Activation of Wnt canonical pathway is transduced through Frizzled (FZD) family receptors and LRP5/LRP6 coreceptor to the β-catenin signaling cascade (Bhanot *et al.*, 1996; Pinson *et al.*, 2000). In the presence of canonical Wnt signal, FZD binds to Dishevelled (DVL) and LRP5/6 to AXIN-FRAT to form a complex. β-catenin is protected from phosphorylation (Tolwinski *et al.*, 2003) and the stabilized β-catenin translocates from the cytoplasm to the nucleus to activate the transcription of Wnt responsive genes by binding with T-cell factor/lymphoid enhancer factor (TCF/LEF) family transcription factors. Activation of these tissue-specific Wnt target genes is involved in the development of human tumors, including breast, colon, and other cancers (Jones and Kemp, 2008; Lee *et al.*, 1995; Ojalvo *et al.*, 2010).

To investigate the therapeutic targets for TNBC, microarray has been performed to identify the genes that may be involved in the tumorigenesis of TNBC. FZD7 is differentially expressed in TNBC which raises the possibility that aberrant Wnt signaling might be critical for TNBC development. In this chapter we will address the role that FZD7 plays in cell proliferation of TNBC and its mechanism.

2. FZD7 plays a critical role in cell proliferation of TNBC

Basal-like breast cancer is categorized as TNBC because almost all basal-like breast cancers do not have hormone receptor expression and HER2 overexpression (Perou *et al.*, 2000; Sotiriou *et al.*, 2003). Although aberrant Wnt signaling activation has been observed in breast cancer (Brown, 2001; Turashvili *et al.*, 2006), the correlation of Wnt signaling with TNBC has rarely been investigated. However, canonical Wnt pathway activation in basal-like tumor has been observed (DiMeo *et al.*, 2009; Lindvall *et al.*, 2009). Recently, we performed Human Gene Array ST-1.0 (Affymetrix) in 19 breast tumor samples of five triple negative and 14 non-triple negative breast cancers (non-TNBC). Identification of the differentially expressed genes was carried out under the criteria of 1.5 fold up-regulated in TNBC with p-value less than 0.01. FZD7 as well as other two Wnt pathway genes were found to be overexpressed in TNBC tissues. Among these genes, FZD7 showed the greatest change as compared to other genes (Table 1). Although other Frizzled, such as FZD3 and FZD5 showed high level expression in TNBC tissues, it was not significantly higher ($p>0.05$). This result suggested that overexpression of FZD3 and FZD5 in the TNBC samples used in our microarray study may have been due to the variation of individual samples, but not from overall upregulation of FZD3 and FZD5 in TNBC.

Log2Ratio	P-value	Symbol	Description	Chromosome	GenBank
1.30663	0.0023467	FZD7	frizzled homolog 7 (Drosophila)	2	NM_003507
1.07657	0.0047925	TCF7	transcription factor 7 (T-cell specific, HMG-box)	5	NM_003202
0.866995	0.0083258	LRP6	low density lipoprotein receptor-related protein 6	12	NM_002336

Table 1. FZD7 and other Wnt pathway genes were up-regulated in TNBC.

2.1 FZD7 is up-regulated in TNBC and its derived cell lines

Aberrant Wnt signaling in TNBC has been noted by a few research groups. Dr. Bu and his team reported that LRP6 overexpression is found in a subtype of breast tumor that is ER-negative and Her2-negative (Liu *et al.*, 2010). This is consistent with our microarray result. Benefiting from free access to the public database, we analyzed FZD7 expression in a larger human breast tumor cohort study reported by Finak *et al* (20). We found that FZD7 mRNA expression was significantly higher in the TNBC samples ($n=14$) as compared to non-TNBC samples ($n=109$; $P=0.0017$, Wilcoxon Test) (Figure 1A). We further evaluated the FZD7 expression using breast tumor tissues. In Fig 1B, the overexpression of FZD7 was observed in all TNBC samples, whereas the other four non-TNBC tissues with equal differentiation/stage minimally expressed FZD7. To validate the FZD7 overexpression in TNBC, immunohistochemistry staining was performed in 20 formalin-fixed paraffin-embedded breast tumor slides. It was found that 67% of TNBC expressed FZD7; while only 5% non-TNBC weakly expressed FZD7 (Fig. 1C). FZD7 expression in various breast cancer cell lines was also assessed (Fig. 1D). Among the seven cell lines investigated, MDA-MB-231 and BT-20 cell lines expressed high levels of FZD7, while the other five cell lines either had no or limited FZD7 expression. While the MDA-MB-231 and BT-20 cell lines were known to be TNBC-derived, all other cell lines were either derived from normal breast tissue (MCF

10A) or non-TNBC tissues. Notably, FZD7 is the most abundant FZD in TNBC cell lines: MDA-MB-231 and BT-20 (Fig. 1E).

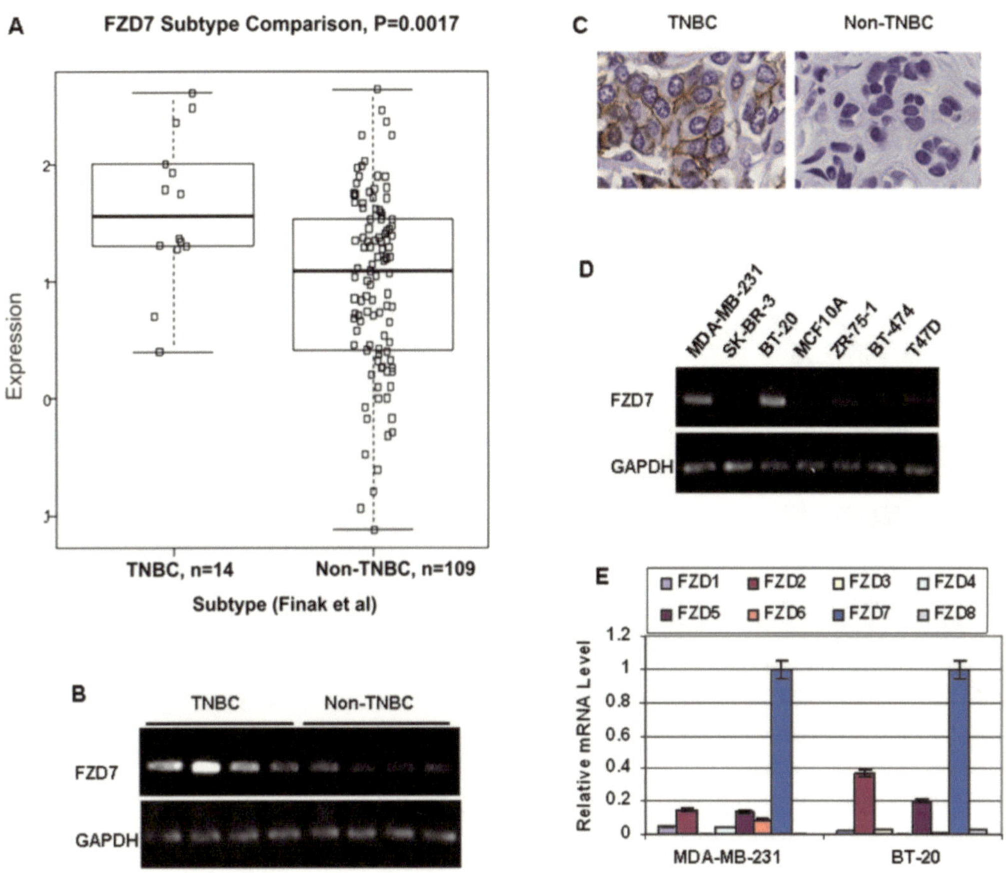

Fig. 1. FZD7 expression in TNBC tissues and TNBC cell lines.

2.2 FZD7shRNA suppressed tumor transformation in TNBC cell lines MDA-MB-231 and BT-20

To evaluate the function of FZD7 in TNBC cells, FZD7shRNA or its control GFPshRNA lentivirus were transduced into TNBC-derived cell lines MDA-MB-231 and BT-20, and were selected with puromycin. Effective knockdown of FZD7 in MDA-MB-231 and BT-20 cells was found in FZD7shRNA lentivirus transduced cells. It was observed that FZD7 expression was reduced by 95% to 97.5% at the mRNA level (Fig.23A, left panel) and almost completely inhibited the protein expression (Fig. 2A, right panel). Specific inhibition of FZD7 expression without affecting the other members of the FZD family was confirmed by RT-PCR in MDA-MB-231(Fig. 2B) and in BT-20 cells (Fig. 2C).

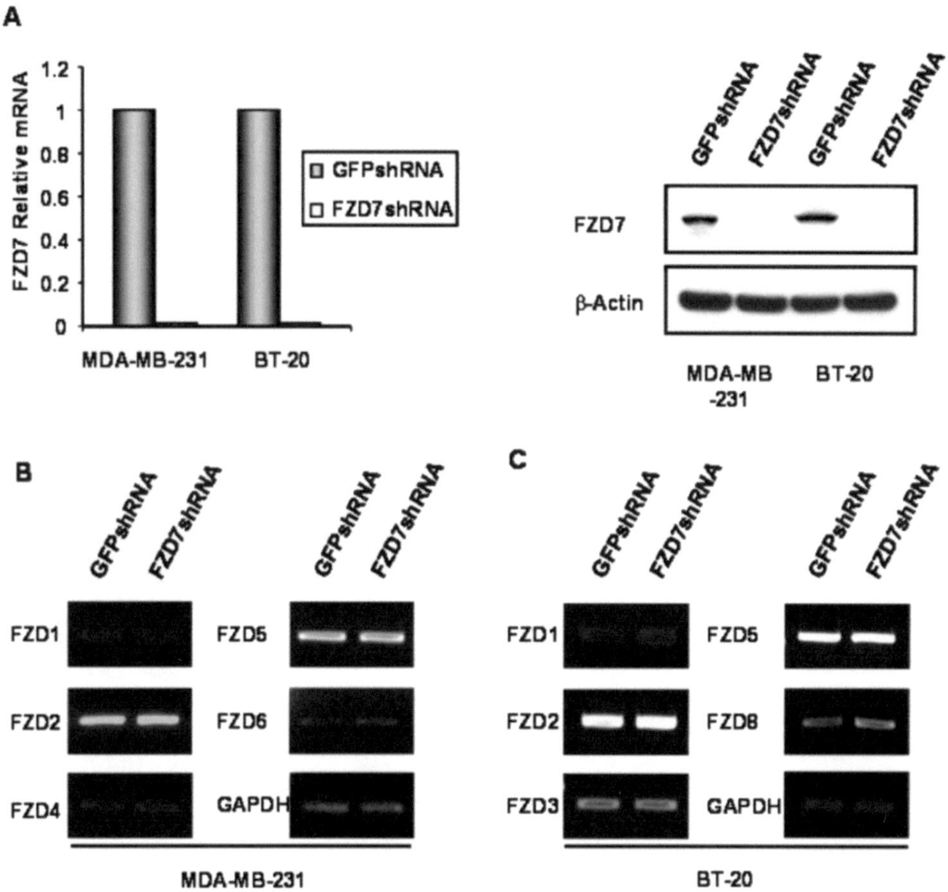

Fig. 2. FZD7 knockdown in MDA-MB-231 and BT-20 cells.

2.2.1 FZD7 is required for cell growth in TNBC cells

Frizzled family gene is commonly up-regulated in various tumors from different organs. Wnt signaling initiated from these genes induce acceleration of cell growth in these tumor cells. Comparisons were made with regards to the rate of cell growth of FZD7shRNA and GFPshRNA lentivirus infected MDA-MB-231 cells. As shown in Fig. 3 left panel, cell growth significantly slowed in FZD7shRNA transduced MDA-MB-231 cells as compared to that of GFPshRNA infected MDA-MB-231 cells. When both cell lines were treated with FZD7 ligand Wnt3a, significant cell growth acceleration was observed in GFPshRNA transduced MDA-MB-231 cells. However, there was no growth advantage seen in FZD7shRNA transduced MDA-MB-231 cells. To determine if the FZD7shRNA alone is sufficient for the growth inhibition, MDA-MB-231/GFPshRNA cells and MDA-MB-231/FZD7shRNA cells were treated with LRP6 inhibitor DKK1 to block the LRP6 signal. As indicated in Fig 3 right panel, there is no significant change in the suppression of cell growth by double treatment with FZD7shRNA and DKK1 as compared with FZD7shRNA treatment alone in MDA-MB-231 cells. In each panel of Fig 3, FZD7 suppressed cells with FZD7shRNA transduction showed significant growth retardation ($P<0.05$). The data indicates that FZD7 plays a critical role in cell growth of TNBC.

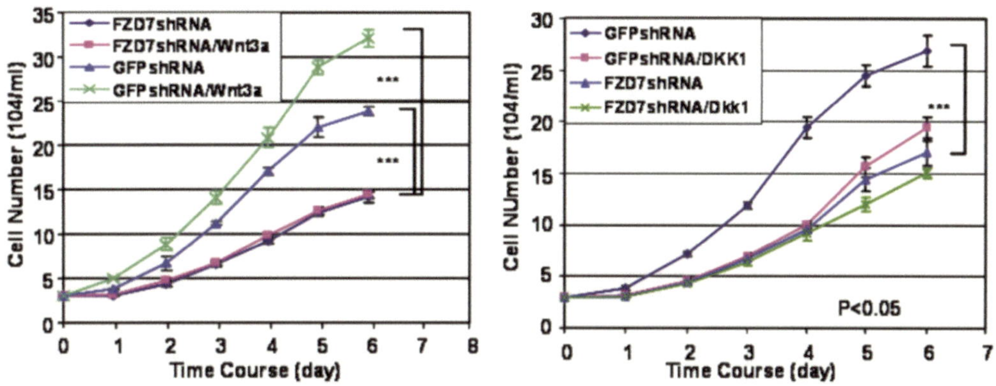

Fig. 3. FZD7 regulated cell growth in MDA-MB-231 cells.

2.2.2 FZD7 plays an important role in cell motility and invasion

We have noted that FZD7 enhances cell growth in TNBC. We then asked whether FZD7 is involved in cell motility and invasion of TNBC. We evaluated the invasive ability of the cells with or without FZD7 by using an invasion assay. MDA-MB-231 and BT-20 cells that express GFPshRNA actively migrated into the bottom layer of the membrane of the insert chamber after overnight culture. A representative area from each well for each cell line cultured was analyzed. The number of invasive cells in the membrane was quantified using the Image-Pro 6.3 software. As shown in Fig. 4A, MDA-MB-231 and BT20 cells treated with

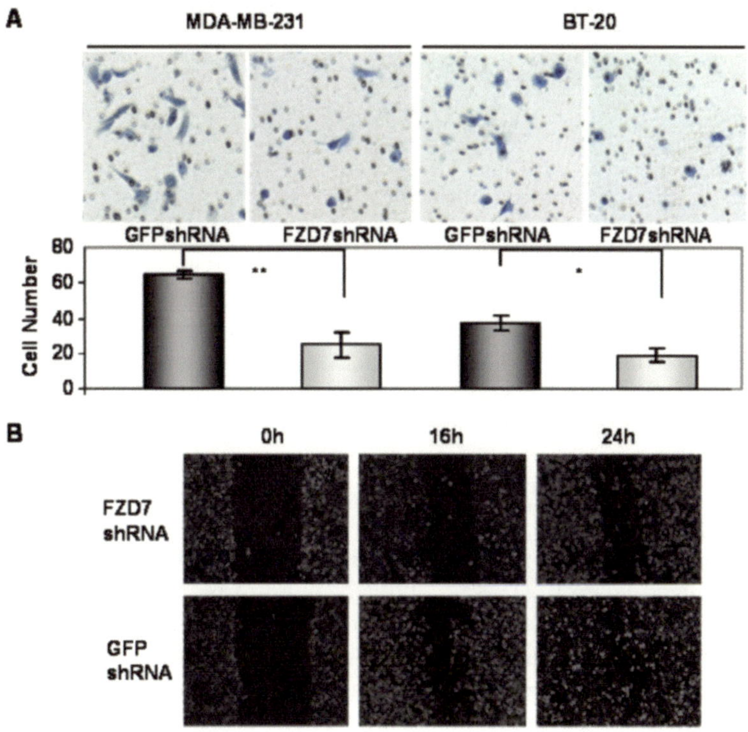

Fig. 4. FZD7 increased cell migration in TNBC.

GFPshRNA virus showed aggressive migration from the metrigel to the membrane. The numbers of cells in the membrane of MDA-MB-231/GFPshRNA and BT-20/GFPshRNA cells were 2.6 and 1.9 times higher than those of MDA-MB-231/FZD7shRNA and BT-20/FZD7shRNA cells respectively. To address the effect of FZD7 in cell motility, we performed a wound healing assay. MDA-MB-231/GFPshRNA cells migrated to the wound area within 16 hours and completely closed the wound within 24 hours; whereas with FZD7 inhibited cells, the wound remained open even after 24 hours of observation (Fig. 4B). These results suggested that FZD7 exert positive effect on cell migration in TNBC.

2.2.3 FZD7 modulated cell tumorigenicity in TNBC

It has been shown that FZD7 is involved in not only enhanced cell growth, but also enhanced cell migration, raising the possibility that FZD7 might be a regulator for cell tumorigenicity in TNBC. To verify this hypothesis, colony formation assay was performed on both FZD7 expressing and FZD7 suppressed MDA-MB-231 cells. It was found that more than twice the number of colonies was observed in GPFshRNA expressing cells as compared to MDA-MB-231/FZD7shRNA cells (Fig. 5). These results indicated that FZD7 is a key factor involved cell colonigenicity in TNBC. Increased colonigenicity in TNBC cells expressing FZD7 lead to accelerated tumor growth in TNBC.

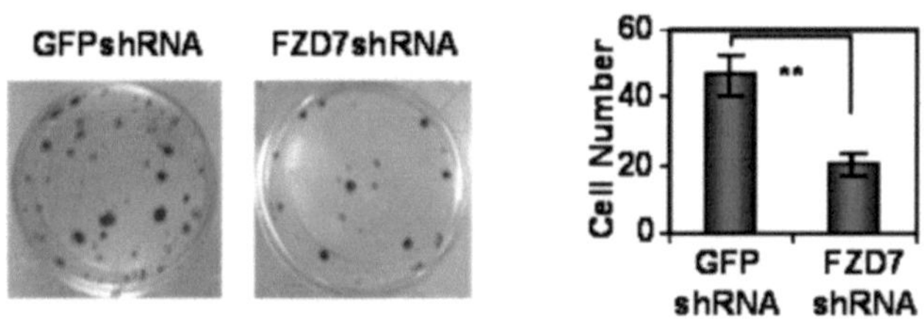

Fig. 5. FZD7 increased cell tumorigenicity in TNBC.

2.3 FZD7 regulated cell transformation through cannonical Wnt signaling pathway

FZD7 is known as the receptor for the Wnt signaling pathway. To investigate if FZD7 affects TNBC tumor cell biology through the canonical Wnt pathway, β-catenin immunofluorescence and DAPI staining was performed to determine the localization of β-catenin thereby confirming the involvement of the Wnt/β-catenin pathway. β-catenin accumulated in the nuclei of MDA-MB-231 cells transduced with GFPshRNA (Figure 5A). However, in cells in which FZD7 expression was suppressed by FZD7shRNA, β-catenin staining was attenuated in the nuclei and remained in the cytoplasm. Furthermore, assessment of TCF7 promoter activity by dual luciferase assay revealed that the promoter activity of TCF7 declined by approximately 50% in FZD7 inhibited MDA-MB-231 and BT-20 cells (Figure 5B).

We then assessed whether expression of target genes of the Wnt pathway (e.g., Cyclin D1 and C-myc) changed when FZD7 was inhibited. Western blot analysis revealed decreased expression of Cyclin D1 and C-myc, downstream components of the Wnt pathway, in MDA-MB-231 and BT-20 cells in which FZD7 was knocked down as compared to GFPshRNA-expressing control cells (Figure5C). To evaluate whether overexpression of FZD7 was sufficient to trigger Wnt/β-catenin signaling, FZD7 tagged with GFP was transiently expressed in MCF7 cells, which expresses low levels of FZD7. MDA-MB-231 cells served as control. Approximately 70% to 80% of transfected cells were GFP-positive, indicating that FZD7 should have been overexpressed. However, overexpression of FZD7 did not activate the Wnt canonical pathway (Figure 5D), and did not appear to generate a significant cell proliferation benefit (Figure 5E).

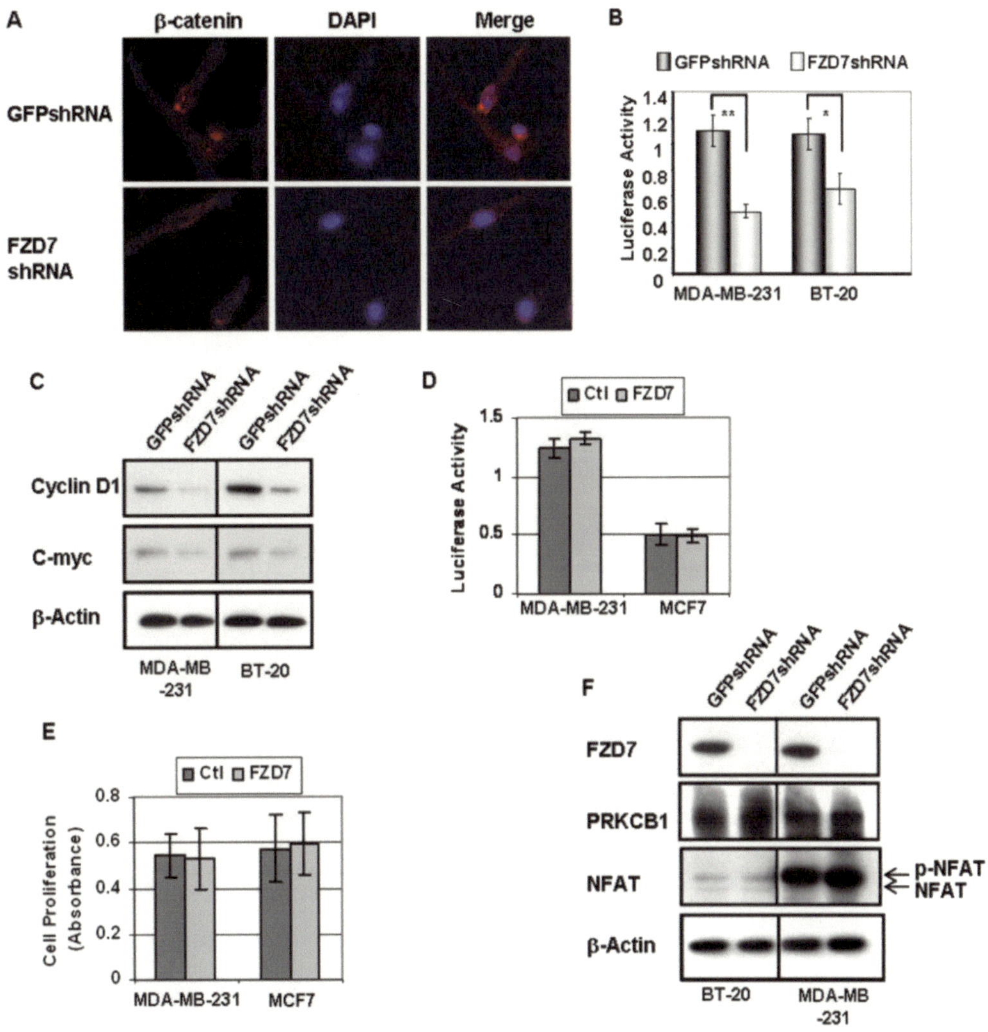

Fig. 6. FZD7 regulated cell transformation through Wnt canonical pathway in TNBC.

In our microarray data, we noticed that two genes, FZD and PKCB1, along the noncanonical Wnt/Ca^{2+} pathway were upregulated in TNBC. In the Wnt/Ca^{2+} pathway, Wnt binds to FZD to initiate signaling that results in the stimulation of protein kinase C (PKC) and the release of intracellular Ca^{2+}. Increased concentrations of Ca^{2+} induce dephosphorylation of NFAT (nuclear factor of activated T-cells), which promotes its translocation to the nucleus where it can activate the transcription of target genes of the Wnt/Ca^{2+} pathway. However, when FZD7 was inhibited in MDA-MB-231 and BT-20 cells, expression of PKCB1 and the phosphorylation status of NFAT did not change (Figure 7), suggesting that FZD7 does not have a role in Wnt/Ca^{2+} signaling in TNBC. Taken together, these data provide strong evidence that Wnt/β-catenin, but not Wnt/Ca^{2+} signaling is active in TNBC, and that blocking the Wnt canonical pathway leads to tumor cells losing their tumorigenicity.

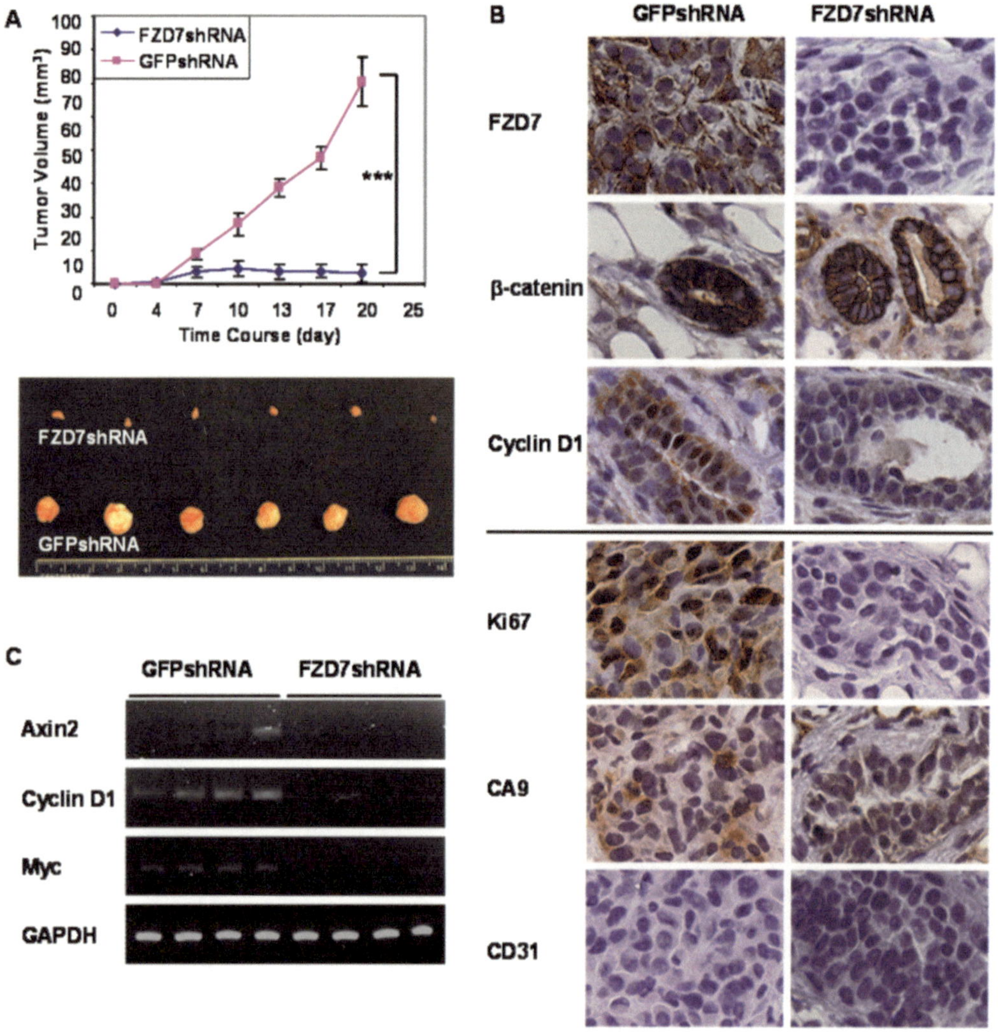

Fig. 7. FZD7 knockdown suppressed tumor growth *in vivo*.

2.4 FZD7shRNA suppresses tumor growth in vivo

To explore whether the Wnt pathway contributes to the tumorigenesis of TNBC in vivo, MDA-MB-231 cells with FZD7shRNA or GFPshRNA were inoculated into NOD-SCID IL2rg female null mice. FZD7shRNA blocked the Wnt signal in MDA-MB-231 cells and induced significant ($p<0.001$) suppression of tumor growth in vivo. Moreover, growth arrest has been observed in MDA-MB-231/FZD7shRNA cell-derived tumors after 1 week of inoculation (Fig. 6A). Gross tissue was harvested and processed with immunohistochemistry (IHC) staining of Wnt pathway gene FZD7, β-catenin, and Wnt pathway target gene Cyclin D1 (Fig. 6B). In Fig. 5B left panel, the GFPshRNA control group tumor showed normal FZD7 expression, β-catenin locatization in the nucleus, and Cyclin D1 expression. In tumors with FZD7shRNA shown in the right panel, most cells expressed β-catenin in the cytoplasm and did not express Cyclin D1. This result is consistent with the in vitro findings and confirms that FZD7shRNA induces growth retardation via the Wnt canonical signal. Furthermore, the tumors with FZD7 or FZD7 suppression were characterized. Hypoxia cell marker CA9, angiogenesis marker CD31 and cell proliferation marker Ki67 in the cells were stained (Fig. 6B). The data revealed that Ki67 expression was significantly increased in FZD7 expressed tumor but not in FZD7 inhibited tumor. CA9 was weakly expressed in both FZD7 expressed tumor and FZD7 suppressed tumor. CD31 was not detected in either tumor. These findings indicate that the activation of Wnt signal in TNBC induces cell proliferation, but may not directly involve cell hypoxia and angiogenesis.

3. Conclusion

TNBC has been a particular focus of attention because it has no confirmed therapeutic molecular target and poor prognosis. Basal-like breast cancer is categorized as TNBC because almost all basal-like breast cancers have no hormone receptor expression and HER2 overexpression (Perou *et al.*, 2000; Sotiriou *et al.*, 2003). Although aberrant Wnt signaling activation has been observed in breast cancer (Brown, 2001; Turashvili *et al.*, 2006), the correlation of Wnt signaling with TNBC has rarely been investigated. However, canonical Wnt pathway activation in basal-like tumor has been observed (DiMeo *et al.*, 2009; Lindvall *et al.*, 2009). More recently, LRP6 overexpression was found in a subtype of breast tumor that is ER-negative and Her2-negative (Liu *et al.*, 2010). This is consistent with our microarray results. In our study, downregulation of FZD7 to inactivate the Wnt signaling in triple negative breast cell line, MDA-MB-231 and BT-20 resulted in impaired cell growth and tumor transformation. The essential role that canonical Wnt signaling plays in TNBC makes it the most attractive therapeutic stratagem in TNBC (Yang *et al.*, 2011). Targeting Wnt pathway genes as novel pharmacological agent for other neoplasms has been investigated and great effect has been observed (Yang *et al.*, 2008). Wnt pathway receptor FZD7 and LRP6 are cell surface antigens. Our data together with other recent findings suggest that with the inhibition of either of these two genes, Wnt signaling pathway will be blocked and Wnt signal-mediated cell proliferation will be suppressed (Bafico *et al.*, 2001). SiRNA or antibodies against these mRNAs or proteins will provide strong blocking of canonical Wnt signaling in TNBC cells. Small molecules that inhibit the biological functions of these two genes may also be powerful drugs for treatment of TNBC. Notably, any agents that increase the phosphorylation activity of CK1 and GSK3 or block β-catenin nuclear accumulation will be possible therapeutic approaches for TNBC.

Constitutive expression of Wnt signaling enhances the self-renewal of mammary progenitor cells, and continuous stimulation of this pathway leads to the formation of breast tumor (Jones and Kemp, 2008; Lindvall *et al.*, 2007). Mouse model study indicated that breast cancers that arise from stem-progenitor cells undergo transformation through deregulation of the Wnt signal, while epithelial cell derived breast tumors are triggered by oncogenic activation of HER2 (Li and Rosen, 2005). We also noticed that breast cell lines expressing high levels of HER2 usually express low levels of FZD7 (data not shown). The association of Wnt signaling and HER2 in breast tumor development will be further explored.

Wnt signaling pathway is a highly conserved pathway. Three signaling branches have been identified: canonical Wnt pathway (Wnt/β-catenin pathway), non-canonical pathway (including planar cell polarity pathway), and Wnt/Ca^{2+} pathway (Komiya and Habas, 2008). We have observed that two genes, FDZ and PKC, along the Wnt/Ca^{2+} pathway were upregulated in TNBC. Addressing the significance of this branch in TNBC in the future remains important.

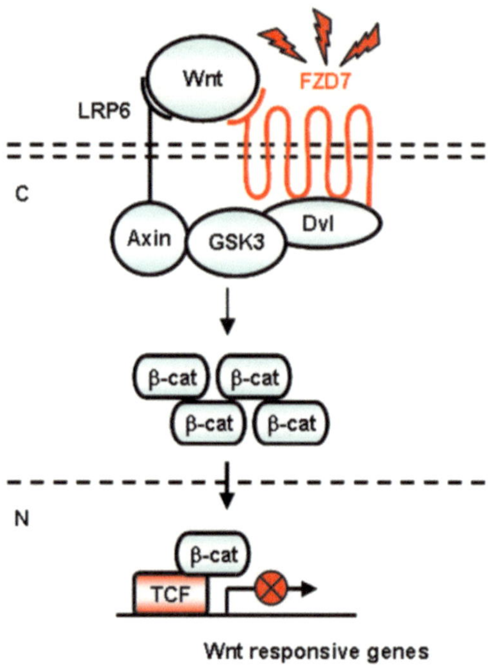

Fig. 8. FZD7 as a target for TNBC.

4. Acknowledgement

We thank Mariko Lee in the Light Microscopy and Digital Imaging Core for assistance with immunofluorescence and IHC microscopy, Arthur Li in the Division of Information Science for statistical analysis, and Yan Wang in the Division of Comparative Medicine for tumor inoculation, tumor measurement and tumor collection. We thank Dr. Keely Walker and Mansze Kong for critical editing of the manuscript.

5. References

Amir E, Ocana A, Freedman O, Clemons M, Seruga B (2010). Chemotherapy: dose-dense treatment for triple-negative breast cancer. *Nat Rev Clin Oncol* 7: 79-80.

Anders CK, Carey LA (2009). Biology, metastatic patterns, and treatment of patients with triple-negative breast cancer. *Clin Breast Cancer* 9 Suppl 2: S73-81.

Bafico A, Liu G, Yaniv A, Gazit A, Aaronson SA (2001). Novel mechanism of Wnt signalling inhibition mediated by Dickkopf-1 interaction with LRP6/Arrow. *Nat Cell Biol* 3: 683-6.

Bhanot P, Brink M, Samos CH, Hsieh JC, Wang Y, Macke JP *et al* (1996). A new member of the frizzled family from Drosophila functions as a Wingless receptor. *Nature* 382: 225-30.

Brown AM (2001). Wnt signaling in breast cancer: have we come full circle? *Breast Cancer Res* 3: 351-5.

Clevers H (2006). Wnt/beta-catenin signaling in development and disease. *Cell* 127: 469-80.

DiMeo TA, Anderson K, Phadke P, Fan C, Perou CM, Naber S *et al* (2009). A novel lung metastasis signature links Wnt signaling with cancer cell self-renewal and epithelial-mesenchymal transition in basal-like breast cancer. *Cancer Res* 69: 5364-73.

Gluz O, Liedtke C, Gottschalk N, Pusztai L, Nitz U, Harbeck N (2009). Triple-negative breast cancer--current status and future directions. *Ann Oncol* 20: 1913-27.

Gonzalez-Angulo AM, Morales-Vasquez F, Hortobagyi GN (2007). Overview of resistance to systemic therapy in patients with breast cancer. *Adv Exp Med Biol* 608: 1-22.

Jones KA, Kemp CR (2008). Wnt-induced proteolytic targeting. *Genes Dev* 22: 3077-81.

Kassam F, Enright K, Dent R, Dranitsaris G, Myers J, Flynn C *et al* (2009). Survival outcomes for patients with metastatic triple-negative breast cancer: implications for clinical practice and trial design. *Clin Breast Cancer* 9: 29-33.

Komiya Y, Habas R (2008). Wnt signal transduction pathways. *Organogenesis* 4: 68-75.

Lee FS, Lane TF, Kuo A, Shackleford GM, Leder P (1995). Insertional mutagenesis identifies a member of the Wnt gene family as a candidate oncogene in the mammary epithelium of int-2/Fgf-3 transgenic mice. *Proc Natl Acad Sci U S A* 92: 2268-72.

Li Y, Rosen JM (2005). Stem/progenitor cells in mouse mammary gland development and breast cancer. *J Mammary Gland Biol Neoplasia* 10: 17-24.

Lindvall C, Bu W, Williams BO, Li Y (2007). Wnt signaling, stem cells, and the cellular origin of breast cancer. *Stem Cell Rev* 3: 157-68.

Lindvall C, Zylstra CR, Evans N, West RA, Dykema K, Furge KA *et al* (2009). The Wnt co-receptor Lrp6 is required for normal mouse mammary gland development. *PLoS One* 4: e5813.

Liu CC, Prior J, Piwnica-Worms D, Bu G (2010). LRP6 overexpression defines a class of breast cancer subtype and is a target for therapy. *Proc Natl Acad Sci U S A* 107: 5136-41.

MacDonald BT, Tamai K, He X (2009). Wnt/beta-catenin signaling: components, mechanisms, and diseases. *Dev Cell* 17: 9-26.

Ojalvo LS, Whittaker CA, Condeelis JS, Pollard JW (2010). Gene expression analysis of macrophages that facilitate tumor invasion supports a role for Wnt-signaling in mediating their activity in primary mammary tumors. *J Immunol* 184: 702-12.

Perez EA, Moreno-Aspitia A, Aubrey Thompson E, Andorfer CA (2010). Adjuvant therapy of triple negative breast cancer. *Breast Cancer Res Treat*.

Perou CM, Sorlie T, Eisen MB, van de Rijn M, Jeffrey SS, Rees CA *et al* (2000). Molecular portraits of human breast tumours. *Nature* 406: 747-52.

Pinson KI, Brennan J, Monkley S, Avery BJ, Skarnes WC (2000). An LDL-receptor-related protein mediates Wnt signalling in mice. *Nature* 407: 535-8.

Rahman M, Pumphrey JG, Lipkowitz S (2009). The TRAIL to targeted therapy of breast cancer. *Adv Cancer Res* 103: 43-73.

Reya T, Clevers H (2005). Wnt signalling in stem cells and cancer. *Nature* 434: 843-50.

Silver DP, Richardson AL, Eklund AC, Wang ZC, Szallasi Z, Li Q *et al* (2010). Efficacy of neoadjuvant Cisplatin in triple-negative breast cancer. *J Clin Oncol* 28: 1145-53.

Sotiriou C, Neo SY, McShane LM, Korn EL, Long PM, Jazaeri A *et al* (2003). Breast cancer classification and prognosis based on gene expression profiles from a population-based study. *Proc Natl Acad Sci U S A* 100: 10393-8.

Tolwinski NS, Wehrli M, Rives A, Erdeniz N, DiNardo S, Wieschaus E (2003). Wg/Wnt signal can be transmitted through arrow/LRP5,6 and Axin independently of Zw3/Gsk3beta activity. *Dev Cell* 4: 407-18.

Turashvili G, Bouchal J, Burkadze G, Kolar Z (2006). Wnt signaling pathway in mammary gland development and carcinogenesis. *Pathobiology* 73: 213-23.

Yang SH, Andl T, Grachtchouk V, Wang A, Liu J, Syu LJ *et al* (2008). Pathological responses to oncogenic Hedgehog signaling in skin are dependent on canonical Wnt/beta3-catenin signaling. *Nat Genet* 40: 1130-5.

Yang L, Wu X, Wang Y, Zhang K, Wu J *et al* (2011). FZD7 Plays a Critical Role in Cell Proliferation in Triple Negative Breast Cancer. *Oncogene*. 2011 May 2. Epub ahead of print.

28

Dysregulation of Wnt Signaling in Breast Cancer

Taj D. King and Yonghe Li
Department of Biochemistry and Molecular Biology
Drug Discovery Division
Southern Research Institute
Birmingham, AL
USA

1. Introduction

The Wnt signaling pathway is a significant pathway that consists of two sub-categories: (1) the canonical Wnt/β-catenin signaling pathway and (2) the non-canonical Wnt signaling pathway. A well-programmed crosstalk exists between canonical and non-canonical Wnt pathways, which enable them to regulate stem cell renewal, cell proliferation, migration, and differentiation. Wnt signals are transduced via the interaction between cell surface receptors and secreted Wnt ligands and Wnt agonists, which subsequently activate downstream proteins that regulate cytoskeletal rearrangement, transcription, and cell cycle. Aberrant Wnt signaling is involved in the development of a variety of cancers, including breast cancer.

Breast cancer is the most invasive form of cancer in women and is the second leading cause of death in women in industrialized nations. Three distinct biomarkers including the estrogen receptor (ER), progesterone receptor (PR), and the human epidermal growth factor receptor 2 (HER-2) are used to determine breast cancer therapy (Nguyen et al., 2010). Anti-ER and HER2 therapies have benefitted a subset of breast cancer patients (Carter et al., 1992; Arteaga, 2003). However, the genetic diversity of this disease varies greatly in that the pathological hallmarks are distinct in each case. Recent discoveries in stem cell research have shown that breast cancer stem cells may be responsible for the aggressiveness of some breast cancers and may contribute to their resistance to chemotherapy and radiation treatment (Diehn et al., 2009; Li et al., 2008b). Wnt signaling is important in stem cell biology and can lead to tumor formation when aberrantly activated. Therefore, it is essential to understand the intrinsic mechanisms of the Wnt signaling pathway to elucidate candidate proteins within this pathway that may serve as potential targets for breast cancer therapy.

2. The Wnt signaling pathways

At the heart of the canonical Wnt pathway is the stabilization of cytosolic β-catenin, which enters the nucleus and activates Wnt target genes by binding to transcription factors of the T-cell factor and the lymphoid enhancing factor (TCF/LEF) family (Kohn and Moon, 2005; McDonald et al., 2009). Wnts are secreted glycoproteins that can bind to low-density lipoprotein receptor-related protein 5 (LRP5) or LRP6 and seven transmembrane receptors of the Frizzled (Fz) family. In the absence of Wnt ligands, β-catenin is phosphorylated by a multi-protein complex that marks it for ubiquitination and degradation by the proteasome (Fig. 1A). This β-catenin degradation complex contains the adenomatous polyposis coli (APC) tumor suppressor, the scaffold protein Axin, the glycogen synthase kinase 3β (GSK3β), and the casein kinase 1 (Ck1). The action of this complex is inhibited upon binding of Wnt to its receptors (Fig. 1B). A variety of Wnt/β-catenin target genes have been identified, which include those that regulate cell proliferation, embryonic developmental and tumor progression (Kohn and Moon, 2005; McDonald et al., 2009).

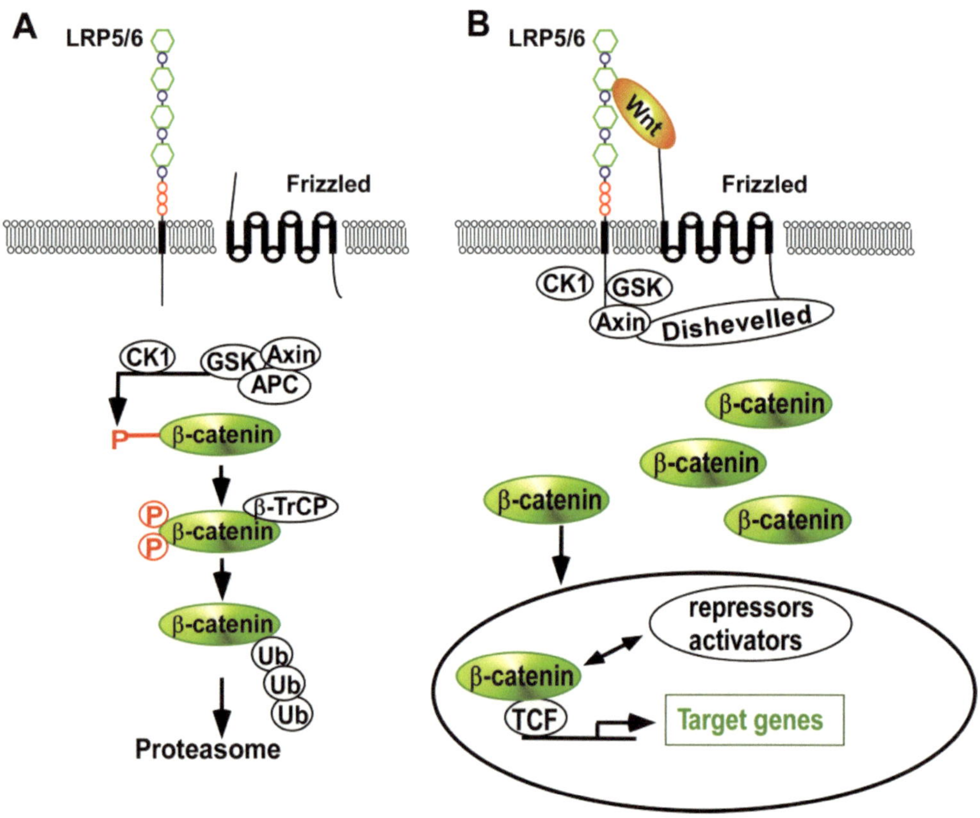

Fig. 1. The canonical Wnt signaling cascade, simplified. (A) In the absence of interaction between Wnts and receptors, β-catenin levels are efficiently regulated by a complex containing APC, axin, and GSK3β. This complex promotes phosphorylation of β-catenin by Ck1 and GSK3β. Phosphorylated β-catenin becomes multi-ubiquitinated (Ub) and subsequently degraded by the 26S proteasome. (B) In the presence of Wnts, phosphorylation and degradation of β-catenin are blocked which allows the association of β-catenin with TCF transcription factors. The TCF:β-catenin complexes bind to DNA and activate Wnt target genes together with various transcriptional repressors or activators.

The non-canonical Wnt signaling pathway, which operates independently of downstream β-catenin activation, consists of the Wnt/Ca^{2+}, Wnt/Planar Cell Polarity (PCP), and Wnt/ROR2 pathway. There are several excellent reviews that discuss the non-canonical Wnt signaling pathway extensively (Kohn and Moon, 2005; Siefert and Mlodzik, 2007; Wang and Nathans,

2007b; Schulte, 2010). The Wnt/Ca^{2+} and the Wnt/PCP pathways are activated via the interaction of Wnt5a and Wnt11 with their Fz co-receptor. This interaction elicits downstream increases in intracellular Ca^{2+} flux (Wnt/Ca^{2+}) and Dishevelled (Dvl)-mediated downstream activation of Rac, Rho, and Jun N-terminal kinase (Wnt/PCP), which ultimately regulate cell motility and orientation. The Wnt/ROR2 pathway requires the interaction of Wnt-5a with ROR2, which activates downstream signaling events that regulate cell motility. Some non-canonical Wnt signaling pathways, including the Wnt/ Ca^{2+} and the Wnt/ROR2 pathways, antagonize canonical Wnt signaling (discussed in more detail below).

2.1 Wnt receptors frizzled protein and LRP5/6

The frizzled (Fz) gene product, originally discovered in *D. melanogaster,* is required for the development of cuticle wing hairs (Vinson and Adler, 1987; Vinson et al., 1989). The Fz receptor consists of 10 mammalian isoforms that contain an N-terminal signal peptide, an extracellular cysteine-rich domain (CRD), a seven-pass transmembrane domain, and an intracellular C-terminal domain, which contains the KTxxxW motif. The CRD of the Fz receptor interacts with the homologous CRD of Wnt proteins (Schulte, 2010). The Fz receptor also interacts with R-spondin (Kazanankaya et al., 2004; Kim et al., 2005; Nam et al., 2006; Wei et al., 2007), Norrin (Smallwood et al., 2007), and secreted frizzled-related proteins (Rattner et al., 1997; Kawano and Kypta, 2003; Bafico et al., 1999). The Fz receptor transduces Wnt signals in a solitary manner or through collaboration with other co-receptors. The Fz receptor forms a ternary complex with Wnt and LRP5/6 to activate the canonical Wnt signaling pathway, which activates β-catenin transcriptional activity (Tamai et al., 2000; Wehrli et al., 2000).

Experiments performed in Drosophila (Wehrli et al., 2000), Xenopus (Tamai et al., 2000) and mice (Pinson et al., 2000) demonstrated that LRP5/6 (termed Arrow in Drosophila) acts as a co-receptor for Wnts, which interact with both Fz and LRP5/6 to activate the canonical Wnt signaling pathway. LRP5/6 appears to transduce the Wnt/β-catenin signal by binding and recruiting Axin to the cell membrane (Mao et al., 2001a; Tolwinski et al., 2003; Liu et al., 2003; Tamai et al., 2004). It has been demonstrated that a PPSPXS motif, which is reiterated five times in the LRP6 intracellular domain and is conserved between LRP5, LRP6, and their Drosophila homolog, Arrow, is sequentially phosphorylated by GSK3β and CK1 upon Wnt stimulation (Tamai et al., 2004, Brennan et al., 2004; Zeng et al., 2005; Davidson et al., 2005). Phosphorylation of the PPSPXS motif provides a docking site for Axin binding (Tamai et al., 2004; Brennan et al., 2004; Zeng et al., 2005; Davidson et al., 2005).

LRP5 and LRP6 are two members of the expanding low density lipoprotein receptor (LDLR) family. The mesoderm development protein (Mesd) and the receptor associated protein (RAP) are two specialized molecular chaperones for members of the LDLR family. Mesd is particularly important for the Wnt co-receptors LRP5 and LRP6, while RAP is critical for other members of the LDLR family such as LRP1 and LRP2 (Culi and Mann, 2003; Hsieh et al., 2003; Culi et al., 2004; Li et al., 2005c; Koduri et al., 2007; Li et al., 2006a). Mesd was discovered due to its requirement for the folding of LRP5 and LRP6 (Culi and Mann, 2003; Hsieh et al., 2003). In mice, the consequences of Mesd deficiency resemble what is seen in Wnt3-deficient mutants (Hsieh et al., 2003). Similar to other ER chaperones, Mesd also carries an endoplasmic reticulum (ER) retention signal (KDEL in Drosophila, REDL in mammals) at its carboxyl terminus and localizes to the ER (Culi and Mann, 2003). All members of the LDLR family have at least one six-bladed β-propeller domain, which is followed by an epidermal growth factor (EGF) repeat (Bu, 2009). Mesd is specifically required for the maturation of these β-propeller/EGF modules through the secretory pathway (Culi et al., 2004). In the absence of Mesd, LRP5 and LRP6 form aggregates in the ER and fail to reach the cell surface (Culi and Mann, 2003; Hsieh et al., 2003; Culi et al., 2004; Li et al., 2005c; Koduri et al., 2007; Li et al., 2006a).

LRP5/6 does not contain CRD domains, but Wnt binds to their β-propeller domains, which are sufficient to transduce Wnt signals (Hey et al., 1998; Liu et al., 2009; Bourhis et al., 2010). Although controversial, the receptor tyrosine kinase-like orphan receptors, ROR1/2 and RYK, can autonomously transduce Wnt signals or serve as co-receptors with Fz to transduce Wnt signals. Similar to the Fz receptor, ROR1/2 possesses a CRD that binds to Wnt proteins, which stimulate receptor dimerization and subsequent activation (Liu et al., 2008; Minami et al., 2010). ROR2 forms a complex with Fz, Wnt, and Cthrci, a Wnt co-factor, to activate the Wnt/Planar Cell Polarity pathway (Yamamoto et al., 2008). Conversely, another study showed that ROR2 cooperates with Fz2 to mediate Wnt-3a-induced β-catenin activation (Li et al., 2008a). Similar to the ROR1/2 kinase, the RYK tyrosine kinase can form a complex with Fz and Wnt-3a to activate downstream β-catenin signaling (Lu et al., 2004) or it can interact with Wnt-5a independent of Fz cooperation to activate non-canonical Wnt signaling (Li et al., 2009). These results suggest that the Fz receptor can act autonomously or in cooperation with other receptors to regulate canonical and non-canonical Wnt signaling pathways.

2.2 Wnt agonists

The mammalian proto-oncogene *int-1* and its *D. melanogaster* counterpart, *wingless*, were discovered prior to the Fz receptors (Nusse and Varmus, 1982; Cabrera et al., 1987; Rijseuijk et al., 1987). The nomenclature was later changed to Wnt, which is an acronym derived from *wingless* and *int-1* (Nusse et al., 1991). Wnts are highly conserved secreted glycoproteins that regulate cell growth and homeostasis in a variety of organ systems. This family of proteins consists of 19 cysteine-rich members that serve as ligands for the Fz receptor (Schulte, 2010). Members of this family can be classified based on their ability to transform epithelial cells. For example, Wnt-1, Wnt-2, Wnt-3, and Wnt-3a are considered to be transforming Wnts; Wnt-6 and Wnt-7a are weakly transforming Wnts; Wnt-4, Wnt-5a, Wnt-5b, and Wnt-7b are non-transforming Wnts (Shimizu et al., 1997). Wnt proteins are palmitoylated (Takada et al., 2006) prior to secretion from the cell via the Wntless/Evi seven-pass transmembrane protein (Banziger et al., 2006; Bartscherer et al., 2006). Following secretion from cells, Wnt proteins interact with the CRD of 10 known mammalian Fz receptors (Schulte, 2010) as well as the extracellular domain of the LRP5/6 receptor (Pinson et al., 2000; Tamai et al., 2000; Wehrli et al., 2000) to activate the canonical Wnt/β-catenin signaling pathway. Wnt proteins also activate non-canonical Wnt signaling via their interaction with Fz (Schulte, 2010), ROR1/2 (Liu et al., 2008; Minami et al., 2010; Li et al., 2008a; Yamamoto et al., 2008), and RYK (Lu et al., 2004; Li et al., 2009). The interaction of Wnt proteins with these receptors enables them to regulate a variety of cellular events including differentiation, proliferation, migration, and tumorigenesis.

R-spondins

R-spondins (Rspo) are a family of secreted proteins that activate Wnt/β-catenin signaling. This family consists of four members (Rspo1-4) that share 40-60% homology and are structural similar (Kazanskaya et al., 2004). Rspo proteins contain a signal peptide at the N-terminus, which is followed by a highly conserved CRD and a thrombospondin motif. The

C-terminus is of varying length between the different isoforms of Rspo proteins, but it is positively charged (Kim et al., 2006). Rspo proteins are expressed simultaneously with Wnt proteins during mouse development, suggesting that they may play an important role in facilitating Wnt/β-catenin signaling (Nam et al., 2006). The action of Rspo proteins on Wnt/β-catenin signaling requires Wnt receptors Fz and LRP5/6; however, the direct binding between Rspo and LRP5/6 is still controversial (Kazanankaya et al., 2004; Kim et al., 2005; Nam et al., 2006; Wei et al., 2007; Li et al. 2010). Furthermore, unlike the Wnt ligands, Rspo proteins do not form a ternary complex with Fz and LRP6 (Nam et al., 2006), suggesting that the mechanistic action of Rspo on Wnt/β-catenin signaling activation is not identical to that of Wnt. One plausible mechanism is that Rspo blocks Dkk1-mediated antagonization of Wnt/β-catenin signaling by interfering with the interaction of Dkk1 with the Kremen and LRP6 receptors (Kim et al., 2008).

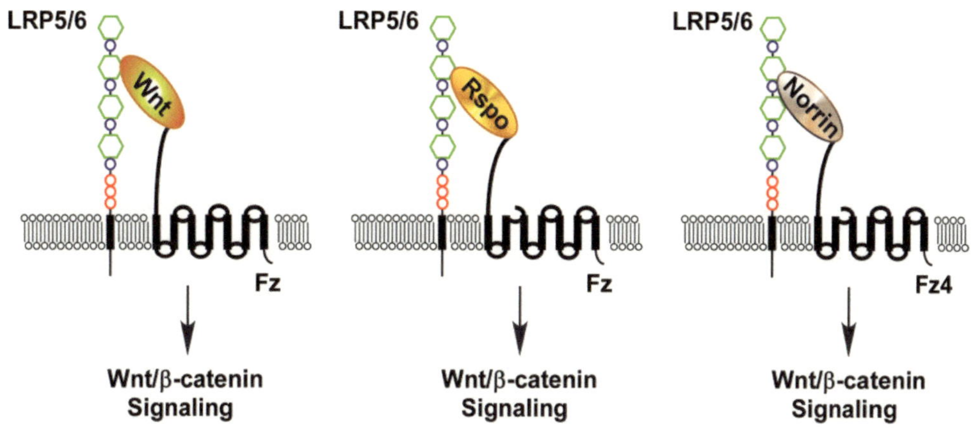

Fig. 2. Secreted Wnt agonists. Wnts are the primary agonists of Wnt/β-catenin signaling by binding to LRP5/6 and Fz to form a complex with LRP5/6 and Fz. Both Rspos and Norrin may act similarly to Wnt, but Norrin specifically binds to Fz4.

Norrin

Norrie disease is a severe X-linked trait that causes impaired retinal development. The clinical features of this malady include blindness, mental retardation, deafness, microcephaly, and hypogonadism (Hendrickx and Leyns, 2008). Mutations in the Norrie disease protein (Norrin) contribute to the pathology of this disease (Berger et al., 1992; Chen et al., 1992). Norrin specifically interacts with the CRD of Fzd4 and the extracellular domain of LRP5/6 receptors, which activates Wnt/β-catenin signaling (Xu et al., 2004; Smallwood et al., 2007). These findings are interesting because Norrin does not share any structural homology with Wnts (Xu et al., 2004). These results are evident of the diverse and complex nature of the regulation of Wnt signaling to promote development and tumor progression.

2.2.1 Wnt antagonists

Dickkopf

Dickkopf (Dkk; German, big head, stubborn) proteins are a family of secreted glycoproteins that function as regulators of Wnt signaling. Dkks consists of four isoforms in vertebrates

(Dkk1-4). Dkk1, 2, and 4 contain a Dkk_N domain (also known as CRD1) near the N-terminus and a colipase fold (also known as CRD2) near the C-terminus. Dkk3 also contains a Dkk_N domain, but the N-terminal soggy domain and the C-terminal colipase fold flank the Dkk_N domain (Niehrs, 2006). The colipase fold is necessary for Dkk1, Dkk2, and Dkk4 to inhibit Wnt signaling (Brott and Sokol, 2002; Li et al., 2002; Mao and Niehrs, 2003). The structural divergence of Dkk3 from the other three Dkk family members is a contributing factor to its functional divergence (Glinka et al., 1998; Krupnik et al., 1999; Mao et al., 2001b). Dkk1 functions solely as an inhibitor of canonical Wnt signaling (Glinka et al., 1998). Dkk1 antagonizes Wnt/β-catenin signaling by binding directly to the YWTD type β-propeller domain of LRP6 and prevents Fz-LRP6 complex formation in response to Wnt. Furthermore, Dkk1 interacts with another transmembrane protein, Kremen. The LRP6-Dkk1-Kremen complex is internalized, thus removing LRP6 from the cell surface (Bafico et al., 2001; Mao et al., 2001b; Semenov et al., 2001; Davidson et al., 2002; Mao et al., 2002; Mao and Niehrs, 2003). Dkk2 can activate Wnt/β-catenin signaling by interacting with Fz (Wu et al., 2000) or LRP6 (Brott and Sokol, 2002). Conversely, depending on the cell type, Dkk2 can inhibit Wnt-Fz-mediated β-catenin activation in the absence of LRP5/6 (Wu et al., 2000; Li et al., 2002; Mao and Niehrs, 2003; Caricasole et al., 2003). Furthermore, Dkk2 can inhibit LRP6 mediated Wnt/β-catenin signaling in the presence of the Kremen2 receptor by inducing the internalization of LRP6 (Mao and Niehrs, 2003). The dichotomy between Dkk1 and Dkk2 regulation of canonical Wnt signaling is due to the structure and function of the two CRDs of Dkk1 and Dkk2. The colipase fold of Dkk1 and Dkk2 can activate LRP6-mediated β-catenin activation, and the Dkk_N domain inhibits the action of the colipase fold of Dkk1, but is neutral on Dkk2 (Li et al., 2002; Brott and Sokol, 2002). Therefore, the structural divergence of the Dkk family of proteins enables them to regulate Wnt/β-catenin signaling differentially.

Schlerostin

Schlerosteosis is an autosomal recessive disorder that causes severe skeletal outgrowth in the skull and mandible. Mutations in the schlersotin (SOST) gene, which is located on chromosome 17q11.2, contribute to the pathology of this disease (Balemans et al., 2001; Brunkow et al., 2001). The SOST gene encodes a 24 kDa secreted glycoprotein that contains a cysteine knot-like domain (Balemans et al., 2001; Brunkow et al., 2001). SOST binds to LRP5/6 and inhibits the interaction of Wnts with LRP5/6, thus inhibiting Wnt/β-catenin signaling (Li et al., 2005b; Ott et al., 2005; Semenov et al., 2005; Semenov and He, 2006). Furthermore, SOST fails to interact with LRP5 carrying the G170V mutation, which is observed in patients with high bone density (Ellies et al., 2006; Semenov and He, 2006).

Secreted frizzled-related proteins

The secreted frizzled related proteins (sFRPs) are soluble secreted proteins (sFRP1-5) that interact with Wnt and Fz proteins, which prevent the binding of Wnts to the Fz receptors. The sFRPs are structurally related to the Wnt-binding domain of the Fz receptor in that their N-terminal domain, which contains the CRD, shares 30-50% sequence homology with that of the Fz receptors (Rattner et al., 1997; Kawano and Kypta, 2003). sFRPs antagonize Wnt signaling by interacting with Wnt ligands via the CRD (Lin `et al., 1997). Furthermore, Uren et al. (2000) showed that mutations in the CRD of sFRP1 abrogate its interaction with *Drosophila* Wg. The same group also showed that the C-terminal domain of sFRP1 interacts with Wnt proteins and that low and high levels of sFRP1 potentiates and inhibits Wg signaling, respectively (Uren et al., 2000). sFRP1 can dimerize or interact with the Fz receptor to form a non-functional complex (Bafico et al., 1999), suggesting that the mechanistic actions of sFRP-induced inhibition of Wnt signaling are broad.

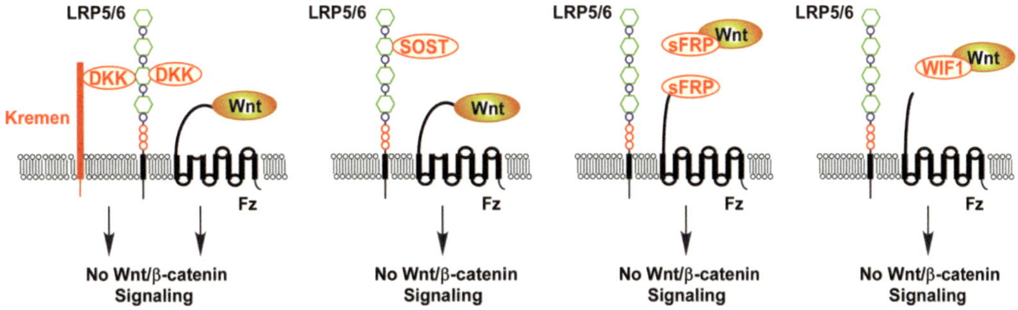

Fig. 3. Secreted Wnt antagonists. By binding to LRP5 or LRP6, Dkk and Sclerostin disrupt Wnt-induced Fz-Wnt-LRP complex and inhibit Wnt/β-catenin signaling. Furthermore, Dkk interacts with another transmembrane protein, Kremen. The LRP-Dkk-Kremen complex is internalized, thus removing LRP5/6 from the cell surface. WIF1 and sFRPs function as inhibitors of Wnt/β-catenin signaling by directly binding to Wnt or both Wnt and Fz.

Wnt inhibitory factor-1

Wnt inhibitory factor-1 (WIF1), another secreted protein that binds to Wnt ligands, is highly conserved in vertebrates, and it was originally discovered as an expressed tag from the human retina (Hsieh et al., 1999). WIF1 consists of an N-terminal signal sequence, a unique WIF domain, and five EGF-like repeats (Hsieh et al., 1999). WIF1 is structurally related to the extracellular domain of RYK (Patthy, 2000; Liepinsh et al., 2006). WIF1 can directly bind Wnt proteins to inhibit Wnt/β-catenin signaling (Hsieh et al., 1999). Furthermore, WIF1 can inhibit Wnt-3a-mediated β-catenin/TCF/LEF transcriptional activity (Surmann-Schmitt et al., 2009) and regulate its own expression through a negative feedback mechanism (Licchesi et al., 2010).

3. Dysregulation of Wnt signaling in breast cancer

Although genetic mutations of APC or β-catenin are rarely observed in certain cancers (e.g. breast cancer), there is compelling evidence that implicates aberrant Wnt/β-catenin signaling in breast cancer development. For example, only 6% of breast tumors contain mutations in the APC gene (Jonsson et al., 2000), which is mutated or deleted in 80% of colon tumors (Kinzler and Vogelstein, 1996). No mutations occur in the amino terminal of β-catenin, which contains the CK1 and GSK3β phosphorylation sites (Jonsson et al., 2000). However, elevated β-catenin expression in breast cancer tissue correlates with a decreased survival rate of breast cancer patients (Jonsson et al., 2000; Dolled-Filhart et al., 2006; Lopez-Knowles et al., 2010; Zardawi et al., 2009; Khramtsov et al., 2010). Cyclin D1 levels are also elevated in 50% of patients with breast cancer (Gillet et al., 1994; Bartkova et al., 1994). Indeed, the cyclin D1 promoter region contains a TCF4-binding site, which is regulated by β-catenin (Tetsu and McCormick, 1999; Shtutman et al., 1999). Elevated β-catenin expression (not due to CTNNB1 activating mutations) and activation is also associated with triple-negative breast cancer and poor clinical prognosis (Geyer et al., 2011). Since elevated expression of β-catenin and subsequent aberrant activation of Wnt/β-catenin signaling in breast cancer development is not due to genetic mutations in APC and β-catenin, dysregulation of this pathway likely occurs at the cell surface or at the level of epigenetic regulation.

3.1 Wnt agonists in mammary gland development and breast cancer

There is compelling evidence that Wnt ligands are involved in the activation of the canonical Wnt signaling pathway during breast cancer development. Wnt1 and Wnt2, the founding members of the Wnt gene family (Nusse and Varmus, 1982; Peters et al., 1983), are tumorigenic. Furthermore, fusion of the Wnt1 allele with the MMTV long terminal repeat and subsequent generation of MMTV-Wnt1 transgenic mice causes mammary gland hyperplasia and increases adenocarcinomas in mice (Tsukamoto et al., 1988). The transforming capability of Wnt genes in mammary epithelial cells is also increased following the insertion of the MMTV (Blasband et al., 1992; Wong et al., 1994). Additionally, the upregulation and transforming capability of several Wnt genes occur in human primary tumors (Dale et al., 1996; Lejeune et al., 1995; Bui et al., 1997). Recently, Oloumi et al. (2010) reported that the rate of mammary tumor growth is significantly increased in Wnt1 and integrin-linked kinase double transgenic mice. Moreover, crosstalk between the Wnt1 and integrin-liked kinase pathways upregulate FOXA1 and estrogen receptor transcription factors, which accelerate breast cancer development (Oloumi et al., 2010). These results implicate Wnt1 in breast cancer development and suggest that Wnt1 may serve as a potential therapeutic target to combat certain forms of breast cancer. Indeed, RNA inhibition of Wnt1 mRNA expression or inhibition of Wnt1 with an anti-Wnt1 antibody induces apoptosis in a variety of cancer cell lines (e.g. breast cancer) that overexpress Wnt1 (He et al., 2004). Other Wnt proteins, including Wnt10b and Wnt11, are also implicated in breast cancer tumorigenesis. A previous study showed that Wnt10b overexpression induced by the MMTV promoter facilitates mammary gland development and tumor formation in male and female mice (Lane and Leder, 1997). A recent study also showed that the estrogen-related receptor-α and β-catenin synergistically induce the expression of Wnt11, which facilitates breast cancer migration (Dwyer et al., 2010). This study is compelling because it suggests that combinational therapy could utilize synthetic drugs to target the estrogen-related receptor-α/β-catenin complex and antibodies to target Wnt11 in order to treat estrogen-dependent breast cancer.

Increasing evidence suggests that non-canonical Wnt signaling also plays a role in mammary gland and breast cancer development. Roarty and Serra (2007) showed that Wnt-5a is necessary for normal ductal extension and branching. According to previous studies, Wnt-5a activates the Wnt/Ca^{2+} signaling pathway, which antagonizes canonical Wnt signaling by inhibiting the downstream transcriptional activity of β-catenin (Ishitani et al., 2003; Topol et al., 2003; Nemeth et al., 2007). However, a previous study also showed that Wnt-5a can inhibit or activate β-catenin transcriptional activity (Mikels and Nusse, 2006). This dichotomy is likely due to the availability of cell surface receptors in different cell types. Although controversial, most studies suggest that Wnt-5a likely acts as a tumor suppressor. In one study, Wnt-5a mRNA levels are upregulated 10- and 4-fold in benign and invasive tumors, respectively, compared to that in normal breast tissue (Lejeune et al., 1995).

It is possible that Wnt-5a may facilitate breast cancer tumorigenesis in a subset of breast cancers given that Wnt-5a can also activate canonical Wnt signaling and that its mRNA levels are increased in some breast tumors. However, several studies have shown that Wnt-5a levels are low in breast cancer tumors and that low Wnt-5a expression may serve as a prognostic indicator of shorter survival rates in some breast cancer patients (Jonsson et al., 2002; Dejmek et al., 2005; Leris et al., 2005). Furthermore, loss of Wnt-5a in normal mouse mammary glands increases canonical Wnt signaling and stimulates mammary tumorigenesis (Roarty et al., 2009). These results suggest that Wnt-5a is generally anti-tumorigenic and can be supported by previous studies, which showed that Wnt-5a enhances β-catenin/E-cadherin complex formation via a Ca^{2+}-dependent mechanism in human breast epithelial cells (Medrek et al., 2009) and that low Wnt-5a expression enhances migration of ductal breast epithelial cells (Jonsson and Andersson, 2001).

Although there is no direct evidence that implicates Norrin in breast cancer tumorigenesis, there is some evidence that suggests that some members of the R-spondin family of proteins may be involved in the pathogenesis of breast cancer and other forms of cancer. For example, MMTV increases R-spo2 expression in mouse mammary tumors following its insertion into the Int7 locus (Lowther et al., 2005), therefore, implicating hRspo2 in mammary tumorigenesis.

3.2 Wnt receptors in mammary gland development and breast cancer

The Wnt co-receptor, LRP5, plays an important role in mammary gland development and in breast cancer. Loss of LRP5 delays mammary gland development and mouse mammary tumor virus (MMTV)-Wnt1-induced tumor formation in mice (Lindvall et al., 2006). Furthermore, a truncated form of LRP5 (LRP5Δ), which is expressed in breast tumors and breast cancer cell lines, could be implicated in mammary gland tumorigenesis (Bjorklund et al., 2009). LRP6 also plays a pivotal role in mammary gland development and breast cancer. Mammary gland development and MMTV-Wnt1-induced mammary tumorigenesis are delayed in $LRP6^{+/-}$ mice (Lindvall et al., 2009). LRP6 expression is also upregulated in basal-like human breast cancer samples (Lindvall et al., 2009). MMTV constructs are also utilized to assess the role of Wnt receptors in mammary development and breast cancer. In fact, MMTV-LRP6 transgenic mice develop hyperplasia in their mammary glands due to LRP6-mediated Wnt/β-catenin signaling (Zhang et al., 2010). LRP6 expression is also upregulated in a variety of human breast cancer cell lines, including the basal-like cell line, MDA-MB-231 (Liu et al., 2010). Transcriptional knockdown of LRP6 mRNA in MDA-MB-231 cells significantly decreases Wnt signaling, cell proliferation, and tumor growth in SCID mouse models. Furthermore, *in vivo* administration of an LRP6 antagonist, Mesd, markedly suppressed growth of MMTV-Wnt1 tumors without causing undesirable side effects (Liu et al., 2010). These results suggest that LRP5 and LRP6 are involved in breast cancer development and that these receptors can serve as therapeutic targets for the treatment of breast cancer.

The other Wnt co-receptor, Fz, is also involved in the development of breast cancer. Previously, Saitoh et al. (2002) showed that Fz10 and Wnt2 mRNAs are synchronously upregulated by β-estradiol treatment in human breast cancer MCF-7 cells, suggesting that increased Fz10 and Wnt2 expression might stimulate breast cancer production. A subsequent study discovered that Fz1 and Fz2 levels are upregulated in advanced infiltrating ductal breast carcinoma (Milovanovic et al., 2004). Furthermore, Benhaj et al.

(2006) showed that most of the Fz receptors, except Fz9 and Fz10, are expressed in human mammary epithelial cells and most breast cancer cell lines. A recent study discovered that thiazolidinediones, which possess antitumor effects in breast cancer cells, abrogate Wnt/β-catenin signaling by negatively regulating the expression of the Wnt co-receptors, Fz1 and LRP6, in human breast cancer MDA-MB-231 and T47D cells (Wang et al., 2009). Another study showed that the anti-helminthic drug, niclosamide, targets the Fz1 receptor by inducing its internalization through endocytosis, which subsequently inhibits Wnt/β-catenin signaling (Chen et al., 2009). Overall, these results suggest that the Fz receptor may also serve as a potential target for breast cancer therapy.

3.3 Inactivation of Wnt antagonists in breast cancer

Mounting evidence suggests that the frequent occurrence of epigenetic silencing of tumor suppressor genes augments the development and progression of cancer (Ting et al., 2006). Epigenetic silencing of genes occurs via hypermethylation of CpG dinucleotides in promoter regions of genes or histone modifications (Veeck and Esteller, 2010). For example, sFRP1 mRNA is absent in invasive breast carcinomas (Suzuki et al., 2008; Ugolini et al., 1999, 2001). This is likely due to the hypermethylation of the promoter region of sFRP1 in breast carcinomas (Lo et al., 2006; Veeck et al., 2006). The promoter regions of sFRP2 and sFRP5 are also hypermethylated at a higher frequency than sFRP1 or Dkk1 in several breast cancer cell lines (Suzuki et al., 2008). Furthermore, transcriptional knockdown of sFRP1 robustly increases Wnt signaling in breast cancer cells (Suzuki et al., 2008). A recent study showed that stable overexpression of sFRP1 in human breast cancer MDA-MB-231 cells blocks canonical Wnt signaling with ensuing decreases in cell proliferation and suppression of tumor growth and metastasis in xenograft mouse models (Matsuda et al., 2009). These results suggest that sFRP1 and sFRP5 expression is essential to suppress tumor growth and metastasis. Indeed, sFRP1 hypermethylation in breast cancer tissue is associated with decreased patient survival (Veeck et al., 2006; Veeck et al., 2008). Promoter hypermethylation of sFRP2 also occurs frequently in breast cancer, but it is not associated with patient clinical outcomes (Veeck et al., 2008). Interestingly, sFRP2 is highly expressed in canine mammary tumors and tumor cell lines (Lee et al., 2003, 2004) and its levels correlate with those of β-catenin; however, there is no correlation between the levels of sFRP2 or β-catenin with that of cyclin D1. These results suggest, in part, that sFRP2 may serve as a diagnostic marker for breast cancer in humans and dogs, although the mechanistic action of increased sFRP2 expression in canine mammary tumors remains to be elucidated. Another Wnt antagonist, WIF1, is also reduced in 60% of breast carcinomas (Wissmann et al., 2003). A subsequent study supports the previous finding showing that WIF1 downregulation via hypermethylation of its promoter occurs frequently in breast cancer (Ai et al., 2006). Overall, these studies suggest that epigenetic silencing of Wnt antagonists may be a cause for aberrant Wnt/β-catenin signaling, which ultimately results in the development and progression of breast cancer.

3.4 Dkk1 in breast cancer osteolytic bone metastasis

Bone is an active tissue maintained by a balance of cellular activities. The osteoblasts are responsible for bone formation. Osteoblasts synthesize and secrete most proteins of the bone extracellular matrix (ECM) and express proteins that are necessary and sufficient to induce mineralization of the ECM. The osteoclasts are multinucleated cells responsible for bone resorption. Importantly, the differentiation of osteoclasts is regulated by osteoblasts (Karsenty et al., 2002). Receptor activator of NF-kappaB ligand (RANKL) and macrophage-colony-stimulating factor (M-CSF), both of which are expressed by osteoblastic cells, promote osteoclast differentiation through interaction with their cognate signaling receptors (RANK and c-fms, respectively) (Lacey et al., 1998; Yasuda et al., 1998). This process is regulated by a variety of factors that are produced by osteoblasts, stromal cells, fibroblasts, and lymphocytes. Critically, the secreted decoy receptor of RANKL, osteoprotegerin (OPG), binds to and inhibits the activity of RANKL. OPG inhibits osteoclast formation both *in vitro* and *in vivo* (Simonet et al., 1997). The requirement for RANKL, RANK and OPG in the control of osteoclast formation is well established (Suda et al., 1999).

In recent years, Wnt/β-catenin signaling has been shown to play a substantial role in the control of bone development and remodeling (for review, see Krishnan et al., 2006). Analyses of patients with the *LRP5/6* gene mutations and *LRP5/6* knockout mice revealed that the Wnt coreceptors LRP5 and LRP6 play a pivotal role in bone metabolism (Boyden et al., 2002; Gong et al., 2001; Little et al., 2002; Van Wesenbeeck et al., 2003; Ai et al., 2005; Kato et al., 2002; Fujino et al., 2003; Kelly et al., 2004; van Meurs et al., 2006; Holmen et al., 2004; Kokubu et al., 2004). Loss-of-function mutations of human *LRP5* are associated with the recessive disorder osteoporosis-pseudoglioma syndrome, whereas gain-of-function mutations of human *LRP5* (e.g., G171V) reduce binding affinity of LRP5 for DKK1 and cause high bone mass (HBM) diseases (Boyden et al., 2002; Gong et al., 2001; Little et al., 2002; Van Wesenbeeck et al., 2003; Ai et al., 2005). Direct roles of Wnt/β-catenin signaling in the regulation of bone formation and bone mass are further supported by animal model studies by altered expression of Wnt/β-catenin signaling inhibitors (Bodine et al., 2004; Li et al., 2006b; Morvan et al., 2006; Wang et al., 2007a; Yu et al., 2005). Wnt proteins have also been shown to be important for osteoblastogenesis and bone formation (Zhang et al., 2004; Li et al., 2005a; Bennett et al., 2005). Furthermore, modulation of Wnt/β-catenin signaling in mesenchymal progenitors and osteoblasts reveals that this pathway controls osteoblast differentiation and is critical for bone homeostasis during postnatal life (Day et al., 2005; Glass et al., 2005; Hill et al., 2005; Holmen et al., 2005; Hu et al., 2005). Using a multipotent mesenchymal cell line, OPG expression was found to be upregulated by Wnt/β-catenin signaling in an in vitro screen for Wnt-regulated genes (Jackson et al., 2005). Moreover, cellular and molecular studies demonstrated that OPG is a direct target gene of the β-catenin-TCF complex in osteoblasts (Glass et al., 2005).

Bone metastasis is a frequent complication of cancer. Several tumors show a particular predilection for metastasis to bone, including breast, prostate, and lung cancer and multiple myeloma (Yoneda et al., 1998; Mundy, 2002; Roodman, 2004; Kozlow and Guise, 2005). In the case of breast cancer, up to 70% of patients with advanced disease develop osteolytic bone metastases, which are a common cause of morbidity and sometimes mortality (Yoneda, 1998). Tumor cells, osteoblasts, osteoclasts, and bone matrix are the four components of a vicious cycle necessary for the initiation and development of bone metastases. Cancer cells are known to produce a variety of stimulators of bone resorption, such as parathyroid hormone related protein (PTHrP) and transforming growth factor (TGF-β). The secretion of some but not all of these factors by cancer cells regulates RANKL and OPG expression in osteoblasts. RANKL stimulates osteoclastic bone resorption by binding to its receptor RANK on osteoclast precursors, while OPG is the secreted decoy receptor of RANKL, and binds to and inhibits the activity of RANKL (Yoneda et al., 1998; Mundy, 2002; Roodman, 2004; Kozlow and Guise, 2005).

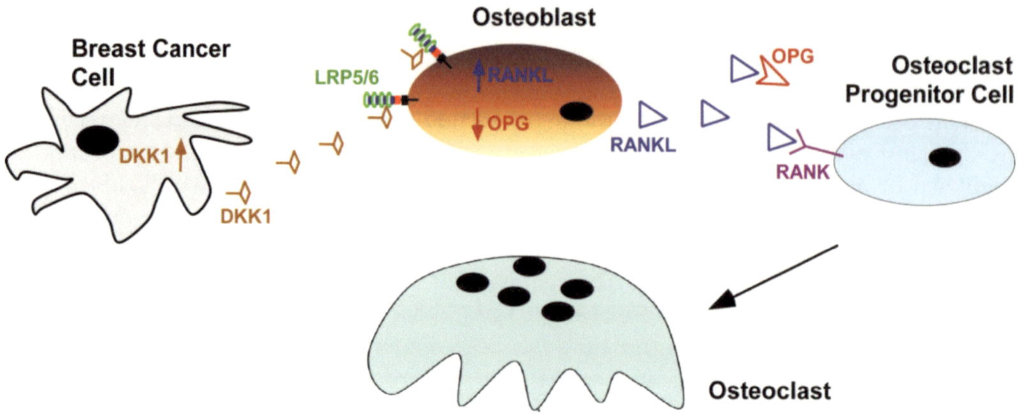

Fig. 4. Model depicting the roles of breast cancer cell-produced DKK1 on osteoclast formation. DKK1 is a Wnt/β-catenin signaling target gene in breast cancer cells. Breast cancer cells with overactivated Wnt/β-catenin signaling produce DKK1. DKK1 secreted by tumor cells blocks Wnt/β-catenin signaling in osteoblasts in a paracrine fashion, resulting in increases RANKL and decreases OPG activity. By decreasing the ratio of OPG to RANKL, DKK1 promotes osteoclastogenesis.

As described above, DKK1 is a specific antagonist of the Wnt/β-catenin signaling pathway. Interestingly, studies also suggested that DKK1 is a direct downstream target of Wnt/β-catenin signaling (Niida et al., 2004; Gonzalez-Sancho et al., 2005; Chamorro et al., 2005). Activation of Wnt/β-catenin signaling by Wnt1 or ectopic expression of active β-catenin, TCF4 or LRP6 mutants induces transcription of the human *Dkk1* gene in several cell line models *in vitro*. Multiple β-catenin/TCF4 binding sites in the *Dkk1* gene promoter region contribute to this activation (Niida et al., 2004; Gonzalez-Sancho et al., 2005; Chamorro et al., 2005). Furthermore, as mentioned above, aberrant Wnt/β-catenin signaling is involved in breast cancer development and progression. Indeed, Dkk1 is highly expressed in several breast cancer cell lines, including the MDA-MB-231 (osteolytic) and MCF-7 (osteolytic and osteoblastic) cell lines (Forget et al., 2007; Pinzone et al., 2009; Bu et al., 2008). Additionally, serum Dkk1 levels were elevated in patients with metastasized breast cancer in the bone compared to patients who were in complete remission (Voorzanger-Rousselot et al., 2007). Dkk1-mediated bone metastasis in breast cancer patients is likely to occur as a result of Dkk1 acting as a molecular switch, which decreases osteoblastogenesis and increases osteolysis (Fig. 4). The mechanistic actions of Dkk1-mediated bone metastasis in breast cancer patients is likely due to the ability of Dkk1 to abrogate Wnt/β-catenin signaling in osteoblasts, which causes a significant decrease in OPG and increase in RANKL levels, thus shifting the balance in the OPG:RANKL ratio (Bu et al., 2008). Increases in RANKL promote osteoclastogenesis and thus, metastasis of breast cancer mesenchymal stem cells into the bone (Pinzone et al., 2009).

3.5 Wnt/β-catenin signaling in breast cancer EMT

Cellular diversity is essential for the development and sustenance of eukaryotic organisms. Epithelial and mesenchymal cells represent two phenotypic distinctions of early organisms. Epithelial cells possess tight junctions, gap junctions, E-cadherins, and epithelial integrins, which foster intercellular communication and fusion with other cells and the extracellular matrix. They also maintain the integrity and regulate the internal environment of an organism (Micalizzi et al., 2010). Mesenchymal cells, which produce the extracellular matrix that supports epithelial cells, are motile compared to their epithelial counterpart (Hay, 2005). Mammalian development is a dynamic process that involves the interconversion between epithelial and mesenchymal cells known as Epithelial-Mesenchymal Transition (EMT) and Mesenchymal-Epithelial Transition (MET) (Micalizzi et al., 2010). The EMT plays a pivotal role in wound healing, fibrosis, and cancer metastasis (Lopez-Novoa and Nieto, 2009). The EMT consists of three types, which include development (type I), fibrosis and wound healing (type II), and cancer (type III) (Kalluri and Weinberg, 2009). Oncogenic EMT is characterized by the loss of the classical epithelial apico-basal polarity, destruction of tight junctions and adherens junctions, and the downregulation of cytokeratins followed by the upregulation of vimentin, a Type III intermediate filament that is expressed in mesenchymal cells (Steinert and Roop, 1988; Ikenouchi et al., 2003; Kokkinos et al., 2007).

Normal epithelial cells are transformed into more invasive mesenchymal cells due to the disintegration of E-cadherin. E-cadherin is a transmembrane glycoprotein that mediates cell-cell contact between epithelial cells. The cytoplasmic domain of E-cadherin interacts with α-, β, and γ-catenin. Under normal cellular conditions, β-catenin forms a complex with E-cadherin to maintain epithelial cell adhesion (Gottardi et al., 2001). However, during epithelial transformation, β-catenin dissociates from the E-cadherin complex and translocates to the nucleus where it synergizes with TCF/LEF1 to induce the expression of downstream target genes (Behrens et al., 1996). The upregulation of β-catenin transcriptional activity induces the expression of vimentin in breast cancer cells, which is a key mediator in EMT (Gilles et al., 2003). The snail and slug zinc-finger transcription factors, which are E-cadherin repressors, are associated with EMT and upregulation of these proteins in breast cancer correlates with poor prognosis of breast cancer patients (Blanco et al., 2002; Moody et al., 2005; Martin et al., 2005). Indeed, aberrant Wnt/β-catenin signaling increases Snail activity (Yook et al., 2006). Other proteins that contribute to the invasive properties of epithelial cells including matrix metalloproteinase-7, CD44, uPAAR, slug, and the γ2 chain of laminin-5 are also downstream target genes of β-catenin (Brabletz et al., 1999; Wielenga et al., 1999; Mann et al., 1999; Hlubek et al., 2001). Overall, dysfunction of the Wnt/β-catenin signaling pathway is intricately involved in regulating the EMT of breast cancer.

3.6 Wnt/β-catenin signaling in breast cancer stem cells

Stem cells are cells that have the capacity to propagate or differentiate into distinct cell types that form mature tissue (Seaberg and Kooy, 2003). Stem cells may lay dormant and accumulate mutations over a long period of time, which ultimately results in the formation of tumors due to aberrant activation of signaling pathways that regulate stem cell continuity and differentiation (Sell, 2004). Previously, stem cells were isolated from human breast cancer tissue, suggesting that cancer stem cells (CSCs) may be involved in the development of breast cancer (Al-Hajj et al., 2003). Breast CSCs are characterized by the expression of cell surface markers including stem cell antigen-1 (Welm et al., 2002), CD44+/CD24-, aldehyde dehydrogenase-1 (ALDH1), ESA, PROCR, CD133, and CXCR4 (Nguyen et al., 2010). Another indicator of breast CSCs is their ability to efflux Hoechst 33342 dye (Alvi et al., 2003; Hirschmann-Jax et al., 2004; Ho et al., 2007). ALDH is a detoxifying enzyme, which oxidizes intracellular aldehydes (Duester, 2000; Magni et al., 1996; Sophos and Vasiliou,

2003; Yoshida et al., 1998). CD44+/CD24- breast CSCs, which express pro-invasive genes, usually display poor prognosis (Sheridan et al., 2006). A recent study showed that metastatic breast cancer in xenograft mouse models display high ALDH1 activity, which may serve as a predictor of poor patient survival (Charafe-Jauffret et al., 2010). Furthermore, breast CSCs positive for ALDH1 but not CD44+/CD24- are resistant to chemotherapy (Tanei et al., 2009), suggesting that ALDH1 expression may be essential for breast CSC propagation and contribute to drug resistance in some breast cancer types. Indeed, ALDH1-positive tumors are more likely to be ER-, PR-, and HER2+ and exhibit poor prognosis (Morimoto et al., 2009). However, the involvement of ALDH1 in breast CSC development is still controversial. One study showed that there is no correlation between ALDH1 expression and ER and PR status and poor patient survival (Restkova et al., 2010). Furthermore, Restkova et al. (2010) showed that ALDH1 is highly expressed in the stroma of breast cancer tumors and is associated with increased survival.

The Wnt/β-catenin signaling pathway plays an important role in stem cell survival by maintaining their continuity and undifferentiated state (Ling et al., 2009). Aberrant Wnt/β-catenin signaling, which may be induced by mutations in the stem cell genome, contributes to the development and progression of breast CSCs. For example, previous studies show that β-catenin positively regulates the expression of CD44 and CD24 (Wielenga et al., 1999, 2000; Shulewitz et al., 2006). Furthermore, increased cytoplasmic and nuclear localization of β-catenin in basal-like breast cancer overlaps with CD44+/CD24- staining, which suggest that CSC populations exist in basal-like/triple negative breast tumors (Khramtsov et al., 2010). The canonical Wnt signaling co-receptor, LRP6 is overexpressed in triple-negative breast cancer (Liu et al., 2010) and facilitates the metastasis of triple-negative breast tumors (DiMeo et al., 2009). Expression of Wnt1 and stabilized β-catenin (ΔN89β-catenin) under the MMTV promoter induces Wnt/β-catenin signaling in distinct progenitor compartments in mouse mammary tumors (Teissedre et al. 2009). Wnt/β-catenin signaling also mediates the radiation resistance of mouse mammary progenitor cells (Chen et al., 2007; Woodward et al., 2007). These results suggest that aberrant Wnt/β-catenin converts normal mammary stem cells into CSCs by altering their self-renewal and differentiation capabilities.

4. Conclusion

Aberrant activation of the Wnt/β-catenin signaling pathway can lead to tumor formation. While genetic mutations of certain intracellular components of the Wnt/β-catenin pathway, such as *APC* and *CTNNB1*, are significant contributing factors for colorectal cancers, they are typically not the predominate mechanism associated with breast cancer. Instead, it is clear that dysregulation of cell surface Wnt/β-catenin signaling components leads to aberrant activation of this pathway in breast cancer. Studies in the past years have demonstrated that Wnt/β-catenin signaling play a critical role in breast development and progression. Therefore, disruption of Wnt/β-catenin signaling at the cell surface represents a great opportunity to develop novel drugs for breast cancer prevention and therapy (Ettenberg et al., 2010; Gong et al., 2010; Liu et al., 2010).

5. Acknowledgment

Research in authors' laboratory is supported by a grant from the National Institutes of Health (R01CA124531).

6. References

Ai L, Tao Q, Zhong S, Fields CR, Kim WJ, Lee MW, Cui Y, Brown KD, and Robertson KD. 2006. Inactivation of Wnt inhibitory factor-1 (WIF1) expression by epigeneticsilencing is a common event in breast cancer. *Carcinogenesis.* 27 (7): 1341-1348.

Ai M, Holmen SL, van Hul W, Williams BO, and Warman ML. 2005. Reduced affinity to and inhibition by DKK1 form a common mechanism by which high bone mass-associated missense mutations in LRP5 affect canonical Wnt signaling. *Mol Cell Biol* 25 (12): 4946-4955.

Al-Hajj M, Wicha MS, Benito-Hernandez A, Morrison SJ, and Clarke MF. 2003. Prospectiveidentification of tumorigenic breast cancer cells. *Proc Natl Acad Sci U S A.* 100 (7): 3983-3988.

Alvi AJ, Clayton H, Joshi C, Enver T, Ashworth A, Vivanco MM, Dale TC, and SmalleyMJ. 2002. Functional and molecular characterisation of mammary side population cells. *Breast Cancer Res* 5 (1): R1-R8.

Arteaga CL. 2003. Trastuzumab, an appropriate first-line single-agent therapy for HER2-overexpressing metastatic breast cancer. *Breast Cancer Res* 5 (2): 96-100.

Bafico A, Gazit A, Pramila T, Finch PW, Yaniv A, and Aaronson SA. 1999. Interaction of frizzled related protein (FRP) with Wnt ligands and the frizzled receptor suggests alternative mechanisms for FRP inhibition of Wnt signaling. *J Biol Chem* 274 (23): 16180-16187.

Bafico A, Liu G, Yaniv A, Gazit A, and Aaronson SA. 2001. Novel mechanism of Wntsignalling inhibition mediated by Dickkopf-1 interaction with LRP6/Arrow. *Nat Cell Biol.* 3 (7): 683-686.

Balemans W, Ebeling M, Patel N, Van Hul E, Olson P, Dioszegi M, Lacza C, WuytsW, Van Den Ende J, Willems P, Paes-Alves AF, Hill S, Bueno M, Ramos FJ, TacconiP, Dikkers FG, Stratakis C, Lindpaintner K, Vickery B, Foernzler D, and Van Hul W. 2001. Increased bone density in sclerosteosis is due to the deficiency of a novel secreted protein (SOST). *Hum Mol Genet* 10 (5): 537-543.

Bänziger C, Soldini D, Schütt C, Zipperlen P, Hausmann G, and Basler K. 2006. Wntless, a conserved membrane protein dedicated to the secretion of Wnt proteins from signaling cells. *Cell* 125 (3): 509-522.

Bartkova J, Lukas J, Müller H, Lützhøft D, Strauss M, and Bartek J. 1994. Cyclin D1 protein expression and function in human breast cancer. *Int J Cancer* 57 (3): 353-361.

Bartscherer K, Pelte N, Ingelfinger D, and Boutros M. 2006. Secretion of Wnt ligands requires Evi, a conserved transmembrane protein. *Cell* 125 (3): 523-533.

Behrens J, von Kries JP, Kühl M, Bruhn L, Wedlich D, Grosschedl R, and Birchmeier W. 1996. Functional interaction of beta-catenin with the transcription factor LEF-1. *Nature* 382 (6592): 638-642.

Bennett CN, Longo KA, Wright WS, Suva LJ, Lane TF, Hankenson KD, and MacDougald OA. 2005. Regulation of osteoblastogenesis and bone mass by Wnt10b. *Proc Natl Acad Sci U S A* 102 (9): 3324-3329.

Benhaj K, Akcali KC, and Ozturk M. 2006. Redundant expression of canonical Wnt ligands in human breast cancer cell lines. *Oncol Rep* 15 (3): 701-707.

Berger W, Meindl A, van de Pol TJ, Cremers FP, Ropers HH, Döerner C, Monaco A, Bergen AA, Lebo R, Warburgh M, et al. 1992. Isolation of a candidate gene for Norriedisease by positional cloning. *Nat Genet* 2(1): 84.

Björklund P, Svedlund J, Olsson AK, Akerström G, and Westin G. 2009. The internally truncated LRP5 receptor presents a therapeutic target in breast cancer. *PLoS One* 4(1): e4243.

Blanco MJ, Moreno-Bueno G, Sarrio D, Locascio A, Cano A, Palacios J, and Nieto MA. 2002. Correlation of Snail expression with histological grade and lymph node status in breast carcinomas. *Oncogene* 21(20): 3241-3246.

Blasband A, Schryver B, and Papkoff J. 1992. The biochemical properties and transforming potential of human Wnt-2 are similar to Wnt-1. *Oncogene* 7 (1): 153-161.

Bodine PV, Zhao W, Kharode YP, Bex FJ, Lambert AJ, Goad MB, Gaur T, Stein GS, Lian JB, and Komm BS. 2004. The Wnt antagonist secreted frizzled-related protein-1 is a negative regulator of trabecular bone formation in adult mice. *Mole Endocrinol* 18 (5): 1222–1237.

Bourhis E, Tam C, Franke Y, Bazan JF, Ernst J, Hwang J, Costa M, Cochran AG, and Hannoush RN. 2010. Reconstitution of a frizzled8.Wnt3a. LRP6 signaling complex reveals multiple Wnt and Dkk1 binding sites on LRP6. *J Biol Chem* 285 (12): 9172-9179.

Boyden LM, Mao J, Belsky J, Mitzner L, Farhi A, Mitnick MA, Wu D, Insogna K, and Lifton RP. 2002. High bone density due to a mutation in LDL-receptor-related protein 5. *N Engl J Med* 346 (20): 1513-1521.

Brabletz T, Jung A, Dag S, Hlubek F, and Kirchner T. 1999. β-Catenin regulates the expression of the matrix metalloproteinase-7 in human colorectal cancer. *Am J Pathol* 155(4): 1033-1038.

Brennan K, Gonzalez-Sancho JM, Castelo-Soccio LA, Howe LR, and Brown AM. 2004. Truncated mutants of the putative Wnt receptor LRP6/Arrow can stabilize beta-catenin independently of Frizzled proteins. *Oncogene* 23: 4873-4884.

Brott BK and Sokol SY. 2002. Regulation of Wnt/LRP signaling by distinct domains of Dickkopf proteins. *Mol Cell Biol* 22 (17): 6100-6110.

Brunkow ME, Gardner JC, Van Ness J, Paeper BW, Kovacevich BR, Proll S, Skonier JE, Zhao L, Sabo PJ, Fu Y, Alisch RS, Gillett L, Colbert T, Tacconi P, Galas D,Hamersma H, Beighton P, and Mulligan J. 2001. Bone dysplasia sclerosteosis results from loss of the SOST gene product, a novel cystine knot-containing protein. *Am J Hum Genet* 68(3): 577-589.

Bu G, Lu W, Liu CC, Selander K, Yoneda T, Hall C, Keller ET, and Li Y. 2008. Breast cancer-derived Dickkopf1 inhibits osteoblast differentiation and osteoprotegerin expression: implication for breast cancer osteolytic bone metastases. *Int J Cancer* 123 (5): 1034-1042.

Bu G. 2009. Apolipoprotein E and its receptors in Alzheimer's disease: pathways, pathogenesis and therapy. *Nat Rev Neurosci* 10 (5): 333-344.

Bui TD, Rankin J, Smith K, Huguet EL, Ruben S, Strachan T, Harris AL, and Lindsay S. 1997. A novel human Wnt gene, WNT10B, maps to 12q13 and is expressed in human breastcarcinomas. *Oncogene* 14(10): 1249-1253.

Cabrera CV, Alonso MC, Johnston P, Phillips RG, and Lawrence PA. 1987. Phenocopies induced with antisense RNA identify the wingless gene. *Cell* 50 (4): 659-663.

Chamorro MN, Schwartz DR, Vonica A, Brivanlou AH, Cho KR, and Varmus HE. 2005. FGF-20 and DKK1 are transcriptional targets of beta-catenin and FGF-20 is implicated in cancer and development. *EMBO J* 24 (1): 73-84.

Caricasole A, Ferraro T, Iacovelli L, Barletta E, Caruso A, Melchiorri D, Terstappen GC, and Nicoletti F. 2003. Functional characterization of WNT7A signaling in PC12 cells: interaction with A FZD5 x LRP6 receptor complex and modulation by Dickkopf proteins. *J Biol Chem* 278 (39): 37024-37031.

Carter P, Presta L, Gorman CM, Ridgway JB, Henner D, Wong WL, Rowland AM, Kotts C, Carver ME, and Shepard HM. 1992. Humanization of an anti-p185HER2 antibody for human cancer therapy. *Proc Natl Acad Sci U S A* 89 (10): 4285-4289.

Charafe-Jauffret E, Ginestier C, Iovino F, Tarpin C, Diebel M, Esterni B, Houvenaeghel G, Extra JM, Bertucci F, Jacquemier J, Xerri L, Dontu G, Stassi G,Xiao Y, Barsky SH, Birnbaum D, Viens P, and Wicha MS. 2010. Aldehyde dehydrogenase 1-positive cancer stem cells mediate metastasis and poor clinical outcome ininflammatory breast cancer. *Clin Cancer Res* 16 (1): 45-55.

Chen ZY, Hendriks RW, Jobling MA, Powell JF, Breakefield XO, Sims KB, and Craig IW. 1992. Isolation and characterization of a candidate gene for Norrie disease. *Nat Genet* 1 (3): 204-208.

Chen MS, Woodward WA, Behbod F, Peddibhotla S, Alfaro MP, Buchholz TA, and Rosen JM. 2007. Wnt/beta-catenin mediates radiation resistance of Sca1+ progenitors in animmortalized mammary gland cell line. *J Cell Sci* 120 (3): 468-477.

Chen M, Wang J, Lu J, Bond MC, Ren XR, Lyerly HK, Barak LS, and Chen W. 2009. The anti-helminthic niclosamide inhibits Wnt/Frizzled1 signaling. Biochemistry 48(43): 10267-10274.

Culi J and Mann RS. 2003. Boca, an endoplasmic reticulum protein required for wingless signaling and trafficking of LDL receptor family members in Drosophila. *Cell* 112 (3): 343-354.

Culi J, Springer TA, and Mann RS. 2004. Boca-dependent maturation of beta-propeller/EGF modules in low-density lipoprotein receptor proteins. *EMBO J* 23 (6): 1372-1380.

Dale TC, Weber-Hall SJ, Smith K, Huguet EL, Jayatilake H, Gusterson BA, Shuttleworth G, O'Hare M, and Harris AL. 1996. Compartment switching of WNT-2 expression inhuman breast tumors. *Cancer Res* 56 (19): 4320-4323.

Davidson G, Mao B, del Barco Barrantes I, and Niehrs C. 2002. Kremen proteins interact with Dickkopf1 to regulate anteroposterior CNS patterning. *Development* 129 (24): 5587-5596.

Davidson G, Wu W, Shen J, Bilic J, Fenger U, Stannek P, Glinka A, and Niehrs C. 2005. Casein kinase 1 gamma couples Wnt receptor activation to cytoplasmic signal transduction. *Nature* 438 (7069): 867-872.

Day TF, Guo X, Garrett-Beal L, and Yang Y. 2005. Wnt/beta-catenin signaling in mesenchymal progenitors controls osteoblast and chondrocyte differentiation during vertebrate skeletogenesis. *Dev Cell* 8 (5): 739-750.

Dejmek J, Leandersson K, Manjer J, Bjartell A, Emdin SO, Vogel WF, Landberg G, and Andersson T. 2005. Expression and signaling activity of Wnt-5a/discoidin domainreceptor-1 and Syk plays distinct but decisive roles in breast cancer patient survival. *Clin Cancer Res.* 11 (2 Pt 1): 520-528.

Diehn M, Cho RW, Lobo NA, Kalisky T, Dorie MJ, Kulp AN, Qian D, Lam JS, AillesLE, Wong M, Joshua B, Kaplan MJ, Wapnir I, Dirbas FM, Somlo G, Garberoglio C, Paz B, Shen J, Lau SK, Quake SR, Brown JM, Weissman IL, Clarke MF. 2009. Association of reactive oxygen species levels and radioresistance in cancer stem cells. *Nature* 458 (7239): 780-783.

DiMeo TA, Anderson K, Phadke P, Fan C, Perou CM, Naber S, and Kuperwasser C. 2009. A novel lung metastasis signature links Wnt signaling with cancer cell self-renewaland epithelial-mesenchymal transition in basal-like breast cancer. *Cancer Res* 69 (3): 5364-5373.

Dolled-Filhart M, McCabe A, Giltnane J, Cregger M, Camp RL, and Rimm DL. 2006. Quantitative in situ analysis of beta-catenin expression in breast cancer shows decreased expression is associated with poor outcome. *Cancer Res* 66 (10); 5487-5494.

Duester G. 2000. Families of retinoid dehydrogenases regulating vitamin A function: production of visual pigment and retinoic acid. *Eur J Biochem* 267(14): 4315-4324.

Dwyer MA, Joseph JD, Wade HE, Eaton ML, Kunder RS, Kazmin D, Chang CY, and McDonnell DP. 2010. WNT11 expression is induced by estrogen-related receptor alpha and beta-catenin and acts in an autocrine manner to increase cancer cell migration. *Cancer Res* 70(22): 9298-9308.

Ellies DL, Viviano B, McCarthy J, Rey JP, Itasaki N, Saunders S, and Krumlauf R. 2006. Bone density ligand, Sclerostin, directly interacts with LRP5 but not LRP5G171Vto modulate Wnt activity. *J Bone Miner Res* 21 (11): 1738-1749.

Ettenberg SA, Charlat O, Daley MP, Liu S, Vincent KJ, Stuart DD, Schuller AG, Yuan J, Ospina B, Green J, Yu Q, Walsh R, Li S, Schmitz R, Heine H, Bilic S, Ostrom L, Mosher R, Hartlepp KF, Zhu Z, Fawell S, Yao YM, Stover D, Finan PM, Porter JA, Sellers WR, Klagge IM, and Cong F. 2010. Inhibition of tumorigenesis driven bydifferent Wnt proteins requires blockade of distinct ligand-binding regions byLRP6 antibodies. *Proc Natl Acad Sci U S A* 107(35): 15473-15478.

Forget MA, Turcotte S, Beauseigle D, Godin-Ethier J, Pelletier S, Martin J, Tanguay S, and Lapointe R. 2007. The Wnt pathway regulator DKK1 is preferentially expressedin hormone-resistant breast tumours and in some common cancer types. *Br J Cancer* 96 (4): 646-653.

Fujino T, Asaba H, Kang MJ et al. 2003. Low-density lipoprotein receptor-related protein 5 (LRP5) is essential for normal cholesterol metabolism and glucose-induced insulin secretion. *Proc Natl Acad Sci U S A*. 100: 229-234.

Geyer FC, Lacroix-Triki M, Savage K, Arnedos M, Lambros MB, MacKay A, Natrajan R, and Reis-Filho JS. 2011. β-Catenin pathway activation in breast cancer is associatedwith triple-negative phenotype but not with CTNNB1 mutation. *Mod Pathol* 24 (2): 209-231.

Gilles C, Polette M, Mestdagt M, Nawrocki-Raby B, Ruggeri P, Birembaut P, and Foidart JM. 2003. Transactivation of vimentin by beta-catenin in human breast cancercells. *Cancer Res* 63 (10): 26658-26664.

Gillett C, Fantl V, Smith R, Fisher C, Bartek J, Dickson C, Barnes D, and Peters G. 1994. Amplification and overexpression of cyclin D1 in breast cancer detected byimmunohistochemical staining. *Cancer Res* 54 (7): 1812-1817.

Glass DA 2nd, Bialek P, Ahn JD, Starbuck M, Patel MS, Clevers H, Taketo MM, Long F, McMahon AP, Lang RA, and Karsenty G. 2005. Canonical Wnt signaling in differentiated osteoblasts controls osteoclast differentiation. *Dev Cell* 8 (5): 751-764.

Glinka A, Wu W, Delius H, Monaghan AP, Blumenstock C, and Niehrs C. 1998. Dickkopf-1 is a member of a new family of secreted proteins and functions in head induction. *Nature* 391(6665): 357-362.

Gong Y, Slee RB, Fukai N, Rawadi G, Roman-Roman S, Reginato AM, Wang H, Cundy T, Glorieux FH, Lev D, Zacharin M, Oexle K, Marcelino J, Suwairi W, Heeger S, Sabatakos G, Apte S, Adkins WN, Allgrove J, Arslan-Kirchner M, Batch JA, Beighton P, Black GC, Boles RG, Boon LM, Borrone C, Brunner HG, Carle GF, Dallapiccola B, De Paepe A, Floege B, Halfhide ML, Hall B, Hennekam RC, Hirose T, Jans A, Jüppner H, Kim CA, Keppler-Noreuil K, Kohlschuetter A, LaCombe D, Lambert M, Lemyre E, Letteboer T, Peltonen L, Ramesar RS, Romanengo M, Somer H, Steichen-Gersdorf E, Steinmann B, Sullivan B, Superti-Furga A, Swoboda W, van den Boogaard MJ, Van Hul W, Vikkula M, Votruba M, Zabel B, Garcia T, Baron R, Olsen BR, Warman ML; and Osteoporosis-Pseudoglioma Syndrome Collaborative Group. 2001. LDL receptor-related protein 5 (LRP5) affects bone accrual and eye development. *Cell* 107 (4): 513-523.

Gong Y, Bourhis E, Chiu C, Stawicki S, DeAlmeida VI, Liu BY, Phamluong K, Cao TC, Carano RA, Ernst JA, Solloway M, Rubinfeld B, Hannoush RN, Wu Y, Polakis P, and Costa M. 2010. Wnt isoform-specific interactions with coreceptor specify inhibition or potentiation of signaling by LRP6 antibodies. *PLoS One* 5 (9): e12682.

González-Sancho JM, Aguilera O, García JM, Pendás-Franco N, Peña C, Cal S, García de Herreros A, Bonilla F, and Muñoz A. 2005. The Wnt antagonist DICKKOPF-1 gene is a downstream target of beta-catenin/TCF and is downregulated in human colon cancer. *Oncogene* 24 (6): 1098-1103.

Gottardi CJ and Gumbiner BM. 2001. Adhesion signaling: how beta-catenin interacts with its partners. *Curr Biol* 11 (19): R792-R794.

Hay ED. 2005. The mesenchymal cell, its role in the embryo, and the remarkablesignaling mechanisms that create it. *Dev Dyn* 233 (3): 706-720.

He B, You L, Uematsu K, Xu Z, Lee AY, Matsangou M, McCormick F, and Jablons DM. 2004. A monoclonal antibody against Wnt-1 induces apoptosis in human cancer cells. *Neoplasia* 6 (1): 7-14.

He X, Semenov M, Tamai K, and Zeng X. 2004. LDL receptor-related proteins 5 and 6 in Wnt/beta-catenin signaling: arrows point the way. *Development* 131 (8): 1663-1677.

Hendrickx M and Leyns L. 2008. Non-conventional Frizzled ligands and Wnt receptors. *Dev Growth Differ* 50 (4): 229-243.

Hey PJ, Twells RC, Phillips MS, Yusuke Nakagawa, Brown SD, Kawaguchi Y, Cox R, Guochun Xie, Dugan V, Hammond H, Metzker ML, Todd JA, and Hess JF. 1998. Cloning of a novel member of the low-density lipoprotein receptor family. *Gene* 216 (1): 103-111.

Hill TP, Spater D, Taketo MM, Birchmeier W, and Hartmann C. 2005. Canonical Wnt/beta-catenin signaling prevents osteoblasts from differentiating into chondrocytes. *Dev Cell* 8 (5): 727-738.

Hirschmann-Jax C, Foster AE, Wulf GG, Nuchtern JG, Jax TW, Gobel U, Goodell MA, and Brenner MK. 2004. A distinct "side population" of cells with high drug effluxcapacity in human tumor cells. *Proc Natl Acad Sci U S A* 101 (39): 14228-14233.

Hlubek F, Jung A, Kotzor N, Kirchner T, and Brabletz T. 2001. Expression of the invasion factor laminin gamma2 in colorectal carcinomas is regulated by beta-catenin.*Cancer Res* 61 (22): 8089-8093.

Ho MM, Ng AV, Lam S, and Hung JY. 2007. Side population in human lung cancer cell lines and tumors is enriched with stem-like cancer cells. *Cancer Res* 67 (10): 4827-4833.

Holmen SL, Giambernardi TA, Zylstra CR, Buckner-Berghuis BD, Resau JH, Hess JF, Glatt V, Bouxsein ML, Ai M, Warman ML, and Williams BO. 2004. Decreased BMD and limb deformities in mice carrying mutations in both Lrp5 and Lrp6. *J Bone Miner Res* 19 (12): 2033-2040.

Holmen SL, Zylstra CR, Mukherjee A, Sigler RE, Faugere MC, Bouxsein ML, Deng L, Clemens TL, and Williams BO. 2005. Essential role of beta-catenin in postnatal bone acquisition. *J Biol Chem* 280: 21162-21168.

Hsieh JC, Kodjabachian L, Rebbert ML, Rattner A, Smallwood PM, Samos CH, Nusse R, Dawid IB, and Nathans J. 1999. A new secreted protein that binds to Wnt proteins andinhibits their activities. *Nature* 398 (6726): 431-436.

Hsieh JC, Lee L, Zhang L, Wefer S, Brown K, DeRossi C, Wines ME, Rosenquist T, and Holdener BC. 2003. Mesd encodes an LRP5/6 chaperone essential for specification of mouse embryonic polarity. *Cell* 112 (3): 355-367.

Hu H, Hilton MJ, Tu X, Yu K, Ornitz DM, and Long F. 2005. Sequential roles of Hedgehog and Wnt signaling in osteoblast development. *Development* 132 (1): 49-60.

Ikenouchi J, Matsuda M, Furuse M, and Tsukita S. 2003. Regulation of tight junctions during the epithelium-mesenchyme transition: direct repression of the geneexpression of claudins/occludin by Snail. *J Cell Sci* 116 (Pt 10): 1959-1967.

Ishitani T, Kishida S, Hyodo-Miura J, Ueno N, Yasuda J, Waterman M, Shibuya H, Moon RT, Ninomiya-Tsuji J, and Matsumoto K. 2003. The TAK1-NLK mitogen-activated proteinkinase cascade functions in the Wnt-5a/Ca(2+) pathway to antagonize Wnt/beta-catenin signaling. *Mol Cell Biol* 23 (1): 131-139.

Jackson A, Vayssiere B, Garcia T, Newell W, Baron R, Roman-Roman S, and Rawadi G. 2005. Gene array analysis of Wnt-regulated genes in C3H10T1/2 cells. *Bone* 36 (4): 585-598.

Jönsson M, Borg A, Nilbert M, and Andersson T. 2000. Involvement of adenomatous polyposis coli (APC)/beta-catenin signalling in human breast cancer. *Eur J Cancer.* 36 (2): 242-248.

Jönsson M and Andersson T. 2001. Repression of Wnt-5a impairs DDR1 phosphorylation and modifies adhesion and migration of mammary cells. *J Cell Sci* 114 (Pt 11): 2043-2053.

Jönsson M, Dejmek J, Bendahl PO, and Andersson T. 2002. Loss of Wnt-5a protein is associated with early relapse in invasive ductal breast carcinomas. *Cancer Res* 62 (2): 409-416.

Kalluri R, and Weinberg RA. 2009. The basics of epithelial-mesenchymal transition. *J Clin Invest* 119 (6): 1420-1428.

Kazanskaya O, Glinka A, del Barco Barrantes I, Stannek P, Niehrs C, and Wu W. 2004. R-Spondin2 is a secreted activator of Wnt/beta-catenin signaling and is required for Xenopus myogenesis. *Dev Cell* 7 (4): 525-534.

Karsenty G, and Wagner EF. 2002. Reaching a genetic and molecular understanding of skeletal development. *Dev Cell* 2 (4): 389-406.

Kato M, Patel MS, Levasseur R, Lobov I, Chang BH, Glass DA 2nd, Hartmann C, Li L, Hwang TH, Brayton CF, Lang RA, Karsenty G, and Chan L. 2002. Cbfa1-independent decrease in osteoblast proliferation, osteopenia, and persistent embryonic eye vascularization in mice deficient in LRP5, a Wnt coreceptor. *J. Cell Biol* 157 (2): 303-314.

Kawano Y and Kypta R. 2003. Secreted antagonists of the Wnt signalling pathway. *J Cell Sci* 116 (13): 2627-2634.

Kelly OG, Pinson KI, and Skarnes WC. 2004. The Wnt co-receptors LRP5 and LRP6 are essential for gastrulation in mice. *Development* 131 (12): 2803-2815.

Khramtsov AI, Khramtsova GF, Tretiakova M, Huo D, Olopade OI, and Goss KH. 2010. Wnt/beta-catenin pathway activation is enriched in basal-like breast cancers and predicts poor outcome. *Am J Pathol* 176 (6): 2911-2920.

Kim KA, Kakitani M, Zhao J, Oshima T, Tang T, Binnerts M, Liu Y, Boyle B, Park E, Emtage P, Funk WD, Tomizuka K. 2005. Mitogenic influence of human R-spondin1 on the intestinal epithelium. *Science* 309(5738): 1256-1259.

Kim KA, Zhao J, Andarmani S, Kakitani M, Oshima T, Binnerts ME, Abo A, Tomizuka K, and Funk WD. 2006. R-Spondin proteins: a novel link to beta-catenin activation. *Cell Cycle* 5 (1): 23-26.

Kim KA, Wagle M, Tran K, Zhan X, Dixon MA, Liu S, Gros D, Korver W, Yonkovich S, Tomasevic N, Binnerts M, and Abo A. 2008. R-Spondin family members regulate the Wntpathway by a common mechanism. *Mol Biol Cell* 19 (6): 2588-2596.

Kinzler KW and Vogelstein B. 1996. Lessons from hereditary colorectal cancer. *Cell* 87 (2); 159-70.

Koduri V and Blacklow SC. 2007. Requirement for natively unstructured regions of mesoderm development candidate 2 in promoting low-density lipoprotein receptor-related protein 6 maturation. *Biochemistry.* 46 (22): 6570-6577.

Kohn AD and Moon RT. 2005. Wnt and calcium signaling: beta-catenin-independent pathways. *Cell Calcium* 38 (3-4): 439-446.

Kokkinos MI, Wafai R, Wong MK, Newgreen DF, Thompson EW, and Waltham M. 2007. Vimentin and epithelial-mesenchymal transition in human breast cancer--observations invitro and in vivo. *Cells Tissues Organs* 185 (1-3): 191-203.

Kokubu C, Heinzmann U, Kokubu T, Sakai N, Kubota T, Kawai M, Wahl MB, Galceran J, Grosschedl R, Ozono K, Imai K. 2004. Skeletal defects in ringelschwanz mutant mice reveal that Lrp6 is required for proper somitogenesis and osteogenesis. *Development* 131 (21): 5469-5480.

Kozlow W, and Guise TA. 2005. Breast cancer metastasis to bone: mechanisms of osteolysis and implications for therapy. *J. Mammary Gland Biol Neoplasia* 10 (2): 169-180.

Krishnan V, Bryant HU, and Macdougald OA. 2006. Regulation of bone mass by Wnt signaling. *J Clin Invest* 116 (5): 1202-1209.

Krupnik VE, Sharp JD, Jiang C, Robison K, Chickering TW, Amaravadi L, Brown DE, Guyot D, Mays G, Leiby K, Chang B, Duong T, Goodearl AD, Gearing DP, SokolSY, and

McCarthy SA. 1999. Functional and structural diversity of the human Dickkopf genefamily. *Gene* 238 (2): 301-313.

Lacey DL, Timms E, Tan HL, Kelley MJ, Dunstan CR, Burgess T, Elliott R, Colombero A, Elliott G, Scully S, Hsu H, Sullivan J, Hawkins N, Davy E, Capparelli C, Eli A, Qian YX, Kaufman S, Sarosi I, Shalhoub V, Senaldi G, Guo J, Delaney J, Boyle WJ. 1998. Osteoprotegerin ligand is a cytokine that regulates osteoclast differentiation and activation. *Cell* 93 (2): 165-176.

Lane TF and Leder P. 1997. Wnt-10b directs hypermorphic development and transformation in mammary glands of male and female mice. *Oncogene* 15 (18): 2133-2144.

Lejeune S, Huguet EL, Hamby A, Poulsom R, and Harris AL. 1995. Wnt5a cloning, expression, and up-regulation in human primary breast cancers. *Clin Cancer Res* 1 (2): 215-222.

Leris AC, Roberts TR, Jiang WG, Newbold RF, and Mokbel K. 2005. WNT5A expression in human breast cancer. *Anticancer Res* 25 (2A): 731-734.

Li L, Mao J, Sun L, Liu W, and Wu D. 2002. Second cysteine-rich domain of Dickkopf-2 activates canonical Wnt signaling pathway via LRP-6 independently of dishevelled.*J Biol Chem* 277(8): 5977-5981.

Li X, Liu P, Liu W, Maye P, Zhang J, Zhang Y, Hurley M, Guo C, Boskey A, Sun L, Harris SE, Rowe DW, Ke HZ, and Wu D. 2005a. Dkk2 has a role in terminal osteoblast differentiation and mineralized matrix formation. *Nat Genet* 37 (9): 945-952.

Li X, Zhang Y, Kang H, Liu W, Liu P, Zhang J, Harris SE, and Wu D. 2005b. Sclerostin binds to LRP5/6 and antagonizes canonical Wnt signaling. *J Biol Chem* 280 (20): 19883-19887.

Li Y, Chen J, Lu W, McCormick LM, Wang J, and Bu G. 2005c. Mesd binds to mature LDL-receptor-related protein-6 and antagonizes ligand binding. *J Cell Sci* 118 (22): 5305-5314.

Li Y, Lu W, He X, and Bu G. 2006a. Modulation of LRP6-mediated Wnt signaling by molecular chaperone Mesd. *FEBS Lett* 580 (22): 5423-5428.

Li J, Sarosi I, Cattley RC, Pretorius J, Asuncion F, Grisanti M, Morony S, Adamu S, Geng Z, Qiu W, Kostenuik P, Lacey DL, Simonet WS, Bolon B, Qian X, Shalhoub V, Ominsky MS, Zhu Ke H, Li X, and Richards WG. 2006b. Dkk1-mediated inhibition of Wnt signaling in bone results in osteopenia. *Bone* 39 (4): 754-766.

Li C, Chen H, Hu L, Xing Y, Sasaki T, Villosis MF, Li J, Nishita M, Minami Y, and Minoo P. 2008a. Ror2 modulates the canonical Wnt signaling in lung epithelial cells through cooperation with Fzd2. *BMC Mol Biol* 23: 9-11.

Li X, Lewis MT, Huang J, Gutierrez C, Osborne CK, Wu MF, Hilsenbeck SG, Pavlick A, Zhang X, Chamness GC, Wong H, Rosen J, Chang JC. 2008b. Intrinsic resistance of tumorigenic breast cancer cells to chemotherapy. *J Natl Cancer Inst* 100 (9): 672-679.

Li L, Hutchins BI, and Kalil K. 2009. Wnt5a induces simultaneous cortical axon outgrowth and repulsive axon guidance through distinct signaling mechanisms. *J Neurosci* 29 (18): 5873-5883.

Li Y, Lu W, King TD, Liu CC, Bijur GN, and Bu G. 2010. Dkk1 stabilizes Wnt co-receptor LRP6: implication for Wnt ligand-induced LRP6 down-regulation. *PLoS One* 5 (6): e11014.

Licchesi JD, Van Neste L, Tiwari VK, Cope L, Lin X, Baylin SB, and Herman JG. 2010. Transcriptional regulation of Wnt inhibitory factor-1 by Miz-1/c-Myc. *Oncogene* 29 (44): 5923-5934.

Liepinsh E, Bányai L, Patthy L, and Otting G. 2006. NMR structure of the WIF domain of the human Wnt-inhibitory factor-1. *J Mol Biol* 357 (3): 942-950.

Lin K, Wang S, Julius MA, Kitajewski J, Moos M Jr, and Luyten FP. 1997. The cysteine-rich frizzled domain of Frzb-1 is required and sufficient for modulationof Wnt signaling. *Proc Natl Acad Sci U S A* 94 (21): 11196-11200.

Lindvall C, Evans NC, Zylstra CR, Li Y, Alexander CM, and Williams BO. 2006. The Wnt signaling receptor Lrp5 is required for mammary ductal stem cell activity andWnt1-induced tumorigenesis. *J Biol Chem* 281 (46): 35081-35087.

Lindvall C, Zylstra CR, Evans N, West RA, Dykema K, Furge KA, and Williams BO. 2009. The Wnt co-receptor Lrp6 is required for normal mouse mammary gland development. *PLoSOne* 4 (6): e5813.

Little RD, Carulli JP, Del Mastro RG, Dupuis J, Osborne M, Folz C, Manning SP, Swain PM, Zhao SC, Eustace B, Lappe MM, Spitzer L, Zweier S, Braunschweiger K, Benchekroun Y, Hu X, Adair R, Chee L, FitzGerald MG, Tulig C, Caruso A, Tzellas N, Bawa A, Franklin B, McGuire S, Nogues X, Gong G, Allen KM, Anisowicz A, Morales AJ, Lomedico PT, Recker SM, Van Eerdewegh P, Recker RR, and Johnson ML. 2002. A mutation in the LDL receptor-related protein 5 gene results in the autosomal dominant high-bone-mass trait. *Am J Hum Genet* 70 (1): 11-19.

Liu G, Bafico A, Harris VK, and Aaronson SA. 2003. A novel mechanism for Wnt activation of canonical signaling through the LRP6 receptor. *Mol Cell Biol* 23 916): 5825 -5835.

Liu Y, Rubin B, Bodine PV, and Billiard J. 2008. Wnt5a induces homodimerization andactivation of Ror2 receptor tyrosine kinase. *J Cell Biochem* 105 (2): 497-502.

Liu CC, Pearson C, and Bu G. 2009. Cooperative folding and ligand-binding properties of LRP6 beta-propeller domains. *J Biol Chem* 284 (22): 15299-15307.

Liu CC, Prior J, Piwnica-Worms D, and Bu G. 2010. LRP6 overexpression defines a class of breast cancer subtype and is a target for therapy. *Proc Natl Acad Sci U S A* 107 (11): 5136-5141.

Lee JL, Chang CJ, Chueh LL, and Lin CT. 2003. Expression of secreted frizzled-related protein 2 in a primary canine mammary tumor cell line: a candidate tumor markerfor mammary tumor cells. *In Vitro Cell Dev Biol Anim* 39 (5-6): 221-227.

Lee AY, He B, You L, Dadfarmay S, Xu Z, Mazieres J, Mikami I, McCormick F, and Jablons DM. 2004. Expression of the secreted frizzled-related protein gene family is downregulated in human mesothelioma. *Oncogene* 23 (39): 6672-6676.

Ling L, Nurcombe V, and Cool SM. 2008. Wnt signaling controls the fate of mesenchymal stem cells. *Gene* 433 (1-2): 1-7.

Lo PK, Mehrotra J, D'Costa A, Fackler MJ, Garrett-Mayer E, Argani P, and Sukumar S. 2006. Epigenetic suppression of secreted frizzled related protein 1 (SFRP1) expression in human breast cancer. *Cancer Biol Ther* 5 (3): 281-286.

López-Knowles E, Zardawi SJ, McNeil CM, Millar EK, Crea P, Musgrove EA, Sutherland RL, and O'Toole SA. 2010. Cytoplasmic localization of beta-catenin is a marker of poor outcome in breast cancer patients. *Cancer Epidemiol Biomarkers Prev* 19 (1): 301-309.

López-Novoa JM and Nieto MA. 2009. Inflammation and EMT: an alliance towards organ fibrosis and cancer progression. *EMBO Mol Med* 1 (6-7): 303-314.

Lowther W, Wiley K, Smith GH, and Callahan R. 2005. A new common integration site, Int7, for the mouse mammary tumor virus in mouse mammary tumors identifies a gene whoseproduct has furin-like and thrombospondin-like sequences. *J Virol* 79 (15): 10093-10096.

Lu W, Yamamoto V, Ortega B, and Baltimore D. 2004. Mammalian Ryk is a Wnt coreceptor required for stimulation of neurite outgrowth. *Cell* 119 (1): 97-108.

MacDonald BT, Tamai K, and He X. 2009. Wnt/beta-catenin signaling: components, mechanisms, and diseases. *Dev Cell* 17 (1): 9-26.

Mao J, Wang J, Liu B, Pan W, Farr GH 3rd, Flynn C, Yuan H, Takada S, Kimelman D, Li L, and Wu D. 2001a. Low-density lipoprotein receptor-related protein-5 binds to Axin and regulates the canonical Wnt signaling pathway. *Mol Cell* 7 (4): 801-809.

Mao B, Wu W, Li Y, Hoppe D, Stannek P, Glinka A, and Niehrs C. 2001b. LDL-receptor-related protein 6 is a receptor for Dickkopf proteins. *Nature* 411 (6835): 321-325.

Mao B, Wu W, Davidson G, Marhold J, Li M, Mechler BM, Delius H, Hoppe D, Stannek P, Walter C, Glinka A, and Niehrs C. 2002. Kremen proteins are Dickkopf receptorsthat regulate Wnt/beta-catenin signalling. *Nature* 417 (6889): 664-667.

Mao B and Niehrs C. 2003. Kremen2 modulates Dickkopf2 activity during Wnt/LRP6 signaling. *Gene* 302 (1-2): 179-183.

Magni M, Shammah S, Schiró R, Mellado W, Dalla-Favera R, and Gianni AM. 1996. Induction of cyclophosphamide-resistance by aldehyde-dehydrogenase gene transfer. *Blood* 87 (3): 1097-1103.

Mann B, Gelos M, Siedow A, Hanski ML, Gratchev A, Ilyas M, Bodmer WF, Moyer MP, Riecken EO, Buhr HJ, and Hanski C. 1999. Target genes of beta-catenin-Tcell-factor/lymphoid-enhancer-factor signaling in human colorectal carcinomas. *Proc Natl Acad Sci U S A* 96 (4): 1603-1608.

Martin TA, Goyal A, Watkins G, and Jiang WG. 2005. Expression of the transcription factors snail, slug, and twist and their clinical significance in human breast cancer. *Ann Surg Oncol* 12 (6): 488-496.

Matsuda Y, Schlange T, Oakeley EJ, Boulay A, and Hynes NE. 2009. WNT signaling enhances breast cancer cell motility and blockade of the WNT pathway by sFRP1 suppressesMDA-MB-231 xenograft growth. *Breast Cancer Res* 11(3): R32.

Medrek C, Landberg G, Andersson T, and Leandersson K. 2009. Wnt-5a-CKI{alpha} signaling promotes {beta}-catenin/E-cadherin complex formation and intercellular adhesion in human breast epithelial cells. *J Biol Chem* 284 (16): 10968-10979.

Micalizzi DS, Farabaugh SM, and Ford HL. 2010. Epithelial-mesenchymal transition in cancer: parallels between normal development and tumor progression. *J MammaryGland Biol Neoplasia* 15 (2): 117-134.

Mikels AJ and Nusse R. 2006. Purified Wnt5a protein activates or inhibits beta-catenin-TCF signaling depending on receptor context. *PLoS Biol* 4 (4): e115.

Minami Y, Oishi I, Endo M, and Nishita M. 2010. Ror-family receptor tyrosine kinases in noncanonical Wnt signaling: their implications in developmental morphogenesis and human diseases. *Dev Dyn* 239 (1): 1-15.

Milovanovic T, Planutis K, Nguyen A, Marsh JL, Lin F, Hope C, and Holcombe RF. 2004. Expression of Wnt genes and frizzled 1 and 2 receptors in normal breast epithelium and infiltrating breast carcinoma. *Int J Oncol* 25 (5): 1337-1342.

Moody SE, Perez D, Pan TC, Sarkisian CJ, Portocarrero CP, Sterner CJ, Notorfrancesco KL, Cardiff RD, and Chodosh LA. 2005. The transcriptional repressor Snail promotes mammary tumor recurrence. *Cancer Cell* 8 (3): 197-209.

Morimoto K, Kim SJ, Tanei T, Shimazu K, Tanji Y, Taguchi T, Tamaki Y, Terada N, and Noguchi S. 2009. Stem cell marker aldehyde dehydrogenase 1-positive breast cancersare characterized by negative estrogen receptor, positive human epidermal growth factor receptor type 2, and high Ki67 expression. *Cancer Sci* 100 (6): 1062-1068.

Morvan F, Boulukos K, Clément-Lacroix P, Roman Roman S, Suc-Royer I, Vayssière B, Ammann P, Martin P, Pinho S, Pognonec P, Mollat P, Niehrs C, Baron R, Rawadi G. 2006. Deletion of a single allele of the Dkk1 gene leads to an increase in bone formation and bone mass. *J Bone Miner Res* 21 (6): 934-945.

Mundy GR. 2002. Metastasis to bone: causes, consequences and therapeutic opportunities. *Nat Rev Cancer* 2: 584-593.

Nam JS, Turcotte TJ, and Yoon JK. 2006. Dynamic expression of R-spondin family genes in mouse development. *Gene Expr Patterns* 7 (3): 306-312.

Nemeth MJ, Topol L, Anderson SM, Yang Y, and Bodine DM. 2007. Wnt5a inhibits canonical Wnt signaling in hematopoietic stem cells and enhances repopulation. *Proc NatlAcad Sci U S A* 104 (39): 15436-15441.

Niehrs C. 2006. Function and biological roles of the Dickkopf family of Wnt modulators. *Oncogene* 25 (57): 7469-7481.

Niida A, Hiroko T, Kasai M, Furukawa Y, Nakamura Y, Suzuki Y, Sugano S, Akiyama T. 2004. DKK1, a negative regulator of Wnt signaling, is a target of the beta-catenin/TCF pathway. *Oncogene* 23 (52): 8520-8526.

Nguyen NP, Almeida FS, Chi A, Nguyen LM, Cohen D, Karlsson U, and Vinh-Hung V. 2010. Molecular biology of breast cancer stem cells: potential clinical applications. *Cancer Treat Rev* 36 (6): 485-491.

Nusse R, Brown A, Papkoff J, Scambler P, Shackleford G, McMahon A, Moon R, and Varmus H. 1991. A new nomenclature for int-1 and related genes: the Wnt gene family. *Cell* 64 (2): 231.

Nusse R and Varmus HE. 1982. Many tumors induced by the mouse mammary tumor virus contain a provirus integrated in the same region of the host genome. *Cell* 31 (1): 99-109.

Oloumi A, Maidan M, Lock FE, Tearle H, McKinney S, Muller WJ, Aparicio SA, and Dedhar S. 2010. Cooperative signaling between Wnt1 and integrin-linked kinase induces accelerated breast tumor development. *Breast Cancer Res* 12 (3): R38.

Ott SM. 2005. Sclerostin and Wnt signaling--the pathway to bone strength. *J Clin Endocrinol Metab* 90 (12): 6741-6743.

Patthy L. 2000. The WIF module. *Trends Biochem Sci* 25 (1): 12-23.

Peters G, Brookes S, Smith R, and Dickson C. 1983. Tumorigenesis by mouse mammary tumor virus: evidence for a common region for provirus integration in mammary tumors. *Cell* 33 (2): 369-377.

Pinson KI, Brennan J, Monkley S, Avery BJ, and Skarnes WC. 2000. An LDL-receptor-related protein mediates Wnt signalling in mice. *Nature* 407 (6803): 535-538.

Pinzone JJ, Hall BM, Thudi NK, Vonau M, Qiang YW, Rosol TJ, and Shaughnessy JD Jr. 2009. The role of Dickkopf-1 in bone development, homeostasis, and disease. *Blood* 113 (3): 517-525.

Rattner A, Hsieh JC, Smallwood PM, Gilbert DJ, Copeland NG, Jenkins NA, and Nathans J. 1997. A family of secreted proteins contains homology to the cysteine-rich ligand-binding domain of frizzled receptors. *Proc Natl Acad Sci U S A* 94 (7): 2859-2863.

Resetkova E, Reis-Filho JS, Jain RK, Mehta R, Thorat MA, Nakshatri H, and Badve S. 2010. Prognostic impact of ALDH1 in breast cancer: a story of stem cells and tumormicroenvironment. *Breast Cancer Res Treat* 123 (1): 97-108.

Rijsewijk F, Schuermann M, Wagenaar E, Parren P, Weigel D, and Nusse R. 1987. The Drosophila homolog of the mouse mammary oncogene int-1 is identical to the segment polarity gene wingless. *Cell* 50 (4): 649-657.

Roarty K, Baxley SE, Crowley MR, Frost AR, and Serra R. 2009. Loss of TGF-beta or Wnt5a results in an increase in Wnt/beta-catenin activity and redirects mammary tumour phenotype. *Breast Cancer Res* 11 (2): R19.

Roarty K and Serra R. 2007. Wnt5a is required for proper mammary gland development and TGF-beta-mediated inhibition of ductal growth. *Development* 134 (21): 3929-3939.

Roodman GD. 2004. Mechanisms of bone metastasis. *N Engl J Med* 350: 1655-1664.

Saitoh T, Mine T, and Katoh M. 2002. Up-regulation of Frizzled-10 (FZD10) by beta-estradiol in MCF-7 cells and by retinoic acid in NT2 cells. *Int J Oncol* 20 (1): 117-120.

Schulte G. 2010. International Union of Basic and Clinical Pharmacology. LXXX. The class Frizzled receptors. *Pharmacol Rev* 62 (4): 632-667.

Seaberg RM and van der Kooy D. 2003. Stem and progenitor cells: the premature desertion of rigorous definitions. *Trends Neurosci* 26 (3): 125-131.

Seifert JR and Mlodzik M. 2007. Frizzled/PCP signalling: a conserved mechanism regulating cell polarity and directed motility. *Nat Rev Genet* 8 (2): 126-138.

Sell S. 2004. Stem cell origin of cancer and differentiation therapy. *Crit Rev Oncol Hematol* 51 (1): 1-28.

Semënov MV, Tamai K, Brott BK, Kühl M, Sokol S, and He X. 2001. Head inducer Dickkopf-1 is a ligand for Wnt coreceptor LRP6. *Curr Biol* 11 (12): 951-961.

Semënov M, Tamai K, and He X. 2005. SOST is a ligand for LRP5/LRP6 and a Wnt signaling inhibitor. *J Biol Chem* 280 (29): 26770-26775.

Semenov MV and He X. 2006. LRP5 mutations linked to high bone mass diseases cause reduced LRP5 binding and inhibition by SOST. *J Biol Chem* 281 (50): 38276-3884.

Sheridan C, Kishimoto H, Fuchs RK, Mehrotra S, Bhat-Nakshatri P, Turner CH, Goulet R Jr, Badve S, and Nakshatri H. 2006. CD44+/CD24- breast cancer cells exhibitenhanced invasive properties: an early step necessary for metastasis. *Breast Cancer Res* 8 (5): R59.

Shimizu H, Julius MA, Giarré M, Zheng Z, Brown AM, and Kitajewski J. 1997. Transformation by Wnt family proteins correlates with regulation of beta-catenin. *Cell Growth Differ* 8 (12): 1349-1358.

Shtutman M, Zhurinsky J, Simcha I, Albanese C, D'Amico M, Pestell R, and Ben-Ze'ev A. 1999. The cyclin D1 gene is a target of the beta-catenin/LEF-1 pathway. *Proc NatlAcad Sci U S A* 96 (10): 5522-5527.

Shulewitz M, Soloviev I, Wu T, Koeppen H, Polakis P, and Sakanaka C. 2006. Repressor roles for TCF-4 and Sfrp1 in Wnt signaling in breast cancer. *Oncogene* 25 (31): 4361-4369.

Simonet WS, Lacey DL, Dunstan CR, Kelley M, Chang MS, Lüthy R, Nguyen HQ, Wooden S, Bennett L, Boone T, Shimamoto G, DeRose M, Elliott R, Colombero A, Tan HL, Trail G, Sullivan J, Davy E, Bucay N, Renshaw-Gegg L, Hughes TM, Hill D, Pattison W, Campbell P, Sander S, Van G, Tarpley J, Derby P, Lee R, and Boyle WJ. 1997. Osteoprotegerin: A novel secreted protein involved in the regulation of bone density. *Cell* 89 (2): 309-319.

Smallwood PM, Williams J, Xu Q, Leahy DJ, and Nathans J. 2007. Mutational analysis of Norrin-Frizzled4 recognition. *J Biol Chem* 282 (6): 4057-4068.

Sophos NA and Vasiliou V. 2002. Aldehyde dehydrogenase gene superfamily: the 2002 update. *Chem Biol Interact* 143-144: 5-22.

Steinert PM and Roop DR. 1988. Molecular and cellular biology of intermediate filaments. *Annu Rev Biochem* 57: 593-625.

Suda T, Takahashi N, Udagawa N, Jimi E, Gillespie MT, and Martin TJ. 1999. Modulation of osteoclast differentiation and function by the new members of the tumor necrosis factor receptor and ligand families. *Endocr Rev* 20 (3): 345-357.

Surmann-Schmitt C, Widmann N, Dietz U, Saeger B, Eitzinger N, Nakamura Y, Rattel M, Latham R, Hartmann C, von der Mark H, Schett G, von der Mark K, and StockM. 2009. Wif-1 is expressed at cartilage-mesenchyme interfaces and impedes Wnt3a-mediated inhibition of chondrogenesis. *J Cell Sci* 122 (Pt 20): 3627-3637.

Suzuki H, Toyota M, Carraway H, Gabrielson E, Ohmura T, Fujikane T, Nishikawa N, Sogabe Y, Nojima M, Sonoda T, Mori M, Hirata K, Imai K, Shinomura Y, Baylin SB, and Tokino T. 2008. Frequent epigenetic inactivation of Wnt antagonist genes in breast cancer. *Br J Cancer* 98 (6): 1147-1156.

Takada R, Satomi Y, Kurata T, Ueno N, Norioka S, Kondoh H, Takao T, and Takada S. 2006. Monounsaturated fatty acid modification of Wnt protein: its role in Wntsecretion. *Dev Cell* 11 (6): 791-801.

Tamai K, Semenov M, Kato Y, Spokony R, Liu C, Katsuyama Y, Hess F, Saint-Jeannet JP, and He X. 2000. LDL-receptor-related proteins in Wnt signal transduction. *Nature*. 407 (6803): 530-535.

Tamai K, Zeng X, Liu C, Zhang X, Harada Y, Chang Z, and He X. 2004. A mechanism for Wnt coreceptor activation. *Mol Cell* 13 (1): 149-156.

Tanei T, Morimoto K, Shimazu K, Kim SJ, Tanji Y, Taguchi T, Tamaki Y, and Noguchi S. 2009. Association of breast cancer stem cells identified by aldehyde dehydrogenase 1expression with resistance to sequential Paclitaxel and epirubicin-based chemotherapy for breast cancers. *Clin Cancer Res* 15 (12): 4234-4241.

Teissedre B, Pinderhughes A, Incassati A, Hatsell SJ, Hiremath M, and Cowin P. 2009. MMTV-Wnt1 and -DeltaN89beta-catenin induce canonical signaling in distinctprogenitors and differentially activate Hedgehog signaling within mammary tumors. *PLoS One* 4 (2): e4537.

Tetsu O and McCormick F. 1999. Beta-catenin regulates expression of cyclin D1 in colon carcinoma cells. *Nature* 398 (6726): 422-426.

Ting AH, McGarvey KM, and Baylin SB. 2006. The cancer epigenome--components and functional correlates. *Genes Dev* 20 (23): 3215-3231.

Tolwinski NS, Wehrli M, Rives A, Erdeniz N, DiNardo S, and Wieschaus E. 2003. Wg/Wnt signal can be transmitted through arrow/LRP5,6 and Axin independently of Zw3/Gsk3beta activity. *Dev Cell* 4 (3): 407-418.

Topol L, Jiang X, Choi H, Garrett-Beal L, Carolan PJ, and Yang Y. 2003. Wnt-5a inhibits the canonical Wnt pathway by promoting GSK-3-independent beta-catenin degradation. *J Cell Biol* 162 (5): 899-908.

Tsukamoto AS, Grosschedl R, Guzman RC, Parslow T, and Varmus HE. 1988. Expression of theint-1 gene in transgenic mice is associated with mammary gland hyperplasia and adenocarcinomas in male and female mice. *Cell* 55 (4): 619-625.

Ugolini F, Adélaïde J, Charafe-Jauffret E, Nguyen C, Jacquemier J, Jordan B, Birnbaum D, and Pébusque MJ. 1999. Differential expression assay of chromosome arm 8p genesidentifies Frizzled-related (FRP1/FRZB) and Fibroblast Growth Factor Receptor 1 (FGFR1) as candidate breast cancer genes. *Oncogene* 18 (10): 1903-1910.

Ugolini F, Charafe-Jauffret E, Bardou VJ, Geneix J, Adélaïde J, Labat-Moleur F, Penault-Llorca F, Longy M, Jacquemier J, Birnbaum D, and Pébusque MJ. 2001. WNT pathway and mammary carcinogenesis: loss of expression of candidate tumor suppressor gene SFRP1 in most invasive carcinomas except of the medullary type. *Oncogene* 20 (41): 5810-5817.

Uren A, Reichsman F, Anest V, Taylor WG, Muraiso K, Bottaro DP, Cumberledge S, and Rubin JS. 2000. Secreted frizzled-related protein-1 binds directly to Wingless and is abiphasic modulator of Wnt signaling. *J Biol Chem* 275 (6): 4374-4382.

Van Meurs JB, Rivadeneira F, Jhamai M, Hugens W, Hofman A, van Leeuwen JP, Pols HA, and Uitterlinden AG. 2006. Common genetic variation of the low-density lipoprotein receptor-related protein 5 and 6 genes determines fracture risk in elderly white men. *J Bone Miner Res* 21 (1): 141-150.

Van Wesenbeeck L, Cleiren E, Gram J, Beals RK, Bénichou O, Scopelliti D, Key L, Renton T, Bartels C, Gong Y, Warman ML, De Vernejoul MC, Bollerslev J, and Van Hul W. 2003. Six novel missense mutations in the LDL receptor-related protein 5 (LRP5) gene in different conditions with an increased bone density. *Am J Hum Genet* 72 (3): 763-771.

Veeck J, Geisler C, Noetzel E, Alkaya S, Hartmann A, Knüchel R, and Dahl E. 2008. Epigenetic inactivation of the secreted frizzled-related protein-5 (SFRP5) genein human breast cancer is associated with unfavorable prognosis. *Carcinogenesis* 29 (5): 991-998.

Veeck J, Niederacher D, An H, Klopocki E, Wiesmann F, Betz B, Galm O, Camara O, Dürst M, Kristiansen G, Huszka C, Knüchel R, and Dahl E. 2006. Aberrant methylation ofthe Wnt antagonist SFRP1 in breast cancer is associated with unfavourable prognosis. *Oncogene* 25 (24): 3479-3488.

Veeck J, Noetzel E, Bektas N, Jost E, Hartmann A, Knüchel R, and Dahl E. 2008. Promoter hypermethylation of the SFRP2 gene is a high-frequent alteration and tumor-specific epigenetic marker in human breast cancer. *Mol Cancer* 7: 83.

Veeck J and Esteller M. 2010. Breast cancer epigenetics: from DNA methylation to microRNAs. *J Mammary Gland Biol Neoplasia* 15 (1): 5-17.

Vinson CR and Adler PN. 1987. Directional non-cell autonomy and the transmission of polarity information by the frizzled gene of Drosophila. *Nature* 329 (6139): 549-551.

Vinson CR, Conover S, and Adler PN. 1989. A Drosophila tissue polarity locus encodes a protein containing seven potential transmembrane domains. *Nature* 338 (6212): 63-64.

Voorzanger-Rousselot N, Goehrig D, Journe F, Doriath V, Body JJ, Clézardin P, and Garnero P. 2007. Increased Dickkopf-1 expression in breast cancer bone metastases. *Br J Cancer* 97 (7): 964-970.

Wang FS, Ko JY, Lin CL, Wu HL, Ke HJ, and Tai PJ. 2007a. Knocking down dickkopf-1 alleviates estrogen deficiency induction of bone loss. A histomorphological study in ovariectomized rats. *Bone* 40 (2): 485-492

Wang Y and Nathans J. 2007b. Tissue/planar cell polarity in vertebrates: new insights and new questions. *Development* 134 (4): 647-658.

Wang PS, Chou FS, Bloomston M, Vonau MS, Saji M, Espinosa A, and Pinzone JJ. 2009. Thiazolidinediones downregulate Wnt/beta-catenin signaling via multiplemechanisms in breast cancer cells. *J Surg Res* 153 (2): 210-216.

Wehrli M, Dougan ST, Caldwell K, O'Keefe L, Schwartz S, Vaizel-Ohayon D, Schejter E, Tomlinson A, and DiNardo S. 2000. Arrow encodes an LDL-receptor-related protein essential for Wingless signaling. *Nature* 407 (6803): 527-530.

Wei Q, Yokota C, Semenov MV, Doble B, Woodgett J, and He X. 2007. R-spondin1 is a high affinity ligand for LRP6 and induces LRP6 phosphorylation and beta-catenin signaling. *J Biol Chem* 282 (21): 15903-15911.

Welm BE, Tepera SB, Venezia T, Graubert TA, Rosen JM, and Goodell MA. 2002. Sca-1(pos) cells in the mouse mammary gland represent an enriched progenitor cell population. *Dev Biol* 245 (1): 42-56.

Wielenga VJ, Smits R, Korinek V, Smit L, Kielman M, Fodde R, Clevers H, and Pals ST. 1999. Expression of CD44 in Apc and Tcf mutant mice implies regulation by the WNTpathway. *Am J Pathol* 154 (2): 515-523.

Wielenga VJ, van der Neut R, Offerhaus GJ, and Pals ST. 2000. CD44 glycoproteins in colorectal cancer: expression, function, and prognostic value. *Adv Cancer Res* 77: 169-187.

Wissmann C, Wild PJ, Kaiser S, Roepcke S, Stoehr R, Woenckhaus M, Kristiansen G, Hsieh JC, Hofstaedter F, Hartmann A, Knuechel R, Rosenthal A, and Pilarsky C. 2003. WIF1, a component of the Wnt pathway, is down-regulated in prostate, breast, lung, and bladder cancer. *J Pathol* 201 (2): 204-212.

Wong GT, Gavin BJ, and McMahon AP. 1994. Differential transformation of mammary epithelial cells by Wnt genes. *Mol Cell Biol* 14 (9): 6278-6286.

Woodward WA, Chen MS, Behbod F, Alfaro MP, Buchholz TA, and Rosen JM. 2007. WNT/beta-catenin mediates radiation resistance of mouse mammary progenitor cells. *Proc Natl Acad Sci U S A.* 104 (2): 618-623.

Wu W, Glinka A, Delius H, and Niehrs C. 2000. Mutual antagonism between dickkopf1 and dickkopf2 regulates Wnt/beta-catenin signalling. *Curr Biol* 10 (24): 1611-1614.

Xu Q, Wang Y, Dabdoub A, Smallwood PM, Williams J, Woods C, Kelley MW, Jiang L, Tasman W, Zhang K, and Nathans J. 2004. Vascular development in the retina and innerear: control by Norrin and Frizzled-4, a high-affinity ligand-receptor pair. *Cell* 116 (6): 883-895.

Yamamoto S, Nishimura O, Misaki K, Nishita M, Minami Y, Yonemura S, Tarui H, and Sasaki H. 2008. Cthrc1 selectively activates the planar cell polarity pathway of Wnt signaling by stabilizing the Wnt-receptor complex. *Dev Cell* 15 (1): 23-36.

Yasuda H, Shima N, Nakagawa N, Yamaguchi K, Kinosaki M, Mochizuki S, Tomoyasu A, Yano K, Goto M, Murakami A, Tsuda E, Morinaga T, Higashio K, Udagawa N, Takahashi N, and Suda T. 1998. Osteoclast differentiation factor is a ligand for osteoprotegerin/osteoclastogenesis-inhibitory factor and is identical to TRANCE/RANKL. *Proc Natl Acad Sci. U S A* 95 (7): 3597-3602.

Yoneda T. 1998. Cellular and molecular mechanisms of breast and prostate cancer metastasis to bone. *Eur J Cancer* 34 (2): 240-245.

Yook JI, Li XY, Ota I, Hu C, Kim HS, Kim NH, Cha SY, Ryu JK, Choi YJ, Kim J, Fearon ER, and Weiss SJ. 2006. A Wnt-Axin2-GSK3beta cascade regulates Snail1 activity inbreast cancer cells. *Nat Cell Biol* 8 (12): 1398-1406.

Yoshida A, Rzhetsky A, Hsu LC, and Chang C. 1998. Human aldehyde dehydrogenase gene family. *Eur J Biochem* 251 (3): 549-557.

Yu HM, Jerchow B, Sheu TJ, Liu B, Costantini F, Puzas JE, Birchmeier W, and Hsu W. 2005. The role of Axin2 in calvarial morphogenesis and craniosynostosis. *Development* 132 (8): 1995-2005.

Zardawi SJ, O'Toole SA, Sutherland RL, and Musgrove EA. 2009. Dysregulation of Hedgehog, Wnt and Notch signalling pathways in breast cancer. *Histol Histopathol* 24 (3): 385-398.

Zeng X, Tamai K, Doble B, Li S, Huang H, Habas R, Okamura H, Woodgett J, and He X. 2005. A dual-kinase mechanism for Wnt co-receptor phosphorylation and activation. *Nature* 438 (7069): 873-877.

Zhang Y, Wang Y, Li X, Zhang J, Mao J, Li Z, Zheng J, Li L, Harris S, and Wu D. 2004. The LRP5 high-bone-mass G171V mutation disrupts LRP5 interaction with Mesd. *Mol Cell Biol* 24 (11): 4677-4684.

Zhang J, Li Y, Liu Q, Lu W, and Bu G. 2010. Wnt signaling activation and mammary gland hyperplasia in MMTV-LRP6 transgenic mice: implication for breast cancertumorigenesis. *Oncogene* 29 (4): 539-549.

29

Interactions of STAP-2 with BRK and STAT3/5 in Breast Cancer Cells

Osamu Ikeda, Yuichi Sekine and Tadashi Matsuda
Department of Immunology, Graduate School of Pharmaceutical Sciences, Hokkaido University, Sapporo, Japan

1. Introduction

A number of molecular markers have recently been identified that may have prognostic value in breast cancer, and among the most notable of these are the estrogen receptor (ER) and the progesterone receptor (PR). ER/PR-positive breast cancer patients (60–80%) are hormone-responsive and therefore have a significantly better prognosis compared with ER/PR-negative patients (Clark and McGuire, 1983; Early Breast Cancer Trialists' Collaborative Group, 2005; Thorpe, 1988). However, approximately 50% of patients with advanced disease do not respond to endocrine therapy (Normanno et al., 2005).

Another well-known prognostic marker is epidermal growth factor receptor-2 (ErbB2; also known as HER2), which is a member of the epidermal growth factor receptor (EGFR) family. In approximately 30% of human breast cancers, ErbB2 is present at levels significantly above those found in normal cells (Hynes and Stern, 1994; Stern, 2000; Yarden, 2001). Recent studies have indicated that ErbB2 plays important roles in malignant transformation and tumorigenesis (Hudziak et al., 1987; Slamon et al., 1987, 1989). Therefore, breast cancer tumors that involve large amounts of ErbB2 protein are correlated with poor clinical outcomes (Menard et al., 2001). Herceptin (also known as Trastuzumab), a humanized monoclonal antibody against the extracellular domain of ErbB2, is used to treat patients expressing high levels of ErbB2. Although Herceptin significantly decreases the rates of breast cancer recurrence and mortality (Piccart-Gebhart et al., 2005; Slamon et al., 2001; Ward et al., 2009), almost 50% of patients with the ErbB2-amplified tumors do not respond to this treatment and develop resistance to the drug (Slamon et al., 2006).

Conversely, tumors with neither hormone receptor expression nor ErbB2 amplification are classified as triple-negative (TN) tumors (Sorlie et al., 2003). TN tumors are an aggressive subtype of breast cancer that account for approximately 15% of breast cancer cases. The TN tumor shows a higher histologic grade, and a worse prognosis compared with that of hormone receptor-positive or ErbB2-positive tumors (Dent et al., 2007; Liedtke et al., 2008). Therapeutically, despite being highly chemosensitive, their progression-free time is generally short (Dent et al., 2007; Liedtke et al., 2008), and TN tumors develop resistance to endocrine therapy and Herceptin, illustrating the urgent need for novel therapeutic strategies. Recently, new potential therapeutic targets for this type of breast cancer have been discovered, including poly-(ADP-ribose)-polymerase 1

(Bryant et al., 2005; Evers et al., 2008; Tutt et al., 2009), vascular endothelial growth factor receptor (Mendel et al., 2003), EGFR (Corkery et al., 2009; Pal and Mortimer, 2009), SRC tyrosine kinase (Conlin and Seidman, 2008; Finn, R.S., 2007), mammalian target of rapamycin (Saal et al., 2005), heat shock protein 90 (Caldas-Lopes et al., 2009), breast tumor kinase (BRK) and signal transducing adaptor protein-2 (STAP-2) (Mitchel et al., 2000; Ikeda et al., 2009, 2010, 2011).
STAP-2 is a recently identified adaptor protein, which contains pleckstrin homology (PH) and Src homology 2 (SH2)-like domains, as well as a signal transducer and activator of transcription 3 (STAT3)-binding motif in its C-terminal region (Minoguchi et al., 2003). Importantly, human STAP-2 was originally identified as BKS and is a substrate for BRK, a non-receptor protein tyrosine kinase (PTK) known alternatively as protein tyrosine kinase 6 (PTK6) (Mitchell et al., 2000). BRK is highly expressed in human breast cancer cells (Barker et al., 1997). Recently, STAP-2, STAT3, and STAT5A/B have been identified as BRK substrates. However, the molecular mechanism by which the STAP-2-BRK-STAT3/5 axis participates in the tumorigenesis in breast cancer remains poorly characterized. In this review, we focus on the STAP-2-BRK-STAT3/5 axis as a potential therapeutic target and/or prognostic marker and demonstrate a functional link between STAP-2 and BRK/STAT3/5-mediated transcriptional activation and cell growth in human breast cancer cells.

2. STAP-2

2.1 Structure and expression

Human STAP-2 is the first identified substrate for the BRK non-receptor tyrosine kinase (Mitchell et al., 2000). We also cloned murine STAP-2 as a c-*fms* interacting protein (Minoguchi et al., 2003). PTKs play an important role in regulating cell growth, differentiation, and transformation. Activated receptor tyrosine kinases trans-phosphorylate several tyrosines in their cytoplasmic domains, providing recognition sites for various adaptor and effector proteins in multiple signal transduction pathways. Adaptor proteins often function as inter- or intra-molecular bridges and thereby play an important role in the assembly of larger protein complexes or in the stabilization of certain conformational states. They also utilize their functional domains, such as SH2 and SH3 domains, to mediate interactions that link various proteins involved in signal transduction.
STAP-1 was cloned as a c-kit-interacting protein and bears high sequence and structural similarity to its sister protein, STAP-2 (Masuhara et al., 2000) (Fig. 1A). Both STAP-1 and STAP-2 contain an N-terminal PH domain and a region weakly related to an SH2 domain (overall 33% amino acid identity). The N-terminal PH domains of the STAP proteins share 36% amino acid identity and 58% similarity. In the absence of stimulation, over-expressed STAP-2 protein localizes throughout the cytoplasm and nucleus in A431 epidermoid carcinoma cells, but translocates to the plasma membrane following stimulation of EGFR. A mutant STAP-2 lacking the N-terminal PH domain (ΔPH) fails to localize at the plasma membrane, demonstrating that the PH domain of STAP-2 is necessary and sufficient for plasma membrane recruitment by EGFR stimulation.
The central region of STAP-2 is distantly related to the SH2 domain. This region of STAP-2 shares 40% sequence identity with that of STAP-1 and 29% sequence identity with the SH2 domain of human phospholipase C-γ2. However, STAP-2 has a C-terminal proline-rich

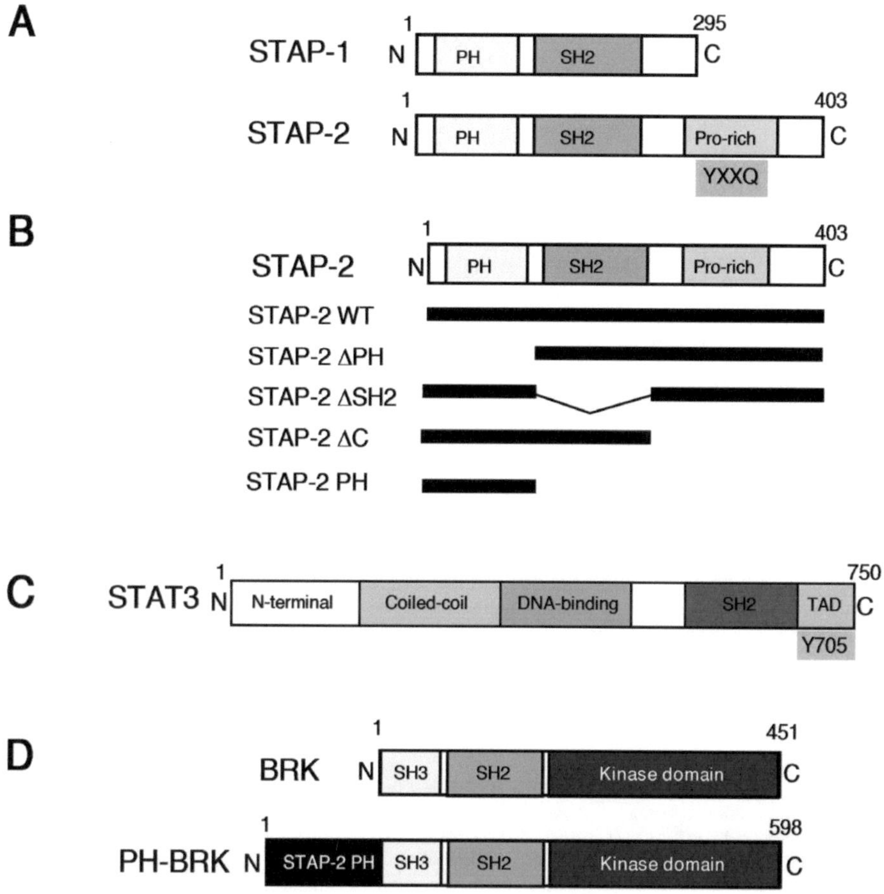

Fig. 1. Schematic diagrams of the domain structures of the STAP-1 (A), STAP-2 (A, B), STAT3 (C), BRK and the STAP-2 PH-BRK fusion protein (D).

region and a STAT3-binding motif, YXXQ, both of which are absent from STAP-1. Cytokine receptors commonly utilize a YXXQ motif in their cytoplasmic regions to recruit and activate STAT3 (Hirano et al., 2000). STAP-2 is expressed in a variety of tissues and cells such as lymphocytes, macrophages and hepatocytes (Minoguchi et al., 2003), and its abundant expression pattern (Fig. 2A) suggests that STAP-2 influences a variety of signaling or transcriptional molecules. STAP-1, however, shows a more restricted expression pattern, being located predominantly in hematopoietic cells (Masuhara et al., 2000). Notably, STAP-2 is constitutively expressed in macrophages, and the 5′ region of the STAP-2 genomic sequence contains several potential binding sites for c-Rel, AP-1, p65/NF-κB and STATs. In the murine myeloid leukemia cell line, M1, STAP-2 mRNA expression is strongly induced by LIF in parallel with its differentiation into macrophages. These expression patterns of STAP-2 support a paradigm whereby STAP-2 in macrophages mediates signals for acute-phase responses after infection. Indeed, LPS- or IL-6-stimulated induction of acute phase protein genes was significantly decreased in STAP-2-deficient hepatocytes (Minoguchi et al., 2003).

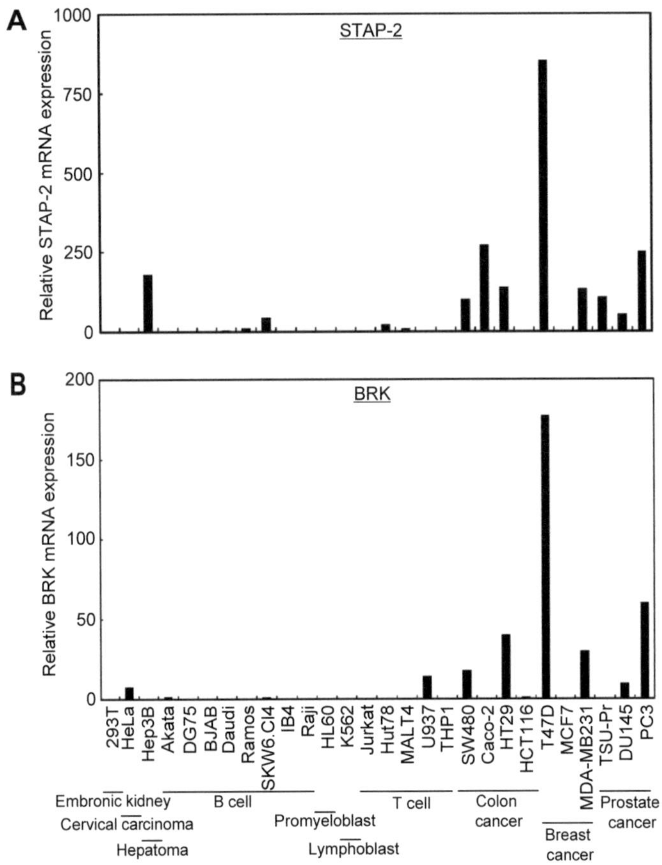

Fig. 2. Expression profile of STAP-2 and BRK. Expression of STAP-2 and BRK in a variety of human cell lines (A, B). Total RNA samples isolated from these cells were also subjected to quantitative real-time PCR analysis using *STAP-2* and *BRK* primers. Data represent the levels of these mRNA normalized to that of an *ACTIN* internal control and are expressed relative to the value of 293T samples. Shown is a representative experiment, which was repeated at least three times with similar results.

2.2 Interacting proteins

Recently, many STAP-2 binding partners have been identified. As summarized in Table 1, STAP-2 interacts with, and modulates the function of, several signaling molecules including STAT3/5- (Minoguchi et al., 2003; Sekine et al., 2005), FcεRI- (Yamamoto et al., 2003), M-CSFR/c-FMS- (Ikeda et al., 2007) and Toll-like receptor-mediated signals (Sekine et al., 2006). STAP-2 interacts with STAT3 through the C-terminal YXXQ motif and enhances STAT3 transcriptional activity. STAP-2 also interacts with STAT5 through its PH and SH2-like domains. It is noteworthy that thymocytes and peripheral T cells from STAP-2-deficient mice show enhanced IL-2- or TCR-dependent cell growth (Sekine et al., 2005). STAP-2 positively regulates LPS/TLR4-mediated signals in macrophages. STAP-2, particularly its SH2-like domain, binds to both MyD88 and IKK-α/β, but not to TRAF6 or IRAK1, and forms a functional complex composed of MyD88-STAP-2-IKK- α/β. These interactions augment MyD88- and/or IKK–α/β-dependent signals, leading to enhancement of NF-κB activity (Sekine et al., 2006).

Interacting protein	Domain or region	References
BRK	PH, (SH2-like)	Ikeda et al., 2009, 2010, 2011; Mitchel et al., 2000
STAT3	YXXQ motif, (SH2-like)	Ikeda et al., 2010; Minoguchi et al., 2003
STAT5A/B	PH, SH2-like	Sekine et al., 2005
c-Fms	PH, (SH2-like)	Ikeda et al., 2007
PLCγ1/2	SH2-like, C-terminal	Yamamoto et al., 2003
MyD88	SH2-like	Sekine et al., 2006
IKKα/β	SH2-like	Sekine et al., 2006
LMP1	PH, SH2-like	Ikeda et al., 2008
TRAF1	Not determined	Ikeda et al., 2008
TRAF3	PH, SH2-like	Ikeda et al., 2008
FAK	SH2-like	Sekine et al., 2007
Cbl	PH, SH2-like	Sekine et al., 2007
Vav1	SH2-like, C-terminal	Sekine et al., 2009
Rac1	Not determined	Sekine et al., 2009

Table 1. STAP-2 interacting proteins.

M-CSFR/c-FMS directly interacts with the PH domain of STAP-2 independently following M-CSF-stimulation (Ikeda et al., 2007). STAP-2 regulates M-CSF-induced tyrosine phosphorylation of M-CSFR/c-FMS as well as the activation of Akt and extracellular signal regulated kinase. In addition, over-expression of STAP-2 results in the impairment of migration in response to M-CSF and of the wound-healing process in macrophages. This demonstrates that STAP-2 directly binds to M-CSFR/c-FMS and interferes with PI3K signaling, leading to macrophage motility. In T cells, STAP-2 enhances Cbl-dependent degradation of FAK and downregulates integrin/FAK-mediated cell adhesion to fibronectin (Sekine et al., 2007). Furthermore, STAP-2 constitutively interacts with, and enhances the tyrosine phosphorylation of, a GDP/GTP exchange factor, Vav1, and also binds to a small GTPase, Rac1 (Sekine et al., 2009). These interactions control chemokine-induced chemotaxis of T cells.

STAP-2 also interacts with Epstein-Barr virus (EBV)-derived latent membrane protein 1 (LMP1) and negatively regulates LMP1-induced NF-κB activation (Ikeda et al., 2008). EBV is linked to the development of multiple malignancies, including post-transplant lymphoma, Hodgkin disease, and nasopharyngeal carcinoma (Thorley-Lawson, 2001). EBV-LMP1 is expressed in many EBV-associated tumor cells and is responsible for most of their altered cellular growth properties (Brinkmann and Schulz, 2006). STAP-2 associates with LMP1 through the PH and SH-2-like domains, and this interaction occurs physiologically in EBV-positive human B cells. STAP-2 regulates LMP1-mediated NF-κB signaling through direct or indirect interactions with TRAF3 and TRADD. Importantly, STAP-2 mRNA is induced by expression of LMP1 in human B cells, and transient expression of STAP-2 in EBV-positive human B cells decreases cell growth. These data suggest that STAP-2 responds to EBV infection and acts as an endogenous negative regulator of EBV-LMP1-mediated signaling through TRAF3 and TRADD.

3. BRK

3.1 Structure and expression

BRK was originally isolated from a metastatic breast carcinoma (Mitchell et al., 1994). An identical protein was independently cloned as a highly-expressed protein tyrosine kinase, PTK6, from human melanocytes (Lee et al., 1993). In addition, *Ptk6* (previously termed Sik), a cDNA for the mouse ortholog that has 80% amino acid identity to BRK/PTK6, was also cloned from mouse intestinal crypt cells (Siyanova et al., 1994). BRK displays approximately 56% homology to the kinase domain of c-Src and a similar domain arrangement (Serfas and Tyner, 2003). BRK is a 451 amino acid protein that contains an SH3 domain, an SH2 domain and a tyrosine kinase catalytic domain, but lacks an N-terminal myristoylation site for membrane targeting (Serfas and Tyner, 2003). BRK is expressed in many malignancies, such as colon and prostate tumors and metastatic melanomas (Derry et al., 2003; Easty et al., 1997; Llor et al., 1999; Schmandt et al., 2006). BRK expression is also detected in a large proportion of human mammary gland tumors, but is not expressed in normal mammary gland (Barker et al., 1997). In normal tissues, BRK expression is developmentally regulated and restricted to differentiating epithelial cells in a range of tissues including small intestine and colon (Vasioukhin et al., 1995; Haegebarth et al., 2005, 2006) (Fig. 2B).

3.2 Substrates, interacting proteins and activation

Several BRK-interacting proteins or substrates have been identified (Table 2). BRK substrates include RNA-binding proteins (Sam68 (Coyle et al., 2003; Derry et al., 2000; Lukong et al., 2005), SLM-1/2 (Haegebarth et al., 2004), and the polypyrimidine tract-binding protein-associated splicing factor (PSF) (Lukong et al., 2009)), transcription factors (STAT3 (Liu et al., 2006) and STAT5A/B (Weaver and Silva, 2007)), adaptor molecules (STAP-2) (Mitchell et al., 2000), and a variety of signaling molecules (paxillin (Chen et al., 2004), p190RhoGAP (Shen et al., 2008), kinesin-associated protein 3A (KAP3A) (Lukong and Richard, 2008), Akt (Zhang et al., 2005), β-catenin (Palka-Hamblin et al., 2010), and ARAP1 (Arf-GAP, Rho-GAP, ankyrin repeat and PH domain-containing protein 1; also known as centaurin δ-2) (Kang et al., 2010)). Although BRK expression is known to induce tyrosine phosphorylation in some of these, similar actions in others have yet to be confirmed.

Sam68 is the most extensively studied BRK substrate. BRK expression suppressed cell proliferation through EGFR-mediated phosphorylation of Sam68 in a human breast cancer cell line (Coyle et al., 2003; Derry et al., 2000; Lukong et al., 2005). Similarly, BRK phosphorylates the Sam68-like mammalian proteins, SLM-1 and SLM-2, and negatively regulates their RNA-binding functions (Haegebarth et al., 2004). Downstream of EGFR, PSF is a BRK substrate, and this tyrosine phosphorylation of PSF induces cytoplasmic relocalization, impairment of its binding to polypyrimidine RNA, and cell cycle arrest (Lukong et al., 2009). Furthermore, BRK expression promotes cell migration and tumor invasion by phosphorylating the focal adhesion protein, paxillin, followed by activation of the small GTPase, Rac1, *via* the function of CrkII (Chen et al., 2004). BRK also phosphorylates p190RhoGAP-A (regulating the small GTPases, RhoA and Ras, and promoting breast malignancy) (Shen et al., 2008); a kinesin-2 subunit, KAP3A (promoting cell migration) (Lukong and Richard, 2008); and Akt (regulating basal Akt activity in normal cells) (Zhang et al., 2005).

Substrate	Function	Phosphorylation site	References
SAM68	Cell cycle	Y345, Y434, Y440	Coyle et al., 2003; Derry et al., 2000; Lukong et al., 2005
SLM-1/SLM-2	Not validated	Not determined	Haegebarth et al., 2004
PSF	Cell cycle	C-terminus	Lukong et al., 2009
STAT3	Cell cycle	Y705	Liu et al., 2006
STAT5A/B	Cell cycle	Y694/Y699	Weaver and Silva, 2007
STAP-2/BKS	Cell growth	Y250	Ikeda et al., 2009; Mitchel et al., 2000
Paxillin	Migration	Y31, Y118	Chen et al., 2004
p190RhoGAP	Migration	Y1109	Shen et al., 2008
KAP3A	Migration	C-terminus	Lukong and Richard, 2008
Akt	Intestinal epithelial cell differentiation	Not determined	Zhang et al., 2005
beta-catenin	Cell growth	Y64, Y142, Y331, Y333	Palka-Hamblin et al., 2010
ARAP1/centaurin-2	Regulation of EGFR internalization	Y231	Kang et al., 2010
BRK	Regulation of kinase activity	Y13, Y61, Y66, Y114, Y342, Y351	Qiu and Miller, 2002

Table 2. BRK substrates.

Mice deficient in the BRK murine ortholog, Sik, show increased cell proliferation, decreased apoptosis, and increased levels of activated Akt in the small intestine (Haegebarth et al., 2006), suggesting a role for BRK in differentiation of epithelial cells of the small intestine. This is further implied by the evidence that BRK directly phosphorylates and inhibits β-catenin, interrupting T-cell factor-mediated transcription in the intestine, and indicating that BRK may be a negative regulator of the Wnt-signaling pathway (Palka-Hamblin et al., 2010).

BRK may contribute to tumorigenesis by modulating EGF/EGFR signaling. It phosphorylates ARAP1, which results sequentially in inhibition of EGFR internalization, increased duration of EGF/EGFR signaling, and increased oncogenic capacity (Kang et al., 2010). Importantly, over-expression of BRK sensitizes human mammary epithelial cells to EGF and/or heregulin stimuli, and increases anchorage-independent growth (Kamalati et al., 1996, 2000), while down-regulation of BRK also influences EGF- and heregulin-induced cell proliferation. These observations suggest that BRK is involved in signaling induced by members of the EGFR family (Ostrander et al., 2007). Notably, BRK interacts with additional ErbB family members (ErbB2, ErbB3, and ErbB4) as well as EGFR (ErbB1) (Kamalati et al., 1996; Aubele et al., 2007; Xiang et al., 2008). BRK is co-amplified with ErbB2 to promote proliferation and confer resistance to lapatinib, an ErbB2 kinase inhibitor in breast cancer (Xiang et al., 2008), suggesting that BRK is a potential target in ErbB2-positive breast cancer.

As mentioned above, BRK kinase activity is promoted by ligands for the ErbB receptor, such as EGF and heregulin. However, it is also activated by the expression of ErbB2 even in the absence of ligands, and by other stimuli such as IGF-1 (Qiu et al., 2005), calcium and ionomycin (Vasioukhin and Tyner, 1997; Wang et al., 2005), fetal bovine serum (Zhang et al., 2005), and osteopontin (Chakraborty et al., 2008). BRK activation occurs under the conditions already described, but also during keratinocyte differentiation, together with upregulation of expression (Wang et al., 2005).

The mechanism of regulation of BRK kinase activity is similar to SRC family kinases, with some notable differences. Structural studies reveal that BRK is autophosphorylated at Tyr-13, 61, 66, 114, 351 and 342 (Qiu and Miller, 2002). Tyr-342 (Y342 in BRK and Y416 in SRC) resides within the kinase activation loop, and phosphorylation of this residue increases kinase activity of wild-type (WT) BRK. However, mutation of Tyr-342 to alanine (Y342A) blocks activation of BRK (Qiu and Miller, 2002). In addition, mutation of the C-terminal residue Tyr-447 (Y447 in BRK and Y527 in SRC) to Phe (Y447F) results in a constitutively active kinase (Kamalati et al., 1996). Trp-184 (W184 in BRK and W260 in SRC) lies within the SH2-kinase linker region and, in contrast to SRC family enzymes, has been shown to interact intramolecularly with residues in the BRK kinase domain. The conserved Trp184 to Ala (W184A) mutation completely inhibits kinase activity (Kim and Lee, 2005), as does the substitution of Lys-219 (K219 in BRK and K295 in SRC) with Met (K219M), which destroys the putative ATP binding site of BRK (Kamalati et al., 1996).

Unlike SRC family kinases, BRK lacks myristoylation signals for membrane targeting, allowing it some freedom in its subcellular localization and broadening its range of substrates and interacting proteins. Several studies demonstrate that the function of BRK varies between cell types and may be dependent on expression levels, kinase activity, interaction with substrates or other binding proteins and, significantly, on intracellular localization. Indeed, oncogenic functions of BRK are enhanced by targeting it to the plasma membrane but are abolished if it is modified to remain in the nucleus (Ie Kim and Lee, 2009). BRK expression is detected in both the cytoplasm and nucleus in the normal intestine, skin and oral epithelium, and in breast and colon tumors (Brauer and Tyner, 2010). In normal differentiated prostate epithelium and in well-differentiated prostate tumors, it is detected in the nucleus, but is absent from the nuclei of poorly-differentiated tumors, which may implicate it in differentiation of the prostate (Derry et al., 2003). At the present time, it is not clear how intracellular localization of BRK is regulated. Therefore, further studies are required to confirm the significance of BRK subcellular localization. Indeed, BRK does not contain any nuclear localization or export signal, suggesting that interaction with substrates such as STAP-2 or other interacting proteins may be important in regulating its distribution.

4. Signal transducer and activator of transcription (STAT) 3/5

The signal transducer and activator of transcription (STAT) family is known to mediate cell proliferation, differentiation and survival in immune responses, hematopoiesis, neurogenesis and many other biological processes (Darnell et al., 1994; Ihle, 1996; O'Shea, 1997). Seven different STAT genes have currently been identified in mammals. The encoded proteins vary in length between 750–850 amino acid residues and share 20–50% amino acid sequence identity. As shown in Fig. 1, notable features of STAT proteins are the STAT family DNA binding domain, an SH2 domain and a major tyrosine phosphorylation site at Y705 (STAT3). In general, STAT proteins bind as dimers to DNA target sites with a nine-base-pair (bp) consensus sequence, TTCCGGGAA, and binding constants in the nanomolar range. In unstimulated cells, STATs are present as monomers in the cytoplasm. STATs are activated by phosphorylation at tyrosine residues, which leads to the formation of dimers *via* reciprocal interactions between the SH2 domain of one monomer and the phosphorylated tyrosine of the other. Dimers then translocate to the nucleus where they recognize specific DNA-binding sites and induce target gene transcription. Tyrosine phosphorylation of STATs (Y705 in STAT3, and Y694/Y699 in STAT5A/B, respectively) is normally a transient and tightly regulated process. However, in tumor cells, constitutive activation of STATs is linked to persistent activity of tyrosine kinases, including Janus kinases, Src, EGFR, Bcr-Abl, and many others. These kinases might be activated by cytokines or by structural alterations. For instance, EGFR over-expression and activation may underlie STAT activation in breast, lung and head and neck cancer (Zhang et al., 2004). Constitutive activation or dysregulated expression of STATs is detected in primary tumors and cancer cell lines, including leukemia, multiple myeloma, lymphomas, melanoma and cancers of the breast, skin, lung, ovaries, pancreas, prostate, kidney, thyroid, and head and neck (Desrivieres et al., 2006). Persistent signaling of specific STATs, particularly STAT3 and STAT5, has been demonstrated to directly contribute to oncogenesis by stimulating cell proliferation and preventing apoptosis (Bowman et al., 2000).

5. Interactions of STAP-2 with BRK and STAT3/5

5.1 BRK, STAP-2 and STAT3/5

STAP-2 is the first BRK interacting protein identified and shown to be phosphorylated. STAT3 and STAT5, which play crucial roles in cell proliferation and differentiation, are also believed to be activated by BRK (Liu et al., 2006; Weaver and Silva, 2007). Our previous studies demonstrate that STAP-2 interacts with and influences several signaling molecules, including STAT3 and STAT5. Furthermore, both STATs play fundamental roles in the normal growth and development of the mammary gland (Hennighausen et al., 1997), and are often over-expressed or constitutively-activated in breast cancer tumors (Bowman et al., 2000). It is therefore of key importance to clarify the interactions between BRK, STAP-2, and STAT3/5.

5.2 STAT3/5 activation by BRK and STAP-2

We attempted to elucidate the roles of STAP-2 in BRK-mediated transcriptional activation of STAT3/5 in breast cancer cells. Transient transfection experiments using expression of luciferase (Luc) reporter genes driven by STAT3 (STAT3-Luc) and STAT5 (STAT5-Luc) showed that STAP-2 enhances BRK-mediated activation of STAT3 and STAT5. We showed that co-expression of STAP-2 and BRK increases BRK-mediated STAT3/5 activation compared with BRK expression alone, and small-interfering RNA or short-hairpin RNA-mediated reduction of endogenous STAP-2 expression strongly decreases BRK-mediated STAT3/5 activation in T47D human breast cancer cells. To further clarify the molecular mechanisms underlying BRK/STAP-2-mediated STAT3/5 activation in breast cancer cells, we tested the effect of STAP-2 on BRK-mediated phosphorylation of STAT3/5, which is an important step for transcriptional activation. Phosphorylation of STAT3/5 is markedly enhanced in MCF7 human breast cancer cells overexpressing STAP-2. In addition, constitutive phosphorylation of STAT3/5 in control T47D cells is markedly reduced in STAP-2 knockdown cell clones. These results indicate that STAP-2 plays important roles in BRK-mediated tyrosine phosphorylation of STAT3/5 in breast cancer cells.

5.3 Molecular interactions among STAP-2, STAT3, STAT5 and BRK

We previously reported that STAP-2 binds to several functional molecules. For example, the SH2 domain of STAP-2 interacts with MyD88 and IKKs (Sekine et al., 2006), and the PH and SH2 domains of STAP-2 mediate its association with STAT5 (Sekine et al., 2005), LMP1 and TRAF3 (Ikeda et al., 2008). To assess the functional relationships among BRK, STAP-2 and STAT3/5, we determined the domains of STAP-2 responsible for BRK-mediated STAT3/5 activation. The BRK-mediated STAT3/5-Luc activity is significantly and dose-dependently enhanced by expression of STAP-2 WT and, to a slightly lesser degree, by expression of the mutant STAP-2 ΔSH2 and STAP-2 ΔC genes, which lack the SH2 domain and the C-terminal domain, respectively. Importantly, however, STAP-2 ΔPH (lacking the PH domain) does not elevate STAT3/5-Luc activity mediated by BRK. Similarly, enhanced phosphorylation of

STAT3/5 by BRK is observed in the presence of a construct encoding just the STAP-2 PH domain (STAP-2 PH). These findings indicate that the PH domain of STAP-2 plays an essential role in the BRK-mediated STAT3/5 activation. However, BRK-mediated STAT3/5 phosphorylation is incomplete in the presence of the STAP-2 PH domain compared to that induced by STAP-2 WT, indicating that other domains of STAP-2 may be required for full BRK-mediated STAT3/5 phosphorylation.

5.4 BRK kinase activity and intracellular localization

Aside from differences in phosphorylation profiles, further differences between STAP-2 WT and STAP-2 ΔPH were confirmed with confocal microscopy experiments. STAP-2 WT is distributed throughout the cytoplasm and nucleus, but STAP-2 ΔPH is located mainly in the cytoplasm. Interestingly, BRK distribution is largely consistent with that of STAP-2, being localized in the nucleus only in the presence of STAP-2 WT, and localizing entirely in the cytoplasm when the PH domain of STAP-2 is disrupted (i.e. in the presence of STAP-2 ΔPH). From this, we can conclude that STAP-2, *via* its PH domain, affects BRK distribution, probably because of its effects on the activation state of BRK. To clarify the effect of the STAP-2 PH domain on BRK activation, we used a STAP-2 PH-BRK fusion protein (PH-BRK), in which BRK is fused to the N terminus of STAP-2 PH. PH-BRK shows robust kinase activity compared with BRK WT and induces marked activation and tyrosine phosphorylation of STAT3 in breast cancer cells. Moreover, PH-BRK is mainly localized in the nucleus, although BRK is localized throughout the cytoplasm and nucleus. Therefore, the STAP-2 PH domain controls the kinase activity and localization of BRK and thus regulates BRK-mediated STAT3 activation. Similarly, PH-BRK also activates STAT5 (data not shown).

5.5 Cell growth

STAP-2 knockdown T47D clones grow more slowly than control T47D cells. Reducing the expression of BRK, STAT3, STAT5b, or STAP-2 expression in T47D cells using siRNA causes a significant decrease in cell growth, indicating that these proteins play important roles in T47D cell growth. It is noteworthy that growth is decreased to similar extents in these four T47D cell types. This may suggest that BRK-induced cell growth in T47D cells is largely dependent on STAT3/5 and STAP-2. Notably, the expression of several genes in the STAT3/5-mediated signaling pathway, including SOCS3, C/EBPδ, cyclin D1, and c-Myc, is also reduced by STAP-2 knockdown in T47D cells. Taken together, BRK/STAT3/5-mediated proliferation is a major mechanism for breast cancer cell growth, and STAP-2 plays essential roles in this process.

6. Conclusion

Activation of STAT3/5 by BRK is a critical event during the process of BRK-mediated tumorigenesis in breast cancer cells. Our manipulation of STAP-2 expression revealed essential roles of STAP-2 in this process through complex interactions between BRK, STAP-2 and STAT3/5. In particular, experiments using deletion mutants indicated that the PH domain of STAP-2 is involved in multiple processes including binding between BRK and STAP-2, activation and phosphorylation of STAT3/5, and activation of BRK. These findings suggest a model for how STAP-2 cooperates with BRK to enhance breast cancer growth. Our proposed mechanisms are now illustrated in Fig. 3. Taken together, STAP-2 plays crucial

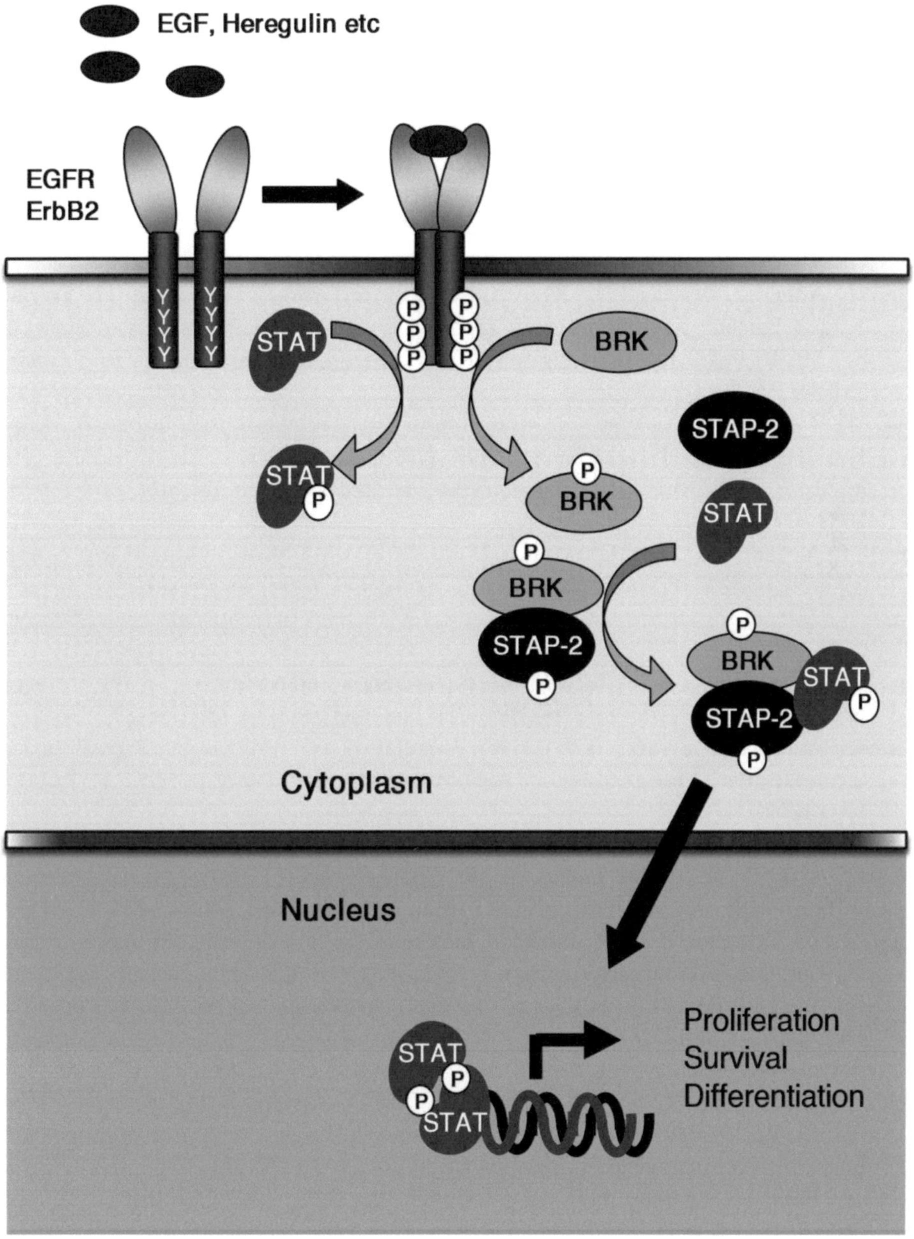

Fig. 3. Schematic showing the proposed function of STAP-2 in BRK-mediated STAT signaling. STAT activation occurs as shown *via* growth factor receptor signaling (EGFR), or nonreceptor tyrosine kinase signaling (BRK). BRK is not required when STATs bind directly to EGFR for activation (upper left), but BRK enhances activation of STATs phosphorylated by EGFR-activated BRK (upper right). In this pathway, STAP-2 can form complex with BRK and STAT, leading to activation of both BRK and STAT. Once activated, STATs dimerize and translocate to the nucleus where they activate the transcription of genes involved in proliferation, survival, and differentiation.

roles in both the BRK/STAT3 and BRK/STAT5 axes, which are major events for BRK-induced breast cancers. Our findings regarding BRK/STAP-2 interactions will therefore be helpful in developing breast cancer treatments. Furthermore, the synergistic effects of BRK and STAP-2 on STAT3/5 activation suggest that evaluating the expression of BRK together with STAP-2 may provide more useful prognostic scores for the outcomes of breast carcinomas than by measuring BRK expression alone.

7. References

Aubele, M., Auer, G., Walch, A.K., Munro, A., Atkinson, M.J., Braselmann, H., Fornander, T., and Bartlett, J.M. (2007). PTK (protein tyrosine kinase)-6 and HER2 and 4, but not HER1 and 3 predict long-term survival in breast carcinomas. *Br J Cancer,* 96, 801-807.

Aubele, M., Walch, A.K., Ludyga, N., Braselmann, H., Atkinson, M.J., Luber, B., Auer, G., Tapio, S., Cooke, T., and Bartlett, J.M. (2008). Prognostic value of protein tyrosine kinase 6 (PTK6) for long-term survival of breast cancer patients. *Br J Cancer,* 99, 1089-1095.

Barker, K.T., Jackson, L.E., and Crompton, M.R. (1997). BRK tyrosine kinase expression in a high proportion of human breast carcinomas. *Oncogene,* 15, 799-805.

Bowman, T., Garcia, R., Turkson, J., and Jove, R. (2000). STATs in oncogenesis. *Oncogene,* 19, 2474-2488.

Brauer, P.M., and Tyner, A.L. (2010). Building a better understanding of the intracellular tyrosine kinase PTK6 - BRK by BRK. *Biochim Biophys Acta,* 1806, 66-73.

Brinkmann, M.M., and Schulz, T.F. (2006). Regulation of intracellular signalling by the terminal membrane proteins of members of the Gammaherpesvirinae. *J Gen Virol,* 87, 1047-1074.

Bryant, H.E., Schultz, N., Thomas, H.D., Parker, K.M., Flower, D., Lopez, E., Kyle, S., Meuth, M., Curtin, N.J., and Helleday, T. (2005). Specific killing of BRCA2-deficient tumours with inhibitors of poly(ADP-ribose) polymerase. *Nature,* 434, 913-917.

Caldas-Lopes, E., Cerchietti, L., Ahn, J.H., Clement, C.C., Robles, A.I., Rodina, A., Moulick, K., Taldone, T., Gozman, A., Guo, Y., Wu, N., de Stanchina, E., White, J., Gross, S.S., Ma, Y., Varticovski, L., Melnick, A., and Chiosis, G. (2009). Hsp90 inhibitor PU-H71, a multimodal inhibitor of malignancy, induces complete responses in triple-negative breast cancer models. *Proc Natl Acad Sci U S A,* 106, 8368-8373.

Chakraborty, G., Jain, S., and Kundu, G.C. (2008). Osteopontin promotes vascular endothelial growth factor-dependent breast tumor growth and angiogenesis via autocrine and paracrine mechanisms. *Cancer Res,* 68, 152-161.

Chen, H.Y., Shen, C.H., Tsai, Y.T., Lin, F.C., Huang, Y.P., and Chen, R.H. (2004). Brk activates rac1 and promotes cell migration and invasion by phosphorylating paxillin. *Mol Cell Biol,* 24, 10558-10572.

Clark, G.M., and McGuire, W.L. (1983). Prognostic factors in primary breast cancer. *Breast Cancer Res Treat,* 3 Suppl, S69-72.

Conlin, A.K., and Seidman, A.D. (2008). Beyond cytotoxic chemotherapy for the first-line treatment of HER2-negative, hormone-insensitive metastatic breast cancer: current status and future opportunities. *Clin Breast Cancer,* 8, 215-223.

Corkery, B., Crown, J., Clynes, M., and O'Donovan, N. (2009). Epidermal growth factor receptor as a potential therapeutic target in triple-negative breast cancer. *Ann Oncol,* 20, 862-867.

Coyle, J.H., Guzik, B.W., Bor, Y.C., Jin, L., Eisner-Smerage, L., Taylor, S.J., Rekosh, D., and Hammarskjold, M.L. (2003). Sam68 enhances the cytoplasmic utilization of intron-containing RNA and is functionally regulated by the nuclear kinase Sik/BRK. *Mol Cell Biol,* 23, 92-103.

Darnell, J.E., Jr., Kerr, I.M., and Stark, G.R. (1994). Jak-STAT pathways and transcriptional activation in response to IFNs and other extracellular signaling proteins. *Science,* 264, 1415-1421.

Dent, R., Trudeau, M., Pritchard, K.I., Hanna, W.M., Kahn, H.K., Sawka, C.A., Lickley, L.A., Rawlinson, E., Sun, P., and Narod, S.A. (2007). Triple-negative breast cancer: clinical features and patterns of recurrence. *Clin Cancer Res,* 13, 4429-4434.

Derry, J.J., Prins, G.S., Ray, V., and Tyner, A.L. (2003). Altered localization and activity of the intracellular tyrosine kinase BRK/Sik in prostate tumor cells. *Oncogene,* 22, 4212-4220.

Derry, J.J., Richard, S., Valderrama Carvajal, H., Ye, X., Vasioukhin, V., Cochrane, A.W., Chen, T., and Tyner, A.L. (2000). Sik (BRK) phosphorylates Sam68 in the nucleus and negatively regulates its RNA binding ability. *Mol Cell Biol,* 20, 6114-6126.

Desrivieres, S., Kunz, C., Barash, I., Vafaizadeh, V., Borghouts, C., and Groner, B. (2006). The biological functions of the versatile transcription factors STAT3 and STAT5 and new strategies for their targeted inhibition. *J Mammary Gland Biol Neoplasia,* 11, 75-87.

Early Breast Cancer Trialists' Collaborative Group. (2005). Effects of chemotherapy and hormonal therapy for early breast cancer on recurrence and 15-year survival: an overview of the randomised trials. *Lancet,* 365, 1687-1717.

Easty, D.J., Mitchell, P.J., Patel, K., Florenes, V.A., Spritz, R.A., and Bennett, D.C. (1997). Loss of expression of receptor tyrosine kinase family genes PTK7 and SEK in metastatic melanoma. *Int J Cancer,* 71, 1061-1065.

Evers, B., Drost, R., Schut, E., de Bruin, M., van der Burg, E., Derksen, P.W., Holstege, H., Liu, X., van Drunen, E., Beverloo, H.B., Smith, G.C., Martin, N.M., Lau, A., O'Connor, M.J., and Jonkers, J. (2008). Selective inhibition of BRCA2-deficient mammary tumor cell growth by AZD2281 and cisplatin. *Clin Cancer Res,* 14, 3916-3925.

Finn, R.S., Dering, J., Ginther, C., Wilson, C.A., Glaspy, P., Tchekmedyian, N., Slamon, D.J. (2007). Dasatinib, an orally active small molecule inhibitor of both the src and abl kinases, selectively inhibits growth of basal-type/"triple-negative" breast cancer cell lines growing in vitro. *Breast Cancer Res Treat,* 105:319-26.

Haegebarth, A., Bie, W., Yang, R., Crawford, S.E., Vasioukhin, V., Fuchs, E., and Tyner, A.L. (2006). Protein tyrosine kinase 6 negatively regulates growth and promotes enterocyte differentiation in the small intestine. *Mol Cell Biol,* 26, 4949-4957.

Haegebarth, A., Heap, D., Bie, W., Derry, J.J., Richard, S., and Tyner, A.L. (2004). The nuclear tyrosine kinase BRK/Sik phosphorylates and inhibits the RNA-binding activities of the Sam68-like mammalian proteins SLM-1 and SLM-2. *J Biol Chem,* 279, 54398-54404.

Haegebarth, A., Nunez, R., and Tyner, A.L. (2005). The intracellular tyrosine kinase Brk sensitizes non-transformed cells to inducers of apoptosis. *Cell Cycle*, 4, 1239-1246.

Hennighausen, L., Robinson, G.W., Wagner, K.U., and Liu, X. (1997). Developing a mammary gland is a stat affair. *J Mammary Gland Biol Neoplasia*, 2, 365-372.

Hirano, T., Ishihara, K., and Hibi, M. (2000). Roles of STAT3 in mediating the cell growth, differentiation and survival signals relayed through the IL-6 family of cytokine receptors. *Oncogene*, 19, 2548-2556.

Hudziak, R.M., Schlessinger, J., and Ullrich, A. (1987). Increased expression of the putative growth factor receptor p185HER2 causes transformation and tumorigenesis of NIH 3T3 cells. *Proc Natl Acad Sci U S A*, 84, 7159-7163.

Hynes, N.E., and Stern, D.F. (1994). The biology of erbB-2/neu/HER-2 and its role in cancer. *Biochim Biophys Acta*, 1198, 165-184.

Ie Kim, H., and Lee, S.T. (2009). Oncogenic functions of PTK6 are enhanced by its targeting to plasma membrane but abolished by its targeting to nucleus. *J Biochem*, 146, 133-139.

Ihle, J.N. (1996). STATs and MAPKs: obligate or opportunistic partners in signaling. *Bioessays*, 18, 95-98.

Ikeda, O., Miyasaka, Y., Sekine, Y., Mizushima, A., Muromoto, R., Nanbo, A., Yoshimura, A., and Matsuda, T. (2009). STAP-2 is phosphorylated at tyrosine-250 by Brk and modulates Brk-mediated STAT3 activation. Biochem Biophys Res Commun, *384*, 71-75.

Ikeda, O., Mizushima, A., Sekine, Y., Yamamoto, C., Muromoto, R., Nanbo, A., Oritani, K., Yoshimura, A., and Matsuda, T. (2011). Involvement of STAP-2 in Brk-mediated phosphorylation and activation of STAT5 in breast cancer cells. *Cancer Sci*, 102, 756-761.

Ikeda, O., Sekine, Y., Kakisaka, M., Tsuji, S., Muromoto, R., Ohbayashi, N., Oritani, K., Yoshimura, A., and Matsuda, T. (2007). STAP-2 regulates c-Fms/M-CSF receptor signaling in murine macrophage Raw 264.7 cells. *Biochem Biophys Res Commun*, 358, 931-937.

Ikeda, O., Sekine, Y., Mizushima, A., Nakasuji, M., Miyasaka, Y., Yamamoto, C., Muromoto, R., Nanbo, A., Oritani, K., Yoshimura, A., and Matsuda, T. (2010). Interactions of STAP-2 with Brk and STAT3 participate in cell growth of human breast cancer cells. *J Biol Chem*, 285, 38093-38103.

Ikeda, O., Sekine, Y., Yasui, T., Oritani, K., Sugiyma, K., Muromoto, R., Ohbayashi, N., Yoshimura, A., and Matsuda, T. (2008). STAP-2 negatively regulates both canonical and noncanonical NF-kappaB activation induced by Epstein-Barr virus-derived latent membrane protein 1. *Mol Cell Biol*, 28, 5027-5042.

Kamalati, T., Jolin, H.E., Fry, M.J., and Crompton, M.R. (2000). Expression of the BRK tyrosine kinase in mammary epithelial cells enhances the coupling of EGF signalling to PI 3-kinase and Akt, via erbB3 phosphorylation. *Oncogene*, 19, 5471-5476.

Kamalati, T., Jolin, H.E., Mitchell, P.J., Barker, K.T., Jackson, L.E., Dean, C.J., Page, M.J., Gusterson, B.A., and Crompton, M.R. (1996). Brk, a breast tumor-derived non-receptor protein-tyrosine kinase, sensitizes mammary epithelial cells to epidermal growth factor. *J Biol Chem*, 271, 30956-30963.

Kang, S.A., Lee, E.S., Yoon, H.Y., Randazzo, P.A., and Lee, S.T. (2010). PTK6 inhibits down-regulation of EGF receptor through phosphorylation of ARAP1. *J Biol Chem,* 285, 26013-26021.

Kim, H., and Lee, S.T. (2005). An intramolecular interaction between SH2-kinase linker and kinase domain is essential for the catalytic activity of protein-tyrosine kinase-6. *J Biol Chem,* 280, 28973-28980.

Lee, S.T., Strunk, K.M., and Spritz, R.A. (1993). A survey of protein tyrosine kinase mRNAs expressed in normal human melanocytes. *Oncogene,* 8, 3403-3410.

Liedtke, C., Mazouni, C., Hess, K.R., Andre, F., Tordai, A., Mejia, J.A., Symmans, W.F., Gonzalez-Angulo, A.M., Hennessy, B., Green, M., *et al.* (2008). Response to neoadjuvant therapy and long-term survival in patients with triple-negative breast cancer. *J Clin Oncol,* 26, 1275-1281.

Liu, L., Gao, Y., Qiu, H., Miller, W.T., Poli, V., and Reich, N.C. (2006). Identification of STAT3 as a specific substrate of breast tumor kinase. *Oncogene,* 25, 4904-4912.

Llor, X., Serfas, M.S., Bie, W., Vasioukhin, V., Polonskaia, M., Derry, J., Abbott, C.M., and Tyner, A.L. (1999). BRK/Sik expression in the gastrointestinal tract and in colon tumors. *Clin Cancer Res* 5, 1767-1777.

Lukong, K.E., Huot, M.E., and Richard, S. (2009). BRK phosphorylates PSF promoting its cytoplasmic localization and cell cycle arrest. *Cell Signal* 21, 1415-1422.

Lukong, K.E., Larocque, D., Tyner, A.L., and Richard, S. (2005). Tyrosine phosphorylation of sam68 by breast tumor kinase regulates intranuclear localization and cell cycle progression. *J Biol Chem,* 280, 38639-38647.

Lukong, K.E., and Richard, S. (2008). Breast tumor kinase BRK requires kinesin-2 subunit KAP3A in modulation of cell migration. *Cell Signal,* 20, 432-442.

Masuhara, M., Nagao, K., Nishikawa, M., Sasaki, M., Yoshimura, A., and Osawa, M. (2000). Molecular cloning of murine STAP-1, the stem-cell-specific adaptor protein containing PH and SH2 domains. *Biochem Biophys Res Commun,* 268, 697-703.

Menard, S., Fortis, S., Castiglioni, F., Agresti, R., and Balsari, A. (2001). HER2 as a prognostic factor in breast cancer. *Oncology,* 61 Suppl 2, 67-72.

Mendel, D.B., Laird, A.D., Xin, X., Louie, S.G., Christensen, J.G., Li, G., Schreck, R.E., Abrams, T.J., Ngai, T.J., Lee, L.B., Murray, L.J., Carver, J., Chan, E., Moss, K.G., Haznedar, J.O., Sukbuntherng, J., Blake, R.A., Sun, L., Tang, C., Miller, T., Shirazian, S., McMahon, G., and Cherrington, J.M. (2003). In vivo antitumor activity of SU11248, a novel tyrosine kinase inhibitor targeting vascular endothelial growth factor and platelet-derived growth factor receptors: determination of a pharmacokinetic/pharmacodynamic relationship. Clin *Cancer Res,* 9, 327-337.

Minoguchi, M., Minoguchi, S., Aki, D., Joo, A., Yamamoto, T., Yumioka, T., Matsuda, T., and Yoshimura, A. (2003). STAP-2/BKS, an adaptor/docking protein, modulates STAT3 activation in acute-phase response through its YXXQ motif. *J Biol Chem,* 278, 11182-11189.

Mitchell, P.J., Barker, K.T., Martindale, J.E., Kamalati, T., Lowe, P.N., Page, M.J., Gusterson, B.A., and Crompton, M.R. (1994). Cloning and characterisation of cDNAs encoding a novel non-receptor tyrosine kinase, brk, expressed in human breast tumours. *Oncogene,* 9, 2383-2390.

Mitchell, P.J., Sara, E.A., and Crompton, M.R. (2000). A novel adaptor-like protein which is a substrate for the non-receptor tyrosine kinase, BRK. *Oncogene,* 19, 4273-4282.

Normanno, N., Di Maio, M., De Maio, E., De Luca, A., de Matteis, A., Giordano, A., and Perrone, F. (2005). Mechanisms of endocrine resistance and novel therapeutic strategies in breast cancer. *Endocr Relat Cancer,* 12, 721-747.

O'Shea, J.J. (1997). Jaks, STATs, cytokine signal transduction, and immunoregulation: are we there yet? *Immunity,* 7, 1-11.

Ostrander, J.H., Daniel, A.R., Lofgren, K., Kleer, C.G., and Lange, C.A. (2007). Breast tumor kinase (protein tyrosine kinase 6) regulates heregulin-induced activation of ERK5 and p38 MAP kinases in breast cancer cells. *Cancer Res,* 67, 4199-4209.

Pal, S.K., and Mortimer, J. (2009). Triple-negative breast cancer: novel therapies and new directions. *Maturitas,* 63, 269-274.

Palka-Hamblin, H.L., Gierut, J.J., Bie, W., Brauer, P.M., Zheng, Y., Asara, J.M., and Tyner, A.L. (2010). Identification of beta-catenin as a target of the intracellular tyrosine kinase PTK6. *J Cell Sci,* 123, 236-245.

Petro, B.J., Tan, R.C., Tyner, A.L., Lingen, M.W., and Watanabe, K. (2004). Differential expression of the non-receptor tyrosine kinase BRK in oral squamous cell carcinoma and normal oral epithelium. *Oral Oncol,* 40, 1040-1047.

Piccart-Gebhart, M.J., Procter, M., Leyland-Jones, B., Goldhirsch, A., Untch, M., Smith, I., Gianni, L., Baselga, J., Bell, R., Jackisch, C., Cameron, D., Dowsett, M., Barrios, C.H., Steger, G., Huang, C.S., Andersson, M., Inbar, M., Lichinitser, M., Láng, I., Nitz, U., Iwata, H., Thomssen, C., Lohrisch, C., Suter, T.M., Rüschoff, .J, Suto, T., Greatorex, V., Ward, C., Straehle, C., McFadden, E., Dolci, M.S., and Gelber, R.D.; Herceptin Adjuvant (HERA) Trial Study Team. (2005). Trastuzumab after adjuvant chemotherapy in HER2-positive breast cancer. *N Engl J Med,* 353, 1659-1672.

Qiu, H., and Miller, W.T. (2002). Regulation of the nonreceptor tyrosine kinase Brk by autophosphorylation and by autoinhibition. *J Biol Chem,* 277, 34634-34641.

Qiu, H., Zappacosta, F., Su, W., Annan, R.S., and Miller, W.T. (2005). Interaction between Brk kinase and insulin receptor substrate-4. *Oncogene,* 24, 5656-5664.

Saal, L.H., Holm, K., Maurer, M., Memeo, L., Su, T., Wang, X., Yu, J.S., Malmstrom, P.O., Mansukhani, M., Enoksson, J., Hibshoosh, H., Borg, A., and Parsons, R. (2005). PIK3CA mutations correlate with hormone receptors, node metastasis, and ERBB2, and are mutually exclusive with PTEN loss in human breast carcinoma. *Cancer Res,* 65, 2554-2559.

Schmandt, R.E., Bennett, M., Clifford, S., Thornton, A., Jiang, F., Broaddus, R.R., Sun, C.C., Lu, K.H., Sood, A.K., and Gershenson, D.M. (2006). The BRK tyrosine kinase is expressed in high-grade serous carcinoma of the ovary. *Cancer Biol Ther,* 5, 1136-1141.

Sekine, Y., Ikeda, O., Tsuji, S., Yamamoto, C., Muromoto, R., Nanbo, A., Oritani, K., Yoshimura, A., and Matsuda, T. (2009). Signal-transducing adaptor protein-2 regulates stromal cell-derived factor-1 alpha-induced chemotaxis in T cells. *J Immunol,* 183, 7966-7974.

Sekine, Y., Tsuji, S., Ikeda, O., Sugiyma, K., Oritani, K., Shimoda, K., Muromoto, R., Ohbayashi, N., Yoshimura, A., and Matsuda, T. (2007). Signal-transducing adaptor protein-2 regulates integrin-mediated T cell adhesion through protein degradation of focal adhesion kinase. *J Immunol,* 179, 2397-2407.

Sekine, Y., Yamamoto, C., Ikeda, O., Muromoto, R., Nanbo, A., Oritani, K., Yoshimura, A., and Matsuda, T. (2009). The protein content of an adaptor protein, STAP-2 is controlled by E3 ubiquitin ligase Cbl. *Biochem Biophys Res Commun*, 384, 187-192.

Sekine, Y., Yamamoto, T., Yumioka, T., Sugiyama, K., Tsuji, S., Oritani, K., Shimoda, K., Minoguchi, M., Yoshimura, A., and Matsuda, T. (2005). Physical and functional interactions between STAP-2/BKS and STAT5. *J Biol Chem*, 280, 8188-8196.

Sekine, Y., Yumioka, T., Yamamoto, T., Muromoto, R., Imoto, S., Sugiyma, K., Oritani, K., Shimoda, K., Minoguchi, M., Akira, S., Yoshimura, A., and Matsuda, T. (2006). Modulation of TLR4 signaling by a novel adaptor protein signal-transducing adaptor protein-2 in macrophages. *J Immunol*, 176, 380-389.

Serfas, M.S., and Tyner, A.L. (2003). Brk, Srm, Frk, and Src42A form a distinct family of intracellular Src-like tyrosine kinases. *Oncol Res*, 13, 409-419.

Shen, C.H., Chen, H.Y., Lin, M.S., Li, F.Y., Chang, C.C., Kuo, M.L., Settleman, J., and Chen, R.H. (2008). Breast tumor kinase phosphorylates p190RhoGAP to regulate rho and ras and promote breast carcinoma growth, migration, and invasion. *Cancer Res*, 68, 7779-7787.

Siyanova, E.Y., Serfas, M.S., Mazo, I.A., and Tyner, A.L. (1994). Tyrosine kinase gene expression in the mouse small intestine. *Oncogene*, 9, 2053-2057.

Slamon, D.J., Clark, G.M., Wong, S.G., Levin, W.J., Ullrich, A., and McGuire, W.L. (1987). Human breast cancer: correlation of relapse and survival with amplification of the HER-2/neu oncogene. *Science*, 235, 177-182.

Slamon, D.J., Godolphin, W., Jones, L.A., Holt, J.A., Wong, S.G., Keith, D.E., Levin, W.J., Stuart, S.G., Udove, J., Ullrich, A., *et al.* (1989). Studies of the HER-2/neu proto-oncogene in human breast and ovarian cancer. *Science*, 244, 707-712.

Slamon, D.J., Leyland-Jones, B., Shak, S., Fuchs, H., Paton, V., Bajamonde, A., Fleming, T., Eiermann, W., Wolter, J., Pegram, M., Baselga, J., and Norton, L. (2001). Use of chemotherapy plus a monoclonal antibody against HER2 for metastatic breast cancer that overexpresses HER2. *N Engl J Med*, 344, 783-792.

Slamon, D.J., Romond, E.H., and Perez, E.A. (2006). Advances in adjuvant therapy for breast cancer. *Clin Adv Hematol Oncol*, 4, suppl 1, 4-9; discussion suppl 10; quiz 12 p following suppl 10.

Sorlie, T., Tibshirani, R., Parker, J., Hastie, T., Marron, J.S., Nobel, A., Deng, S., Johnsen, H., Pesich, R., Geisler, S., Demeter, J., Perou, C.M., Lønning, P.E., Brown, P.O., Børresen-Dale, A.L., and Botstein, D. (2003). Repeated observation of breast tumor subtypes in independent gene expression data sets. *Proc Natl Acad Sci U S A*, 100, 8418-8423.

Stern, D.F. (2000). Tyrosine kinase signalling in breast cancer: ErbB family receptor tyrosine kinases. *Breast Cancer Res*, 2, 176-183.

Thorley-Lawson, D.A. (2001). Epstein-Barr virus: exploiting the immune system. *Nat Rev Immunol*, 1, 75-82.

Thorpe, S.M. (1988). Estrogen and progesterone receptor determinations in breast cancer. Technology, biology and clinical significance. *Acta Oncol*, 27, 1-19.

Tutt, A., Robson, M., Garber, J.E., Domchek, S.M., Audeh, M.W., Weitzel, J.N., Friedlander, M., Arun, B., Loman, N., Schmutzler, R.K., Wardley, A., Mitchell, G., Earl, H., Wickens, M., and Carmichael, J. (2010). Oral poly(ADP-ribose) polymerase inhibitor olaparib in patients with BRCA1 or BRCA2 mutations and advanced breast cancer: a proof-of-concept trial. *Lancet,* 376, 235-244.

Vasioukhin, V., Serfas, M.S., Siyanova, E.Y., Polonskaia, M., Costigan, V.J., Liu, B., Thomason, A., and Tyner, A.L. (1995). A novel intracellular epithelial cell tyrosine kinase is expressed in the skin and gastrointestinal tract. *Oncogene,* 10, 349-357.

Vasioukhin, V., and Tyner, A.L. (1997). A role for the epithelial-cell-specific tyrosine kinase Sik during keratinocyte differentiation. *Proc Natl Acad Sci U S A,* 94, 14477-14482.

Wang, T.C., Jee, S.H., Tsai, T.F., Huang, Y.L., Tsai, W.L., and Chen, R.H. (2005). Role of breast tumour kinase in the in vitro differentiation of HaCaT cells. *Br J Dermatol,* 153, 282-289.

Ward, S., Pilgrim, H., and Hind, D. (2009). Trastuzumab for the treatment of primary breast cancer in HER2-positive women: a single technology appraisal. *Health Technol Assess,* 13 Suppl *1*, 1-6.

Weaver, A.M., and Silva, C.M. (2007). Signal transducer and activator of transcription 5b: a new target of breast tumor kinase/protein tyrosine kinase 6. *Breast Cancer Res,* 9, R79.

Xiang, B., Chatti, K., Qiu, H., Lakshmi, B., Krasnitz, A., Hicks, J., Yu, M., Miller, W.T., and Muthuswamy, S.K. (2008). Brk is coamplified with ErbB2 to promote proliferation in breast cancer. *Proc Natl Acad Sci U S A,* 105, 12463-12468.

Yamamoto, T., Yumioka, T., Sekine, Y., Sato, N., Minoguchi, M., Yoshimura, A., and Matsuda, T. (2003). Regulation of FcepsilonRI-mediated signaling by an adaptor protein STAP-2/BSK in rat basophilic leukemia RBL-2H3 cells. *Biochem Biophys Res Commun,* 306, 767-773.

Yarden, Y. (2001). Biology of HER2 and its importance in breast cancer. *Oncology,* 61 Suppl 2, 1-13.

Zhang, P., Ostrander, J.H., Faivre, E.J., Olsen, A., Fitzsimmons, D., and Lange, C.A. (2005). Regulated association of protein kinase B/Akt with breast tumor kinase. *J Biol Chem,* 280, 1982-1991.

Zhang, Q., Thomas, S.M., Xi, S., Smithgall, T.E., Siegfried, J.M., Kamens, J., Gooding, W.E., and Grandis, J.R. (2004). SRC family kinases mediate epidermal growth factor receptor ligand cleavage, proliferation, and invasion of head and neck cancer cells. *Cancer Res,* 64, 6166-6173.

30

Histamine and Breast Cancer: A New Role for a Well Known Amine

Graciela Cricco[1], Nora Mohamad[1], María Soledad Sáez[1], Eduardo Valli[1,2], Elena Rivera[1] and Gabriela Martín[1,2]
[1]*Laboratory of Radioisotopes, School of Pharmacy and Biochemistry, University of Buenos Aires*
[2]*Scientific and Technical Research National Council (CONICET) Argentina*

1. Introduction

Metastases are the most devastating aspect of cancer since most deaths from cancer are related to them. The ability of tumors to invade the neighboring extracellular matrix, which is primarily accompanied by augmented matrix metalloproteinases (MMPs) production and cell migration, is critical for metastases.

After surgical removal of primary breast tumors, malignant cells may still remain and radiotherapy is an efficient modality to reduce the risk of local recurrence. However, proliferative, invasive, and metastatic capacities can be increased in the surviving tumor cells of irradiated breast and other neoplasias (Baluna et al, 2006; Tsukamoto et al, 2007; Tsutsumi et al, 2009). To improve the efficacy of radiotherapy, this phenomenon must be further studied to elaborate therapeutic modalities to prevent radiation enhancement of cancer cell invasion.

Histamine is an endogenous biogenic amine extensively distributed throughout the organism which exerts multiple functions in physiologic and pathophysiological processes by stimulation of four G-protein coupled receptors (H1, H2, H3 and H4 histamine receptors) with different tissue expression patterns and functions. It is well known that diverse tumoral tissues and cell lines express the different histamine receptors through which histamine brings about its effects on cell proliferation, differentiation, survival and death. A great deal of evidence shows a relevant role of histamine in tumor progression, however controversial results are published depending on the cell type and the histamine receptor subtype that is activated (Blaya et al, 2010; Francis et al, 2009; Parsons & Ganellin, 2006; Soule et al, 2010). It has also been determined that numerous tumour tissues and cell lines express L-histidine decarboxylase, the histamine-synthesizing enzyme, and contain high levels of endogenous histamine which released to the extracellular media may exert its effects via a paracrine or autocrine regulation (Falus et al, 2001; Pós et al, 2004; Rivera et al, 2000). Additionally some effects on tumor growth may be mediated by histamine regulation of angiogenesis and immunity (Lázár-Molnár et al, 2002; Tomita et al, 2003).

Our research team has demonstrated the expression of histamine membrane receptors and their association to different signalling pathways in breast cancer biopsies and a large number of transformed cell lines, being our works the first ones to report the presence of H3 and H4 receptors linked to cell proliferation in breast and pancreatic cancer cell lines. We determined that histamine can modulate not only cell proliferation but differentiation, apoptosis and secretion of different growth factors (Cricco et al, 2006, 2008; Medina et al, 2006, 2008, 2009; Rivera et al, 2000, 2004). We have demonstrated that the highly invasive and metastatic breast cancer cell line MDA-MB 231 expresses the four known types of histamine receptors through which histamine differentially regulates cell proliferation in a dose dependent way. At concentrations over 10 μM a significant decrease in clonogenic growth was observed, while at concentrations lower than 0.5 μM proliferation was increased. The negative effect on proliferation was associated with the induction of arrest in G2/M phase of cell cycle, differentiation and a significant augmentation of apoptotic death (Medina et al, 2006).

Histamine and antihistamines have a modulatory effect on epithelial and endothelial cell adhesion and on the expression of different MMPs (Asano et al, 2004; Ciprandi et al, 2003; Gschwandtner et al, 2008). It has also been described a stimulatory action on migration of fibroblasts, haematopoyetic and immune cells, mainly via H4 receptors (Gschwandtner et al, 2010; Kohyama et al, 2010). However most of these reports refer to normal cells, existing less information regarding to tumor cells. Recently we have demonstrated the ability of HA to modulate MMPs, tissue inhibitors of matrix metalloproteinases (TIMPs) and cell adhesion in the breast cancer cell lines HBL-100 and MDA-MB 231 (Genre et al, 2009). We have also determined the upregulation of MMP2 and cell migration in the pancreatic carcinoma cell line PANC-1 by histamine (Cricco et al, 2006).

Reactive oxygen species (ROS) such as superoxide anion and hydrogen peroxide (H2O2) are continuously produced as by-products of aerobic metabolism primarily in the mitochondria and other cellular sources. In addition, external agents like ultraviolet radiation and ionizing radiation also increase intracellular ROS levels. Under physiologic conditions cells are protected against oxidative stress by an interacting network of antioxidant enzymes like superoxide dismutases, catalase and glutathion peroxidase. Though ROS may induce cellular damage when there is an imbalance between their generation and scavenging, numerous studies support the role of ROS as essential participants in cell signaling depending on their concentration, timing and location (Thannickal and Fanburg, 2000).

The aim of the present study was to investigate the role of HA and HA receptors activation in early cellular events involved in metastatic capacity, such as expression and activity of matrix metalloproteinases MMP2 and MMP9, cell migration and invasion in MDA-MB 231 cells. Since ionizing radiation may affect metastatic competence depending upon cell type and irradiation characteristics, and given that histamine increases MDA-MB 231 cells intrinsic sensibility to ionizing radiation by downregulating catalase activity and enhancing H2O2 intracellular levels at the same doses that inhibit cell proliferation (Medina et al, 2006), the possible interaction between histamine treatment and irradiation was also evaluated. The identification of drugs that can both regulate tumor cell survival and metastatic ability will help to delineate more effective strategies for therapeutic intervention in malignant diseases.

2. Effects of histamine and histamine receptor agonists upon matrix metalloproteinases MMP2 and MMP9

MMP2 and MMP9, also called gelatinase A and gelatinase B respectively, belong to a large family of zinc-dependent endopeptidases formed by more than 20 members which participate in the proteolysis of basement membrane and extracellular matrix proteins, collagen and fibronectin. MMPs are involved in normal tissue remodeling events like wound healing, bone resorption and mammary involution. Their anomalous expression is associated to various pathological processes including inflammation and cancer (Freije et al, 2003). MMPs are secreted in a latent zymogen form (proenzyme). The inactive enzyme conformation is maintained due to thiol interactions between cysteine residues in the prodomain and the zinc atom present in the catalytic site of all MMPs. *In vitro*, MMPs activation can occur when the prodomain is cleaved by other proteases or when the zinc-cysteine bound is interrupted (Van Wart & Birkedal-Hansen, 1990).

Regulation of MMPs occurs on three levels: alteration of gene expression, activation of latent zymogens and inhibition by TIMPs. This regulation is tightly controlled in normal states while it is altered during tumor cell progression, being a critical step for cancer invasion and metastases (Chakraborti et al, 2003). Initially, it was believed that the major role of MMPs in metastases was to facilitate the breakdown of physical barriers. At present, it is widely accepted that MMPs may have a more complex role making important contributions at other steps in the metastatic process (Chabottaux & Noel, 2007). *In vitro* and *in vivo* studies demonstrate an entire correlation between MMP2, MMP9 and TIMPs expression and metastasis (Baum et al, 2007; Chambers & Matrisian, 1997; Duffy et al, 2008; John & Tuszynski, 2001; Wroblewski et al, 2002). Accordingly, MMP2 and MMP9 have been associated with breast cancer development and tumor progression (Köhrmann et al, 2009). An elevated activity of gelatinases in plasma and sera of patients with breast cancer confirms the role of these enzymes in the development of such tumors though clinical correlation with parameters like tumor grade and stage, size and lymph node involvement is still fragmentary (Decokc et al 2005; La Rocca et al, 2004; Stankovic et al, 2010).

In a previous work we determined a dissimilar role of histamine in the modulation of gelatinolytic activities and cell adhesion in mammary cell lines with different tumorigenic capacity (Genre et al, 2009), To further investigate histamine action and also histamine receptors implicated in breast cancer invasiveness we conducted *in vitro* experiments employing different doses of histamine and histamine receptor agonists and antagonists (listed in Table 1) in MDA-MB 231 cell line (ATCC HTB-26). Cells were cultured in RPMI supplemented with 10% fetal bovine serum, L-glutamine (0.3 g/L) and gentamicin (0.04 g/L) under standard conditions of 5% CO_2 and temperature of 37°C.

Ligand	Characteristic	References
2-(3-trifluoromethylphenil)histamine dimaleate (Sigma Aldrich)	H1 histamine receptor agonist	Leschke et al (1995). Synthesis and histamine H1 receptor agonist activity of a series of 2-phenylhistamines, 2-heteroarylhistamines, and analogues. *J Med Chem*, Vol. 38, No8, (April 1995), pp. 1287-1294, ISSN 0022-2623
Amthamine dihydrobromide (Tocris)	H2 histamine receptor agonist	Eriks el al (1992). Histamine H2 -receptor agonists -synthesis, in vitro pharmacology, and qualitative structure activity relationships of substituted 4-(2-Aminoethyl)thiazoles and 5-(2-Aminoethyl)thiazoles. *J Med Chem*, Vol. 35, No17, (August 1992), pp. 3239-3246, ISSN:0022-2623

Table 1. Histamine receptor agonists and antagonists employed in this study. (Continued)

Ligand	Characteristic	References
R(alpha) methylhistamine dihydrobromide (Tocris)	H3 histamine receptor agonist	Leurs el al (1995). The medicinal chemistry and therapeutic potential of ligands for the histamine H3 receptor. *Prog Drug Res,* Vol. 45, pp.107-165, ISSN 0071-786X
VUF 8430 dihydrobromide (Tocris)	H4 histamine receptor agonist	Lim et al (2006). Discovery of S-(2-guanidylethyl)-isothiourea (VUF 8430) as a potent nonimidazole histamine H4 receptor agonist. *J Med Chem,* Vol.49, No.23, (November 2006), pp. 6650-6651, ISSN 0022-2623
Clobenpropit dihydrobromide (Tocris)	H4 histamine receptor agonist and H3 histamine receptor antagonist	Liu et al (2001). Cloning and pharmacological characterization of a fourth histamine receptor (H_4) expressed in bone marrow. *Mol Pharmacol,* Vol.59, No3, (March 2001), pp 420-426, ISSN 0026-895X
Ranitidine hydrochloride (Sigma Aldrich)	H2 histamine receptor antagonist	Brittain & Daly (1981) A review of the animal pharmacology of ranitidine -a new, selective histamine H_2-antagonist. *Scand J Gastroenterol, Suppl,* Vol.69, (June 1981), pp. 1-9, ISSN 0085-5928
JNJ7777120 (Johnson & Johnson)	H4 histamine receptor antagonist	Jablanowski et al (2003). The first potent and selective non-imidazole human histamine H_4 receptor antagonists. *J Med Chem,* Vol. 6, No19, (September 2003), pp. 3957-3960. Sep 11;46(19):3957-60, ISSN 0022-2623

Table 1. Histamine receptor agonists and antagonists employed in this study.

2.1 Evaluation of matrix metalloproteinases activity

MMP2 and MMP9 gelatinolytic activity was evaluated by zymography, a powerful electrophoretic technique for identifying proteolytic activity of enzymes separated in polyacrylamide gels under nonreducing conditions. Cells were cultured in serum-free RPMI medium for 24h in absence or presence of treatments. Conditioned media mixed with non-reducing buffer were electrophoresed in 7% SDS-polyacrylamide gel containing 1% of gelatin. Gels were then rinsed, incubated (48h at 37°C) and subsequently stained (0.1% Coomasie Brilliant Blue). Activity of lytic bands was determined by densitometry (Image J 1.42q, NIH, US).

There was a biphasic effect when cells were cultured with histamine concentrations varying from 0.1 μM to 20 μM. A significant increase in the activity of MMP2 and MMP9 pro and active forms was observed with 0.5 μM histamine (low dose) while a dramatic reduction in the activity of MMP2 and MMP9 (pro and active forms) occurred with histamine over 10 μM (high doses) as shown in Figure 1.

Testing H1, H2, H3 and H4 histamine receptor agonists we could observe that activities of both MMPs were differentially modulated. 10 μM H2 agonist amthamine evoked the reduction in lytic bands induced by high doses of histamine while 10 μM H4 agonists VUF 8430 and clobenpropit produced a significant rise of MMP2 and MMP9 activities as low doses of histamine did (Figure 2). The increase and decrease in gelatinolytic activities produced by histamine were blocked by the specific H4 antagonist JNJ7777120 (10 μM) and H2 antagonist ranitidine (10 μM) respectively (data not shown). In addition, no significant changes in both activities were determined employing H1 and H3 histamine agonists so that they were no longer tested in current assays.

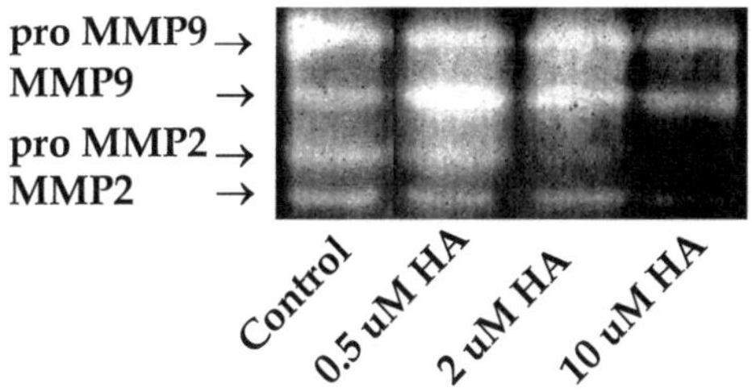

Fig. 1. Effect of histamine on MMP2 and MMP9 gelatinolytic activity. Activity was evaluated by zymography after 24h of treatment with different concentrations of histamine in serum free RPMI medium. The figure shows a representative gel.

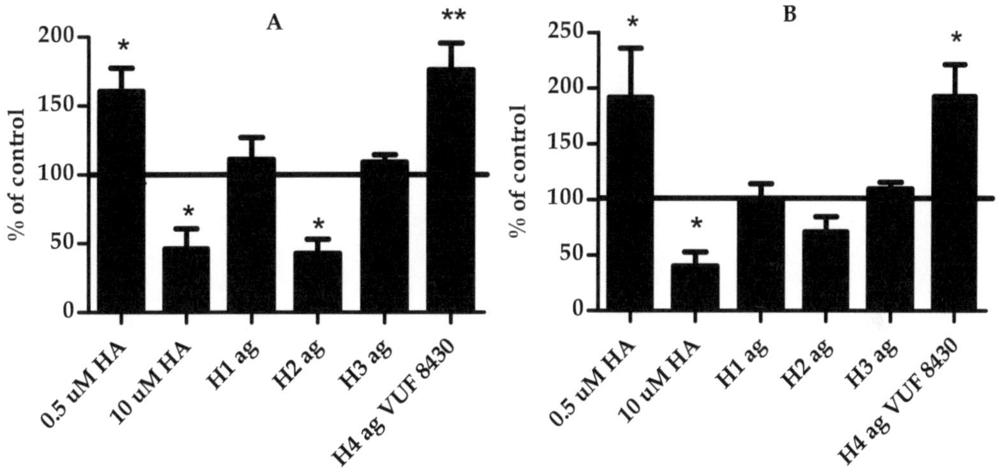

Fig. 2. Effect of histamine and histamine receptor agonists on MMPs gelatinolytic activity. A: MMP2 zymography. B: MMP9 zymography. Activity of lytic bands for each treatment was determined by densitometry and normalized to control values. Bars show the means ± SEM of three experiments run in triplicates. $^{*}p<0.05$ and $^{**}p<0.01$ vs control. One way Anova, Dunnet post test.

2.2 Determination of MMP2 and MMP9 mRNA steady state levels

MMP2 and MMP9 mRNA steady state levels were evaluated in cell cultures after 24h treatments using RT-PCR. Total RNA was extracted with Trizol®. Retrotranscription was carried out with MMLV enzyme. DNA was amplifyed by PCR and products were run in 2% agarose gels containing ethidium bromide. Semiquantification using GAPDH as housekeeping gene was performed with the Image J 1.42q (NIH, US) software.

	Primer sequence 5´-3´	PCR product size (bp)
MMP2	*s* ACC CAT TTA CAC CTA CAC CAA G *a* GTA TAC CGC ATC AAT CTT TTC CG	306
MMP9	*s* CCC ATT TCG ACG ATG AC *a* GGC ACT GAG GAA GAA TGA TCT AAG	639
GAPDH	s GCA GGG GGG AGC CAA AAG GG *a* TGC CAG CCC CAG CGT CAA AG	566

Table 2. Sequence of primers used in PCR reactions.

A significant reduction of mRNA steady states levels of both MMPs was observed when MDA-MB 231 cells were treated with histamine concentrations over 10 μM in agreement to our previous report (Genre et al, 2009), being this effect reproduced by 10 μM amthamine. On the other hand, there was an important increase in mRNA expression when these cells received 0.5 μM HA (low dose of HA) or H4 agonist VUF 8430 (Figure 3). Similar results were obtained employing the H4 agonist clobenpropit.

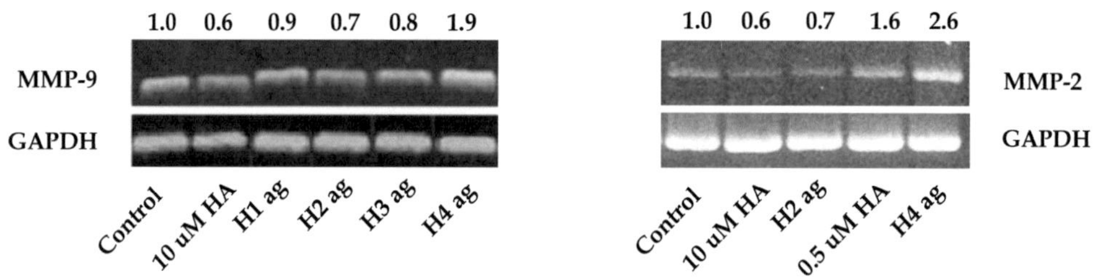

Fig. 3. mRNA expression of MMPs in MDA-MB231 cells. MMP2 and MMP9 mRNA steady state levels were determined by RT-PCR after 24h treatment with histamine and histamine receptor agonists. Figure shows representative gels for PCR products. The numbers above represent for each treatment the relative expression to controls of MMPs normalized to GAPDH.

2.3 Immunodetection of MMP2 and MMP9

Protein expression determination was performed by immunocytochemistry. MDA-MB 231 cells were grown on coverglasses and after 24h treatment cells were fixed, permeabilized and endogenous peroxidase was inhibited. Cells were incubated for 18h at 4°C with anti-MMP9 Ab (1/50, Calbiochem) or anti-MMP2 Ab (1/50, Cell Signalling) and for 2h with horse radish peroxidase conjugated anti-rabbit IgG (1/100, Sigma-Aldrich). This was followed by diaminobencidine and hematoxylin staining and observation by optical microscope.

Immunocytochemical staining supported the results of RT-PCR. A higher cytoplasmatic expression of MMP9 was seen when cells were treated with 0.5 μM histamine or H4 agonists. In turn a lower expression of MMP9 was detected in the presence of 10 μM histamine or H2 agonist (Figure 4). Similar results were obtained for MMP2 (data not shown).

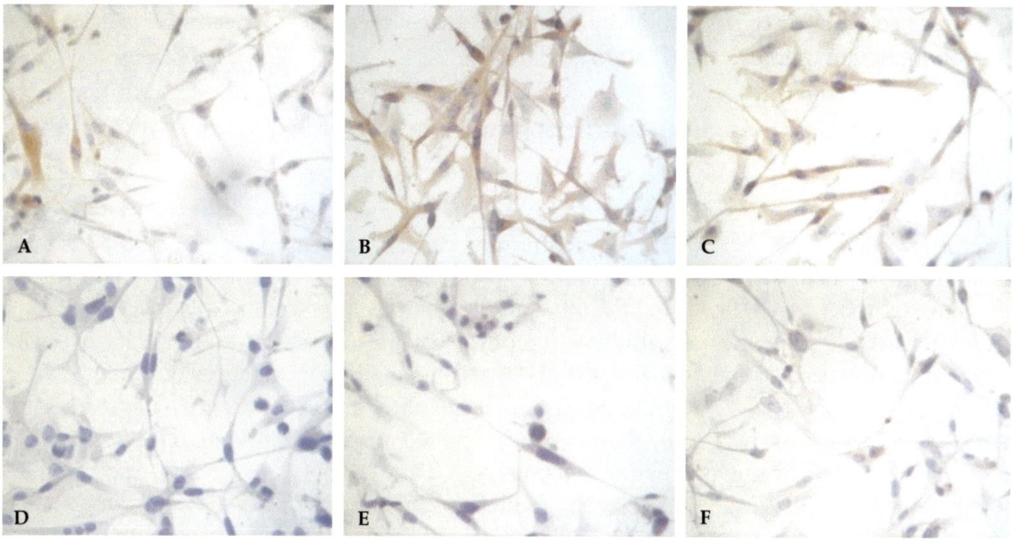

Fig. 4. Action of histamine and histamine receptor agonists on MMP2 and MMP9 protein expression in MDA-MB 231 cells. Expression was evaluated by immunocytochemistry. A: control, B: 0.5 µM HA, C: H4 agonist VUF 8340, D: negative control, E: 10 µM HA, F: H2 agonist. Photographs correspond to MMP9 expression. 400x magnification. Similar results were obtained for MMP2 expression.

Our research indicates that the mRNA and protein expression patterns of MMP2 and MMP9 were dose-dependently modified by HA through H2 and H4 receptors in MDA-MB 231 cells. Additionally, changes in gelatinolytic activity of MMP2 and MMP9 were registered in parallel to these results suggesting that an increment in protein expression may account for the increase in gelatinolytic activity.

These data constitute the first report about histamine-induced MMPs enhancement through H4 receptors in breast tumor cells. Most of *in vitro* reports upon histamine and MMPs modulation are related to inflammatory and allergic processes via H1 and H2 receptors and more recently via H4 receptors. Asano and coworkers showed that fexofenadine hydrochloride, a selective H1 receptor antagonist, may inhibit mRNA and protein expression of MMP2 and MMP9 in nasal fibroblasts and thereby possibly reduce the severity of allergic rhinitis, characterized by remodeling of the nasal wall and eosinophil and mast cell infiltration (Asano et al, 2004). It has been reported the histamine-induced production of MMP2 through H1 and H2 receptors in microvascular endothelial cells is associated to angiogenic processes (Doyle & Haas, 2009). An increase in mRNA level, protein expression and gelatinolytic activity of MMP9 is observed in human keratinocytes via H1 receptors stimulation in skin remodelling and fibrosis (Gschwandtner et al, 2008). Moreover, the *in vitro* production of other MMPs as MMP3, MMP8 and MMP13 is stimulated by histamine in human articular chondrocytes and rheumatoid synovial fibroblasts (Tetlow & Woolley, 2002; 2004). Modulation of mRNA for MMP1 by histamine has also been described in human corneal epithelial cells (Sharif et al, 1998). Regarding tumor cells, we have reported that histamine is able to reduce cell adhesion and to enhance the gelatinolytic activity of MMP2 in the pancreatic cancer cell line PANC-1 (Cricco et al, 2006). Furthermore, tranilast an antiallergic compound used clinically to control atopic and fibrotic disorders exerts its action by reducing the expression and activity of MMP2 in human malignant glioma cells (Platten et al, 2001).

3. Histamine and histamine agonists modulate MDA-MB 231 cells migration and invasion

In view of current results on MMP2 and MMP9 expression and activity we explored the migratory capacity of MDA-MB 231 mammary cells. Directed migration is an essential component of cell invasion during tumor progression and metastasis. The migratory response of MDA-MB 231 cells to histamine and histamine agonists was investigated using a 24-well transwell unit with polyethylene terephthalate (PET) membranes having a pore size of 8.0 μm (BD Falcon, Basel, Switzerland). For invasion assay the upper part of the transwell was coated with Matrigel®, a synthetic basement membrane (BD Biosciences, Bedford, MA). A fixed number of cells (1.10^4/chamber) was plated on the transwell. The medium in compartments of the lower chambers contained 2% FBS plus treatments. Inserts were incubated for 6 h at 37ºC. Non migrating cells on the upper surface of membranes were gently scrubbed with a cotton swab. Cells migrated or invading the lower surface of the membrane were fixed with methanol, and stained with hematoxilin. Ten random fields were counted under a light microscope at 50x magnification.

Histamine exerted a dual action on the migratory behavior of cells. It is improved by doses of histamine lower than 1 μM and reduced by concentrations over 10 μM (Figure 5). The stimulatory response disclosed by histamine was evoked by the H4 agonists and prevented by the specific H4 antagonist. On the other hand, histamine-induced inhibitory effect on cell motility was mimicked by the H2 agonist while relapsed by ranitidine. H1 agonist and H3 agonist did not modify cell migration; consequently they were not longer tested.

In addition similar results were displayed by histamine and histamine agonists when invasiveness was evaluated, as depicted in Figure 6. These results are in full concordance with those obtained for MMPs, reinforcing the idea that histamine may have a key role as mediator of MDA-MB 231 cells invasive ability.

A body of evidence shows a chemotactic response of inflammatory and immune cells to histamine. Because of its preferential expression in immunocompetent cells, the H4 receptor is closely related with the regulatory functions of histamine during the immune response. It has been published that histamine mediates chemotaxis via the H4 receptor in mast cells, in human monocyte-derived dendritic cells and in eosinophils, related to immune and inflammatory disorders (Baumer et al, 2008; Gutzmer et al, 2005; Hofstra et al, 2003; Ling et al, 2004; Thurmond et al, 2004). Barnad et al (2007) proved that exposure to histamine cause eosinophils to migrate from the bloodstream to the inflammatory focus into tissues, inducing actin polymerization through the H4 receptor. Histamine also activates signaling pathways typical of chemotaxis inducing migratory responses in T lymphocytes, via the H4 receptor (Truta-Feles K et al, 2010). Besides this chemotactic action in immune cells it has also been reported that histamine promotes invasiveness specifically through activation of H1 receptor in human cytotrophoblasts required to initiate blastocyst implantation (Liu et al, 2004).

Regarding tumor cells it has been reported that histamine acts as a chemoattractant for human carcinoma and melanoma cells via H1 receptor stimulation (Blaya et al, 2010; Tilly et al, 1990). Accordingly, the antiallergic compound tranilast inhibits cell migration and invasion in human malignant glioma cells blocking H1 receptors (Platten et al, 2001). A divergent response (stimulatory or inhibitory) on the migration rate of SW756 cervical carcinoma cells has been disclosed by histamine acting on H1 receptor or H4 receptor, respectively (Rudolph et al, 2008). However, as far as we know, our work is the first report about histamine-modulated migration and invasion through H4 and H2 receptors in breast tumor cells.

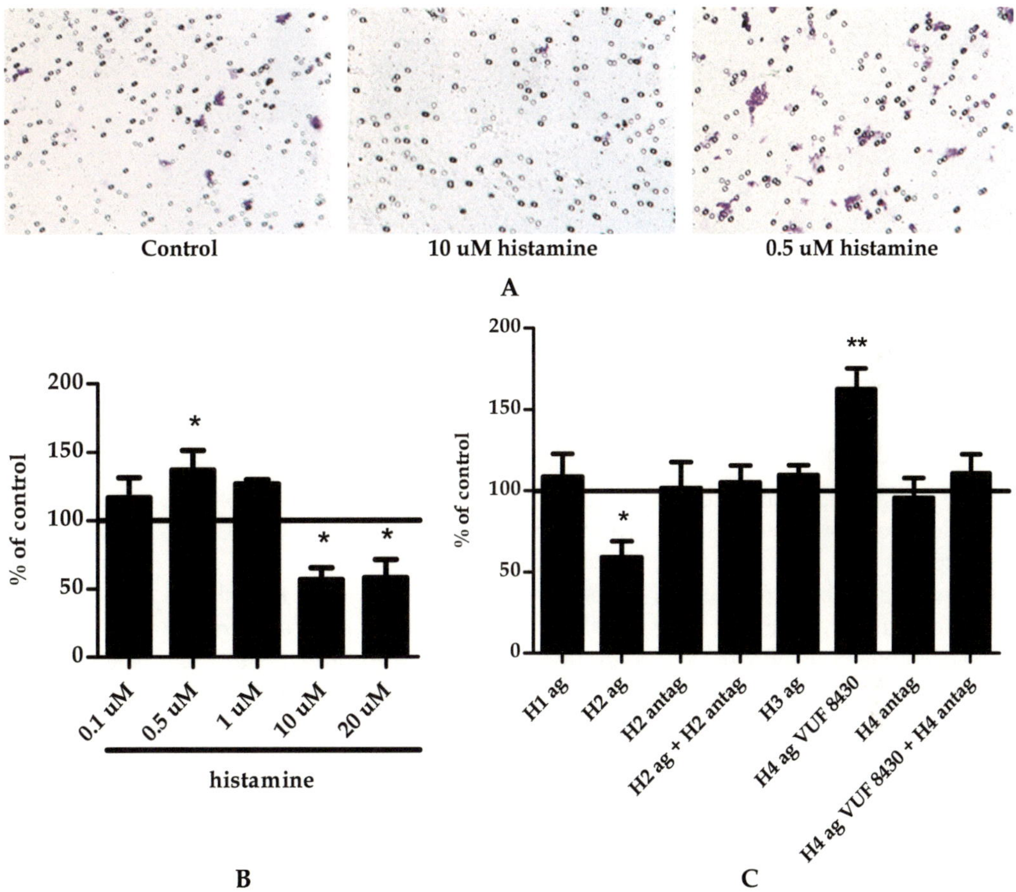

Fig. 5. Histamine induced migration of MDA-MB 231 cells. Migration was evaluated by using transwell units with 8 µm pore size PET membranes. A: Photographs are representative of random fields observed at 50x magnification. B-C: Bars show the means ± SEM of three experiments run in duplicates. Results are expressed for each treatment as the number of cells on the lower side of membranes normalized to control values. B: Concentration-response curve of histamine. C: Effect of histamine receptor agonists and antagonists on cell migration. $^{*}p<0.05$ and $^{**}p<0.01$ vs control. One way ANOVA, Dunnet post test.

4. H202 involvement in histamine actions

Many cell surface receptors produce transient levels of ROS (specifically H2O2) when are activated by peptide growth factors, cytokines and ligands of G protein-coupled receptors

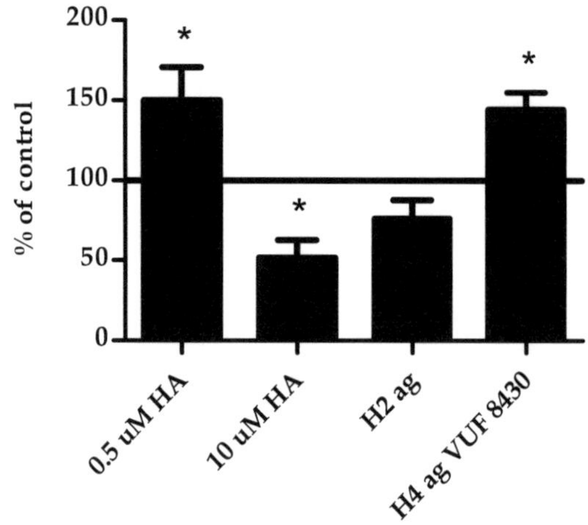

Fig. 6. Effect of histamine and histamine receptor agonists on cell invasion. Invasion was evaluated by using transwell units with 8 µm pore size PET membranes coated with Matrigel®. Bars show the means ± SEM of three experiments run in duplicates. Results are expressed for each treatment as the number of cells invading the lower side of membranes normalized to control values. *$p<0.05$ vs control. One way Anova, Dunnet post test.

(GPCRs) like histamine receptors (Rhee et al, 2000). In a previous work we reported that high doses of histamine enhance H2O2 intracellular levels in MDA-MB 231 cells (Medina et al, 2006).

ROS will contribute to various aspects of malignant tumors, including carcinogenesis, aberrant growth and metastasis which is a complex process including epithelial-mesenchymal transition (EMT), migration, invasion of the tumor cells and angiogenesis around the tumor lesion (Pani et al, 2009). Significant amounts of ROS are able to kill cancer cells through their oxidative action. At lower concentrations, however, ROS work as second messengers in signal transduction, and activate a variety of proteins or upregulate their transcription. The ROS-regulated genes relevant to EMT and metastasis include EGF, EGFR, VEGF, E-cadherin, integrin and MMPs (Nishikawa 2008; Wu, 2006).

In order to explore the effect of ROS on cellular events related to invasiveness of MDA-MB 231 cells we conducted the following experiments.

4.1 Measurement of ROS levels

The fluorescent dye dichlorofluorescein diacetate (DFH-DA) is an important tool to indicate oxidations in cells and is one of a very few markers available for measuring intracellular ROS levels in live cells. DFH-DA is a non polar and non fluorescent compound that freely diffuses through cell membranes. Once it enters the cells, its ester moiety is cleaved by intracellular esterases, and then DFH is retained in the cells. Oxidation of DFH by ROS yields a fluorescent species that can be detected by flow cytometry.

In order to investigate the effect of ROS on cellular events related to invasiveness we measured the steady state levels of ROS employing 5 µM DFH-DA dye in MDA-MB 231 cells after 1h treatment with histamine, histamine agonists and antagonists. Exogenous catalase (125 IU/mL) was added 15 minutes before treatments to metabolize intracellular H2O2 levels.

Histamine augmented intracellular steady state of ROS levels in a dose-dependent manner (Tabla 3). Histamine in low concentration and 10 μM H4 agonists increased intracellular ROS levels up to 135%, while high doses of histamine and 10 μM H2 agonists augmented them up to 190%. When exogenous catalase was added to histamine-treated cells there was a significant reduction of ROS levels almost to control value confirming that intracellular H2O2 was the major species involved since H2O2 is the only substrate for catalase.

Treatment	mean fluorescence (% respect of control values)
0.5 μM HA	123 ± 5
5 μM HA	140 ± 8*
20 μM HA	184 ± 10**
H4 agonist	135 ± 9*
H2 agonist	190 ± 15**
catalase	83 ± 6
catalase + 10 μM HA	120 ± 7
catalase + 0.5 μM HA	105 ± 6

Table 3. Effect of histamine, histamine receptor agonists and catalase on ROS levels in MDA-MB 231 cells. ROS levels were assessed by flow cytometry using DFH-DA, a specific fluorescent dye, and mean fluorescence values for each treatment were normalized to controls. Table show the means ± SEM of three experiments run in duplicates *$p<0.05$ and **$p<0.01$ vs control. One way Anova, Dunnet post test.

4.2 Gelatinolytic activity is modified by endogenous and exogenous H2O2 levels

MDA-MB 231 cells were treated with different concentrations of exogenous H2O2 and assayed by zymography. A biphasic response of MMP2 and MMP9 was observed depending on the H2O2 concentration added, as shown in Figure 7. Results indicate that different thresholds of H2O2 may be required for enhancing or inhibiting MMPs activities.

A link between ROS and MMPs has been widely discussed. Evidence supports that activation of proenzymes (MMP1, MMP2, MMP7 and MMP9) is regulated by ROS through interactions with thiol groups (Nelson & Melendez, 2004). It has been reported that higher doses of H2O2 may alter signal transduction pathways leading to protein degradation (Rhee et al, 2003). Our data are in agreement with Rajagopalan and coworkers who demonstrated ROS-induced activation of MMP2 at low doses of exogenous H2O2 (4 μM) and inactivation at higher doses (10–50 μM) in macrophage-derived foam cells when they studied the stability of atherosclerotic plaques (Rajagopalan et al, 1996). Suppression of MMP2 activity by H2O2 in a dose- and time-dependent manner was also observed during acute ulceration being reverted by antioxidants (Ganguly et al, 2006). However, most of reports inform about a positive modulation of MMP2 and MMP9 in response to oxidative stress in different tissues and cell lines including mammary cells (Mori et al, 2004).

Addition of exogenous catalase to tumor mammary cells half an hour before treatments was able to impede both the increase and decrease in gelatinolytic activities disclosed by histamine and histamine agonists confirming that intracellular H2O2 levels were involved in the modulation of enzymatic activity of both MMPs (Figure 8).

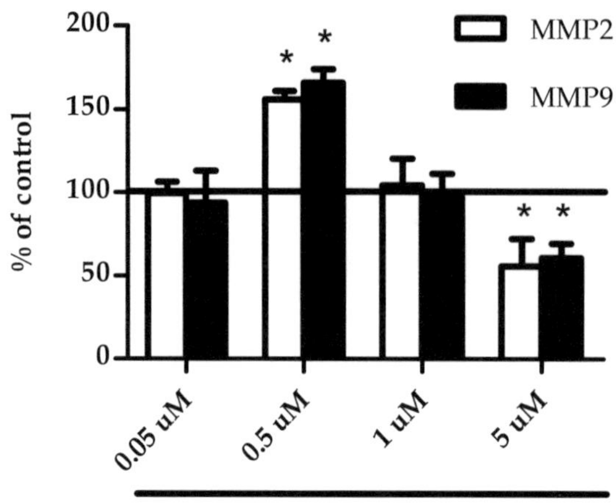

Fig. 7. Action of exogenous H2O2 on MMP2 and MMP9 gelatinolytic activity. Concentration-response curve obtained by zymography. Activity of lytic bands for each treatment was determined by densitometry and normalized to control values. Bars show the means ± SEM of three experiments run in triplicates *$p<0.05$ vs control. Two way Anova, Bonferroni post test.

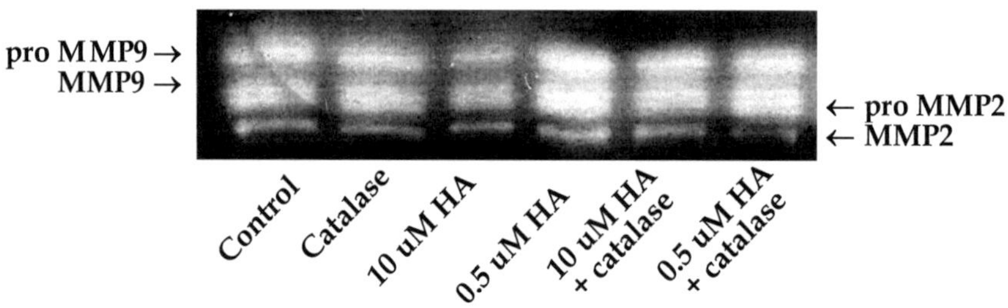

Fig. 8. Effect of catalase on histamine-regulated gelatinolytic activity of MMP2 and MMP9. Activity was evaluated by zymography after 24 h of treatment in serum free RPMI medium. Figure shows a representative gel.

4.3 Cell migration is influenced by H2O2 levels

In order to correlate H2O2 levels with the migratory capacity in MDA-MB 231 cells, we assayed different H2O2 concentrations using transwells. Cell migration was modified by exogenous H2O2 in a dose dependent manner (Figure 9A). It was significantly stimulated by low doses while inhibited by high ones. Considering that histamine and histamine agonists differentially modulate intracellular H2O2 as shown in table 3, our research suggests that the magnitude of these rises in histamine-treated cells may therefore be essential for the migratory and invasive behavior. This possibility is supported by the results obtained when exogenous catalase (125 IU/mL) was added to cell cultures (Figure 9B).

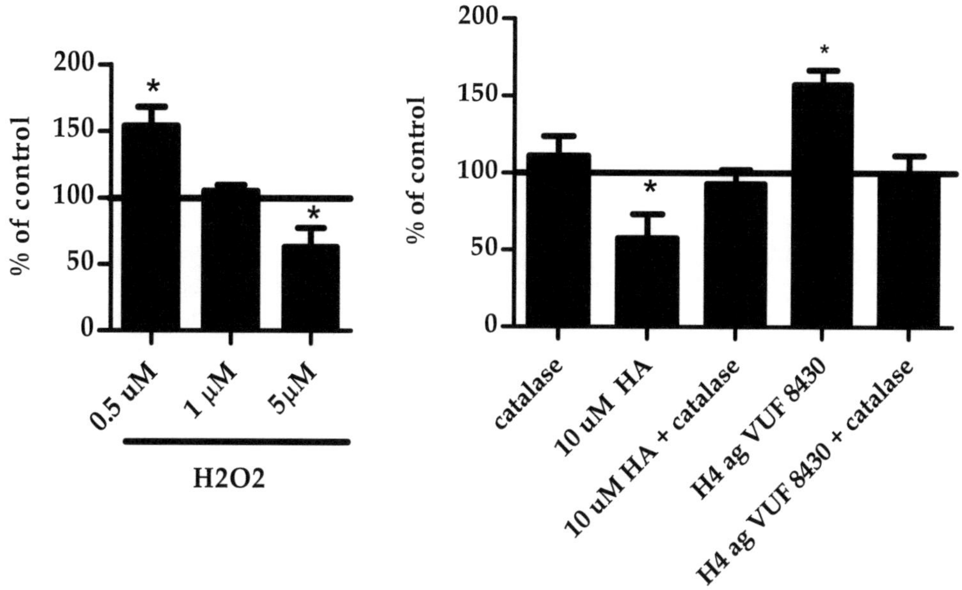

A B

Fig. 9. Effect of H2O2 on migration of MDA-MB 231 cells. Migration was evaluated by using transwell units with 8 um pore size PET membranes. Bars show the means ± SEM of three experiments run in duplicates. Results are expressed for each treatment as the number of cells counted on the lower side of membranes normalized to control values. A: Concentration-response curve for exogenous H2O2. B: Effect of catalase on histamine induced-cell migration. *$p<0.05$ vs control. One way ANOVA, Dunnet post test.

Overall, our data strongly support the hypothesis that ROS are involved in histamine-induced modulation of MMP2 and MMP9, which are assumed to play a critical role in tumor invasion. Divergent migration and invasion responses (stimulatory or inhibitory) to histamine may be due to changes in the cellular redox balance through H2 and H4 receptor activation as in the case of MMPs. Likely, when H2O2 is produced at high concentrations in MDA-MB 231 cells, it may be capable to affect enzymatic activities by altering signaling pathways and even cause cellular damage. Many elements in the process leading to cell migration are considered to be redox-sensitive (Pani et al, 2009; Svineng et al, 2008). ROS modify the activity of several key enzymes, resulting in the reorganization of actin cytoskeleton, adhesion and stimulation of migration. There is evidence that ROS can regulate such critical target molecules as PKC, MAPK, PI3K, tyrosine phospatases, PTEN, Src and focal adhesion kinase (FAK) (Rhee et al, 2000, 2003).

Preliminary results obtained in our laboratory show an increase in c-Src phosphorylation in the presence of low doses of histamine or H2O2 exogenously added suggesting a possible role of this kinase in MDA-MB 231 cells migration induced by histamine (data not shown).

4.4 Determination of catalase activity

We have previously reported that histamine in a high concentration inhibits catatase activity in MDA-MB 231 cells (Medina et al, 2006). To further correlate catalase activity with the intracellular H2O2 levels generated by histamine and histamine agonists treatments, we measured the endogenous enzymatic activity spectrophotometrically. Briefly, cells were treated for 24h, scrapped and collected in potassium phosphate buffer 50 mM pH 7.0. This was followed by sonic disruption. Protein concentration was determined by Bradford assay. Catalase activity was determined using whole cell homogenates by measuring the exponential decay of 20 mM H2O2 ($\Delta\varepsilon_{240} = 43.6\ M^{-1}\ cm^{-1}$) at 25°C monitored at 240 nm. Specific activity was expressed as the number of catalase units per mg of protein. One catalase unit is defined as the amount of catalase that breaks 1 µmol of H2O2 down per minute, at 25°C and pH 7.

There was a reduction of the enzymatic activity when cells were cultured in the presence of 0.5 µM histamine or H4 agonists, being this reduction more significant at higher doses of histamine or with H2 agonists (Figure 10). Data indicate that the modulation of catalase activity in our experimental conditions is critical in the control of endogenous H2O2 levels which in turn trigger different biological responses. In this sense, other authors have demonstrated in colon and liver tumor cells that high basal levels of ROS are mainly controlled by catalase (Laurent et al, 2005). Expression of catalase is known to be regulated at message, protein and activity levels. Soluble factors from tumor cells as TNF alpha have been suggested to be repressors of catalase expression, and cell signaling molecules as PKA, PKC and Casein Kinase II have been reported to elevate catalase activity *in vitro* (Nishikawa 2002; Reimer el 1994; Yano & Yano, 2002). Histamine could act at any of these levels (Baker et al, 2002; Igaz et al, 2001; Leurs et al, 2009; Steffel el al, 2006)

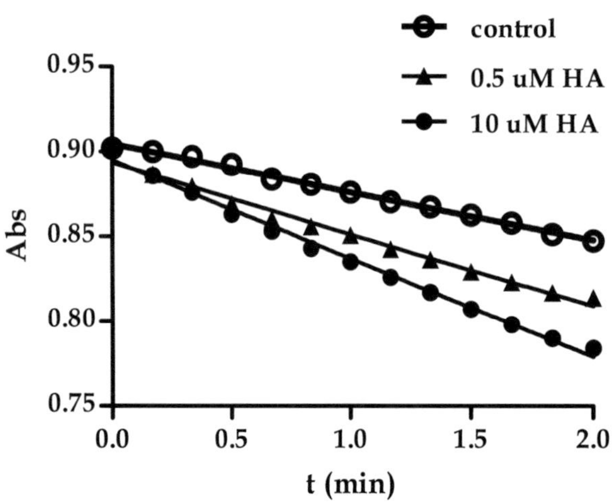

Treatment	Catalase activity (IU/mg protein)
control	10.8 ± 0.9
0.5 µM HA	8.5 ± 0.8*
10 µM HA	5.4 ± 0.6*
H2 agonist	6.2 ± 0.7*
H4 agonist	8.1 ± 0.9*

Fig. 10. Effect of histamine and histamine receptor agonists on catalase activity. Activity was evaluated spectrophotometrically by measuring the extinction of the H202, the substrate of catalase enzyme. Slopes of straight lines fit by linear regression represent the rate of extinction and are correlated with enzymatic activity. Embedded table shows catalase activities for histamine and histamine receptor agonists. Results are expressed as means ± SEM of two experiments run in duplicates. *$p<0.05$ vs control. One way Anova. Dunnet post test.

5. Ionizing radiation enhances the activity of MMPs and cell migration – Interaction between histamine and ionizing radiation

The mechanisms that control the therapeutic efficacy of radiotherapy have classically focused on the ability of ionizing radiation to kill cancer cells while sparing normal tissues. Radiation therapy after surgery consists typically of irradiation of the breast with 50-60 gray, delivered over 6 weeks in 2 gray fractions. Fractionation allows time to normal cells to recover, to tumor cells to reenter to radio-sensitive phase of the cell cycle and to hypoxic tumor areas to re-oxygenate and as a result become more responsive to ionizing radiation.

Sensitivity of tumor cells to ionizing radiation is crucial to outline the probability of local control and finally of cure of cancers by radiotherapy. Many factors are involved in affecting susceptibility of tumor cells to ionizing radiation and the generation of ROS as a result of photon irradiation accounts for approximately 75% of radiation-induced damage. ROS production occurs within seconds of starting radiation treatment and this initial redox perturbation has important implications in terms of the final cellular response to ionizing radiation.

As already mentioned we have previously demonstrated that histamine is able to increment MDA-MB 231 cells intrinsic radiosensitivity by downregulating catalase activity and increasing H2O2 intracellular levels at the same doses that inhibits cell proliferation. Recently we have established a radioprotective role of histamine on bone marrow against cellular damage induced by ionizing radiation (Medina et al, 2010). We have also proved that histamine prevents radiation-induced toxicity on small intestine by modulating the antioxidant enzymes expression and by suppressing apoptosis and increasing proliferation of damaged intestinal mucosa (Medina et al, 2007). Intracellular ROS concentration is critical for cell growth and survival; in normal cells ROS levels are kept low, but quite the opposite in tumor cells high levels of ROS close to the threshold of cytotoxicity are related to cell proliferation. Thus drugs that modulate antioxidant enzymes may differentially affect normal and neoplastic cells growth and death. In view of these antecedents, we proposed to study the interaction between histamine and ionizing radiation on the proinvasive ability of this cell line. MDA-MB 231 cells were gamma irradiated with a 2 gray dose using an IBL 437C, H type irradiator in presence or absence of histamine or histamine agonists. After irradiation culture media were conditioned for 24 h and then zymographies were carried out; migration assays were immediately performed. Ionizing radiation increased ROS levels in irradiated control cells and a rise in MMPs activity and cell migration was also found compared to non irradiated control cells (Figure 11). This effect observed on cellular events related to MDA-MB 231 invasiveness was counteracted when irradiated cells were treated with high doses of histamine or with H2 agonist, which may be due to the largest amount of ROS generated in these conditions.

The effects of irradiation on malignant biological behaviors of cells surviving irradiation have been reported for a variety of tumor cells. Many of these reports provide evidence that irradiated tumor cells acquire malignant potency through increased motility and invasiveness, up-regulation of MMPs, as well as an enhanced capacity for adhesion. The activation of different signal transduction cascades including stress kinases, the PI3K/Akt/NF-kB pathway or the c-Src is implicated in these radiation-induced responses. The same signaling mechanisms are engaged in ROS mediated actions on invasive capacity (Cheng el al, 2006; Hwang et al, 2006; Jung et al, 2007; Wild-Bold el al 2006). Current studies

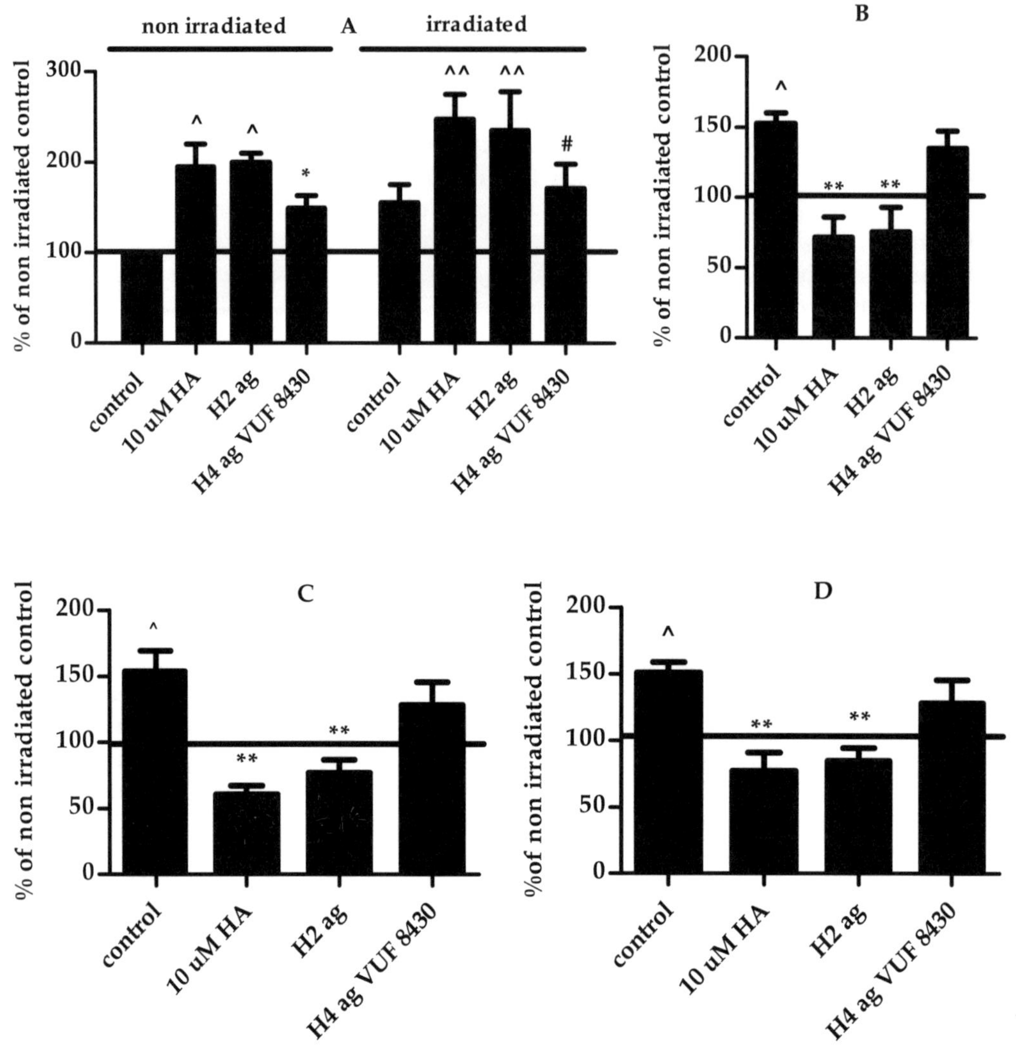

Fig. 11. Effect of ionizing radiation on MDA-MB 231 cells. A: ROS levels induced by histamine and histamine receptor agonists. B: Effect of histamine and histamine receptor agonists on cell migration of irradiated cells. C: Effect of histamine and histamine receptor agonists on MMP2 gelatinolytic activity of irradiated cells. D: Effect of histamine and histamine receptor agonists on MMP9 gelatinolytic activity of irradiated cells. Bars represent the means ± SEM of at least three experiments run in duplicates ^ $p<0.05$ and ^^$p<0.01$ vs non irradiated control, *$p<0.05$ vs 10 µM HA and vs control, **$p<0.01$ vs control, # $p<0.05$ vs 10 µM HA. Two way Anova, Bonferroni post test.

in our laboratory are intended to confirm the crucial role of distinct levels of ROS generated in the opposite responses of MDA-MB 231 cells to different histamine concentrations and ionizing radiation, and to identify the signaling pathways concerned.

6. Conclusions

Understanding the molecular mechanisms of metastases is one of the most relevant issues in cancer research. New growths (metastases) at distant sites from the primary tumor require a number of steps to be completed successfully. Tumor cells must bind to one or more components of the basement membrane or extracellular matrix, degrade them to migrate, intravasate in blood and lymphatic vessels and finally extravasate to be seeded at distant locations. MMP2 and MMP9 are mainly involved in these processes, being abundantly expressed in various malignant tumors.

In the last decade a subcutaneous formulation of histamine dihydrochloride has been used as an adjuvant with interleukin-2 therapy for the potential treatment of metastatic melanoma, acute myelogenous leukemia and renal cell carcinoma, mainly based upon its action on immunity (Perz & Ho, 2008). Our research provides novel evidence for a possible use of histamine as a pharmacological agent with low side effects that targets oncogenic pathways which may regulate breast tumor cell proliferation and/or survival and simultaneously may control invasion and metastasis.

Radiotherapy is a highly effective modality for locoregional treatment of breast tumors and other cancers. Despite the fact that it has been classically considered to exert its therapeutic effect by killing tumor cells, clinical and experimental evidence indicates that results extend beyond cancer cell death pointing out that ionizing radiation might promote a metastatic behavior of cancer cells. Our current results also open a perspective for the potential use of histamine to improve radiotherapy efficacy not only increasing intrinsic radiosensitivity of breast tumor cells specifically, but wielding an effect on the possible development of radio-induced metastases.

In view that a shift in the paradigm from a population-based to a personalized patient-based treatment emerges as a near step in cancer therapy correlating molecular expression signatures with treatment outcomes, the determination of histamine receptors in patient tumors seems feasible and may help design more effective therapies.

7. Acknowledgements

This work was supported by grants from the University of Buenos Aires (UBACYT B029), from the National Agency for Scientific and Technological Promotion (PICT 01022) and from the EU-FP7 COST Action BM0806 (Recent advances in histamine receptor H4R research). We thank Dr Nicholas Carruthers from Johnson & Johnson for the H4 antagonist JNJ7777120.

8. References

Asano, K., Kanai, K. & Suzaki, H. (2004). Suppressive activity of fexofenadine hydrochloride on metalloproteinase production from nasal fibroblasts in vitro. *Clin Exp Allergy*, Vol.34, No.12, (December 2004), pp 1890-1898, ISSN 0954-7894

Bakker, R., Timmerman, H. & Leurs, R. (2002). Histamine receptors: specific ligands, receptor biochemistry, and signal transduction. *Clin Allergy Immunol*, Vol.17, (2002) pp 27-64, ISSN 1075-7910

Baluna, R., Eng, T. & Thomas, C. (2006). Adhesion molecules in radiotherapy. *Radiat Res*, Vol.166, No.6, (December 2006), pp 819-831, ISSN 0033-7587

Barnard R., Barnard, A., Salmon, G., Wai, L. & Sreckovic, S. (2008). Histamine-Induced Actin Polymerization in Human Eosinophils: An Imaging Approach for Histamine H4 Receptor. *Cytometry A.*, Vol.73, No.4, (April 2008), pp 299-304, ISSN 1552-4930

Baum, O., Hlushchuk, R., Forster, A., Greiner, R., Clézardin, P., Zhao, Y., Djonov, V & Gruber, G. (2007). Increased invasive potential and up-regulation of MMP-2 in MDA-MB-231 breast cancer cells expressing the beta3 integrin subunit. *Int J Oncol*, Vol.30, No.2, (February 2007), pp 325-332, ISSN 1019-6439

Bäumer, W., Wendorff, S., Gutzmer, R., Werfel, T., Dijkstra, D., Chazot, P., Stark, H. & Kietzmann, M. (2008). Histamine H4 receptors modulate dendritic cell migration through skin--immunomodulatory role of histamine. *Allergy*, Vol.63, No.10, (October 2008), pp 1387-1394, ISSN 1398-9995

Blaya, B., Nicolau-Galmés, F., Jangi, S., Ortega-Martínez, I., Alonso-Tejerina, E., Burgos-Bretones, J., Pérez-Yarza, G., Asumendi, A. & Boyano, M. (2010). Histamine and histamine receptor antagonists in cancer biology. *Inflamm Allergy Drug Targets*, Vol.9, No.3, (July 2010), pp 146-157, ISSN 1871-5281

Ciprandi, G., Tosca, M., Cosentino, C., Riccio, A., Passalacqua, G. & Canonica, G. (2003). Effects of fexofenadine and other antihistamines on components of the allergic response: adhesion molecules. *J Allergy Clin Immunol*, Vol.112, No.4 Suppl, (October 2003), pp S78-82, ISSN 0091-6749

Chakraborti, S., Mandal, M., Das, S., Mandal, A. & Chakraborti, T. (2003). Regulation of matrix metalloproteinases: an overview. *Mol Cell Biochem*, Vol.253, No.1-2, (November 2003), pp 269-285, ISSN 0300-8177

Chambers, A. & Matrisian, L. (1997). Changing views of the role of matrix metalloproteinases in metastasis. *J Natl Cancer Inst*, Vol. 3, No.89(17), (September 1997), pp 1260-1270, Review, ISSN 0027-8874

Cheng, J., Chou, C., Kuo, M. & Hsieh, C. (2006). Radiation-enhanced hepatocellular carcinoma cell invasion with MMP-9 expression through PI3K/Akt/NF-jB signal transduction pathway. *Oncogene*, Vol.25, No.53, (November 2006), pp 7009–7018, ISSN 0950-9232

Cricco, G., Núñez, M., Medina, V., Garbarino, G., Mohamad, N., Gutiérrez, A., Cocca, C., Bergoc, R., Rivera, E. & Martín, G. (2006). Histamine modulates cellular events involved in tumour invasiveness in pancreatic carcinoma cells. *Inflamm Res*, Vol.55, Suppl 1, (April 2006), pp S83-S84, ISSN 1023-3830

Cricco, G., Martín, G., Medina, V., Núñez, M., Mohamad, N., Croci, M., Crescenti, E., Bergoc, R. & Rivera, E. (2006) Histamine inhibits cell proliferation and modulates the expression of Bcl-2 family proteins via the H2 receptor in human pancreatic cancer cells. *Anticancer Res*, Vol.26, No.6B, (November-December 2006), pp 4443-4450, ISSN 0250-7005

Cricco, G., Mohamad, N., Sambuco, L., Genre, F., Croci, M., Gutiérrez, A., Medina, V., Bergoc, R., Rivera, E. & Martín, G. (2008). Histamine regulates pancreatic carcinoma cell growth through H3 and H4 receptors.G. *Inflamm Res*. Vol.57, Suppl 1, (March 2008), pp S23-S24, ISNN 1023-3830

Decock, J., Hendrickx, W., Wildiers, H., Christiaens, M., Neven, P., Drijkoningen, M. & Paridaens, R. (2005). Plasma gelatinase levels in patients with primary breast cancer in relation to axillary lymph node status, Her2/neu expression and other clinicopathological variables. *Clinical Exp Metastasis,* Vol.22, No.6, (October 2005), pp 495-502, ISSN 0262-0898

Doyle, J. & Haas, T. (2009). Differential role of beta-catenin in VEGF and histamine-induced MMP-2 production in microvascular endothelial cells. *J Cell Biochem,* Vol.15, No.107(2), (May 2009) pp 272-83, ISSN 0730-2312

Duffy, M., McGowan, P. & Gallagher, W. (2008). Cancer invasion and metastasis: changing views. *J Pathol.* Vol.214, No.3, (February 2008), pp 283-293, ISSN 0022-3417

Falus, A., Hegyesi, H., Lázár-Molnár, E., Pós, Z., László, V. & Darvas, Z. (2001). .Paracrine and autocrine interactions in melanoma: histamine is a relevant player in local regulation. *Trends Immunol,* Vol.22, No.12, (December 2001), pp 648-652, ISSN 1471-4906

Francis, H., Onori, P., Gaudio, E., Franchitto, A., DeMorrow, S., Venter, J., Kopriva, S., Carpino, G., Mancinelli, R., White, M., Meng, F., Vetuschi, A., Sferra, R. & Alpini. (2009). H3 histamine receptor-mediated activation of protein kinase Calpha inhibits the growth of cholangiocarcinoma in vitro and in vivo. *Mol Cancer Res,*Vol.7, No.10, (October 2009), pp 1704-1713, ISSN 1541-7786

Freije, J., Balbín, M., Pendás, A., Sánchez, L., Puente, X. & López-Otín, C. (2003). Matrix metalloproteinases and tumor progression. *Adv Exp Med Biol,* Vol.532, (2003), pp 91-107, ISSN 0065-2598

Ganguly, K., Kundu, P., Banerjee, A., Reiter, R. & Swarnakar, S. (2006). Hydrogen peroxide-mediated downregulation of matrix metalloprotease-2 in indomethacin-induced acute gastric ulceration is blocked by melatonin and other antioxidants. *Free Radic Biol Med,* Vol.41, No.6, (September 2006), pp 911-925, ISSN 0891-5849

Genre, F., Valli, E., Medina, V., Gutiérrez, A., Sambuco, L., Rivera, E., Cricco, G. & Martín, G. (2009). Effect of histamine on the expression of metalloproteinases and cell adhesion in breast cancer cell lines. *Inflamm Res,*Vol.58, Suppl 1, (April 2009), 55-56, ISSN 1023-3830

Gschwandtner, M., Purwar, R., Wittmann, M., Bäumer, W., Kietzmann, M., Werfel, T. & Gutzmer, R. (2008). Histamine upregulates keratinocyte MMP-9 production via the histamine H1 receptor. *J Invest Dermatol,* Vol.128, No.12, (December 2008), pp 2783-2791, ISSN 0022-202X

Gschwandtner, M., Rossbach, K., Dijkstra, D., BäμMer, W., Kietzmann, M., Stark, H., Werfel, T. & Gutzmer, R. (2010). Murine and human Langerhans cells express a functional histamine H4 receptor: modulation of cell migration and function. *Allergy,* Vol.65, No.7, (July 2010), pp 840-849, ISSN 0105-4538

Gutzmer, R., Diestel, C., Mommert, S., Köther, B., Stark, H., Wittmann, M. & Werfel, T. (2005). Histamine H4 receptor stimulation suppresses IL-12p70 production and mediates chemotaxis in human monocyte-derived dendritic cells. *J Immunol,* Vol.174, No.9, (May 2005), pp 5224-5232, ISSN 0022-1767

Hwang, S., Jung, J., Jeong, J., Kim, Y., Oh, E., Kim, T., Kim, J., Cho, K. & Han, I. (2006). Dominant-negative Rac increases both inherent and ionizing radiation-induced cell migration in C6 rat glioma cells. *Int J Cancer,* Vol. 118, No.8, (April 2006), pp 2056–2063, ISSN 0020-7136

Hofstra, C., Desai, P., Thurmond, R. & Fung-Leung, W. (2003). Histamine H4 receptor mediates chemotaxis and calcium mobilization of mast cells. *J Pharmacol Exp Ther*, Vol.305, No.3, (June 2003), pp1212-1221, ISSN 0022-3565

Igaz, P., Novák, I., Lázaár, E., Horváth, B., Héninger, E. & Falus A. (2001). Bidirectional communication between histamine and cytokines. *Inflamm Res,* Vol.50, No.3, (March 2001), pp 123-128, Review, ISSN 1023-3830

John, A. & Tuszynski, G. (2001). The role of matrix metalloproteinases in tumor angiogenesis and tumor metastasis. *Pathol Oncol Res,* Vol.7, No.1, (February 2001), pp 14-23, ISSN 1219-4956

Jung, J., Hwang, S., Hwang, J., Oh, E., Park, S. & Han, I. (2007). Ionising radiation induces changes associated with epithelial-mesenchymal transdifferentiation and increased cell motility of A549 lung epithelial cells. *Eur J Cancer,* Vol.43, No.7, (May 2007), pp 1214-1224, ISSN 1359-6349

Kattan, Z., Minig, V., Leroy, P., Dauça, M. & Becuwe P. (2008). Role of manganese superoxide dismutase on growth and invasive properties of human estrogen-independent breast cancer cells. *Breast Cancer Res Treat,* Vol.108, No.2, (March 2008), pp 203-215, ISSN 0167-6806

Köhrmann, A., Kammerer, U., Kapp, M., Dietl, J. & Anacker J. (2009). Expression of matrix metalloproteinases (MMPs) in primary human breast cancer and breast cancer cell lines: New findings and review of the literature. *BMC Cancer,* Vol.9, No.188, (June 2009), ISSN 1471-2407

Kohyama, T., Yamauchi, Y., Takizawa, H., Kamitani, S., Kawasaki, S. & Nagase, T. (2010). Histamine stimulates human lung fibroblast migration. *Mol Cell Biochem,* Vol 337. No.1-2, (April 2010), pp 77-81, ISSN 0300-8177

La Rocca, G., Pucci-Minafra, I., Marrazzo, A., Taormina, P. & Minafra, S. (2004). Zymographic detection and clinical correlations of MMP-2 and MMP-9 in breast cancer sera. *British J Cancer, Vol.*90, No.7, (April 2004), 1414–1421, ISSN 0007-0920

Laurent, A., Nicco, C., Chéreau, C., Goulvestre, C., Alexandre, J., Alves, A., Lévy, E., Goldwasser, F., Panis, Y., Soubrane , O., Weill, B. & Batteux, F. (2005). Controlling tumor growth by modulating endogenous production of reactive oxygen species. Cancer Res, Vol.65, No.3, (February 2005), pp 948-956, ISSN 0008-5472

Lázár-Molnár, E., Hegyesi, H., Pállinger, E., Kovács, P., Tóth, S., Fitzsimons, C., Cricco, G., Martin, G., Bergoc, R., Darvas, Z., Rivera, E. & Falus A. (2002). Inhibition of human primary melanoma cell proliferation by histamine is enhanced by interleukin-6. *Eur J Clin Invest,* Vol.32, No.10, (October 2002), pp 743-749, ISSN 0014-2972

Leurs, R., Chazot, P., Shenton, F., Lim, H. & de Esch, I. (2009). Molecular and biochemical pharmacology of the histamine H4 receptor. *Br J Pharmacol,* Vol.157, No.1, (May 2009), pp 14-23, ISSN 0007-1188

Ling, P., Ngo, K., Nguyen, S., Thurmond, R., Edwards, J., Karlsson, L. & Fung-Leung, W. (2004). Histamine H4 receptor mediates eosinophil chemotaxis with cell shape change and adhesion molecule upregulation. *Br J Pharmacol.* Vol.142, No.1, (May 2004), pp 161-171, ISSN 0007-1188

Liu, Z., Kilburn, B., Leach, R., Romero, R., Paria, B. & Armant, D. (2004). Histamine enhances cytotrophoblast invasion by inducing intracellular calcium transients through the histamine type-1 receptor. *Mol Reprod Dev,* Vol.68, No3, (July 2004), pp 345-353, ISSN 1040-452X

McArdle, F., Pattwell, D., Vasilaki, A., McArdle, A. & Jackson, M. (2005). Intracellular generation of reactive oxygen species by contracting skeletal muscle cells. *Free Radic Biol Med,* Vol.39, No.5, (September 2005), pp 651-657, ISSN 0891-5849

Medina, V., Cricco, G., Nuñez, M., Martín, G., Mohamad, N., Correa-Fiz, F., Sanchez-Jimenez, F., Bergoc, R. & Rivera, E. (2006). Histamine-mediated signaling processes in human malignant mammary cells. *Cancer Biol Ther,* Vol.5, No.11, (Nov 2006), p 1462-1471, ISSN 1538-4047

Medina, V., Croci, M., Mohamad, N., Massari, N., Garbarino, G., Cricco, G., Núñez, M., Martín, G., Crescenti, E., Bergoc, R. & Rivera, E. (2007). Mechanisms underlying the radioprotective effect of histamine on small intestine. *Int J Radiat Biol,*Vol.83, No.10, (October 2007), pp 653-63, ISSN 0955-3002

Medina, V., Croci, M., Crescenti, E., Mohamad, N., Sanchez-Jiménez, F., Massari, N., Nuñez, M., Cricco, G., Martin, G., Bergoc, R. & Rivera, E. (2008). The role of histamine in human mammary carcinogenesis: H3 and H4 receptors as potential therapeutic targets for breast cancer treatment. *Cancer Biol Ther,* Vol.7, No.1, (January 2008), pp 28-35, ISNN 1538-4047

Medina, V., Massari, N., Cricco, G., Martín, G., Bergoc, R. & Rivera, E. (2009). Involvement of hydrogen peroxide in histamine-induced modulation of WM35 human malignant melanoma cell proliferation. *Free Radic Biol Med.* Vol.46, No.11, (June 2009), pp 1510-1515, ISSN 0891-5849

Medina, V., Croci, M., Carabajal, E., Bergoc, R. & Rivera, E. (2010). Histamine protects bone marrow against cellular damage induced by ionising radiation.*Int J Radiat Biol,* Vol.86, No.4, (April 2010), pp 283-290, ISSN 0955-3002

Mori, K., Shibanuma, M. & Nose, K. (2004). Invasive potential induced under long-term oxidative stress in mammary epithelial cells. *Cancer Res,* Vol.64, No.20, (October 2004), pp 7464-72, ISSN 0008-5472

Murthy, S., Ryan, A., He, C., Mallampalli, R. & Carter, A. (2010). Rac1-mediated mitochondrial H2O2 generation regulates MMP-9 gene expression in macrophages via inhibition of SP-1 and AP-1. *J Biol Chem,* Vol.285, No.32, (August 2010), pp 25062-25073, ISSN 0021-9258

Nelson, K. & Melendez, J. (2004). Mitochondrial redox control of matrix metalloproteinases. *Free Radic Biol Med,*Vol. 37, No.6, (September 2004), pp 768-84, ISSN 0891-5849

Nishikawa, M. (2008). Reactive oxygen species in tumor metastasis. *Cancer Lett,* Vol.266, No.1, (July 2008), pp 53-59, ISSN 0304-3835

Pani, G., Giannoni, E., Galeotti, T. & Chiarugi, P. (2009). Redox-Based Escape Mechanism from Death: The Cancer Lesson. *Antioxidants & Redox Signaling,* Vol.11, No.11, (November 2009), pp 2791-2806, ISSN 1523-0864

Parsons, M. & Ganellin, C. Histamine and its receptors. (2006). *Br J Pharmacol,* Vol.147, Suppl.1, (Jan 2006), pp S127-S135, ISSN 0007-1188

Perz, J. & Ho, A. (2008).Histamine dihydrochloride for the treatment of acute myeloid leukemia, malignant melanoma and renal cell carcinoma. *Future Oncol,* Vol.4, No.2, (April 2008), pp 169-177, ISSN 1479-6694

Platten, M., Wild-Bode, C., Wick, W., Leitlein, J., Dichgans, J. & Weller, M. (2001). N-[3,4-dimethoxycinnamoyl]-anthranilic acid (tranilast) inhibits transforming growth factor-beta relesase and reduces migration and invasiveness of human malignant glioma cells. *Int J Cancer*, Vol.93, No.1, (July 2001), pp 53-61, ISSN 0020-7136

Pos, Z., Hegyesi, H. & Rivera, E. (2004). Histamine and cell proliferation, In: *Histamine biology and medical aspects,* A. Falus (Ed), 199-225, SpringMed Publishing Ltd, ISBN 3-8055-7715-X, Budapest, Hungary

Rajagopalan, S., Meng, X., Ramasamy, S., Harrison, G. &. Galis, Z. (1996). Reactive Oxygen Species Produced by Macrophage-derived Foam Cells Regulate the Activity of Vascular Matrix Metalloproteinases In Vitro Implications for Atherosclerotic Plaque Stability. *J Clin Invest*, Vol.98, No.11, (December 1996), pp 2572–2579, ISSN 0021-9738

Reimer, D., Bailley, J. & Singh, S. (1994). Complete cDNA and 5' genomic sequences and multilevel regulation of the mouse catalase gene. *Genomics*, Vol.21, No.2, (May 1994), pp 325-336, ISSN 0888-7543

Rhee, S., Bae, Y., Lee, S. & Kwon, J. (2000). Hydrogen Peroxide: A Key Messenger That Modulates Protein Phosphorylation Through Cysteine Oxidation, 10.10.2010, Available from htpp//www.stke.org/cgi/content/full/OC_sigtrans;2000/53/pe1

Rhee, S., Chang, T., Bae, Y., Lee, S. & Kang, S. (2003). Cellular regulation by hydrogen peroxide. *J Am Soc Nephrol,* Vol.14, No.8 Suppl 3, (August 2003), pp S211-215, ISSN 1046-6673

Rivera, E., Cricco, G., Engel, N., Fitzsimons, C., Martín, G. & Bergoc, R. (2000). Histamine as an autocrine growth factor: an unusual role for a widespread mediator. *Semin Cancer Biol,* Vol.10, No.1, (February 2000), pp 15-23, ISSN 1044-579X

Rudolph, M., Boza, Y., Yefi, R., Luza, S., Andrews, E., Penissi, A., Garrido, P. & Rojas, I. (2008). The influence of mast cell mediators on migration of SW756 cervical carcinoma cells. *J Pharmacol Sci,* Vol.106, No.2, (February 2008), pp 208-218, ISSN 1347-8613

Sharif, N., Wiernas, T., Howe, W., Griffin, B., Offord, E. & Pfeifer, A. (1998). Human corneal epithelial cell functional responses to inflammatory agents and their antagonists. *Invest Ophthalmol Vis Sci.* Vol.39, No13, (December 1998), pp 2562-2571, ISSN 1552-5783

Soule, B., Simone, N., DeGraff ,W., Choudhuri, R., Cook, J. & Mitchell J. (2010). Loratadine dysregulates cell cycle progression and enhances the effect of radiation in human tumor cell lines. *J Radiat Oncol,* Vol.5, No8, (February 2010), ISSN 0360-3016

Stankovic, S., Konjevic, G., Gopcevic, K., Jovic, V., Inic, M. & Jurisic, V. (2010)., Activity of MMP-2 and MMP-9 in sera of breast cancer patients. *Pathol Res Pract,* Vol.206, No.4, (April 2010), pp 241-247, ISSN 0344-0338

Steffel, J., Arnet, C., Akhmedov, A., Iseli, S., Lüscher, T. & Tanner FC. (2006). Histamine differentially interacts with tumor necrosis factor-alpha and thrombin in endothelial tissue factor induction: the role of c-Jun NH2-terminal kinase. *J Thromb Haemost*, Vol.4, No.11, (November 2006), pp 2452-2460, ISSN 1538-7933

Svineng, G., Ravuri, C., Rikardsen O., Huseby, N. & Winberg, J. (2008). The role of reactive oxygen species in integrin and matrix metalloproteinase expression and function. *Connect Tissue Res.* Vol.49, No.3, (2008), pp 197-202, ISSN 0300-8207

Tetlow, L. & Woolley, D. (2002). Histamine stimulates matrix metalloproteinase-3 and -13 production by human articular chondrocytes in vitro. *Ann Rheum Dis,* Vol.61, No8, (August 2002), pp 737-740, ISSN 1468-2060

Tetlow, L. & Woolley, D. (2004). Effect of histamine on the production of matrix metalloproteinases-1, -3, -8 and -13, and TNFalpha and PGE(2) by human articular chondrocytes and synovial fibroblasts in vitro: a comparative study. *Virchows Arch.* Vol.445, No5, (November 2004), pp 485-490, ISSN 1432-2307

Thannickal, V. & Fanburg, B. (2000). Reactive oxygen species in cell signaling. *Am J Physiol Lung Cell Mol Physiol,* Vol.279, No.6, (December 2000), pp L1005-L1028, ISSN 1040-0605

Thurmond, R., Desai, P., Dunford, P., Fung-Leung, W., Hofstra, C., Jiang, W., Nguyen, S., Riley, J., Sun, S., Williams, K., Edwards, J. & Karlsson, L. (2004). A potent and selective histamine H4 receptor antagonist with anti-inflammatory properties . *J Pharmacol Exp Ther.*; Vol.309, No.1, (April 2004), pp 404-413, ISSN 0022-3565

Tilly, B., Tertoolen, L., Remorie, R., Ladoux, A., Verlaan, I., de Laat, S. & Moolenaar, W. (1990). Histamine as a growth factor and chemoattractant for human carcinoma and melanoma cells: action through Ca2(+)-mobilizing H1 receptors. *J Cell Biol,* Vol.110, No.4, (April 1990), pp 1211-1215, ISSN 0021-9525

Tomita, K., Izumi, K. & Okabe, S. (2003). Roxatidine- and cimetidine-induced angiogenesis inhibition suppresses growth of colon cancer implants in syngeneic mice. *J Pharmacol Sci,* Vol.93, No.3, (November 2003), pp 321-30, ISSN 1347-8613

Truta-Feles, K., Lagadari, M., Lehmann, K., Berod, L., Cubillos, S., Piehler, S., Herouy, Y., Barz, D., Kamradt, T., Maghazachi, A. & Norgauer, J. (2010). Histamine modulates γδ-T lymphocyte migration and cytotoxicity, via Gi and Gs protein-coupled signalling pathways. *Br J Pharmacol,* Vol.161, No.6, (November 2010), pp 1291-1300, ISSN 0007-1188

Tsukamoto, H., Shibata, K., Kajiyama, H., Terauchi, M., Nawa, A. & Kikkawa, F. (2007). Irradiation-induced epithelial-mesenchymal transition (EMT) related to invasive potential in endometrial carcinoma cells. *Gynecol Oncol,* Vol.107,No.3, (December 2007), pp 500-504, ISSN 0090-8258

Tsutsumi, K., Tsuda, M., Yazawa, N., Nakamura, H., Ishihara, S., Haga, H., Yasuda, M., Yamazaki, R., Shirato, H., Kawaguchi, H., Nishioka, T. & Ohba, Y. (2009). Increased motility and invasiveness in tumor cells that survive 10 Gy irradiation. *Cell Struct Funct,* Vol.34, No.2, (July 2009), pp 89-96, ISSN 0386-7196

Van Wart, H. & Birkedal-Hansen, H. (1990). The cysteine switch: a principle of regulation of metalloproteinase activity with potential applicability to the entire matrix metalloproteinase gene family. *Proc Natl Acad Sci USA,* Vol.87, No.14, (July 1990), pp 5578–5582, ISSN 0027-8424

Wroblewski, L., Pritchard, D., Carter, S. &, Varro A. (2002). Gastrin-stimulated gastric epithelial cell invasion: the role and mechanism of increased matrix metalloproteinase 9 expression. *Biochem J,* Vol.365, Pt 3, (August 2002), pp 873-879, ISSN 0264-6021

Wild-Bode, C., Weller, M., Rimner, A., Dichgans, J. & Wick, W. (2001). Sublethal Irradiation Promotes Migration and Invasiveness of Glioma Cells: Implications for Radiotherapy of Human Glioblastoma. *Cancer Res,* Vol.61, No. 6, (March 2001), pp 2744-2750, ISSN 0008-5472

Wu, W. (2006). The signaling mechanism of ROS in tumor progression. *Cancer Metastasis Rev.* Vol.25, No.4, (December 2006), pp 695-705, ISSN 0167-7659

Yano, S. & Yano, N. (2002). Regulation of catalase enzyme activity by cell signaling molecules. *Mol Cell Biochem,* Vol.240, No1-2, (November 2002), pp 119-130, ISNN 0300-8177

31

$1,25(OH)_2D_3$ and Cyclooxygenase-2: Possible Targets for Breast Cancer?

M. Thill[1], S. Becker[1], D. Fischer[1], K. Diedrich[1], D. Salehin[2] and M. Friedrich[2]
[1]*Department of Obstetrics and Gynecology, University Schleswig-Holstein, Campus Luebeck, Luebeck*
[2]*Department of Gynecology and Obstetrics, Helios Hospital Krefeld, Krefeld*
Germany

1. Introduction

Currently, breast cancer is the most common malignancy in women. In the U.S. in 2005, approximately 211.240 patients were newly diagnosed with primary breast cancer and 58.490 women were diagnosed with ductal carcinoma in situ (DCIS). Of these, 58.490 deaths are estimated. Therefore breast cancer takes second place following only behind lung cancer [1,2,3]. Because of this, it is necessary to develop new strategies and treatment options that may improve the prognosis.

Besides the classic histo-pathological parameters used to estimate the prognosis of malignant diseases, the identification of additional molecular prognostic parameters would be very helpful in planning treatment by evaluating protein or mRNA expression in tumor tissue. One of these potential molecular prognostic parameters might be the cyclooxygenase-2 (COX-2) [4, 5]. New treatment strategies using compounds that attack well defined proteins in the tumor require verification of the expression of these target proteins. Many similarities exist between tumor tissue and inflammatory modified tissue and normally, inflammatory reaction is self limiting, however, in tumor tissue the inflammatory reaction is persistent. An increased angiogenesis and an elevated production of cytokines, chemokines and proteases lead to good conditions for cell proliferation and invasion in the tumor tissue [6].

Targeted strategies might eliminate this inflammatory reaction that promotes tumor growth and tumorigenesis and there is already promising data around the use of COX-2-inhibitors. The antiproliferative effects of vitamin D may be another starting point; however the data on vitamin D intake or to the exertion of vitamin D analogs is occasionally inconsistent.

The important role that vitamin D and calcium adopt in the human metabolism was recognized as early as the nineteen-twenties as it was used to prevent the bone disease, rickets which was widespread in children at that time [7]. In the last 20 years non-classical effects of vitamin D and its influence on physiology followed because it's potentially anticarcinogen impacts made it more and more interesting. Besides stable calcium-homeostasis by the renal expressed 1-α-hydroxylase functionality, extra renal expressed 1-α-hydroxylase also is also known to have antiproliferative and immune-modulating features

[8-10]. This fact has led to the development of new treatment strategies in the clinical use of $1,25(OH)_2D_3$ (calcitriol). The goal was to affect and treat cancer, psoriasis, autoimmune diseases and host-graft-rejection [11-14]. Implementation of these new treatment options in vivo was conspicuously hindered as $1,25(OH)_2D_3$ has a potentially hypercalcaemic side effect. Finally the application of synthetic $1,25(OH)_2D_3$ analogs led to several successful results due to its less calciotropic effects [15, 16]. The implementation of vitamin D, primarily cancer and autoimmune diseases appears to play a more preventative role as opposed to therapeutic [17, 18].

Observational studies showed an association between vitamin D intake and $25(OH)_2D_3$ plasma levels as well as a reduced risk of breast cancer [19, 20]. Studies that tried to elucidate the correlation between sunlight and cancer prevention demonstrated that long sunlight exposure was associated with a low rate of primary breast cancer and consecutively a low mortality rate [21-24]. $1,25(OH)_2D_3$ is the biologically active form of vitamin D that binds as a ligand to the nuclear vitamin D receptor (VDR) of the genes that are important for vitamin D metabolism (1-α-hydroxylase, 24-hydroxylase) [25]. $1,25(OH)_2D_3$ and its analogs are able to inhibit the proliferation of breast cancer cells in vitro and in vivo [26-29].

2. Prostaglandin metabolism

The cyclooxygenase system consists of two different isoenzymes, COX-1 and COX-2. This system is an integral part of the prostaglandin syntethase complex and is involved controlling inflammatory processes (**1**). After transformation of arachidonic acid to prostaglandin G_2 (PGG_2), a glutathione dependent peroxidase converts PGG_2 to PGH_2 by an oxi- and peroxidation. PGH_2 acts as basic substrate for the synthesis of different prostaglandins by the microsomal and cytosolic prostaglandin synthase, which are tissue- and cell-specific. Based on the cellular enzyme setting, different prostaglandins are synthesized in different tissues where they act in an auto- or paracrine manner [30]. Prostaglandin E_2 (PGE_2) is one of the best known prostaglandins and is generated by the prostaglandin E synthase. These consist of three different forms: two microsomal prostaglandin E synthases and the cytosolic prostaglandin synthase E [31].

The 15-hydroxyprostaglandin dehydrogenase (15-PGDH) belonging to the oxidoreductases family, inactivates all generated prostaglandins by oxidation to 15-keto metabolites which then have greatly reduced biological activity [32].

3. PG-receptors

The physiological effects of many prostaglandins are mediated by binding to G protein coupled receptors. These effects regulate inflammatory mediations, control hormone regulation, constrict or dilate in vascular smooth muscle cells and regulate calcium movement and their specific receptors activate signal transduction pathways which could induce chronic processes like angiogenesis. For example, PGE_2 interacts with four cell surface receptors - EP_{1-4} and the EP_2 receptor subtype is involved in the G_s/cAMP/proteinkinase which is a-signalling pathway leading to an increased VEGF expression. PGJ_2 and PGA_2 interact with nuclear receptors, belonging to the peroxisome proliferator-activated receptors (PPARs) family. After dimerization with the 9-cis-Retinoid receptor (RXR) and then binding to a sequence specific responsive element located at the promoter of its target gene, they directly induce gene expression [33].

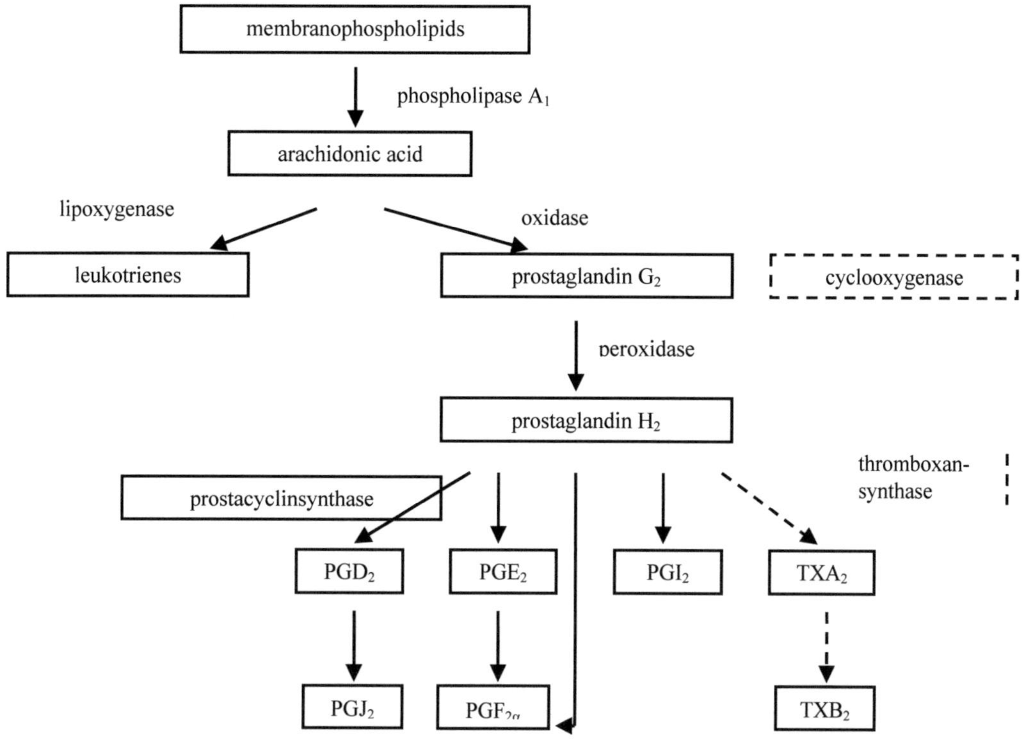

Fig. 1. Prostaglandin metabolism.

4. Isoenzymes COX-1 und COX-2

COX-1 is ubiquitary and not a relevant prognostic factor [34]. In contrast, the COX-2 enzyme is not constitutively expressed. The COX-2 gene expression is stimulated by many growth factors, cytokines and prostaglandins and is associated with inflammation [35]. COX-2 is predominantly a pro inflammatory enzyme but late in the inflammatory phase, the enzyme is involved in limiting inflammation.

Studies with COX-1 and COX-2 knockout mice lead to new consolidated findings about the function of these enzymes concerning ovarian functionality and reproduction as well as cardiovascular development [36 - 39]. The COX enzymes are the main target of non-steroidal anti inflammatory drugs (NSAID) where isoenzymes specifically inhibit the biological activity of COX enzymes. Celecoxib and rofecoxib are selective COX-2 inhibitors whereas acetylsalicylic acid, ibuprofen and indomethacin are non-specific and target both isoenzymes.

5. Role of COX-2 in carcinogenesis

The cyclooxygenases, especially COX-2, play an important role in the development and progression of malignant tumours. The over expression of COX-2 is associated with the differentiation of tumor cells by several mechanisms [40] and can be detected in various epithelial carcinomas such as in colon [41, 42], gastric [43] and esophageal cancers [44] as well as in prostate [45], liver, pancreas and lung cancers [46]. One of the mechanisms that are modulated during carcinogenesis is the neoangiogenesis [47 – 55].

Epidemiological studies have shown that a continuous intake of NSAIDs protects against the incidence of breast cancer [56-58].
Increased PGE_2 levels can be detected in cultivated human breast cancer cell lines as well as in invasive human breast cancer cells [59-62] and are associated with both a negative hormone receptor status and an escalated mestastic potential [59].
As mentioned previously, PGE_2 is the ligand for at least four cell surface receptors - EP_{1-4} and several studies have presented the impact of the EP_1-receptor in carcinogenesis of colon and breast cancer [63]. A blockage of the EP_2-receptor leads to a reduction and a diminishment of intestinal polyposis in $APC^{\Delta 716}$-knock-out mice [64]. There was an increased detection of EP_2- and EP_4-receptors in the breast tumors of COX-2-MMTV mice; therefore, it appears that the EP-receptors play an important role in mediating PG functions and in promoting carcinogenesis.

6. Role of 15-PGDH in carcinogenesis

Increased PGE_2 levels in context to mammary carcinomas are associated with an enhanced cell proliferation, invasiveness, resistance to apoptosis and angiogenesis [65, 66]. The regulation of plasma PGE_2 level results from its synthesis and its biological inactivation through 15-PGDH, the key enzyme for the biological inactivation of PGs [32]. Recent studies hypothesized 15-PGDH as a tumor suppressor gene in correlation to colon, bladder and bronchial carcinomas [67-69]. Wolf and co-workers [70] assumed antiproliferative effects of 15-PGDH in breast cancer cells. The estrogen receptor (ER) positive and well differentiated MCF-7 breast cancer cell line had an increased 15-PGDH expression compared to poorly differentiated, ER negative MDA-MB-231 cells, which express COX-2 and lead to primary breast cancer. Different studies reported that MCF-7 cells are the only breast cancer cell line with an enhanced 15-PGDH expression and low levels of 15-PGDH are accompanied by poorly prognostic factors [70]. This data attended by a microarray analysis of van't Veer and co-workers [71] supports the advice that a loss of 15-PGDH expression plays a pivotal role in the development of poorly differentiated mammary carcinomas. Data generated from genetically modified MDA-MB-231 cells that over express the enzyme and MCF-7 where 15-PGDH was knockout, corroborates the hypothesis that 15-PGDH acts as a tumor suppressor gene in breast cancer [70]. MDA-MB-231 cells showed a decreased invasiveness similar to studies in colon [67] and bronchial carcinomas [68]. Yan and co-workers [67] reported that 15-PGDH is naturally expressed in colon tissues and was dramatically reduced in colon carcinomas. The reconstitution of 15-PGDH in immunodeficiency mice prevented the colon cancer cells from generating tumors and so the authors concluded, that 15-PGDH acts as tumor suppressor and inhibits the angiogenic and proliferative effects of COX-2 in vivo.

7. COX-2 expression in breast cancer

Experimental immunochemical studies of COX-2 expression in breast cancer have produced varying and sometimes controversial and inconsistent data. Generally the consensus is that COX-2 is expressed by invasive ductal and lobular carcinoma and that the proportion of COX-2 positive tumors varies between studies (Table 1). In studies where poor prognostic tumor characteristics were examined, a correlation was found between prognostic parameters such as hormone receptor negativity, HER2 positivity, increased tumor size, high nuclear grade, development of distant metastases and a reduced survival rate (Table 1) [5]. Moreover COX-2 expression correlates with aromatase expression.

An explanation for the variable findings of COX-2 protein expression may be caused by the different scoring systems and cut-offs used for COX-2 immunoreactivity.
Half and co-workers [72] examined immonochemical human breast cell lines of normal and neoplastic breast tissue and detected a COX-2 expression in breast cancer cells in 43%, in DCIS in 62.5% and benign breast cells had a COX-2 expression in 81%. The more elevated COX-2 expression in DCIS in terms of a premalignant lesion might mean that an up-regulation or over-expression of COX-2 occurs relatively early in the carcinogenesis of breast cancer [72]. Contrary to Half and co-workers [72], Denkert and co-workers [73] could not detect a COX-2 expression in benign breast tissue and this may support the partially conflicting data. Denkert and co-workers [73] detected a COX-2 expression in 41% in invasive ductal breast cancer, however detected it in only 14% of invasive lobular tumors and 21% in other breast carcinomas (Table1). The COX-2 expression was associated with positive axillary lymph nodes (>50% node positive, just 16% in node negative breast cancer), extensive tumor growth (58% in tumors >20mm, in 24% in tumors <20mm), poor nuclear grading, vascular invasion and hormone receptor negativity.
Not all the studies have determined a correlation between COX-2 expression and clinicopathological parameters. Half and co-workers [72] could not demonstrate a significant correlation but Ristimäki and co-workers [74] certainly did show a significant correlation between COX-2 expression and hormone receptor negativity, extensive tumor growth, high nuclear grading and HER2 positivity. In a recently published paper by Singh-Ranger and co-workers [75], a correlation to distant metastases was described and Nassar and co-workers [76] demonstrated a correlation to nuclear grading and tumor size; however a correlation to important clinical goals such as eradicating the disease and enhancing overall survival rate have not yet been found.
Therefore COX-2 over-expression correlates in a different manner depending upon its aggressiveness the invasive potential of tumor cells, and then consequently exhibiting a higher incidence of distant metastases [40].

Refe-rence	N =	COX-2 positive (%)			Correlation of COX-2 expression and clinicopathological parameters						
		Carcinoma	DCIS	Benign tissue	Angio-genesis	HR-status	HER2	Grading	Age	Node +	Big tumor
[77]	44	2/44 (4,5%)	-	-	Not examined						
[78]	27	7/17 (42%)	8/10 (80%)	-	Not examined						
[72]	106	18/42 (43%)	10/16 (63%)	39/48 (81%)	-	No	No	-	-	-	-
[73]	221	80/221 (36%)	-	0%	Yes	Yes	-	Yes	No	Yes	Yes
[79]	46	50%	-	-	Yes	No	No	No	No	Yes	
[74]	1576	589/1576 (37,4%)	-	-	-	Yes	Yes	Yes	-	Yes	Yes
[80]	106	90/106 (85%)	-	-	No	No	No	No	No	No	No
[81]	128	41%	-	-	Yes	-	-	Yes	-	Yes	Yes
[82]	192	40,6%	-	-	-	Yes	Yes	Yes	-	-	Yes
[83]	65	41/65 (63%)	-	-	-	Yes	Yes	-	-	-	-
[76]	43	41/43 (95%)	-	-	-	No	No	Yes	-	-	Yes

Table 1. Immunochemical examinations of COX-2 expression and correlation with selected clinicopathological parameters in breast tissue.

Transcriptional studies have also revealed a distinct variation in their results regarding COX-2 expression. The detection rate varies between 50 and 100% in the literature (Table 2). There is a comparable relationship between COX-2 immunoreactivity and mRNA expression in tumor tissue [77]. Zhao and co-workers [84] demonstrated an increased mRNA expression in hormone receptor positive breast cancer; a result that was confirmed by Singh and co-workers [85] in breast cancer with positive progesterone receptors. However, only a small number of studies have examined the correlation between mRNA expression and clinico-pathological parameters. These results are summarized in Table 2.

Reference	N =	COX-2-mRNA positive (%)	Clinicopathological correlation of COX-2 with						
			Angio-genesis	HR-status	HER2	Grading	Age	Node +	Big tumor
[86]	40	40/40 (100%)	Not examined						
[72]	9	9/9 (100%)	Not examined						
[87]	7	7/7 (100%)	-	-	-	-	-	-	-
[88]	20	10/20 (50%)	-	-	-	-	-	-	-
[85]	18	18/18 (100%)	Not examined	Yes (PR)	Not examined				
[84]	30	27/30 (90%)	-	Yes (ER+)	-	Not examined			

Table 2. COX-2 mRNA expression and correlation with selected clinicopathological parameters in breast cancer.

These results are contrary to the immunochemically evaluated data, which show an association to hormone receptor negative tumors. This could be explained because before the genetic information of COX-2 is translated into a biologically active protein, COX-2 mRNA is post transcriptionally modified in the nucleus. Thus, we speculate that the COX-2 mRNA is destabilised by its AU rich sequences and no COX-2 protein is generated. Therefore, the correlation between the hormone receptor status and COX-2 mRNA levels is not obvious in studies where the COX-2 protein expression was investigated [5]. There are some well known factors which affect the COX-2 mRNA levels like interleukin-1 stabilises the highly unstable COX-2 mRNA transcript [89], however steroids may destabilise the COX-2 mRNA [90]. Furthermore, it might be possible that genetically different subtypes of breast cancer express COX-2 and are then associated with both hormone receptor-negative and receptor-positive tumors [91]. Additionally, Ristimäki and co-workers [74] reported that hormone receptor-positive patients who express COX-2 had a poor survival rate.

7.1 COX-2 and hormone receptors

There is concurrent evidence about the interaction of PGE_2/COX-2 and the estrogen receptor signalling pathway. For example, COX-2 expression is correlated with the expression of the aromatase [92] and in vitro studies support this data. It has been shown that COX-2 promotes the aromatase transcription, whereas COX-2 inhibitors diminish it [93]. Based on the elevated synthesis of prostaglandins in cells that express COX-2, the aromatase expression and activity is increased in breast cells [94, 95]. Expression of aromatase leads to estrogen production and from cell line studies; we know that hormone receptor expression can be induced by sex steroid hormones [96]. All the data supports the

close correlation between COX-2 and hormone receptors. Wolf and co-workers [70] reported a link between the estrogen signalling pathway and 15-PGDH by a negative feedback mechanism. High levels of this hormone reduced the 15-PGDH expression but the activity of the ERE (estrogen responsive element) and the activity of the aromatase increased.
New studies suggest a synergism between selective COX-2 and aromatase inhibitors.

7.2 Results from in vivo studies

The impact of COX-2 in carcinogenesis of breast tumors has been shown in transgenic mice models [97]. It has been reported that the over-expression of COX-2 in breast tissues is associated with decreased BAX and Bcl-xL (pro apoptotic) and increased Bcl-2 (anti apoptotic) protein levels. Therefore, the author suggested that induction of carcinogenesis is COX-2 dependent [97]. In contrast, the resistance to apoptosis is associated with increased COX-2 levels [98]. The importance of COX-2 in correlation to the tumor formation has been investigated in COX-2 knockout mice. The COX-2 knockout mice lead to an 86% reduction of intestinal adenoids [99].

7.3 COX-2 and tumorigenesis

The expression of COX-2 is regulated by post-transcriptional and -translational mechanisms. Different cytokines, growth factors and oncogenes have been shown to induce the COX-2 expression which is associated with carcinogenesis [46, 100].

7.3.1 Influence of COX-2 on angiogenesis and apoptosis

Angiogenesis is the development of new blood vessels and is an important factor in tumor proliferation, invasion and metastasis. Davies and co-workers [101] showed a significant positive correlation between COX-2 expression and the endothelial surface marker CD31. Other reports confirmed a positive correlation between COX-2 and the vascular endothelial growth factor (VEGF) [102, 103]. During carcinogenesis COX-2 modulates the neoangiogenesis and seems to stimulate the production of proangiogenic factors such as VEGF, basic fibroblast growth factor (bFGF), transforming growth factor 1 (TGF1), platelet derived growth factor (PDGF) and endothelin [104, 105]. The application of selective COX-2 inhibitors decreased the angiogenesis in different vivo models [106]. Recently, an angiogenesis independent mechanism, so called Vasculogenic Mimicry (VM), was described where poorly differentiated breast cancer cells were nourished without the mechanisms of classic neoangiogenesis [107-109]. VM is a phenomenon of vessel formation of epithelial tumor cells without any participation of endothelial cells and itis a mechanism independent of or simultaneous to neoangiogenesis thus ensuring the tumor perfusion [110]. Hence, the VM might be an important factor for new antiangiogenic therapeutical approaches. The existence of VM in breast cancer patients is associated with a poor 5-year survival rate compared to patients without. [111]. Basu and co-workers [112] reported that highly invasive MDA-MB-231 breast cancer cells and the less invasive subtype MDA-MB-435 cells that over express COX-2, formed new micro vessels. In contrast, non-invasive MCF-7- and ZR-75-1-breast cancer cells which had a lower COX-2 expression did not. The application of the COX-2 inhibitor celecoxib (40 und 60 µmol/l, $p>0.001$), inhibits the formation of new vessels. This effect was restored with PGE_2. This data was confirmed by an in vivo xenograft model. VEGF, GRO, IL-6, IL-8, TIMP1, TIMP2 were the main angiogenic proteins which were inhibited by celecoxib [112].

7.4 Breast cancer and NSAIDs

The rationale for using NSAIDs is their non-selective (ASS, ibuprofen etc.) or selective (COX-2 inhibitors such as celecoxib) suppression of the COX-system. In a meta-analysis consisting of 14 epidemiological studies (6 cohort studies and 8 case control studies) breast cancer risk was reduced by 18% due to constant intake of NSAIDs [113]. An extensive Canadian study including 5882 patients reported a reduction of breast cancer incidence by 24% due to the NSAIDs intake for 2 - 5 years [58]. Another case control study demonstrated a 40% reduction after 5 years of NSAIDs intake [57]. These results seemingly justify the preventive use of NSAIDs, however, contrarian results were delivered by the Nurses Health Study. This trial showed no difference during the intake of ASS (100mg) in neither women with breast cancer nor in healthy women [114]. On the contrary it was in patients with colon cancer who led the continuous intake of NSAIDs to a reduction of incidence in 40-50% [56, 115, 116].

Data of animal models supports the use of selective COX-2 inhibitors both for the therapeutic and preventive uses. For instance, the use of celecoxib in rats led to an averaged downsizing of breast tumor volume by 32%, however, a tumor volume enlargement of 518% was observed in the control group [117]. Harris and co-workers [118] examined the influence of celecoxib in 120 rats. Three groups of rats were formed. In one group the food was enriched with celecoxib. The other two groups obtained either ibuprofen or nothing. After seven days 7,12-Dimethylbenz(a)anthracene (DMBA) was applied intragastrically and the described food was continued for another 105 days. A distinct reduction in tumor incidence, variety and tumor volume was shown in the celecoxib treated group [118]. In a recently published paper Barnes and co-workers [119] could induce breast tumors in mice by injecting estrogen-positive MCF7/HER2-18- and estrogen-negative MDAMB231 breast cancer cells. The application of celecoxib resulted in a significant growth reduction of the MCF7/HER-18 tumors (58.7%) and the MDAMB231 tumors (46.3%) in comparison to the control group. Therefore, celecoxib dropped the COX-2 expression and enhanced the apoptosis significantly [119]. Yoshinaka and co-workers [120] also showed that the use of celecoxib significantly reduced tumor sizes, increased apoptosis and that a reduced DNA synthesis in the tumor tissue of mice induced breast carcinomas. Moreover the neoangiogenesis was influenced as VEGF-A-mRNA levels were found to be reduced [120].

7.5 COX-2-inhibitors in systemic treatment

Several studies have evaluated the significance of COX-2 inhibitors in combination with systemic treatment. A phase II study observed a clinical benefit of 47.5% for the combination of capecitabine and celecoxib in patients with metastatic breast cancer. The combination was well tolerated [121].

Recently published data about COX-2 and its significance on the aromatase and influence on the female hormonal balance are of strong interest. Besides finding an increased effect on estrogen synthesis in malignant breast tissue, a strong correlation between COX-2 and aromatase mRNA expression were found. This data supports the assumption that COX-2 is able to regulate aromatase activity in breast tissue [92]. A possible synergism between COX-2 and aromatase-inhibitors is even more interesting and so a prospective randomised phase III multicenter trial (REACT-trial) was conducted that included primary breast cancer patients in order to evaluate the combination of celecoxib and exemestane, an aromatase

inhibitor, in an adjuvant setting. The combination of celecoxib and exemestane was already well tolerated and had shown a clinical benefit of 74% [122] or had led to a benefit extension (median 96.6 weeks vs. 49.1 weeks) in patients with metastatic breast cancer [123].
Other malignancies were also proven on the benefit of selective and non-selective COX-2 inhibitors in combination with other compounds such as chemotherapy [124, 125], tyrosinekinase inhibitors [126] and other new approaches [127]. Some of them are encouraging, like the results of the ASCENT trial [124] and some are disappointing. Further work is required to establish how NSAIDs can be best applied for therapeutic benefit.

8. Vitamin D

8.1 Vitamin D metabolism

Vitamin D, a secosteroid hormone, is assimilated by food (milk, fish, liver), multi-vitamin preparations and dietary supplements [128]. Vitamin D is also synthesised from 7-dehydrocholesterol and provitamin D3 after skin exposure with sunlight (ultraviolet spectrum 290-315nm) [129]. Based on its animal or herbal origin, there are two existing vitamin D metabolites: cholecalciferol (vitamin D_3) and ergocalciferol (vitamin D_2) [17], which is less efficient in increasing the 25-hydroxyvitaminD [$25(OH)_2D_3$] serum levels [130]. Cholecalciferol attains to the liver through the bloodstream and is transformed to $25(OH)_2D_3$ (25-hydroxyvitamin D_3, calcediol, 25-hydroxycholecalciferol) by a hydroxylation on the C25 position [131, 132]. $25(OH)_2D_3$, a circulating metabolite, correlates with the vitamin D balance. The hydroxylation of cholecalciferol on the C25 position is inadequately regulated. $25(OH)_2D_3$ level increased with the vitamin D intake, therefore, the $25(OH)_2D_3$ serum level is normally used as an indicator of the vitamin D balance [133]. The serum level range of $25(OH)_2D_3$ is between 10 and 50 ng/ml and round about 30pg/ml for $1,25(OH)_2D_3$ [134]. $25(OH)_2D_3$ is renally converted to the biologically active metabolite 1,25-dihydroxycholecalciferol [1,25(OH)2D3] by the 1-α-hydroxylase (CYP27B1). $1,25(OH)_2D_3$ is 100-1000 fold more active than the other natural metabolites [135]. The 1-α-hydroxylase, a mitochondrial enzyme, which belongs to the P450 enzyme family is located in the renal proximal tubule. Besides the renal expression of the enzyme, many studies reported an extra renal expression of 1-α-hydroxylase and thus an extra renal synthesis of $1,25(OH)_2D_3$. This enzyme has been detected in many cell types and tissues, e.g. prostate, breast, lung, pancreas, parathyroid and monocytes [136]. The extra renal synthesised $1,25(OH)_2D_3$ has cell specific functions and as a result acts as local auto- and paracrine factors. In this context, many extra renal effects of $1,25(OH)_2D_3$, e.g. cell cycle arrest, induction of apoptosis and cell differentiation, have been reported [136]. The fine tuned activity of 1-α-hydroxylase correlates inversely with the calcium metabolism and thus the circulating levels of $1,25(OH)_2D_3$ correlates inversely with the ingested amount of calcium [137]. $1,25(OH)_2D_3$ Serum levels are maintained in pmol/l range by a classic negative feedback mechanism. The decrease of calcium or phosphate levels leads to an increase of the 1-α-hydroxylase activity and an enhanced synthesis of $1,25(OH)_2D_3$ which in turn promotes the intestinal resorption of calcium and phosphate and the calcium mobilisation from the bones. The activity of 1-α-hydroxylase decreased with increasing $1,25(OH)_2D_3$ levels, which leads to 24 hydroxylase activation. This enzyme degrades $1,25(OH)_2D_3$ to its inactive metabolite $24,25(OH)_2D_3$ [138, 139], which is subsequently converted to calcitroic acid and excreted. Hence, the nutritive intake of calcium directly regulates 1-α-hydroxylase activity and indirectly modifies parathormone levels. This hormone produced in the parathyroids increases the phosphate excretion in the proximal tubule but promotes the sodium, potassium and calcium resorbtion in the distal tubule. Under normocalcemic conditions, the activity of 1-α-hydroxylase is inhibited. These regulations are necessary to synthesize $1,25(OH)_2D_3$ even though much is needed to cover the calcium and phosphate demand and to avoid a $1,25\ (OH)_2D_3$ intoxication [139]. The circulating vitamin D level depends on many different factors such as: the vitamin D content in either the ingested nutrition or the dietary supplements, and the endogenous production and degeneration via vitamin D metabolising enzymes. A simplified scheme of vitamin D metabolism is presented in figure (**2**).

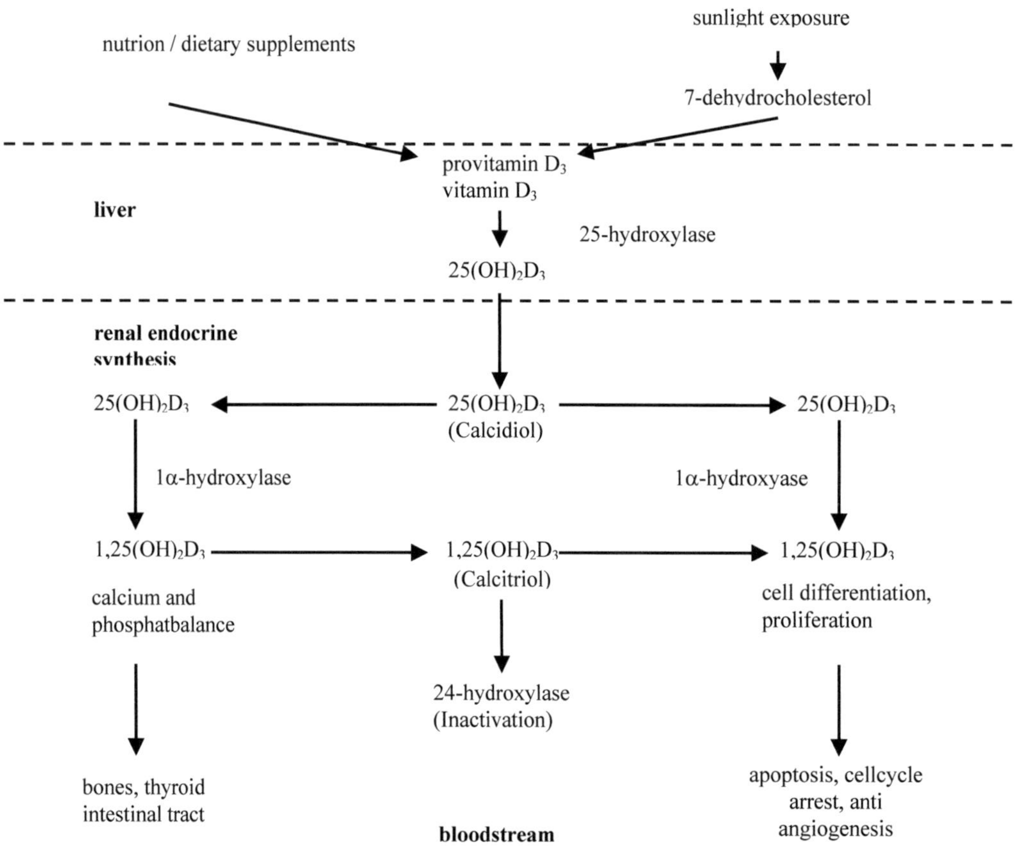

Fig. 2. Simplified scheme of the vitamin D metabolism. Vitamin D (food intake, synthesis in skin) is metabolised in liver to $25(OH)_2D_3$, then via the renal 1-α-hydroxylase (endocrine signalling pathway or extra renal in tissues (autocrine/paracrine signalling pathway) to $1,25(OH)_2D_3$.

8.2 Extrarenal vitamin D metabolizing enzymes

The biologically active metabolite is produced after a series of hydroxylations through cytochrome P450 enzymes which belong to the cytochrome p450 super family. The different enzymes are handled as follows:

8.2.1 1-α-hydroxylase (CYP27B1)

The 25-hydroxyvitamin-D_3-[$25(OH)_2D_3$]1-α-hydroxylase (1-α-hydroxylase) is encoded by the CYP27b1 gene and catalyzes the synthesis of $1,25(OH)_2D_3$ from $25(OH)_2D_3$. $1,25(OH)_2D_3$ is the most important regulator of the enzyme that leads to a decreased enzyme expression. The regulation of the extra renal 1-α-hydroxylase depends on local factors like cytokines (interleukins, interferones and tumor necrosis) and growth. The optimal $1,25(OH)_2D_3$-level tuning mechanism is not yet completely understood [139]. The reduced expression of the enzyme suggests the involvement of a negative vitamin D responsive element (VDRE) and Turunen and co-workers [140] showed that the enzyme's response to $1,25(OH)_2D_3$ is a cell specific event with participation of many VDREs. The suppression of cell proliferation, the induction of apoptotic events and the modulation of immune responses are counted among the classical features of $1,25(OH)_2D_3$. After binding to the vitamin D receptor, $1,25(OH)_2D_3$ is able to arrest the cell cycle of a tumor cell in the G1-G0 phase via specific mechanisms [139]. In prostate and colon cancer the tumor protective effects of vitamin D is correlated to vitamin D deficiency [141]. Much data reports that both the renal and extra renal 1-α-hydroxylase are based on the expression of the same gene product. In contrast to the renal 1-α-hydroxylase, the extra renal enzyme is not subjected to the auto regulation as mentioned above [136, 142]. Therefore the enzyme's tissue specific expression might be a key mechanism in connecting the vitamin D metabolism to the anticarcinogenic effects of $1,25(OH)_2D_3$.

Although the enzyme's cytokine and growth factor related regulation is not completely understood, it has been shown that different cytokines stimulate the 1-α-hydroxylase in different cell types [139, 143-146]. Another potential mechanism of gene regulation is the incidence of different gene polymorphisms [147] and inactive variants due to alternative splicing of the 1-α-hydroxylase mRNA. But this mechanism's function is not completely clarified. Alternative splicing within the post transcriptional modification is a normal process of gene expression in breast cancer cells and based on the pre mRNA, different mature mRNAs are generated when introns or exons are deleted or added. Thus, the translation of these mRNAs leads to different enzyme proteins, however, mis-spliced mRNAs are usually quickly degraded although it appears that this mechanism has failed in various cells. It has been reported that different protein variants of 1-α-hydroxylase might have diverse biological functions. Fischer and co-workers [148] showed 6 different variants of the enzyme in MCF10F via nested touchdown PCR, but in MCF-7, these variants appeared weakly expressed. Based on this data, the authors concluded that because alternative splicing regulates the level of the active enzyme extrarenaly it therefore regulates the local production of $1,25(OH)_2D_3$ [149]. The activity of the extrarenally expressed 1-α-hydroxylase is an important factor of the tumor pathophysiology because of an accumulation of $1,25(OH)_2D_3$ in many tissues. Studies of prostate [150, 151], colon [152-154] and breast cancer [148, 155, 156] have shown the expression of 1-α-hydroxylase in healthy as well as in malignant tissues. Thus, $1,25(OH)_2D_3$, which is produced extrarenally might have autocrine behaviour to protect cells against transformation and supports the suggestion of its carcinoprotective effects. Accordingly, low 1-α-hydroxylase levels correlate with the risk of prostate-, colon- [157] or breast cancer [158, 159]. Moreover, the extra renal production of $1,25(OH)_2D_3$ inhibits cell proliferation and promotes cell differentiation in xenograft models [160]. Besides the expression of the 1-α-hydroxylase in breast [155, 161], endometrial [162], cervical and ovarian carcinomas [163], the induction of the enzyme has also been shown in lymphomas [164] and dysgerminomas [165]. In these reports, the local synthesis of 1,25$(OH)_2D_3$ was mediated by the 1-α-hydroxylase expression of tumor associated macrophages. The expression of the enzyme mammary gland tissue occurs in lobules and ductus, primarily in the cancer tissue and invasive tumor cells and inflammatory infiltrate. Thus, it might be possible that the enzyme activity and the vitamin D receptor (VDR) expression are considerably higher than in the benign tissue compared to aggressive tumor cell lines (MCF-7res, MDA-MB231) [166]. Townsend and co-workers [166] compared breast cancer and benign tissue samples via reverse transcription PCR. They reported a 27-fold induction of the 1-α-hydroxylase expression and 7-fold induction of the VDR expression in tumor samples. Because 80% of the tumor tissues had an increased 1-α-hydroxylase und VDR, they concluded that there was a closed coupling of both gene products. These results are in compliance with Segersten and co-workers [161]. The capacity of 1-α-hydroxylase to synthesize 1,25$(OH)_2D_3$ within the mammary gland parenchyma results in, on the one hand, the available amount of 25$(OH)_2D_3$, and is dependent on sun light exposure and the season [167-170] - normally there is no definite correlation between 25$(OH)_2D_3$ and 1,25$(OH)_2D_3$ – yet on the other hand, the level of the extra renal production of 1,25$(OH)_2D_3$ is limited by the expression of the 1,25$(OH)_2D_3$- decomposing enzyme 24-hydroxylase, which is stimulated by 1,25$(OH)_2D_3$ in VDR expressing tissues. Based on the missing correlation of 24-hydroxylase and VDR or the 1-α-hydroxylase in breast cancer tissues, it seems that 24-hydroxylase is independently regulated. Kemmis and co-workers [171] demonstrated the expression of a functioning VDR and an inhibition of proliferation via 1,25$(OH)_2D_3$ in benign breast cells and MCF-7. The VDR expression in HMEC breast cells was higher than in MCF7 cells. Furthermore, the authors showed an expression of 25$(OH)_2D_3$ metabolizing 1-α-hydroxylase and 24-hydroxylase in these cell types, whereas the 1-α-hydroxylase expression was higher in MCF-7. In contrast to renal HKC8 cells, the expression of 1-α-hydroxylase was not inhibited by 1,25$(OH)_2D_3$. Based on the strong induction of the 24-hydroxylase through the 1,25$(OH)_2D_3$ application, the authors showed that MCF7 cells were more sensitive in response to 1,25$(OH)_2D_3$ compared to HKC-8 and HMEC cells. From this data, they concluded that there is a functional vitamin D receptor as well as intact signalling transduction pathways in MCF-7 cells. The data suggests that the synthesis of 1,25$(OH)_2D_3$ and the activation of the VDR inhibits the cell proliferation in breast cells. Thus, the treatment of benign breast cells with 25$(OH)_2D_3$ leads to an activation of the VDR transcription and the regulation of its target genes (CYP27B1, CYP24) and finally to an inhibition of cell proliferation. According to that, CYP27B1 lords it over CYP24 which means a transformation of 25$(OH)_2D_3$ to 1,25$(OH)_2D_3$. Kemmis and co-workers [171] have shown for the first time that physiological 1,25$(OH)_2D_3$ levels (30-100nmol/L) are able to inhibit cell proliferation in benign HMEC cells and in MCF7 breast cancer cells. Interestingly, aging process and the associated lack of estrogens correlate with decreased 25$(OH)_2D_3$ levels. The reason is that the ability of estrogen to stimulate the renal CYP27B1 activity [172]. Accordingly, the lack of estrogens leads to decreased 1,25$(OH)_2D_3$ levels and presents the highest risk for breast cancer in postmenopausal women [273].

8.2.2 24-hydroxylase (CYP24)

The 25-hydroxyvitamine D_3-24 hydroxylase (24-OHase, 24-hydroxylase) encoded by the CYP224 gene is induced by 1,25$(OH)_2D_3$ in breast cell lines where the enzyme is time and dose dependently stimulated by 1,25$(OH)_2D_3$ [174]. An increased enzyme expression in ovarian, cervical and breast cancer compared to healthy tissue samples has been shown by immunochemistry and real time PCR [163]. In contrast, Townsend and co-workers [166] showed a 4-fold increase of the enzyme expression in malignant breast tissues compared to healthy tissue samples using the same technique. Additionally, the expression of 24 hydroxylase increased in breast cancer cells foremost in hormone resistant MCF-7 Res and the aggressive MDA-MB231 cells compared to benign MCF-12A cells [166]. Kemmis and co-workers [171] reported the highest 24 hydroxylase expression in MCF-7 cells and Segersten and co-workers [161] showed a 2-fold enzyme expression in tumor tissues compared to benign tissue samples. The authors concluded that the conversion of $1,25(OH)_2D_3$ into the inactive metabolite $1,24,25(OH)_3D_3$ is significantly higher in malignant tissues. Furthermore Townsend and co-workers [166] detected the enzyme only in breast cancers with an increased 1-α-hydroxylase and VDR expression. Further analysis showed that in a healthy tissue sample expression of 24-hydroxylase correlated with both 1α-hydroxylase and VDR. There was not such a correlation in breast tumors. Hypothetically, the 24 hydroxylase acts as a part of a well organized feedback mechanism and is transcriptionally modulated to increase the local $1,25(OH)_2D_3$ and VDR level [166]. The synthesis of $1,25(OH)_2D_3$ via the 1-α-hydroxylase has been shown in benign and malignant mammary gland tissues but this mechanism's efficiency in tumor tissues might be affected by a dysregulated 24 hydroxylase expression.

8.3 Vitamin D-receptor (VDR / mVDR)

The vitamin D receptor (VDR) is an ubiquitary expressed steroid hormone receptor. Like other steroid, thyroid and retinoid receptors, the VDR is a member of the nuclear hormone receptor family. The receptor binds to its ligand $1,25(OH)_2D_3$, interacts with other receptors by dimerization and binds as homodimers or heterodimers to specific DNA sequences. So called vitamin D responsive elements (VDRE) recruit additional co-activators (such as SRC-1, GRIP-1/TIF2, ACTR) and interact with the transcriptional processing order to initiate or inhibit the transcription of its target genes [25]. It is well known, that steroid receptors consist of different variants with distinct specificities. Sunn and co-workers [175] described an N-terminal variant of the VDR. $1,25(OH)_2D_3$ mediates its genomic effects as a VDR ligand and via the directed binding to the VDRE [176]. Besides its function in bone metabolism and in the calcium/phosphate balance, the VDR interacts with different signalling pathways, e.g. with p21, a cyclin dependent kinase inhibitor which is involved in cell cycle regulation and inhibition of the cancer cell proliferation [26]. There are some suggestions about the existence of a membrane VDR (mVDR) [177]. The mVDR mediates its signals through the change of the intracellular calcium concentrations and through interactions with the protein kinase C and enzymes of the MAPK family [178-183]. Although the mVDR seems unrelated to the nuclear VDR, Marcinkowska and co-workers [184] reported an interaction of both receptors. The function of this mechanism is not clearly defined and the cloning of the mVDR has failed until today.

Many studies reported that extra renal VDR expression is associated with the non-classical effects of $1,25(OH)_2D_3$. The VDR expression has been shown in healthy breast tissues and in more than 80% of the breast cancer tissues [185]. The natural ligand of the VDR, $1,25(OH)_2D_3$ and many new developed synthetic vitamin D analogues inhibit cell proliferation and induce apoptosis in breast cancer cell lines [186, 187]. Furthermore, in animal models, vitamin D analogues retard the tumor growth and lead to a regression of breast tumors [12].

8.4 Vitamin D-receptor gene polymorphism

The gene that encodes the VDR has various polymorphisms. It has been hypothesised that the genetic VDR polymorphism influences the breast cancer risk due to its potential effects on VDR gene expression and protein function [188, 189]. Many polymorphisms of the VDR gene have been identified and several, such as FOK1, Bsm1, APA1, TAQ1 and Poly(A) are well analysed [190, 191]. The studies that were conducted had conflicting results [191]. Curran and co-workers [192] showed a significant association of the VDR polymorphism APA1 und TAQ with the breast cancer risk. A significant increased breast cancer risk in women with the ff genotype FOK1 was observed by Chen and co-workers [193]. Sinotte and co-workers [194] detected a significant link between familial breast cancer disposition and FOK1. Other data came from Trabert and co-workers [195] who found a correlation between a higher breast cancer risk and the genotype Bsm1 bb in postmenopausal women although there is also published data without any evidence for a link between VDR polymorphisms and breast cancer risk [196-199]. An analysis of the last 13 published studies in which different VDR polymorphisms and its relation to breast cancer were examined leads to the suggestion that the modification of breast cancer risk is associated with certain VDR polymorphisms and therefore $1,25(OH)_2D_3$ might modify the risk of breast cancer [200]. A recently published paper by McCullough and co-workers [201] presented certain VDR gene polymorphisms associated with a decreased breast cancer risk in women who ingested high doses of calcium (no calcitriol) concluding that nutritive influences might modify the link between gene polymorphisms and breast cancer. This data could shed light on breast cancer risk evaluation or could even be used in a predictive manner to answer the question about which women are strongly endangered to develop distant metastases.

9. Calcium

Like vitamin D, humans ingest calcium through food or dietary supplements. 99% of calcium is bound as hydroxyl phosphatide in bones and teeth [202]. Only 1% calcium is extracellularly located. Plasma levels of calcium (Ca^{2+}) are limited by the intestinal absorption, the renal secretion and the reabsorption. Additionally, the skeletal calcium storage and resorption keep the plasma levels of calcium in a closed range (3.5–5mmol/l) [202].

10. Vitamin D, calcium and breast cancer risk

10.1 Dietary and supplemental vitamin D intake

For $1,25(OH)_2D_3$ several studies have shown both an antiproliferative effect and an inhibition of angiogenesis in malignant and healthy breast cancer cells [17, 185, 203-206]. In mouse models, an increased intake of vitamin D led to the suppression of epithelial hyperproliferation and tumorigenesis of the mammary gland that was caused by rich nutrition [207, 208].

Last but not least, it has been proven by the First National Health and Nutrition Examination Survey Epidemiologic Follow-Up Study that sunlight exposure is inversely correlated with breast cancer risk [209, 210]. In this study, the female population in the north-eastern parts of the U.S. have a higher risk of contracting breast cancer compared to the other states of the U.S. This leads to the suggestion that sunlight induced vitamin D production has a positive influence in avoiding breast cancer [20].

In contrast, in the Nurses' Health Study, there was an inverse association between vitamin D intake and breast cancer risk among premenopausal women but no association among postmenopausal women [20]. Consistent with this observation, a study published a few years ago was based on the Cancer Prevention Study II Nutrition Cohort and observed no associations between breast cancer and total and dietary vitamin D intakes among postmenopausal women [211]. Another Italian study recently showed an inverse association between vitamin D intake (in the study >143 IU) and breast cancer in 2569 breast cancer patients [212]. Two other studies that concentrated on vitamin D deficiency and its susceptibility for breast cancer incidence approved that a deficiency conditional on nutrition in adolescence does not lead to an increased breast cancer risk [213, 214].
The proper dose of vitamin D remains unclear and a recommendation does not exist, however a meta-analysis gives evidence towards a dose of >400 IU per day to reduce breast cancer risk [213].

10.2 Role of vitamin D in breast cancer

To date, there have been several epidemiologic studies of the association between vitamin D and breast cancer risk, however, their results have not been consistent. Several studies observed an association between $25(OH)_2D_3$ plasma levels and breast cancer incidence [19, 215-217]. The predictive value of $25(OH)_2D_3$ plasma levels depends upon the time they have been measured. Plasma levels that have been measured within a few years before breast cancer diagnosis are less predictive than plasma level measured many years before [217]. Furthermore, plasma levels that have been measured around 15 years before diagnosis do not have any aetiological value for the genesis of breast cancer [216].
Bertone-Johnson and co-workers [217] found a marginally significant reduction of breast cancer risk in women >60 years who had elevated $25(OH)_2D_3$ and $1,25(OH)_2D_3$ plasma levels. In contrast, published data by Shin and co-workers [20] demonstrated a significantly decreased breast cancer incidence in premenopausal, but not in postmenopausal women, who had continuous vitamin D intake.
Furthermore, a case control study observed that women with plasma $25(OH)_2D_3$ concentration <50nmol/l had >5 times higher risk of breast cancer than those with plasma concentrations exceeding >150 nmol/l [158]. Janowsky and co-workers [19] also showed an inverse association between $1,25(OH)_2D_3$ plasma levels to the point of diagnosis and breast cancer risk in patients with breast cancer. However, there was no difference in $1,25(OH)_2D_3$ plasma levels between patients with breast cancer and those with DCIS. The authors suggested that the grade of invasion was not correlated with the extent of $1,25(OH)_2D_3$ level. Another nested case-control study with 96 breast cancer cases and 96 controls found no association between prediagnostic $1,25(OH)_2D_3$ levels and levels at the time of diagnosis and breast cancer risk among postmenopausal women [216].
The circulating concentration of $25(OH)_2D_3$ is considered to be an excellent measure of the availability of vitamin D from the diet, supplements and from synthesis in the skin [218]. Its potential importance in breast carcinogenesis is due to the fact that $25(OH)_2D_3$ can be metabolised to $1,25(OH)_2D_3$ by 1-α-hydroxylase in breast tissue [155]. Thus, $25(OH)_2D_3$ levels may be more representative of intracellular levels of $1,25(OH)_2D_3$ than circulating levels of $1,25(OH)_2D_3$ [217].
To date, no studies have been published investigating intracellular or tissue levels of $1,25(OH)_2D_3$ and $25(OH)_2D_3$ in association with breast cancer risk.

10.3 Dietary and supplemental calcium intake

Many studies about the importance of calcium and its association to breast cancer have already been published. Most of them are case-control studies and nearly all of them are relatively small and there is insufficient documentation regarding risk factors for breast cancer in multivariate analyses.

Calcium is participating on carcinogenesis via regulation of cell proliferation, differentiation and apoptosis [219-221]. Cell proliferation and differentiation of breast cells can be increased by elevated calcium levels [208, 222, 223]. Boyapati and co-workers [224] observed a non-significant inverse association between calcium intake and breast cancer risk among pre- and postmenopausal women but the Nurses' Health Study has shown this association only for premenopausal women [20].

The anti-carcinogenic effects of calcium are last but not least, mediated by vitamin D, therefore calcium is one of the key mediators of the vitamin D induced apoptosis in breast cancer cells [208].

11. Calcitriol and prostaglandins in cancer

The stimulation of the renal calcitriol [$1,25(OH)_2D_3$] synthesis in vitro is well known as well as the inhibition of acetysalicylic acid as a non-selective NSAID [225]. This justifies the clinical use of NSAIDs in treating arthritis for example. Hayes and co-workers [226] observed an inhibition of calcitriol synthesis caused by PGE_1 and PGE_2 in synovial fluid macrophages from arthritic joints and with that he proved the link between vitamin D and prostaglandin metabolism. Several published studies have proven the anti-carcinogenic effects shown in different signalling pathways on prostate cancer cells [227-229]. The team around David Feldman examined the influence of calcitriol in established human prostate cancer cell lines (androgen dependent LNCaP cells and androgen independent PC-3 cells) and in primary normal prostatic epithelial cells derived from normal and cancerous human prostate tissue. They showed that calcitriol regulates biologically active prostaglandin levels and prostaglandin actions by three mechanisms: calcitriol suppresses the COX-2 expression and moreover it up-regulates the expression of 15-PGDH. This dual influence of calcitriol was associated with a decrease of PGE_2 secretion in prostate cancer cells. Calcitriol reduces the mRNA expression of prostaglandin receptors EP_2 and FP, additionally a mechanism to inhibit the biological activity of prostaglandins.

The combination of calcitriol and NSAIDs led to a significant growth inhibition in prostate cancer cells via its synergistic effects. These findings might postulate that calcitriol and NSAIDs are definitely a useful combination in chemo preventive and/or therapeutic strategies in prostate cancer [230]. Unpublished own data support these results as we showed an inverse correlation between VDR- and COX-2 expression in breast cancer cells and a downregulation of COX-2 and an upregulation of 15 PGDH by calcitriol. Therefore we propose that these findings and suggest a possible link between VDR, associated target genes and the prostaglandin metabolism.

12. Concluding remarks

In conclusion, there is promising preclinical data inhibiting COX-2 in breast cancers, therefore the chance exists to innovatively disturb carcinogenesis of those gynecological oncological neoplasms Phase II trials have already been conducted to clear the safety of a celecoxib treatment in metastatic breast cancer. Furthermore, calcitriol and calcium have shown anti-carcinogenic effects in experimental studies and several epidemiological studies have demonstrated an inverse association between vitamin D and calcium intake and breast cancer. Other studies have detected an inverse association between plasma and serum levels and breast cancer risk. Experimental studies support the hypothesis that the reduction of breast cancer risk is more significant among premenopausal women than among postmenopausal women and mPGES-1 and EP receptors might be important targets for the development of new anti inflammatory and antiproliferative tumor therapies.

Questions that remain unanswered are: has calcitriol as antiproliferative effects in breast cancer as was proven in prostate cancer? Does a link exist between vitamin D and prostaglandin metabolism in breast cancers? These questions have to be answered as the increasing incidence of breast cancer have yet to be solved. Innovative treatment strategies fall on fruitful ground. Thus we need further studies that elucidate the importance of COX-2 inhibitors in the preventive as well as in the adjuvant settings in breast cancers and finally that will evaluate the promising importance in the neoangiogenesis in detail.

13. Acknowledgments

The authors declare no conflict of interest relevant to this article.

14. Abbreviations

bFGF	=	basic fibroblast growth factor
COX	=	cyclooxygenase
DCIS	=	ductal carcinoma in situ
DMBA	=	Dimethylbenz(a)anthracene
ER	=	estrogen receptor
ERE	=	estrogen responsive element
FIGO	=	Fédération Internationale de Gyneécologie et d'Obstétrique
GRO	=	growth related protein
HER2	=	human epidermal growth factor receptor 2
IL	=	interleukin
NSAID	=	non-steroidal anti-inflammatory drug
mPGES-1	=	microsomalmicrosomal prostaglandin E synthase-1
mRNA	=	messenger ribonucleic acid
PCR	=	polymerase chain reaction
PDGF	=	platelet derived growth factor
PG	=	prostaglandin
PGDH	=	prostaglandin dehydrogenase
PPAR	=	peroxisomes proliferator-activated receptor
TGF1	=	transforming growth factor 1
TIMP	=	tissue inhibitor of matrix metalloproteinase
VDR	=	vitamin D receptor
VDRE	=	vitamin D responsive element
VEGF	=	vascular endothelial growth factor
VM	=	vasculogenic mimicry

15. References

[1] American Cancer Society. *Cancer facts and figures 2005*. Atlanta, American Cancer Society 2005, p. 9. (http://www.cancer.org/downloads/STT/CAFF2005f4PWSecured.pdf)

[2] Ozols, R. F.; Rubins, S. C.; Dembo, A. J.; Robboy, S. In *Gynecologic oncology: Epithelial ovarian cancer*; Hoskins, W. J.; Perez, C. A.; Young, R. C.; Ed.; Lippincott Williams & Wilkins: Philadelphia, 1992 pp. 731-781.

[3] FIGO (International Federation of Gynecology and Obstetrics) annual report on the results of treatment in gynecological cancer. *Int. J. Gynaecol. Obstet.* 2003, *83 Suppl 1: ix-xxii*, 1-229.

[4] Ferrandina, G.; Lauriola, L.; Zannoni, G. F.; Fagotti, A.; Fanfani, F.; Legge, F.; Maggiano, N.; Gessi, M.; Mancuso, S.; Ranelletti, F. O.; Scambia, G. Increased cyclooxygenase-2 (COX-2) expression is associated with chemotherapy resistance and outcome in ovarian cancer patients. *Ann. Oncol.* 2002, *13*, 1205-1211.

[5] Singh-Ranger, G.; Salhab, M.; Mokbel, K. The role of cyclooxygenase-2 in breast cancer: review. Breast Cancer Res. Treat. 2008, 109(2), 189-198.

[6] Coussens, L. M.; Werb, Z. *Inflammation and cancer. Nature* 2002, *420(6917)*, 860-867.

[7] Park, E. The etiology of rickets. *Physiol. Rev.* 1923 (Baltimore) iii, 106-163.

[8] Deluca, H. F.; Cantorna, M. T. Vitamin D: its role and uses in immunology. *FASEB J.* 2001, *15*, 2579-2585.

[9] Guyton, K. Z.; Kensler, T. W.; Posner, G. H. Vitamin D and vitamin D analogs as cancer chemopreventive agents. *Nutr. Rev.* 2003, *61*, 227-238.

[10] Jones, G.; Strugnell, S. A.; Deluca, H. F. Current understanding of the molecular actions of vitamin D. *Physiol. Rev.* 1998, *78*, 1193-1231.

[11] Adorini L. Immunomodulatory effects of vitamin D receptor ligands in autoimmune diseases. *Int. Immunopharmacol.* 2002, *2*, 1017-1028.

[12] Colston, K. W.; Hansen, C. M. Mechanisms implicated in the growth regulatory effects of vitamin D in breast cancer. *Endocr. Relat. Cancer* 2002, *9(1)*, 45-59.

[13] Johnson, C. S.; Hershberger, P. A.; Trump, D. L. Vitamin D-related therapies in prostate cancer. *Cancer Metastasis Rev.* 2002, *21*, 147-158.

[14] Mathieu, C.; Adorini, L. The coming of age of 1,25-dihydroxyvitamin D_3 analogs as immunomodulatory agents. *Trends Mol. Med.* 2002, *8*, 174-179.

[15] O'Kelly, J.; Koeffler, H. P. Vitamin D analogs and breast cancer. *Recent Results Cancer Res.* 2003, *164*, 333-348.

[16] van den Bemd, G. J.; Chang, G. T. Vitamin D and vitamin D analogs in cancer treatment. *Curr. Drug Targets* 2002, *3*, 85-94.

[17] Welsh, J.; Wietzke, J. A.; Zinser, G. M.; Byrne, B.; Smith, K.; Narvaez, C. J. Vitamin D_3 receptor as a target for breast cancer prevention. *J. Nutr.* 2003, *133*, 2425-2433S.

[18] Garland, C. F.; Garland, F. C.; Gorham, E. D. Calcium and vitamin D. Their potential roles in colon and breast cancer prevention. *Ann. N. Y. Acad. Sci.* 1999, *889*, 107-119.

[19] Janowsky, E. C.; Lester, G. E.; Weinberg, C. R.; Millikan, R. C.; Schildkraut, J. M.; Garrett, P. A.; Hulka, B. S. Association between low levels of 1,25-dihydroxyvitamin D and breast cancer risk. *Public Health Nutr.* 1999, *2*, 283-291.

[20] Shin, M. H.; Holmes, M. D.; Hankinson, S. E.; Wu, K.; Colditz, G. A.; Willett, W. C. Intake of dairy products, calcium, and vitamin D and risk of breast cancer. J. *Natl. Cancer Inst.* 2002, *94*, 1301-1311.

[21] Studzinski, G. P.; Moore, D. C. Sunlight—can it prevent as well as cause cancer? *Cancer Res.* 1995, *55*, 4014–4022.

[22] Gorham, E. D.; Garland, F. C.; Garland, C. F. Sunlight and breast cancer incidence in the USSR. *Int. J. Epidemiol.* 1990, *19*, 820–824.

[23] Garland, F. C.; Garland, C. F.; Gorham, E. D.; Young J. F. Geographic variation in breast cancer mortality in the United States: a hypothesis involving exposure to solar radiation. *Prev. Med.* 1990, *19*, 614–622.

[24] Blot, W. J.; Fraumeni J. F. Jr.; Stone B. J. Geographic patterns of breast cancer in the United States. *J. Natl. Cancer. Inst.* 1977, *59*, 1407–1411.

[25] Malloy, P. J.; Pike, J. W.; Feldman, D. The vitamin D receptor and the syndrome of hereditary 1,25-dihydroxyvitamin D-resistant rickets. *Endocr. Rev.* 1999, *20*, 156-188.

[26] Liu, M.; Lee, M. H.; Cohen, M.; Bommakanti, M.; Freedman, L. P. Transcriptional activation of the Cdk inhibitor p21 by vitamin D_3 leads to the induced differentiation of the myelomonocytic cell line U937. *Genes Dev.* 1996, *10*, 142–153.

[27] Polly, P.; Carlberg, C.; Eisman, J. A.; Morrison, N. A. Identification of a vitamin D_3 response element in the fibronectin gene that is bound by a vitamin D_3 receptor homodimer. *J. Cell. Biochem.* 1996, *60*, 322–333.

[28] Polly, P.; Carlberg, C.; Eisman, J. A.; Morrison, N. A. 1α,25-dihydroxyvitamin D_3 receptor as a mediator of transrepression of retinoid signaling. *J. Cell. Biochem.* 1997, *67*, 287–296.

[29] Berger, U.; Wilson, P.; McClelland, R. A.; Colston, K.; Haussler, M. R.; Pike, J. W.; Coombes, R. C. Immunocytochemical detection of 1,25-dihydroxyvitamin D receptors in normal human tissues. J. *Clin. Endocrinol. Metab.* 1988, *67*, 607–613.

[30] Stack, E.; DuBois, R. N. Regulation of cyclo-oxygenase-2. *Best Pract. Res. Clin. Gastroenterol.* 2001, *15 (5)*, 787-800.

[31] Murakami, M.; Kudo, I. Recent advances in molecular biology and physiology of the prostaglandin E2-biosynthetic pathway. *Prog. Lipid. Res.* 2004, *43(1)*, 3-35.

[32] Anggard, E. The biological activities of three metabolites of prostaglandin E_1. *Acta Physiol. Scand.* 1966, *66*, 509–510.

[33] Tsuboi, K.; Sugimoto, Y.; Ichikawa, A. Prostanoid receptor subtypes. *Prostaglandins Other Lipid. Mediat.* 2002, *68-69*, 535–556.

[34] Williams, C. S.; DuBois, R. N. Prostaglandin endoperoxide synthase: why two isoforms? *Am. J. Physiol.* 1996, *270*, 393-400.

[35] Herschman, H. R. Prostaglandin synthase 2. *Biochim. Biophys. Acta.* 1996, *1299(1)*, 125-140.

[36] Langenbach, R.; Morham, S. G.; Tiano, H. F.; Loftin, C. D.; Ghanayem, B. I.; Chulada, P. C.; Mahler, J. F.; Lee, C. A.; Goulding, E. H.; Kluckman, K. D.; Kim, H. S.; Smithies, O. Prostaglandin synthase 1 gene disruption in mice reduces arachidonic acid-induced inflammation and indomethacin-induced gastric ulceration. *Cell* 1995, *83(3)*, 483-492.

[37] Lim, H.; Paria, B. C.; Das, S. K.; Dinchuk, J. E.; Langenbach, R.; Trzaskos, J. M.; Dey, S. K. Multiple female reproductive failures in cyclooxygenase 2-deficient mice. *Cell* 1997, *91(2)*, 197-208.

[38] Davis, B.J.; Lennard, D. E.; Lee, C. A.; Tiano, H. F.; Morham, S. G.; Wetsel, W. C.; Langenbach, R. Anovulation in cyclooxygenase-2 deficient mice is restored by prostaglandin E2 and interleukin-1 beta. *Endocrinology* 1999, *140(6)*, 2685–2695.

[39] Loftin, C. D.; Trivedi, D. R.; Tiano, H. F.; Clark, JA.; Lee, C. A.; Epstein, J. A.; Morham, S. G.; Breyer, M. D.; Nguyen, M.; Hawkins, BM. Failure of ductus arteriosus closure and remodelling in neonatal mice deficient in cyclooxygenase-1 and -2. *Proc. Natl. Acad. Sci. U.S.A.* 2001, *98(3)*, 1059–1064

[40] Rozic, J. G.; Chakraborty, C.; Lala, P. K. Cyclooxygenase inhibitors retard murine mammary tumor progression by reducing tumor cell migration, invasiveness and angiogenesis. *Int. J. Cancer.* 2001, *93*, 497-506.

[41] Eberhart, C. E.; Coffey, R. J.; Radhika, A.; Giardiello, F. M.: Ferrebach, S.; Dubois, R. N. Up-regulation of cyclooxygenase gene expression in human colorectal adenomas and adenocarcinomas. *Gastroenterology* 1994, *107*, 1183-1188.

[42] Sinicrope, F. A.; Lemoine, M.; Xi, L.; Lynch, P. M.; Cleary, K. R.; Shen, Y.; Frazier, M. L. Reduced expression of cyclooxygenase 2 proteins in hereditary nonpolyposis colorectal cancers relative to sporadic cancers. *Gastroenterology* 1999, *117*, 350-358.

[43] Ristimaki, A.; Honkanen, N.; Jankala, H.; Sipponen, P.; Harkonen, M. Expression of cyclooxygenase-2 in human gastric carcinoma. *Cancer Res.* 1997, *57*, 1276-1280.

[44] Zimmermann, K. C.; Sarbia, M.; Weber, A.; Bochard, F.; Gabbert, H. E.; Schror, K. Cyclooxygenase-2 expression in human esophageal carcinoma. *Cancer Res.* 1999, *5*, 198-204.

[45] Swami, S.; Krishnan, A. V.; Moreno, J.; Bhattacharyya, R. B.; Peehl, D.; Feldman, D. Calcitriol and enistein actions to inhibit the prostaglandin pathway: potential combination therapy to treat prostate cancer. *J. Nutr.* 2007, *137*, 205S-210S.

[46] Subbaramaiah, K.; Dannenberg, A. J. Cyclooxygenase 2: a molecular target for cancer prevention and treatment. Trends. *Pharmacol. Sci.* 2003, *24*, 96–102.

[47] Heinonen, P. K.; Metsa-Ketela, T. Prostaglandin and thromboxane production in ovarian cancer tissue. *Gynecol. Obstet. Invest.* 1984, *18(5)*, 225-229.

[48] Ylikorkala, O.; Kauppila, A.; Viinikka, L. Prostacyclin and thromboxane in ovarian cancer: effect of cytostatics and prostaglandin synthesis inhibitors. *Gynecol. Oncol.* 1983, *16(3)*, 340-345.

[49] Munkarah, A. R.; Morris, R.; Baumann, P.; Deppe, G.; Malone, J.; Diamond, M. P.; Saed, G. M. Effects of prostaglandin E(2) on proliferation and apoptosis of epithelial ovarian cancer cells. *J. Soc. Gynecol. Investig.* 2002, *9(3)*, 168-173.

[50] Gupta, R. A.; Tejada, L. V.; Tong, B. J.; Das, S. K.; Morrow, J. D.; Dey, S. K.; DuBois, R. N. Cyclooxygenase-1 is overexpressed and promotes angiogenic growth factor production in ovarian cancer. *Cancer Res.* 2003, *63(5)*, 906-911.

[51] Ali-Fehmi, R.; Morris, R. T.; Bandyopadhyay, S.; Che, M.; Schimp, V.; Malone, J.M. Jr.; Munkarah, A. R. Expression of cyclooxygenase-2 in advanced stage ovarian serous carcinoma: correlation with tumor cell proliferation, apoptosis, angiogenesis, and survival. *Am. J. Obstet. Gynecol.* 2005, *192(3)*, 819-825.

[52] Daikoku, T.; Wang, D.; Tranguch, S.; Morrow, J. D.; Orsulic, S.; DuBois, R. N.; Dey, S. K. Cyclooxygenase-1 is a potential target for prevention and treatment of ovarian epithelial cancer. *Cancer Res.* 2005, *65(9)*, 3735-3744.

[53] Dore, M.; Cote, L. C.; Mitchell, A.; Sirois, J. Expression of prostaglandin G/H synthase type 1, but not type 2, in human ovarian adenocarcinomas. *J. Histochem. Cytochem.* 1998, *46(1)*, 77-84.

[54] Daikoku, T.; Tranguch, S.; Trofimova, I. N.; Dinulescu, D. M.; Jacks, T.; Nikitin, A. Y.; Connolly, D. C.; Dey, S.K. Cyclooxygenase-1 is overexpressed in multiple

genetically engineered mouse models of epithelial ovarian cancer. *Cancer Res.* 2006, *66(5)*, 2527-2531.

[55] Rodriguez-Burford, C.; Barnes, M; N.; Oelschlager, D. K.; Myers, R. B.; Talley, L. I.; Partridge, E. E.; Grizzle, W. E. Effects of nonsteroidal anti-inflammatory agents (NSAIDs) on ovarian carcinoma cell lines: preclinical evaluation of NSAIDs as chemopreventive agents. *Clin. Cancer Res.* 2002, *8(1)*, 202-209.

[56] Schreinemachers, D. M., Everson, R. B. Aspirin use and lung, colon, and breast cancer. Incidence in a prospective study. *Epidemiology* 1994, *5*, 138-146.

[57] Harris, R. E., Namboodiri, K. K., Farrar, W. B. Non-steroidal anti-inflammatory drugs and breast cancer. *Epidemiology* 1996, *7*, 203-205.

[58] Sharp, C. R., Collet, J. P., McNutt, M., Belzile, E., Boivin, J. F., Hanley, J. A. Nested case control study of the effect of non-steroidal anti-inflammatory drugs on breast cancer risk and stage. *Br. J. Cancer* 2000, *83*, 112-120.

[59] Liu, X.; Rose, D. Differential expression and regulation of cyclooxygenase-1 and -2 in two human breast cancer cell lines. *Cancer Res.* 1996, *56*, 5125-5127.

[60] Schrey, M. P.; Patel, K. V. Prostaglandin E_2 production and metabolism in human breast cancer cells and breast fibroblasts. Regulation by inflammatory mediators. *Br. J. Cancer* 1995, *72*, 1412-1419.

[61] Rolland, P. H.; Martin, P. M.; Jacquemier, J.; Rolland, A.; Toga, M. Prostaglandins in human breast cancer: evidence suggesting that elevated prostaglandin production is a marker of high metastatic potential for neoplastic cells. *J. Natl. Cancer Inst. (Bethesda)* 1980, *64*, 1061-1070.

[62] Karmali, R. A.; Welts, S.; Thaler, H. T.; Lefevre, F. Prostaglandins in breast cancer. Relationship to disease stage and hormone status. *Br. J. Cancer* 1983, *48*, 689-696.

[63] Kawamori, T.; Wakabayashi, K. COX-2 and prostanoid receptors: good targets for chemoprevention. *J. Environ. Pathol. Toxicol. Oncol.* 2002, *21(2)*, 149-153.

[64] Sonoshita, M.; Takaku, K.; Sasaki, N.; Sugimoto, Y.; Ushikubi, F.; Narumiya, S.; Oshima, M.; Taketo, M. M. Acceleration of intestinal polyposis through prostaglandin receptor EP2 in Apc(Delta 716) knockout mice. *Nat. Med.* 2001, *7*, 1048–1051.

[65] Zha, S.; Yegnasubramanian, V.; Nelson, W. G.; Isaacs, W. B.; De Marzo, A. M. Cyclooxygenases in cancer: progress and perspective. *Cancer Lett.* 2004, *215*, 1–20.

[66] Chang, S. H.; Liu, C. H.; Conway, R.; Han, D. K.; Nithipatikom, K.; Trifan, O. C.; Lane, T. F.; Hla, T. Role of prostaglandin E2-dependent angiogenic switch in cyclooxygenase 2-induced breast cancer progression. *Proc. Natl. Acad. Sci. U S A* 2004, *101*, 591–596.

[67] Yan, M.; Rerko, R. M.; Platzer, P.; Dawson, D.; Willis, J.; Tong, M.; Lawrence, E.; Lutterbaugh, A.; Lu, S.; Lu, S.; Willson, J. K.; Luo, G.; Hensold, J.; Tai, H. H.; Wilson, K.; Markowitz, S. D. 15-Hydroxyprostaglandin dehydrogenase, a COX-2 oncogene antagonist, is a TGF-beta-induced suppressor of human gastrointestinal cancers. *Proc. Natl. Acad. Sci. USA* 2004, *101*, 17468–17473.

[68] Ding, Y.; Tong, M.; Liu, S.; Moscow, J. A.; Tai, H. H. NAD^+-linked 15-hydroxyprostaglandin dehydrogenase (15-PGDH) behaves as a tumor suppressor in lung cancer. *Carcinogenesis* 2005, *26*, 65–72.

[69] Gee, J. R.; Montoya, R. G.; Khaled, H. M.; Sabichi, A. L.; Grossman, H. B. Cytokeratin 20, AN43, PGDH, and COX-2 expression in transitional and squamous cell carcinoma of the bladder. *Urol. Oncol.* 2003, *21*, 266–270.

[70] Wolf, I.; O'Kelly, J.; Rubinek, T.; Tong, M.; Nguyen, A.; Lin, B. T.; Tai, H. H.; Karlan, B. Y.; Koeffler, H. P. 15-hydroxyprostaglandin dehydrogenase is a tumor suppressor of human breast cancer. *Cancer Res.* 2006, *66(15)*, 7818-7823.

[71] van 't Veer, L. J.; Dai, H.; van de Vijver, M. J.; He, Y. D.; Hart, A. A.; Mao, M.; Peterse, H. L.; van der Kooy, K.; Marton, M. J.; Witteveen, A. T.; Schreiber, G. J.; Kerkhoven, R. M.; Roberts, C.; Linsley, P. S.; Bernards, R.; Friend, S. H. Gene expression profiling predicts clinical outcome of breast cancer. *Nature* 2002, *415*, 530–536.

[72] Half, E.; Tang, X. M.; Gwyn, K.; Sahin, A.; Wathen, K.; Sinicrope, F. A. Cyclooxygenase-2 expression in human breast cancers and adjacent ductal carcinoma in situ. *Cancer Res.* 2002, *62*, 1676–1681.

[73] Denkert, C.; Winzer, K. J.; Müller, B. M.; Weichert, W.; Pest, S.; Köbel, M.; Kristiansen, G.; Reles, A.; Siegert, A.; Guski, H.; Hauptmann, S. Elevated expression of cyclooxygenase-2 is a negative prognostic factor for disease free survival and overall survival in patients with breast carcinoma. *Cancer* 2003, *97(12)*, 2978-2987.

[74] Ristimäki, A.; Sivula, A.; Lundin, J.; Lundin, M.; Salminen, T.; Haglund, C.; Joensuu, H.; Isola, J. Prognostic significance of elevated cyclooxygenase-2 expression in breast cancer. *Cancer Res.* 2002, *62*, 632–635.

[75] Singh Ranger, G.; Thomas, V.; Jewell, A.; Mokbel, K. Elevated cyclooxygenase-2 expression correlates with distant metastases in breast cancer. *Anticancer Res.* 2004, *24(4)*, 2349–2351.

[76] Nassar, A.; Radhakishnan, A.; Cabero, I. A.; Cotsonis, G.; Cohen, C. COX-2 expression in invasive breast cancer: Correlation with prognostic parameters and outcome. Appl. Immunohistochem. *Mol. Morphol.* 2007, *15(3)*, 255-259.

[77] Hwang, D., Scollard, D., Byrne, J., Levine, E. Expression of cyclooxygenase-1 and cyclooxygenase-2 in human breast cancer. *J. Natl. Cancer Inst.* 1998, *90*, 455-460.

[78] Soslow, R., Dannenberg, A., Rush, D., Woerner, B. M., Khan, K. N., Masferrer, J., Koki, A. COX-2 is expressed in human pulmonary, colonic, and mammary tumors. *Cancer* 2000, 2637-2645.

[79] Costa, C.; Soares, R.; Reis-Filho, J. S.; Leitão, D.; Amendoeira, I., Schmitt, F. C. Cyclooxygenase 2 expression is associated with angiogenesis and lymph node metastasis in human breast cancer. *J. Clin. Pathol.* 2002, *55*, 429-434.

[80] Kelly, L. M.; Hill, A. D. K.; Kennedy, S.; Connolly, E. M.; Ramanath, R.; The, S.; Dijkstra, B.; Purcell, R.; McDermott, E. W.; O'Higgins, N. Lack of prognostic effect of COX-2 expression in primary breast cancer on short term follow-up. *Eur. J. Surg. Oncol.* 2002, *29*, 707–710.

[81] Lim, S. C. Role of COX-2, VEGF and cyclin D1 in mammary infiltrating duct carcinoma. *Oncol. Rep.* 2003, *10 (5)*, 1241-1249.

[82] Wülfing, P.; Diallo, R.; Müller, C.; Wülfing, C.; Poremba, C.; Heinecke, A.; Rody, A.; Greb, R. R.; Böcker, W.; Kiesel, L. Analysis of cyclooxygenase-2 expression in human breast cancer: high throughput tissue microarray analysis. *J. Cancer Res. Clin. Oncol.* 2003, *129*, 375-382.

[83] Boland, G. P.; Butt, I. P.; Prasad, R.; Knox, W. F.; Bundred, N. J. COX-2 expression is associated with an aggressive phenotype in ductal carcinoma in situ. *Br. J. Cancer* 2004, *90*, 423–429.

[84] Zhao, X. Q.; Pang, D.; Xue, Y. Expression of the cyclooxygenase-2 gene in human breast carcinoma. *Zhongua Wai Ke Za Zhi* 2003, *41(6)*, 427–429.

[85] Singh Ranger, G.; Kirkpatrick, K. L.; Clark, G. M.; Mokbel, K. Cyclooxygenase-2 (COX-2) mRNA expression correlates with progesterone receptor positivity in human breast cancer. *Curr. Med. Res. Opin.* 2003, *19(2)*, 131–134.

[86] Kirkpatrick, K.; Ogunkolade, W.; Bustin, S.; Jenkins, P.; Ghilchik, M.; Mokbel, K. The mRNA expression of cyclooxygenase-2 and vascular endothelial growth factor in human breast cancer. *Breast Cancer Res. Treat.* 2001, *69(3)*, 373.

[87] Watanabe, O.; Shimizu, T.; Imamura, H.; Kinoshita, J.; Utada, Y.; Okabe, T.; Kimura, K.; Hirano, A.; Yoshimatsu, K.; Aiba, M.; Ogawa, K. Expression of cyclooxygenase-2 in malignant and benign breast tumours. *Anticancer Res.* 2003, *23(4)*, 3215–3221.

[88] Yoshimura, N.; Sano, H.; Okamoto, M.; Akioka, K.; Ushogome, H.; Kadotani, Y.; Yoshimura, R.; Nobori, S.; Higuchi, A.; Ohmori, Y.; Nakamura, K. Expression of cyclooxygenase-1 and -2 in human breast cancer. *Surg. Today* 2003, *33*, 805–811.

[89] Ristimäki, A.; Garfinkel, S.; Weesendorf, J.; Maciag, T.; Hla, T. Induction of cyclooxygenase-2 by interleukin-1 alpha. Evidence for post-transcriptional regulation. *J. Biol. Chem.* 1994, *269(16)*, 11769-11775.

[90] Evett, G. E.; Xie, W.; Chipman, J. G.; Robertson, D. L.; Simmons, D. L. Prostaglandin GH Synthase isoenyme 2 expression in fibroblasts: regulation by dexamethasone, mitogens and oncogenes. *Arch. Biochem. Biophys.* 2003, *306*, 169–177.

[91] Sorlie, T.; Perou, C. M.; Tibshirani, R. Gene expression patterns of breast carcinomas distinguish tumor subclasses with clinical implications. *PNAS USA* 2001, *98*, 10869–10874.

[92] Salhab, M.; Singh-Ranger, G.; Mokbel, R.; Jouhra, F.; Jiang, W.G.; Mokbel, K. Cyclooxygenase-2 mRNA expression correlates with aromatase expression in human breast cancer. *J. Surg. Oncol.* 2007, *96(5)*, 424-428.

[93] Diaz-Cruz, E. S.; Shapiro, C. L.; Brueggemeier, R. W. Cyclooxygenase inhibitors suppress aromatase expression and activity in breast cancer cells. *J. Clin. Endocrinol. Metab.* 2005, *90*, 2563–2570.

[94] Richards, J. A.; Petrel, T. A.; Brueggemeier, R. W. Signaling pathways regulating aromatase and cyclooxygenases in normal and malignant breast cells. *J. Steroid. Biochem. Mol. Biol.* 2002, *80*, 203–212.

[95] Brueggemeier, R. W.; Richards, J. A.; Petrel, T. A. Aromatase and cyclooxygenases: enzymes in breast cancer. *J. Steroid. Biochem. Mol. Biol.* 2003, *86*, 501–507.

[96] Vienonen, A.; Syvala, H.; Miettinen, S.; Tuohimaa, P.; Ylikomi, T. Expression of progesterone receptor isoforms A and B is differentially regulated by estrogen in different breast cancer cell lines. *J. Steroid. Biochem. Mol. Biol.* 2002, *80*, 307–313.

[97] Liu, C. H., Chang, S., Narko, K., Trifan, O. C., Wu, M., Smith, E., Haudenschild, C., Lane, T. F., Hla, T. Overexpression of cyclooxygenase-2 is sufficient to induce tumorigenesis in transgenic mice. *J. Biol. Chem.* 2001, *276*, 18563-18569.

[98] Tsujii, M.; DuBois, R. N. Alterations in cellular adhesion and apoptosis in epithelial cells overexpressing prostaglandin endoperoxide synthase 2. *Cell* 1995, *93*, 705-716.

[99] Oshima, M., Dinchuk, J. E., Kargman, S. L., Oshima, H., Hancock, B., Kwong, E., Trzaskos, J. M., Evans, J. F., Taketo, M. M. Suppression of intestinal polyposis in Apc716 knockout mice by inhibition of cyclooxygenase-2 (COX-2). *Cell* 1996, *80*, 803-809.

[100] Mestre, J. R.; Subbaramaiah, K.; Sacks, P. G.; Schantz, S. P.; Tanabe, T.; Inoue, H.; Dannenberg, A. J. Retinoids suppress epidermal growth factor-induced

transcription of cyclooxygenase-2 in human oral squamous carcinoma cells. *Cancer Res.* 1991, *57(14)*, 2890–2895.

[101] Davies, G.; Salter, J.; Hills, M.; Martin, L.-A.; Sacks, N.; Dowsett, M. Correlation between cyclooxygenase-2 expression and angiogenesis in human breast cancer. *Clin. Cancer Res.* 2003, *9*, 2651-2656.

[102] Lim, S. C.; Park, S. Y.; Do, N. Y. Correlation of cyclooxygenase-2 pathway and VEGF expression in head and neck squamous cell carcinoma. *Oncol. Rep.* 2003, *10 (5)*, 1073-1079.

[103] Chu, J.; Lloyd, F. L.; Trifan, O. C.; Knapp, B.; Rizzo, M. T. Potential involvement of the cyclooxygenase-2 pathway in the regulation of tumor-associated angiogenesis and growth in pancreatic cancer. *Mol. Cancer Ther.* 2003, *(1)*, 1-7.

[104] Tsujii, M.; Kawano, S.; Tsujii, S.; Sawaoka, H.; Hori, M.; DuBois, N. Cyclooxygenase regulates angiogenesis induced by colon cancer cells. *Cell* 1998, *93*, 705-716.

[105] Gately, S. The contributions of cyclooxygenase-2 to tumour angiogenesis. *Cancer Metastasis Rev.* 2001, *19(1–2)*, 19–27.

[106] Daniel, T. O.; Liu, H.; Morrow, J. D.; Crews, B. C.; Marnett, L.J. Thromboxane A2 is a mediator of cyclooxygenase-2-dependent endothelial migration and angiogenesis. *Cancer Res.* 1999, *59*, 4574-4577.

[107] Pezzella, F.; Pastorino, U.; Tagliabue, E.; Andreola, S.; Sozzi, G.; Gasparini, G.; Menard, S,.; Gatter, K. C.; Harris, A. L.; Fox, S.; Buyse, M.; Pilotti, S.; Pierotti, M.; Rilke, F. Non-small-cell lung carcinoma tumor growth without morphological evidence of neo-angiogenesis. *Am. J. Pathol.* 1997, *151*, 1417-1423.

[108] Maniotis, A. J.; Folberg, R.; Hess, A.; Seftor, E. A.; Gardner, L. M.; Pe'er, J.; Trent, J. M.; Meltzer, P. S.; Hendrix, M. J. Vascular channel formation by human melanoma cells in vivo and in vitro: vasculogenic mimicry. *Am. J. Pathol.* 1999, *155*, 739-752.

[109] Shirakawa, K.; Shibuya, M.; Heike, Y.; Takashima, S.; Watanabe, I.; Konishi, F.; Kasumi, F.; Goldman, C. K.; Thomas, K. A.; Bett, A.; Terada, M.; Wakasugi, H. Tumor-infiltrating endothelial cells and endothelial precursor cells in inflammatory breast cancer. *Int. J. Cancer* 2002, *99*, 344-351.

[110] Hendrix, M. J.; Seftor, E. A.; Hess, A. R.; Seftor, R. E. Vasculogenic mimicry and tumour-cell plasticity: lessons from melanoma. *Nat. Rev. Cancer* 2003, *3*, 411-421.

[111] Shirakawa, K.; Kobayashi, H.; Heike, Y.; Kawamoto, S.; Brechbiel, M. W.; Kasumi, F.; Iwanaga, T.; Konishi, F.; Terada, M;, Wakasugi, H. Hemodynamics in vasculogenic mimicry and angiogenesis of inflammatory breast cancer xenograft. *Cancer Res.* 2002, *62*, 560–566.

[112] Basu, G. D.; Liang, W. S.; Stephan, D. A.; Wegener, L. T.; Conley, C. R; Pockaj, B. A.; Mukerjee, P. A novel role for cyclooxygenase-2 in regulating vascular channel formation by human breast cancer cells. *Breast Cancer Res.* 2006, *8(6)*, R69.

[113] Khuder, S.A.; Mutgi, A. B. Breast cancer and NSAID use: a metaanalysis. *Br. J. Cancer.* 2001, *84*, 1188–1192.

[114] Egan, K., Stampfer, M., Giovannucci, E., Rosner, B., Colditz, G. Prospective study of regular aspirin use and the risk of breast cancer. *J. Natl. Cancer Inst.* 1996, (Bethesda), *88*, 988-993.

[115] Rosenberg, L.; Palmer, J. R.; Zauber, A. G.; Warshaver, M. E.; Stolley, P.D.; Shapiro, S. A hypothesis: nonsteroidal anti-inflammatory drugs reduce the incidence of large-bowel cancer. *J. Natl. Cancer Inst.* 1991, *83*, 355-358.

[116] Thun, M. J.; Namboodiri, M. M.; Heath, C. W. Jr. Aspirin use and reduced risk of fatal colon cancer. *N. Engl. J. Med.* 1991, *325*, 1593-1596.

[117] Alshafie, G. A., Abou-Issa, H., Seibert, K., Harris, R. Chemotherapeutic evaluation of celecoxib, a cyclooxygenase-2 inhibitor, in rats mammary tumor model. *Oncol. Rep.* 2000, *7*, 1377-1381.

[118] Harris, R. E.; Alshafie, G. A.; Abou-Issa, H.; Seibert, K. Chemoprevention of breast cancer in rats by celecoxib, a cyclooxygenase 2 inhibitor. *Cancer Res.* 2000, *60*, 2101-2103.

[119] Barnes, N. L.; Warnberg, F.; Farnie, G.; White, D.; Jiang, W.; Anderson, E.; Bundred, N. J. Cyclooxygenase-2 inhibition: effects on tumour growth, cell cycling and lymphangiogenesis in a xenograft model of breast cancer. *Br. J. Cancer* 2007, *96(4)*, 575-582.

[120] Yoshinaka, R.; Shibata, M. A.; Morimoto, J.; Tanigawa, N.; Otsuki, Y. COX-2 inhibitor celecoxib suppresses tumor growth and lung metastasis of a murine mammary cancer. *Anticancer Res.* 2006, *26(6B)*, 4245-4254.

[121] Fabi, A.; Metro, G.; Papaldo, P.; Mottolese, M.; Melucci, E.; Carlini, P.; Sperduti, I.; Russillo, M.; Gelibter, A.; Ferretti, G.; Tomao, S.; Milella, M.; Cognetti, F. Impact of celecoxib on capecitabine tolerability and activity in pretreated metastatic breast cancer: results of a phase II study with biomarker evaluation. *Cancer Chemother. Pharmacol.* 2008, *62(4)*, 717-725.

[122] Canney, P. A.; Machin, M. A.; Curto, J. A feasibility study of the efficacy and tolerability of the combination of Exemestane with the COX-2 inhibitor Celecoxib in post-menopausal patients with advanced breast cancer. *Eur. J. Cancer* 2006, *42(16)*, 2751-2756.

[123] Dirix, L. Y.; Ignacio, J.; Nag, S.; Bapsy, P.; Gomez, H.; Raghunadharao, D.; Paridaens, R.; Jones, S.; Falcon, S.; Carpentieri, M.; Abbattista, A.; Lobelle, J. P. Treatment of advanced hormone-sensitive breast cancer in postmenopausal women with exemestane alone or in combination with celecoxib. *J. Clin. Oncol.* 2008, *10, 26(8)*, 1253-1259.

[124] Beer, T. M.; Ryan, C. W.; Venner, P. M.; Petrylak, D. P.; Chatta, G. S.; Ruether, J. D.; Chi, K. N.; Young, J.; Henner, W.D.; ASCENT(AIPC Study of Calcitriol ENhancing Taxotere) Investigators. Intermittent chemotherapy in patients with metastatic androgen-independent prostate cancer: results from ASCENT, a double-blinded, randomized comparison of high-dose calcitriol plus docetaxel with placebo plus docetaxel. *Cancer* 2008, *112(2)*, 326-330.

[125] Dragovich, T.; Burris, H. 3rd, Loehrer, P.; Von Hoff, D. D.; Chow, S.; Stratton, S.; Green, S.; Obregon, Y.; Alvarez, I.; Gordon, M. Gemcitabine plus celecoxib in patients with advanced or metastatic pancreatic adenocarcinoma: results of a phase II trial. *Am. J. Clin. Oncol.* 2008, *31(2)*, 157-162.

[126] Agarwala, A.; Fisher, W.; Bruetman, D.; McClean, J.; Taber, D.; Titzer, M.; Juliar, B.; Yu, M.; Breen, T.; Einhorn, L. H.; Hanna, N. Gefitinib plus celecoxib in chemotherapy-naïve patients with stage IIIB/IV non-small cell lung cancer: a phase II study from the Hoosier Oncology Group. *J. Thorac. Oncol.* 2008, *3(4)*, 374-379.

[127] Xiao, H.; Zhang, Q.; Lin, Y.; Reddy, B. S.; Yang, C. S.; Combination of atorvastatin and celecoxib synergistically induces cell cycle arrest and apoptosis in colon cancer cells. *Int. J. Cancer* 2008, *122(9)*, 2115-2124.

[128] Giovanucci, E. The epidemiology of vitamin D and cancer incidence and mortality: a review (United States). *Cancer causes control* 2005, *16*, 83-95.

[129] Holick, M. F. Sunlight and vitamin D for bone health and prevention of autoimmune diseases, canc ers, and cardiovascular disease. *Am. J. Clin. Nutr.* 2004, *80*, 1678–1688S.

[130] Trang, H. M.; Cole, D. E.; Rubin, L. A.; Pierratos, A.; Siu, S.; Vieth, R. Evidence that vitamin D_3 increases serum 25-hydroxyvitamin D more efficiently than does vitamin D2. *Am. J. Clin. Nutr.* 1998, *68*, 854–858.

[131] Hollis, B. W.; Wagner, C. L. Normal serum vitamin D levels. *N. Engl. J. Med.* 2005, *352(5)*, 515-516.

[132] Reichrath, J. Vitamin D and the skin: an ancient friend, revisited. *Experimental Dermatology* 2007, *16(7)*, 618-625

[133] Holick, M. F. The cutaneous photosynthesis of previtamin D3: a unique photoendocrine system. *J. Invest. Dermatol.* 1981, *77*, 51-58.

[134] Feskanich, D.; Ma, J.; Fuchs, C. S.; Kirkner, G. J.; Hankinson, S. E.; Hollis, B. W.; Giovannucci, E. L. Plasma vitamin D metabolites and risk of colorectal cancer in women. *Cancer Epidemiol. Biomarkers Prev.* 2004, *13(9)*, 1502-1508.

[135] Ohyama, Y., Yamasaki, T. Eight cytochrome P450s catalyze vitamin D metabolism. *Front. Biosci.* 2004, *9*, 3007-3018.

[136] Hewison, M.; Zehnder, D.; Chakraverty, R.; Adams, J. S. Vitamin D and barrier function: a novel role for extra-renal 1α-hydroxylase. *Mol. Cell Endocrinol.* 2004, *215*, 31–38.

[137] Bell, N. H. Renal and nonrenal 25-hydroxyvitamin D-1α-hydroxylases and their clinical significance. *J. Bone Miner. Res.* 1998, *13*, 350–353.

[138] Omdahl, J. L.; Morris, H. A.; May, B. K. Hydroxylase enzymes of the vitamin D pathway: expression, function, and regulation. *Annu. Rev. Nutr.* 2002, *22*, 139-166.

[139] Dusso, A. S.; Brown, A. J.; Slatopolsky, E. Vitamin D. *Am. J. Physiol. Renal Physiol.* 2005, *289(1)*, F8-28.

[140] Turunen, M. M.; Dunlop, T. W.; Carlberg, C.; Väisänen, S. Selective use of multiple vitamin D response elements underlies the 1 alpha,25-dihydroxyvitamin D3-mediated negative regulation of the human CYP27B1 gene. *Nucleic Acids Res.* 2007, *35(8)*, 2734-2747.

[141] Zitterman, A. Vitamin D in preventive medicine: are we ignoring the evidence? *Br. J Nutr.* 2003, *89*, 552-572.

[142] Hewison, M.; Zehnder, D.; Bland, R.; Stewart, P. M. 1α-Hydroxylase and the action of vitamin D. *J. Mol. Endocrinol.* 2000, *25*, 141–148.

[143] Zehnder, D.; Bland, R.; Chana, R. S.; Wheeler, D. C.; Howie, A. J.; Williams, M. C.; Stewart, P. M.; Hewison, M. Synthesis of 1,25-dihydroxyvitamin D(3) by human endothelial cells is regulated by inflammatory cytokines: a novel autocrine determinant of vascular cell adhesion. *J. Am. Soc. Nephrol.* 2002, *13(3)*, 621-629.

[144] Stoffels, K.; Overbergh, L.; Giulietti, A.; Verlinden, L.; Bouillon, R.; Mathieu, C. Immune regulation of 25-hydroxyvitamin-D3-1alpha-hydroxylase in human monocytes. J. *Bone Miner. Res.* 2006, *21(1)*, 37-47.

[145] Overbergh, L.; Stoffels, K.; Waer, M.; Verstuyf, A.; Bouillon, R.; Mathieu, C. Immune regulation of 25-hydroxyvitamin D-1alpha-hydroxylase in human monocytic THP1

cells: mechanisms of interferon-gamma-mediated induction. *J. Clin. Endocrinol. Metab.* 2006, *91(9)*, 3566-3574.

[146] Stoffels, K.; Overbergh, L.; Bouillon, R.; Mathieu, C. Immune regulation of 1alpha-hydroxylase in murine peritoneal macrophages: unravelling the IFNgamma pathway. *J. Steroid. Biochem. Mol. Biol.* 2007, *103(3-5)*, 567-571.

[147] Lopez, E. R,; Zwermann, O.; Segni, M.; Meyer, G.; Reincke, M.; Seissler, J.; Herwig, J.; Usadel K. H.; Badenhoop, K. A promoter polymorphism of the CYP27B1 gene is associated with Addison's disease, Hashimoto's thyroiditis, Graves' disease and type 1 diabetes mellitus in Germans. *Eur. J. Endocrinol.* 2004, *151*, 193–197.

[148] Fischer, D.; Seifert, M.; Becker, S.; Ludders, D.; Cordes, T.; Reichrath, J.; Friedrich, M. 25-Hydroxyvitamin D3 1alpha-hydroxylase splice variants in breast cell lines MCF-7 and MCF-10. *Cancer Genomics Proteomics* 2007, *4(4)*, 295-300.

[149] Cordes, T.; Diesing, D.; Becker, S.; Fischer, D.; Diedrich, K.; Friedrich, M. Expression of splice variants of 1alpha-hydroxylase in mcf-7 breast cancer cells. *J. Steroid. Biochem. Mol. Biol.* 2007, *103(3-5)*, 326-329.

[150] Barreto, A. M.; Schwartz, G. G.; Woodruff, R.; Cramer, S. D. 25-Hydroxyvitamin D_3, the prohormone of 1,25-dihydroxyvitamin D_3, inhibits the proliferation of primary prostatic epithelial cells. *Cancer Epidemiol. Biomarkers Prev.* 2000, *9*, 265–270.

[151] Schwartz, G. G.; Whitlatch, L. W.; Chen, T. C.; Lokeshwar, B. L.; Holick, M. F. Human prostate cells synthesize 1,25-dihydroxyvitamin D_3 from 25-hydroxyvitamin D_3. *Cancer Epidemiol. Biomarkers Prev.* 1998, *7*, 391–395.

[152] Tangpricha, V.; Flanagan, J. N.; Whitlatch, L. W.; Tseng, C. C.; Chen, T. C.; Holt, P. R.; Lipkin, M. S.; Holick, M. F. 25-Hydroxyvitamin D-1α-hydroxylase in normal and malignant colon tissue. *Lancet* 2001, *357*, 1673–1674.

[153] Bareis, P.; Bises, G.; Bischof, M. G.; Cross, H. S.; Peterlik, M. 25-hydroxy-vitamin D metabolism in human colon cancer cells during tumor progression. *Biochem. Biophys. Res. Commun.* 2001, *285*, 1012–1017.

[154] Ogunkolade, B. W.; Boucher, B. J.; Fairclough, P. D.; Hitman, G. A.; Dorudi, S.; Jenkins, P. J.; Bustin, S. A. Expression of 25-hydroxyvitamin D-1-α-hydroxylase mRNA in individuals with colorectal cancer. *Lancet* 2002, *359*, 1831–1832.

[155] Friedrich, M.; Diesing, D.; Cordes, T.; Fischer, D.; Becker, S.; Chen, T. C. Flanagan, J. N.; Tangpricha, V.; Gherson, I.; Holick, M. F.; Reichrath, J. Analysis of 25-hydroxyvitamin D3-1alpha-hydroxylase in normal and malignant breast tissue. *Anticancer Res.* 2006, *26(4A)*, 2615-2620.

[156] Garland, C. F.; Comstock, G. W.; Garland, F. C.; Helsing, K. J.; Shaw, E. K.; Gorham, E. D. Serum 25-hydroxyvitamin D and colon cancer: eight-year prospective study. *Lancet* 1989, *2*, 1176–1178.

[157] Holt, P. R.; Arber, N.; Halmos, B.; Forde, K.; Kissileff, H.; McGlynn, K. A.; Moss, S. F.; Kurihara, N.; Fan, K. Colonic epithelial cell proliferation decreases with increasing levels of serum 25-hydroxy vitamin D. *Cancer Epidemiol. Biomarkers Prev.* 2002, *11*, 113–119.

[158] Lowe, L. C.; Guy, M.; Mansi, J. L.; Peckitt, C.; Bliss, J.; Wilson, R. G.; Colston, K. W. Plasma 25-hydroxy vitamin D concentrations, vitamin D receptor genotype and breast cancer risk in a UK Caucasian population. *Eur. J. Cancer* 2005, *41*, 1164–1169.

[159] Berube, S.; Diorio, C.; Verhoek-Oftedahl, W.; Brisson, J. Vitamin D, calcium and mammographic breast densities. *Cancer Epidemiol. Biomarkers Prev.* 2004, *13*, 1466–1472.

[160] Huang, D. C.; Papavasiliou, V.; Rhim, J. S.; Horst, R. L.; Kremer, R. Targeted disruption of the 25-hydroxyvitamin D3 1alpha-hydroxylase gene in ras-transformed keratinocytes demonstrates that locally produced 1alpha,25-dihydroxyvitamin D3 suppresses growth and induces differentiation in an autocrine fashion. *Mol. Cancer Res.* 2002, *1*, 56–67.

[161] Segersten, U.; Holm, P. K.; Björklund, P.; Hessman, O.; Nordgren, H.; Binderup, L.; Akerström, G.; Hellman, P.; Westin, G. 25-Hydroxyvitamin D3 1alpha-hydroxylase expression in breast cancer and use of non-1alpha-hydroxylated vitamin D analogue. *Breast Cancer Res.* 2005, *7(6)*, 980-986.

[162] Agic, A.; Xu, H.; Altgassen, C.; Noack, F.; Wolfler, M. M.; Diedrich, K.; Friedrich, M.; Taylor, R. N.; Hornung, D. Relative expression of 1,25-dihydroxyvitamin D3 receptor, vitamin D 1 alpha-hydroxylase, vitamin D 24-hydroxylase, and vitamin D 25-hydroxylase in endometriosis and gynecologic cancers. *Reprod. Sci.* 2007, *14(5)*, 486-497.

[163] Friedrich, M.; Rafi, L.; Mitschele, T.; Tilgen, W.; Schmidt, W.; Reichrath, J. Analysis of the vitamin D system in cervical carcinomas, breast cancer and ovarian cancer. *Recent Results Cancer Res.* 2003, *164*, 39-46.

[164] Hewison, M.; Kantorovich, V.; Liker H. R.; van Herle, A. J.; Cohan, P.; Zehnder, D.; Adams, J. S. Vitamin D-mediated hypercalcemia in lymphoma: evidence for hormone production by tumoradjacent macrophages. *J. Bone Miner. Res.* 2003, *18*, 579-582.

[165] Evans, K. N.; Taylor, H.; Zehnder, D.; Kilby, M. D.; Bulmer, J. N.; Shah, F.; Adams, J. S.; Hewison, M. Increased expression of 25-hydroxyvitamin D-1α-hydroxylase in dysgerminomas: a novel form of humoral hypercalcemia of malignancy. *Am. J. Pathol.* 2004, *165*, 807–813.

[166] Townsend, K.; Banwell, C. M.; Guy, M.; Colston, K. W.; Mansi, J. L.; Stewart, P. M.; Campbell, M. J.; Hewison, M. Autocrine metabolism of vitamin D in normal and malignant tissue. *Clin. Cancer Res.* 2005, *11(9)*, 3579-3586.

[167] Ainsleigh, H. G. Beneficial effects of sun exposure on cancer mortality. *Prev. Med.* 1993, *22*, 132-140.

[168] Gorham, E. D.; Garland, F. C.; Garland, C. F. Sunlight and breast cancer incidence in the USSR. *Int. J. Epidemiol.* 1990, *19*, 820–824.

[169] Garland, F. C.; Garland, C. F.; Gorham, E. D.; Young, J. F. Geographic variation in breast cancer mortality in the United States: a hypothesis involving exposure to solar radiation. *Prev. Med.* 1990, *19*, 614–622.

[170] Grant, W. B. An estimate of premature cancer mortality in the U.S. due to inadequate doses of solar ultraviolet-B radiation. *Cancer* 2002, *94*, 1867–1875.

[171] Kemmis, C. M.; Salvador, S. M.; Smith, K. M.; Welsh, J. Human mammary epithelial cells express CYP27B1 and are growth inhibited by 25-hydroxyvitamin D-3, the major circulating form of vitamin D-3. *J. Nutr.* 2006, *136*, 887-892.

[172] Holick, M. F.; Siris, E. S.; Binkley, N.; Beard, M. K.; Khan, A.; Katzer, J. T.; Petruschke, R. A.; Chen, E.; de Papp, A. E. Prevalence of vitamin D inadequacy among

postmenopausal women. North American women receiving osteoporosis therapy. *J. Clin. Endocrinol. Metabo.* 2005, *90*, 3215-3224.

[173] Sowers, M. R.; Wallace, R. B.; Hollis, B. W.; Lemke, J. H. Parameters related to 25-OH-D levels in a population-based study of women. *Am. J. Clin. Nutr.* 1986, *43*, 621–628.

[174] Diesing, D.; Cordes, T.; Fischer, D.; Diedrich, K.; Friedrich, M. Vitamin D--metabolism in the human breast cancer cell line MCF-7. *Anticancer Res.* 2006, *26(4A)*, 2755-2759.

[175] Sunn, K. L.; Cock, T. A.; Crofts, L. A.; Eismann, J. A.; Gardiner, E. M. Novel N-terminal variant of human VDR. *Mol. Endocrinol.* 2001, *15(9)*, 1599-1609.

[176] Tsai, M. J.; O'Malley, B. W. Molecular mechanisms of action of steroid/thyroid receptor superfamily members. *Annu. Rev. Biochem.* 1994, *63*, 451–486.

[177] Nemere, I.; Szego, C. M. Early actions of parathyroid hormone and 1,25-dihydroxycholecalciferol on istolated epithelial cells from rat intestine. *Endocrinology* 1981, *108*, 1450-1462.

[178] Studzinski, G. P.; McLane, J. A.; Uskokovic, M. R. Signaling pathways for vitamin D-induced differentiation: implications for therapy of proliferative and neoplastic diseases. *Crit. Rev. Eukaryot. Gene Expr.* 1993, *4*, 279-312.

[179] Marcinkowska, E.; Wiedlocha, A.; Radzikowsi, C. 1,25-dihydroxyvitamin D_3 induced activation and subsequent nuclear translocation of MAPK is upstream regulated by PKC in HL-60 cells. *Biochem. Biophys. Res. Commun.* 1997, *241*, 410-426.

[180] Marcinkowska, E.; Wiedlocha, A.; Radzikowski, C. Evidence that phosphatidylinositol 3-kinase and p70S6Kprotein are involved in differentiation of HL-60 cells induced by calcitriol. *Anticancer Res.* 1998, *18*, 3507-3514.

[181] Marcinkowska, E. Evidence that activation of MEK1,2/erk1,2 signal transduction pathway is necessary for calcitriol-induced differentiation of HL-60 cells. *Anticancer Res.* 2001, *21*, 499-504.

[182] Mehta, R. G.; Mehta, R. R. Vitamin D and cancer. *J. Nutr. Biochem.* 2002, *13*, 252–264.

[183] Boland, R.; De Boland, A. R.; Buitrago, C.; Morelli, S.; Santillan, G.; Vazque, G.; Capiati, D.; Baldi, C. Non-genomic stimulation of tyrosine phosphorylation cascades by 1,25(OH)(2)D(3) by VDR-dependent and –independent mechanisms in muscle cells. *Steroids* 2002, *67*, 477-482.

[184] Marcinkowska, E.; Wiedlocha, A. Steroid signal transduction activated at the cell membrane: from plants to animal. *Acta Biochimica Polonica* 2002, *49*, 735-745.

[185] Colston, K. W.; Berger, U.; Coombes, R. C. Possible role for vitamin D in controlling breast cancer cell proliferation. *Lancet* 1989, *1*, 188–191.

[186] James, S. Y.; Mackay, A. G.; Colston, K. W. Vitamin D derivatives in combination with 9-cis retinoic acid promote active cell death in breast cancer cells. *J. Mol. Endocrinol.* 1995, *14(3)*, 391-394.

[187] Welsh, J. E. Induction of apoptosis in breast cancer cells in response to vitamin D and antiestrogens. *Biochem. Cell. Biol.* 1995, *72(11–12)*, 537-545.

[188] Berger, U.; Wilson, P.; McClelland, R. A.; Colston, K.; Haussler, M. R.; Pike, J. W.; Coombes, R. C. Immunocytochemical determination of estrogen receptor, progesterone receptor, and 1,25-dihydroxyvitamin D_3 receptor in breast cancer and relationship to prognosis. *Cancer Res.* 1991, *51*, 239–244.

[189] Welsh, J. Targets of vitamin D receptor signaling in the mammary gland. *J. Bone Miner. Res.* 2007, *22 Suppl 2*, V86-90.

[190] Uitterlinden, A. G.; Fang, Y.; Van Meurs, J. B.; Pols, H. A.; Van Leeuwen, J. P. Genetics and biology of vitamin D receptor polymorphisms. *Gene* 2004, *338(2)*, 143-156.

[191] Guy, M.; Lowe, L. C.; Bretherton-Watt, D.; Mansi, J. L.; Peckitt, C.; Bliss, J.; Wilson, R. G.; Thomas, V.; Colston, K. W. Vitamin D receptor gene polymorphisms and breast cancer risk. *Clin. Cancer Res.* 2004, *15, 10(16)*, 5472-5481.

[192] Curran, J. E.; Vaughan, T.; Lea, R. A.; Weinstein, S. R.; Morrison, N. A.; Griffiths, L. R. Association of A vitamin D receptor polymorphism with sporadic breast cancer development. *Int. J. Cancer* 1999, *83*, 723–726.

[193] Chen, W. Y.; Bertone-Johnson, E. R.; Hunter, D. J.; Willett, W. C.; Hankinson, S. E. Associations between polymorphisms in the vitamin D receptor and breast cancer risk. Cancer Epidemiol. *Biomarkers Prev.* 2005, *14(10)*, 2335-2339.

[194] Sinotte, M.; Rousseau, F.; Ayotte, P.; Dewailly, E.; Diorio, C.; Giguere, Y.; Berube, S.; Brisson, J. Vitamin D receptor polymorphisms (FokI, BsmI) and breast cancer risk: association replication in two case-control studies within French Canadian population. *Endocr. Relat. Cancer.* 2008, *15(4)*, 975-83.

[195] Trabert, B.; Malone, K. E.; Daling, J. R.; Doody, D. R.; Bernstein, L.; Ursin, G.; Marchbanks, P. A.; Strom, B. L.; Humphrey, M. C.; Ostrander, E. A. Vitamin D receptor polymorphisms and breast cancer risk in a large population-based case-control study of Caucasian and African-American women. *Breast Cancer Res.* 2007, *9(6)*, R84.

[196] Lundin, A. C.; Soderkvist, P.; Eriksson, B.; Bergman-Jungestrom, M.; Wingren, S. Association of breast cancer progression with a vitamin D receptor gene polymorphism. South-East Sweden Breast Cancer Group. *Cancer Res.* 1999, *59*, 2332–2334.

[197] Ruggiero, M.; Pacini, S.; Aterini, S.; Fallai, C.; Ruggiero, C.; Pacini, P. Vitamin D receptor gene polymorphism is associated with metastatic breast cancer. *Oncol. Res.* 1998, *10*, 43–46.

[198] Dunning, A. M.; McBride, S.; Gregory, J.; Durocher, F.; Foster, N. A.; Healy, C. S.; Smith, N.; Pharoah, P. D.; Luben, R. N.; Easton, D. F.; Ponder, B. A. No association between androgen or vitamin D receptor gene polymorphisms and risk of breast cancer. *Carcinogenesis* 1999, *20*, 2131–2135.

[199] Newcomb, P. A.; Kim, H.; Trentham-Dietz, A.; Farin, F.; Hunter, D.; Egan, K. M. Vitamin D receptor polymorphism and breast cancer risk. *Cancer Epidemiol. Biomarkers Prev.* 2002, *11*, 1503–1504.

[200] Cui, Y.; Rohan, T. E. Vitamin D, Calcium, and breast cancer risk: A review. *Cancer Epidemiol. Biomarkers Prev.* 2006, *15(18)*, 1427-1437.

[201] McCullough, M. L.; Stevens, V. L.; Diver, W. R.; Feigelson, H. S.; Rodriguez, C.; Bostick, R. M.; Thun, M. J.; Calle, E. E. Vitamin D pathway gene polymorphisms, diet, and risk of postmenopausal breast cancer: a nested case-control study. *Breast Cancer Res.* 2007, *9(1)*, R9.

[202] Cashman, K. D. Calcium intake, calcium bioavailability and bone health. *Br. J. Nutr.* 2002, *87 Suppl 2*, S169–177.

[203] Welsh, J. Vitamin D and breast cancer: insights from animal models. *Am. J. Clin. Nutr.* 2004, *80*, 1721–1724S.

[204] Mantell, D. J.; Owens, P. E.; Bundred, N. J.; Mawer, E. B.; Canfield, A. E. 1α,25-Dihydroxyvitamin D(3) inhibits angiogenesis in vitro and in vivo. *Circ. Res.* 2000, *87*, 214–220.

[205] Saez, S.; Falette, N.; Guillot, C.; Meggouh, F.; Lefebvre, M. F.; Crepin, M.; William, L. McGuire. Memorial Symposium. $1,25(OH)2D_3$ modulation of mammary tumor cell growth in vitro and in vivo. *Breast Cancer Res. Treat.* 1993, *27*, 69–81.

[206] Eisman, J. A.; Sutherland, R. L.; McMenemy, M. L.; Fragonas, J. C.; Musgrove, E. A.; Pang, G. Y. Effects of 1,25-dihydroxyvitamin D3 on cell-cycle kinetics of T 47D human breast cancer cells. *J. Cell. Physiol.* 1989, *138(3)*, 611-616.

[207] Jacobson, E. A.; James, K. A.; Newmark, H. L.; Carroll, K. K. Effects of dietary fat, calcium, and vitamin D on growth and mammary tumorigenesis induced by 7,12-dimethylbenz(a)anthracene in female Sprague-Dawley rats. *Cancer Res.* 1989, *49*, 6300–6303.

[208] Xue, L.; Lipkin, M.; Newmark, H.; Wang, J. Influence of dietary calcium and vitamin D on diet-induced epithelial cell hyperproliferation in mice. *J. Natl. Cancer Inst.* 1999, *91*, 176–181.

[209] John, E. M.; Schwartz, G. G.; Dreon, D. M.; Koo, J. Vitamin D and breast cancer risk: the NHANES I epidemiologic follow-up study, 1971-1975 to 1992. National Health and Nutrition Examination Survey. *Cancer Epidemiol. Biomarkers Prev.* 1999, *8*, 399–406.

[210] Knight, J. A.; Lesosky, M.; Barnett, H.; Raboud, J. M.; Vieth, R. Vitamin D and reduced risk of breast cancer: A population-based control study. *Cancer Epidemiol. Biomarkers Prev.* 2007, *16*, 422-429.

[211] McCullough, M. L.; Rodriguez, C.; Diver, W. R.; Feigelson, H. S.; Stevens, V. L.; Thun, M. J.; Calle, E. E. Dairy, calcium, and vitamin D intake and postmenopausal breast cancer risk in the Cancer Prevention Study II Nutrition Cohort. Cancer Epidemiol. *Biomarkers Prev.* 2005, *14*, 2898–2904.

[212] Rossi, M.; McLaughlin, J. K.; Lagiou, P.; Bosetti, C.; Talamini, R.; Lipworth, L.; Giacosa, A.; Montella, M.; Franceschi, S.; Negri, E.; La Vecchia, C. Vitamin D intake and breast cancer risk: a case-control study in Italy. *Ann. Oncol.* 2009, *20(2)*, 374-378.

[213] Frazier, A. L.; Ryan, C. T.; Rockett, H.; Willett, W. C.; Colditz, G. A. Adolescent diet and risk of breast cancer. *Breast Cancer Res.* 2003, *5*, R59–64.

[214] Frazier, A. L.; Li, L.; Cho, E.; Willett, W. C.; Colditz, G. A. Adolescent diet and risk of breast cancer. *Cancer Causes Control* 2004, *15*, 73–82.

[215] Gissel, T.; Rejnmark, L.; Mosekilde, L.; Vestergaard P. Intake of vitamin D and risk of breast cancer--a meta-analysis. *J. Steroid. Biochem. Mol. Biol.* 2008, *111(3-5)*, 195-199.

[216] Hiatt, R. A.; Krieger, N.; Lobaugh, B.; Drezner, M. K.; Vogelman, J. H.; Orentreich, N. Prediagnostic serum vitamin D and breast cancer. *J. Natl. Cancer Inst.* 1998, *90*, 461–463.

[217] Bertone-Johnson, E. R.; Chen, W. Y.; Holick, M. F.; Hollis, B. W.; Colditz, G. A.; Willett, W. C.; Hankinson, S. E. Plasma 25-hydroxyvitamin D and 1,25-dihydroxyvitamin D and risk of breast cancer. *Cancer Epidemiol. Biomarkers Prev.* 2005, *14*, 1991–1997.

[218] Mawer, E. B.; Walls, J.; Howell, A.; Davies, M.; Ratcliffe, W. A.; Bundred, N. J. Serum 1,25-dihydroxyvitamin D may be related inversely to disease activity in breast cancer patients with bone metastases. *J. Clin. Endocrinol. Metab.* 1997, *82*, 118–122.

[219] Whitfield, J. F.; Boynton, A. L.; MacManus, J. P.; Sikorska, M.; Tsang, B. K. The regulation of cell proliferation by calcium and cyclic AMP. *Mol. Cell Biochem.* 1979, *27*, 155-179.

[220] Mathiasen, I. S.; Sergeev, I. N.; Bastholm, L.; Elling, F.; Norman, A. W.; Jaattela, M. Calcium and calpain as key mediators of apoptosis-like death induced by vitamin D compounds in breast cancer cells. *J. Biol. Chem.* 2002, *277*, 30738–30745.

[221] Sergeev, I. N. Calcium as a mediator of 1,25-dihydroxyvitamin D_3-induced apoptosis. *J. Steroid. Biochem. Mol. Biol.* 2004, *89–90*, 419–425.

[222] McGrath, C. M.; Soule, H. D. Calcium regulation of normal human mammary epithelial cell growth in culture. *In Vitro* 1984, *20*, 652–662.

[223] Russo, J.; Russo, I. H. The pathway of neoplastic transformation of human breast epithelial cells. *Radiat. Res.* 2001, *155*, 151–154.

[224] Boyapati, S. M.; Shu, X. O.; Jin, F.; Dai, Q.; Ruan, Z.; Gao, Y. T.; Zheng, W. Dietary calcium intake and breast cancer risk among Chinese women in Shanghai. *Nutr. Cancer* 2003, *46*, 38–43.

[225] Wark, J. D.; Larkins, R. G.; Eisman, J. A.; Wilson, K. R. Regulation of 25-hydroxyvitamin-D-la-hydroxylase in chick isolated renal tubules: effects of prostaglandin E2, frusemide and acetylsalicylate. Clin. Sci. 1981, 62, 53-59.

[226] Hayes, M. E.; Rai, A.; Cooper, R. G.; Bayley, D.; Freemont, A. J.; Mawer, E. B. Inhibition by prostaglandin E1 and E2 of 1,25-dihydroxyvitamin D3 synthesis by synovial fluid macrophages from arthritic joints. *Ann. Rheum. Dis.* 1992, *51*, 632-637.

[227] Miller, G. J. Vitamin D and prostate cancer: biologic interactions and clinical potentials. *Cancer Metastasis Rev.* 1998, *17*, 353–360.

[228] Konety, B. R.; Getzenberg, R. H. Vitamin D and prostate cancer. Urol *Clin. North Am.* 2002, *29*, 95–106.

[229] Zhuang, S. H.; Burnstein, K. L. Antiproliferative effect of 1α,25-dihydroxyvitamin D3 in human prostate cancer cell line LNCaP involves reduction of cyclin-dependent kinase 2 activity and persistent G1 accumulation. Endocrinology 1998, 139, 1197–1207.

[230] Moreno, J.; Krishnan, A. V.; Swami, S.; Nonn, L.; Peehl, D. M.; Feldman, D. Regulation of prostaglandin metabolism by calcitriol attenuates growth stimulation in prostate cancer cells. *Cancer Res.* 2005, *65(17)*, 7917-7925.

32

Calcium, Ca^{2+}-Sensing Receptor and Breast Cancer

Chunfa Huang[1,2,3,4] and R. Tyler Miller[1,2,4]
[1]*Louis Stokes Cleveland Veteran Affairs Medical Center,*
[2]*Departments of Medicine,*
[3]*Case Comprehensive Cancer Center, Case Western Reserve University,*
[4]*Rammelkamp Center for Research and Education, MetroHealth System Campus,*
Cleveland, Ohio,
United States of America

1. Introduction

Breast cancer is the most commonly diagnosed cancer and one of the leading causes of cancer-associated death among women worldwide. Each year, more than one million new cases of breast cancer are diagnosed worldwide, and an estimated 370,000 women die from breast cancer (1, 2). Ca^{2+} as an important nutrient from dairy products functions as an important signalling messenger from the beginning to the end of our life, and plays a critical role in many physiological processes such as gene transcription, cell growth, proliferation, migration, differentiation and apoptosis (3-11). Many of these processes are associated with tumorigenesis and cancer progression. Dysregulation of calcium homeostasis and signaling causes many human diseases, including mammary gland pathophysiology and breast cancer (3, 4, 5 and 9).

2. Ca^{2+} and breast cancer

Ca^{2+} is a ubiquitous cellular signal which has been strongly implicated in triggering and regulating various cell functions by Ca^{2+}-regulated proteins and their signaling pathways (3-11). The concentration of free extracellular Ca^{2+} (Ca_o^{2+}) in our serum is kept constant by processing that constantly feeds Ca^{2+} into, and withdraws it from the extracellular fluid, such as dietary calcium intake and bone calcium turnover (5-7). Decreases in the concentration of free Ca_o^{2+} in plasma (hypocalcemia) result in increased neuromuscular irritability and tetany. Increases in total serum Ca_o^{2+} (hypercalcemia) can result in fatigue, depression, mental confusion, anorexia, nausea, vomiting, constipation, reversible renal tubular defects, increased urination, alteration in the electrocardiogram (a short QT interval), and cardiac arrhythmias as well as renal insufficiency and calcification in the kidney, skin, vessels, lungs, heart and stomach. There is a ~12,000-fold Ca^{2+}-gradient between intracellular (~100 nM) and extracellular (~1.2 mM) free Ca^{2+} concentrations in cells. To maintain this Ca^{2+} gradient, cells chelate, compartmentalize, or remove Ca^{2+} from the cytoplasm (3). Regulation of cellular processes via Ca^{2+}-signaling such as binding of Ca^{2+} to proteins, change of intracellular Ca^{2+} (Ca_i^{2+}) concentrations, and modification of other protein functions by Ca^{2+} have been shown to play important roles in cancer initiation, tumor formation, tumor progression, metastasis, invasion and angiogenesis (12-14). For instance, Ca^{2+} can activate transcription factors such as nuclear factor of activated T cells (NFAT) resulting in modulation of cellular transcription (11), regulate cell proliferation promoting cancer cell progression (4, 9, 12), and modulate poly-(ADP-ribose) polymerase-1 (PARP1), mitochondrial membrane permeabilization and DNA damage leading to apoptosis and necrosis (10, 13). By mobilizing the release of Ca_i^{2+} from endoplasmic reticulum, angiogenic factors such as vascular endothelial growth factor can increase Ca_i^{2+} that in turn promote angiogenesis (14), Ca^{2+} signaling also plays an important role in cellular motility such as during tumor invasion and metastasis (4, 5, 9, 12).

2.1 Ca^{2+} intake and breast cancer risk

Calcium is a threshold nutrient and is the most abundant mineral element in the body. Dietary calcium has an important impact on bone metabolism and bone health, and is also among a number of nutritional factors suggested to be associated with cancer. Higher intakes of Ca^{2+} are reported to increase the risk of prostate cancer (15, 16) and lung cancer (17), and to reduce the risk of ovarian cancer and colorectal cancers (18, 19). Many epidemiological studies around the world that evaluated the association between Ca^{2+} intake and the risk of breast cancer have been published (20-32). Table I summaries thirteen studies from eight countries during the last five years. Most of these epidemiological studies indicate no significant association between Ca^{2+} intake and the risk of breast cancer, and some of these investigations show a negative association (20-32). Epidemiologic studies suggest that higher intake of Ca^{2+} may not be associated with breast tumorigenesis.

Studies	Calcium	Breast cancer risk	References
Chinese women	Food	No association/reduction	20, 21
Norwegian women	Dairy product	No significant association	22
Canadian women	Food and supplements	No association	23
German women	Food	No association	24
Swedish women	Food	No association	25
American women	Food and supplements	No association/modest reduction	26-30
Japanese women	Food and supplements	Reduction	31
French women	Food	Negative association	32

Table 1. Calcium intake and breast cancer risk.

2.2 Serum Ca^{2+} and breast cancer risk

As one of many nutrients in dairy products, it is difficult to study the role of calcium intake in breast cancer risk. Serum calcium is maintained within a fairly narrow range from 8.5 to 10 .5 mg/dl (2 .2 to 2 .7 mmol/L). Given the emerging interest in the potential role of Ca^{2+} in the etiology of breast cancer, several investigations focus on analyzing the relationship between the levels of serum calcium and the risk of breast cancer. In 2007, the first cohort study of 7847 women performed by Almquist et al. (33) evaluated serum calcium in relation to breast cancer risk. They found a positive association between total calcium and breast cancer risk among overweight postmenopausal women. In follow-up studies in which 462 women were diagnosed with incident breast cancer, they found that serum calcium levels in premenopausal and overweight women were positively associated with increased tumor aggressiveness as determined by a higher risk of nodal metastasis (34, 35). Recently, these results were supported by Martin et al. who also found that serum calcium levels among postmenopausal women are positively associated with incident breast cancer in white women (36), while another study found no association between total serum calcium and breast cancer risk among postmenopausal women (37). Although more studies on the relationship between serum calcium and breast cancer risk are necessary, hypercalcemia defined as an abnormal elevation in serum calcium levels is a frequent complication of breast cancer (38-41). This suggests the Ca_o^{2+} could play an important role in the regulation of breast cancer progression.

2.3 Bone metastasis of breast cancer cells and Ca^{2+} release

Hypercalcemia, which has been found in 30-40% of breast cancer patients, is the most frequent metabolic complication of breast cancer (38-41). In a significant minority of patients, cancer-induced hypercalcemia is caused by systemic secretion of parathyroid hormone-related protein (PTHrP) by cancer cells, and PTHrP causes increased bone resorption and enhances renal retention of calcium (42, 43). Most commonly, hypercalcemia occurs in patients with multiple bone metastases. Breast cancer cell metastases to bone often cause bone destruction or osteolysis, and leads to the release of growth factors from the bone matrix (e.g., transforming growth factor, insulin-like growth factor, basic fibroblast growth factor), and the release of large quantities of Ca^{2+} into the bone microenvironment (44-49). The growth factors can stimulate breast cancer cell proliferation (47), while Ca^{2+} also plays an important role in crosstalk between tumor cells and bone microenvironment to promote a vicious cycle of tumor cell growth and bone destruction.

3. Ca^{2+}-sensing receptor and breast cancer

Recent studies have demonstrated that some G protein coupled receptors (GPCR) such as endothelin receptors, chemokine receptors and lysophosphatidic acid receptors play an important role in tumorigenesis and metastasis of multiple human cancers (50-52). Some other GPCRs, for instance neuropeptide receptors, adenosine A_{2B} receptor, P_{2Y} receptor, bradykinin receptor, thrombin receptor, metabotropic glutamate receptors, estrogen receptor, and EGF-like module containing mucin-like hormone receptor 2 are also expressed at a significantly higher level in cancer tissues and have been implicated in cancer progression (53-57). The Ca^{2+}-sensing receptor (CaR) has a characteristic seven transmembrane domain GPCR structure and was initially characterized as a sensor for modulating parathyroid hormone and calcitonin release in response to change in blood Ca^{2+} levels (58). The metastasis of breast cancer cells to bone result in osteolysis and lead to the release of large quantities of Ca^{2+} into the bone microenvironment (45, 46). This Ca_o^{2+} can be a primary signaling molecule and act through the CaR that directly regulates multiple signaling pathways involved in breast cancer cell growth, proliferation, differentiation, apoptosis and migration (58, 59), and through the Ca^{2+} channels which elevate intracellular Ca^{2+} (Ca_i^{2+}) levels to modulate Ca^{2+}-dependent proteins (60).

3.1 CaR expression and breast cancer

3.1.1 Up-regulation of CaR expression in breast cancer cells and specimens

The CaR is expressed in the epithelial ducts of the normal human breast, and the level of expression is associated with mammary gland development, with lower levels in pregnancy and involution, low levels before pregnancy and higher levels with lactation (61). These physiological changes in CaR expression are involved in the control of PTHrP secretion that feeds back to regulate Ca^{2+} influxes to the mammary glands. These influxes regulate the proliferation of normal mammary epithelial cells. During lactation, bone loss is rapid and completely reversible upon weaning, and large amounts of calcium are transferred into milk, placing nursing mothers under calcemic stress. Bone turnover increases and bone mass decreases, presumably to free skeletal calcium for milk production (62, 63). It is known that the receptor is also expressed in breast carcinomas and breast cancer cell lines (64). Using an anti-CaR antibody with peptide blocking to demonstrate specificity, we (65) recently reported that the levels of CaR expression are significantly increased in breast cancer cell lines compared to nonmalignant breast cell lines (Fig. 1). Mihai et al. analyzed the relationship between the levels of CaR expression and bone metastases in 108 breast cancer patients, and found that patients with higher CaR expression are more likely to develop bone metastases (66). The higher Ca_o^{2+} concentration in the erosion sites of breast cancer metastasis and up-regulation of CaR expression in breast cancer cells could lead to cell signaling abnormalities. This suggests the potential changes in CaR-mediated signaling in breast cancer cells.

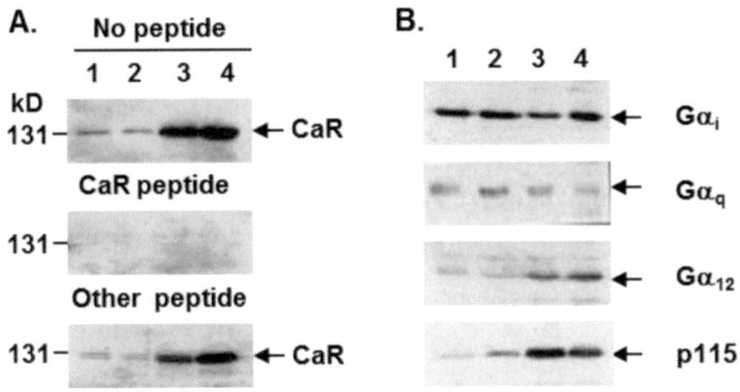

Fig. 1. **Expression of CaR, G protein and p115RhoGEF in normal breast cells and breast cancer cells.** Equal amounts of protein from Hs 578Bst (lane 1), MCF-10A (lane 2), MDA-MB-231 (lane 3) and MCF-7 cell (lane 4) lysates were processed for immunoblotting using antibodies against different proteins as shown on the right. A) Peptide blocking: anti-CaR antibody incubated with no peptide (top) immunogenic peptide (middle) or non-specific peptide (bottom); B) $G\alpha_i$ (top), $G\alpha_q$ (upper middle) $G\alpha_{12}$ (lower middle) and p115RhoGEF (p115, bottom).

3.1.2 Alteration of other CaR-signaling components in breast cancer

Like other GPCRs, the CaR signaling cascade contains four major components: receptor, G protein (heterotrimeric $\alpha\beta\gamma$), regulators of G-protein signaling (RGS) protein, and effectors (67). Current evidence shows that the CaR couples to G_s, G_i, G_q, and $G_{12/13}$ and can be regulated by RGS4 and p115-RhoGEF (58, 65, 68, and 69). Kelly et al. (70) recently reported that expression of $G\alpha_{12}$ is significantly up-regulated in the earliest stages of breast cancer by immunohistochemical detection, and that the inhibition of $G\alpha_{12}$ signaling reduces the metastatic dissemination of breast cancer cells in an animal model. $G\alpha_{12/13}$ acts through p115RhoGEF, a RGS protein with GAP activity for the $G\alpha_{12/13}$ subunits and guanine nucleotide exchange activity for the small G protein Rho (67). To explore the role of CaR-mediated signaling in breast cancer cells, we compared the levels of G protein ($G\alpha_i$, $G\alpha_q$ and $G\alpha_{12}$) and p115RhoGEF expression in two nonmalignant breast cell lines (Hs 578Bst and MCF-10A) and two breast cancer cell lines (MDA-MB-231, estrogen receptor/progesterone receptor negative and highly invasive, and MCF-7, estrogen receptor/progesterone receptor positive and weakly invasive), and found that the levels of $G\alpha_{12}$ and p115RhoGEF expression are dramatically up-regulated in two breast cancer cell lines (Fig. 1). Up-regulation of CaR, $G\alpha_{12}$ and p115RhoGEF expression in breast cancer cells indicates a potential signaling role in breast tumorigenesis and cancer progression.

3.2 CaR signaling in breast cancer cells

3.2.1 CaR signaling regulates the activation of choline kinase in breast cancer cells

Alteration in choline phospholipid metabolism as detected by nuclear magnetic resonance is a common feature of breast and many other cancer cells or tumors (71-76). Evidence from animal and cell studies as well as preclinical and clinical studies shows significant increases in phosphocholine (P-cho) levels in a range of human tumors (breast, colon, prostate, lung, neuroblastoma and lymphomas, etc) (77-82). Choline kinase (ChoK), the enzyme expressed in various tissues and that catalyzes the phosphorylation of choline to P-cho, is the first phosphorylation reaction in the CDP-choline pathway for the biosysthesis of phosphatidylcholine (83). Based on increased ChoK expression and activity in cancer cells and tumors, and increased ChoK activity in *ras* transformed cells (77-82, 84), ChoK has been proposed to play a role in the onset or progression of human cancer (breast, colon, prostate and lung, etc) and to be a target for developing anti-tumor drugs and an avenue for pharmaceutical therapy. Earlier studies also showed that various growth factors such as epidermal growth factor, fibroblast growth factor, platelet-derived growth factor, insulin-dependent growth factor and vascular endothelial growth factor enhance ChoK activity during tumor formation (85-87).

Because overexpression of the CaR-signaling components (Fig. 1 and refs 65, 66, 70) and increases of ChoK activity and P-cho production (72, 77-82) have consistently been observed in breast cancer cells and breast tumors, and metastasis of breast cancer cells to bone leads to the release of large quantities of Ca^{2+} (45, 46), it is possible that up-regulation of CaR signaling leads to a significantly altered choline phospholipid metabolism which regulates breast cancer cell proliferation. To evaluate the roles of Ca^{2+}- and CaR-regulated ChoK in breast cancer cells, we (65) recently prelabeled Hs 578Bst cells, MCF-10A cells, MDA-MB-231 cells and MCF-7 cells with [^{3}H]choline to study Ca^{2+}-induced ChoK activation and P-cho production, and found that Ca^{2+}-induced [^{3}H]P-cho production was significantly increased in breast cancer cells compared to the nonmalignant breast cells in time- or dose-dependent manners. Using an anti-CaR antibody to block Ca_o^{2+} binding to the CaR and siRNA to silence CaR gene expression, we further demonstrated that [^{3}H]P-cho production in response to Ca_o^{2+}-stimulation was CaR-dependent. By analyzing cellular lipid profiles and using siRNA to silence ChoK expression, we defined that the production of [^{3}H]P-cho was primarily related to CaR-induced ChoK activation. Treatment of the cells with either pertussis toxin or C_3 exoenzyme, and co-immunoprecipiation of $G\alpha_{12}$ with the CaR, we found that the enhancement of ChoK activation and P-cho production in breast cancer cells occurs via a CaR-$G\alpha_{12}$-Rho signaling pathway.

3.2.2 CaR signaling regulates breast cancer cell proliferation

Because the CaR stimulates ChoK activation in breast cancer cells, understanding ChoK activation and P-cho production in the regulation of cell proliferation is very important. Glunde et al. (81) recently knocked down ChoK expression by transfecting ChoK-specific siRNA and short hairpin RNA into breast cancer cells and found that down-regulation of ChoK expression reduced cell proliferation measured by proliferating cell nuclear antigen and Ki-67, and induced cell differentiation measured by cytosolic lipid droplet formation and expression of galectin-3. Shah et al. (82) showed that overexpression of ChoK in human breast cancer cells increases invasiveness and drug resistance. Overexpression of ChoK in HEK 293 cells leads to up-regulation of cyclin D1 and cyclin D3 expression and down-regulation of TGFβ receptor1, cyclin G2, cyclin-dependent kinase inhibitor 1A (p21, Cip1) and 1B (p27, Kip1) expression, which is involved in the regulation of TGFβ signaling (88). These data suggest that up- or down-regulation of ChoK expression and activity is associated with cell proliferation. Furthermore, the increase of cellular P-cho observed in cancer cells and tissues (71-79) indicates that P-cho produced by ChoK activation may play an important role in the regulation of cell function. Earlier studies in cell models showed direct evidence that treatment of fibroblasts with P-cho increases DNA synthesis and the effect is enhanced with other agonists such as ATP and insulin (89). Up-regulation of ChoK activation and P-cho production in human breast cancer cells and tumors indicates that CaR-ChoK signaling plays an important role in promoting breast cancer cell proliferation.

P-cho could stimulate breast cancer cell proliferation. Many recent studies show that several synthetic alkylphosphocholines (edelfosine, miltefosine and perifosine), P-cho analogs, have been developed as a new class of anti-cancer agents. These P-cho analogs act on cellular membranes rather than the DNA, and disturb signal transduction including the inhibition of phosphatidylcholine synthesis, the inhibition of the MAP-kinase/ERK proliferative and phosphatidylinositol 3-kinase/ Akt survival pathways, the stimulation of the Stress-activated protein kinase/JNK cell death pathway, and the inhibition of cell attachment, spreading, and migration (90-94). P-cho analogs as a class of anti-tumor drugs have been used more and more in clinical studies, but exploring the molecular mechanism of how they interact with cancer cells continues.

The CaR, through the $G\alpha_{12}$-p115RhoGEF-ChoK signaling pathway, connects to the synthesis of choline-containing phospholipids and the proliferation of breast cancer cells. Recently, studies also showed that the CaR plays a role in epidermal growth factor receptor (EGFR) transactivation to regulate cell proliferation. Using H-500 rat Leydig cancer cells as a model for humoral hypercalcemia of malignancy, Tfelt-Hansen et al. showed that treatment of H-500 cells with Ca_o^{2+} stimulates PTHrP release leading to CaR-induced activation of ERK1/2 and stimulation of cellular proliferation through the transactivation of the EGFR (95, 96). El Hiani et al. further reported that high Ca_o^{2+} induced CaR activation leads to breast cancer cell proliferation, and the inhibition of EGFR kinase reduced the activation of ERK1/2, and breast cancer cell proliferation (97). This cross-talk between the CaR and the EGFR in the regulation of cell proliferation was also found in Rat-1 fibroblasts (98). All these data indicate that the CaR can act through EGFR transactivation to regulate breast cancer cell proliferation.

Bone tissue is the most common organ targeted by breast cancer cells where metastasis can directly or indirectly stimulate osteoclast-mediated bone resorption. Tumor-induced osteolysis leads to the release of large quantities of calcium. The local Ca^{2+} level at resorption sites has been reported to rise as high as 40 mM (46). Hence, metastatic breast cancer cells could be faced with abnormally high Ca^{2+} concentrations. One recent report showed that the high Ca^{2+} concentrations through the CaR signaling pathway stimulate PTHrP expression and secretion in MCF-7 and MDA-MB-231 breast cancer cells (64). Tumor-cell derived PTHrP enhances bone remodeling and release of numerous biological factors, facilitates skeletal progression by directly stimulating tumor cell proliferation (99, 100), and promotes homotypic aggregation of breast cancer cells in suspension and three-dimensional cultures (101-103). This suggests that the Ca_o^{2+} and CaR in the bone environment can regulate a signaling network through different cell types to promote breast cancer cell proliferation.

3.2.3 CaR signaling regulates breast cancer cell migration

Elevated Ca_o^{2+} concentrations stimulate PTHrP secretion from various normal and malignant cells. PTHrP plays a central role in the development of breast cancer metastases to bone, and skeletal metastases of breast cancers express more PTHrP and maintains at the levels higher than those in normal breast epithelial cells, primary breast cancers, or nonskeletal metastases (42). By transfection of vector, mutated and wild-type PTHrP into breast cancer cells (MCF-7), the study showed that wild-type PTHrP-overexpressing cells increased cell laminin, adhesion, migration, and Matrigel invasion. Overexpression of wild-type PTHrP also increased the cell surface expression of the pro-invasive integrins $\alpha6$ and $\beta4$ (104). Using Boyden Chamber and Scratch Wound migration assays, Saidak et al. (105) showed direct evidence that Ca_o^{2+} at concentrations of 2.5 mM and 5 mM induces cell migration compared to basal levels for several breast cancer cell lines. The highly bone metastatic breast cancer cells strongly respond to elevated concentrations of Ca_o^{2+} in the migration assays. Knockdown of the CaR by siRNA resulted in an inhibition of Ca_o^{2+}-induced migration, indicating the involvement of this receptor in the effect. All these data indicate that Ca_o^{2+} acts through the CaR to promote breast cancer cell migration.

Cell migration is required for cancer cells to spread, invasion and metastasis, and metastasis of cancer cells is significantly associated with increased mortality and reduced treatment effectiveness. Cell migration is achieved through dynamic remodeling of filamentous actin and of focal adhesion sites. Tu et al. (106) demonstrated the involvement of the CaR in the activation of E-cadherin signaling. Using human epidermal keratinocytes as a cell model, silencing CaR expression blocks the Ca_o^{2+}-induced formation of adherens junctions, and the association of phosphoinositide 3-kinase (PI3K) with the E-cadherin-catenin complex. Ca_o^{2+} does not stimulate tyrosine phosphorylation of β-, γ-, and p120-catenin and Fyn in the CaR-deficient keratinocytes. Further studies find that Rho GTPase is a part of the CaR-mediated signaling cascade regulating cell adhesion. Ca_o^{2+}-induced Rho activation requires a direct interaction between CaR and filamin A (107). The CaR regulated E-cadherin cell membrane localization and complex formation of E-cadherin and β-catenin was also reported in human colon carcinoma cells (108). CaR-specific siRNA and the CaR antagonist (NPS2390) can partially inhibit wound repair of human bronchial epithelial cells, and these signaling pathway(s) are associated with phospholipase C which can be blocked by U73122 and ERK1/2 which can be inhibited by PD 98059 (109). Ca_o^{2+} acts through the CaR to stimulate migration of osteoclast precursor RAW 264.7cells via the PI3K/Akt pathway but not the MAPK (ERK, p38 and JNK) pathways (110). In Boyden Chamber and Scratch Wound migration assays, Saidak et al. reported that inhibition of either ERK1/2 by U0126 or phospholipase Cβ by U73122 led to an abolition of the Ca_o^{2+}-induced migration of breast cancer cells (105). These data suggest that the CaR can regulate cell migration, however, the details of the CaR-induced breast cancer cell migration remain largely unknown.

4. Future perspective

Cloning of the CaR has provided a molecular tool to study the receptor-mediated signaling and -associated human diseases including breast cancer. Until now, most of the studies have focused on how the CaR is associated with the characteristic abnormalities in the functions of the parathyroids and kidneys, and which signaling pathways of the CaR are involved in the regulation of cell functions (Fig. 2) by CaR overexpression and RNA interference. Much remains to be learned, such as CaR expression in other tissues, including tumor tissues and the pathways that are regulated in the tissues by identifying single-nucleotide polymorphisms (SNP) in the CaR, determining whether gain or loss of function SNPs in the CaR lead to tumorigenesis and cancer progression, and by analyzing the role of CaR-mediated signaling in CaR-associated tumorigenesis and progression to develop potent and specific CaR antagonists that would be extremely useful in cancer therapy. In addition, the CaR and perhaps other sensors for calcium or other agonists for the CaR, and transactivation of other receptors such as EGF receptor by the CaR in the cells will likely regulate a wide variety of cellular functions via different signaling pathways. Therefore, understanding system biology and signalling networks controlled by CaR-signaling is important for the potential cancer therapy.

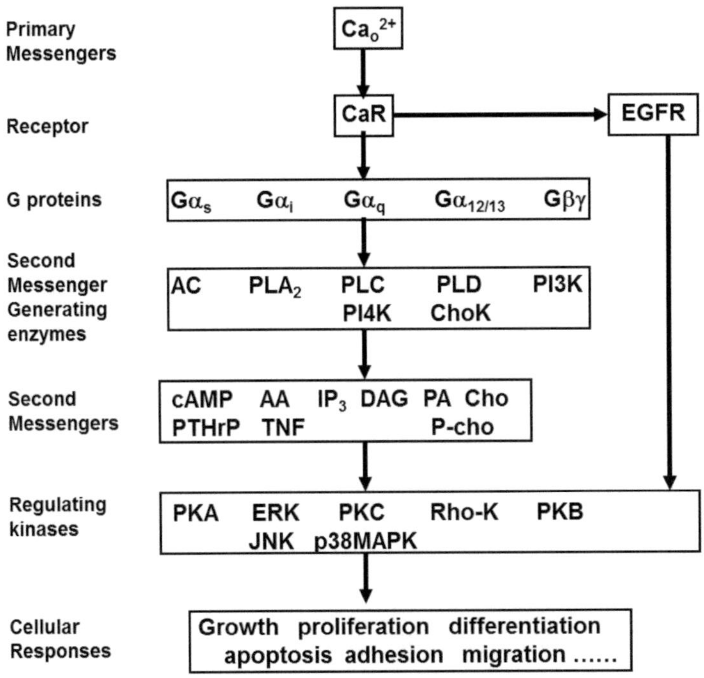

Fig. 2. **A schematic diagram of CaR-mediated signaling pathways.** Many of these signaling pathways were identified in different cell lines and heterologous expression systems, and may not all exist in breast cancer cells. CaR, Ca^{2+}-sensing receptor; EGFR, epidermal growth factor receptor; AC, adenyl cyclase; ChoK, choline kinase; PLC, phospholipase C; PLA_2, phospholipase A_2; PLD, phospholipase D; PI3K, phosphatidylinositol-3 kinase; PI4K, phosphatidylinositol-4-kinase; PKA, protein kinase A; PKB, protein kinase B; PKC, protein kinase C; Rho-K, Rho kinases; p38MAPK, p38 mitogen-activated protein kinases; JNK, c-Jun N-terminal kinases; ERK, extracellular-signal-regulated kinases.

5. References

[1] Jemal A, Siegel R, Ward E, Hao Y-p, Xu J-q, Murray T, Thun MJ. Cancer statistics, 2008. CA Cancer J Clin. 2009;58:71–96.

[2] Jemal A, Center MM, DeSantis C, Ward EM. Global patterns of cancer incidence and mortality rates and trends. Cancer Epidemiol Biomarkers Prev. 2010;19:1893-907.

[3] Clapham D. Calcium signaling. Cell. 2007;131:1047–58.

[4] Whitfield JF. Calcium, calcium-sensing receptor and colon cancer. Cancer Lett. 2009;275:9-16.

[5] Peterlik M, Grant WB, Cross HS. Calcium, vitamin D and cancer. Anticancer Res. 2009;29:3687-98.

[6] VanHouten JN. Calcium sensing by the mammary gland. J Mammary Gland Biol Neoplasia. 2005;10:129-39.

[7] Abrams SA. Calcium turnover and nutrition through the life cycle. Proc Nutr Soc. 2001;60:283-9.

[8] Rizzuto R, Pozzan T. Microdomains of intracellular Ca2+: molecular determinants and functional consequences. Physiol Rev. 2006;86:369-408.

[9] Saidak Z, Mentaverri R, Brown EM. The role of the calcium-sensing receptor in the development and progression of cancer. Endocrinol Rev 2009;30:178–95.

[10] Block GJ, DiMattia GD, Prockop DJ. Stanniocalcin-1 regulates extracellular ATP-induced calcium waves in human epithelial cancer cells by stimulating ATP release from bystander cells. PLoS ONE 2010;5:e10237.

[11] West AE, Chen WG, Dalva MB, Dolmetsch RE, Kornhauser JM, Shaywitz AJ, Takasu MA, Tao X, Greenberg ME. Calcium regulation of neuronal gene expression. Proc Natl Acad Sci U S A. 2001;98:11024-31.

[12] Parkash J, Asotra K. Calcium wave signaling in cancer cells. Life Sci. 2010;87:587-95.

[13] Contreras L, Drago I, Zampese E, Pozzan T. Mitochondria: the calcium connection. Biochim Biophys Acta. 2010;1797:607-18.

[14] Munaron L, Fiorio PA. Endothelial calcium machinery and angiogenesis: understanding physiology to interfere with pathology. Curr Med Chem 2009;16:4691–703.

[15] Butler LM, Wong AS, Koh WP, Wang R, Yuan JM, Yu MC. Calcium intake increases risk of prostate cancer among Singapore Chinese. Cancer Res. 2010;70:4941-8.

[16] Newmark HL, Heaney RP. Dairy products and prostate cancer risk. Nutr Cancer. 2010;62:297-9.

[17] Mahabir S, Forman MR, Dong YQ, Park Y, Hollenbeck A, Schatzkin A. Mineral intake and lung cancer risk in the NIH-American Association of Retired Persons Diet and Health study. Cancer Epidemiol Biomarkers Prev. 2010;19:1976-83.

[18] Toriola AT, Surcel HM, Calypse A, Grankvist K, Luostarinen T, Lukanova A, Pukkala E, Lehtinen M. Independent and joint effects of serum 25-hydroxyvitamin D and calcium on ovarian cancer risk: a prospective nested case-control study. Eur J Cancer. 2010;46:2799-805.

[19] Huncharek M, Muscat J, Kupelnick B. Colorectal cancer risk and dietary intake of calcium, vitamin D, and dairy products: a meta-analysis of 26,335 cases from 60 observational studies. Nutr Cancer. 2009;61:47-69.

[20] Zhang CX, Ho SC, Fu JH, Cheng SZ, Chen YM, Lin FY. Dairy products, calcium intake, and breast cancer risk: a case-control study in china. Nutr Cancer. 2011;63:12-20.

[21] Chen P, Hu P, Xie D, Qin Y, Wang F, Wang H. Meta-analysis of vitamin D, calcium and the prevention of breast cancer. Breast Cancer Res Treat. 2010;121:469-77.

[22] Hjartåker A, Thoresen M, Engeset D, Lund E. Dairy consumption and calcium intake and risk of breast cancer in a prospective cohort: the Norwegian Women and Cancer study. Cancer Causes Control. 2010;21:1875-85.

[23] Anderson LN, Cotterchio M, Vieth R, Knight JA. Vitamin D and calcium intakes and breast cancer risk in pre- and postmenopausal women. Am J Clin Nutr. 2010;91:1699-707.

[24] Abbas S, Linseisen J, Chang-Claude J. Dietary vitamin D and calcium intake and premenopausal breast cancer risk in a German case-control study. Nutr Cancer. 2007;59:54-61

[25] Larsson SC, Bergkvist L, Wolk A. Long-term dietary calcium intake and breast cancer risk in a prospective cohort of women. Am J Clin Nutr. 2009;89:277-82.

[26] Chlebowski RT, Johnson KC, Kooperberg C, Pettinger M, Wactawski-Wende J, Rohan T, Rossouw J, Lane D, O'Sullivan MJ, Yasmeen S, Hiatt RA, Shikany JM, Vitolins M, Khandekar J, Hubbell FA; Women's Health Initiative Investigators. Calcium plus vitamin D supplementation and the risk of breast cancer. J Natl Cancer Inst. 2008;100:1581-91.

[27] Rohan TE, Negassa A, Chlebowski RT, Ceria-Ulep CD, Cochrane BB, Lane DS, Ginsberg M, Wassertheil-Smoller S, Page DL. A randomized controlled trial of calcium plus vitamin D supplementation and risk of benign proliferative breast disease. Breast Cancer Res Treat. 2009;116:339-50.

[28] Lin J, Manson JE, Lee IM, Cook NR, Buring JE, Zhang SM. Intakes of calcium and vitamin D and breast cancer risk in women. Arch Intern Med. 2007;167:1050-9.

[29] Cui Y, Rohan TE. Vitamin D, calcium, and breast cancer risk: a review. Cancer Epidemiol Biomarkers Prev. 2006;15:1427-37.

[30] McCullough ML, Rodriguez C, Diver WR, Feigelson HS, Stevens VL, Thun MJ, Calle EE. Dairy, calcium, and vitamin D intake and postmenopausal breast cancer risk in the Cancer Prevention Study II Nutrition Cohort. Cancer Epidemiol Biomarkers Prev. 2005;14:2898-904.

[31] Kawase T, Matsuo K, Suzuki T, Hirose K, Hosono S, Watanabe M, Inagaki M, Iwata H, Tanaka H, Tajima K. Association between vitamin D and calcium intake and breast cancer risk according to menopausal status and receptor status in Japan. Cancer Sci. 2010;101:1234-40.

[32] Kesse-Guyot E, Bertrais S, Duperray B, Arnault N, Bar-Hen A, Galan P, Hercberg S. Dairy products, calcium and the risk of breast cancer: results of the French SU.VI.MAX prospective study. Ann Nutr Metab. 2007;51:139-45.

[33] Almquist M, Manjer J, Bondeson L, Bondeson AG. Serum calcium and breast cancer risk: results from a prospective cohort study of 7,847 women. Cancer Causes Control. 2007;18:595-602.

[34] Almquist M, Anagnostaki L, Bondeson L, Bondeson AG, Borgquist S, Landberg G, Malina J, Malm J, Manjer J. Serum calcium and tumour aggressiveness in breast cancer: a prospective study of 7847 women. Eur J Cancer Prev. 2009;18:354-60.
[35] Almquist M, Bondeson AG, Bondeson L, Malm J, Manjer J. Serum levels of vitamin D, PTH and calcium and breast cancer risk-a prospective nested case-control study. Int J Cancer. 2010;127:2159-68.
[36] Martin E, Miller M, Krebsbach L, Beal JR, Schwartz GG, Sahmoun AE. Serum calcium levels are elevated among women with untreated postmenopausal breast cancer. Cancer Causes Control. 2010;21:251-7.
[37] Sprague BL, Skinner HG, Trentham-Dietz A, Lee KE, Klein BE, Klein R. Serum calcium and breast cancer risk in a prospective cohort study. Ann Epidemiol. 2010;20:82-5.
[38] Santarpia L, Koch CA, Sarlis NJ. Hypercalcemia in cancer patients: pathobiology and management. Horm Metab Res. 2010;42:153-64.
[39] DeMauro S, Wysolmerski J. Hypercalcemia in breast cancer: an echo of bone mobilization during lactation? J Mammary Gland Biol Neoplasia. 2005;10:157-67.
[40] Stewart AF. Clinical practice. Hypercalcemia associated with cancer. N Engl J Med. 2005;352:373-9.
[41] Hickey RC, Samaan NA, Jackson GL. Hypercalcemia in patients with breast cancer. Osseous metastases, hyperplastic parathyroid tissue, or pseudohyperparathyroidism? Arch Surg 1981;116:545–52.
[42] Guise TA. Molecular mechanisms of osteolytic bone metastases. Cancer. 2000;88:2892-8.
[43] Kingsley LA, Fournier PG, Chirgwin JM, Guise TA. Molecular biology of bone metastasis. Mol Cancer Ther. 2007;6:2609-17.
[44] Guise TA, Kozlow WM, Heras-Herzig A, Padalecki SS, Yin JJ, Chirgwin JM. Molecular mechanisms of breast cancer metastases to bone. Clin Breast Cancer. 2005;5:S46-53.
[45] Montcourrier P, Silver I, Farnoud R, Bird I, Rochefort H. Breast cancer cells have a high capacity to acidify extracellular milieu by a dual mechanism. Clin Exp Metastasis. 1997;15:382-92.
[46] Silver IA, Murrills RJ, Etherington DJ. Microelectrode studies on the acid microenvironment beneath adherent macrophages and osteoclasts. Exp Cell Res. 1988;175:266-76.
[47] Hynes NE, Watson CJ. Mammary gland growth factors: roles in normal development and in cancer. Cold Spring Harb Perspect Biol. 2010;2:a003186.
[48] Akhtari M, Mansuri J, Newman KA, GuiseTM, Seth P. Biology of breast cancer bone metastasis. Cancer Biol Ther. 2008;7:3-9.
[49] Käkönen SM, Mundy GR. Mechanisms of osteolytic bone metastases in breast carcinoma. Cancer. 2003;97:834-9
[50] Gohji K, Kitazawa S, Tamada H, Katsuoka Y et al. Expression of endothelin receptor a associated with prostate cancer progression. J Urol. 2001;165:1033–6.
[51] Kawada K, Hosogi H, Sonoshita M, et al. Chemokine receptor CXCR3 promotes colon cancer metastasis to lymph nodes. Oncogene. 2007;26:4679-88.

[52] Xie Y, Gibbs TC, Mukhin YV, et al. Role for 18:1 lysophosphatidic acid as an autocrine mediator in prostate cancer cells. J Biol Chem. 2002;277:32516-26.

[53] Li S, Huang S, Peng SB. Overexpression of G protein-coupled receptors in cancer cells: involvement in tumor progression. Int J Oncol. 2005;27:1329-39.

[54] Taub JS, Guo R, Leeb-Lundberg LM, et al. Bradykinin receptor subtype 1 expression and function in prostate cancer. Cancer Res. 2003;63:2037–2041.

[55] Chay CH, Cooper CR, Gendernalik JD, et al. A functional thrombin receptor (PAR1) is expressed on bone-derived prostate cancer cell lines. Urology. 2002;60:760-5.

[56] Davies JQ, Lin HH, Stacey M, Yona S, Chang GW, Gordon S, Hamann J, Campo L, Han C, Chan P, Fox SB. Leukocyte adhesion-GPCR EMR2 is aberrantly expressed in human breast carcinomas and is associated with patient survival. Oncol Rep. 2011;25:619-27.

[57] Carmeci C, Thompson DA, Ring HZ, Francke U, Weigel RJ. Identification of a gene (GPR30) with homology to the G-protein-coupled receptor superfamily associated with estrogen receptor expression in breast cancer. Genomics. 1997;45:607-17.

[58] Hofer AM, Brown EM. Extracellular Ca2+ sensing and signalling. Nat Rev Mol Cell Biol. 2003;4:530-8.

[59] Riccardi D, Finney BA, Wilkinson WJ, Kemp PJ. Novel regulatory aspects of the extracellular Ca2+-sensing receptor, CaR. Pflugers Arch. 2009;458:1007-22.

[60] Buraei Z, Yang J. The ß subunit of voltage-gated Ca2+ channels. Physiol Rev. 2010;90:1461-506.

[61] VanHouten J, Dann P, McGeoch G, Brown EM, Krapcho K, Neville M, Wysolmerski JJ. The calcium-sensing receptor regulates mammary gland parathyroid hormone-related protein production and calcium transport. J Clin Invest. 2004;113:598–608.

[62] Kovacs CS. Calcium and bone metabolism in pregnancy and lactation. J Clin Endocrinol Metab 2001;86:2344–8.

[63] Kalkwarf HJ, Specker BL. Bone mineral changes during pregnancy and lactation. Endocrine. 2002;17:49–53.

[64] Sanders JL, Chattopadhyay N, Kifor O, Yamaguchi T, Butters RR, Brown EM. Extracellular calcium-sensing receptor expression and its potential role in regulating parathyroid hormone-related peptide secretion in human breast cancer cell lines. Endocrinology. 2000;141:4357-64.

[65] Huang C, Hydo LM, Liu S, Miller RT. Activation of choline kinase by extracellular Ca2+ is Ca2+-sensing receptor, G□12 and Rho-dependent in breast cancer cells. Cell Signal. 2009;21:1894-900.

[66] Mihai R, Stevens J, McKinney C, Ibrahim NB. Expression of the calcium receptor in human breast cancer--a potential new marker predicting the risk of bone metastases. Eur J Surg Oncol. 2006;32:511-5.

[67] Ross EM, Wilkie TM. GTPase-activating proteins for heterotrimeric G proteins: regulators of G protein signaling (RGS) and RGS-like proteins. Annu Rev Biochem. 2000;69:795–827.

[68] Huang C, Hujer KM, Wu Z, Miller RT. The Ca2-+-sensing receptor couples to G□12/13 to activate phospholipase D in Madin-Darby canine kidney cells. Am J Physiol. 2004;286:C22-30.

[69] Mamillapalli R, Wysolmerski J. The calcium-sensing receptor couples to Galpha(s) and regulates PTHrP and ACTH secretion in pituitary cells. J Endocrinol. 2010;204:287-97.

[70] Kelly P, Moeller BJ, Juneja J, Booden MA, Der CJ, Daaka Y, Dewhirst MW, Fields TA, Casey PJ. The G12 family of heterotrimeric G proteins promotes breast cancer invasion and metastasis. Proc Natl Acad Sci U S A. 2006;103:8173-8.

[71] Glunde K, Ackerstaff E, Mori N, Jacobs MA, Bhujwalla ZM. Choline phospholipid metabolism in cancer: consequences for molecular pharmaceutical interventions. Mol Pharm. 2006;3:496-506.

[72] Aboagye EO, Bhujwalla ZM. Malignant transformation alters membrane choline phospholipid metabolism of human mammary epithelial cells. Cancer Res. 1999;59:80-84.

[73] Glunde K, Jie C, Bhujwalla ZM. Molecular causes of the aberrant choline phospholipid metabolism in breast cancer. Cancer Res. 2004;64:4270-6.

[74] Iorio E, Mezzanzanica D, Alberti P, Spadaro F, Ramoni C, D'Ascenzo S, Millimaggi D, Pavan A, Dolo V, Canevari S and Podo F. Alterations of choline phospholipid metabolism in ovarian tumor progression. Cancer Res. 2005;65:9369-76.

[75] Daly PF, Lyon RC, Faustino PJ, Cohen JS. Phospholipid metabolism in cancer cells monitored by 31P NMR spectroscopy. J Biol Chem. 1987;262:14875-8.

[76] Ackerstaff E, Pflug BR, Nelson JB, Bhujwalla ZM. Detection of increased choline compounds with proton nuclear magnetic resonance spectroscopy subsequent to malignant transformation of human prostatic epithelial cells. Cancer Res. 2001;61:3599-603.

[77] Ramírez de Molina A, Gutiérrez R, Ramos MA, Silva JM, Silva J, Bonilla F, Sánchez JJ, Lacal JC. Increased choline kinase activity in human breast carcinomas: clinical evidence for a potential novel antitumor strategy. Oncogene. 2002;21:4317-22.

[78] Eliyahu G, Kreizman T, Degani H. Phosphocholine as a biomarker of breast cancer: molecular and biochemical studies. Int J Cancer. 2007;120:1721-30

[79] Ramírez de Molina A, Báñez-Coronel M, Gutiérrez R, Rodríguez-González A, Olmeda D, Megías D, Lacal JC. Choline kinase activation is a critical requirement for the proliferation of primary human mammary epithelial cells and breast tumor progression. Cancer Res. 2004;64:6732-9.

[80] Janardhan S, Srivani P, Sastry GN. Choline kinase: an important target for cancer. Curr Med Chem. 2006;13:1169-86

[81] Glunde K, Raman V, Mori N, Bhujwalla ZM. RNA interference-mediated choline kinase suppression in breast cancer cells induces differentiation and reduces proliferation. Cancer Res 2005;65:11034-43.

[82] Shah T, Wildes F, Penet MF, Winnard PT Jr, Glunde K, Artemov D, Ackerstaff E, Gimi B, Kakkad S, Raman V, Bhujwalla ZM. Choline kinase overexpression increases invasiveness and drug resistance of human breast cancer cells. NMR Biomed. 2010;23:633-42.

[83] Vance DE. In Vance DE and Vance JE Editors: Biochemistry of Lipids, Lipoproteins and Membranes. 4th Edition. Netherland: Elsevier Science B.V. 2002;pp205-232.
[84] Ramírez de Molina A, Penalva V, Lucas L, Lacal JC. Regulation of choline kinase activity by Ras proteins involves Ral-GDS and PI3K. Oncogene. 2002;21:937-46.
[85] Uchida T. Stimulation of phospholipid synthesis in HeLa cells by epidermal growth factor and insulin: activation of choline kinase and glycerophosphate acyltransferase. Biochim Biophys Acta. 1996;1304:89-104.
[86] Cuadrado A, Carnero A, Dolfi F, Jiménez B, Lacal JC. Phosphorylcholine: a novel second messenger essential for mitogenic activity of growth factors. Oncogene. 1993;8:2959-68.
[87] Chung T, Huang JS, Mukherjee JJ, Crilly KS, Kiss Z. Expression of human choline kinase in NIH 3T3 fibroblasts increases the mitogenic potential of insulin and insulin-like growth factor I. Cell Signal. 2000;12:279-88.
[88] Ramírez de Molina A, Gallego-Ortega D, Sarmentero-Estrada J, Lagares D, Gómez Del Pulgar T, Bandrés E, García-Foncillas J, Lacal JC. Choline kinase as a link connecting phospholipid metabolism and cell cycle regulation: implications in cancer therapy. Int J Biochem Cell Biol. 2008 ;40:1753-63.
[89] Chung T, Crilly KS, Anderson WH, Mukherjee JJ, Kiss Z. ATP-dependent choline phosphate-induced mitogenesis in fibroblasts involves activation of pp70 S6 kinase and phosphatidylinositol 3'-kinase through an extracellular site. Synergistic mitogenic effects of choline phosphate and sphingosine 1-phosphate. J Biol Chem. 1997;272:3064-72.
[90] Vink SR, van Blitterswijk WJ, Schellens JH, Verheij M. Rationale and clinical application of alkylphospholipid analogues in combination with radiotherapy. Cancer Treat Rev. 2007;33:191-202.
[91] Gills JJ, Dennis PA. Perifosine: update on a novel Akt inhibitor. Curr Oncol Rep. 2009;11:102-10.
[92] Martelli AM, Papa V, Tazzari PL, Ricci F, Evangelisti C, Chiarini F, Grimaldi C, Cappellini A, Martinelli G, Ottaviani E, Pagliaro P, Horn S, Bäsecke J, Lindner LH, Eibl H, McCubrey JA. Erucylphosphohomocholine, the first intravenously applicable alkylphosphocholine, is cytotoxic to acute myelogenous leukemia cells through JNK- and PP2A-dependent mechanisms. Leukemia. 2010;24:687-98.
[93] Königs SK, Pallasch CP, Lindner LH, Schwamb J, Schulz A, Brinker R, Claasen J, Veldurthy A, Eibl H, Hallek M, Wendtner CM. Erufosine, a novel alkylphosphocholine, induces apoptosis in CLL through a caspase-dependent pathway. Leuk Res. 2010;34:1064-9.
[94] Chakrabandhu K, Huault S, Hueber AO. Distinctive molecular signaling in triple-negative breast cancer cell death triggered by hexadecylphosphocholine (miltefosine). FEBS Lett. 2008;582:4176-84.
[95] Tfelt-Hansen J, Chattopadhyay N, Yano S, Kanuparthi D, Rooney P, Schwarz P, Brown EM. Calcium-sensing receptor induces proliferation through p38 mitogen-activated protein kinase and phosphatidylinositol 3-kinase but not extracellularly regulated kinase in a model of humoral hypercalcemia of malignancy. Endocrinology. 2004;145:1211-7.

[96] Yano S, Macleod RJ, Chattopadhyay N, Tfelt-Hansen J, Kifor O, Butters RR, Brown EM. Calcium-sensing receptor activation stimulates parathyroid hormone-related protein secretion in prostate cancer cells: role of epidermal growth factor receptor transactivation. Bone. 2004;35:664-72.

[97] El Hiani Y, Lehen'kyi V, Ouadid-Ahidouch H, Ahidouch A. Activation of the calcium-sensing receptor by high calcium induced breast cancer cell proliferation and TRPC1 cation channel over-expression potentially through EGFR pathways. Arch Biochem Biophys. 2009;486:58-63.

[98] Tomlins SA, Bolllinger N, Creim J, Rodland KD. Cross-talk between the calcium-sensing receptor and the epidermal growth factor receptor in Rat-1 fibroblasts. Exp Cell Res. 2005;308:439-45.

[99] Hoey RP, Sanderson C, Iddon J, Brady G, Bundred NJ, Anderson NG. The parathyroid hormone-related protein receptor is expressed in breast cancer bone metastases and promotes autocrine proliferation in breast carcinoma cells. Br J Cancer. 2003;88:567–73.

[100] Cataisson C, Lieberherr M, Cros M, Gauville C, Graulet AM, Cotton J, Calvo F, de Vernejoul MC, Foley J, Bouizar Z. Parathyroid hormone-related peptide stimulates proliferation of highly tumorigenic human SV40-immortalized breast epithelial cells. J Bone Miner Res. 2000;15:2129–39.

[101] Shen X, Falzon M. PTH-related protein modulates PC-3 prostate cancer cell adhesion and integrin subunit profile. Mol Cell Endocrinol. 2003;199:165–77.

[102] Ahlstrom M, Pekkinen M, Riehle U, Lamberg-Allardt C. Extracellular calcium regulates parathyroid hormone-related peptide expression in osteoblasts and osteoblast progenitor cells. Bone. 2008;42:483-90.

[103] Dittmer A, Schunke D, Dittmer J. PTHrP promotes homotypic aggregation of breast cancer cells in three-dimensional cultures. Cancer Lett. 2008;260:56-61.

[104] Shen X, Qian L, Falzon M. PTH-related protein enhances MCF-7 breast cancer cell adhesion, migration, and invasion via an intracrine pathway. Exp Cell Res. 2004;294:420-33.

[105] Saidak Z, Boudot C, Abdoune R, Petit L, Brazier M, Mentaverri R, Kamel S. Extracellular calcium promotes the migration of breast cancer cells through the activation of the calcium sensing receptor. Exp Cell Res. 2009;315:2072-80.

[106] Tu CL, Chang W, Xie Z, Bikle DD. Inactivation of the calcium sensing receptor inhibits E-cadherin-mediated cell-cell adhesion and calcium-induced differentiation in human epidermal keratinocytes. J Biol Chem. 2008;283:3519-28.

[107] Tu CL, Chang W, Bikle DD. The Calcium-Sensing Receptor-Dependent Regulation of Cell-Cell Adhesion and Keratinocyte Differentiation Requires Rho and Filamin A. J Invest Dermatol. 2011 PMID:21209619

[108] Wang X, Chen W, Singh N, Promkan M, Liu G. Effects of potential calcium sensing receptor inducers on promoting chemosensitivity of human colon carcinoma cells. Int J Oncol. 2010;36:1573-80.

[109] Milara J, Mata M, Serrano A, Peiró T, Morcillo EJ, Cortijo J. Extracellular calcium-sensing receptor mediates human bronchial epithelial wound repair. Biochem Pharmacol. 2010;80:236-46.

[110] Boudot C, Saidak Z, Boulanouar AK, Petit L, Gouilleux F, Massy Z, Brazier M, Mentaverri R, Kamel S. Implication of the calcium sensing receptor and the Phosphoinositide 3-kinase/Akt pathway in the extracellular calcium-mediated migration of RAW 264.7 osteoclast precursor cells. Bone. 2010;46:1416-23.

33

Signal Transduction Pathways Mediated by Unsaturated Free Fatty Acids in Breast Cancer Cells

Eduardo Perez Salazar, Luis Castro-Sanchez and Pedro Cortes-Reynosa
Cell Biology Department, Cinvestav-IPN, Mexico City, Mexico

1. Introduction

Breast cancer is the most common cancer of women, and its incidence is especially rising in developing countries and representing 23% of all female cancers around the world. The geographical variation at incidence is highest in the developed world and lowest in the developing countries. However, the breast cancer incidence has shown an alarming increasing trend in recent years. It is estimated that more than one million women are diagnosed with mammary cancer every year, and more than 400,000 will die worldwide from this disease and 55% related deaths, occur in low and middle income countries. Therefore, it is estimated that 1.7 million women will be diagnosed with this malignant disease in 2020 (Curado et al., 2009; El Saghir et al., 2007; Porter, 2008).

The normal mammary contains lobules and ducts that consist of a bi-layered luminal epithelium associated with myoepithelial cells and surrounded by the basement membrane (BM) that separates the epithelium from the stroma. Breast cancer is a genetically and genomically heterogeneous disease that initiates in a premalignant lesion, denominated atypical ductal hyperplasia (ADH), characterized by abnormal growth of cell layers within the duct or lobule. ADH is thought to be precursor of ductal carcinoma in situ (DCIS), which is a non-invasive lesion that contains abnormal cells (Hansen and Bissell, 2000). The transformation of mammary epithelial cells is an accumulation of epigenetic and genetic alterations with changes in the interactions within the microenvironment to give rise to metastatic breast cancer. During these multisteps, the control of different cellular process become deregulated, such as proliferation, survival, differentiation and migration and aberrant tumour-stromal cell interactions facilitate this process by initiating a desmoplastic response with significant matrix remodeling and progressive stiffening of the stroma (Paszek and Weaver, 2004; Van't Veer and Weigelt, 2003; Weigelt et al., 2005; Nguyen and Massague, 2007). In the metastasis, cells detach from the primary tumour and must invade through BM, enter the vasculature (intravasate), survive in lymphatic o circulatory system, exit into vasculature (extravasate) and establish a new tumor in a foreign microenvironment. Some of the components that are required for the malignant process are well established, as well as the breast cancer higher risk-markers in the women. However, there are differences in the risk to acquire breast cancer, between premenopausal and postmenopausal women. Early age at the onset of menarche, late age at first childbirth, the nulliparity and shorter duration of lactation are markers of increased risk in the etiology of premenopausal breast cancer. These factors are not associated with breast cancer in postmenopausal women (McPherson et al., 2000; Chambers et al., 2002; McGee et al., 2006; Gout and Huot, 2008). Nevertheless, the dietary factors associated with higher intake of fat and abdominal fat accumulation increase the risk of breast cancer in postmenopausal women and leads to increased synthesis of estrogen, higher levels of estrogens and free fatty acids (FFAs) in blood (Boyd et al., 2003: Hankinson et al., 1998). The aim of the chapter is describe the signal transduction pathways mediated by three unsaturated free fatty acids (oleic, arachidonic and linoleic acid) and their role in cellular processes that participate in proliferation and invasion.

2. Free fatty acids and breast cancer

Breast cancer is the most frequently diagnosed malignant neoplasia worldwide and is a health problem in women of developed and emergent countries, where lately has been observed an increase in frequency and mortality. Particularly, breast cancer incidence in western women is approximately five times greater than that in Asian women, however when low-risk ethnic groups migrate to the west, their incidence of postmenopausal breast cancer rises progressively in successive generations, suggesting that environmental or lifestyle factors rather than genetic factors are important (Sakamoto and Sugano, 1991; Ferlay et al., 2007).

Diet has been prominent among the potential environmental factors, because numerous studies in women using different study designs and different geographical areas have been carried out to establish the relationship between diet and breast cancer. The results have shown that obesity and certain dietary factor such as a higher intake of fatty acids (FAs) and meats seem to increase the risk of breast cancer (Boyd et al., 2003; Lahmann et al., 2004; Carmichael, 2006). Actually, it is clear that a combination of high total energy intake and inadequate physical exercise allows genetically susceptible individuals to become obese, while the increased metabolic activity in their enlarged adipose deposits releases an excess of compounds, including FFAs (Proietto et al., 1999).

The unsatured FAs are divided in monounsatured (MUFA) and polyunsaturated (PUFA). The principal sources of MUFAs are vegetable oils and meat, while PUFAs are mostly found in eggs, fish and seafoods. PUFAs are classified into two families -n-3 and n-6 PUFAs, the n-3 include eicosapentaenoic acid (EPA), docosahexaenoic acid (DHA), α-linoleic acid (ALA) and steridonic acid (SA), while n-6 including linoleic acid (LA), arachidonic acid (AA), docosapentaenoic acid (DPA) and γ-linoleic acid (GLA). It has been suggested that these exogenous FAs may participate in the etiology, evolution and/or progression of breast cancer, whereas epidemiological studies demonstrated that both the amount of fat and the type of FA present in the diet affect the tumorigenesis, cancer growth and metastasis process (Goodstine et al., 2003; Bartsch et al., 1999; Welsch, 1992).

Oleic acid (OA) is the most abundant dietary MUFA, and it has an inverse relationship with breast cancer (Franceschi et al., 1996; London et al., 1993; Voorrips et al., 2002; Wirfalt et al., 2002; Gaard et al., 1995). In addition, epidemiological studies show that olive oil, with high content of OA, presents preventive properties to the acquisition of breast cancer (Trichopoulou et al., 1995; Owen et al., 2000; Wahrburg and Assmann, 2001). In contrast, some studies show a positive correlation between MUFA and breast cancer (London et al., 1993; Wirfalt et al., 2002; Gaard et al., 1995).

The PUFAs ALA, EPA and DHA function as inhibitors of the progression of human breast cancer, whereas n-6 PUFA, LA is a stimulator of this disease (Rose et al., 1994; Rose et al.,

1995; Rose et al., 1997; Menendez et al., 2006). The n-3 PUFAs mechanism by which may low the breast cancer risk is through an inhibition on biosynthesis of AA-derived eicosanoids, which are linked to inflammation and carcinogesis processes. The PUFAs n-3 are incorporated into membrane phospholipids, where they partially replace the AA, and it suppresses the biosynthesis of AA-derived eicosanoids, and stimulates the EPA-derived 3-series prostanoids and 5-series leukotrienes synthesis (Crawford et al., 2000).

Her-2/*neu* overexpression induces aggressive breast carcinoma and low sensibility to chemotherapy and anti-estrogens therapy (Crawford et al., 2000 Hudelist et al., 2003;). ALA, EPA, DHA, GLA and OA are dietary fatty acids with a protector effect to the breast cancer adquisition, the mechanism involved is the downregulation of Her-2/*neu* in SK-Br3 and BT-474 human breast cancer cell lines. In contrast, LA induces tumorigenesis by an increase on Her-2/*neu* (Menendez et al., 2006). In addition, stearic acid a satured FA in the western diet has been found to have "anti-cancer properties" both *in vivo* and *in vivo* (Wickramasinghe et al., 1996; Hardy et al., 2003; Singh et al., 1995; Tinsley et al., 1981).

3. Peroxisome proliferator-activated receptors (PPARs)

3.1 Definition

Peroxisome proliferator-activated receptors (PPARs) are regulators of lipid metabolism and their main function is to allow the release of fatty acids from plasmatic transport proteins, and promote the cellular uptake. These receptors are transcription factors that belong to the nuclear hormone receptor superfamily, and are activated by lipids from the diet or from intracellular signaling pathways, which include saturated and unsaturated fatty acids, and fatty acids derivates. PPARs are classified in three groups namely, PPARα (NR1C1); PPARβ/δ (NR1C2) and PPARγ (NR1C3). PPARα is expressed in tissues with high fatty acid metabolism, including liver, kidney, small intestine, heart, brown adipose tissue and muscle. It regulates the expression of enzymes that participate in the mitochondrial and peroxisomal fatty acid oxidation. PPARβ/δ is expressed ubiquitously, regulates the β-oxidation and plays an important role in energy consumption in peripheral tissues. PPARγ presents two isoforms that differ at their N terminus, δ1 and δ2, and is expressed in white and brown adipose tissue, intestine, brain, vascular cells, skeletal muscle and some immune cells. It promotes lipid storage, because it regulates the differentiation of adipocytes. In addition, PPARα and PPARβ regulate the expression of lipoprotein lipase (LPL) and fatty acid translocase, which induce fatty acid release from lipoproteins, and the uptake of cholesterol and fatty acids respectively (Feige et al., 2006; Michalik et al., 2006).

3.2 Structure

PPARs isotypes have a protein domain organization common to nuclear receptor superfamily (Figure 1). N-terminal A/B domain contains the ligand-independent activation function 1 (AF1). The C-terminal domain presents the DNA-binding domain, consisting of two zinc-finger motifs that is a hallmark of nuclear receptors, and targets the receptor to specific DNA sequences. D domain is the hinge region, and confers structure flexibility to the receptor dimmers, allowing them to bind with several specific DNA sequences. The C-terminal E/F domain contains the ligand binding domain (LBD), and a ligand-dependent activation function 2 (AF2). This domain also exposes the main surfaces for dimerization and for the cofactors interaction (co-activators or co-repressors). The LBD consists of 12 α helices and 4 β sheets that delineate a Y-shape hydrophobic pocket, representing the ligand-binding cavity.

The transcription activity of PPARs is mediated by the formation of heterodimmers with the retinoic X receptors (RXR, NR2B). RXRs present three isoforms, resulting in different combinations of heterodimers, which influence the recognition of target gene promoters. Heterodimmers bind to specific response elements namely PPARs response elements (PPREs), which consist on one direct repeat of AGGTCA consensus sequence spaced by a nucleotide. However, PPAR-RXR complex formation does not require ligand and DNA binding activity (Feige et al., 2006).

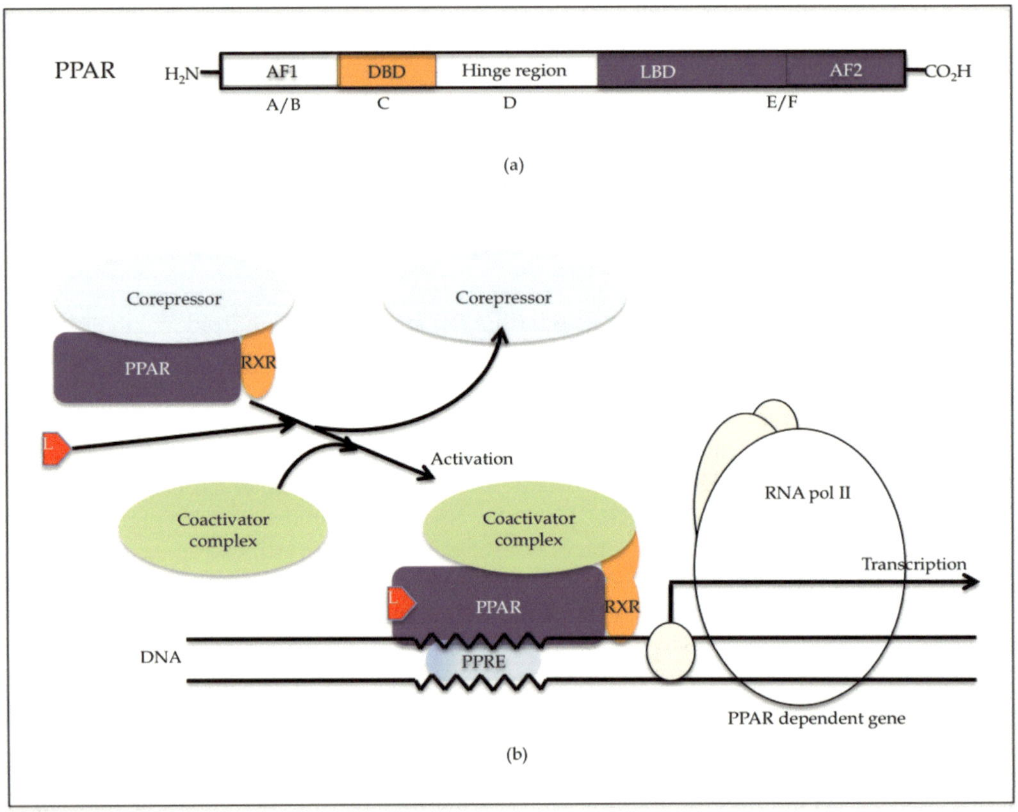

Fig. 1. General features and architecture domains in human PPARs. (a) Schematic representation of PPAR domains: A/B domain, contains a ligand-independent activation function 1 (AF1), C domain, contains the DNA-binding domain (DBD), D domain contains the hinge region and the C-terminal includes the E/F domain with the ligand-binding domain and the ligand-dependent activation domain (AF2). (b) General mechanism of genomic expression by PPAR/RXR heterodimers. Upon ligand (L) binding to PPAR through the LBD domain, the PPAR associates with coactivator to turn on target genes via the PPAR response element (PPRE) located in the promoter of target genes.

3.3 PPARs and breast cancer

Peroxisome proliferators are a variety of compounds that bind to PPARs and induce DNA replication and proliferation in rodent hepatocytes, while PPARα long-term activation promotes the development of hepatocarcinomas in rodent liver (Michalik et al., 2004, Peters et al., 2005). However the participation of PPARs in the promotion and development of human cancers is unclear. PPRAα expression in humans is less than rats and its activation induces a reduced transcription response, and it has not involved in hepatocytes proliferation. In humans, PPARβ/δ is highly expressed in colorectal cancer and is implicated at its carcinogenesis and metastasis. However, PPARα and PPARβ/δ have not been implicated in breast cancer. PPARγ is expressed in a variety of tumor including breast cancer. PPARγ activation by using troglitazone and GW7845 ligands prevents preneoplastic mammary lesion in rats (Mehta et al., 2000; Suh et al., 1999). In human breast cancer cells, PPARγ activation by exogenous ligands prevents growth, induces apoptosis, and promotes changes in epithelial gene expression accompanied with a less malignant state. In addition, overexpression of PPARγ decreases proliferation and induces apoptosis in the absence of exogenous ligands (Meng et al., Yin et al., 2001; Elstner et al., 1998; Mueller et al., 1998).

4. GPR40 and GPR120

G-protein coupled receptors (GPCRs) are the largest membrane receptor family in the human genome. These receptors mediate a great variety of cell functions including proliferation, survival, immune response, blood pressure regulation, cardiac and smooth muscle contraction and have been implicated in cancer progression and metastasis. GPCRs present a common structure constituted for a single peptide chain that traverse the membrane seven times, exposing three loops on either side of the membrane, with the N-terminus toward outside and the C-terminal on the cytosolic face of the plasma membrane. GPCR activation is mediated by ligands binding to its extracellular domain that induces conformational changes, allowing the cytosolic domain bind to G protein associated with the inner face of plasma membrane. G proteins are heterotrimers which contain three subunits namely α, β and γ. The ligand binding to GPCR promotes G protein activation, which is mediated for the dissociation of GDP bound to the Gα subunit and its replacement with GTP, and then leads to dissociation of Gα from Gβγ subunits. However, this activation is short because GTP bound to Gα is hydrolyzed to GDP in seconds. Gα-GTP and Gβγ subunits complexes induce several signal transduction pathways that is determined for the ligands. G-protein α-subunits present a great variety of effectors (Table 1), and they have been classified in four main families (G_s, $G_{i/0}$, $G_{q/11}$, $G_{12/13}$). The βγ subunits transmit signals independently of α-subunits and second messengers, some of the functions mediated by these subunits including regulation of ligand receptor affinity and receptor phosphorylation (Hardy et al., 2005; Yonezawa et al., 2004; Ichimura et al., 2009).
FFAs stimulate PPARs and mediate the transcription of genes involved in glucose and lipid metabolism. However, several biological effects such as proliferation are independent of PPARs and are mediated by GPCRs. The non-esterified (free) fatty acid receptor 1 (FFAR1) or GPR40 (G-protein-coupled receptor 40) is a GPCR located on chromosome 19q13.1 that is activated by medium and long chain saturated and unsaturated FFAs. FFAR1 is expressed in the pancreas (α cells in islets and insulin-secreting β cells), K and L cells of small and large intestine and mononuclear peripheral blood cells. FFAR1 is coupled with both $G\alpha_{i/0}$ and $G\alpha_{q/11}$. GPR120 is a GPCR located on chromosome 10q23.33 that is activated by saturated FFAs with a carbon chain length of 14 - 18, and with saturated FFAs with a chain length of 16-22. In addition, GPR120 is expressed in the intestine, adypocites, taste buds, monocytes and lung, and is coupled with $G\alpha_{q/11}$ (Ichimura et al., 2009)

G protein family	Members	Effects	Associated effector protein	2nd messenger or downstream effectors
G_s	G_s and G_{olf}	Up	Adenylyl cyclase Ca^{2+} channel	cAMP Ca^{2+}
		Down	Na+ channel	Change in membrane potential
$G_{i/o}$	G_{i1}, G_{i2}, G_{o1}, G_{o2}, G_z, G_t and G_{gus}	Up	K^+ channel Phospholipase C	Change in membrane potential IP_3 and DAG
		Down	Adenylyl cyclase Ca^{2+} channel	cAMP Ca^{2+}
$G_{q/11}$	G_q, G_{11}, G_{14} and $G_{15/16}$	Up	Phospholipase C	IP_3 and DAG
$G_{12/13}$	G_{12} and G_{13}	Up	Small GTPases RhoA	MAPK (Mitogen-activated protein kinase) cascades and monomeric G-proteins (Ras, Rac and Rho)

Table 1. Properties and effectors of G protein family. Keys: Up= Stimulation; Down= Inhibition; IP_3: Inositol 1,4,5-triphosphate; DAG= 1,2-diacylglycerol; cAMP= cyclic AMP.

In breast cancer cells, have been reported the expression of FFAR1 and GPR120 as well as their expression in human mammary non-tumorigenic epithelial cells MCF10A. Furthermore, oleic acid induces an increase in cellular Ca^{2+} concentrations and proliferation through a FFAR1-dependent pathway in breast cancer cells (Hardy et al., 2005, Yonezawa et al., 2004).

5. Signal transduction pathways mediated by oleic and arachidonic acids in breast cancer cells

5.1 Signal transduction pathways mediated by oleic acid in breast cancer cells

OA is an essential FFA monounsaturated and one of the most abundant fatty acids in plasma. However, little is known about the signal transduction pathways mediated by OA in breast cancer cells. The Src family has an important role in a great variety of cell functions, including cell cycle progression, growth, survival and migration. Src kinases are involved in breast cancer, because in breast tumors and human mammary carcinoma cell lines, Src kinase activity is enhanced relative to that in normal breast tissue, while in breast cancer cells the activated Src increases the adhesion, survival and integrin expression (Park et al., 2004; Parsons and Parsons, 1997; Rosen et al., 1986). In breast cancer cells MDA-MB-231, OA induces Src activation, given by its phosphorylation at tyrosine (Tyr)-418, as well as ERK1/2 activation, given by its phosphorylation at threonine (Thr)-202 and Tyr-204, and ERK1/2 activation is dependent on Src kinase activity. In contrast, OA induces only ERK 1 activation in mammary non-tumorigenic epithelial cells MCF10A (Soto-Guzman et al., 2008).

Transactivation of epidermal growth factor receptor (EGFR) induced by GPCRS occurs via activation of metalloproteinases (MMPs) and subsequent release of EGF-like ligands, such as HB-EGF, from growth factors precursors in the plasma membrane. Furthermore, it has been proposal that Src family kinases also are mediators of GPCR-induced EGFR transactivation, because Src induces EGFR tyrosine phosphorylation after stimulation of LPA and α2A-adregernic receptors coupled with Gi, whereas angiotensin II promotes the association of Src with Shc, Grb2 and EGFR, and then Src activated phosphorylates EGFR at

Tyr-845 and Tyr-1101. In addition, it has been reported that the mechanism of MMPs activation requires Src kinase activation (Prenzel et al., 1999; Fischer et al., 2003). In MDA-MB-231 cells, ERK1/2 activation induced by OA requires EGFR and MMPs activations. These findings show that ERK1/2 activation induced by OA requires EGFR transactivation and they suggest that Src and/or MMPs activities mediate EGFR transactivation.

The AP-1 transcription factor consists of homo- or hetero-dimers of proteins encoded by the *fos* and *jun* gene families, and their combination determine the genes that are regulated. AP-1 participates in fundamental cellular processes and control cellular responses including proliferation, differentiation, oncogenic transformation, apoptosis and metastasis (Eferl and Wagner, 2003; Tulchinsky, 2000; Shaulian and Karin, 2001). In MCF7 cells, an overexpression of c-Jun enhances motility and invasion, whereas Fra-2, a member of Fos family, plays a pivotal role in cell invasion and motility in MCF7 and MDA-MB-231 breast cancer cells (Smith et al., 1999; Rinehart-Kim et al., 2000; Milde-Langosch et al., 2008; Milde-Langosch et al., 2004). In addition, OA induces AP-1-DNA complex formation through an ERK1/2, Src and MMPs-dependent pathway, as well as, it requires EGFR transactivation in MCF7 breast cancer cells. Mammary non-tumorigenic epithelial cells MCF10A present a constitutive AP-1-DNA binding activity and OA stimulation does not induce an increase on AP-1-DNA complex formation (Soto-Guzman et al., 2008). These findings strongly suggest that AP-1 activation induced by OA promotes the invasion process by the expression of genes regulated for AP-1, including MMP-1, MMP-3, MMP-9, ARP2/3 and p41Bm CapG. Furthermore, AP-1-DNA binding activity induced by OA is restricted to breast cancer cells (Bahassi el et al., 2004; Benbow and Brinckerhoff, 1997; Lee et al., 1987).

In breast cancer cells MCF7 and MDA-MB-231, OA induces cell proliferation and it is mediated at least in part through FFAR1, epidermal growth factor receptor (EGFR), PI3K, phospholipase C (PLC), Src, MMPs, MEK1/2 and ERK1/2. However, OA does not induce cell proliferation in mammary non-tumorigenic epithelial cells MCF10A. These findings suggest that cell proliferation induced by OA is a restricted process in breast cancer cells. OA signaling is coupled with GPCR activation via Gi/Go proteins, because inhibition of Gi/Go proteins prevents cell proliferation, an increase in cellular Ca^{2+} concentration and ERK1/2 activation. However, the participation of GPR120 remains to be investigated, because it is able to bind medium chain FFA, such as OA (Soto-Guzman et al., 2008; Hardy et al., 2005; Yonezawa et al., 2004).

Cancer metastasis involves several steps including cell detachment, migration, invasion, intravasation, extravasation and proliferation in distal sites. Focal adhesion kinase (FAK) is a non-receptor tyrosine kinase that localizes to focal adhesions and is activated by diverse signaling molecules that mediate cell growth and differentiation including growth factors, Src family kinases members, bioactive lipids and extracellular matrix (ECM) components. FAK is a critical signaling molecule involved in the various stages of tumorigenesis and metastasis processes through regulation of migration, cell survival, proliferation, spreading, invasion and metastasis. In breast cancer tumors, FAK gene is amplified, its protein is overexpressed and FAK expression correlates with increased invasion and metastasis tumors. In addition, tumor cells overexpressing FAK have a tendency to invade surrounding tissues and metastasize *in vivo*, where FAK induces the formation of podosomes and invadopodia that promote an invasive cell phenotype (Hsia et al., 2003; Parsons et al., 2000; Parsons, 2003; Zhao and Guan, 2009; Cance et al., 2000). In MDA-MB-231 breast cancer cell cultures, OA induces FAK activation, given by its phosphorylation at Tyr-397, migration and invasion (Navarro-Tito et al., 2010; Soto-Guzman et al., 2010).

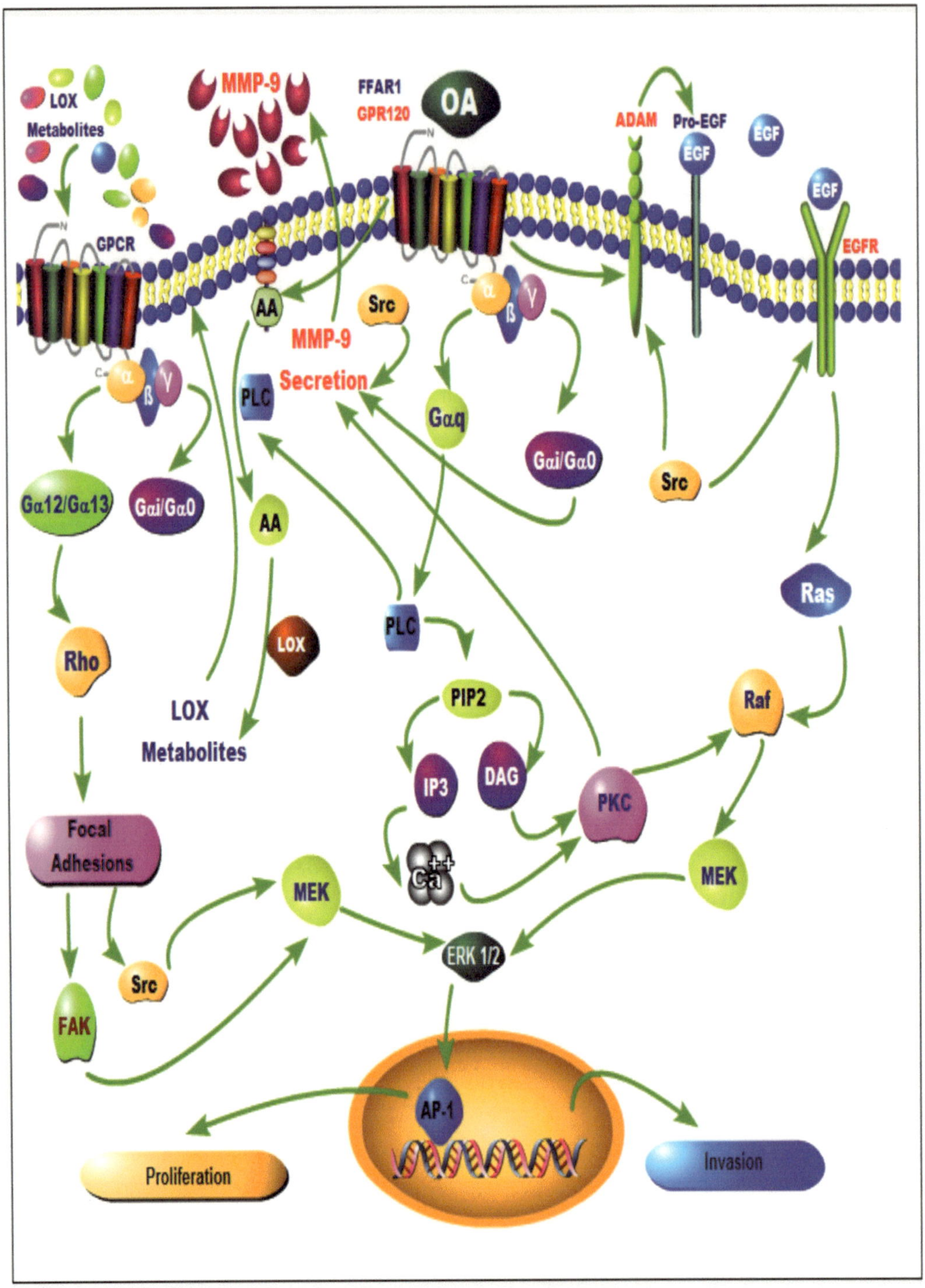

Fig. 2. Overview of the signal transduction pathways mediated by OA in breast cancer cells.

A model of reciprocal catalytic activation between FAK and Src kinases has been proposal, where phosphorylation of FAK at Tyr-397 creates a high affinity-binding site recognized by the SH2 domain of Src family kinases, and it leads to the recruitment and activation of Src through FAK, accompanied with formation of FAK–Src complex. Src family kinases associated with FAK, phosphorylate FAK at additional tyrosine residues, such as Tyr-576 and Tyr-577, inducing a maximal FAK kinase activity. Then, maximal activity of FAK stimulates an intermolecular phosphorylation between FAK molecules at Tyr-397, leading to signal amplification (Owen et al., 1999; Salazar and Rozengurt, 2001). In line with this model, OA mediates FAK activation in a fashion dependent of Src kinase activity in MDA-MB-231 breast cancer cells (Navarro-Tito et al., 2010).

AA is one of the major polyunsaturated fatty acids present in mammalian cell membrane phospholipids. AA is mainly produced from membrane glycerophospholipids in the nuclear envelope and from plasma membrane via the activity of cytosolic phospholypase A2 (cPLA2). Alternatively, phospholipase C (PLC) produces AA, by metabolize phosphatidylinositol and phosphatidylinositol phosphate to inositol phosphates (IP3) and diacylglycerol (DAG). DAG is metabolized by DAG lipase to 2-arachidonyl-glycerol (2-AG) and then AA is released from 2-AG by monoacylglycerol lipase or fatty acid amidohydrolase. Free AA is enzymatically metabolized by three major pathways: lipoxygenases (LOXs), cyclooxygenases (COXs) and cytochrome P450 epoxygenases (CYP). LOXs pathway produces several hydroperoxyeicosatetraenoic acids (HPETEs) and hydroxyeicosatetraenoics acids (HETEs), while COXs pathway is mediated by two enzymes, namely COX-1 and COX-2, these enzymes produce PGG2 and PGH2, which are subsequently converted into prostaglandins (PGs) and thromboxanes (TXs). CYP pathway produces HETEs and epoxides. AA and its metabolites are involved in biological processes, including chemotaxis, inflammation, angiogenesis, cell survival, mitogenesis and apoptosis (Brash, 2001; Piomelli, 1993; Harizi et al., 2008). In line with this notion, OA mediates the AA production via PLC/DAG lipase/monoacylglycerol lipase or fatty acidamidohydrolase and then AA is metabolized through LOXs and their metabolites mediate FAK activation and cell migration in MDA-MB-231 breast cancer cells. In addition, a positive feedback between ERK1/2 activation and COXs/LOXs metabolites maintains proliferation and migration in high metastatic potential breast cancer cells (You et al., 2009; Navarro-Tito et al., 2010).

LOXs are a family of nonheme iron dioxygenases including 5-, 8- 12- and 15-LOX, whose main products are 5(S)-, 8(S), 12(S)- and 15(S)-HETE, respectively. Among them, 12(S)-HETE promotes the formation of focal adhesion plaques via a *Pertussis toxin* (PTX) sensitive pathway, leading to enhance adhesion to fibronectin in murine B16 amelanotic melanoma cells, whereas it stimulates ERK1/2 phosphorylation through a PTX sensitive pathway in prostate cancer cells. 12(S)-HETE acts on target cells through a GPCR coupled with Gi/Go proteins (Harizi et al., 2008, McCabe et al., 2006, Liu et al., 1995). In breast cancer cells MDA-MB-231, OA promotes FAK activation and migration in a fashion dependent on LOX metabolites and a GPCR coupled with Gi/Go (Navarro-Tito et al., 2010). These findings strongly suggest that OA induces FAK phosphorylation and cell migration via the production of 12(S)-HETE, which is secreted into the extracellular space and activates a GPCR coupled with Gi/Go and/or G12/G13.

MMPs are a family of zinc-dependent endopeptidases that collectively are capable of degrading all ECM components. However, MMPs substrates also include other proteins such as MMPs, proteinase inhibitors, growth factors, growth factors binding proteins, chemokines, cytokines, cell surface receptors and cell adhesion molecules. MMPs have been implicated in several aspects of tumor progression, including cell migration, angiogenesis, tumor cell growth and invasion through BM, and interstitial matrices. MMPs gene family is composed of at least 20 members and is subgrouped into different types based on sequence characteristic and substrate specificity. Particularly, MMP-2 (gelatinase A) and MMP-9 (gelatinase B) are associated with tumor progression and metastasis due to their ability to degrade type IV collagen, the main component of BM, and their elevated expression in malignant tumors. In breast cancer, these gelatinases are highly expressed and is suggested that play an important role in breast cancer invasion, metastasis and angiogenesis (Pellikainen et al., 2004; Duffy et al., 2000; Egeblad and Werb, 2002; Curran and Murray, 1999).

Increased levels of PKC are associated with malignant transformation in breast cancer cells lines and a positive correlation between elevated PKC levels and invasive potential of breast cancer cell lines is suggested. In line with these notions, OA promotes MMP-9 secretion an invasion through a PKC-dependent pathway in MDA-MB-231 breast cancer cells. However, OA is not able to produce invasion in the non-invasive MCF7 breast cancer cells. Human mammary non-tumorigenic epithelial cells MCF10A present a constitutive secretion of MMP-9 and OA does not induce an increase on its secretion, and does not promote MMP-9 secretion in non-tumorigenic epithelial cells MCF12A (Soto-Guzman et al., 2010). These findings strongly suggest that MMP-9 secretion induced by OA is restricted to breast cancer cells and therefore OA may contribute to invasiveness and metastasis process in breast cancer cells (Soto-Guzman et al., 2010).

EGFR and Her-2 overexpression correlates with a reduction on survival and induction of invasion and metastasis in malignante breast cancer. In MDA-MB-231 breast cancer cells, OA promotes MMP-9 secretion and invasion trough an EGFR and Src-dependent pathway (Soto-Guzman et al., 2010). Since, Src family kinases are mediators of GPCR-induced EGFR transactivation, and that OA induces Src activation, it is propose that OA mediates MMP-9 secretion and invasion through and EGFR transactivation-dependent pathway. OA also mediates invasion through a Gi/Go coupled pathway and MMPs activity. It suggests that OA induces invasion via FFAR1 coupled with Gi/Go and/or GPR120 activation and support the proposal that OA mediates invasion via EGFR transactivation. Furthermore, during invasion process, cells induce the formation of invadopodia protrusions, which are actin and proteins associated with MMPs.

5.2 Signal transduction pathways mediated by arachidonic acid in breast cancer cells

AA is a common dietary n-6 cis polyunsaturated fatty acid that is present in an esterified form in cell membrane phospholipids, however AA might be also present in the extracellular microenvironment. AA and its metabolites are implicated in a variety of biological processes including chemotaxis, signal transduction and inflammatory diseases such as artherosclerosis, cancer and rheumatoid arthritis (Brash, 2001).

In MDA-MB-231 breast cancer cells, AA stimulates adhesion to type IV collagen through a 15(S)-lipoxygenase pathway (Palmantier et al., 1996; Nony et al., 2005). AA also induces FAK activation and cell migration via a GPCR couple to Gi/Go and through a LOXs and Src activity-dependent pathway (Navarro-Tito et al., 2008). It suggests that FFAR1 and GPR120 do not participate in the signal transduction pathways and in the cellular processes induced by AA.

The Src family kinases have been implicated in cellular pathways mediated by AA, because AA induces Src activation and cell migration in MDA-MB-231 breast cancer cells. FAK activation is dependent on Src kinase activity; it is agreement with the model of reciprocal catalytic activation of FAK and Src kinases (Navarro-Tito et al., 2008).

Epithelial to mesenchymal transition (EMT) is the process by which epithelial cells are transdifferentiated to a more mesenchymal state. EMT is an essential process during early stages of normal embryonic development, and wound repair. EMT is characterized by the loss of epithelial properties, including cell-cell contacts and baso-apical polarity, accompanied by the acquisition of mesenchymal markers, such as vimentin expression, smooth-muscle actin, N-cadherin, specific myosin isoforms, fibronectin, MMPs, and then cells undergo major changes in their cytoskeleton that enable acquire a mesenchymal appearance with an increase in motility and invasiveness. EMT has been implicated in the progression toward an advanced cancer phenotype, because EMT may endow cancer cells with enhanced motility and invasiveness, and therefore cells acquire the ability to execute the multiple steps of the invasion-metastasis cascade (Hay, 2005; Thiery and Sleeman, 2006; Thiery, 2002; Huber et al., 2005).

Classical cadherins are transmembrane adhesion receptors that mediate cell-cell adhesion through their extracellular domains and connect to the actin microfilaments indirectly via α- and β-catenin in the cytoplasm. They promote the formation of stable cell-cell contacts and the development of adherens junctions. EMT induces disassembled of adherens junctions and the actin cytoskeleton reorganizes from an epithelial cortical alignment associated with cell-cell junctions into actin stress fibers, anchored to focal adhesion complexes. Loss of Ecadherin expression is considered as a hallmark event of EMT, because reduction on E-cadherin levels induces the disruption of epithelial cell-cell contacts that initiates a series of signaling events and a major cytoskeletal reorganization (Halbleib and Nelson, 2006; Gumbiner, 2005; Tepass et al., 2000). E-cadherin expression is negatively regulated by several zinc-finger transcription factors, including Snail1, Snail2, Twist and ZEB1/ZEB2, each of which binds to E-boxes on E-cadherin promoter and represses its transcription (Baranwal and Alahari, 2009; Cano et al., 2000). In mammary epithelial cells MCF10A, AA does not induce a reduction of E-cadherin levels and it does not induce an increase of Snail1, Snail2, Twist and ZEB1 transcription factors. However, AA induces the release of E-cadherin from adherens junctions (Martinez-Orozco et al., 2010).

During EMT, the decrease in epithelial traits is accompanied by acquisition of mesenchymal characteristics including increased expression of smooth-muscle actin, vimentin, fibronectin, MMPs and N-cadherin. Vimentin and N-cadherin are expressed in cells of mesenchymal origin; however they also are expressed in epithelial cells when they become involved in physiological or pathological processes that require epithelial cell migration, such as tumor invasion. Moreover, a reduction on E-cadherin levels and/or release from adherens junctions has been associated with the *novo* vimentin expression and with the metastatic conversion of epithelial cells (Thiery, 2003; Gavert and Ben-Ze'ev, 2008; Gilles et al., 2003; Hazan et al., 2000; Nieman et al., 1999). In line with this notion, AA induces an increase on vimentin and N-cadherin expressions in MCF10A cells (Martinez-Orozco et al., 2010). In addition, vimentin only is expressed in invasive breast cancer cell lines, while its expression in MCF10A and breast cancer cells enhances the migration capacity of these cells (Bindels et al., 2006; Gilles et al., 1999; Hendrix et al., 1996).

The NFkB transcription factor is implicated in cell proliferation, migration, oncogenesis and EMT. NFkB mediates EMT by transcription regulation of Snail1, Snail2, Twist and ZEB1, which are repressor of E-cadherin, claudins and occludins genes. NFkB also promotes the expression of other genes implicated in the EMT process, such as vimentin and MMP-9, whereas it can increase MMP-2 activity by inducing the expression of MT1-MMP (Huber et al., 2004; Karin et al., 2002; Bolos et al., 2003; Cano et al., 2000; Min et al., 2008; Han et al., 2001). In mammary epithelial cells MCF10A, AA induces the NFkB activation and MMP-9 secretion (Martinez-Orozco et al., 2010). These findings suggest that NFkB participates in vimentin expression, secretion and/or expression of MMP-9, and promoting EMT process. In addition, MMPs are implicated in EMT during embryogenesis as well as in early and late stages of cancer progression, angiogenesis and metastasis. Particularly, MMP-9, MMP-13 and MMP-17 have been associated with breast cancer progression, whereas in intestinal epithelial cells, MEK1 and EGF plus TGF-β mediate EMT with an increase on MMP-9 secretion and an increase in the expression of MMP-3, MMP-9, MMP-10 and MMP-14. In line with notion, AA induces MMP-9 secretion in MCF10A cells (Lemieux et al., 2009; Uttamsingh et al., 2008; Duong and Erickson, 2004; Egeblad and Werb, 2002; Nielsen et al., 2001).

EMT is associated with decreased epithelial type cytokeratins (CKs), such as 8 and 18. Breast carcinomas usually retain the expression of epithelial type CKs, but they also express a CKs pattern of myoepithelial cells (Hollier et al., 2009; Wetzels et al., 1991; Malzahn et al., 1998). In mammary epithelial cells MCF10A, AA promotes an increase of CK5 and CK8 expression, strongly suggesting that AA induces an EMT process and therefore an increase in the migratory ability (Martinez-Orozco et al., 2010). It has been reported that the expression pattern of CK5, CK8, CK14 and CK17 are useful in distinguishing benign from invasive breast carcinomas (Otterbach et al., 2000; Takei et al., 1995; Jarasch et al., 1988).

EMT is induced by a variety of cellular growth factors and signaling pathways. These pathways have common targets, such as FAK and Src. FAK and Src represent key players in the regulation of cell matrix interactions and focal contacts formation and mediate a variety of cell functions, such as migration, survival, invasiveness and EMT (Cicchini et al., 2008; Grunert et al., 2003; Mandal et al., 2008; Parsons and Parsons, 1997; Slack et al., 2001; Avizienyte et al., 2002). In murine met hepatocyte (MMH) cells stimulated with TGF-β, FAK activity and its signaling are required for transcriptional up-regulation of mesenchymal and invasiveness markers and delocalization of membrane-bound E-cadherin (Cicchini et al., 2008). In the human embryonic carcinoma cell line NT2/D1 and mouse mammary epithelial cells NmuMG, TGF-β promotes EMT in a fashion dependent on FAK and Src kinase activity and the up-regulatin of caveolin-1 (Bailey and Liu, 2008). In addition, Src family members co-localize with E-cadherin at the sites of cell-cell adhesion in non-migrating epithelial cells, and its activation is required to disrupt cadherin-dependent cell-cell contacts in normal human keratinocytes. In KM12C colon cancer cells, Src induces E-cadherin deregulation through specific integrin signaling and the Src-dependent tyrosine phosphorylation of FAK at peripheral integrin-dependent protrusions (Calautti et al., 1998; Avizienyte et al., 2002; Owens et al., 2000). In line with this notion, AA induces Src and FAK activation and cell migration in MCF10A cells. Cell migration is dependent on Src activity (Martinez-Orozco et al., 2010). Taken together these findings demonstrate that AA induces an epithelial-to-mesenchymal-like transition in MCF10A cells, and they suggest that AA may promote invasion and metastasis in breast cancer.

5.3 Signal transduction pathways mediated by linoleic acid in breast cancer cells

LA is the major PUFA in the most diet and is required for the biosynthesis of eicosanoids. LA is able to induce inappropriate inflammatory responses that contribute to various chronic diseases, including cancer. The signal transduction pathways mediated by LA in breast cancer cells has not been studied in detail and we actually have a little bit of information. In human breast cancer cells, LA induces expression of plasminogen activator protein-1, proliferation migration and invasion, while LA promotes an increase of intracellular Ca^{2+} levels and proliferation in bovine mammary epithelial cells (Yonezawa et al., 2008; Reyes et al., 2004; Byon et al., 2009).

6. Conclusions

The research in the field of signal transduction pathways mediated by FFAs in mammary epithelial cells delineates a new role for FFAs in the invasion and progression of breast cancer. The findings show that FFAs induces activation of protein kinases cascades and transcription factors in cell cultures of mammary epithelial cells, which promote cellular processes including growth, migration, invasion and EMT. Therefore, FFAs may play an important role in the invasion, progression and metastasis processes in breast cancer.

7. References

Avizienyte, E., Wyke, A. W., Jones, R. J., McLean, G. W., Westhoff, M. A., Brunton, V. G. & Frame, M. C. (2002). Src-induced de-regulation of E-cadherin in colon cancer cells requires integrin signalling. *Nat Cell Biol, 4*, 632-638.

Bahassi el, M., Karyala, S., Tomlinson, C. R., Sartor, M. A., Medvedovic, M. & Hennigan, R. F. (2004). Critical regulation of genes for tumor cell migration by AP-1. *Clin Exp Metastasis, 21*, 293-304.

Bailey, K. M. & Liu, J. (2008). Caveolin-1 up-regulation during epithelial to mesenchymal transition is mediated by focal adhesion kinase. *J Biol Chem, 283*, 13714-13724.

Baranwal, S. & Alahari, S. K. (2009). Molecular mechanisms controlling E-cadherin expression in breast cancer. *Biochem Biophys Res Commun, 384*, 6-11.

Bartsch, H., Nair, J. & Owen, R. W. (1999). Dietary polyunsaturated fatty acids and cancers of the breast and colorectum: emerging evidence for their role as risk modifiers. *Carcinogenesis, 20*, 2209-2218.

Benbow, U. & Brinckerhoff, C. E. (1997). The AP-1 site and MMP gene regulation: what is all the fuss about? *Matrix Biol, 15*, 519-526.

Bindels, S., Mestdagt, M., Vandewalle, C., Jacobs, N., Volders, L., Noel, A., van Roy, F., Berx, G., Foidart, J. M. & Gilles, C. (2006). Regulation of vimentin by SIP1 in human epithelial breast tumor cells. *Oncogene, 25*, 4975-4985.

Bolos, V., Peinado, H., Perez-Moreno, M. A., Fraga, M. F., Esteller, M. & Cano, A. (2003). The transcription factor Slug represses E-cadherin expression and induces epithelial to mesenchymal transitions: a comparison with Snail and E47 repressors. *J Cell Sci, 116*, 499-511.

Boyd, N. F., Stone, J., Vogt, K. N., Connelly, B. S., Martin, L. J. & Minkin, S. (2003). Dietary fat and breast cancer risk revisited: a meta-analysis of the published literature. *Br J Cancer, 89*, 1672-1685.

Brash, A. R. (2001). Arachidonic acid as a bioactive molecule. *J Clin Invest, 107*, 1339-1345.

Byon, C. H., Hardy, R. W., Ren, C., Ponnazhagan, S., Welch, D. R., McDonald, J. M. & Chen, Y. (2009). Free fatty acids enhance breast cancer cell migration through plasminogen activator inhibitor-1 and SMAD4. *Lab Invest, 89*, 1221-1228.

Calautti, E., Cabodi, S., Stein, P. L., Hatzfeld, M., Kedersha, N. & Paolo Dotto, G. (1998). Tyrosine phosphorylation and src family kinases control keratinocyte cell-cell adhesion. *J Cell Biol, 141*, 1449-1465.

Cance, W. G., Harris, J. E., Iacocca, M. V., Roche, E., Yang, X., Chang, J., Simkins, S. & Xu, L. (2000). Immunohistochemical analyses of focal adhesion kinase expression in benign and malignant human breast and colon tissues: correlation with preinvasive and invasive phenotypes. *Clin Cancer Res, 6*, 2417-2423.

Cano, A., Perez-Moreno, M. A., Rodrigo, I., Locascio, A., Blanco, M. J., del Barrio, M. G., Portillo, F. & Nieto, M. A. (2000). The transcription factor snail controls epithelial-mesenchymal transitions by repressing E-cadherin expression. *Nat Cell Biol, 2*, 76-83.

Carmichael, A. R. (2006). Obesity as a risk factor for development and poor prognosis of breast cancer. *BJOG, 113*, 1160-1166.

Cicchini, C., Laudadio, I., Citarella, F., Corazzari, M., Steindler, C., Conigliaro, A., Fantoni, A., Amicone, L. & Tripodi, M. (2008). TGFbeta-induced EMT requires focal adhesion kinase (FAK) signaling. *Exp Cell Res, 314*, 143-152.

Crawford, M., Galli, C., Visioli, F., Renaud, S., Simopoulos, A. P. & Spector, A. A. (2000). Role of plant-derived omega-3 fatty acids in human nutrition. *Ann Nutr Metab, 44*, 263-265.

Curado, M. P., Voti, L. & Sortino-Rachou, A. M. (2009). Cancer registration data and quality indicators in low and middle income countries: their interpretation and potential use for the improvement of cancer care. *Cancer Causes Control, 20*, 751-756.

Curran, S. & Murray, G. I. (1999). Matrix metalloproteinases in tumour invasion and metastasis. *J Pathol, 189*, 300-308.

Chambers, A. F., Groom, A. C. & MacDonald, I. C. (2002). Dissemination and growth of cancer cells in metastatic sites. *Nat Rev Cancer, 2*, 563-572.

Duffy, M. J., Maguire, T. M., Hill, A., McDermott, E. & O'Higgins, N. (2000). Metalloproteinases: role in breast carcinogenesis, invasion and metastasis. *Breast Cancer Res, 2*, 252-257.

Duong, T. D. & Erickson, C. A. (2004). MMP-2 plays an essential role in producing epithelial-mesenchymal transformations in the avian embryo. *Dev Dyn, 229*, 42-53.

Eferl, R. & Wagner, E. F. (2003). AP-1: a double-edged sword in tumorigenesis. *Nat Rev Cancer, 3*, 859-868.

Egeblad, M. & Werb, Z. (2002). New functions for the matrix metalloproteinases in cancer progression. *Nat Rev Cancer, 2*, 161-174.

El Saghir, N. S., Khalil, M. K., Eid, T., El Kinge, A. R., Charafeddine, M., Geara, F., Seoud, M. & Shamseddine, A. I. (2007). Trends in epidemiology and management of breast cancer in developing Arab countries: a literature and registry analysis. *Int J Surg, 5*, 225-233.

Elstner, E., Muller, C., Koshizuka, K., Williamson, E. A., Park, D., Asou, H., Shintaku, P., Said, J. W., Heber, D. & Koeffler, H. P. (1998). Ligands for peroxisome proliferator-activated receptorgamma and retinoic acid receptor inhibit growth and induce apoptosis of human breast cancer cells in vitro and in BNX mice. *Proc Natl Acad Sci U S A, 95*, 8806-8811.

Feige, J. N., Gelman, L., Michalik, L., Desvergne, B. & Wahli, W. (2006). From molecular action to physiological outputs: peroxisome proliferator-activated receptors are nuclear receptors at the crossroads of key cellular functions. *Prog Lipid Res, 45*, 120-159.

Ferlay, J., Autier, P., Boniol, M., Heanue, M., Colombet, M. & Boyle, P. (2007). Estimates of the cancer incidence and mortality in Europe in 2006. *Ann Oncol, 18*, 581-592.

Fischer, O. M., Hart, S., Gschwind, A. & Ullrich, A. (2003). EGFR signal transactivation in cancer cells. *Biochem Soc Trans, 31*, 1203-1208.

Franceschi, S., Favero, A., Decarli, A., Negri, E., La Vecchia, C., Ferraroni, M., Russo, A., Salvini, S., Amadori, D., Conti, E., Montella, M. & Giacosa, A. (1996). Intake of macronutrients and risk of breast cancer. *Lancet, 347*, 1351-1356.

Gaard, M., Tretli, S. & Loken, E. B. (1995). Dietary fat and the risk of breast cancer: a prospective study of 25,892 Norwegian women. *Int J Cancer, 63*, 13-17.

Gavert, N. & Ben-Ze'ev, A. (2008). Epithelial-mesenchymal transition and the invasive potential of tumors. *Trends Mol Med, 14*, 199-209.

Gilles, C., Polette, M., Mestdagt, M., Nawrocki-Raby, B., Ruggeri, P., Birembaut, P. & Foidart, J. M. (2003). Transactivation of vimentin by beta-catenin in human breast cancer cells. *Cancer Res, 63*, 2658-2664.

Gilles, C., Polette, M., Zahm, J. M., Tournier, J. M., Volders, L., Foidart, J. M. & Birembaut, P. (1999). Vimentin contributes to human mammary epithelial cell migration. *J Cell Sci, 112 (Pt 24)*, 4615-4625.

Goodstine, S. L., Zheng, T., Holford, T. R., Ward, B. A., Carter, D., Owens, P. H. & Mayne, S. T. (2003). Dietary (n-3)/(n-6) fatty acid ratio: possible relationship to premenopausal but not postmenopausal breast cancer risk in U.S. women. *J Nutr, 133*, 1409-1414.

Gout, S. & Huot, J. (2008). Role of cancer microenvironment in metastasis: focus on colon cancer. *Cancer Microenviron, 1*, 69-83.

Grunert, S., Jechlinger, M. & Beug, H. (2003). Diverse cellular and molecular mechanisms contribute to epithelial plasticity and metastasis. *Nat Rev Mol Cell Biol, 4*, 657-665.

Gumbiner, B. M. (2005). Regulation of cadherin-mediated adhesion in morphogenesis. *Nat Rev Mol Cell Biol, 6*, 622-634.

Halbleib, J. M. & Nelson, W. J. (2006). Cadherins in development: cell adhesion, sorting, and tissue morphogenesis. *Genes Dev, 20*, 3199-3214.

Han, Y. P., Tuan, T. L., Wu, H., Hughes, M. & Garner, W. L. (2001). TNF-alpha stimulates activation of pro-MMP2 in human skin through NF-(kappa)B mediated induction of MT1-MMP. *J Cell Sci, 114*, 131-139.

Hankinson, S. E., Willett, W. C., Manson, J. E., Colditz, G. A., Hunter, D. J., Spiegelman, D., Barbieri, R. L. & Speizer, F. E. (1998). Plasma sex steroid hormone levels and risk of breast cancer in postmenopausal women. *J Natl Cancer Inst, 90*, 1292-1299.

Hansen, R. K. & Bissell, M. J. (2000). Tissue architecture and breast cancer: the role of extracellular matrix and steroid hormones. *Endocr Relat Cancer, 7*, 95-113.

Hardy, S., El-Assaad, W., Przybytkowski, E., Joly, E., Prentki, M. & Langelier, Y. (2003). Saturated fatty acid-induced apoptosis in MDA-MB-231 breast cancer cells. A role for cardiolipin. *J Biol Chem, 278*, 31861-31870.

Hardy, S., St-Onge, G. G., Joly, E., Langelier, Y. & Prentki, M. (2005). Oleate promotes the proliferation of breast cancer cells via the G protein-coupled receptor GPR40. *J Biol Chem, 280*, 13285-13291.

Harizi, H., Corcuff, J. B. & Gualde, N. (2008). Arachidonic-acid-derived eicosanoids: roles in biology and immunopathology. *Trends Mol Med, 14*, 461-469.

Hay, E. D. (2005). The mesenchymal cell, its role in the embryo, and the remarkable signaling mechanisms that create it. *Dev Dyn, 233*, 706-720.

Hazan, R. B., Phillips, G. R., Qiao, R. F., Norton, L. & Aaronson, S. A. (2000). Exogenous expression of N-cadherin in breast cancer cells induces cell migration, invasion, and metastasis. *J Cell Biol, 148*, 779-790.

Hendrix, M. J., Seftor, E. A., Chu, Y. W., Trevor, K. T. & Seftor, R. E. (1996). Role of intermediate filaments in migration, invasion and metastasis. *Cancer Metastasis Rev, 15*, 507-525.

Hollier, B. G., Evans, K. & Mani, S. A. (2009). The epithelial-to-mesenchymal transition and cancer stem cells: a coalition against cancer therapies. *J Mammary Gland Biol Neoplasia, 14*, 29-43.

Hsia, D. A., Mitra, S. K., Hauck, C. R., Streblow, D. N., Nelson, J. A., Ilic, D., Huang, S., Li, E., Nemerow, G. R., Leng, J., Spencer, K. S., Cheresh, D. A. & Schlaepfer, D. D. (2003). Differential regulation of cell motility and invasion by FAK. *J Cell Biol, 160*, 753-767.

Huber, M. A., Azoitei, N., Baumann, B., Grunert, S., Sommer, A., Pehamberger, H., Kraut, N., Beug, H. & Wirth, T. (2004). NF-kappaB is essential for epithelial-mesenchymal transition and metastasis in a model of breast cancer progression. *J Clin Invest, 114*, 569-581.

Huber, M. A., Kraut, N. & Beug, H. (2005). Molecular requirements for epithelial-mesenchymal transition during tumor progression. *Curr Opin Cell Biol, 17*, 548-558.

Hudelist, G., Kostler, W. J., Attems, J., Czerwenka, K., Muller, R., Manavi, M., Steger, G. G., Kubista, E., Zielinski, C. C. & Singer, C. F. (2003). Her-2/neu-triggered intracellular tyrosine kinase activation: in vivo relevance of ligand-independent activation mechanisms and impact upon the efficacy of trastuzumab-based treatment. *Br J Cancer, 89*, 983-991.

Ichimura, A., Hirasawa, A., Hara, T. & Tsujimoto, G. (2009). Free fatty acid receptors act as nutrient sensors to regulate energy homeostasis. *Prostaglandins Other Lipid Mediat, 89*, 82-88.

Jarasch, E. D., Nagle, R. B., Kaufmann, M., Maurer, C. & Bocker, W. J. (1988). Differential diagnosis of benign epithelial proliferations and carcinomas of the breast using antibodies to cytokeratins. *Hum Pathol, 19*, 276-289.

Karin, M., Cao, Y., Greten, F. R. & Li, Z. W. (2002). NF-kappaB in cancer: from innocent bystander to major culprit. *Nat Rev Cancer, 2*, 301-310.

Lahmann, P. H., Hoffmann, K., Allen, N., van Gils, C. H., Khaw, K. T., Tehard, B., Berrino, F., Tjonneland, A., Bigaard, J., Olsen, A., Overvad, K., Clavel-Chapelon, F., Nagel, G., Boeing, H., Trichopoulos, D., Economou, G., Bellos, G., Palli, D., Tumino, R., Panico, S., Sacerdote, C., Krogh, V., Peeters, P. H., Bueno-de-Mesquita, H. B., Lund, E., Ardanaz, E., Amiano, P., Pera, G., Quiros, J. R., Martinez, C., Tormo, M. J., Wirfalt, E., Berglund, G., Hallmans, G., Key, T. J., Reeves, G., Bingham, S., Norat, T., Biessy, C., Kaaks, R. & Riboli, E. (2004). Body size and breast cancer risk: findings from the European Prospective Investigation into Cancer And Nutrition (EPIC). *Int J Cancer, 111*, 762-771.

Lee, W., Mitchell, P. & Tjian, R. (1987). Purified transcription factor AP-1 interacts with TPA-inducible enhancer elements. *Cell, 49*, 741-752.

Lemieux, E., Bergeron, S., Durand, V., Asselin, C., Saucier, C. & Rivard, N. (2009). Constitutively active MEK1 is sufficient to induce epithelial-to-mesenchymal transition in intestinal epithelial cells and to promote tumor invasion and metastasis. *Int J Cancer, 125*, 1575-1586.

Liu, B., Khan, W. A., Hannun, Y. A., Timar, J., Taylor, J. D., Lundy, S., Butovich, I. & Honn, K. V. (1995). 12(S)-hydroxyeicosatetraenoic acid and 13(S)-hydroxyoctadecadienoic acid regulation of protein kinase C-alpha in melanoma cells: role of receptor-mediated hydrolysis of inositol phospholipids. *Proc Natl Acad Sci U S A, 92*, 9323-9327.

London, S. J., Sacks, F. M., Stampfer, M. J., Henderson, I. C., Maclure, M., Tomita, A., Wood, W. C., Remine, S., Robert, N. J., Dmochowski, J. R. & et al. (1993). Fatty acid composition of the subcutaneous adipose tissue and risk of proliferative benign breast disease and breast cancer. *J Natl Cancer Inst, 85*, 785-793.

Malzahn, K., Mitze, M., Thoenes, M. & Moll, R. (1998). Biological and prognostic significance of stratified epithelial cytokeratins in infiltrating ductal breast carcinomas. *Virchows Arch, 433*, 119-129.

Mandal, M., Myers, J. N., Lippman, S. M., Johnson, F. M., Williams, M. D., Rayala, S., Ohshiro, K., Rosenthal, D. I., Weber, R. S., Gallick, G. E. & El-Naggar, A. K. (2008). Epithelial to mesenchymal transition in head and neck squamous carcinoma: association of Src activation with E-cadherin down-regulation, vimentin expression, and aggressive tumor features. *Cancer, 112*, 2088-2100.

Martinez-Orozco, R., Navarro-Tito, N., Soto-Guzman, A., Castro-Sanchez, L. & Perez Salazar, E. (2010). Arachidonic acid promotes epithelial-to-mesenchymal-like transition in mammary epithelial cells MCF10A. *Eur J Cell Biol, 89*, 476-488.

McCabe, N. P., Selman, S. H. & Jankun, J. (2006). Vascular endothelial growth factor production in human prostate cancer cells is stimulated by overexpression of platelet 12-lipoxygenase. *Prostate, 66*, 779-787.

McGee, S. F., Lanigan, F., Gilligan, E. & Groner, B. (2006). Mammary gland biology and breast cancer. Conference on Common Molecular Mechanisms of Mammary Gland Development and Breast Cancer Progression. *EMBO Rep, 7*, 1084-1088.

McPherson, K., Steel, C. M. & Dixon, J. M. (2000). ABC of breast diseases. Breast cancer-epidemiology, risk factors, and genetics. *BMJ, 321*, 624-628.

Mehta, R. G., Williamson, E., Patel, M. K. & Koeffler, H. P. (2000). A ligand of peroxisome proliferator-activated receptor gamma, retinoids, and prevention of preneoplastic mammary lesions. *J Natl Cancer Inst, 92*, 418-423.

Menendez, J. A., Vazquez-Martin, A., Ropero, S., Colomer, R. & Lupu, R. (2006). HER2 (erbB-2)-targeted effects of the omega-3 polyunsaturated fatty acid, alpha-linolenic acid (ALA; 18:3n-3), in breast cancer cells: the "fat features" of the "Mediterranean diet" as an "anti-HER2 cocktail". *Clin Transl Oncol, 8*, 812-820.

Meng, J., Ding, Y., Shen, A., Yan, M., He, F., Ji, H., Zou, L., Liu, Y., Wang, Y., Lu, X. & Wang, H. Overexpression of PPARgamma can down-regulate Skp2 expression in MDA-MB-231 breast tumor cells. *Mol Cell Biochem, 345*, 171-180.

Michalik, L., Auwerx, J., Berger, J. P., Chatterjee, V. K., Glass, C. K., Gonzalez, F. J., Grimaldi, P. A., Kadowaki, T., Lazar, M. A., O'Rahilly, S., Palmer, C. N., Plutzky, J., Reddy, J. K., Spiegelman, B. M., Staels, B. & Wahli, W. (2006). International Union of Pharmacology. LXI. Peroxisome proliferator-activated receptors. *Pharmacol Rev, 58*, 726-741.

Michalik, L., Desvergne, B. & Wahli, W. (2004). Peroxisome-proliferator-activated receptors and cancers: complex stories. *Nat Rev Cancer, 4*, 61-70.

Milde-Langosch, K., Janke, S., Wagner, I., Schroder, C., Streichert, T., Bamberger, A. M., Janicke, F. & Loning, T. (2008). Role of Fra-2 in breast cancer: influence on tumor cell invasion and motility. *Breast Cancer Res Treat, 107*, 337-347.

Milde-Langosch, K., Roder, H., Andritzky, B., Aslan, B., Hemminger, G., Brinkmann, A., Bamberger, C. M., Loning, T. & Bamberger, A. M. (2004). The role of the AP-1 transcription factors c-Fos, FosB, Fra-1 and Fra-2 in the invasion process of mammary carcinomas. *Breast Cancer Res Treat, 86*, 139-152.

Min, C., Eddy, S. F., Sherr, D. H. & Sonenshein, G. E. (2008). NF-kappaB and epithelial to mesenchymal transition of cancer. *J Cell Biochem, 104*, 733-744.

Mueller, E., Sarraf, P., Tontonoz, P., Evans, R. M., Martin, K. J., Zhang, M., Fletcher, C., Singer, S. & Spiegelman, B. M. (1998). Terminal differentiation of human breast cancer through PPAR gamma. *Mol Cell, 1*, 465-470.

Navarro-Tito, N., Robledo, T. & Salazar, E. P. (2008). Arachidonic acid promotes FAK activation and migration in MDA-MB-231 breast cancer cells. *Exp Cell Res, 314*, 3340-3355.

Navarro-Tito, N., Soto-Guzman, A., Castro-Sanchez, L., Martinez-Orozco, R. & Salazar, E. P. (2010). Oleic acid promotes migration on MDA-MB-231 breast cancer cells through an arachidonic acid-dependent pathway. *Int J Biochem Cell Biol, 42*, 306-317.

Nguyen, D. X. & Massague, J. (2007). Genetic determinants of cancer metastasis. *Nat Rev Genet, 8*, 341-352.

Nielsen, B. S., Rank, F., Lopez, J. M., Balbin, M., Vizoso, F., Lund, L. R., Dano, K. & Lopez-Otin, C. (2001). Collagenase-3 expression in breast myofibroblasts as a molecular marker of transition of ductal carcinoma in situ lesions to invasive ductal carcinomas. *Cancer Res, 61*, 7091-7100.

Nieman, M. T., Prudoff, R. S., Johnson, K. R. & Wheelock, M. J. (1999). N-cadherin promotes motility in human breast cancer cells regardless of their E-cadherin expression. *J Cell Biol, 147*, 631-644.

Nony, P. A., Kennett, S. B., Glasgow, W. C., Olden, K. & Roberts, J. D. (2005). 15S-Lipoxygenase-2 mediates arachidonic acid-stimulated adhesion of human breast carcinoma cells through the activation of TAK1, MKK6, and p38 MAPK. *J Biol Chem, 280*, 31413-31419.

Otterbach, F., Bankfalvi, A., Bergner, S., Decker, T., Krech, R. & Boecker, W. (2000). Cytokeratin 5/6 immunohistochemistry assists the differential diagnosis of atypical proliferations of the breast. *Histopathology, 37*, 232-240.

Owen, J. D., Ruest, P. J., Fry, D. W. & Hanks, S. K. (1999). Induced focal adhesion kinase (FAK) expression in FAK-null cells enhances cell spreading and migration requiring both auto- and activation loop phosphorylation sites and inhibits adhesion-dependent tyrosine phosphorylation of Pyk2. *Mol Cell Biol, 19*, 4806-4818.

Owen, R. W., Giacosa, A., Hull, W. E., Haubner, R., Wurtele, G., Spiegelhalder, B. & Bartsch, H. (2000). Olive-oil consumption and health: the possible role of antioxidants. *Lancet Oncol, 1*, 107-112.

Owens, D. W., McLean, G. W., Wyke, A. W., Paraskeva, C., Parkinson, E. K., Frame, M. C. & Brunton, V. G. (2000). The catalytic activity of the Src family kinases is required to disrupt cadherin-dependent cell-cell contacts. *Mol Biol Cell, 11*, 51-64.

Palmantier, R., Roberts, J. D., Glasgow, W. C., Eling, T. & Olden, K. (1996). Regulation of the adhesion of a human breast carcinoma cell line to type IV collagen and vitronectin: roles for lipoxygenase and protein kinase C. *Cancer Res, 56*, 2206-2212.

Park, H. B., Golubovskaya, V., Xu, L., Yang, X., Lee, J. W., Scully, S., 2nd, Craven, R. J. & Cance, W. G. (2004). Activated Src increases adhesion, survival and alpha2-integrin expression in human breast cancer cells. *Biochem J, 378*, 559-567.

Parsons, J. T. (2003). Focal adhesion kinase: the first ten years. *J Cell Sci, 116*, 1409-1416.

Parsons, J. T., Martin, K. H., Slack, J. K., Taylor, J. M. & Weed, S. A. (2000). Focal adhesion kinase: a regulator of focal adhesion dynamics and cell movement. *Oncogene, 19*, 5606-5613.

Parsons, J. T. & Parsons, S. J. (1997). Src family protein tyrosine kinases: cooperating with growth factor and adhesion signaling pathways. *Curr Opin Cell Biol, 9*, 187-192.

Paszek, M. J. & Weaver, V. M. (2004). The tension mounts: mechanics meets morphogenesis and malignancy. *J Mammary Gland Biol Neoplasia, 9*, 325-342.

Pellikainen, J. M., Ropponen, K. M., Kataja, V. V., Kellokoski, J. K., Eskelinen, M. J. & Kosma, V. M. (2004). Expression of matrix metalloproteinase (MMP)-2 and MMP-9 in breast cancer with a special reference to activator protein-2, HER2, and prognosis. *Clin Cancer Res, 10*, 7621-7628.

Peters, J. M., Cheung, C. & Gonzalez, F. J. (2005). Peroxisome proliferator-activated receptor-alpha and liver cancer: where do we stand? *J Mol Med, 83*, 774-785.

Piomelli, D. (1993). Arachidonic acid in cell signaling. *Curr Opin Cell Biol, 5*, 274-280.

Porter, P. (2008). "Westernizing" women's risks? Breast cancer in lower-income countries. *N Engl J Med, 358*, 213-216.

Prenzel, N., Zwick, E., Daub, H., Leserer, M., Abraham, R., Wallasch, C. & Ullrich, A. (1999). EGF receptor transactivation by G-protein-coupled receptors requires metalloproteinase cleavage of proHB-EGF. *Nature, 402*, 884-888.

Proietto, J., Filippis, A., Nakhla, C. & Clark, S. (1999). Nutrient-induced insulin resistance. *Mol Cell Endocrinol, 151*, 143-149.

Reyes, N., Reyes, I., Tiwari, R. & Geliebter, J. (2004). Effect of linoleic acid on proliferation and gene expression in the breast cancer cell line T47D. *Cancer Lett, 209*, 25-35.

Rinehart-Kim, J., Johnston, M., Birrer, M. & Bos, T. (2000). Alterations in the gene expression profile of MCF-7 breast tumor cells in response to c-Jun. *Int J Cancer, 88*, 180-190.

Rose, D. P., Connolly, J. M. & Liu, X. H. (1994). Effects of linoleic acid on the growth and metastasis of two human breast cancer cell lines in nude mice and the invasive capacity of these cell lines in vitro. *Cancer Res, 54*, 6557-6562.

Rose, D. P., Connolly, J. M. & Liu, X. H. (1995). Effects of linoleic acid and gamma-linolenic acid on the growth and metastasis of a human breast cancer cell line in nude mice and on its growth and invasive capacity in vitro. *Nutr Cancer, 24*, 33-45.

Rose, D. P., Connolly, J. M. & Liu, X. H. (1997). Fatty acid regulation of breast cancer cell growth and invasion. *Adv Exp Med Biol, 422*, 47-55.

Rosen, N., Bolen, J. B., Schwartz, A. M., Cohen, P., DeSeau, V. & Israel, M. A. (1986). Analysis of pp60c-src protein kinase activity in human tumor cell lines and tissues. *J Biol Chem, 261*, 13754-13759.

Sakamoto, G. & Sugano, H. (1991). Pathology of breast cancer: present and prospect in Japan. *Breast Cancer Res Treat, 18 Suppl 1*, S81-83.

Salazar, E. P. & Rozengurt, E. (2001). Src family kinases are required for integrin-mediated but not for G protein-coupled receptor stimulation of focal adhesion kinase autophosphorylation at Tyr-397. *J Biol Chem, 276*, 17788-17795.

Shaulian, E. & Karin, M. (2001). AP-1 in cell proliferation and survival. *Oncogene, 20*, 2390-2400.

Singh, R. K., Hardy, R. W., Wang, M. H., Williford, J., Gladson, C. L., McDonald, J. M. & Siegal, G. P. (1995). Stearate inhibits human tumor cell invasion. *Invasion Metastasis, 15*, 144-155.

Slack, J. K., Adams, R. B., Rovin, J. D., Bissonette, E. A., Stoker, C. E. & Parsons, J. T. (2001). Alterations in the focal adhesion kinase/Src signal transduction pathway correlate with increased migratory capacity of prostate carcinoma cells. *Oncogene, 20*, 1152-1163.

Smith, L. M., Wise, S. C., Hendricks, D. T., Sabichi, A. L., Bos, T., Reddy, P., Brown, P. H. & Birrer, M. J. (1999). cJun overexpression in MCF-7 breast cancer cells produces a tumorigenic, invasive and hormone resistant phenotype. *Oncogene, 18*, 6063-6070.

Soto-Guzman, A., Navarro-Tito, N., Castro-Sanchez, L., Martinez-Orozco, R. & Salazar, E. P. (2010). Oleic acid promotes MMP-9 secretion and invasion in breast cancer cells. *Clin Exp Metastasis, 27*, 505-515.

Soto-Guzman, A., Robledo, T., Lopez-Perez, M. & Salazar, E. P. (2008). Oleic acid induces ERK1/2 activation and AP-1 DNA binding activity through a mechanism involving Src kinase and EGFR transactivation in breast cancer cells. *Mol Cell Endocrinol, 294*, 81-91.

Suh, N., Wang, Y., Williams, C. R., Risingsong, R., Gilmer, T., Willson, T. M. & Sporn, M. B. (1999). A new ligand for the peroxisome proliferator-activated receptor-gamma

(PPAR-gamma), GW7845, inhibits rat mammary carcinogenesis. *Cancer Res, 59,* 5671-5673.

Takei, H., Iino, Y., Horiguchi, J., Kanoh, T., Takao, Y., Oyama, T. & Morishita, Y. (1995). Immunohistochemical analysis of cytokeratin #8 as a prognostic factor in invasive breast carcinoma. *Anticancer Res, 15,* 1101-1105.

Tepass, U., Truong, K., Godt, D., Ikura, M. & Peifer, M. (2000). Cadherins in embryonic and neural morphogenesis. *Nat Rev Mol Cell Biol, 1,* 91-100.

Thiery, J. P. (2002). Epithelial-mesenchymal transitions in tumour progression. *Nat Rev Cancer, 2,* 442-454.

Thiery, J. P. (2003). Epithelial-mesenchymal transitions in development and pathologies. *Curr Opin Cell Biol, 15,* 740-746.

Thiery, J. P. & Sleeman, J. P. (2006). Complex networks orchestrate epithelial-mesenchymal transitions. *Nat Rev Mol Cell Biol, 7,* 131-142.

Tinsley, I. J., Schmitz, J. A. & Pierce, D. A. (1981). Influence of dietary fatty acids on the incidence of mammary tumors in the C3H mouse. *Cancer Res, 41,* 1460-1465.

Trichopoulou, A., Katsouyanni, K., Stuver, S., Tzala, L., Gnardellis, C., Rimm, E. & Trichopoulos, D. (1995). Consumption of olive oil and specific food groups in relation to breast cancer risk in Greece. *J Natl Cancer Inst, 87,* 110-116.

Tulchinsky, E. (2000). Fos family members: regulation, structure and role in oncogenic transformation. *Histol Histopathol, 15,* 921-928.

Uttamsingh, S., Bao, X., Nguyen, K. T., Bhanot, M., Gong, J., Chan, J. L., Liu, F., Chu, T. T. & Wang, L. H. (2008). Synergistic effect between EGF and TGF-beta1 in inducing oncogenic properties of intestinal epithelial cells. *Oncogene, 27,* 2626-2634.

Van't Veer, L. J. & Weigelt, B. (2003). Road map to metastasis. *Nat Med, 9,* 999-1000.

Voorrips, L. E., Brants, H. A., Kardinaal, A. F., Hiddink, G. J., van den Brandt, P. A. & Goldbohm, R. A. (2002). Intake of conjugated linoleic acid, fat, and other fatty acids in relation to postmenopausal breast cancer: the Netherlands Cohort Study on Diet and Cancer. *Am J Clin Nutr, 76,* 873-882.

Wahrburg, U. & Assmann, G. (2001). Properties of olive oil. *Lancet, 357,* 1626.

Weigelt, B., Peterse, J. L. & van 't Veer, L. J. (2005). Breast cancer metastasis: markers and models. *Nat Rev Cancer, 5,* 591-602.

Welsch, C. W. (1992). Relationship between dietary fat and experimental mammary tumorigenesis: a review and critique. *Cancer Res, 52,* 2040s-2048s.

Wetzels, R. H., Kuijpers, H. J., Lane, E. B., Leigh, I. M., Troyanovsky, S. M., Holland, R., van Haelst, U. J. & Ramaekers, F. C. (1991). Basal cell-specific and hyperproliferation-related keratins in human breast cancer. *Am J Pathol, 138,* 751-763.

Wickramasinghe, N. S., Jo, H., McDonald, J. M. & Hardy, R. W. (1996). Stearate inhibition of breast cancer cell proliferation. A mechanism involving epidermal growth factor receptor and G-proteins. *Am J Pathol, 148,* 987-995.

Wirfalt, E., Mattisson, I., Gullberg, B., Johansson, U., Olsson, H. & Berglund, G. (2002). Postmenopausal breast cancer is associated with high intakes of omega6 fatty acids (Sweden). *Cancer Causes Control, 13,* 883-893.

Yin, F., Wakino, S., Liu, Z., Kim, S., Hsueh, W. A., Collins, A. R., Van Herle, A. J. & Law, R. E. (2001). Troglitazone inhibits growth of MCF-7 breast carcinoma cells by targeting G1 cell cycle regulators. *Biochem Biophys Res Commun, 286*, 916-922.

Yonezawa, T., Haga, S., Kobayashi, Y., Katoh, K. & Obara, Y. (2008). Unsaturated fatty acids promote proliferation via ERK1/2 and Akt pathway in bovine mammary epithelial cells. *Biochem Biophys Res Commun, 367*, 729-735.

Yonezawa, T., Katoh, K. & Obara, Y. (2004). Existence of GPR40 functioning in a human breast cancer cell line, MCF-7. *Biochem Biophys Res Commun, 314*, 805-809.

You, J., Mi, D., Zhou, X., Qiao, L., Zhang, H., Zhang, X. & Ye, L. (2009). A positive feedback between activated extracellularly regulated kinase and cyclooxygenase/ lipoxygenase maintains proliferation and migration of breast cancer cells. *Endocrinology, 150*, 1607-1617.

Zhao, J. & Guan, J. L. (2009). Signal transduction by focal adhesion kinase in cancer. *Cancer Metastasis Rev, 28*, 35-49.

34

Adrenoceptors and Breast Cancer: Review Article

Roisman Reuth[1], Alex Beny[2], Reznick Abraham Zeev[3], Klemm Ofer[1], Raphaeli Guy[1] and Roisman Isaac[1]
[1]*Carmel College, Haifa,*
[2]*Rambam Medical Center, Haifa,*
[3]*Rapapport Faculty of Medicine, Technion - Israel Institute of Technology, Haifa, Israel*

Dedicated to Mrs. Minka Klavins and Prof. Janis V. Klavins
Albert Einstein College of Medicine, New York, NY, USA

1. Introduction

The incidence of breast cancer has increased greatly in Israel over the past decade. It is estimated that in Israel in 2009 approximately 4800 new patients will suffer from breast cancer. Despite recent advances in the diagnosis and treatment of breast cancer, this disease continues to be a major cause of death. One of the biggest challenges in breast cancer treatment is bone metastasis. Breast cancer cells are capable of migrating to the bone marrow and utilizing the marrow microenvironment to remain quiescent. The preprotachykinin-1 (PPT-I) gene encodes for the tachykinin peptides, which interact with neurokinin (NK) receptors. Studies have correlated this interaction with breast cancer cells integration into the bone marrow and breast cancer progression [(1)].

Environmental and psychological stresses have been shown to be associated with an increased incidence of cancer in man and animals. Stress-induced neuron chemical hormonal and immunological changes have been shown to influence tumor development. Stress may promote mammary carcinogenesis by affecting the neuroendocrine system and I or immune function. Neuroendocrine affects may involve changes in adrenocortical steroids or opioid peptides which may exert their effects by altering immune functions [(2)].

One of the risk factors for breast cancer is the increased amount of adipose tissue after menopause which elevates estradiol production.

The adrenergic system plays a role in regulating energy balance through thermogensis and lipid mobilization from brown or white adipose tissues [(3)].

The human fat cells are equipped with adrenergic receptors (adreno receptors) β1, β2 (ADRB1/2) and β3 (ADRB3) [(4)].

2. Physiology

The degree of affinity for adrenaline (epinephrine) is $\beta2 > \beta1 > \beta3$ and the noradrenaline (norephinephrine) it is $\beta1 \geq \beta2 > \beta3$ [(5)].

Norepinephrine, epinephrine and dopamine are members of biogenic amines. They share a common precursor - tyrosine. It is converted to L-dopa by tyrosine hydroxylase and L-dopa is converted to dopamine by dopa decarboxylase. In the nerve terminal dopamine is converted to norepinepherine.
If phenylethanol - N - methyl transferase (PNMT) is present norepinephrine is methylated to epinephrine. Adrenergic neurons secrete norepinephrine because they contain dopamine β hydroxylase.
Adreno receptors may be activated by norepinephrine, which is released from adrenergic neurons, or by epinephrine, which is secreted into the circulation by the adrenal medulla. Among the sympathetic adrenoreceptors, receptor type is related to function [6].
In addition to their role as neurotransmitters and stress hormones, catecholamines play a trophic role in the control of cell replication and differentiation in target cells that express adrenergic receptors. In some cell lines, β -adrenergic stimulation elicits a small, promotional effect on cell replication, whereas in others, stimulation of these receptors and the consequent rise in intracellular cAMP levels inhibits mitosis. β -adrenoreceptors on cancer cells, thus, recapitulate both the promotional and inhibitory roles of these receptors in cell replication seen in the development of normal cells.

2.1 Location and mechanism of autonomic action

Adrenoreceptor type	Target organ	Mechanism of action
α1	Vascular smooth muscle, skin, renal and splanchnic gastrointestinal tract, bladder sphincter, iris, radial muscle, sphincters	IP_3, increase of intracellular $[Ca^{2+}]$
α2	Gastrointestinal tract wall, presynaptic adrenergic neurons	Inhibition of adenylyl cyclase, decrease cAMP
β1	Heart, salivary gland, adipose tissue, kidney	stimulation of adenylyl cyclase, increase cAMP
β2	Va Vascular smooth muscle of skeletal muscle, GI wall, GI bladder wall, bronchioles	stimulation of adenylyl cyclase, increase cAMP

The β -adrenergic agonist isoproterenol, stimulates mammary epithelial cell division in vitro, as well as the development of end bud structures in the mammary gland of ovary ectomized mice from which arise the mammary carcinoma induced by administration of dimethylbenz (α) anthracene (DMBA). Specific β -adrenergic receptors of the β2 subtype are present in epithelial cell membranes from lactating mammary gland tissue.
The hormonal modulations of receptors which affect uterine contractility correlates with the onset of psychological responses of the uterus such as contraction and relaxation. In analogy with the uterus the regulation of the physiological status of the mammary gland is achieved by modification of endocrine, autonomic and mechanical factors during adolescence, the menstrual cycle, pregnancy parturition and lactation. The mammary gland, as other paired endocrine glands (adrenals, ovaries and testes), receives sympathetic innervations.
High levels of β -adrenergic receptors are measured as palpable mammary tumors, reaching a maximal concentration well before the actual increase in tumor mass. The hormone

sensitivity of the tumoral β -adrenergic receptor is further confirmed by the high receptor concentration measured in progressing mammary tumors.
Stress effects may involve ACTH, glucocorticoids, catecholamines, prolactin, opioids and immunosuppression, all factors crucially involved in tumor growth.
Catecholestrogens, their receptors, together with their catabolizing enzyme, catecholo-methyltransferease(COMT), are locally formed in both normal and neoplastic mammary tissues. COMT levels are significantly increased in the cytosol of malignant tumor cells than in the cytosol of benign tumor or normal cells (7).

2.2 Adrenoceptors and cancer

Recent studies in human cancer cell lines in animal models have shown that the growth of adenocarcinomas of the lungs, pancreas and colon are under β -adrenergic control (8-12).
The expression of β -adrenergic receptors has been correlated with the over-expression of the arachidonic acid-metabolizing enzymes cyclooxygenase-2 (COX-2) and lipoxygenases (LOX) in adenocarcinomas of lungs, colon, prostate and pancreas. Inhibitors of these enzymes have been identified as cancer preventive agents in animal models.

2.3 Adrenoceptors and breast cancer

Many of breast adenocarcinomas over express COX-2 and / or LOX (13).
This may say that a subset of breast cancers may also be under β adrenergic control.
Studies have demonstrated that three estrogen-responsive and three non-estrogen responsive human cell lines derived from breast adenocarcinoma show a reduction in DNA synthesis in response to beta-blockers or inhibitors of the arachidonic acid- metabolizing enzymes COX-2 and 5-LOX.
Another study analysis by reverse transcription polymerase chain reaction (RT-PCR) revealed expression of β_2-adrenergic receptors in all six breast cancer cell lines tested (MDA-MB-361, ZR-75-l, MCF-7, MDA-MB-453, MDA-MB-468, MDA-MB-4355).
β_1 receptors were not found in two estrogen non-responsive cell lines (MDA-MB*4355*, MDA-MB-453 (14).
It was found that the second messenger cAMP may be a growth promoter for mouse, rat and human mammary epithelioma (15, 16).
The effects of cAMP observed in malignant cells are involved in redifferentiation amounting to renormalization of number of properties including morphology, adhesive properties, lectin agglutination, cell movement and biochemical functions (17).
A correlation between β adreno receptor (β -AR) stimulation and estrogen and progesterone receptor functions was found in human breast cancer (18).
β_2-adrenergic stimulation induced cell proliferation in hormone-dependent human breast cancer cell line (C6-5), but without involving the female steroid hormone receptor system (18).
In C6-5 cells, the presence of functional β -AR's could be reasonable related to cell proliferation when exposed to different concentrations of clenbuterol, a β_2-AR agonist showed increased cell proliferation without involving significantly lower than that induced by oestradiol β adreno receptor-mediated inhibition of DNA synthesis was not shared by another cancer cell line, C6 rat glioma, that expresses a different β -receptor subtype a lower levels whereas found that MDA-MB-231 cells express β_2-receptors exclusively, C6 cell express primarily the β_1 subtype (19).
In mammary tissue there are data that support a role of catecholamines in the control of many cellular activities. Initial experiments indicate epinephrine sensitive adenylate cyclase

activities in 7, 12 - dimethylbenz (α) anthracene - induced mammary carcinoma. Two groups have demonstrated the presence of β -adrenergic receptors (β -AR) from mammary glands of lactating rats. β -adrenergic compounds stimulated the enzyme leading to the generation of cAMP and its activation was completely abolished by the β -AR blocking drug propranolol.

β -adrenergic - related increases in cAMP formation undoubtedly influence lactose production by the acinar secretory end pieces. The initial response to β -AR is usually an increase in adenylate cyclase activity resulting in an increased cellular cAMP concentration.

Among the epithelial, endocrine, and secretory cancer cell lines that express adrenoreceptors, MDA-MB-231 human breast cancer cells exhibit comparatively high concentrations. It is thus of critical interest that stimulation of these receptors leads to immediate inhibition of DNA synthesis and, with prolonged exposure, reductions in the total number of cancer cells: inhibition of DNA synthesis is a reliable predictor of chemotherapeutic responses in breast cancer cells.

In prostate or breast cancer cells stimulated by EGF or androgen or estradiol, small peptides (6-10 amino acids) derived from ER or AR sequences involved in the receptor interaction with Src, prevent AR/ER/Src association, Src/Erk pathway stimulation, cyclin D1 expression and DNA synthesis. The peptide action is restricted to cells expressing the steroid receptors and to signals mediated by these receptors. Remarkably, the peptides do not modify. Although there has been no systematic screening of breast cancer cell lines for β -adrenergic expression these receptors have identified in both estrogen-dependent type and estrogen-independent type, including C6-5, BF 20, T47-D, VHB-1 and MCF-7. Regardless of the ancillary mechanisms involved in β -receptor – mediated inhibition of mitosis in MDA-MB-231 breast cancer cells, the fact that inhibition does not disappear with receptor down regulation and desensitization raises the possibility for therapeutic strategies employing receptor agonists, alone or in combination with glucocorticoids and phosphodiesterase inhibitors [(20)].

Screening of human cancers for the presence of β -adrenoreceptors or other cAMP –linked neurotransmitter receptors may establish new treatment strategies.

β -adrenergic receptors (β -AR's) were identified in CG-5 breast cancer cells using a radiometric assay. The total β -AR concentration was measured using the highly potent β -adrenergic antagonist CGP 12 177, and the densities of β -AR subtypes were discriminated in the presence of highly selective unlabelled ligands (CGP 207 12A and ICI 118551).

The second messenger cAMP was found to be a growth promoter for mouse, rat and human mammary epithelioma and its levels are elevated in several breast carcinomas.

The effects of cAMP observed in malignant cells are often involved in redifferentiation, amounting to apparent renormalization of a number of properties including morphology, adhesive properties, lectin agglutination, cell movement and biochemical functions. A correlation between β -AR stimulation and estrogen and progesterone receptor functions was found in human breast cancer.

It was observed that β_2-adrenergic stimulation induced cell proliferation in a hormone-dependent human breast cancer cell line (CG-5), but without involving the female steroid hormone receptor system.

CG-5 cells (mammary breast cell cancer cell line) contain measurable concentrations of specific β AR's coupled to adenylate cyclase. The characteristics of these β -AR's, identified by binding and competition assays, are those of β_1-AR and β_2 -AR subtypes. β_2-AR concentration is significantly higher than β_1-AR concentration in CG-5 cell membranes.

Negligible concentrations of β -AR's were found in MCF-7 breast cancer cells from which CG-5 cells are derived. In C6-5 cells the presence of functional β -AR's could be reasonably related to cell proliferation when exposed to different concentrations of clenbuterol, a β_2-AR agonist, showed increased cell proliferation without involving steroid hormone receptors.
Although the enhancement of CG-5 cell growth was significantly lower than that induced by estradiol the presence of functional β -AR's (with the prevalence of the β 2-AR subtype) in tumor cell line suggests that β -adrenergic stimulation and resulting cAMP production may be responsible for CG-5 cell proliferation.
Medroxyprogesterone acetate (MPA) is one of the most widely used compounds in the endocrine therapy of advanced breast cancer in women. The mechanisms underlying the antitumor activity of MPA are poorly understood. This steroid presents a high affinity for progesterone (PgR) as well as for androgen (AR) and glucocorticoid receptors (GR) in human mammary tumors.
The most easily explained effects of MPA are related to its glucocorticoid-like action.
Suppression of adrenal function by MPA is believed to be caused both by an inhibitory action at the pituitary level and by direct inhibition of steroidogenesis.
In addition to ER and PgR, which are the most widely used markers of differentiated endocrine functions in breast cancer; AR and GR (Glucocorticoid receptors) are present in a substantial number of mammary tumors and established cell lines. The ZR-75-1 human breast cancer cell line is an unusually appropriate system to study the direct effect of MPA on cell growth. ZR-75-1 cells contain functional receptors for estrogens, androgens, progestins and glucocorticoids. Progestins inhibit ZR-75-1 cell proliferation exclusively in presence of estrogens and in absence of insulin.
MPA further decreased the growth of ZR-75- 1 cells co-incubated with maximally inhibitory concentrations of either 5 alpha-dihydrotestosterone ((DHT) or dexamethasone (DEX) although at about 300-fold higher MPA concentrations with DHT-treated than with DEX-treated ZR-75-1 cells, thus demonstrating a highly predominant androgenic effect. The main action of MPA on ZR-75-1 human breast cancer cell growth is due to its androgen receptor-mediated inhibitory action.
The majority of breast cancer are adenocarcinomas and many of them over express cyclooxygenase - 2 (COX-2) [(9)] and/or lipoxygenases (LOX). This raises the possibility that comparable to findings in adenocarcinomas of the lungs, pancreas, colon and prostate, and a subset of breast cancer may also be under beta adrenergic control. Studies have demonstrated that three estrogen-responsive and three non-estrogen responsive human cell lines derived from breast adenocarcinomas demonstrated a significant reduction in DNA synthesis in response to beta-blockers or inhibitors of the arachidonic acid metabolizing enzymes COX-2 [(9)] and LOX-5.
Analysis by reverse transcription polymerase chain reaction (RT-PCR) revealed expression of β_2-adrenergic receptors in all six breast cancer cell tested (MDA-MB- 361, ZR-75-1, MCF-7, MDA-MB -453, MDA-MB-468, MDA-MB-435S) whereas β_1 receptors were not found in two estrogen non-responsive cell lines (MDA-MB-435S, MDA-MB-453).
Expression of mRNA that encodes a G-protein coupled inward by rectifying potassium channel 1 (GIRK1) [(7)] has been shown in 40% breast cancer samples. This expression of GIRK1 was associated with a more aggressive clinical behavior. Previous studies indicated that the beta-adrenergic agonist isoproterenol stimulates growth. GIRK currents have been shown to be increased in cells stimulated with the beta-adrenergic agonist isoproterenol in rat atrial myocytes transferred with β_1 or β_2 receptors. Two po1ymorphisms in the β_2 or β_3

adrenergic receptors were found to be correlated with decreased risk for breast cancer, suggesting an important role of this receptor family in the genesis of breast cancer.
In C6-5 cells [16, 19] the presence of functional β -AR's could be reasonable related to cell proliferation when exposed to different concentration of clenbuterol, a β_2-AR agonist showed increased cell proliferation without involving significantly lower than that induced by estradiol β adreno receptor-mediated inhibition of DNA synthesis was not shared by another cancer cell line, C6 rat glioma, that expresses a different β -receptor subtype a lower levels whereas [20] found that MOA-MB-23 1 cells express β_2-receptors exclusively, C6 cell express primarily the β_1 subtype.
There is increasing evidence that describes a histamine role in normal and cancer cell proliferation. To better understand the importance of histamine in breast cancer development, the expression of histamine H3 (H3R) and H4 (H4R) receptors and their association with proliferating cell nuclear antigen (PCNA), histidine decarboxylase (HDC) and histamine content were explored in mammary biopsies. Additionally, we investigated whether H3R and H4R were implicated in the biological responses triggered by histamine in MDA-MB-231[20] breast cancer cells.
Centrally assess estrogen receptor (ER) and progesterone receptor (PgR) levels by immunohistochemistry and investigate their predictive value for benefit of chemo-endocrine compared with endocrine adjuvant therapy alone in two randomized clinical trials for node-negative breast cancer.
Low levels of ER and PgR are predictive of the benefit of adding chemotherapy to endocrine therapy. Low PgR may add further predictions among pre-and perimenopausal but not postmenopausal patient whose tumors express ER.
The majority of all breast cancers are hormone responsive, traditionally defined by he expression of oestogen receptor (ER) alpha and/or progesterone receptors. In contrast to ERalpha, the clinical significance of the relatively recently identified ERbeta is still unclear.
ERalpha and ERbeta seem to be differentially associated to clinicopathological parameters, and this would support the fact that they might have different functions in vivo.
In prostate or breast cancer cells stimulated by EGF or androgen or estradiol, small peptides (6-10 amino acids) derived from ER or AR sequences involved in the receptor interaction with Src, prevent AR/ER/Src association, Src/Erk pathway stimulation, cyclin D1 expression and DNA synthesis. The peptide action is restricted to cells expressing the steroid receptors and to signals mediated by these receptors. Remarkably, the peptides do no modify!
Epidermal growth factor (EGF), transforming growth factor-alpha (TGFalpha), amphiregulin (AREG), betacellulin (BTC), heparin-binding EGF-like growth factor (HB-EGF),epiregulin (EREG) and neuregulins1-4 (NRG1-4) were quantified in 363 tumors by real-time reverse transcription-polymerase chain reaction using TaqMan probes.
Paget's disease (PD) of the breast as well as the vulva is a rare condition, therefore anti-hormonal therapy is not indicated. The high frequency of Her-2/neu and COX-2 overexpression, however, suggests that these molecules could be therapeutically relevant in patients with PD.
Epidemiological evidence indicates that the association between body weight and breast cancer risk may differ across menopausal status as well as the estrogen receptor (ER) and progesterone receptor (PR) tumor status.
The relation between body weight and breast cancer risk is critically dependent on the tumor's ER/PR status and the woman's menopausal status. Body weith control is the effective strategy for preventing ER+PR+ tumors after menopause.

ErbB3 transactivation can make tumor cells resistance to ErbB1/ErbB2 targeting drugs. This urges for a reliable method to determine cel surface ErbB3 levels, but their hands iodinated NRG1 beta is unstable and tends to underestimate the umber of ErbB3 receptors in a radio-receptor assay.

Furthermore, they show by differential competition with unlabled NRG/YYDLL and betacellulin that the number of ErbB3 and ErbB4 receptors can be quantified separately on cultured human breast cancer cells.

Esterogen receptor (ER) antagonists have been widely used for breast cancer treatment, but the efficacy and drug resistance remain to be clinical concerns. The purpose of this study was to determine whether the extracts of coptis, an anti-inflammatory herb, improve the anticancer efficacy of ER antagonists, Their results showed that the combined treatment of ER antagonists and the crude extract of coptis or its purified compound berberine conferred synergetic growth inhibitory effect on MCF-7 cells (ER+), but not on MDA-MB-231 cells (R-). Similar results were observed in the combined treatment of fulvestrant, a specific aromatase antagonist. Analysis of the expression of breast cancer related genes indicated the EGFR, HER2, bci-2, and COX-2 were significantly downregulated, while IFN-beta and p21 were remarkably upregulated by herberine.

The negative association between he oestrogen receptor (ER) and the human epidermal growth factor 2 (HER-2) in breast cancer travels in both directions. ER+ tumors are less likely HER-2+ and HER-2+ are less likely ER+. Studies the age-related immunohistochemical (IHC) expression of ER, HER-2 in 2,227 tumors using age as a continuous variable [21].

Estrogen receptors (ERs) are overexpressed in human breast cancers (BCs) and associated with differentiated tumors and with a more favorable prognosis [22-34].

Paradoxically, ERs mediate the mitogenic action of estrogens in human BC cells and the efficacy of antiestrogens in adjuvant therapy of primary tumors. The exact mechanism underlying the ER protection against cancer progression to metastasis remains to be investigated. They show that ERs decrease invasiveness of BC cells. Detailed studies revealed that the unliganded and the E2-activated ERs decrease cancer cell invasion in vitro through two distinct mechanisms. In the presence of ligand, ERalpha inhibits invasion through a mechanism requiring the functional ERalpha domains involved in the transcriptional activation of target genes.

Hormone receptors play important roles in breast cancer. The expression of hormone receptors in breast cancer was investigated to evaluate the importance of hormone receptors in the clinicopathology of breast cancer.

Androgen receptor (AR), estrogen receptor (ER) and progesterone receptor (PR) expression characteristics were evaluated using immunohistochemistry stain, comparing patient age, tumor size and axillary lymph node status for 23 pure mucinous and 105 non-mucinous infiltrating ductal carcinomas in the human female breast.

Findings revealed that mucinous carcinoma samples from the breast show distinct clinicopathologic and hormone receptor expression features compared to non-mucinous carcinoma.

There is increasing evidence that describes a histamine role in normal and cancer cell proliferations. To better understand the importance of histamine in breast cancer development, the expression of histamine H3 (H3R) nad H4 (H4R) receptors and their association with proliferating cell nuclear antigen (PCNA), histidine decarboxylase (HDC) and histamine content were explored in mammary biopsies. Additionally, we investigated whether H3R and H4R were implicated in the biological MDA-MB-231 breast cancer cells.

β -adrenergic receptors (β -AR's) were identified in C6-5 breast cancer cells using a radiometric assay. The total β -AR concentration was measured using the highly potent β -adrenergic antagonist CGP 12 177, and the densities of β -AR subtypes were discriminated in the presence of highly selective unlabelled ligands (CGP 20712A and ICI 118551).
The second messenger cAMP was found to be a growth promoter for mouse, rat and human mammary epithelioma and its levels are elevated in several breast carcinomas.
It was observed that β_2-adrenergic stimulation induced cell proliferation in a hormone dependent human breast cancer cell line (CG-5), but without involving the female steroid hormone receptor system. CG-5 cells (mammary breast cell cancer cell line) contain measurable concentrations of specific β AR's coupled to adenylate cyclase. The characteristics of these β -AR's, identified by binding and competition assays, are those of β_1-AR and β_2-AR subtypes. β_2-AR concentration is significantly higher than β_1-AR concentration in CG-5 cell membranes. Negligible concentrations of β –AR's were found in MCF-7 breast cancer cells from which CG-5 cells are derived.
Although the enhancement of CG-5 cell growth was significantly lower than that induced by estradiol the presence of functional β -AR's (with the prevalence of the β_2- subtype AR) in tumor cell line suggests that β -adrenergic stimulation and resulting cAMP production may be responsible for CG-S cell proliferation.
Medroxyprogesterone acetate (MPA) is one of the most widely used compounds in the endocrine therapy of advanced breast cancer in women.
The mechanisms underlying the antitumor activity of MPA are poorly understood.
This steroid presents a high affinity for progesterone (PgR) as well as for androgen (AR) and glucocorticoid receptors (GR) in human mammary tumors.
The most easily explained effects of MPA are related to its glucocorticoid-like action.
Suppression of adrenal function by MPA is believed to be caused both by an inhibitory action at the pituitary level and by direct inhibition of steroidogenesis.
In addition to ER and PgR, which are the most widely used markers of differentiated endocrine functions in breast cancer; AR and GR are present in a substantial number of mammary tumors and established cell lines. The ZR-75-1 human breast cancer cell line is an unusually appropriate system to study the direct effect of MPA on cell growth. ZR-75-1 cells contain functional receptors for estrogens, androgens progestins and glucocorticoids. Progestins inhibit ZR-75- 1 cell proliferation exclusively in presence of estrogens and in absence of insulin.
MPA further decreased the growth of ZR-75-1 cells co-incubated with maximally inhibitory concentrations of either 5 alpha-dihydrotestosterone (DHT) or dexamethasone (DEX) at about 300-fold higher MPA concentrations with DHT-treated than with DEX-treated ZR-75-1 cells, thus demonstrating a highly predominant androgenic effect. The main action of MPA on ZR-75-1 human breast cancer cell growth is due to its androgen receptor-mediated inhibitory action.

3. Summary

In normal and malignant mammary tissues there are data supporting a role for catecholeamines in the control of many cellular activities. The presence of functional β-AR's in human mammary cell lines has been described. All six breast cell lines express either GIRK2 or GIRK4 indicating that functional GIRK potassium channels are possible in these cancer cell lines. The direct control of cell proliferation shown in vitro could eventually open new avenues for adjuvant therapies in the treatment of breast diseases.

4. References

[1] Reddy BY, Trzaska KA, Murthy RG, et al. Neurokinin receptors as potential targets in breast cancer treatment. Curr Drug Discov Technol, 2008; 5:15-19
[2] Tejwani GA, Gudehithlu KP, Hanissian SH, et al. Facilitation of dimethylbenz[α]antracene- induced rat mammary tumorigensis by restraint stress: role of β-endorphin, prolactin and naltrexone. Carcinogenesis, 1991; 12:637-641.
[3] Lafontan M, Berlan M. Fat cell adrenergic receptors and the control of white and brown fat cell function. J Lipid Res. 1993; 34:1057-1091.
[4] Huang XE, Hamajima N, Sito T, et al. Possible association of beta2- and beta3-adrenergic receptor gene polymorphism with susceptibility to breast cancer. Breast Cancer Res. 2001; 3: 264-269. Epub 2001 Apr 26.
[5] Arch JR, Kaumann AJ. Beta 3 and atypical beta-adrenoceptors. Med Res Rev. 1993; 13:663-729.
[6] Marchetti B, Spinola PG, Pelletier G, et al. A potential role for catecholamines in the development and progression of carcinogen-induced mammary tumors: hormonal control of beta-adrenergic receptors and correlation with tumor growth. J Steroid Biochem Mol Biol. 1991; 38:307-320.
[7] Plummer HK, Yu Q, Cakir Y, et al. Expression of inwardly rectifying potassium channels (GIRKs) and beta-adrenergic regulation of breast cancer cell lines. BMC Cancer. 2004;4:93
[8] Schuller HM, Tithof PK, Williams M, et al. The tobacco-specific carcinogen 4-(methylnitrosamino)-1-(3-pyridyl)-1-butanone is a beta-adrenergic agonist and stimulates DNA synthesis in lung adenocarcinoma via beta-adrenergic receptor-mediated release of arachidonic acid. Cancer Res. 1999; 59:4510-4515.
[9] Schuller HM, Plummer HK, Bochsler PN, et al. Co-expression of beta adrenergic receptors and cyclooxygenase-2 in pulmonary adenocarcinoma. Int J Oncol. 2001; 19:445-449.
[10] Schuller HM, Porter B, Riechert A. Beta-adrenergic modulation of NNK-induced lung carcinogenesis in hamsters. J Cancer Res Clin Oncol.2000; 126:624-630.
[11] Masur K, Niggemann B, Zanker KS, et al. Norepinephrine-induced migration of SW 480 colon carcinoma cells is inhibited by beta-blockers. Cancer Res. 2001; 61:2866-2869.
[12] Weddle DL, Tithoff P, Williams M, et al. Beta-adrenergic growth regulation of human cancer cell lines derived from pancreatic ductal carcinoma. Carcinogenesis. 2001; 22: 473-479.
[13] Parrett ML, Harris RE, Joarder FS, et al. Cyclooxygenase-2 gene expression in human breast cancer. Int J Oncology. 1997; 10:503-507.
[14] Cakir Y, Plummer HK, Tithof PK, et al. Beta-adrenergic and arachidonic acid-mediated growth regulation of human breast cancer cell lines. Int J Oncol. 2002; 21:153-157.
[15] Yang Y, Guzman R, Richards J, et al. Growth factor- and cyclic nucleotide-induced proliferation of normal and malignant mammary epithelial cells in primary culture. Endocrinology. 1980; 107:35-41.
[16] Badino GR, Novelli A, Girardi C, et al. Evidence for functional beta-adenoceptors subtypes in CG-5 breast cancer cell. Pharmacol Res. 1996; 33:255-260.
[17] Yabushita H, Sartorelli AC. Effects of sodium butyrate, dimethylsulfoxide and dibutyryl cAMP on the poorly differentiated ovarian adenocarcinoma cell line AMOC-2. Oncol Res.1993; 5:173-182.
[18] Draoui A, Vandewalle B, Hornez L, et al. Beta-adrenergic receptors in human breast cancer: identification, characterization and correlation with progesterone and estradiol receptors. Anticancer Res. 1991; 11:677-680.

[19] Re G, Badino P, Girardi C, et al. Effects of beta-2 agonist (clenbuterol) on cultured human (CG-5) breast cancer cells. Pharmacol Res. 1992; 26:377-384.

[20] Slotkin TA, Zhang J, Dancel R, et al. Beta-adrenoceptor signaling and its control of cell replication in MDA-MB-231 human breast cancer cells. Breast Cancer Res Treat. 2000; 60:153-166.

[21] Neven P, Van Calster B, Van den Bempt I, et al. Age interacts with the expression of steroid and HER-2 receptors in operable invasive breast cancer. Breast Cancer Res Treat. 2008; 110:153-159.

[22] Maynadier M, Nirdé P, Ramirez JM, et al. Role of estrogens and their receptors in adhesion and invasiveness of breast cancer cells. Adv Exp Med Biol. 2008; 617: 485-489.

[23] Cho LC, Hsu YH. Expression of androgen, estrogen and progesterone receptors in mucinous carcinoma of the breast. Kaohsiung Med Sci. 2008; 24: 227-232.

[24] Medina V, Croci M, Crescenti E, et al. The role of histamine in human mammary carcinogenesis: H3 and H4 receptors as potential therapeutic targets for breast cancer treatment. Cancer Biol Ther. 2008; 7: 28-35.

[25] Subbaramaiah K, Hudis C, Chang SH, et al. EP2 and EP4 receptors regulate aromatase expression in human adipocytes and breast cancer cells. Evidence of a BRCA1 and p300 exchange. J Biol Chem. 2008; 283: 3433-3444.

[26] Viale G, Regan MM, Maiorano E, et al. Chemoendocrine compared with endocrine adjuvant therapies for node-negative breast cancer: predictive value of centrally reviewed expression of estrogen and progesterone receptors – International Breast Cancer Study Group. J Clin Oncol. 2008; 26: 1404-1410.

[27] Borgquist S, Holm C, Stendahl M, et al. Oestrogen receptors alpha and beta show different association to clinicopathological parameters and their co-expression might predict a better response to endocrine treatment in breast cancer. Clin Pathol. 2008; 61: 197-203.

[28] Auricchio F, Migliaccio A, Castoria G. Sex-steroid hormones and EGF signalling in breast and prostate cancer cells: targeting the association of Src with steroid receptors. Steroids. 2008; 73: 880-884.

[29] Révillion F, Lhotellier V, Hornez L, et al. ErbB/HER ligands in human breast cancer; and relationships with their receptors the bio-pathological features and prognosis. Ann Oncol. 2008;19:73-80.

[30] Horn LC, Purz S, Krumpe C, et al. COX-2 and Her-2/neu are overexpressed in Paget's disease of the vulva and the breast: results of a preliminary study. Arch Gynecol Obstet. 2008; 277: 135-138.

[31] Dawood S, Broglio K, Kau SW, et al. Triple receptor-negative breast cancer: the effect of race on response to primary systemic treatment and survival outcomes. J Clin Oncol. 2009; 27:220-226.

[32] Suzuki R, Orsini N, Saji S, et al. Body weight and incidence of breast cancer defined by estrogen and progesterone receptor status - a meta-analysis. Int J Cancer. 2009; 124: 698-712.

[33] Van der woning SP and van Zoelen EJ. Quantification of $ErbB_3$ receptor density on human breast cancer cells, using a stable radio-labeled mutant of NRG1beta. Biochem Biophys Res Commun. 2009; 378: 285-289.

[34] Lui J, He C, Zhou K, et al. Coptis extracts enhance the anticancer effect of estrogen receptor antagonists on human breast cancer cells. Biochem Biophys Res Commun. 2009; 378: 174-178.

35

Steroid Receptor Coactivators and Their Expression, Regulation and Functional Role in Endocrine Responsive and Resistant Breast Cancer

Line L. Haugan Moi[1,3], Marianne Hauglid Flågeng[1], Ingvild S. Fenne[1], Jennifer Gjerde[1], Ernst A. Lien[1,2] and Gunnar Mellgren[1,2]
[1]*Institute of Medicine, University of Bergen*
[2]*The Hormone Laboratory, Haukeland University Hospital*
[3]*Department of Clinical Pathology, University Hospital of North Norway*
Norway

1. Introduction

Breast cancer is the most frequent malignancy and one of the leading causes to cancer related deaths in women. Most human breast cancers express the estrogen receptor (ER) which belongs to the family of nuclear receptors and is a ligand-regulated transcription factor. It is well established that the natural ligand of ER, estrogen, has pro-carcinogenic and growth promoting effects in the mammary epithelium by stimulating proliferation and leaving the cells prone to mutations during cell cycle progression (Foster et al., 2001). Endocrine treatment of hormone sensitive breast cancer targets the estrogen activity in breast cancer cells by blocking the ER with a selective ER modulator (SERM) such as tamoxifen or inhibiting estrogen synthesis using aromatase inhibitors such as anastrozole or letrozole. Endocrine treatment decreases mortality, prolongs disease-free survival and can even reduce the incidence of breast cancer in women at increased risk (Cuzick et al., 2003). Approximately 70 % of women with ER positive tumors respond to endocrine therapy, but resistance do occur, either *de novo* or develop over time. The molecular mechanism involved in endocrine resistance is one of the central areas of breast cancer research.

The trancriptional activity of the ER is not only regulated by its ligands, but also by the level and activity of coregulator proteins. Nuclear receptor coactivators serve as adapters between the receptor and the trancriptional machinery. They possess diverse enzymatic acitivities such as histone acetyltransferase, histone methyltransferase, chromatin remodeling and ubiquitin-conjugation activity and are involved in every step of ER regulated transcription, from chromatin remodeling to transcriptional termination. The members of the p160 family of coactivators are some of the best studied coactivators. These steroid receptor coactivators (SRCs) are small proteins of 160 kDa with similar structural and functional properties, and include SRC-1, SRC-2/transcription intermediary factor-2 (TIF-2) and SRC-3/amplified in breast cancer 1 (AIB1). The SRCs are not only crucial to ER mediated effects in normal tissue. They have also been shown to be involved in the carcinogenic process and are overexpressed in breast cancer. In addition, the SRCs are of relevance to the tissue-specific effects of tamoxifen and data suggest that they may be important to the cellular sensitivity to endocrine treatment. The SRCs and their expression, regulation and functional role during endocrine treatment in breast cancer *in vitro* and *in vivo* are the focus of this chapter.

2. Expression and functional role of SRCs in breast tissue

The SRCs are genetically distinct, but have structural similarities with 40 - 55 % sequence homology (Xu & Li, 2003). Although the SRCs have similar functional properties, experimental evidence indicates different physiological functions for the SRCs, which in part can be explained by tissue-specific expression levels, different affinities for the various nuclear receptors and variations in post-translational modifications (Chauchereau et al., 2003; Fenne et al., 2008; Hoang et al., 2004; Wu et al., 2004; Xu et al., 2009). In the classical activation of ER-mediated gene transcription, the ligand estradiol (E2) binds to the ER and promotes binding of the ER-E2 complex to the estrogen receptor element (ERE) of the target gene promoter. Here they recruit coregulatory proteins to a multi-subunit complex for gene transcription (Mangelsdorf et al., 1995; Pearce & Jordan, 2004). The ER has an activation function-1 (AF-1) domain in the N-terminus whereas the centrally located DNA-binding domain (DBD) is responsible for specific binding of the ER to EREs on target genes. The dimerization domain contains the ligand binding domain (LBD) and the AF-2. The AF-1 contributes to the constitutive estrogen-independent activation by the receptor and is separated by a hinge region from the AF-2. The SRCs have a basic helix-loop-helix (bHLH) domain, a Per-Arnt-Sim (PAS) domain and a nuclear hormone interaction domain (NID) including three LXXLL-sequences where L is leucine and X any amino acid (Fig. 1).

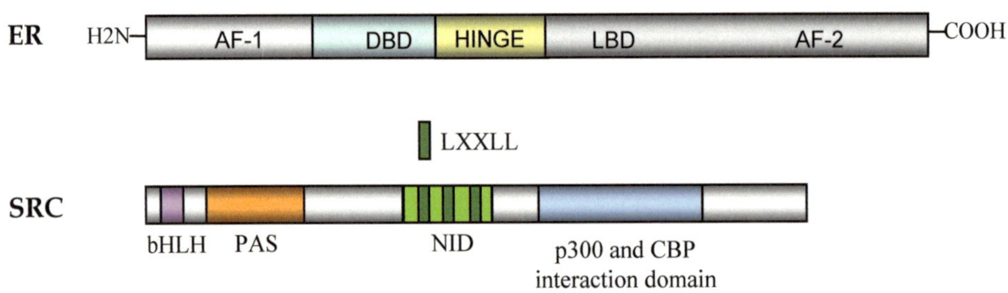

Fig. 1. Schematic presentation of the functional domains of the ER and the SRCs.

Upon ligand binding, the helix 12 of the ER is positioned across the LBD, and together with helices 3-5 form a hydrophobic groove where the LXXLL motifs of coactivators can bind (Heery et al., 1997). The coactivators in the multi-subunit protein complex alter the chromatin structure and facilitate recruitment of the RNA polymerase II and the basal transcriptional machinery in a programmed cyclic manner to initiate transcription of the target gene (Metivier et al., 2003).

The SRC family members are widely expressed and are detected in tissues such as placenta, testis, pancreas, lung, kidney, liver and brain (Xu & O'Malley, 2002; Xu & Li, 2003). The expression levels of the three SRC proteins in normal human breast epithelial cells are variable, but usually very low (Xu et al., 2009). SRCs are known to be overexpressed in several types of human cancers, including breast cancer, where their overexpression is due to enhanced cellular amplification of their genes, and/or by a decrease in the intracellular degradation process of the coactivators (Xu et al., 2009). The SRCs are known to contribute to proliferation and development of breast cancers by mechanisms such as stimulation of the G1 to S phase transition during cell cycle by regulation of expression of mitogenic genes such as *c-MYC* and *cyclin D1* (Dubik & Shiu, 1992; Sabbah et al., 1999).

2.1 SRC-1

SRC-1 was the first nuclear receptor coactivator to be cloned and identified (Onate et al., 1995). The gene is located on the short arm of chromosome 2 at position 2p23 (Carapeti et al., 1998). SRC-1$^{-/-}$ mice show partial steroid hormone resistance and hepatic insufficiency (Xu et al., 1998; Louet et al., 2010). Noteworthy, ovariectomized female SRC-1$^{-/-}$ mice have decreased uterine growth and reduced mammary gland ductal side branching and alveolar formation in response to estrogen compared with wild-type mice, indicating a role of SRC-1 in estrogen-regulated breast development (Xu et al., 1998; Xu & Li, 2003). We found higher SRC-1 mRNA levels by real-time RT-PCR in human breast cancer samples compared to normal breast tissue (Haugan Moi et al., 2010), and the same has been observed at the protein level (Hudelist et al., 2003; Fleming et al., 2004b; Myers et al., 2004). SRC-1 protein expression in breast cancer has been reported to associate positively with human epidermal growth factor receptor 2/neu (HER-2/neu) and negatively with ERβ (Fleming et al., 2004b). *In vitro* studies indicate that SRC-1 plays an important role in ER-mediated growth of breast cancer cells. Overexpression of SRC-1 potentiates E2-stimulated growth of MCF-7 breast cancer cells in accordance with an increase in the expression of estrogen-responsive genes (Tai et al., 2000). SRC-1 has also been reported to specifically promote breast cancer metastasis, possibly by promoting migration and invasion by enhancing PEA3 mediated transcriptional activation of Twist, a master regulator of metastasis (Qin et al., 2009). Furthermore, SRC-1 may promote metastasis in mammary tumors by facilitating Ets-2 mediated HER-2/neu expression and activating colony stimulating factor-1 expression to recruit macrophages to mammary tumors in mice (Wang et al., 2009).

2.2 SRC-2/TIF-2

The human SRC-2/TIF-2 gene is located on the long arm of chromosome 8 at position 8q21 (Kalkhoven et al., 1998). Knock-out experiments indicate that SRC-2/TIF-2 are of special relevance to fertility and fat metabolism where SRC-2/TIF-2$^{-/-}$ mice have defective spermatogenesis, testicular degeneration, placenta hypoplasia, male and female hypofertility, higher lipolysis in white fat, higher energy expenditure in brown fat and resistance to obesity (Gehin et al., 2002; Picard et al., 2002). Increased levels of SRC-2/TIF-2 mRNA have been observed in intraductal and invasive carcinoma compared to normal breast tissue (Kurebayashi et al., 2000; Haugan Moi et al., 2010). Knockdown of SRC-2/TIF-2 has been shown to inhibit growth of MCF-7 breast cancer cells due to decreased cell proliferation, increased apoptosis and reduced ER mediated transcriptional activity (Cavarretta et al., 2002; Karmakar et al., 2009). However, overall SRC-2/TIF-2 is the least studied of the coactivators in breast cancer.

2.3 SRC-3/AIB1

The third member of the SRC family, SRC-3/AIB1, is located on the long arm of chromosome 20 at position 20q12 in humans and was first identified as a gene amplified and overexpressed in several human breast cancer cell lines (Anzick et al., 1997). The *SRC-3/AIB1* gene is found to be amplified in 5-10% of breast cancer cases, and SRC-3/AIB1 are overexpressed at mRNA and protein level in 20-60 % of breast cancer patients (Anzick et al., 1997; Takeshita et al., 1997; Bautista et al., 1998; Murphy et al., 2000; Bouras et al., 2001; List et al., 2001; Hudelist et al., 2003; Zhao et al., 2003). Female SRC-3/AIB1$^{-/-}$ mice have significantly lower levels of estrogen and delayed mammary gland development, indicating a proliferative role of this coactivator in breast tissue (Xu et al., 2000). In transgenic mice, overexpression of SRC-3/AIB1 leads to development of tumors in several organs including breast, in addition to increased expression of the insulin-like growth factor-1 (IGF-1) and activation of intracellular pathways suggesting that SRC-3/AIB1 is acting as an oncogene (Torres-Arzayus et al., 2004). The oncogenic potential of SRC-3/AIB1 has been ascribed to mechanisms such as enhanced interaction between ER and the *cyclin D1* promoter, hence leading to increased levels of cyclin D1 and stimulation of cell cycle progression (Planas-Silva et al., 2001). Conversely, cyclin D1 expression has been shown to be reduced in SRC-3/AIB1 knock-out cells (Karmakar et al., 2009), and mice with reduced SRC-3/AIB1 expression have a decrease in epithelial proliferation associated with a reduction in cyclin expression (Fereshteh et al., 2008). Overexpression of SRC-3/AIB1 also stimulates the Akt signaling pathway which promotes cell growth (Torres-Arzayus et al., 2004; Zhou et al., 2003). Matrix metalloproteinases (MMPs) are zink-dependent enzymes involved in the degradation of extracellular matrix and are essential to the metastatic process. Experimental evidence suggests that SRC-3/AIB1 promotes breast cancer metastasis by stimulating the transcription factor PEA3 to enhance expression of MMP2 and MMP9 (Qin et al., 2008).

2.4 Regulation of SRCs expression during endocrine treatment

Most studies seem to indicate higher levels of the SRCs in malignant breast tumors compared to normal breast tissue. However, the expression levels of the SRCs have been shown to change during endocrine treatment in breast cancer. In a clinical study of preoperative tamoxifen treatment for 4 weeks using tamoxifen doses from 1 to 20 mg/daily, we found the mRNA levels of all three SRCs to be significantly upregulated in tamoxifen treated normal and malignant breast tissue compared to samples from untreated patients. The increase in coactivator mRNA expression was especially evident for SRC-3/AIB1 (Haugan Moi et al., 2010). In a clinical study on neoadjuvant treatment with aromatase inhibitors in locally advanced breast cancer, we also found the mRNA levels of coactivators in tumors to increase during treatment, especially for SRC-1 (Flågeng et al., 2009). This is in line with *in vitro* studies. E2 has been shown to repress SRC-3/AIB1 mRNA and protein expression in MCF-7 human breast cancer cells primarily by suppressing SRC-3/AIB1 gene transcription (Lauritsen et al., 2002). Conversely, total SRC-3/AIB1 mRNA levels were increased when MCF-7 breast cancer cells were treated with the antiestrogen 4-hydroxytamoxifen. 4-hydroxtamoxifen has also been shown to increase the stability and hence steady-state levels of SRC-1 and SRC-3/AIB1 proteins in a MCF-7 breast cancer-derived cell line (Lonard et al., 2004). We also found an increase in the mRNA levels of HER-2/neu and a positive correlation between SRC-1 and HER-2/neu in human breast tissue treated with aromatase inhibitors. This finding is interesting in light of *in vitro* assays suggesting that ER and HER-2/neu compete for the coactivator SRC-1. Under antiestrogenic conditions, SRC-1 will be released from the ER and may instead bind to the HER-2/neu enhancer and facilitate transcription of HER-2/neu, leading to increased expression of HER-2/neu under estrogen deprived conditions (Newman et al., 2000).

3. SRCs and endocrine treatment in breast cancer: Molecular mechanisms

The regulation of SRCs during endocrine treatment is especially interesting since the coactivators are directly involved in the molecular mechanisms underlying the antiestrogenic effects. The natural ligand of ER, estrogen, is converted from androgens by the enzyme aromatase. Endocrine treatment of ER positive breast cancer includes aromatase inhibitors or the SERM tamoxifen. Aromatase inhibitors block the synthesis of estrogens by binding to and suppressing the aromatase enzyme that converts androgens to estrogens. Tamoxifen binds to the ER and functions as an antagonist in breast tissue and prevents estrogen from binding to the ER. The net effect of both therapeutic regiments is to block ER-dependent transcriptional regulation of genes and prevent proliferation (Fig. 2).

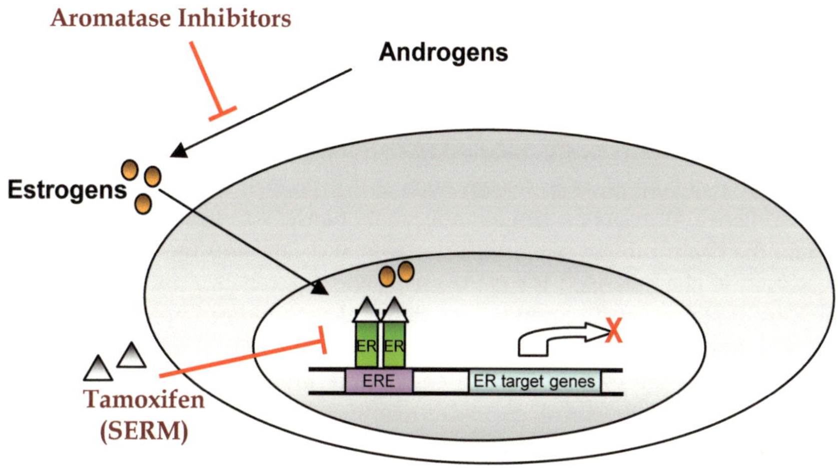

Fig. 2. Schematic presentation of the mechanisms of action of endocrine treatment in breast cancer using tamoxifen or aromatase inhibitors.

3.1 The SERM tamoxifen

Tamoxifen is a synthetic estrogen antagonist which has been in clinical use for over 30 years. While the success of tamoxifen in breast cancer therapy is based on its ER antagonistic effects in malignant breast tissue, tamoxifen demonstrates ER agonistic effects in other organ systems such as bone and liver. ER appears to bind to corepressors in the presence of SERMs in breast tissue, while coactivator recruitment is favored when E2 is bound to ER. Upon binding to ER, SERMs inhibit ER transcriptional activity by competing with E2 for the binding site and by blocking the AF-2 activity of ER (Shiau et al., 1998; Brzozowski et al., 1997). The potent ER antagonistic metabolite 4-hydroxytamoxifen induces a displacement and rotation of the receptor's helix 12. The helix 12 then binds to the hydrophobic pocket via a sequence resembling the NR box of the coactivators, and thereby inhibits coactivator recruitment (Brzozowski et al., 1997; Shiau et al., 1998). The binding of 4-hydroxytamoxifen instead favors recruitment of the two corepressors silencing mediator for retinoid and thyroid hormone receptor (SMRT) and nuclear receptor corepressor (NCoR). These corepressors are associated with histone deacetylase activity and inhibit ER regulated gene transcription (Webb et al., 2003; Fleming et al., 2004a).

However, tamoxifen may exert ER agonistic effects depending on the coactivator context. For example, it has been shown that overexpression of SRC-3/AIB1 and the growth factor HER-2/neu increases the ER agonistic properties of tamoxifen (Shou et al., 2004) and that tamoxifen resistance develops when SRC-3/AIB1 is high and the transcriptional repressor paired box 2 (PAX2) is low in breast cancer cells (Hurtado et al., 2008). Elevated expression of SRC-1 in the uterine derived Ishikawa cell line increases the agonist behavior of 4-hydroxytamoxifen, whereas lower expression of SRC-1 in MCF-7 cells contributed to an ER-antagonistic behavior of tamoxifen (Shang & Brown., 2002). Studies have shown that the estrogenic effects of tamoxifen can be mediated by the constitutive active AF-1 domain of ER which can be stimulated by several mechanisms, including high levels of coactivators (Webb et al., 1998). Hence, the levels of SRCs may determine the response to tamoxifen treatment, at least *in vitro*.

3.2 Aromatase inhibitors

Aromatase inhibitors work by blocking the estrogen synthesis and depriving the breast cancer cells of this important growth factor. In premenopausal women, estrogens are primarily synthesized by the granulose cells in the ovaries, but aromatase activity and conversion of androgens to estrogens also take place in tissues such as subcutaneous fat, breast tissue and bone which are the primary sources of estrogens after menopause. Aromatase is a cytochrome P450 enzyme where the haem protein binds the androgen and catalyzes the formation of the phenolic A-ring which is characteristic for estrogens. Type 1 aromatase inhibitors such as formestane and exemestane, also known as steroidal inhibitors, are analogues to androstenedione and work by competitive binding to the active site of aromatase. Type 2 aromatase inhibitors include the first generation compound aminoglutethimide, the second generation drug fadrozole and the third generation compounds anastrozole and letrozole, which are widely used clinically. These non-steroidal aromatase inhibitors work by binding to an iron atom in the haem group of aromatase and have proved very effective in inhibiting aromatase activity. In the absence of agonist, the ER will be locacted in the cytoplasm associated with heat shock protein (hsp), and dimerization, conformational changes and coactivator recruitment will be inhibited, hence leading to reduced transcription of ER-regulated genes. However, resistance to aromatase inhibitors does occur. In the frequently used cellular model system for resistance to aromatase inhibitors, breast cancer cells are grown in estrogen-deprived conditions for 1-6 months. These long-term estrogen deprived cells (LTED) develop enhanced sensitivity to E2 (Masamura et al., 1995; Santen et al., 2005). This hypersensitivity is associated with upregulation of ERα and the mitogen activated protein kinases (MAPKs) (Jeng et al., 1998; Jeng et al., 2000). The MAPKs are found downstream of several growth factor receptors including HER-2/neu and could phosphorylate and influence the activity of the SRCs, but also the ER. Accumulated evidence points to an important crosstalk between ER and growth factor pathways where posttranslational modifications of the SRCs are involved. These modifications could influence not only SRC activity, but also the effect of endocrine treatment in breast cancer over time.

4. SRCs and growth factor signaling

4.1 Posttranslational modifications of SRCs with functional aspects

The SRCs are components and targets of multiple cell signaling pathways that modulate their activity. Extracellular stimuli such as hormones, growth factors and cytokines induce a variety of posttranslational modifications of SRCs, including acetylation, methylation, phosphorylation, ubiquitination and sumoylation. These modifications influence the SRCs transcriptional activity and/or the SRC protein levels and stability (Baek & Rosenfeld, 2004; Li & Shang, 2007; Xu et al., 2009).

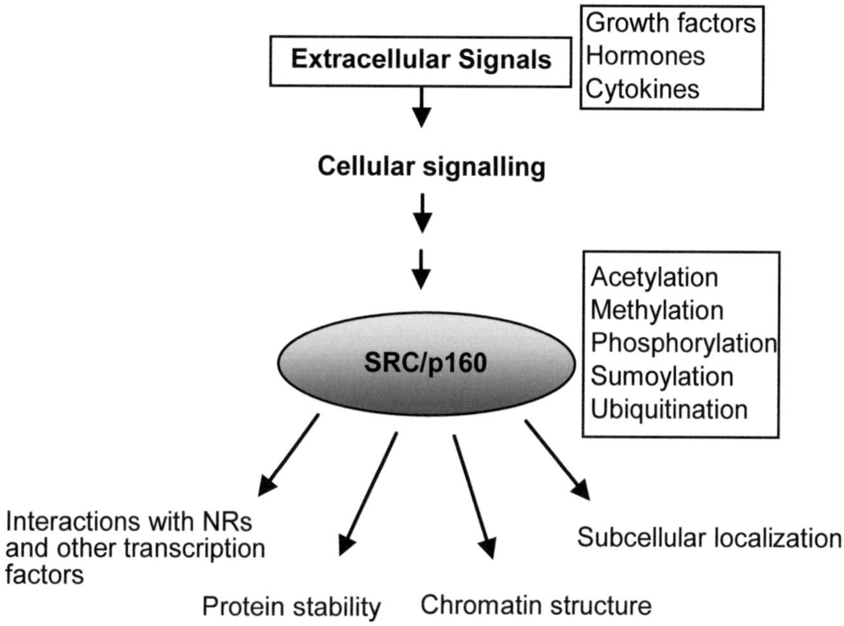

Fig. 3. Functional aspects of posttranslational modifications of the SRCs.

Phosphorylation of coactivators modulates ER-dependent gene transcription by regulating coactivator function in various ways. Three SRC-1 phosphorylation sites with corresponding kinases have been identified (S395, T1179 and S1185), one SRC-2/TIF-2 (S736) and sixteen SRC-3/AIB1 phosphorylation sites (T24, S505, S543, S601, S857, S860, S867, S1033, S1042, S1048, T1059, S1062, T1064, T1067, T1114 and Y1357) (Bulynko & O'Malley, 2011). Comparison of these sites reveals little conservation of sequences among the SRCs, indicating that phosphorylation is a significant determinant of the specificity of the SRCs (Wu et al., 2005).

Phosphorylation may influence the function and acitivity of the SRCs. It is shown *in vitro* using COS-1 cells that positions S395 and T1179/S1185 of SRC-1 are phosphorylated by the MAPK family members ERK1 and ERK2 (Rowan et al., 2000b) where MAPK-mediated phosphorylation on T1179 and S1185 has been shown to increase the affinity of SRC-1 for androgen receptor (AR) in prostate cancer cells (Ueda et al., 2002; Gregory et al., 2004). ERK2 may also phosphorylate SRC-3/AIB1 *in vitro* which stimulates the recruitment of p300 and associated histone acetyltransferase activity (Font de Mora & Brown, 2000). cAMP regulated phosphorylation of SRC-1 occurs through an indirect pathway in which protein kinase A (PKA) induces the activity of ERK1 and ERK2 (Rowan et al., 2000a). SRC-3/AIB1 phosphorylation-defective mutants exhibit reduced ability to interact with ER compared to wild type SRC-3/AIB1, both in the absence and presence of E2 (Wu et al., 2004). Epidermal growth factor (EGF)-induced activation of ER-, progesterone receptor (PR)- and AR-dependent transcription is shown to be regulated through phosphorylation of SRC-2/TIF-2 at S736 by the EGF-activated ERK MAPK and p38MAPK which stimulate SRC-2/TIF-2 coactivator function (Lopez et al., 2001; Gregory et al., 2004; Frigo et al., 2006).

Phosphorylation and dephosphorylation of proteins also regulate the nuclear import and export by modifying the nuclear localization signals (NLS) and nuclear export signals (NES) of the proteins (Whitmarsh & Davis, 2000). The sequence of the bHLH domain of the SRCs has been shown to be important for their nuclear localization. SRC-1 and SRC-3/AIB1 contain a conserved bipartite NLS in their bHLH-PAS domain (Amazit et al., 2003; Li et al., 2007). Furthermore, specific residues in the NLS of SRC-3/AIB1 are identified to signal proteasome-dependent turnover of SRC-3/AIB1 in the nucleus (Li et al., 2007). SRC-1 also contains a non-conserved sequence localized in its C-terminal region that is suggested to serve as a NES. The return of SRC-1 to the cytoplasm is proposed to be involved in termination of hormone action (Amazit et al., 2003).

Phosphorylation does not only influence the activation and subcellular localization of the SRCs, but also regulate the ubiquitination and degradation of the coactivators. Phosphorylated SRCs are suggested to be targets for enzymes in the ubiquitin-proteasome pathway. The ubiquitin-proteasome degradation pathway is regarded as an important mechanism to control the steady state levels of SRCs, thereby modulating growth responses to various growth-promoting factors (Lonard & O'Malley, 2005). Retinoic acid-induced phosphorylation of SRC-3/AIB1 by p38MAPK at S860, and phosphorylation at S505 by Akt/protein kinase B (PKB)-activated glycogen synthase kinase-3 (GSK3) have been shown to mediate SRC-3/AIB1 degradation (Gianni et al., 2006; Wu et al., 2007). On the other hand, atypical PKC-induced phosphorylation of the C-terminal region of SRC-3/AIB1 was reported to increase its stabilization by protecting it from proteasome-mediated degradation leading to an increased estrogen-induced breast cancer cell growth (Yi et al., 2008).

Growth factor pathways regulate SRC function not only through phosphorylation. We found activation of the cAMP/PKA pathway to stimulate association of SRC-2/TIF-2 with an ER-transcription complex prior to its degradation by the ubiquitin-proteasome system (Fenne et al., 2008). MCF-7 breast cancer cells were transfected with an expression plasmid encoding HA-GRIP1, the rodent homologue to SRC-2/TIF-2, along with the luciferase reporter construct ERE-TATA-luc. Cells were treated with cAMP analog and cAMP-elevating agents for different time-lengths and after 48 hours the cells where lysed and subjected to luciferase assay. A time-dependent regulation of cAMP/PKA on SRC-2/TIF-2 coactivator function was observed (Fig. 4A). PKA is activated when hormones bind to a G-protein coupled receptor (GPCR). The activated receptor interacts with adenylyl cyclase (AC) which catalyses the conversion of ATP to cAMP, further activating the cAMP dependent PKA (Fig. 4b). PKA can regulate SRC-2/TIF-2 coactivator function in a time-dependent matter. Short-term treatment stimulated SRC-2/TIF-2 coactivator function, whereas long-term treatments inhibited SRC-2/TIF-2 function due to ubiquitin-proteasome-mediated degradation (Hoang et al., 2004; Fenne et al., 2008).

All three SRCs can also be modified by site-specific sumoylation of lysine residues in their respective NIDs (Kotaja et al., 2002; Chauchereau et al., 2003). Sumoylation of SRC-2/TIF-2 has been shown to increase its coactivation of AR by enhancing their interaction (Kotaja et al., 2002). Conversely, sumoylation of SRC-1 increases its interaction with the PR and leads to prolonged retention of SRC-1 in the nucleus (Chauchereau et al., 2003). In contrast to SRC-1 and SRC-2/TIF-2, sumoylation of SRC-3/AIB1 seems to attenuate its coactivation function (Wu et al., 2006).

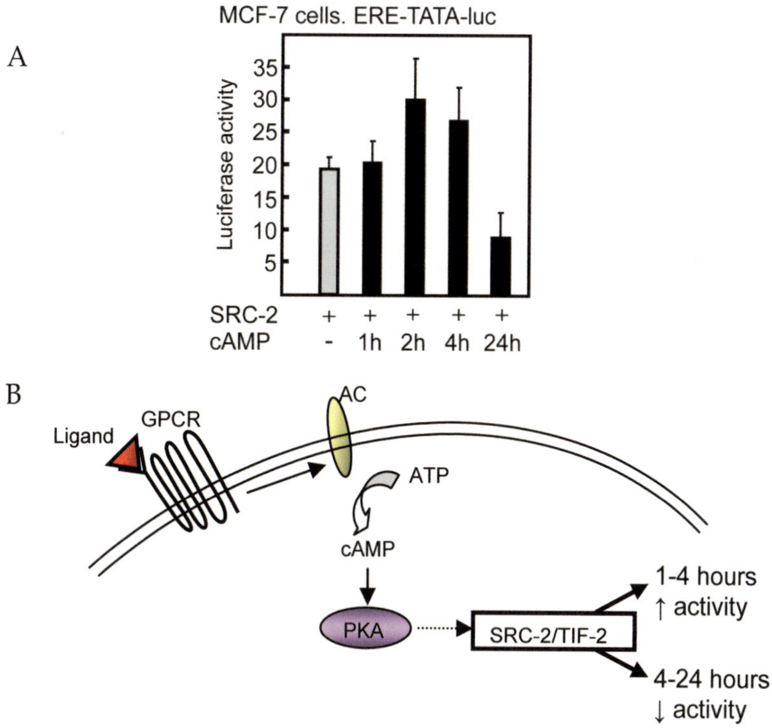

Fig. 4. cAMP-PKA signaling influence SRC-2/TIF-2 function in a time-dependent manner.

4.2 SRCs, growth factor signaling and response to endocrine therapy

The SRCs are regulated by post-translational modifications by kinases found downstream in growth factor signaling pathways often activated in cancers, such as the MAPKs operating downstream of HER-2/neu. Posttranslational modification can stabilize and functionally activate the SRC proteins, a mechanism which has been shown to contribute not only to ER-agonstic effects of tamoxifen, but also to estrogen hypersensitivity and resistance to aromatase inhibitors. *In vitro* it has been shown that tamoxifen resistance with loss of ER antagonistic effects develops when SRC-3/AIB1 is high and the transcriptional repressor PAX2 is low in breast cancer cells (Hurtado et al., 2008). Conversely, dissociation of SRC-3/AIB1 from ER restores tamoxifen's antagonistic effect in resistant breast cancer cells and inhibits further breast cancer cell growth (Planas-Silva et al., 2001; List et al., 2001).

Clinically, studies have shown an association between SRC-1 and reduced disease-free survival in breast cancer patients with locally advanced disease treated with endocrine therapy (Al-azawi et al., 2008; Redmond et al., 2009). During neoadjuvant treatment with aromatase inhibitors, we found higher levels of SRC-1 mRNA levels during treatment, especially in tumors that responded to treatment (Flågeng et al., 2009). Low expression of SRC-1 combined with high ERβ expression has been found to be a good prognostic indicator to endocrine treatment in breast cancers (Myers et al., 2004). However, the clearest association between high levels of SRCs and poor clinical outcome has been found in tumors also overexpressing HER-2/neu. Patients with tumors overexpressing HER-2/neu in combination with SRC-3/AIB1 or SRC-1 undergoing tamoxifen treatment show reduced sensitivity to endocrine therapy, greater risk of disease recurrence and reduced disease-free survival (Fleming et al., 2004b; Osborne et al., 2003). Overexpression of SRC-3/AIB1 and HER-2/neu in breast tumors is associated with disease recurrences and poor prognosis. This could be linked to the HER-2/neu-mediated activation of MAPK and Akt which causes phosphorylation of SRC-3/AIB1 and ER, resulting in transcriptional activation and cell proliferation. Activation of Akt has also been shown to stabilize SRC-3/AIB1 by inhibiting GSK3 (Wu et al., 2007) whereas PKA-induced resistance to tamoxifen is associated with an altered orientation between ER and SRC-1 (Zwart et al., 2007). Overall, the SRCs can be targeted by central growth factor pathways mediating pro-survival signals and stimulating proliferation. The SRCs close functional relationship with the ER makes posttranslational modifications of the SRCs important points of crosstalk between ER and growth factor signaling pathways during endocrine treatment in breast cancer (Fig. 5).

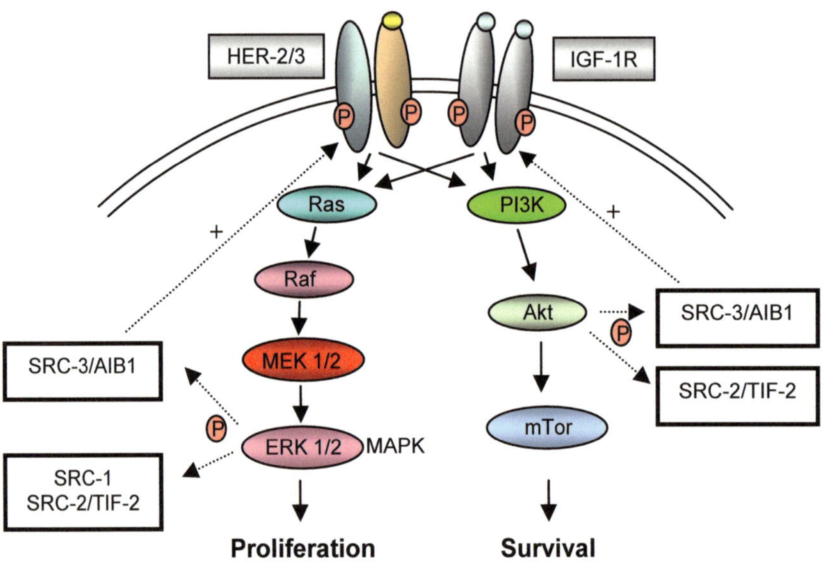

Fig. 5. Cross-talk between growth-factor signaling pathways and SRCs in breast cancer. Ligand-activated growth factor receptor dimers including the human epidermal growth factor receptor-2 and -3 (HER-2/3) and the insulin-like growth factor-1 receptor (IGF-1R) are phosphorylated at intracellular domains and signal both through the MAPK and the phosphatidyl-inositol 3-kinase (PI3K) signaling pathway. ERK 1 and 2 may phosphorylate SRC-1, SRC-2/TIF-2 and SRC-3/AIB1. Akt may phosporylate SRC-2/TIF-2 and SRC-3/AIB1. SRC-3/AIB1 is a modulator increasing the activity and signaling both through HER-2 and IGF-1R leading to cell growth.

5. Conclusion

Most human breast cancers express ER which belongs to the family of nuclear receptors and is a ligand-regulated transcription factor. Endocrine treatment involves blocking the ER with a selective ER modulator such as tamoxifen or inhibiting estrogen synthesis using aromatase inhibitors. The SRCs are crucial to ER mediated effects and their expression level and activity have been shown to dictate the effect of ER on gene expression to a large extent. SRC-1, SRC-2/TIF-2 and SRC-3/AIB1 are expressed in normal and malignant breast tissue where SRC-3/AIB1 is now considered to be an oncogene. SRC-1 and SRC-3/AIB1 may promote metastasis in mammary tumors by enhancing the transcriptional activation of regulators of metastasis such as Twist and MMPs. The expression levels of the SRCs are influenced by endocrine treatment, an observation which may be of relevance to the treatment response to endocrine therapy over time. We found the mRNA levels of the SRCs, especially SRC-3/AIB1, to be significantly upregulated in both normal and malignant breast tissue after 4 weeks of tamoxifen in the 1-20 mg dose range. The mRNA expression of SRC-1 has also been shown to increase significantly in a clinical study of neoadjuvant treatment with aromatase inhibitors for 14-16 weeks, especially in the subgroup of patients achieving an objective treatment response. This is in line with *in vitro* studies in MCF-7 cells showing that estrogens suppress the mRNA levels of SRC-3/AIB1 by suppressing SRC-3/AIB1 gene transcription whereas 4-hydroxytamoxifen increases the SRC-3/AIB1 mRNA expression level. The importance of the expression level and functional activation of the SRCs during endocrine treatment is evident from cellular assays on tamoxifen treatment. High levels of coactivators relative to corepressors may lead to ER agonistic effects by 4-hydroxytamoxifen. Further, posttranslational modification of both coactivators and ER can lead to altered molecular conformations, intracellular relocation, stabilization and ubiquitination which would influence the activity and stability of the SRCs, as shown for the PKA-mediated regulation of SRC-2/TIF-2. In several clinical trials the levels of coactivators have been found of relevance, not only to the response to endocrine treatment, but also to long term clinical outcome. High protein levels of SRC-1 have been shown to be associated with reduced disease-free survival, both in untreated and tamoxifen treated patients, whereas elevated mRNA expression levels of SRC-3/AIB1 have been associated with high tumor grade and shorter disease-free and overall survival. Tumors undergoing tamoxifen therapy and overexpressing HER-2/neu in combination with SRC-3/AIB1 are more likely to be tamoxifen resistant and are associated with reduced disease-free survival. High expression of HER-2/neu in combination with SRC-1 has also been associated with a greater risk of recurrence on endocrine treatment. In summary, SRCs are expressed in normal and malignant breast tissue and they have a crucial role in mediating the effect of endocrine treatment in breast cancer. The expression levels of SRCs are regulated by endocrine treatment and their functional role is modified by posttranslational modifications mediated by growth factor pathways involved in breast cancer development and endocrine resistance. Further research on SRCs and their role in the crosstalk between ER and growth factor pathways during endocrine treatment is important to improve breast cancer therapy.

6. References

Al-azawi, D., McIlroy, M., Kelly, G., Redmond, A.M., Bane, F.T., Cocchiglia, S., Hill, A.D.K. & Young, L.S. (2008). Ets-2 and p160 proteins collaborate to regulate c-Myc in endocrine resistant breast cancer. *Oncogene*, Vol. 27, No. 21, pp. 3021-3031.

Amazit, L., Alj, Y., Tyagi, R.K., Chauchereau, A., Loosfelt, H., Pichon, C., Pantel, J., Foulon-Guinchard, E., Leclerc, P., Milgrom, E. & Guiochon-Mantel, A. (2003). Subcellular localization and mechanisms of nucleocytoplasmic trafficking of steroid receptor coactivator-1. *J Biol Chem*, Vol. 278, No. 34, pp. 32195-32203.

Anzick, S. L., Kononen, J., Walker, R. L., Azorsa, D. O., Tanner, M. M., Guan, X. Y., Sauter, G., Kallioniemi, O. P., Trent ,J. M. & Meltzer, P.S. (1997). AIB1, a steroid receptor coactivator amplified in breast and ovarian cancer. *Science* , Vol. 277, No. 5328, pp. 965-968.

Baek, S.H. & Rosenfeld, M.G. (2004). Nuclear receptor coregulators: their modification codes and regulatory mechanism by translocation. *Biochem Biophys Res Commun,* Vol. 319, No. 3, pp. 707-714.

Bautista, S., Valles, H., Walker, R. L., Anzick, S., Zeillinger, R., Meltzer, P. & Theillet, C. (1998). In breast cancer, amplification of the steroid receptor coactivator gene AIB1 is correlated with estrogen and progesterone receptor positivity. *Clin Cancer Res,* Vol. 4, No. 12, pp. 2925-2929.

Bouras, T., Southey, M. C. & Venter, D.J. (2001). Overexpression of the steroid receptor coactivator AIB1 in breast cancer correlates with the absence of estrogen and progesterone receptors and positivity for p53 and HER2/neu. *Cancer Res,* Vol. 61, No. 3, pp. 903-907.

Brzozowski, A. M., Pike, A. C., Dauter, Z., Hubbard, R. E., Bonn, T., Engstrom, Ohman, O., L., Greene, G. L., Gustafsson, J. A. & Carlquist, M. (1997). Molecular basis of agonism and antagonism in the oestrogen receptor. *Nature,* Vol. 389, No. 6652, pp. 753-758.

Bulynko, Y.A. & O'Malley, B.W. (2011). Nuclear receptor coactivators: structural and functional biochemistry. *Biochemistry,* Vol. 50, No. 3, pp. 313-328.

Carapeti, M., Agular, R.C., Chase, A., Goldman, J.M. & Cross, N.C. (1998). Assignment of the steroid receptor coactivator-1 (SRC-1) gene to human chromosome band 2p23. *Genomics,* Vol. 52, No. 2, pp. 242-244.

Cavarretta, I.T., Mukopadhyay, R., Lonard, D.M., Cowsert, L.M., Bennett, C.F., O'Malley, B.W. & Smith, C.L. (2002). Reduction of coactivator expression by antisense oligodeoxynucleotides inhibits ERalpha transcriptional activity and MCF-7 proliferation. *Mol Endocrinol,* Vol. 16, No. 2, pp. 253-270.

Chauchereau, A., Amazit, L., Quesne, M., Guiochon-Mantel, A. & Milgrom, E. (2003). Sumoylation of the progesterone receptor and of the steroid receptor coactivator SRC-1. *J Biol Chem,* Vol. 278, No. 14, pp. 12335-12343.

Cuzick, J., Powles, T., Veronesi, U., Forbes, J., Edwards, R., Ashley, S. & Boyle, P. (2003). Overview of the main outcomes in breast-cancer prevention trials. *Lancet,* Vol. 361, No. 9354, pp. 296-300.

Dubik, D. & Shiu, R.P. (1992). Mechanism of estrogen activation of c-myc oncogene expression. *Oncogene,* Vol. 7, No. 8, pp. 1587-1594.

Fenne, I.S., Hoang, T., Hauglid, M., Sagen, J.V., Lien, E.A. & Mellgren, G. (2008). Recruitment of coactivator glucocorticoid receptor interacting protein 1 to an estrogen receptor transcription complex is regulated by the 3`,5`-cyclic adenosine 5`-monophosphate-dependent protein kinase. *Endocrinology,* Vol. 148, No. 9, pp. 4336-4345.

Fereshteh, M. P., Tilli, M.T., Kim, S.E., Xu, J., O'Malley, B.W., Wellstein, A., Furth, P.A. & Riegel, A.T. (2008). The nuclear receptor coactivator amplified in breast cancer-1 is required for Neu (ErbB2/HER2) activation, signaling, and mammary tumorigenesis in mice. *Cancer Res,* Vol. 68, No. 10, pp. 3697-3706.

Fleming, F. J., Hill, A. D., McDermott, E.W., O'Higgins, N. J. & Young, L. S. (2004a). Differential recruitment of coregulator proteins steroid receptor coactivator-1 and silencing mediator for retinoid and thyroid receptors to the estrogen receptor-estrogen response element by beta-estradiol and 4-hydroxytamoxifen in human breast cancer. *J Clin Endocrinol Metab,* Vol. 89, No. 1, pp. 375-383.

Fleming, F. J., Myers, E., Kelly, G., Crotty, T. B., McDermott, E.W., O'Higgins, N. J., Hill, A. D. & Young, L. S. (2004b). Expression of SRC-1, AIB1, and PEA3 in HER2 mediated endocrine resistant breast cancer; a predictive role for SRC-1. *J Clin Pathol,* Vol. 57, No. 10, pp. 1069-1074.

Flågeng, M.H., Haugan Moi, L.L., Dixon, J.M., Geisler, J., Lien, E.A., Miller, W.R., Lønning, P.E. & Mellgren, G. (2009). Nuclear receptor co-activators and HER-2/neu are upregulated in breast cancer patients during neo-adjuvant treatment with aromatase inhibitors. *Br J Cancer,* Vol. 101, No. 8, pp. 1253-1260.

Font de Mora, J. & Brown, M. (2000). AIB1 is a conduit for kinase-mediated growth factor signaling to the estrogen receptor. *Mol Cell Biol,* Vol. 20, No. 14, pp. 5041-5047.

Foster, J. S., Henley, D. C., Ahamed, S.& Wimalasena, J. (2001). Estrogens and cell-cycle regulation in breast cancer. *Trends Endocrinol Metab,* Vol. 12, No. 7, pp. 320-327.

Frigo, D.E., Basu, A., Nierth-Simpson, E.N., Weldon, C.B., Dugan, C.M., Elliott, S., Collins-Burow, B.M., Salvo, V.A., Zhu, Y., Melnik, L.I., Lopez, G.N., Kushner, P.J., Curiel, T.J., Rowan, B.G., McLachlan, J.A. & Burow M.E. (2006). p38 mitogen-activated protein kinase stimulates estrogen-mediated transcription and proliferation through the phosphorylation and potentiation of the p160 coactivator glucocorticoid receptor-interacting protein 1. *Mol Endocrinol,* Vol. 20, No. 5, pp. 971-983.

Gehin, M., Mark, M., Dennefeld, C., Dierich, A., Gronemeyer H. & Chambon, P. (2002). The function of TIF2/GRIP1 in mouse reproduction is distinct from those of SRC-1 and p/CIP. *Mol Cell Biol,* Vol. 22, No. 16, pp. 5923-5937.

Gianni, M., Parrella, E., Raska, I. Jr, Gaillard, E., Nigro, E.A., Gaudon, C., Garattini, E. &Rochette-Egly, C. (2006). P38MAPK-dependent phosphorylation and degradation of SRC-3/AIB1 and RARalpha-mediated transcription. *EMBO J,* Vol. 25, No. 4, pp. 739-751.

Gregory C.W., Fei, X., Ponguta, L.A., He, B., Bill, H.M., French, F.S. & Wilson, E.M. (2004). Epidermal growth factor increases coactivation of the androgen receptor in recurrent prostate cancer. *J Biol Chem,* Vol. 279, No. 8, pp. 7119-30.

Haugan Moi, L.L., Flågeng, M.H., Gandini, S., Guerrieri-Gonzaga, A., Bonanni, B., Lazzeroni, M., Gjerde, J., Lien, E.A., DeCensi, A. & Mellgren, G. (2010). Effect of low dose tamoxifen on Steroid Receptor Coactivator 3/Amplified in Breast Cancer 1 in normal and malignant human breast tissue. *Clin Cancer Res,* Vol. 16, No. 7, pp. 2176-2186.

Heery, D. M., Kalkhoven, E., Hoare S. & Parker, M.G. (1997). A signature motif in transcriptional co-activators mediates binding to nuclear receptors. *Nature,* Vol. 387, No. 6634, pp. 733-736.

Hoang, T., Fenne, I. S., Cook, C., Borud, B., Bakke, M., Lien, E.A. & Mellgren, G. (2004). cAMP-dependent protein kinase regulates ubiquitin-proteasome-mediated degradation and subcellular localization of the nuclear receptor coactivator GRIP1. *J Biol Chem,* Vol. 279, No. 47, pp. 49120-49130.

Hudelist, G., Czerwenka, K., Kubista, E., Marton, E., Pischinger, K. & Singer, C. F. (2003). Expression of sex steroid receptors and their co-factors in normal and malignant breast tissue: AIB1 is a carcinoma-specific co-activator. *Breast Cancer Res Treat,* Vol. 78, No. 2, pp. 193-204.

Hurtado, A., Holmes, K. A., Geistlinger, T. R., Hutcheson, I. R., Nicholson, R. I., Brown, M., Jiang, J., Howat, W. J., Ali, S. & Carroll, J. S. (2008). Regulation of ERBB2 by oestrogen receptor-PAX2 determines response to tamoxifen. *Nature,* Vol. 456, No. 7222, pp. 663-666.

Jeng, M. H., Shupnik, M. A., Bender, T. P., Westin, E. H., Bandyopadhyay, D., Kumar, R., Masamura, S. & Santen, R.J. (1998). Estrogen receptor expression and function in long-term estrogen-deprived human breast cancer cells. *Endocrinoloy,* Vol. 139, No.. 10, pp. 4164-4174.

Jeng, M. H., Yue, W., Eischeid, A., Wang, J. P. & Santen. R.J. (2000). Role of MAP kinase in the enhanced cell proliferation of long term estrogen deprived human breast cancer cells. *Breast Cancer Res Treat,* Vol. 62, No. 3, pp. 167-175.

Kalkhoven, E., Valentine, J. E., Heery,D. M. & Parker, M.G. (1998). Isoforms of steroid receptor co-activator 1 differ in their ability to potentiate transcription by the oestrogen receptor. *EMBO J,* Vol. 17, No. 1, pp. 232-243.

Karmakar, S., Foster, E. A. & Smith, C.L. (2009). Unique roles of p160 coactivators for regulation of breast cancer cell proliferation and estrogen receptor-alpha transcriptional activity. *Endocrinology,* Vol. 150, No. 4, pp. 1588-1596.

Kotaja, N., Karvonen, U., Jänne, O.A. & Palvimo, J.J. (2002). The nuclear receptor interaction domain of GRIP1 is modulated by covalent attachment of SUMO-1. *J Biol Chem,* Vol. 277, No. 33, pp. 30283-30288.

Kurebayashi, J., Otsuki, T., Kunisue, H., Tanaka, K., Yamamoto, S. & Sonoo, H. (2000). Expression levels of estrogen receptor-alpha, estrogen receptor-beta, coactivators, and corepressors in breast cancer. *Clin Cancer Res,* Vol. 6, No. 2, pp. 512-518.

Lauritsen, K. J., List, H. J., Reiter, R., Wellstein, A. & Riegel, A.T. (2002). A role for TGF-beta in estrogen and retinoid mediated regulation of the nuclear receptor coactivator AIB1 in MCF-7 breast cancer cells. *Oncogene,* Vol. 21, No. 47, pp. 7147-7155.

Li, C., Wu, R.C., Amazit, L., Tsai, S.Y., Tsai, M.J. & O'Malley, B.W. (2007). Specific amino acid residues in the basic helix-loop-helix domain of SRC-3 are essential for its nuclear localization and proteasome-dependent turnover. *Mol Cell Biol*, Vol. 27, No. 4, pp. 1296-1308.

Li, S. & Shang, Y. (2007). Regulation of SRC family coactivators by post-translational modifications. *Cell Signal,* Vol. 19, No. 6, pp. 1101-12.

List, H. J., Reiter, R., Singh, B., Wellstein, A. & Riegel, A. T. (2001). Expression of the nuclear coactivator AIB1 in normal and malignant breast tissue. *Breast Cancer Res Treat,* Vol. 68, No. 1, pp. 21-28.

Lonard, D. M. & O'Malley, B.W. (2005). Expanding functional diversity of the coactivators. *Trends Biochem Sci,* Vol. 30, No. 3, pp. 126-132.

Lonard, D.M., Tsai, S.Y. & O'Malley, B.W. (2004). Selective estrogen receptor modulators 4-hydroxytamoxifen and raloxifene impact the stability and function of SRC-1 and SRC-3 coactivator proteins. *Mol Cell Biol,* Vol. 24, No. 1, pp. 14-24.

Lopez, G. N., Turck, C. W., Schaufele, F., Stallcup, M.R. & Kushner, P.J. (2001). Growth factors signal to steroid receptors through mitogen-activated protein kinase regulation of p160 coactivator activity. *J Biol Chem,* Vol. 276, No. 25, pp. 22177-22182.

Louet, J. F., Chopra, A. R., Sagen, J. V., An, J., York, B., Tannour-Louet, M.,., Saha, P. K., Stevens, R. D., Wenner, B. R., Ilkayeva, O. R., Bain, J. R., Zhou, S., DeMayo, F., Xu, J., Newgard , C. B. & O'Malley, B.W. (2010). The coactivator SRC-1 is an essential coordinator of hepatic glucose production. *Cell Metab,* Vol. 12, No. 6, pp. 606-618.

Mangelsdorf, D. J., Thummel, C., Beato, M., Herrlich, P., Schutz, G., Umesono, K., Blumberg, B., Kastner, P., Mark, M., Chambon, P. & Evans, R.M. (1995). The nuclear receptor superfamily: the second decade. *Cell,* Vol. 83, No. 6, pp. 835-839.

Masamura, S., Santner, S. J., Heitjan, D. F. & Santen, R. J. (1995). Estrogen deprivation causes estradiol hypersensitivity in human breast cancer cells. *J Clin Endocrinol Metab,* Vol. 80, No. 10, pp. 2918-2925.

Metivier, R., Penot, G., Hubner, M. R., Reid, G., Brand, H., Kos M. & Gannon, F. (2003). Estrogen receptor-alpha directs ordered, cyclical, and combinatorial recruitment of cofactors on a natural target promoter. *Cell,* Vol. 115, No. 6, pp. 751-763.

Murphy, L. C., Simon, S. L., Parkes, A., Leygue, E., Dotzlaw, H., Snell, L., Troup, S., Adeyinka, A. & Watson. P.H. (2000). Altered expression of estrogen receptor coregulators during human breast tumorigenesis. *Cancer Res,* Vol. 60, No. 22, pp. 6266-6271.

Myers, E., Fleming, F. J., Crotty, G., Kelly, E.W., McDermott, J., O'Higgins N., Hill, A. D. & Young, L. S. (2004). Inverse relationship between ER-beta and SRC-1 predicts outcome in endocrine-resistant breast cancer. *Br J Cancer,* Vol. 91, No. 9, pp. 1687-1693.

Newman, S. P., Bates, N. P. , Vernimmen, D., Parker, M. G. & Hurst, H. C. (2000). Cofactor competition between the ligand-bound oestrogen receptor and an intron 1 enhancer leads to oestrogen repression of ERBB2 expression in breast cancer. *Oncogene,* Vol. 19, No. 4, 490-497.

Onate, S.A., Tsai, ., S. Y., Tsai M. J. & O'Malley, B. W. (1995). Sequence and characterization of a coactivator for the steroid hormone receptor superfamily. *Science,* Vol. 270, No. 5240, pp. 1354-1357.

Osborne, C. K., Bardou, V., Hopp, T. A., Chamness, G. C., Hilsenbeck, S. G., Fuqua, S. A., Wong, J., Allred, D. C., Clark, G. M. & Schiff, R. (2003). Role of the estrogen receptor coactivator AIB1 (SRC-3) and HER-2/neu in tamoxifen resistance in breast cancer. *J Natl Cancer Inst,* Vol. 95, No. 5, pp. 353-361.

Pearce, S. T. & Jordan, V.C. (2004). The biological role of estrogen receptors alpha and beta in cancer. *Crit Rev Oncol Hematol*, Vol. 50, No. 1, pp. 3-22.

Picard, F., Gehin, M., Annicotte, J., Rocchi, S., Champy, M. F., O'Malley, B. W., Chambon, P. & Auwerx, J. (2002). SRC-1 and TIF2 control energy balance between white and brown adipose tissues. *Cell,* Vol. 111, No. 7, pp. 931-941.

Planas-Silva, M. D., Shang, Y., Donaher, J. L., Brown, M. &. Weinberg, R. A. (2001). AIB1 enhances estrogen-dependent induction of cyclin D1 expression. *Cancer Res,* Vol. 61, No. 10, pp. 3858-3862.

Qin, L., Liao, L., Redmond, A., Young, L., Yuan, Y., Chen, H., O'Malley, B. W. & Xu, J. (2008). The AIB1 oncogene promotes breast cancer metastasis by activation of PEA3-mediated matrix metalloproteinase 2 (MMP2) and MMP9 expression. *Mol Cell Biol,* Vol. 28, No. 19, pp. 5937-5950.

Qin, L., Liu, Z., Chen, H. & Xu, J. (2009). The steroid receptor coactivator-1 regulates twist expression and promotes breast cancer metastasis. *Cancer Res*, Vol. 69, No. 9, pp. 3819-3827.

Redmond, A. M., Bane, F. T., Stafford, A. T., McIlroy, M., Dillon, M. F., Crotty, T. B., Hill, A. D. & Young, L.S. (2009). Coassociation of estrogen receptor and p160 proteins predicts resistance to endocrine treatment; SRC-1 is an independent predictor of breast cancer recurrence. *Clin Cancer Res*, Vol. 15, No. 6, pp. 2098-2106.

Rowan, B.G., Garrison, N., Weigel, N.L. & O'Malley, B.W. (2000a). 8-Bromo-cyclic AMP induces phosphorylation of two sites in SRC-1 that facilitate ligand-independent activation of the chicken progesterone receptor and are critical for functional cooperation between SRC-1 and CREB binding protein. *Mol Cell Biol*, Vol. 20, No. 23, pp. 8720-8730.

Rowan, B.G., Weigel, N.L. & O'Malley, B.W. (2000b). Phosphorylation of steroid receptor coactivator-1. Identification of the phosphorylation sites and phosphorylation through the mitogen-activated protein kinase pathway. *J Biol Chem*, Vol. 275, No. 6, pp. 4475-4483.

Sabbah, M., Courilleau, D., Mester, J. & Redeuilh, G. (1999). Estrogen induction of the cyclin D1 promoter: involvement of a cAMP response-like element. *Proc Natl Acad Sci U S A*, Vol. 96, No. 20, pp. 11217-11222.

Santen, R. J., Song R. X., Zhang, Z., Kumar, R., Jeng, M. H., Masamura, A., Lawrence Jr., J., Berstein, L. & Yue, W. (2005). Long-term estradiol deprivation in breast cancer cells up-regulates growth factor signaling and enhances estrogen sensitivity. *Endocr Relat Cancer,* Vol. 12, No. Suppl 1, pp. S61-73.

Shang, Y. & Brown, M. (2002). Molecular determinants for the tissue specificity of SERMs. *Science,* Vol. 295, No. 5564, pp. 2465-2468.

Shiau, A. K., Barstad, D., Loria, P. M., Cheng, L., Kushner, P. J., Agard, D. A. & Greene, G.L. (1998). The structural basis of estrogen receptor/coactivator recognition and the antagonism of this interaction by tamoxifen. *Cell*, Vol. 95, No. 7, pp. 927-937.

Shou, J., Massarweh, S., Osborne, C. K., Wakeling, A. E., Ali S., Weiss, H. & Schiff, R. (2004). Mechanisms of tamoxifen resistance: increased estrogen receptor-HER2/neu cross-talk in ER/HER2-positive breast cancer. *J Natl Cancer Inst,* Vol. 96, No. 12, pp. 926-935.

Tai, H., Kubota, N. & Kato, S. (2000). Involvement of nuclear receptor coactivator SRC-1 in estrogen-dependent cell growth of MCF-7 cells. *Biochem Biophys Res Commun*, Vol. 267, No. 1, pp. 311-316.

Takeshita, A., Cardona, G. R., Koibuchi, N., Suen C. S. & Chin, W.W. (1997). TRAM-1, A novel 160-kDa thyroid hormone receptor activator molecule, exhibits distinct properties from steroid receptor coactivator-1. *J Biol Chem*, Vol 272, No. 44, pp. 27629-27634.

Torres-Arzayus, M. I., Font de Mora, J., Yuan, J., Vazquez, F. , Bronson, R., Rue, M., Sellers W. R. & Brown, M. (2004). High tumor incidence and activation of the PI3K/AKT pathway in transgenic mice define AIB1 as an oncogene. *Cancer Cell,* Vol. 6, No. 3, pp. 263-274.

Ueda, T., Mawji, N. R., Bruchovsky, N. & Sadar, M.D. (2002). Ligand-independent activation of the androgen receptor by interleukin-6 and the role of steroid receptor coactivator-1 in prostate cancer cells. *J Biol Chem,* Vol. 277, No. 41, pp. 38087-38094.

Wang, S., Yuan, Y., Liao, L., Kuang, S. Q., Tien, J. C., O'Malley, B. W. & Xu, J. (2009). Disruption of the SRC-1 gene in mice suppresses breast cancer metastasis without affecting primary tumor formation. *Proc Natl Acad Sci U S A*, Vol. 106, No. 1, pp. 151-156.

Webb, P., Nguyen P. & Kushner, P. J. (2003). Differential SERM effects on corepressor binding dictate ERalpha activity in vivo. *J Biol Chem*, Vol. 278, No. 9, pp. 6912-6920.

Webb, P., Nguyen, P., Shinsako, J., Anderson, C., Feng, W., Nguyen, M.P., Chen, D., Huang, S.M., Subramanian, S., McKinerney, E., Katzenellenbogen, B.S., Stallcup, M.R. & Kushner, P.J. (1998). Estrogen receptor activation function 1 works by binding p160 coactivator proteins. *Mol Endocrinol*, Vol. 12, No. 10, pp. 1605-1618.

Whitmarsh, A.J. & Davis, R.J. (2000). Regulation of transcription factor function by phosphorylation. *Cell Mol Life Sci*, Vol. 57, No. 8-9; pp. 1172-1183.

Wu, H., Sun, L., Zhang, Y., Chen, Y., Shi, B., Li, R., Wang, Y., Liang, J., Fan, D., Wu, G., Wang, D., Li, S. & Shang, Y. (2006). Coordinated regulation of AIB1 transcriptional activity by sumoylation and phosphorylation. *J Biol Chem*, Vol. 281, No. 31, pp. 21848-21856.

Wu, R.C., Feng, Q., Lonard, D.M. & O'Malley, B.W. (2007). SRC-3 coactivator functional lifetime is regulated by a phospho-dependent ubiquitin time clock. *Cell*, Vol. 129, No. 6, pp. 1125-1140.

Wu, R. C., Qin, J., Yi, P., Wong, J.S., Tsai, Y., Tsai, M. J. & O'Malley, B.W. (2004). Selective phosphorylations of the SRC-3/AIB1 coactivator integrate genomic reponses to multiple cellular signaling pathways. *Mol Cell*, Vol. 15, No. 6, pp. 937-949.

Wu, R. C., Smith, C.L. & O'Malley, B.W. (2005). Transcriptional regulation by steroid receptor coactivator phosphorylation. *Endocr Rev*, Vol. 26, No. 3, pp. 393-399.

Xu, J. & Li, Q. (2003). Review of the in vivo functions of the p160 steroid receptor coactivator family. *Mol Endocrinol*, Vol. 17, No. 9, pp. 1681-1692.

Xu, J., Liao, L., Ning, G., Yoshida-Komiya, H., Deng, C. & O'Malley, B.W. (2000). The steroid receptor coactivator SRC-3 (p/CIP/RAC3/AIB1/ACTR/TRAM-1) is required for normal growth, puberty, female reproductive function, and mammary gland development. *Proc Natl Acad Sci U S A*,Vol. 97, No. 12, pp. 6379-6384.

Xu, J. & O'Malley, B.W. (2002). Molecular mechanisms and cellular biology of the steroid receptor coactivator (SRC) family in steroid receptor function. *Rev Endocr Metab Disord*, Vol. 3, No. 3, pp. 185-192.

Xu, J., Wu, R. C. & O'Malley, B.W. (2009). Normal and cancer-related functions of the p160 steroid receptor co-activator (SRC) family. *Nat Rev Cancer*, Vol. 9, No. 9, pp. 615-630.

Xu, J., Qiu, Y., DeMayo, F. J., Tsai, S. Y., Tsai, M. J. & O'Malley, B.W. (1998). Partial hormone resistance in mice with disruption of the steroid receptor coactivator-1 (SRC-1) gene. *Science*, Vol. 279, No. 5358, pp. 1922-1925.

Yi, P., Feng, Q., Amazit, L., Lonard, D.M., Tsai, S.Y., Tsai, M.J. & O'Malley, B.W. (2008). Atypical protein kinase C regulates dual pathways for degradation of the oncogenic coactivator SRC-3/AIB1. *Mol Cell*, Vol. 29, No. 4, pp. 465-476.

Zhao, C., Yasui, K., Lee, C. J., Kurioka, H., Hosokawa, Y., Oka, T. & Inazawa, J. (2003). Elevated expression levels of NCOA3, TOP1, and TFAP2C in breast tumors as predictors of poor prognosis. *Cancer*, Vol. 98, No. 1, pp. 18-23.

Zhou, G., Hashimoto, Y., Kwak, I., Tsai, S.Y. & Tsai, M.J. (2003). Role of the steroid receptor coactivator SRC-3 in cell growth. *Mol Cell Biol*, Vol. 23, No. 21, pp. 7742-7755.

Zwart, W., Griekspoor, A., Berno, V., Lakeman, K., Jalink, K., Mancini, M., Neefjes, J., Michalides, R. (2007). PKA-induced resistance to tamoxifen is associated with an altered orientation of ERalpha towards co-activator SRC-1. *EMBO J*, Vol. 26, No. 15, pp.3534-3544.